Peterson's Nursing Programs 2006

OTHER RECOMMENDED TITLES

ARCO Master the Nursing School and Allied Health Entrance Exams
Peterson's Scholarships, Grants & Prizes
Peterson's College Money Handbook

Peterson's Nursing Programs 2006

THOMSON
PETERSON'S™

Australia • Canada • Mexico • Singapore • Spain • United Kingdom • United States

THOMSON
PETERSON'S

About Thomson Peterson's

Thomson Peterson's (www.petersons.com) is a leading provider of education information and advice, with books and online resources focusing on education search, test preparation, and financial aid. Its Web site offers searchable databases and interactive tools for contacting educational institutions, online practice tests and instruction, and planning tools for securing financial aid. Thomson Peterson's serves 110 million education consumers annually.

For more information, contact Thomson Peterson's, 2000 Lenox Drive, Lawrenceville, NJ 08648; 800-338-3282; or find us on the World Wide Web at www.petersons.com/about.

Editor: Joe Krasowski; Production Editor: Linda Seghers; Copy Editors: Bret Bollmann, Jill C. Schwartz, Jim Colbert, Michael Haines, Pam Sullivan, Sally Ross, and Valerie Bolus Vaughan; Research Project Manager: Christine Lucas; Research Associate: Kristina Moran; Programmer: Phyllis Johnson; Manufacturing Manager: Ivona Skibicki; Composition Manager: Linda M. Williams; Client Service Representatives: Mimi Kaufman, Eric Wallace, Jim Swinarski, and Mary Ann Murphy.

ISSN 1073-7820
ISBN 0-7689-1748-4

Printed in the United States of America

10 9 8 7 6 5 4 3 2 1 07 06 05

Eleventh Edition

Contents

Foreword

The American Association of Colleges of Nursing (AACN) is proud to collaborate on *Peterson's Nursing Programs 2006.*

According to the Bureau of Labor Statistics, more than 1 million new and replacement registered nurses will be needed by the year 2012 to fill new positions and vacancies. As registered nurses find employment beyond hospitals in such areas as home care, community health, and long-term care, newly licensed RNs must have the proper education and training to work in these settings. It is vital that those seeking to enter or advance in a nursing career find the appropriate nursing program. This guide allows readers to find the program that best fits their needs, whether beginning a new career in nursing or attempting to advance one.

According to AACN's most recent annual institutional survey, enrollment in entry-level B.S.N. programs continues to climb. Gains were reported in all parts of the country in the 2004–05 academic year, with an overall 14.1 percent increase in enrollments nationwide. Nursing schools are working hard to find creative solutions to expand capacity and recruit new students during this nursing shortage.

Although the health-care environment is complex and dynamic, there continues to be a significant demand for professional-level nurses. The primary route into professional-level nursing is the four-year baccalaureate degree. The professional nurse with a baccalaureate degree is the only basic nursing graduate prepared to practice in all health-care settings, including critical care, public health, primary care, and mental health. In addition, advanced practice nurses (APNs) deliver essential services as nurse practitioners, certified nurse-midwives, clinical nurse specialists, and nurse anesthetists. APNs typically are prepared in master's degree programs, and the demand for their services is expected to increase substantially.

Higher education in nursing expands the gateway to a variety of career opportunities in the health-care field. In addition to providing primary care to patients, graduates can work as case managers for the growing numbers of managed-care companies or can assume administrative or managerial roles in hospitals, clinics, insurance companies, and other diverse settings.

The Nursing School Adviser section of this guide is instructive and invaluable. Whether you are a high school student looking for a four-year program, an RN returning to school, or a professional in another field contemplating a career change, this section will address your concerns. This information presents various nursing perspectives to benefit students from diverse backgrounds.

Peterson's effort in making this guide well organized and convenient to read cannot be overstated. Peterson's has worked with AACN in producing a publication that is comprehensive and user-friendly. Like the previous editions, this edition is a genuine collaborative work, as AACN provided input from start to finish.

AACN's dedication and achievements in advancing the quality of baccalaureate and graduate nursing education are appreciated by Peterson's. We at AACN are fortunate to work with an organization that prides itself on being the leading publisher of education search and selection.

Furthermore, this publication would not be possible without the cooperation of the institutions included in this guide. We acknowledge the time and effort of those who undertook the task of completing and returning the surveys regarding their programs. We certainly appreciate their contribution.

Peterson's Nursing Programs 2006 is the only comprehensive and concise guide to baccalaureate and graduate nursing education programs in the United States and Canada. We hope its contents will serve as the impetus for those looking for a rewarding and satisfying career in health care. AACN is proud to present this publication to the nursing profession and to those who seek to enter it.

—Jean E. Bartels, Ph.D., RN
President, AACN

—Geraldine D. Bednash, Ph.D., RN, FAAN
Executive Director, AACN

A Note from the Peterson's Editors

For more than thirty-five years, Peterson's has given students and parents the most comprehensive, up-to-date information on undergraduate and graduate institutions in the United States, Canada, and abroad.

Peterson's Nursing Programs 2006 provides prospective nursing students with the most comprehensive information on baccalaureate and graduate nursing education in the United States and Canada. Our goal is to help students find the best nursing program for them.

To this end, Peterson's has joined forces with the Association of American Colleges of Nursing (AACN), the national voice for America's baccalaureate- and higher-degree nursing education programs. AACN's educational, research, governmental advocacy, data collection, publications, and other programs work to establish quality standards for bachelor's- and graduate-degree nursing education, assist deans and directors to implement those standards, influence the nursing profession to improve health care, and promote public support of baccalaureate and graduate education, research, and practice in nursing—the nation's largest health-care profession.

For those seeking to enter the nursing profession or to further their nursing careers, *Peterson's Nursing Programs 2006* includes information needed to make important nursing program decisions and to approach the admissions process with knowledge and confidence.

The Nursing School Adviser section includes useful articles to help guide nursing education choices, with information on nursing careers today, selecting a nursing program, financing nursing education, going back to school, and more.

Also found in **The Nursing School Adviser** is the "How to Use This Guide" article, which explains some of the key factors to consider when choosing a nursing program. In addition, it explains how the book is organized and shows you how to maximize your use of *Peterson's Nursing Programs 2006* to its full potential.

If you already have specifics in mind, such as a particular program, turn to the **Quick-Reference Chart.** Here you can search through "Nursing Programs At-a-Glance" for particular degree options offered by specific programs of interest.

In the **Profiles of Nursing Programs** section you'll find expanded and updated nursing program descriptions, arranged alphabetically by state. Each profile provides all of the need-to-know information about accredited nursing programs in the United States and Canada.

If you are looking for additional information, you can turn to the **In-Depth Descriptions of Nursing Programs** section. Here you will find more than 70 two-page narrative descriptions written by admissions deans who chose to provide additional information about their schools and programs.

Finally, turn to the back of the book to find eight **Indexes** listing institutions offering *baccalaureate, master's, concentrations within master's, doctoral, postdoctoral, distance learning,* and *continuing education* programs. The last index lists every college and university contained in the guide along with its corresponding page reference.

Peterson's publishes a full line of resources to help guide you and your family through the admissions process. Peterson's publications can be found at your local bookstore, library, high school guidance office, or online at www.petersons.com. The editors at Peterson's wish you great success in your nursing program search!

THE NURSING SCHOOL ADVISER

Nursing Fact Sheet

Misconceptions about nursing have contributed to misinformation about the profession. Here are the real facts:

- **Nursing is the nation's largest health-care profession, with more than 2.7 million registered nurses nationwide.** Of all licensed RNs, 2.2 million, or 81.7 percent, are employed in nursing.
- **Nursing students account for more than half of all health professions students in the United States.**
- **Nurses comprise the largest single component of hospital staff, are the primary providers of hospital patient care, and deliver most of the nation's long-term care.**
- **Most health-care services involve some form of care by nurses.** Although 60 percent of all employed RNs work in hospitals, many are employed in a wide range of other settings, including private practices, health-maintenance organizations, public health agencies, primary-care clinics, home health care, nursing homes, outpatient surgicenters, nursing school–operated nursing centers, insurance and managed-care companies, schools, mental health agencies, hospices, the military, industry, nursing education, and health care research.
- **Though often collaborative, nursing does not "assist" medicine or other fields.** Nursing operates independent of, not auxiliary to, medicine and other disciplines. Nurses' roles range from direct patient care and case management to establishing nursing practice standards, developing quality assurance procedures, and directing complex nursing-care systems.
- **With more than four times as many RNs in the United States as physicians,** nursing delivers an extended array of health-care services, including primary and preventive care by advanced nurse practitioners in such areas as pediatrics, family health, women's health, and gerontological care. Nursing's scope also includes services by certified nurse-midwives and nurse anesthetists, as well as care in cardiac, oncology, neonatal, neurological, and obstetric/gynecological nursing and other advanced clinical specialties.
- **The primary pathway to professional nursing, as compared to technical-level practice, is the four-year Bachelor of Science in Nursing (B.S.N.) degree.** Registered nurses are prepared through a baccalaureate program; a two- to three-year associate degree in nursing program; or a three-year hospital training program, receiving a hospital diploma. All take the same state licensing exam—the NCLEX-RN®. *(The number of diploma programs has declined steadily—to less than 10 percent of all basic RN education programs—as nursing education has shifted from hospital-operated instruction into the college and university system.)*
- **To meet the more complex demands of today's health-care environment, a federal advisory panel has recommended that at least two thirds of the basic nurse workforce hold baccalaureate or higher degrees in nursing by the year 2010.** Aware of the need, RNs are seeking the B.S.N. degree in increasing numbers. In 1980, almost 55 percent of employed registered nurses held a hospital diploma as their highest educational credential, 22 percent held the bachelor's degree, and 18 percent held an associate degree. By 2000, a diploma was the highest educational credential for only 22.3 percent of employed RNs, while the number with bachelor's degrees had climbed to 32.7 percent, with 34.3 percent holding an associate degree as their top academic preparation. In 2003, 9,856 RNs with diplomas or associate degrees graduated from B.S.N. programs.
- **In 2000, of all employed RNs, 9.6 percent held master's degrees and 0.6 percent held doctoral degrees as their highest educational preparation.** However, the demand for master's- and doctorally prepared nurses for advanced practice, clinical specialties, teaching, and research roles far outstrips the supply.
- **According to the U.S. Bureau of Labor Statistics, registered nursing is the occupation with the largest projected job growth from 2002–12.** Other federal projections indicate that by 2020, the U.S. nursing shortage will grow to more than 800,000 registered nurses. Even as health care continues to shift beyond the hospital to more community-based primary care and other outpatient sites, federal projections say the rising complexity of acute care will see demand for RNs in hospitals climb by 36 percent by the year 2020.

"Your Nursing Career: A Look at the Facts," March 2004. Reprinted with permission from the American Association of Colleges of Nursing.

Counselors of Care in the Modern Health-Care System

Geraldine Bednash, Ph.D., RN, FAAN
Executive Director
American Association of Colleges of Nursing

A Different Era

The nursing profession is alive and reshaping itself. The role of nurses as those who minister exclusively to a patient's basic-care needs has changed. Much of the effectiveness and productivity of the future health-care industry will derive from the training of and services provided by nurses.

Modern nurses take a proactive role in health care by addressing health issues before they develop into problems. They oversee the continued care of patients who have left the health-care facility. Nurses are expected to make complex decisions in areas ranging from patient screening to diagnosis and education. They explore and document the effects of alternative therapies (e.g., guided imagery) and address public health problems, such as teen pregnancy. They explore and understand new technology and how it relates both to patient care and to their own job performance. They work in a variety of settings and are held accountable for their decisions. In today's health-care environment, health-care administrators must recruit nurses with a broad, well-rounded education.

Health-care providers must change the way they administer care. Instead of focusing on the treatment of illness, they must promote wellness. Nurses will oversee patient treatment and medication and must understand the repercussions of these health-care processes for the patient and his or her family.

Cost is the driving force behind this industry-wide transformation. Insurance companies have, for the most part, instigated changes in the way health-care benefits are paid. The old fee-for-service system is no longer the only option. The trend toward managed care, in which a fixed amount of money is allocated for the care of each patient, is changing the way care is provided. It seems that employers of the future will recruit nurses who understand the overall structure of the health-care industry, who possess highly developed critical-thinking skills, and who bring to their positions a well-rounded understanding of the risks and benefits of every health-care decision.

Counselors of Care

Job prospects for graduates of nursing programs are positive. Although many graduates receive associate degrees as registered nurses (RNs), hospital administrators and other employers want applicants with at least a Bachelor of Science in nursing degree.

To practice in a fast-changing health system, entry-level RNs must understand community-based primary care and emphasize health promotion and cost-effective coordinated care—all hallmarks of baccalaureate education. In addition to its broad scientific curriculum and focus on leadership and clinical decision-making skills, a Bachelor of Science in nursing degree education provides specific preparation in community-based care not typically included in associate degree or hospital diploma programs. Moreover, the nurse with a baccalaureate degree is the only basic nursing graduate prepared for all health-care settings—critical care, outpatient care, public health, and mental health—and so has the flexibility to practice in outpatient centers, private homes, and neighborhood clinics where demand is fast expanding as health care moves beyond the hospital to more primary and preventive care throughout the community.

Health-care administrators realize that patients are becoming more sophisticated about the care they receive, requiring an explanation and understanding of their health needs. Nurses will have to be knowledgeable care providers, working with physicians, pharmacists, and public health officials in interdisciplinary settings to satisfy these requirements.

Broader training enables graduates of baccalaureate programs to provide improved and varying types of care, and ensures stability and security in an industry now noted for its instability.

Promising Opportunities

One of the rewards of a baccalaureate education can be a competitive salary. Graduates of four-year degree programs can expect salaries starting around $35,000 per year, a figure that might fluctuate depending on geographic area and, more specifically, by the demand in that area. Obviously, the greater the need for nurses, the higher their salaries.

The baccalaureate degree also serves as a foundation for the pursuit of a master's degree in nursing, which prepares students for the role of advanced practice nurse (APN). Students can earn degrees as clinical nurse specialists in neonatology, oncology, cardiology, and other specialties or as nurse practitioners, nurse-midwives, or nurse anesthetists. Master's-prepared nurses can also enjoy rewarding careers in nursing administration and education.

These programs generally span one to two years. Graduates can expect starting salaries of approximately $50,000 annually in advanced practice nursing settings, and demand for these graduates is expected to be high over the next fifteen years. In some localities, for example, the nurse practitioner may be the sole provider of health care to a family.

Overall Transformation

The nursing field must be transformed to be compatible with the overall changes in the health-care industry. The latest statistics put the average age of nurses at 44, with only 10 percent of nurses under the age of 30. It is projected that over the next ten years much of the nursing population will retire. Employment figures for full-time-equivalent RNs will be about 2.1 million in 2005—a growth of 17 percent above 1995 levels.

The traditional career path of nurses is expected to change. More nurses will enter master's programs directly from baccalaureate programs, and more master's degree graduates will pursue doctoral degrees at a younger age. Since nurses will play a critical role in providing health care, a four-year baccalaureate degree is a crucial first step in preparing nurses to assume increased patient responsibilities within the health-care system.

Creating a Career Destination of Choice: Career Opportunities in a Time of Nursing Shortage

Geraldine Bednash, Ph.D., RN, FAAN
Executive Director
American Association of Colleges of Nursing

The United States is in the midst of a nursing shortage that is expected to intensify as baby boomers age and the need for health care grows. Compounding the problem is the fact that nursing colleges and universities across the country are struggling to maintain enrollment levels, which remain insufficient to meet the projected demand for nursing care.

The American Association of Colleges of Nursing (AACN) is concerned about the nursing shortage and is working with member schools, policy makers, kindred organizations, and the media to bring attention to this health-care crisis. AACN is directing its efforts toward enacting legislation, identifying strategies, and forming collaborations to address the nursing shortage.

Current and Projected Shortage Indicators

- The American College of Healthcare Executives reported in October 2004 that 72 percent of hospital CEOs are experiencing nursing shortages at their facilities.
- According to a July 2002 report by the Health Resources and Services Administration, thirty states were estimated to have shortages of registered nurses (RNs) in the year 2000. The shortage is projected to intensify over the next two decades, with forty-four states plus the District of Columbia expected to have RN shortages by the year 2020.
- According to the National Council of State Boards of Nursing, the number of first-time, U.S.-educated nursing school graduates who took the NCLEX-RN®, the national licensure examination for registered nurses, decreased by 20 percent from 1995–2003. A total of 19,820 fewer students in this category took the exam in 2003 as compared to 1995.
- According to the latest projections from the U.S. Bureau of Labor Statistics published in the February 2004 *Monthly Labor Review,* more than 1 million new and replacement nurses will be needed by 2012. For the first time, the U.S. Department of Labor has identified Registered Nursing as the top occupation in terms of job growth through the year 2012.
- According to American Hospital Association's June 2001 *TrendWatch,* 126,000 nurses are needed to fill vacancies at our nation's hospitals. Today, 75 percent of all hospital vacancies are for nurses.
- According to a study by Dr. Peter Buerhaus and colleagues, published in the *Journal of the American Medical Association* on June 14, 2000, the U.S. will experience a 20 percent shortage in the number of nurses needed in our nation's health-care system by the year 2020. This translates into a shortage of more than 400,000 RNs nationwide.

Contributing Factors Impacting the Nursing Shortage

Enrollment in schools of nursing is not growing fast enough to meet the projected demand for nurses.

- Though AACN reported in December 2003 that enrollments in entry-level baccalaureate programs increased by 16.6 percent over the previous year, this increase is not sufficient to meet the projected demand for nurses. In a report published in the November/December 2003 issue of *Health Affairs,* Dr. Peter Buerhaus and his colleagues found that "because the number of young RNs has decreased so dramatically over the past two decades, enrollments of young people in nursing programs would have to increase at least 40 percent annually to replace

Number of Candidates Taking the NCLEX-RN® Exam
First-Time, U.S.-Educated Candidates Only

Program	1996	1997	1998	1999	2000	2001	2002	2003
Diploma	6,346	5,240	3,978	3,161	2,679	2,310	2,424	2,565
Baccalaureate	32,278	31,828	30,142	28,107	26,048	24,832	25,806	26,630
Associate	55,554	52,396	49,045	45,255	42,665	41,567	42,310	47,423
Total	94,178	89,464	83,165	76,523	71,392	68,709	70,540	76,618

those expected to leave the workforce through retirement."

A shortage of nursing school faculty members is restricting nursing program enrollments.

- According to a survey by the AACN, *2004–2005 Enrollment and Graduations in Baccalaureate and Graduate Programs in Nursing,* U.S. nursing schools turned away 15,944 qualified applicants from entry-level baccalaureate nursing programs in 2003 due to an insufficient number of faculty members, clinical sites, classroom space, clinical preceptors, and budget restraints. In 2002, a total of 5,283 students were turned away from all types of professional nursing programs as well. Almost 76 percent of the nursing schools responding to the 2003 survey pointed to faculty shortages as a reason for not accepting all qualified applicants into entry-level baccalaureate programs. More than 29,000 qualified applicants were turned away from nursing schools due to a shortage of faculty.
- According to a study released by the Southern Regional Board of Education (SREB) in February 2002, a serious shortage of nursing faculty members was documented in sixteen SREB states and the District of Columbia. Survey findings show that the combination of faculty vacancies (432) and newly budgeted positions (350) points to a 12 percent shortfall in the number of nurse educators needed. Unfilled faculty positions, resignations, projected retirements, and the shortage of students being prepared for the faculty role pose a threat to the nursing education workforce over the next five years.

With fewer new nurses entering the profession, the average age of the RN is climbing.

- According to the *National Sample Survey of Registered Nurses* released in February 2002 by the Division of Nursing within the Bureau of Health Professions, the average age of the working registered nurse was 43.3 in March 2000, up from 42.3 in 1996. The RN population under the age of 30 dropped from 25.1 percent of the nursing population in 1980 to 9.1 percent in 2000.
- According to a July 2001 report released by the Government Accounting Office, *Nursing Workforce: Emerging Nurse Shortages Due to Multiple Factors* (GAO-01-944), 40 percent of all RNs will be older than age 50 by the year 2010.

The total population of registered nurses is growing at the slowest rate in twenty years.

- According to the latest *National Sample Survey of Registered Nurses,* the total RN population has increased at every four-year interval in which the survey has been taken since 1980. Although the total RN population increased from 2,558,874 in 1996 to 2,696,540 in 2000, it was the lowest increase (5.4 percent) reported since the survey began in 1980. Of the total RN population in 2000, an estimated 58.5 percent work full-time in nursing, 23.2 percent work part-time, and 18.3 percent are not employed in nursing.

Changing demographics signal a need for more nurses to care for our aging population.

- According to a July 2001 report released by the Government Accounting Office, *Nursing Workforce: Emerging Nurse Shortages Due to Multiple Factors* (GAO-01-944), "a serious shortage of nurses is expected in the future as demographic pressures influence both supply and demand. The future demand for nurses is expected to increase dramatically as the baby boomers reach their 60s, 70s, and beyond."
- According to a May 2001 report, *Who Will Care for Each of Us?: America's Coming Health Care Crisis,* released by the Nursing Institute at the University of Illinois College of Nursing, the ratio of potential caregivers to the people most likely to need care, the elderly population, will decrease by 40 percent between 2010 and 2030. Demographic changes may limit access to health care unless the number of nurses and other caregivers grows in proportion to the rising elderly population.

Job burnout and dissatisfaction are driving nurses to leave the profession.

- According to a study released in the *Journal of the American Medical Association (JAMA)* in October 2002, nurses reported greater job dissatisfaction and emotional exhaustion when they were responsible for more patients than they can safely care for. Lead researcher Dr. Linda Aiken concluded that "failure to retain nurses contributes to avoidable patient deaths."
- According to a study published by Dr. Linda Aiken and colleagues in the May/June 2001 issue of *Health Affairs,* more than 40 percent of nurses working in hospitals reported being dissatisfied with their jobs. The study indicates that 1 out of every 3 hospital nurses under the age of 30 are planning to leave their current job in the next year.

High nurse turnover and vacancy rates are affecting access to health care.

- According to a February 2002 report on health workforce shortages prepared by First Consulting Group for the American Hospital Association and other trade groups, the average nurse vacancy rate in U.S. hospitals was 13 percent. More than one in seven hospitals reported a severe RN vacancy rate of more than 20 percent. High vacancy rates were measured across rural and urban settings and in all regions of the country. Survey respondents indicated that a shortage of personnel is contributing to emergency department overcrowding and ambulance diversions.
- According to the report *Acute Care Hospital Survey of RN Vacancies and Turnover Rates in 2000,* released in January 2002 by the American Organization of Nurse Executives, the average RN turnover rate in acute-care hospitals was 21.3 percent. The average nurse vacancy rate was 10.2 percent, with the highest rates found in critical-care units (14.6 percent) and medical-surgical care

(14.1 percent). Nurse executives surveyed indicated that staffing shortages are contributing to emergency department overcrowding (51 percent) and the need to close beds (25 percent).

Impact of Nurse Staffing on Patient Care

Recent studies point to the connection between adequate levels of registered nurse staffing and safe patient care.

- A shortage of nurses prepared at the baccalaureate level may be affecting health- care quality and patient outcomes. In a study published in the September 24, 2003 issue of the *Journal of the American Medical Association,* Dr. Linda Aiken and her colleagues at the University of Pennsylvania identified a clear link between higher levels of nursing education and better patient outcomes. This extensive study found that surgical patients have a "substantial survival advantage" if treated in hospitals with higher proportions of nurses educated at the baccalaureate or higher degree level. In hospitals, a 10 percent increase in the proportion of nurses holding B.S.N. degrees decreased the risk of patient death and failure to rescue by 5 percent.
- A survey reported in the December 12, 2002 issue of the *New England Journal of Medicine* found that 53 percent of physicians and 65 percent of the public cited the shortage of nurses as a leading cause of medical errors. Overall, 42 percent of the public and more than a third of U.S. doctors reported that they or their family members have experienced medical errors in the course of receiving medical care. The survey was conducted by the Harvard School of Public Health and the Henry J. Kaiser Family Foundation.
- According to a study published in the October 23/30, 2002 issue of the *Journal of the American Medical Association,* more nurses at the bedside could save thousands of patient lives each year. Nurse researchers at the University of Pennsylvania determined that patients who have common surgeries in hospitals with high nurse-to-patient ratios have an up to 31 percent increased chance of dying. Funded by the National Institute for Nursing Research, the study found that every additional patient in an average hospital nurse's workload increased the risk of death in surgical patients by 7 percent. Having too few nurses may actually cost more money given the high costs of replacing burnt-out nurses and caring for patients with poor outcomes.
- In *Health Care at the Crossroads: Strategies for Addressing the Evolving Nursing Crisis,* a report released in August 2002 by the Joint Commission on Accreditation of Healthcare Organizations (JCAHO), the authors found that a shortage of nurses in America's hospitals is putting patient lives in danger. JCAHO examined 1609 hospital reports of patient deaths and injuries since 1996 and found that low nursing-staff levels were a contributing factor in 24 percent of the cases.
- According to a study published in the *New England Journal of Medicine* in May 2002, a higher proportion of nursing care provided by RNs and a greater number of hours of care by RNs per day are associated with better outcomes for hospitalized patients. This extensive study was conducted by Dr. Jack Needleman and Dr. Peter Buerhaus.

Strategies to Address the Nursing Shortage

- The **Call to the Profession** is a group of top leaders from national nursing organizations who are working together to ensure safe, quality nursing care for consumers and a sufficient supply of registered nurses to deliver that care. The group released an action plan called *Nursing's Agenda for the Future* in April 2002.
- The **TriCouncil for Nursing,** an alliance of four autonomous nursing organizations (AACN, ANA, AONE, NLN), each focused on leadership for education, practice, and research, issued a joint policy statement in January 2001 on *Strategies to Reverse the New Nursing Shortage.*
- The **Nurse Reinvestment Act** was signed by the President on August 1, 2002 and has been sent back to Congress for appropriations. Provisions of this new law include scholarship money to attract new students into nursing, a Faculty Loan Cancellation Program to remove financial barriers to faculty careers, funding to promote best practices in nursing care, and public service announcements to champion nursing careers.
- In April 2001, a coalition of twenty-three national nursing organizations issued a joint call to Congress to stem the nursing shortage. The group released a comprehensive plan to address the shortage entitled "Assuring Quality Health Care for the United States: Supporting Nurse Education and Training," which outlined funding priorities and called for new initiatives to recruit and retain nurses.
- Two national media campaigns have been launched to help polish the image of nursing. **Nurses for a Healthier Tomorrow** is a coalition of forty nursing and health-care organizations working together to raise interest in nursing careers among middle school and high school students. The coalition has conducted nationwide focus groups with students ages 6–15 years, secured over $600,000 in sponsorship, launched a Web site, created a televised public service announcement, and designed print ads that can be downloaded for free from the Web. In February 2002, Johnson & Johnson launched the **Campaign for Nursing's Future,** a multimedia initiative to promote careers in nursing that includes paid television commercials, a recruitment video, a Web site, and brochures mailed to schools across the country.

Opportunities Abound in Times of Shortage

There has never been a better time to become a nurse. Salaries are rising, and working conditions are improving in an effort to appeal to new students and retain working RNs in the profession. Nurses are gaining more independence on the job, which enables them to maximize their education and expertise at work. Job security is also extremely high because the projected supply of RNs does not meet the projected demand.

Media coverage of the nursing shortage has also helped showcase the many roles available within the profession. Though there is a great demand for nurses to provide direct care, nurses are also needed as researchers, health-care administrators, policy analysts, and nurse executives. The baccalaureate-prepared nurse enjoys the greatest chance for career advancement as well as the opportunity to move into upper-level roles requiring a master's degree or doctorate.

One of the greatest areas of need is for nursing school faculty members. Nurse educators are the key to preparing new nurses and adapting curricula in response to changing technology and professional practices. The shortage of nurse faculty members hinders the efforts of nursing schools in many parts of the country to expand enrollments in response to the projected shortage.

The nursing shortage has also focused federal attention on the need to remove economic barriers to the profession. This translates into more resources for financial aid—grants, loans, and scholarships. In addition, special programs exist to recruit members of diverse, underrepresented groups into nursing. Be sure to check with the financial aid officers at the schools you wish to attend for the details on specific programs.

RNs Returning to School: Choosing a Nursing Program

Marilyn Oermann, Ph.D., RN, FAAN
Professor
College of Nursing
Wayne State University

If you are thinking about returning to school to complete your baccalaureate degree or to pursue a graduate degree in nursing, you are not alone. Registered nurses (RNs) are returning to school in record numbers, many seeking advancement or transition to new roles in nursing. Over the last two decades, the number of RNs prepared initially in diploma and associate degree in nursing programs who have graduated from baccalaureate nursing degree programs has more than doubled, according to the AACN. There are expanded opportunities for nurses with baccalaureate degrees in nursing. Although the decision to return to school means considerable investment of time, financial resources, and effort, the benefits can be overwhelmingly positive.

Higher education in nursing opens doors to many opportunities for career growth not otherwise available. By continuing your education, you can

- update your knowledge and skills, critical today in light of rapid advances in health care.
- move more easily into a new role within your organization or in other health-care settings.
- pursue a different career path within nursing.

Moreover, returning to school brings personal fulfillment and satisfaction gained through learning more about nursing and the changing health-care system and using that knowledge in the delivery and management of patient care.

More Skills and Flexibility Needed

If you are contemplating returning to school, here are some facts to consider. The health-care system continues to undergo dramatic changes. These changes include hospitalized patients who are more acutely ill; an aging population; technological advances that require highly skilled nursing care; a greater role for nurses in primary care, health promotion, and health education; and the need for nurses to care for patients and families in multiple settings, such as schools, workplaces, homes, clinics, and outpatient facilities, as well as hospitals. With the nursing shortage, nurses are in great demand in hospitals. Moreover, as hospitals continue to become centers for acute and critical care, the nurse's role in both patient care and management of other health-care providers in the hospital has become more complex, requiring advanced knowledge and skills.

Because of the complexity of today's health-care environment, AACN and other leading nursing organizations have called for the baccalaureate degree in nursing as the minimum educational requirement for professional nursing practice. In fact, nurse executives in hospitals have indicated their desire for the majority of nurses on staff to be prepared at least at the baccalaureate level to handle the increasingly complex demands of patient care and management of health-care delivery. The baccalaureate nursing degree is essential for nurses to function in different management roles, move across employment settings, have the flexibility to change positions within nursing, and advance in their career. Baccalaureate nursing degree programs prepare the nurse for a broad role within the health-care system and for practice in hospitals, community settings, home health care, neighborhood clinics, and other outpatient settings where opportunities are expanding. Continuing education provides the means for nurses to prepare themselves for a future role in nursing.

The demand for nurses with baccalaureate and more advanced degrees will continue to grow. There is an excess of nurses prepared at the associate degree level, a mounting shortage of baccalaureate-prepared nurses, and only half as many nurses prepared at master's and doctoral levels as needed. Nurses with baccalaureate nursing degrees are needed in all areas of health care, and the demand for nurses with master's and doctoral preparation for advanced practice, management, teaching, and research will continue.

Identifying Strategies

The decision to return to school marks the beginning of a new phase in your career development. It is essential for you to plan this future carefully. Why are you thinking about returning to school, and what do you want to accomplish by doing so? Understanding why you want to go back to school will help you select the best program for you. Knowing what you want to accomplish will help you to focus on your goals and overcome the obstacles that could prevent you from achieving your full potential.

Even if you decide that additional education will help you reach your professional goals, you may also have a list of reasons why you think you cannot return to school—no time, limited financial resources, fear of failure, and concerns about meeting family responsibilities, among others. If you are concerned about the demands of school combined with existing responsibilities, begin by identifying strategies for incorporating classes and study time into your present schedule or consider taking an online course. Remember, you can start your program with one course and reevaluate your time at the end of the term.

Research and anecdotal evidence from adults returning to college indicate that despite their need to balance school work with a career and, often, family responsibilities, these adult learners experience less stress and manage their lives better than they had thought possible. Many of these adult learners report that the satisfaction gained from their education more than compensates for any added stress. Furthermore, studies of nurses who have returned to school suggest that while their education may create stress for them, most nurses cope effectively with the demands of advanced education.

If costs are of concern, it is best to investigate tuition-reimbursement opportunities where you are employed, scholarships from the nursing program and other nursing organizations, and loans. The financial aid officer at the program you are considering is probably the best available resource to answer your financial assistance questions.

If you are unsure of what to expect when returning to school, remember that such feelings are natural for anyone facing a new situation. If you are motivated and committed to pursuing your degree, you will succeed. Most nursing programs offer resources, such as test-taking skills, study skills, and time-management workshops, as well as assistance with academic problems. You can combine school, work, family, and other responsibilities. Even with these greater demands, the benefits of education outweigh the difficulties.

Clarifying Career Goals

Nursing, unlike many other professions, has a variety of educational paths for nurses returning for advanced education. You should decide if baccalaureate- or graduate-level work is congruent with your career goals. The next step in this process is to reexamine your specific career goals, both immediate and long-term, to determine the level and type of nursing education you will need to meet them. Ask yourself what you want to be doing in the next five to ten years. Discuss your ideas with a counselor in a nursing education program, nurses who are practicing in roles you are considering, and others who are enrolled in a nursing program or who have recently completed a nursing degree.

Baccalaureate degree nursing programs prepare nurses as generalists for practice in all health-care settings. Graduate nursing education occurs at two levels—master's and doctoral. Master's programs vary in length, typically between one and two years. Preparation for roles in advanced practice as nurse practitioners, certified nurse midwives, clinical nurse specialists, certified registered nurse anesthetists, nursing administrators, and nursing educators requires a master's degree in nursing. Many programs meet the needs of RNs by offering options such as accelerated course work, advanced placement, evening and weekend classes, and distance learning courses.

A trend in education for RNs is accelerated programs that combine the baccalaureate and master's nursing programs. These combined programs are designed for RNs without degrees whose career goals involve advanced nursing practice and other roles requiring a master's degree. Nurses who complete these combined programs may be awarded both a baccalaureate and a master's degree in nursing or a master's degree only.

At the doctoral level, nurses are prepared for a variety of roles, including research and teaching. Doctoral programs generally consist of three years of full-time study beyond the master's degree, although some programs admit baccalaureate graduates and include the master's-level requirements and degree within the doctoral program.

Matching a Program to Your Needs

Once you have defined your career goals and the level of nursing education they will require, the next step is matching your needs with the offerings and characteristics of specific nursing programs. Some of the criteria you may want to consider in evaluating potential schools of nursing include the types of programs offered, the length of the program and its specific requirements, the availability of full- and part-time study and number of credits required for part-time study, the flexibility of the program, if distance education courses are available, and the days, times, and sites at which classes and clinical experiences are offered as they relate to your work schedule. Take into consideration the program's accreditation status; faculty qualifications in terms of research, teaching, and practice; and the resources of the school of nursing and of the college/university, such as library holdings, computer services, and statistical consultants. You should also consider the clinical settings used in the curriculum and their relationship to your career goals, as well as the availability of financial aid for nursing students.

Carefully review the admission criteria, including minimum grade point average; scores required on any admission tests, such as the Graduate Record Examinations (GRE) for master's and doctoral programs; and any requirements in terms of work experience. For students returning for a baccalaureate degree, prior nursing knowledge may be validated through testing, transfer of courses, and other mechanisms. Review these options prior to applying to a program.

While the intrinsic quality and characteristics of the program are important, your own personal goals and needs have to be included in your decision. Consider commuting distance, if courses are offered online, costs in relation to your financial resources, program design, and flexibility of the curriculum in relation to your work, family, and personal responsibilities. While the majority of nursing programs offer part-time study, many programs also schedule classes to accommodate work situations.

Many schools offer nursing courses online, and in some places, the entire baccalaureate and master's programs are available through distance learning. The largest enrollment in nursing distance learning is in baccalaureate programs for RNs. Distance learning allows RNs to further their education no matter where they live. Many nurses prefer online courses because they can learn at times convenient for them, especially considering competing demands associated with their jobs, families, and other commitments.

Ensure Your Success

Once you have made the decision to return to school and have chosen the program that best meets your needs, take an additional step to ensure your success. Identify the support you will need, both academic and personal, to be successful in the nursing program. Academic support is provided by the institution and may include tutoring services, learning resource centers, computer facilities, and other resources to support your learning. You should take advantage of available support services and seek out resources for areas in which you are weak or need review. Academic support services, however, need to be complemented by personal support through family, friends, and peers. With a firm commitment to pursuing advanced education, a clear choice of a nursing program to meet your goals, and support from others, you are certain to find success in returning to school.

Baccalaureate Programs

Linda K. Amos, Ed.D., RN, FAAN
Associate Vice President for Health Sciences
Professor of Nursing
University of Utah

The health-care industry has continued to change dramatically over the past few years, transforming the roles and escalating opportunities for nurses. The current shortage of nurses is caused by an increased number of hospitalized patients who are older and more acutely ill, a growing elderly population with multiple chronic health problems, and expanded opportunities in HMOs, home care, occupational health, surgical centers, and other primary-care settings. Expanding technological advances prolonging life require more highly skilled personnel.

The increasing scope of nursing opportunities will grow immensely as nurses become the frontline providers of health care. They are assuming important roles in the provision of managed care, and they will be responsible for coordinating and continuing the care outside traditional health-care facilities. Nurses will play a big role in educating the public and addressing the social and economic factors that impact quality of care.

Worldwide Standards

The nursing student of the future will receive a wealth of information. Understanding the technology used to manage that information will be essential to their ability to track and assess care. In this area, nurses will be able to provide care over great distances. In some areas, care is being managed by the nurse via tele-home health over the Internet. Use of the Internet and other computer-oriented systems are now an integral part of the tools used by nurses. Nurses of the future, therefore, will have to become aware of worldwide standards of care. Nevertheless, the primary job of a nurse will be making sure that the right person is providing the right care at the right cost.

This goal will be accomplished as the industry turns away from the hospital as the center of operation. Nurses will work in a broad array of locations, such as clinics, outpatient facilities, community centers, schools, and even places of business. Hospitals are now places only for the very sick, and the name itself may be changed to acute-care center.

Much of the emphasis in health care will shift to preventive care and the promotion of health. In this system, nurses will take on a broader and more diverse role than in the past.

Unlimited Opportunities, Expanded Responsibilities

The four-year baccalaureate programs in today's nursing colleges provide the educational and experiential base not only for entry-level professional practice, but also as the platform on which to build a career through graduate-level study for roles as advanced practice nurses, such as nurse practitioners, nurse midwives, clinical specialists, and nurse administrators and educators. Nurses at this level can be expected to specialize in oncology, pediatrics, neonatology, obstetrics and gynecology, critical care, infection control, psychiatry, women's health, community health, and neuroscience. The potential and responsibilities at this level are great. Increasingly, many families use the nurse practitioner for all health-care needs. In almost all states, the nurse practitioner can prescribe medications and provide health care for the management of chronic non-acute illnesses and preventive care.

The health care system demands a lot from nurses. The education of a nurse must transcend the traditional areas, such as chemistry and anatomy, to include health promotion, disease prevention, screening, genetic counseling, and immunization. Nurses should understand how health problems may have a social cause, such as poverty and environmental contamination, as well as have insight into human psychology, behavior, cultural mores, and values.

The transformation of the health care system offers unlimited opportunities for nurses at the baccalaureate and graduate levels as care in urban and rural settings becomes more accessible. According to the U.S. Bureau of Labor Statistics, employment of RNs will grow faster than the average for all occupations through 2012, due largely to growing demand in settings such as health maintenance organizations, community health centers, home care, and long-term care. The increased complexity of health problems and increased management of health problems out of the hospitals require highly educated and well-prepared nurses at the baccalaureate and graduate levels. It is an exciting era in nursing, one that holds exceptional promise for nurses with a baccalaureate nursing degree.

The compensation for new nurses is again becoming competitive with that of other industries. Entry-level nurses with baccalaureate degrees in nursing can expect a salary range from about $31,000 to $38,000 per year, depending on geographic location and experience. Five years into their careers, the national average for nurses with four-year degrees is over $40,000 per year, with many earning over $50,000. The current shortage has prompted sign-on bonuses and other incentives to attract and retain staff.

Applying to College

Meeting the school's general entrance requirements is the first step toward a university or college degree in nursing.

Admission requirements may vary, but a high school diploma or equivalent is necessary. Most accredited colleges consider SAT scores along with high school grade point average. A strong preparatory class load in science and mathematics is generally preferred among nursing schools. Students may obtain specific admission information by writing to the schools' nursing departments.

To apply to a nursing school, contact the admission offices of the colleges or universities you are interested in and request the appropriate application forms. With limited spaces in nursing schools, programs are competitive and early submission of an application is recommended.

Accreditation

Accreditation of the nursing program is very important, and it should be considered on two levels—the accreditation of the university or college and the accreditation of the nursing program. Accreditation is a voluntary process in which the school or the program asks for an external review of its programs, facilities, and faculty. For nursing programs, the review is performed by peers in nursing education to ensure program quality and integrity.

Baccalaureate nursing programs have two types of regular systematic reviews. First, the school must be approved by the state board of nursing. This approval is necessary to ensure that the graduates of the program may sit for the licensing examinations offered through the National Council of State Boards of Nursing, Inc. The second is accreditation administered by a nursing accreditation agency that is recognized by the U.S. Department of Education.

Although accreditation is a voluntary process, access to federal loans and scholarships requires accreditation of the program, and most graduate schools only accept students who have earned degrees from accredited schools. Further, accreditation ensures an ongoing process of quality improvement that is based on national standards. Canadian nursing school programs are accredited by the Canadian Association of University Schools of Nursing, and the Canadian programs listed in this book must hold this accreditation. There are two recognized accreditation agencies for baccalaureate nursing programs in the United States: the Commission on Collegiate Nursing Education (CCNE) and the National League for Nursing Accrediting Commission (NLNAC).

Focusing Your Education

Academic performance is not the sole basis of acceptance into the upper level of the nursing program. Admission officers also weigh such factors as student activities, employment, and references. Moreover, many require an interview and/or essay in which the nursing candidate offers a goal statement. This part of the admission process can be completed prior to a student's entrance into the college or university or prior to the student's entrance into the school of nursing itself, depending on the program.

In this interview or essay, students may list career preferences and reasons for their choices. This allows admission officers to assess the goals of students and gain insights into their values, integrity, and honesty. One would expect that a goal statement from a student who is just entering college would be more general than that of a student who has had two years of preprofessional nursing studies. The more experienced student would be likely to have a more focused idea of what is to be gained by an education in nursing; there would be more evidence of the student's values and the ways in which she or he relates them to the knowledge gained from preprofessional nursing classes.

Baccalaureate Curriculum

A standard basic or generic baccalaureate program in nursing is a four-year college or university education that incorporates a variety of liberal arts courses with professional education and training. It is designed for high school graduates with no previous nursing experience.

Currently, there are more than 600 baccalaureate programs in the United States. Of the 498 programs that responded to a fall 2004 survey conducted by the American Association of Colleges of Nursing, total enrollment in all nursing programs leading to a baccalaureate degree was 112,081. A report from the National Advisory Council on Nursing Education recommends that at least two thirds of the nursing workforce hold a baccalaureate degree or higher by 2010, compared to the current 40 percent.

The baccalaureate curriculum is designed to prepare students for work within the growing and changing health-care environment. With nurses taking more of an active role in all facets of health care, they are expected to develop critical-thinking and communication skills in addition to receiving standard nurse training in clinics and hospitals. In a university or college setting, the first two years include classes in the humanities, social sciences, basic sciences, business, psychology, technology, sociology, ethics, and nutrition.

In some programs, nursing classes start in the sophomore year, whereas others have students wait until they are juniors. Many schools require satisfactory grade point averages before students advance into professional nursing classes. On a 4.0 scale, admission into the last two years of the nursing program may require a minimum GPA of 2.5 to 3.0 in preprofessional nursing classes. The national average is about 2.8, but the cutoff level varies with each program.

In the junior and senior years, the curriculum focuses on the nursing sciences and emphasis moves from the classroom to health facilities. This is where students are exposed to clinical skills, nursing theory, and the varied roles nurses play in the health-care system. Courses include nurse leadership, health promotion, family planning, mental health, environmental and occupational health, adult and pediatric care, medical and surgical care, psychiatric care, community health, management, and home health care.

This level of education comes in a variety of settings: community hospitals, clinics, social service agencies, schools, and health-maintenance organizations. Training in diverse settings is the best preparation for becoming a vital player in the growing health care field.

Reentry Programs

Practicing nurses who return to school to earn a baccalaureate degree will have to meet requirements that may include possession of a valid RN license and an associate degree or hospital diploma from an accredited institution. Again, it is best to check with the school's admissions department to determine specifics.

Nurses returning to school will have to consider the rapid rate of change in health care and science. A nurse who passed an undergraduate-level chemistry class ten years ago would probably not receive credit for that class today, due to the growth of knowledge in that and all other scientific fields. The need to reeducate applies not only to practicing nurses returning to school, but also to all nurses throughout their careers.

In the same vein, nurses with diplomas from hospital programs who want to work toward a baccalaureate degree would find themselves in need of meeting the common requirements for more clinical practice as well as developing a deeper understanding of community-based nursing practices, such as health prevention and promotion.

There are colleges and universities available to the RN in search of a baccalaureate that give credit for previous nurse training. These programs are designed to accommodate the needs and career goals of the practicing nurse by providing flexible course schedules and credit for previous experience and education. Some programs lead to a master's-level degree, a process that can take up to three years. Licensed practical nurses (LPNs) can also continue their education through baccalaureate programs.

Nurses thinking of reentering school may also consider other specialized programs. For example, there are programs aimed at enabling a nurse with an A.D.N. degree or an LPN/LVN license to earn a B.S.N. Also, accelerated B.S.N. programs are available for students with degrees in other fields.

Choosing a Program

With more than 600 baccalaureate programs in the United States, some research will reveal which programs match your needs and career objectives.

RN to Baccalaureate Programs Fact Sheet

More than 600 RN to baccalaureate programs are available nationwide, including 169 programs offered in a more intense, accelerated format. Program length varies between one and two years depending upon the school's requirements, program type, and the student's previous academic achievement.

Concerns about the limited availability of RN to baccalaureate programs are unfounded. In fact, there are more RN to baccalaureate programs available than four-year nursing programs (476) or accelerated bachelor's degree programs for non-nursing college graduates (136). Access to RN to baccalaureate programs is further enhanced since many programs are offered completely online or on-site at various health-care facilities.

Enrollment in RN to baccalaureate programs is increasing in response to calls for a more highly educated nursing workforce. From 2002 to 2003, enrollments increased by 8.1 percent, or by 2,215 students, the first such increase in RN to baccalaureate programs in six years.

Hundreds of articulation agreements between A.D.N. and diploma programs and four-year institutions exist nationwide, including some statewide agreements, to facilitate students seeking baccalaureate-level nursing education. Before enrolling in diploma and A.D.N. programs, students are encouraged to check with school administrators to see what articulation agreements exist with baccalaureate degree–granting schools and to determine which course work will be transferable.

If you have no health-care experience, it might be best to gain some insight into the field by volunteering or working part-time in a care facility, such as a hospital or an outpatient clinic. Talking to nurse professionals about their work will also lend insight into how your attributes may apply to the nursing field.

When considering a nursing education, consider your personal needs. Is it best for you to work in a heavily structured environment or one that offers more flexibility in terms of, say, integrating a part-time work schedule into studies? Do you need to stay close to home? Do you prefer to work in a large health-care system, such as a health maintenance organization or a medical center, or do you prefer smaller, community-based operations?

As for nursing programs, it is best to ask the following questions: How involved is the faculty in developing students for today's health-care industry? How strong is the school's affiliation with clinics and hospitals? Is there any assurance that a student will gain an up-to-date educational experience for the current job market? Are a variety of care settings available? How much time in clinics will be needed for graduation? What are the program's resources in terms of computer and science laboratories? Does the school work with hospitals and community-based centers to provide health care? How available is the faculty to oversee a student's curriculum? What kind of student support is available in terms of study groups and audiovisual aids? Moreover, what kind of counseling from faculty members and administrators is available to help students develop well-rounded, effective progress through the program?

Visiting a school and talking to the program's guidance counselors will give you a better understanding of how a particular program or school will fit your needs. You can get a closer look at the faculty, its members' credentials, and the focus of the program. It's also not too early to consider what each program can offer in terms of job placement.

Master's Programs

Kathleen Dracup, D.N.Sc., RN
Professor and Dean
School of Nursing
University of California, San Francisco

The transformation of the health-care system is taking place as you read this, and it can be seen even today in the most common areas.

- A mother brings her child into a clinic for treatment of an earache. Instead of a physician, a nurse practitioner provides the care.
- A patient is readied for surgery. A variety of specialists move about the surgery room, but it's not a specially trained physician administering the anesthetic—it's a certified nurse anesthetist.
- During the recovery from an acute illness, it's decided that the patient no longer needs to stay in the hospital but isn't well enough to return home. It's decided that the best place to continue the recovery is an intermediate-care facility. Who makes that decision? A clinical nurse specialist. Who oversees the physical and emotional rehabilitation programs at this facility? Another clinical nurse specialist.

These health-care professionals are all advanced practice nurses (APNs). All have graduate-level degrees, and they serve as proof that the demand for nurses with master's and doctoral degrees for advanced practice, clinical specialties, teaching, and research will double the supply.

Another study estimated that the U.S. could save as much as $8.75 billion annually if APNs were used appropriately in place of physicians. As more and more of the restrictions on APNs succumb to legislative or economic forces, the demand for graduate-level nurses is expected to remain high.

Educational Core for APN

A master's degree in nursing is the educational core that allows advanced practice nurses to work as nurse practitioners, certified nurse-midwives, clinical nurse specialists, and certified nurse anesthetists.

Nurse practitioners conduct physical exams, diagnose and treat common acute illnesses and injuries, administer immunizations, manage chronic problems such as high blood pressure and diabetes, and order lab services and X rays.

Nurse-midwives provide prenatal and gynecological care, deliver babies in hospitals and private settings such as homes, and follow up with postpartum care.

Clinical nurse specialists provide a range of care in specialty areas, such as oncology, pediatrics, and cardiac, neonatal, obstetric/gynecological, neurological, and psychiatric nursing.

Nurse anesthetists administer anesthesia for all types of surgery in operating rooms, dental offices, and outpatient surgical centers.

Master's degrees in nursing administration or nursing education are also available.

There are more than 330 master's degree programs accredited by the Commission on Collegiate Nursing Education (CCNE) or by the National League for Nursing Accrediting Commission (NLNAC). The wide spectrum of programs includes the Master of Science in Nursing (M.S.N.) degree, Master of Nursing (M.N.) degree, Master of Science (M.S.) degree with a major in nursing, or Master of Arts (M.A.) degree with a nursing major. The specific degrees depend on the requirements set by the college or university or by the faculty of the nursing program. There are accelerated programs for RNs, which allow the nurse with a hospital diploma or associate degree to earn both a baccalaureate and a master's degree in a condensed program. Some schools offer accelerated master's degree programs for nurses with non-nursing degrees and for non-nursing college graduates. There are joint-degree programs, such as a master's in nursing combined with a Master of Business Administration, Master of Public Health, or Master of Hospital Administration.

Master's Curriculum

The master's degree builds on the baccalaureate degree to enable the student to develop expertise in one area. That specialty can range from running a hospital to providing care for prematurely born babies, from researching the effectiveness of alternative therapies to tackling social and economic causes of health problems. It is an opportunity for the student who has assessed his or her personal career goals and matched them to individual, community, and industry needs. What students can do with their APN degrees is limited only by their imagination.

Full-time master's programs consist of eighteen to twenty-four months of uninterrupted study. Many graduate school students, however, fit their master's-level studies around their work schedules, which can extend the time it takes to graduate.

Master's-level study incorporates theories and concepts of nursing science and their applications, along with the management of health care. Research is used to provide a foundation for the improvement of health-care techniques. Students also have the opportunity to develop the knowledge, leadership skills, and interpersonal skills that will enable them to improve the health-care system.

Classroom and clinical work are involved throughout the master's program. In class, students spend less time listening to lectures and taking notes and more time participating in student- and faculty-led seminars and roundtable discussions. Extended clinical work is generally required.

Graduate-level education in many programs includes courses in statistics, research management, health economics, health policy, health-care ethics, health promotion, nutrition, family planning, mental health, and the prevention of family and social violence. When students begin to concentrate their study in their clinical areas, any number of courses that support their chosen specialty may be included. For example, a nurse wanting to specialize in pediatrics may take courses in child development.

A clinical nurse specialist can focus on acute care, geriatrics, adult health, community health, critical care, gerontology, rehabilitation, and cardiovascular, surgical, oncology, maternity/newborn, pediatric, mental/psychiatric, and women's health nursing. Areas of specialization in nurse practitioner programs include acute care, adult health, child care, community health, emergency care, geriatric care, neonatal health, occupational health, and primary care.

Admission Requirements

The admission requirements for master's programs in nursing vary a great deal. Generally, a bachelor's degree from a school accredited by the Commission on Collegiate Nursing Education or by the National League for Nursing Accrediting Commission and a state RN license are required. Scores from the Graduate Record Examinations (GRE) or the Miller Analogies Test (MAT), college transcripts, letters of reference, and an essay are typically required. Nonnurses and nurses with nonnursing degrees have special requirements. The profiles and in-depth descriptions of colleges and universities in this publication will give you an idea of each school's specific requirements.

It is important to remember that admissions officers look at a student's transcripts, clinical work, and letters of reference together. A low grade point average is not an automatic knockout—admissions officers are after a composite package. Also, some specialties require specific courses. Students in the nurse anesthetist program, for instance, must have an upper-level college course in biochemistry.

A Master's That's Best for You

Most nurses who think of entering a master's program already have been practicing nursing. They have a good idea what they want to specialize in before they apply for admission. It is crucial to know what you want to study before you enter a master's program.

The best way to ensure success in a master's program is for you to understand your individual strengths and career desires and then find the faculty and college setting that are best suited to help you develop those strengths. Students must make an effort to educate themselves as to the strength of the faculty in each college's master's program. That's the best thing to look for: a strong faculty in one specialty.

This can be tricky. One university's master's program may be rated reasonably high in all fields. Another program might not be rated as high overall, but its cardiovascular program, for example, may be one of the best due to its access to facilities or the fact that its faculty is in the process of developing an innovative new treatment.

This type of information is not hard for the master's candidate to discover; it just takes time. Such information is available from each school's admissions office, which should be more than happy to promote its nursing faculty and support its opinion with proof, such as the research papers that faculty members have published in journals or the number of degrees each faculty member carries.

This type of research is the best way to find a program that meets your needs. The profiles of master's nursing programs in this book should help. If you can, narrow the list to three or four graduate schools and then write each school's admissions department for catalogs and other information. Visit the schools and take time to talk to a guidance counselor from the nursing program.

Other key questions to consider when applying for a master's program are: Does the school offer financial aid, such as loans, scholarships, fellowships, or teaching posts? How much clinical work is needed? Does the clinical work meet your needs, and does the type of clinical work involved match what you understand the health-care system will be using when you graduate? Is the course work flexible? Can you work part-time and still progress toward a master's degree? This is important to know. A majority of master's program students continue to work while they pursue the degree. Therefore, master's degree programs may present a flexible offering of short courses to meet the student's schedule demands.

Some programs require a thesis, whereas others provide another type of culminating experience, such as a comprehensive examination.

The Master's Trends

Today's master's programs have increased the amount of clinical practice that students engage in so that graduates enter the job market ready for certification. There is also a greater emphasis on applying new research findings to methods of patient care. This might involve students' reading literature about new treatments and then incorporating the appropriate changes.

All master's program candidates should consider courses in cost-benefit analysis. As managed-care systems become predominant in the industry, health-care workers will be asked to justify the expense of their treatment as well as its effectiveness. This leads to the crucial issue of quality. There will always be a strong effort to minimize costs in every health-care procedure, but that cannot compromise the quality of care. It's safe to say that discharging a newborn too soon from a hospital due to shortsightedness can be quite costly.

Depending on the specialty, master's candidates entering the job market may be expected to oversee auxiliary-care providers, such as nurse aides or other unlicensed employees. They may work in a team structure, and, in this capacity, the nurse specialist may be expected to manage, motivate, and steer the group. This requires team-building as well as other management techniques.

While everyone in the health-care facility will have a part in ensuring patient satisfaction, nurses, particularly advanced practice nurses, will shoulder a great deal of this load. Developing interpersonal and communication skills, as well as having an understanding of human behavior, will make it easier for the advanced practice nurse to help patients to understand modern health-care procedures, which no doubt will improve their feelings of satisfaction.

Finally, nurses at all levels should be aware of the need for flexibility. Many health-care organizations are reducing the number of beds in hospitals and transferring the care of a growing number of patients to other types of facilities or settings. In light of this trend, it's best for the master's program student to gain experience in a variety of places, such as homes, clinics, and community-based settings.

The demand for high-quality care will continue to grow. Medical innovations and technological advances will continue. The quality and effectiveness of health care will continue to improve, and nurses with graduate degrees will play an active role in this trend.

The Hot Employment Spots

The health-care industry has undergone such radical transformation in the last five years that administrators feel they cannot predict whether any one geographic region will have more hirings than another. Generally, nurses with master's degrees will be in demand in all regions of the country, in both the U.S. and Canada.

Industry trends indicate that along with continuing opportunities in hospitals, more and more nurses will also work outside the hospital in outpatient clinics and community settings and even in businesses. As patients spend less and less time in hospitals, there is a need for nurse specialists to oversee home-care settings and ensure that the quality of care there is high. In this vein, some nurses are taking the initiative and running their own businesses as health-care providers, offering services as they see fit in whatever locations are appropriate.

RN to Master's Degree Programs Fact Sheet

Currently, there are 137 programs available nationwide to transition RNs with diplomas and associate degrees to the master's degree level. These programs prepare nurses to assume positions requiring graduate preparation, including the advanced practice roles of nurse practitioner, clinical nurse specialist, certified nurse-midwife, and certified registered nurse anesthetist. Master's degree-prepared nurses are in high demand as expert clinicians, nurse executives, clinical educators, health policy consultants, and research assistants.

RN to master's degree programs generally take about three years to complete, with specific requirements varying by institution and the student's previous course work. Although the majority of these programs are offered in traditional classroom settings, some RN to master's programs are offered largely online or in a blended classroom/online format.

The baccalaureate-level content missing from diploma and A.D.N. programs is built into the front end of the RN to master's degree program. Mastery of this upper-level basic nursing content is necessary for students to move on to graduate study. Upon completion, programs award both a baccalaureate and a master's degree.

The number of RN to master's degree programs has doubled within the past ten years, from seventy programs in 1994 to 137 programs today. According to AACN's 2003 survey of nursing schools, twenty-three new RN to master's degree programs are in the planning stages.

Immediate Rewards

Advanced practice nurses right out of school can expect annual salaries ranging from $60,000 to $90,000, depending on geographic location and previous experience. However, some rural county health clinics start their nurse practitioners at salaries as low as $40,000 per year.

Certified nurse anesthetists and certified nurse-midwives, however, draw larger salaries. Nurse-midwives, for example, can draw first-year salaries as high as $90,000 per year. Areas such as the Northeast and the West Coast tend to have nurses in these fields at the higher end of the salary scale. After five years of practice, the salary range for APNs stretches from $60,000 to $100,000 a year. Again, it depends on location. After five years, nurse-midwives earn salaries ranging from $65,000 to $120,000 annually.

The Nurse Ph.D.: A Vital Profession Needs Leaders

Carole A. Anderson, Ph.D., RN, FAAN
Vice Provost for Academic Administration
The Ohio State University

There is no doubt that education is the path for a nurse to achieve greater clinical expertise. At the same time, however, the nursing profession needs more nurses educated at the doctoral level to replenish the supply of faculty and researchers. The national shortage of faculty will soon reach critical proportions, having a significant impact on educational programs and their capacity to educate future generations of nursing students.

Although the number of doctorate programs has continued to increase, the total enrollment of students in these programs has remained fairly constant, resulting in a shortage of newly trained Ph.D.'s to renew faculty ranks. As a result, approximately 50 percent of nursing faculty possess the doctorate as a terminal degree. Furthermore, with many advances being made in the treatment of chronic illnesses, there is a continuing need for research that assists patients in living with their illness. This research requires individual investigators who are prepared on the doctoral level.

One reason there is a lack of nurses prepared at the doctoral level is that, compared to other professions, nurses have more interruptions in their careers. Many in the profession are women who work as nurses while fulfilling responsibilities as wives and mothers. As a result, many pursue their education on a part-time basis. Also, the nursing profession traditionally has viewed clinical experience as being a prerequisite to graduate education. This career path results in fewer individuals completing the doctorate at an earlier stage in their career, thereby truncating their productivity as academics, researchers, and administrators. To reverse this trend, many nursing schools have developed programs that admit students into graduate (doctoral and master's) programs directly from their undergraduate or master's programs.

Nursing Research

When nurses do research for their doctorates, many people tend to think that it focuses primarily on nurses and nursing care. In reality, nurses carry out clinical research in a variety of areas, such as diabetes care, cancer care, and eating disorders.

In the last twenty years advances in medicine have involved, for the most part, advancing treatment, not cures. In other words, no cure for the illness has been discovered, but treatment for that illness has improved. However, sometimes the treatment itself causes problems for patients, such as the unwelcome side effects of chemotherapy. Nurses have opportunities to devise solutions to problems like these through research, such as studies on how to manage the illness and its treatment, thereby allowing individuals to lead happy and productive lives.

The Curricula

Doctoral programs in nursing are aimed at preparing students for careers in health administration, education, clinical research, and advanced clinical practice. Basically, doctoral programs prepare nurses to be experts within the profession, prepared to assume leadership roles in a variety of academic and clinical settings, course work, and research. Students are trained as researchers and scholars to tackle complex health-care questions. Program emphasis may vary from a focus on health education to a concentration on policy research. The majority of doctoral programs confer the Doctor of Philosophy (Ph.D.) degree, but some award the Doctor of Nursing Science (D.N.S. or D.N.Sc.), the Doctor of Science in Nursing (D.S.N.), the Nursing Doctorate (N.D.), and the Doctor of Education (Ed.D.).

Doctoral nursing programs traditionally offer courses on the history and philosophy of nursing and the development and testing of nursing and other health-care techniques, as well as the social, economic, political, and ethical issues important to the field. Data management and research methodology are also areas of instruction. Students are expected to work individually on research projects and complete a dissertation.

Doctoral programs allow study on a full- or part-time basis. For graduate students who are employed and therefore seek flexibility in their schedules, many programs offer courses on weekends and in the evenings.

Admission Requirements

Admission requirements for doctoral programs vary. Generally, a master's degree is necessary, but in some schools a master's degree is completed in conjunction with fulfillment of the doctoral degree requirements. Standard requirements include an RN license, Graduate Record Examinations (GRE) scores, college transcripts, letters of recommendation, and an essay. Students applying for doctoral-level study should have a solid foundation in nursing and an interest in research. Programs are usually the equivalent of three to five years of full-time study.

Selecting a Doctoral Program

Selecting a doctoral program comes down to personal choice. Students work closely with professors, and, thus, the support and mentoring you receive while pursuing your degree is as vital as the quality of the facilities. The most important question is whether there is a "match" between your research interest and faculty research. Many of the same questions you would ask about baccalaureate and master's degree programs apply to doctoral programs. However, in a doctoral program, the contact with professors, the use of research equipment and facilities, and the program's flexibility in allowing you to choose your course of study are critical.

Other questions to consider include: Does the university consider research a priority? Does the university have adequate funding for student research? Many nurses with doctoral degrees make the natural transition into an academic career, but there are many other career options available for nurses prepared at this level. For example, nurses prepared at the doctoral level are often hired by large consulting firms to work with others in designing solutions to health-care delivery problems. Others are hired by large hospital chains to manage various divisions, and some nurses with doctoral degrees are hired to manage complex health-care systems at the executive level. On another front, they conduct research and formulate national and international health-care policy. In short, because of the high level of education and a shortage of nurses prepared at this level, there are a number of options.

Salaries are related to the various positions. Faculty salaries vary by the type of institution and by faculty rank, typically ranging from approximately $50,000 at the assistant professor level to over $100,000 at the professor level. Salaries of nurse executives also vary, with the lowest salaries being in small rural hospitals and the highest being in complex university medical centers. In the latter, average salaries are well over $100,000 and often reach close to $200,000 annually. Consultant salaries are wide-ranging but often consist of a base plus some percentage of work contracted. Clinical and research positions vary considerably by the type of institution and the nature of the work. Needless to say, a doctoral education does provide individuals with a wide range of opportunities, with salaries commensurate with the type and level of responsibilities. Are there opportunities to present research findings at professional meetings? Is scholarship of faculty, alumni, and students presented at regional and national nursing meetings and subsequently published? Has the body of research done at a university enhanced the knowledge of nursing and health care?

AACN Indicators of Quality in Research-Focused Doctoral Programs in Nursing

Schools of nursing must consider the indicators of quality in evaluating their ability to mount research-focused doctoral programs. High-quality programs require a large number of increasingly scarce resources and a critical mass of faculty members and students. The AACN Indicators of Quality in Research-Focused Doctoral Programs in Nursing represent those indicators that should be present in a research-focused program.

There is considerable consensus within the discipline that while there are differences in the purpose and curricula of Ph.D. and Doctor of Nursing/Doctor of Nursing Science programs, most programs emphasize preparation for research. Therefore, AACN recommends continuing with a single set of quality indicators for research-focused doctoral programs in nursing whether the program leads to a Ph.D. or to a Doctor of Nursing or Doctor of Nursing Science degree.

The following indicators apply to the Doctor of Philosophy (Ph.D.) in nursing, Doctor of Nursing Science (D.N.S. or D.N.Sc.), and Doctor of Nursing (N.D.) degrees.

Faculty

I. Represent and value a diversity of backgrounds and intellectual perspectives.

II. Meet the requirements of the parent institution for graduate research and doctoral education; a substantial proportion of faculty hold earned doctorates in nursing.

III. Conceptualize and implement productive programs of research and scholarship that are developed over time and build upon previous work, are at the cutting edge of the field of inquiry, are congruent with research priorities within nursing and its constituent communities, include a substantial proportion of extramural funding, and attract and engage students.

IV. Create an environment in which mentoring, socialization of students, and the existence of a community of scholars is evident.

V. Assist students in understanding the value of programs of research and scholarship that continue over time and build upon previous work.

VI. Identify, generate, and utilize resources within the university and the broader community to support program goals.

VII. Devote a significant proportion of time to dissertation advisement. Generally, each faculty member should serve as the major adviser/chair for no more than 3 to 5 students during the dissertation phase.

Programs of Study

The emphasis of the program of study is consistent with the mission of the parent institution, the discipline of nursing, and the degree awarded. The faculty's areas of expertise and scholarship determine specific foci in the program of study. Requirements and their sequence for progression in the program are clear and available to students in writing. Common elements of the program of study are outlined below.

I. Core and related course content—the distribution between nursing and supporting content is consistent with the mission and goals of the program, and the student's area of focus and course work are included in:

   A. Historical and philosophical foundations to the development of nursing knowledge

   B. Existing and evolving substantive nursing knowledge

   C. Methods and processes of theory/knowledge development

   D. Research methods and scholarship appropriate to inquiry

   E. Development-related to roles in academic, research, practice, or policy environments

II. Elements for formal and informal teaching and learning focus on:

   A. Analytical and leadership strategies for dealing with social, ethical, cultural, economic, and political issues related to nursing, health care, and research

   B. Progressive and guided student scholarship research experiences, including exposure to faculty's interdisciplinary research programs

   C. Immersion experiences that foster the student's development as a nursing leader, scholarly practitioner, educator, and/or nurse scientist

D. Socialization opportunities for scholarly development in roles that complement students' career goals

III. Outcome indicators for the programs of study include:

A. Advancement to candidacy requires faculty's satisfactory evaluation (e.g., comprehensive exam) of the student's basic knowledge of elements I-A through I-E identified above

B. Dissertations represent original contributions to the scholarship of the field

C. Systematic evaluation of graduate outcomes is conducted at regular intervals

D. Within three to five years of completion, graduates have designed and secured funding for a research study, or, within two years of completion, graduates have utilized the research process to address an issue of importance to the discipline of nursing or health care within their employment setting

E. Employers report satisfaction with graduates' leadership and scholarship at regular intervals

F. Graduates' scholarship and leadership are recognized through awards, honors, or external funding within three to five years of completion

Resources

I. Sufficient human, financial, and institutional resources are available to accomplish the goals of the unit for doctoral education and faculty research.

A. The parent institution exhibits the following characteristics:

1) Research is an explicit component of the mission of the parent institution
2) An office of research administration
3) A record of peer-reviewed external funding
4) Postdoctoral programs
5) Internal research funds
6) Mechanisms that value, support, and reward faculty and student scholarship and role preparation
7) A university environment that fosters interdisciplinary research and collaboration

B. The nursing doctoral program exhibits the following characteristics:

1) Research active faculty as well as other faculty experts to mentor students in other role preparations
2) Provide technical support for:
(a) Peer review of proposals and manuscripts in their development phases
(b) Research design expertise
(c) Data management and analysis support
(d) Hardware and software availability
(e) Expertise in grant proposal development and management
3) Procure space sufficient for:
(a) Faculty research needs
(b) Doctoral student study, meeting, and socializing
(c) Seminars
(d) Small-group work

C. Schools of exceptional quality also have:

1) Centers of research excellence
2) Endowed professorships
3) Mechanisms for financial support to allow full-time study
4) Master teachers capable of preparing graduates for faculty roles

II. State-of-the-art technical and support services are available and accessible to faculty, students, and staff for state-of-the-science information acquisition, communication, and management.

III. Library and database resources are sufficient to support the scholarly endeavors of faculty and students.

Students

I. Students are selected from a pool of highly qualified and motivated applicants who represent diverse populations.

II. Students' research goals and objectives are congruent with faculty research expertise and scholarship and institutional resources.

III. Students are successful in obtaining financial support through competitive intramural and extramural academic and research awards.

IV. Students commit a significant portion of their time to the program and complete the program in a timely fashion.

V. Students establish a pattern of productive scholarship, collaborating with researchers in nursing and other disciplines in scientific endeavors that result in the presentation and publication of scholarly work that continues after graduation.

Evaluation

The evaluation plan:

I. Is systematic, ongoing, comprehensive, and focuses on the university's and program's specific mission and goals.

II. Includes both process and outcome data related to these indicators of quality in research-focused doctoral programs.

III. Adheres to established ethical and process standards for formal program evaluation, e.g., confidentiality and rigorous quantitative and qualitative analyses.

IV. Involves students and graduates in evaluation activities.

V. Includes data from a variety of internal and external constituencies.

VI. Provides for comparison of program processes and outcomes to the standards of its parent graduate school/university and selected peer groups within nursing.

VII. Includes ongoing feedback to program faculty, administrators, and external constituents to promote program improvement.

VIII. Provides comprehensive data in order to determine patterns and trends and recommend future directions at regular intervals.

IX. Is supported with adequate human, financial, and institutional resources.

Approved by AACN Membership, November 2001.

Accelerated Nursing Programs

Nancy O. DeBasio, Ph.D., RN
Dean and Professor
Research College of Nursing

The significance of the nursing shortage has reached crisis proportions. No single factor is responsible; it is perhaps the confluence of several critical factors that has contributed to the nursing profession's current state. The aging workforce, the projected need for more than a million new and replacement registered nurses by the year 2012, and the entry of 78 million baby boomers into an already over-taxed health-care delivery system over the next years will require the development and implementation of unique and creative strategies to reach out to new student populations. To further underscore the growing awareness of this shortage and its impact on patient care, several major reports have been issued over the past two years that cite strategies to meet this workforce crisis. The April 2002 American Hospital Association report *In Our Hands,* the Institute of Medicine's *Crossing the Quality Chasm,* the August 2002 Joint Commission's *Healthcare at the Crossroads: Strategies Addressing the Evolving Nursing Crisis,* the Robert Wood Johnson report *Health Care's Human Crisis: The American Nursing Shortage,* and the July 2002 report from the Health Services and Resources Administration (HRSA) titled *Projected Supply, Demand, and Shortages of Registered Nurses: 2000–2020* all point to the necessity of investing time, people, and funding to offer opportunities that will facilitate the growth of the nursing workforce in a format that is attractive, educationally sound, and timely.

What Is an Accelerated Program?

Accelerated programs provide an innovative educational opportunity to non-nurse college graduates. Offered at both the baccalaureate and graduate levels, students build upon their previous undergraduate experience and transition into the nursing role in a shorter timeframe. At the baccalaureate level, the nursing curriculum is developed to reflect course objectives, course content, and clinical learning experiences that are similar to those of the traditional four-year curriculum. However, courses and clinical experiences are offered in an intense full-time format with no breaks between sessions. Generally, accelerated baccalaureate programs run from twelve to eighteen months, depending on the institution. In addition, students must complete necessary science prerequisites—such as anatomy and physiology, chemistry, and microbiology—prior to entering the nursing courses. Some institutions include nursing courses such as nutrition and pathophysiology as prerequisites, which must be successfully completed prior to admission to the fast-track nursing curriculum. Students with prior degrees are generally not required to complete additional liberal arts courses that were components of their previous degree program. Some institutions may require course work specific to the nature of that institution. For example, faith-based programs may require completion of religious studies and theology and philosophy courses prior to enrollment in the nursing curriculum. Due to the intensity of the curricula, students are often interviewed as part of the screening process. Students are evaluated on their ability to learn in a fast-paced environment, to act as social support systems, to cope with a variety of situations, and to understand the format of compressed clinical and classroom instruction. In programs where Web-based education is a significant teaching strategy, students are evaluated on their computer capabilities and their previous exposure to independent, online instruction. Total nursing credit-hour requirements vary from program to program. Generally, students complete between 50 and 60 credit hours in the nursing major itself.

Generic or accelerated master's degree programs may be the programs of choice for individuals who view this level as the natural next step in their higher education. Often career changers might question the rationale for completion of a second baccalaureate degree. In these cases, the generic master's degree would be the preferred option. This choice may also be influenced by one's geographic location and the hiring practices of institutions in that particular region. Yale University initiated the first master's program for non-nurse college graduates in 1974. Entry-level master's programs provide basic nursing curricula, generally in the first year of the program, with the addition of graduate core courses and specialty-specific course work in the remainder of the program. At this time, most programs are approximately three years in length. However, institutions are reevaluating curricula and designing unique models that will meet nursing workforce needs as well as the educational needs of this population of learners. For example, the University of Iowa has recently received approval to award a professional master's degree in nursing and health-care practices that can be completed in four semesters. Some accelerated baccalaureate programs may offer an option where students can take a stated number of graduate credits during their baccalaureate experience that can be applied to completion of a master's degree in nursing.

Is This Career Option for Me?

What are key factors one should consider when evaluating a career change into nursing through an accelerated format? First, how would you evaluate yourself based on the following characteristics that are frequently used to describe these learners: highly motivated; strong academic record; inquisitive, sophisticated follower of higher education; willing to challenge the status quo; assertive; high energy level; confident in your capabilities; committed to an intense, compressed educational experience; and having the desire to have a positive impact on the health of the nation and the global society? Second, are you in a position, financially and emotionally, to attend a rigorous, full-time program of study? Third, are you interested in a career that has a multitude of opportunities—at the bedside or in industry, school nursing, research and development, pharmaceutical sales, home health, hospice care, case management, and long-term care? Are you interested in a career where you can provide care to newborns, mothers, children, and the elderly? Do you have interest in a career where you can continue your education to obtain a master's degree or a doctorate, and then choose to become a nursing educator, administrator, researcher, or provider of primary health care as a nurse practitioner? The opportunities are endless.

Where Can I Find an Accelerated Program?

Accelerated programs are not new to nursing education. However, there has been a significant increase in the number of baccalaureate and generic master's programs since the early 1990s. To date, there are 150 accelerated baccalaureate nursing programs, with forty-six new programs in the planning stages, and forty-one generic master's programs, with twenty in the works. These programs are offered in thirty-seven states and the District of Columbia, with the highest concentrations found in Pennsylvania, California, New York, Massachusetts, Connecticut, Ohio, Indiana, and Virginia.

Hospitals and health systems as well as other practice settings are eager to employ this pool of workers because they have demonstrated a record of success and a well-defined work ethic that facilitates a rapid and smooth transition into highly complex health-care delivery environments.

What You Need to Know About Online Learning

Rosalee C. Yeaworth, Ph.D., RN, FAAN
Professor and Dean Emerita
College of Nursing
University of Nebraska Medical Center

Sue Schmidt, M.A. in Education and Human Development
Designer Web Management
MediaOne

Half a century ago, young women who graduated from high school and chose to enter a nursing program were expected to move into a "nurses' home," which housed not only dormitory-style rooms but also classrooms and faculty offices. Most of the clinical learning was done in apprenticeship style in a single hospital setting. There was no such thing as distance learning.

However, over the course of the past half century, nursing education, like health care and education in general, has changed dramatically, creating a need for educators to implement distance education programs. The demographics of nursing students have changed. Not only is the nursing student far more likely to be a man than fifty years ago, but also the student who once was referred to as "nontraditional" is now becoming the traditional student. These students are mature, employed individuals who have complex family responsibilities and often live or work some distance from the university offering the courses they wish to take. The rapid advances in health-care knowledge and technology have increased the demand for nurses with graduate degrees. All nurses are faced with the need to enhance their knowledge through lifelong education as their roles and expectations change. In addition, a much greater effort is being made to provide education and training to residents in rural settings in the hope that they will continue to live and work in these areas.

Universities are addressing these changing educational needs by using advanced technologies and new communication capabilities. Distance learning offerings are continually enhanced by using new technologies and delivery systems such as the Internet and desktop videoconferencing. These technologies enable universities to reach beyond the boundaries imposed on them by traditional classrooms to deliver educational material to students located in different, noncentralized locations, thus allowing instruction and learning to occur independently of time and place. This model, known as "distributive learning," can be used in combination with traditional classroom-based courses and with traditional distance learning courses, or to create wholly virtual classrooms.

Tools used for distance education include:

E-mail—This is one of the most commonly used communication tools. It allows for a one-to-one exchange of information between the sender and receiver of the e-mail message. Course papers and draft materials may be sent, commented on, and returned as attached documents.

Listservs—This is a one-to-many communication exchange. People subscribe to listservs based on discussion topics that interest them. When a participant on a listserv sends an e-mail to the listserv, the message is copied and sent to all people who have subscribed to it. Listservs are generally free; there is no charge to subscribe.

Discussion Groups—This is a many-to-many communication exchange. E-mail and listservs deliver the messages directly to your electronic mailbox. Discussion groups, on the other hand, are retained in a specified area on the Internet. You must go to the discussion group to post your comments and read and reply to the comments of others. The advantage of a discussion group over e-mail or listservs is that the comments can be viewed easily by all and the sequence of comments and replies posted is readily apparent in its structure.

Chat Rooms—Chat is synchronous communication as the participants are online at the same time talking to each other. E-mail, listservs, and discussion groups, on the other hand, are asynchronous communication. With moderated chat, a moderator views the questions and comments posed by the participants and selects those that will be seen by all participants. After posting the comment or question, the moderator answers it. In a regular chat room, there is no management over what is or is not posted.

Streaming Video—Entire lectures can be delivered using streaming video technology. Even students accessing the material with slower modems can receive clear audio and good video images.

Desktop Videoconferencing—With a small camera mounted on top of the computer, students and faculty members are able to see and talk with each other using desktop videoconferencing software.

Virtual Reality—Student lounges can be constructed visually using virtual reality software. When students want to have a discussion with other students, they literally walk into the lounge as an avatar (a visual image of themselves they have selected) and hold live chat sessions with their fellow classmates.

Web Sites—Components of or the entire course content can be delivered via the Internet through the creation of a Web site. Any or all of the technology tools noted above can be linked through an educational Web site. Among other things, a Web site includes the syllabus, discussion groups, assignments, student lounges, faculty information, resources (including links to Web documents that enrich the course content), lecture notes, and other course components. Traditional distance education tools, such as satellite transmission, videotapes, telephone conferences, correspondence material, and CD-ROM interactive instruction, are also frequently used in conjunction with Web-delivered course material.

The key to using technology successfully is to define your goals and objectives and then decide which technology or combination of technologies will be most effective. Keep in mind that faculty members and students must have the appropriate computer equipment and user knowledge to participate in distance learning. Even though computers today are much more user-friendly, it is important to allot some time for students to become accustomed to using the new technologies necessary for transmitting their course material. Campus information technology services should work closely with the faculty to prepare introductory manuals or self-help materials for students. Information technology specialists should be available to answer technology questions or solve problems so that faculty members can concentrate on the course content questions. Enthusiasm can be dampened if too much time must be devoted to learning the technology or dealing with technology problems.

When deciding to take distance-learning courses, other factors must be considered. What you need to participate in distance learning varies with the sophistication of the tools used by the course instructor. Sending and receiving e-mail, participating in discussion groups, and viewing online syllabi require fairly simple technology. You need a computer with a modem and an Internet service provider (ISP). When selecting an ISP, participants should consider cost, reliability of access, and speed. World Wide Web access provided through your cable provider is generally more expensive but provides significantly faster access to documents. Video streaming and desktop videoconferencing require more sophisticated computer systems. Sometimes, in rural areas, the local telephone company or the Internet or TV provider may be limited in their services. Students may find, for example, that they have to use a teleconference line for sound with desktop videoconferencing. It is important to investigate the technology issues in your area before undertaking a course, because technical limitations can add to the cost and decrease your satisfaction and learning. Access to the campus bookstore and library may be a concern for students who are at considerable distance from the school offering the course. Books and supplies may be ordered online from the bookstore, and journal articles can be made available from the library through electronic reserve. Courses that use electronic reserve usually require a fee to cover copyright costs.

Some advantages of distance learning are:

Student-Centered versus Instructor-Directed Learning—Students take an active role in their own learning experience. They are able to select what material they need to cover more extensively and are given the opportunity for exploration through accessing linked material provided by their instructor. They are also given more opportunity to learn at their own pace and select the time when they are more prepared to effectively view the course material.

Flexibility—Students may work at their own computers on a weekend or the middle of the night, not having to worry about library hours or driving in bad weather. Valuable time can be focused on learning rather than on the logistics of getting to class.

Accessibility—Students who would not be able to attend classes because of geographic proximity or time constraints are now able to participate.

Student Interaction Increases—Interaction increases in a distance learning environment. Students not only listen and take notes, but they also pose ideas to and ask questions of the instructor as well as other students in discussion groups. Interaction is encouraged, and the instructor has a better understanding of what and how the student is learning. In most classroom settings, it is very difficult to get students to discuss a topic. They may ask a question of or make a comment to the instructor, but they seldom interact with classmates about course topics.

Collaboration and Team Problem Solving—Using asynchronous and synchronous communication tools, students can work together on projects much more easily today. It has always been difficult to bring a group together face-to-face to discuss what needs to be done. Through these new communication channels, information can be easily passed among a group, and resources, such as research documents and drafts of works in progress, can be distributed instantly.

Increased Sharing of Knowledge—In the traditional classroom, the instructor is the primary source of information. In distance learning, using tools such as a discussion group, students have a greater opportunity to share their knowledge and experience, allowing the members of the group to learn from each other. In addition, access to the Internet allows students to access the experience and knowledge of others outside their immediate classroom setting.

Immediate Access to Updated Material—Any material or announcements that have been changed can be distributed instantly, reducing distribution costs and providing students with access to the most current information.

Developing Needed Technology Skills—Students are learning technology skills that they can apply later in their work setting.

Some important factors should be considered when deciding if a distance education model is right for you. It has been shown that students can learn course content by distance methods as well as or better than in the traditional classroom setting. Less information is available on socialization issues related to the nurse generalist, specialist, or practitioner roles. Socialization involves internalizing attitudes, values, and norms. The role modeling, mentoring, and collegial friendships may or may not be as adaptable to distance methods. Careful selection of clinical settings for experience, on-site preceptors, requirements for certain on-campus experiences, and group attendance of students and faculty members at regional or national meetings are some methods used to assist socialization.

Distance learning will not suffice for the "college experience" of joining sororities and fraternities and of participating in athletic and social activities that many young undergraduate students desire. On the other hand, for the adult learner with job and family responsibilities, the distance education methodologies can provide the opportunity to participate in educational experiences that might otherwise have been beyond consideration.

When selecting your educational program, you should clearly define your goals for your educational experiences. If you want the opportunity to have clinical experience in a particular setting, to be a research or teaching assistant to a certain person, or to be mentored by a selected expert, then your choice would be an on-site educational environment in a particular setting. However, if you want a degree from a particular institution but do not want to move or travel there, you need to explore the distance learning opportunities offered. You need to remember that it is not an either-or proposition. You may be able to combine traditional classroom-based courses with distance learning for selected courses to optimize your overall educational program.

Distance learning is used by more and more educational institutions to provide both degree and continuing education. Many schools collaborate to offer students a selection of courses taught by different colleges and universities. A recent collaborative effort is the Western Governors University, a virtual university that is a partnership involving eighteen states and approximately 100 participating colleges and universities.

As noted above, the world is changing and so is the way we deliver nursing education. Distance education has opened a world of opportunities to students and faculty members. Students now have the ability to further their education by removing many of the time and access barriers they previously faced. Faculty members are presented with new and exciting challenges as they begin to use innovative technologies in their course delivery. With careful consideration and planning, the outcome will enhance the overall learning experience of both learner and teacher.

The International Nursing Student

For many international students completing baccalaureate, master's, or doctoral nursing programs, their choice of learning institutions is obvious. U.S. and Canadian colleges and universities are considered to offer the finest programs of nursing education available anywhere in the world. U.S. and Canadian nursing programs are renowned for their breadth and flexibility, for the excellence of their basic curriculum structure, and for their commitment to extensive on-site clinical training. Nursing study in the U.S. and Canada also affords students the opportunity for hands-on learning and practice in the world's most technologically advanced health-care systems. For many international nursing students, and especially for students from countries that are medically underserved, these features make U.S. and Canadian nursing programs unsurpassed.

Applying to Nursing School

The application process for international students often involves the completion of two separate written applications. Many colleges screen international candidates with a brief preliminary application requesting basic biographical and educational information. This document helps the admission officer determine whether the student has the minimum credentials for admission before requiring him or her to begin the lengthy process of completing and submitting final application forms.

Final applications to U.S. and Canadian colleges and universities vary widely in length and complexity, just as specific admission requirements vary from institution to institution. However, international nursing students must typically have a satisfactory scholastic record and demonstrated proficiency in English. To be admitted to any postsecondary institution in the United States or Canada, you must have satisfactorily completed a minimum of twelve years of elementary and secondary education. The customary cycle for this education includes a six-year elementary program, a three-year intermediate program, and a three-year postsecondary program, generally referred to as high school in the U.S. In addition, nursing school programs generally require successful completion of several years of high school-level mathematics and science.

The documentation of satisfactory completion of secondary schooling (and university education, in the case of graduate-level applicants) is achieved through submission of school reports, transcripts, and teacher recommendations. Because academic records and systems of evaluation differ widely from one educational system to the next, request that your school include a guide to grading standards. If you have received your secondary education at a school in which English is not the language of instruction, be certain to include official translations of all documents.

International students who have completed some university-level course work in their native country may be eligible to receive credit for equivalent courses at the U.S. or Canadian institution in which they enroll. Under special circumstances, practical nursing experience may also qualify for university credit. Policies regarding the transfer of or qualification for credits based on education or nursing experience outside the U.S. (or Canada for Canadian schools) vary widely, so be certain to inquire about these policies at the universities or colleges that interest you.

Language skills are a key to scholastic success. "The ability to speak, write, and understand English is an important determinant of success," says Joann Weiss, former Director of the Nursing and Latin American Studies dual-degree programs at the University of New Mexico in Albuquerque. Her advice for potential international applicants is simple: "Develop a true command of written and spoken English." English proficiency for students who have not received formal education in English-speaking schools is usually demonstrated via the Test of English as a Foreign Language (TOEFL); minimum test scores of 550 to 580 are commonly required. This policy, as well as the level of proficiency required, varies from school to school, so be sure to investigate each college's policies.

In addition, most universities offer some form of English language instruction for international students, often under the rubric ESL (English as a second language). Students who require additional language study to meet admission requirements or students who wish to deepen their skills in written or verbal English should inquire about ESL program availability.

Many colleges and universities also require that all undergraduate applicants take a standardized test—either the SAT and three SAT Subject Tests or the ACT. Like their U.S. and Canadian counterparts, international applicants to graduate-level nursing programs are required by most institutions to take the standardized Graduate Record Examinations (GRE).

Applicants should also be aware that financial assistance for international students is usually quite limited. To spare international students economic hardship during their schooling in the U.S. or Canada, many colleges and universities require them to demonstrate the availability of sufficient financial resources for tuition and minimum living expenses and supplies. As with so many admission requirements, policies regarding financial aid vary considerably; find out early what the policies are at the colleges that interest you.

Attending School in the U.S. or Canada

Once you are accepted by the college or university of your choice, take full advantage of the academic and personal advising systems offered to international students. Most institutions of higher education in the U.S. and Canada maintain an international student advisory office staffed with trained counselors. In addition to general academic counseling and planning, an international adviser can assist in a broad range of matters ranging from immigration and visa concerns to employment opportunities and health-care issues.

With few exceptions, all university students also obtain specialized academic counseling from an assigned faculty adviser. Faculty advisers monitor academic performance and progress and try to ensure that students meet the institutional requirements for their degree. Faculty advisers are excellent sources of information regarding course selection, and some advisers offer tutorials or special language or educational support to international students.

Although all university students face academic challenges, international students often find life outside the classroom equally demanding. Suddenly introduced into a new culture where the way of life may be dramatically different from that of their native country, international students often face a variety of social, domestic, medical, religious, or emotional concerns. Questions about social conventions, meal preparation, or other personal concerns can often be addressed by your international or faculty adviser.

Lorraine Rudowski, Assistant Professor and International Student Adviser at the College of Nursing and Health Science at George Mason University in Fairfax, Virginia, emphasizes the benefits of a strong relationship with your advisers: "My job as an adviser is to provide comprehensive support to my students—from academic counseling and opportunities for language development to emotional support and guidance to attending parties or other informal social events to ease the sense of social and personal isolation often experienced by foreign students."

Dr. Rudowski says international students would do well to find a sponsor or confidant within the university, someone who understands the conventions of the student's native country. "A culturally sensitive sponsor is better equipped to understand the unique needs of each international student and is much more likely to help students obtain the assistance they need, whether we're talking about religious issues, help with study methods or social skills, or simply knowing how to deal with such everyday chores as cooking and cleaning. All of these matters can be sources of deep concern to international students."

Yet for all the academic, social, and personal challenges facing international nursing students, there is good news. Deans of nursing, professors, and advisers typically praise the motivation and determination of their international students, and international nursing students often boast matriculation rates that match or exceed those of their U.S. and Canadian counterparts.

For more information about the rules and regulations governing international students' entrance to U.S. schools, log on to infoUSA, part of the U.S. Department of State's Web site, at http://usinfo.state.gov/usa/infousa/educ/studyus.htm.

Specialty Nursing Organizations

Academy of Medical Surgical Nurses
East Holly Avenue
Box 56
Pitman, NJ 08071-0056
866-877-AMSN
E-mail: amsn@ajj.com
www.medsurgnurse.org

Air & Surface Transport Nurses Association
7995 East Prentice Avenue
Suite 100
Greenwood Village, CO 80111
800-897-NFNA (toll-free)
Fax: 303-770-1614
E-mail: astna@gwami.com
www.astna.org

American Academy of Ambulatory Care Nursing
East Holly Avenue
Box 56
Pitman, NJ 08071-0056
856-256-2350
E-mail: aaacn@ajj.com
www.aaacn.org

American Association of Critical-Care Nurses (AACN)
101 Columbia
Aliso Viejo, CA 92656-4109
949-362-2000
800-899-2226 (toll-free)
Fax: 949-362-2020
E-mail: info@aacn.org
www.aacn.org

American Association of Diabetes Educators
100 West Monroe Street
Suite 400
Chicago, IL 60603
800-338-3633 (toll-free)
Fax: 312-424-2427
E-mail: aade@aadenet.org
www.aadenet.org

The American Association of Legal Nurse Consultants
401 North Michigan Avenue
Chicago, IL 60611
877-402-2562 (toll-free)
Fax: 312-673-6655
E-mail: info@aalnc.org
www.aalnc.org

American Association of Neuroscience Nurses
4700 West Lake Avenue
Glenview, IL 60025
847-375-4733
888-557-2266 (toll-free)
Fax: 877-734-8677
E-mail: info@aann.org
www.aann.org

American Association of Nurse Anesthetists
222 South Prospect Avenue
Park Ridge, IL 60068-4001
847-692-7050
Fax: 847-692-6968
E-mail: info@aana.com
www.aana.com

American Association of Nurse Attorneys
P.O. Box 515
Columbus, OH 43216-0515
877-538-2262 (toll-free)
Fax: 614-221-2335
E-mail: taana@taana.org
www.taana.org

American Association of Occupational Health Nurses, Inc.
2920 Brandywine Road
Suite 100
Atlanta, GA 30341
770-455-7757
Fax: 770-455-7271
E-mail: aaohn@aaohn.org
www.aaohn.org

American Association of Spinal Cord Injury Nurses
75-20 Astoria Boulevard
Jackson Heights, NY 11370
718-803-3782
Fax: 718-803-0414
E-mail: aascin@unitedspinal.org
www.aascin.org

American College of Nurse-Midwives
8403 Colesville Road
Suite 1550
Silver Spring, MD 20910
240-484-1800
Fax: 240-485-1818
www.midwife.org

American College of Nurse Practitioners
1111 19th Street, NW
Suite 404
Washington, DC 20036
202-659-2190
Fax: 202-659-2191
E-mail: acnp@acnpweb.org
www.nurse.org/acnp

American Holistic Nurses Association
P.O. Box 2130
Flagstaff, AZ 86003-2130
800-278-2462 (toll-free)
E-mail: info@ahna.org
www.ahna.org

American Nephrology Nurses' Association
East Holly Avenue
Box 56
Pitman, NJ 08071-0056
856-256-2320
888-600-ANNA (toll-free)
E-mail: anna@ajj.com
www.annanurse.org

American Psychiatric Nurses Association
1555 Wilson Boulevard
Suite 602
Arlington, VA 22209
703-243-2443
Fax: 703-243-3390
E-mail: inform@apna.org
www.apna.org

American Public Health Association
800 I Street, NW
Washington, DC 20001-3710
202-777-APHA
Fax: 202-777-2534
E-mail: comments@apha.org
www.apha.org

American Radiological Nurses Association
7794 Grow Drive
Pensacola, FL 32514
866-486-2762 (toll-free)
Fax: 850-484-8762
E-mail: arna@puetzamc.com
www.arna.net

American Society of Ophthalmic Registered Nurses
P.O. Box 193030
San Francisco, CA 94119
415-561-8513
E-mail: asorn@aao.org
http://webeye.ophth.uiowa.edu/asorn

American Society for Pain Management Nursing
7794 Grow Drive
Pensacola, FL 32514
888-342-7766 (toll-free)
Fax: 850-484-8762
E-mail: aspmn@puetzamc.com
www.aspmn.org

American Society of PeriAnesthesia Nurses
10 Melrose Avenue
Suite 110
Cherry Hill, NJ 08003-3696
877-737-9696 (toll-free)
Fax: 856-616-9601
E-mail: aspan@aspan.org
www.aspan.org

American Society of Plastic Surgical Nurses
3220 Pointe Parkway
Suite 500
Atlanta, GA 30092
678-966-3065
E-mail: info@aspsn.org
www.aspsn.org

Association for Death Education and Counseling
342 North Main Street
West Hartford, CT 06117-2507
860-586-7503
Fax: 860-586-7550
E-mail: info@adec.org
www.adec.org

Association for Professionals in Infection Control and Epidemiology, Inc.
1275 K Street, NW
Suite 1000
Washington, DC 20005-4006
202-789-1890
Fax: 202-789-1899
E-mail: apicinfo@apic.org
www.apic.org

Association of Nurses in AIDS Care
3538 Ridgewood Road
Akron, OH 44333
800-260-6780 (toll-free)
Fax: 330-670-0109
Email: anac@anacnet.org
www.anacnet.org

Association of Pediatric Oncology Nurses
4700 West Lake Avenue
Glenview, IL 60025
847-375-4724
Fax: 877-734-8755
E-mail: info@apon.org
www.apon.org

Association of Perioperative Registered Nurses
2170 South Parker Road
Suite 300
Denver, CO 80231
800-755-2676 (toll-free)
E-mail: custserv@aorn.org
www.aorn.org

Association of Rehabilitation Nurses
4700 West Lake Avenue
Glenview, IL 60025
800-229-7530 (toll-free)
E-mail: info@rehabnurse.org
www.rehabnurse.org

Association of Women's Health, Obstetric, and Neonatal Nurses
2000 L Street, NW
Suite 740
Washington, DC 20036
800-673-8499 (toll-free in the U.S.)
800-245-0231 (toll-free in Canada)
Fax: 202-728-0575
www.awhonn.org

Dermatology Nurses' Association
Box 56
Pitman, NJ 08071-0056
800-454-4362 (toll-free)
E-mail: dna@ajj.com
http://dna.inurse.com

Developmental Disabilities Nurses Association
1733 H Street
Suite 330, PMB 1214
Blaine, WA 98230
800-888-6733 (toll-free)
Fax: 360-332-2280
E-mail: ddnahq@aol.com
www.ddna.org

Emergency Nurses Association
915 Lee Street
Des Plaines, IL 60016-6569
800-900-9659 (toll-free)
Fax: 847-460-4001
E-mail: educsvs@ena.org
www.ena.org

Hospice and Palliative Nurses Association
Penn Center West One
Suite 229
Pittsburgh, PA 15276
412-787-9301
Fax: 412-787-9305
E-mail: hpna@hpna.org
www.hpna.org

Infusion Nurses Society
220 Norwood Park South
Norwood, MA 02062
781-440-9408
Fax: 781-440-9409
www.ins1.org

International Nurses Society on Addictions
P.O. Box 10752
Raleigh, NC 27605
919-821-1292
Fax: 919-833-5743
E-mail: info@intnsa.org
www.intnsa.org

National Organization of Nurse Practitioner Faculties
1522 K Street, NW
Suite 702
Washington, DC 20005
202-289-8044
Fax: 202-289-8046
E-mail: nonpf@nonpf.org
www.nonpf.com

National Association of Nurse Practitioners in Women's Health
503 Capitol Court, NE
Suite 300
Washington, DC 20002
202-543-9693
Fax: 202-543-9858
Email: info@npwh.org
www.npwh.org

National Association for Home Care & Hospice
228 Seventh Street, SE
Washington, DC 20003
202-547-7424
Fax: 202-547-3540
E-mail: exec@nahc.org
www.nahc.org

National Association of Clinical Nurse Specialists
2090 Linglestown Road
Suite 107
Harrisburg, PA 17110
717-234-6799
Fax: 717-234-6798
E-mail: info@nacns.org
www.nacns.org

National Association of Directors of Nursing Administration in Long-Term Care
10101 Alliance Road
Suite 140
Cincinnati, OH 45242
800-222-0539 (toll-free)
Fax: 513-791-3699
E-mail: info@nadona.org
www.nadona.org

National Association of Neonatal Nurses
4700 West Lake Avenue
Glenview, IL 60025-1485
800-451-3795 (toll-free)
Fax: 888-477-6266
E-mail: info@nann.org
www.nann.org

National Association of Orthopaedic Nurses
401 North Michigan Avenue
Suite 2200
Chicago, IL 60611
800-289-6266 (toll-free)
Fax: 312-527-6658
E-mail: naon@smithbucklin.com
www.orthonurse.org

National Association of Pediatric Nurse Practitioners
20 Brace Road
Suite 200
Cherry Hill, NJ 08034-2633
856-857-9700
Fax: 856-857-1600
E-mail: info@napnap.org
www.napnap.org

National Association of School Nurses
P.O. Box 1300
Scarborough, ME 04070-1300
877-627-6476 (toll-free)
Fax: 207-883-2683
E-mail: nasn@nasn.org
www.nasn.org

National Gerontological Nursing Association
7794 Grow Drive
Pensacola, FL 32514
800-723-0560 (toll-free)
Fax: 850-484-8762
E-mail: ngna@puetzamc.com
www.ngna.org

Oncology Nursing Society
125 Enterprise Drive
Pittsburgh, PA 15275
866-257-4ONS
Fax: 877-369-5497
E-mail: customer.service@ons.org
www.ons.org

Preventive Cardiovascular Nurses Association
613 Williamson Street
Suite 205
Madison, WI 53703
608-250-2440
Fax: 608-250-2410
E-mail: info@pcna.net
www.pcna.net

Respiratory Nursing Society
11 Cornel Road
Latham, NY 12110
518-782-9400
888-330-4767 (toll-free)
Fax: 850-484-8762
E-mail: rns@nysna.org
www.respiratorynursingsociety.org

Society for Vascular Nursing
7794 Grow Drive
Pensacola, FL 32514
888-536-4786 (toll-free)
Fax: 850-484-8762
E-mail: svn@puetzamc.com
www.svnnet.org

Society of Gastroenterology Nurses and Associates
401 North Michigan Avenue
Chicago, IL 60611-4267
800-245-7462 (toll-free)
Fax: 312-527-6658
E-mail: sgna@smithbucklin.com
www.sgna.org

Society of Otorhinolaryngology and Head-Neck Nurses, Inc.
116 Canal Street
Suite A
New Smyrna Beach, FL 32168
386-428-1695
Fax: 386-423-7566
E-mail: info@sohnnurse.com
www.sohnnurse.com

Society of Urologic Nurses and Associates
East Holly Avenue
Box 56
Pitman, NJ 08071
888-827-7862 (toll-free)
E-mail: suna@ajj.com
www.suna.org

Wound, Ostomy and Continence Nurses Society
4700 West Lake Avenue
Glenview, IL 60025
888-224-WOCN (toll-free)
Fax: 866-615-8560
E-mail: info@wocn.org
www.wocn.org

PAYING FOR YOUR NURSING EDUCATION

Whether you are considering a baccalaureate degree in nursing or have completed your undergraduate education and are planning to attend graduate school, finding a way to pay for that education is essential.

The cost to attend college is considerable and is increasing each year at a rate faster than most other products and services. In fact, the cost of a nursing education at a public four-year college can be more than $14,000 per year, including tuition, fees, books, room and board, transportation, and miscellaneous expenses. The cost at a private college or university, at either the graduate or undergraduate level, can be more than $30,000 per year.

This is where financial aid comes in. Financial aid is money made available by the government and other sources to help students who otherwise would be unable to attend college. More than $122 billion in aid is provided to students each year. Most college students in this country receive some form of aid, and all prospective students should investigate what may be available. Most of this aid is given to students because neither they nor their families have sufficient personal resources to pay for college. This type of aid is referred to as need-based aid. Recipients of need-based aid include traditional students just out of high school or college, as well as older, nontraditional students who are returning to college or graduate school.

There is also merit-based aid, which is awarded to students who display a particular ability. Merit scholarships are based primarily on academic merit, but may include other special talents. Many colleges and graduate schools offer merit-based aid in addition to need-based aid to their students. Some schools also offer special assistance to members of underrepresented minority groups.

Types and Sources of Financial Aid

There are three types of aid: scholarships (also known as grants or gift aid), loans, and student employment (including fellowships and assistantships). Scholarships and grants are outright gifts and do not have to be repaid. Loans are borrowed money that must be repaid with interest, usually after graduation. Student employment provides jobs during the academic year for which students are paid. For graduate students, student employment may include fellowships in which students work, receive free or reduced tuition, and are paid a stipend for living expenses.

Most of the aid available to students is need-based and comes from the federal government through six large financial aid programs. Two of these programs are grant-based—Federal Pell Grants and Federal Supplemental Educational Opportunity Grants—and are only available to undergraduate students. Three are loan programs—Federal Perkins Loans, Federal Stafford Loans (subsidized and unsubsidized), and Federal PLUS (Parent Loan for Undergraduate Students) loans—that are provided to both undergraduate and graduate students. The sixth program is a student employment program called the Federal Work-Study Program, which is also awarded to undergraduate and graduate students based on financial need.

Federal Financial Aid Programs

Program	Maximum/year
Federal Pell Grants	$4050 (undergraduate students only)
Federal Supplemental Educational Opportunity Grants (FSEOG)	$4000 (undergraduate students only)
Federal Perkins Loans	$4000 (undergraduate students) $6000 (graduate students)
Federal Stafford/Direct Loans (subsidized)	$2625 (first-year students) $3500 (second-year students) $5500 (third- and fourth-year students) $8500 (graduate students)
Federal Stafford/Direct Loans (unsubsidized)	$2625 (first-year students)* $3500 (second-year students)* $5500 (third- and fourth-year students)* $6625 (independent first-year students)* $7500 (independent second-year students)* $10,500 (independent third- and fourth-year students)* $18,500 (graduate students)*
Federal PLUS Loans	Up to cost of attendance (less other financial aid received)

***These amounts are inclusive of subsidized loans*

The federal government also offers a number of programs especially for nursing students. For example, the U.S. Department of Health and Human Services offers Nursing Student Scholarships, Nursing Student Loans, the Nursing Education Loan Repayment Program, and the

Scholarship for Disadvantaged Students (SDS) program. Some of these programs require that one works in a designated nursing shortage area for a period of time. These programs are administered by the nursing school's financial aid office. For more information, log on to http://bhpr.hrsa.gov/dsa.

The second-largest source of aid is from the colleges and universities themselves. Almost all colleges have aid programs from institutional resources, most of which are grants, scholarships, and fellowships. These can be either need- or merit-based.

A third source of aid is from state governments. Nearly every state provides aid for students attending college in their home state, although most only have programs for undergraduates. Most state aid programs are scholarships and grants, but many states now have low-interest loan and work-study programs. Most state grants and scholarships are not "portable," meaning that they cannot be used outside of your home state of residence.

A fourth source of aid is from private sources such as corporations, hospitals, civic associations, unions, fraternal organizations, foundations, and religious groups that bestow scholarships, grants, and fellowships to students. Most of these are not based on need, although the amount of the scholarship may vary depending upon financial need. The competition for these scholarships can be formidable, but the rewards are well worth the process. Many companies also offer tuition reimbursement to employees and their dependents. Check with the personnel or human resources department at your or your parents' place of employment for benefit and eligibility information.

Eligibility for Financial Aid

Since most of the financial aid that college students receive is need-based, colleges employ a process called "need analysis" to determine student awards. For most applicants, there is one form that the student and parents (if the student is a dependent) fill out on which family income, assets, and household information is reported. This form is the Free Application for Federal Student Aid (FAFSA). The end result of this need analysis is the student's "Expected Family Contribution," or EFC, representing the amount a family should be able to contribute toward educational expenses.

Dependent or Independent

The basic principle of financial aid is that the primary responsibility for paying college expenses resides with the family. In determining your EFC, you will first need to know who makes up your "family." That will tell you whose income is counted when the need analysis is done.

Graduate Students: By definition, all graduate nursing students are considered independent for federal aid purposes. Therefore, only your income and assets (and your spouse's if you are married) count in determining your expected family contribution.

Undergraduate Students: If you are financially dependent upon your parents, then their income and assets, as well as yours, are counted toward the family contribution. But if you are considered independent of your parents, only your income (and your spouse's if you are married) counts in the calculation.

According to the U.S. Department of Education, in order to be considered independent for financial aid, you must meet any ONE of the following:

- You were born before January 1, 1982.
- You are married.
- You are or will be enrolled in a master's or doctoral program (beyond a bachelor's degree) during the 2005–06 school year.
- You have children who receive more than half their support from you.
- You have dependents (other than your children or spouse) who live with you and who receive more than half of their support from you and will continue to receive more than half their support from you through June 30, 2006.
- You are an orphan or ward of the court (or were a ward of the court until age 18).
- You are a veteran of the U.S. Armed Forces. ("Veteran" includes students who attended a U.S. service academy and who were released under a condition other than dishonorable. Also, National Guard and Reserve members who served in combat areas can be classified as independent. Contact your financial aid office for more information.)

If you meet any one of these conditions, you are considered independent and only your income and assets (and your spouse's if you are married) count toward your family contribution. Remember, if you are attending school as a graduate student, you are automatically independent for federal aid consideration.

If there are extraordinary circumstances, the financial aid administrator at the college you will be attending has the authority to make exceptions to your dependency status. You will need to provide extensive documentation of your family situation.

If you are considered an independent student, take your total family income for the previous year, subtract all state and federal taxes paid (including FICA), subtract another $3000 ($6000 if you are married), and divide the result in half. If your family income is less than $50,000, this is your estimated EFC. If your income is greater than $50,000, add 35 percent (12 percent if you have children) of your total assets (bank accounts, stocks, etc.). This result is your estimated EFC. If you are dependent, the EFC formula is more complicated. Check out www.petersons.com/finaid/efcsimplecalc.asp to determine your estimated EFC.

Determining Cost and Need

Now that you know approximately how much you and your family will be expected to contribute toward your college expenses, you can subtract the EFC from the total cost of attending a college or graduate school to determine the amount of need-based financial aid for which you will be eligible. The average costs listed assume that you will be attending nursing school full-time. If you will be attending part-time, you should adjust costs accordingly.

Applying for Financial Aid

After you have subtracted your EFC from the cost of your education and determined your financial need, you will have a better understanding of how much assistance you will need. Even if you do not demonstrate financial need, you are still encouraged to file the FAFSA, as you may be eligible for assistance that is not based on need. The process for applying for aid can be confusing if you are not familiar with completing these types of applications. If you need assistance, you should contact the financial aid office for help.

Undergraduate and graduate students applying for aid must fill out the FAFSA. This application is available in high school guidance offices, college financial aid offices, state education department offices, and many local libraries. You can also file the FAFSA online at www.fafsa.ed.gov. If you file online, you will need to have a Personal Identification Number (PIN). The PIN can easily be obtained at www.pin.ed.gov. Dependent students will need a PIN for themselves and one parent. By filing online, your application is processed faster, and you are far less likely to make major errors. The FAFSA, whether you file a paper application or online, becomes available in November or December, almost a year before the fall term in which you will enroll, but you cannot complete it until after January 1.

If you file a paper application, you and your parents (if appropriate) must sign your completed FAFSA and mail it to a processing center in the envelope provided. Do not send any additional materials, but do make copies of everything you filled out.

The processing center enters the data into a computer that runs the federal methodology of need analysis to calculate your EFC. This center then distributes the information to the schools and agencies you listed on the FAFSA. The actual determination of need and the awarding of aid are handled by each college financial aid office.

It is generally recommended that you complete the FAFSA as soon as possible after January 1. You should check with each college to which you are applying to determine its filing deadline. It is important to meet all college deadlines for financial aid, since there is a limited amount of funds available. However, students who procrastinate can still file for federal aid any time during the year.

What Happens After You Submit the FAFSA?

Two to four weeks after you send in your completed FAFSA, you will receive a Student Aid Report (SAR) that shows the information you reported and your calculated EFC. This is an opportunity for you to make corrections or to have the information sent to any new school you are considering that you did not list on the original FAFSA. The SAR contains instructions on how to make corrections or to designate additional schools. If you provided an e-mail address on the FAFSA, this information will be sent to this address rather than through conventional mail.

At the same time that you receive the SAR, the college(s) you specified also receive the information. The financial aid office at the school may request additional information from you or may ask you to provide documentation verifying the information you reported on the FAFSA. For example, they may ask you for a copy of your (and your parents') income tax return or official forms verifying any untaxed income you or your parents received (e.g., Social Security, disability, or welfare benefits).

Once the financial aid office is satisfied that the information is correct, you will receive a financial aid offer. Many colleges like to make this offer in the spring prior to the fall enrollment so that students have ample opportunity to make their plans. However, some colleges will wait until summer to notify you.

Other Applications

The FAFSA is the required form for applying for federal and most state financial aid programs. Most schools also use the FASFA to determine eligibility for institutional aid; however, some colleges and graduate schools require additional information to determine eligibility for institutional aid. Nearly 500 colleges and universities, plus more than 200 private scholarship programs, employ a form called the Financial Aid PROFILE® from the College Scholarship Service (CSS). While the form is similar to the FAFSA, several additional questions must be answered for colleges that award their own funds. You begin the process in October or November by completing a PROFILE® Registration form on which you designate the schools to which you are applying. A few weeks later, you will receive a customized, individualized application that you complete and send back to CSS, which, in turn, forwards your application information to the schools you selected.

Financial Aid Offer

If you qualify for need-based aid, a college will typically offer a combination of the three types of assistance—

scholarship/grant, loan, and work-study—to meet this need. An offer of aid usually is made after you have been admitted to the college or program. You may accept all or part of the financial aid package. If you will be enrolling part-time (fewer than 12 credits per term), be sure to contact the financial aid office in advance.

If you are awarded Federal Work-Study, the amount you are awarded represents your earnings limit for the academic year under the program. In general, schools assume you will earn this money on an hourly basis, so it cannot be used to pay your term bill charges. On most campuses there are many jobs available for students. Not all of these are limited to students in the Federal Work-Study program. Check with your placement office or financial aid office for more information.

Keep in mind that the student budget used to establish eligibility for financial aid is based on averages. It may not reflect your actual expenses. Student budgets usually reflect most expenses for categories of students (for example, single students living in their parents' home, campus-provided housing, or living in an apartment or house near campus, etc.). But if you have unusual expenses that are not included, you should consult with your school's financial aid office regarding a budget adjustment.

If Your Family or Job Situation Changes

Because a family contribution is based on the previous year's income, many nursing students find they do not qualify for need-based aid (or not enough to pay their full expenses). This is particularly true of older students who were working full-time last year but are no longer doing so or who will not work during the academic year. If this is your situation, you should speak to a counselor in the financial aid office about making an adjustment in your family contribution need analysis. Financial aid administrators may make changes to any of the elements that go into the need analysis if there are conditions that merit a change. Contact the financial aid office for more information.

Still Don't Qualify for Need-Based Aid?

If you still don't qualify for need-based aid but feel you do not have the resources necessary to pay for college or graduate school, you still have several options available.

First, there are two student loan programs for which need is not a consideration. These two programs are the Federal Unsubsidized Stafford Loans and the Unsubsidized Direct Loans. There is also a non-need-based loan program for parents of dependent students called the Federal PLUS loan. If you or your parents are interested in borrowing through one of these programs, you should check with the financial aid office for more information. For many students, borrowing to pay for a nursing education can be an excellent investment in one's future. At the same time, be sure that you do not overburden yourself when it comes to paying back the loans. Before you accept a student loan, the financial aid office will schedule a counseling session to make certain that you know the terms of the loan and that you understand the ramifications of borrowing. If you can do without, it is often suggested that you postpone student loans until they are absolutely necessary.

A second option, if you do not qualify for need-based aid, is to search for scholarships. Be wary of scholarship search companies that promise to find you scholarships but require you to pay a fee. There are many resources that provide lists of scholarships, including the annually published *Peterson's Scholarships, Grants & Prizes,* which are available in libraries, counselors' offices, and bookstores. Non-need scholarships require application forms and are extremely competitive; only a handful of students from thousands of applicants receive awards. Check out opportunities on our site, www.petersons.com.

Another practical option is to work more hours at an existing job or to find a paying position if you do not already have one. The student employment or placement office at your college should be able to help you find a job, either on or off campus. Many colleges have vacancies remaining after they have placed financial aid students in their work-study jobs.

You should always contact the financial aid office at the school you plan to attend for advice concerning sources of college-based and private aid.

Employer-Paid Financial Aid

Bob Atwater is a certified personnel consultant and certified medical staff recruiter and founder of Atwater Consulting & Recruiting in Lilburn, Georgia, a consulting firm for the employment and recruitment of physician assistants, nurse practitioners, certified nurse midwives, nurses, and nursing managers.

Health-care administrators, Atwater says, have coined a phrase to characterize their efforts to meet the growing demand for nurses with better skills and training: "Grow your own."

"Constant training through the course of a nursing career is the only way to keep pace with the technological and medical advances, but it can be a financial burden on the nurse," Atwater says.

That is why many employers now give qualified employees a benefits package that includes a continuing education allowance.

For the employer, this type of benefits package can help to recruit candidates willing to further their careers through education. Administrators feel it is the best way to build a staff of nurses with up-to-date certifications in all areas.

In a constantly expanding field, nurses should be required to continue and update their education. The nurses get a paid education, can keep their job, and work flexible hours while they are going to school. Inquiries about these allowances should be made during an interview with the company's human resources department. Additional information can be obtained from the nursing school, local hospitals in the area, or from other health-care professionals. There are many attractive options available because of the nationwide shortage of qualified nurses. Check with a number of potential employers before agreeing to any long-term contract.

SOURCES OF FINANCIAL AID FOR NURSING STUDENTS

The largest proportion of financial aid for college expenses comes from the federal government and is given on the basis of financial need. Beyond this federal need-based aid, which should always be the primary source of financial aid that a prospective student investigates and which is given regardless of one's field of study, a sizable amount of scholarship assistance specifically meant to help students in nursing programs is also available from government agencies, associations, civic or fraternal organizations, and corporations. These sources of aid can be particularly attractive for students who may not be eligible for need-based aid. The following list presents some of the major sources of financial aid specifically for nursing students. Not listed are scholarships that are specific to individual colleges and universities or limited to residents of a particular place or to individuals who have relatively unusual qualifications. Students seeking financial aid should investigate all appropriate possibilities, including sources not listed here. A student can find this information in libraries, bookstores, and guidance offices guides, including two of Peterson's annually updated publications: *Peterson's College Money Handbook,* for information about undergraduate awards given by the federal government, state governments, and specific colleges, and *Peterson's Scholarships, Grants & Prizes,* for information about awards from private sources.

Students should also check out the many scholarship search engines available on the Web, especially www.petersons.com/finaid and www.petersons.com/bcd and www.aacn.nche.edu/Education/Financialaid.htm.

American Association of Colleges of Nursing (AACN)

Award Name: Campus RN/AACN Scholarship Fund
Program Description: This scholarship program supports students who are seeking a baccalaureate, master's or doctoral degree in nursing. Special consideration will be given to students enrolled in a master's or doctoral program with the goal of pursuing a nursing faculty career, completing an RN to baccalaureate program (B.S.N.), or enrolled in an accelerated baccalaureate or master's degree nursing program.
Application Contact: American Association of Colleges of Nursing
One Dupont Circle, NW
Suite 530
Washington, DC 20036
202-463-6930
Fax: 202-785-8320
E-mail: info@campuscareercenter.com
http://aacn.campusrn.com/scholarships/scholarship_rn.asp

Air Force Institute of Technology

Award Name: Air Force Active Duty Health Professions Loan Repayment Program
Program Description: Program provides up to $29,323 to repay qualified educational loans in exchange for active duty service in the U.S. Army.
Application Contact: Air Force Institute of Technology
AFIT/CIML
2275 D Street
Building 16, Room 120
Wright Patterson AFB, OH 45433-7221
800-543-3490 (toll-free)
E-mail: afit.ciml@afit.edu
http://ci.afit.edu/ciml

American Association of Critical-Care Nurses (AACN)

Award Name: AACN Educational Advancement Scholarships
Program Description: Nonrenewable scholarships for AACN members who are RNs currently enrolled in undergraduate or graduate NLNAC-accredited programs. The undergraduate award is for use in the junior or senior year. Minimum 3.0 GPA.
Application Contact: American Association of Critical-Care Nurses Scholarships
101 Columbia
Aliso Viejo, CA 92656-4109
800-899-2226 (toll-free)
E-mail: info@aacn.org
www.aacn.org

American Cancer Society

Award Name: Scholarships in Cancer Nursing
Program Description: Renewable awards for graduate students in nursing pursuing advanced preparation in cancer nursing: research, education, administration, or clinical practice. Must be U.S. citizen.
Application Contact: American Cancer Society
Extramural Grants Program
1599 Clifton Road, NE
Atlanta, GA 30329-4251
800-ACS-2345
E-mail: grants@cancer.org
www.cancer.org

American Health Care Association

Award Name: Durante Nurse Scholarship
Program Description: For students accepted or enrolled in an accredited LPN/RN program and currently employed by an American Health Care Association nursing facility. Winners must volunteer 25 hours of service to an AHCA facility. Send legal-size self-addressed stamped envelope for application.
Application Contact: American Health Care Association
Durante Nurse Scholarship Program
1201 L Street, NW
Washington, DC 20005
202-898-9352
www.ahca.org/about/scholarship.htm

American Holistic Nurses' Association (AHNA)

Award Name: Charlotte McGuire Scholarship Program
Program Description: Open to any licensed nurse or nursing student pursuing holistic education. Experience in holistic health care or alternative health practices is preferred. Must be an AHNA member with a minimum 3.0 GPA.

Application Contact: Charlotte McGuire Scholarships
American Holistic Nurses' Association
P.O. Box 2130
Flagstaff, AZ 86003-2130
800-278-2462 (toll-free)
E-mail: info@ahna.org
www.ahna.org/edu/assist.html

American Indian Graduate Center (AIGC)

Award Name: AIGC Fellowships
Program Description: Graduate fellowships available for American Indian and Alaska Native students from federally recognized U.S. tribes. Applicants must be pursuing a postbaccalaureate graduate or professional degree as a full-time student at an accredited institution in the U.S., demonstrate financial need, and be enrolled in a federally-recognized American Indian tribe or Alaska Native group or provide documentation of Indian descent.
Application Contact: American Indian Graduate Center Fellowships
American Indian Graduate Center
4520 Montgomery Boulevard, NE
Suite 1B
Albuquerque, NM 87109
800-628-1920 (toll-free)
E-mail: marveline@aigc.com
www.aigc.com

Association of Perioperative Registered Nurses (AORN)

Award Name: AORN Foundation Scholarships
Program Description: Applicant must be an active RN and a member of AORN for twelve consecutive months prior to application. Reapplication for each period is required. For baccalaureate, master's of nursing, or doctoral degree at an accredited institution. Minimum 3.0 GPA required.
Application Contact: AORN Scholarship Committee
2170 South Parker Road
Suite 300
Denver, CO 80231
800-755-2676
E-mail: ibendzsa@aorn.org
www.aorn.org/foundation/scholarship.htm

Bethesda Lutheran Homes and Services, Inc.

Award Name: Nursing Scholastic Achievement Scholarship
Program Description: Award for college nursing students with a minimum 3.0 GPA who are Lutheran and have completed their sophomore year of a four-year nursing program or one year of a two-year program. Must be interested in working with people with developmental disabilities.
Application Contact: Bethesda Lutheran Homes and Services, Inc.
National Christian Resource Center
600 Hoffmann Drive
Watertown, WI 53094
800-369-4636 (toll-free)
E-mail: ncrc@blhs.org
www.blhs.org/youth/scholarships/#apply

Foundation of the National Student Nurses' Association, Inc.

Award Names: Scholarship Program
Program Description: One-time awards available to nursing students in various educational situations: enrolled in programs leading to an RN license, RNs enrolled in programs leading to a B.A. in nursing, enrolled in a state-approved school in a specialty area of nursing, and minority students enrolled in nursing or prenursing programs. High school students are not eligible. Funds for graduate study are available only for a first degree in nursing. Based on financial need, academic ability, and health-related nursing and community activities. Application fee of $10. Send self-addressed stamped envelope with two stamps along with application request.
Application Contact: Scholarship Chairperson
Foundation of the National Student Nurses' Association, Inc.
45 Main Street
Suite 606
Brooklyn, NY 11201
718-210-0705
E-mail: nsna@nsna.org
www.nsna.org/foundation

Heart and Stroke Foundation of Canada

Award Name: Nursing Research Fellowships
Program Description: In-training awards for study in an area of cardiovascular or cerebrovascular nursing. For master's degree candidates, the programs must include a thesis or project requirement.
Application Contact: Heart and Stroke Foundation of Canada
1402-222 Queen Street
Ottawa, Ontario K1P 5V9
Canada
613-569-4361
E-mail: research@hsf.ca
www.hsf.ca/research/guidelines/strategic.html

International Order of the King's Daughters and Sons, Inc.

Award Name: International Order of King's Daughters and Sons Health Scholarships
Program Description: For study in the health fields. No biology, premedical, or veterinary applicants accepted. B.A./B.S. students are eligible in junior year. Medical/dental students must have finished first year of school. Send #10 self-addressed stamped envelope for application and information.
Application Contact: Director
Health Careers Department
P.O. Box 1040
Chautauqua, NY 14722-1040
www.iokds.org/healthcareers.htm

Maternity Center Association

Award Name: Hazel Corbin Grant
Program Description: Applicant must be an RN and accepted into a nurse-midwifery program accredited by the American College of Nurse-Midwives.
Application Contact: Maternity Center Association
281 Park Avenue South
5th floor
New York, NY 10010
212-777-5000
E-mail: info@maternitywise.org
www.maternitywise.org/mca/grants/index.html

National Alaska Native American Indian Nurses Association (NANAINA)

Award Name: NANAINA Merit Awards
Program Description: Annual $500 awards presented to NANAINA members who are enrolled in a U.S. federally- or state-recognized tribe and are enrolled as a full-time undergraduate or graduate nursing student in an accredited or state-approved school of nursing.
Application Contact: Dr. Better Keltner
NANAINA Treasurer
3700 Reservoir Road, NW
Washington DC 20057-1107
888-566-8773
www.nanaina.com

National Association of Hispanic Nurses (NAHN)

Award Name: National Scholarship Awards
Program Description: One-time award to an outstanding Hispanic nursing student. Must have at least a 3.0 GPA and be a member of NAHN. Based on academic merit, potential contribution to nursing, and financial need.

Application Contact: Miriam Gonzales
Awards/Scholarship Committee Chair
1501 16th Street, NW
Washington, DC 20036
202-387-2477
E-mail: info@thehispanicnurses.org
www.thehispanicnurses.org

National Association of Neonatal Nurses (NANN)

Award Name: NANN Scholarships
Program Description: Scholarships for members pursuing a B.S.N. or graduate degree in neonatal nursing or nursing administration.
Application Contact: National Association of Neonatal Nurses
4700 West Lake Avenue
Glenview, IL 60025-1485
800-451-3795 (toll-free)
E-mail: info@nann.org
www.nann.org

National Black Nurses Association, Inc. (NBNA)

Award Names: NBNA Scholarships
Program Description: Scholarships available to nursing students who are members of NBNA and are enrolled in an accredited school of nursing. Must demonstrate involvement in African-American community and present letter of recommendation from local chapter of NBNA.
Application Contact: National Black Nurses Association, Inc.
8630 Fenton Street, Suite 330
Silver Spring, MD 20910-3803
800-575-6298
E-mail: nbna@erols.com
www.nbna.org/scholarship.htm

National Student Nurses Association (NSNA)

Award Name: Educational Advancement Scholarships
Program Description: Scholarships of $1,500 for members of NSNA or American Association of Critical Care Nurses who are not RNs, based on academic achievement and demonstrated commitment to nursing through involvement in student organizations and school and community activities related to health care.
Application Contact: National Student Nurses Association Foundation
45 Main Street
Suite 606
Brooklyn, NY 11201
718-210-0705
E-mail: nsna@nsna.org
www.nsna.org

Nurses' Educational Funds, Inc.

Award Name: Nurses' Educational Fund Scholarships
Program Description: Awards for full-time students at master's level, full-time or part-time at doctoral level, or RNs who are U.S. citizens and members of a national professional nursing association. Application fee: $10.
Application Contact: Nurses' Educational Funds, Inc.
304 Park Avenue South
11th Floor
New York, NY 10010
212-590-2443
E-mail: info@n-e-f.org
www.n-e-f.org

Oncology Nursing Society

Award Name: Scholarships
Program Description: ONF offers nearly a dozen one-time scholarships and awards at all levels of study, with various requirements and purposes, to nursing students who are interested in pursuing oncology nursing. Contact the foundation for details about appropriate awards. Application fee: $5.
Application Contact: Oncology Nursing Society
Development Coordinator
125 Enterprise Drive
RIDC Park West
Pittsburgh, PA 15275-1214
866-257-4667
E-mail: customer.service@ons.org
www.ons.org/awards

United States Air Force Reserve Officer Training Corps

Award Name: Air Force ROTC Nursing Scholarships
Program Description: One- to four-year programs available to students of nursing and high school seniors. Nursing graduates agree to accept a commission in the Air Force Nurse Corps and serve four years on active duty after successfully completing their licensing examination. Must have at least a 2.5 GPA for one- and four-year scholarships or at least a 2.65 GPA for two- and three-year scholarships. Two exam failures result in a four-year assignment as an Air Force line officer.
Application Contact: Air Force ROTC
551 East Maxwell Boulevard
Maxwell AFB, AL 36112-6106
866-423-7682
www.afrotc.com/scholarships/index.htm

United States Army Reserve Officers' Training Corps

Award Name: Army ROTC Nursing Scholarships
Program Description: Two- to four-year programs available to students of nursing and high school seniors. Nursing graduates agree to accept a commission in the Army Nurse Corps and serve in the military for a period of eight years. This may be fulfilled by serving on active duty for two to four years, followed by service in the Army National Guard or the United States Army Reserve or in the Inactive Ready Reserve for the remainder of the eight-year obligation.
Application Contact: Army ROTC Cadet Command
Army ROTC Scholarship
Fort Monroe, VA 23651-1052
800-USA-ROTC
www.goarmy.com/rotc/scholarships.jsp

United States Department of Health and Human Services Bureau of Health Professions

Award Names: Nursing Scholarship
Program Description: Awards for U.S. citizens enrolled or accepted for enrollment as a full- or part-time student in an accredited school of nursing in a professional registered nurse program (baccalaureate, graduate, associate degree, or diploma)
Application Contact: Division of Nursing
Bureau of Health Professions
5600 Fishers Lane, Room 9-35
Parklawn Building
Rockville, MD 20857
301-443-5688
www.bhpr.hrsa.gov/dsa

SEARCHING FOR NURSING SCHOOLS ONLINE

The Internet can be a great tool for students and parents gathering information about nursing programs. There are many worthwhile sites to help guide you through the various aspects of the selection process, including Peterson's Nursing Channel at www.petersons.com/nursing.

The majority of nursing programs maintain Web sites, which often provide vast amounts of admissions information. As you surf the Web for information, keep in mind that Web sites can vary greatly in appearance and quality. While some sites are attractive, easy to navigate, and home to large amounts of useful information, others are unimaginative and complex. Upon arriving at a site, determine the source. Who created the site and why? Is the site user-friendly? Can you find the information you need?

How Peterson's Nursing Channel Can Help

Nursing school is a serious commitment of time and resources. Therefore, it is important to have the most up-to-date information about prospective schools at your fingertips. That is why Peterson's Nursing Channel is a great place to start your nursing program search and selection process.

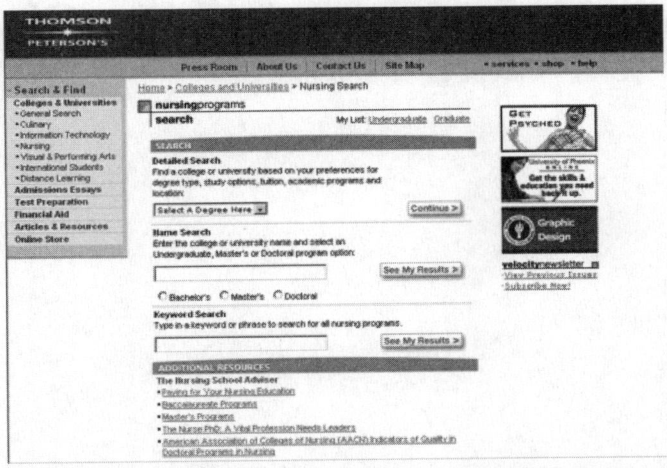

Peterson's Nursing Channel is a comprehensive information resource that will help you make sense of the nursing school admissions process. Peterson's Nursing Channel now offers visitors enhanced search criteria and an easily navigable interface. The Channel is organized into various sections that make finding a program easy and fun. You can search for nursing programs based on:

- *Institution name*
- *Degree type*
- *Study options*
- *Tuition*
- *Academic programs*
- *Location*

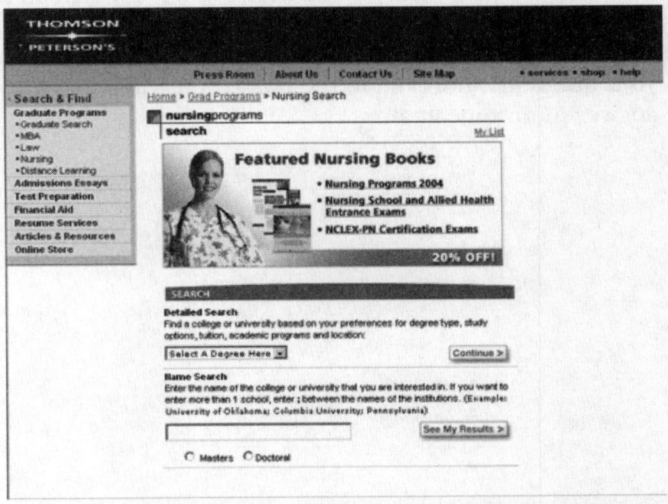

Once you have found the school of your choice, simply click on one of the tabs at the top of the profile to get general information about the institution as a whole. Other tabs include:

- *Students & Faculty*
- *Nursing Program*
- *Campus Life*
- *Financial Aid & Costs*
- *Contact*

Resources

View Descriptions

If the schools you are interested in have provided Peterson's with an **In-Depth Description,** you can do a keyword search on that description. Here, schools are given the opportunity to communicate unique features of their nursing programs to prospective students.

View Announcements

If the schools you are interested in have provided Peterson's with an **Announcement,** you can click on "Announcements" in the "Additional Resources" section of the channel and you will be directed to an alphabetical listing of those schools that provided additional information about their program.

Visit Web Sites

For institutions that have provided information about their Web sites, simply click on the "Visit Web Site" button and be taken directly to that institution's Web page. Once you arrive at the school's Web site, look around and get a feel for the place. Often, schools offer virtual tours of the campus, complete with photos and commentary. If you have any questions about the school, a visit to a school's Web site will often answer these questions.

Send Instant Inquiries

If, after looking at the information provided on Peterson's Nursing Channel and on the school's Web page, you still have questions, you can send an e-mail directly to the admissions department of the school from Peterson's Web site. Just click on the "E-mail Get More Info" button and send your message. In most instances, if you keep your questions short and to the point, you will receive an answer in no time at all.

Add to My List

If you've already narrowed your choices down to one or two schools, or you're just starting from scratch, you'll find the tools you need here. Here you can:

- Save the list of schools you're interested in, which you can then revisit at any time.
- Access all the features of the site.
- Be reminded of important dates and receive notifications when we add new features to the site.

Use the Tools to Your Advantage

Choosing a school is an involved and complicated process. The tools available to you at www.petersons.com/nursing can help you to be more productive in this process. So, what are you waiting for? Fire up the computer. Your future alma mater may be just a click of the mouse away.

How to Use This Guide

The following includes an overview of the various components of *Peterson's Nursing Programs 2006,* along with background information on the criteria used for including institutions and nursing programs in the guide, and explanatory material to help users interpret details presented within the guide.

Profiles of Nursing Programs

The **Profiles of Nursing Programs** section contains detailed profiles of schools that responded to our online survey and the nursing programs they offer. This section is organized geographically; U.S. schools are listed alphabetically by state or territory, followed by Canadian schools listed alphabetically by province.

The profiles contain basic information about the colleges and universities, along with details specific to the nursing school or department, the nursing student body, and the nursing programs offered.

Schools that are members of a consortium appear with an abbreviated profile. The abbreviated profile lists only the school heading and the specific college or university information, followed by a reference line that refers readers to the consortium profile, which contains detailed program information.

An outline of the profile follows. The items of information found under each section heading are defined and displayed. Any item discussed below that is omitted from an individual profile either does not apply to that particular college or university or is one for which no information was supplied. Each profile begins with a heading with the name of the institution (the college or university), the nursing college or unit, the location of the nursing facilities, the school's Web address, and the institution's founding date, specifically the year in which it was chartered or the year when instruction actually began, whichever date is earlier. In most cases, the location is identical to the main campus of the institution. However, in a few instances, the nursing facilities are not located in the same city or state as the main campus of the college or university.

Basic information about the college follows:

Nursing Program Faculty: The total number of full-time and part-time faculty members, followed by, if provided, the percentage of faculty members holding doctoral degrees.

Baccalaureate Enrollment: The total number of matriculated full-time and part-time baccalaureate program students as of fall 2004 is given. This snapshot of the nursing student body indicates the total number of matriculated students, both full-time and part-time, in the baccalaureate-level nursing program; the school's estimate of the percentage of nursing students in each of the following categories is provided, if applicable: women, men, minority, international, and part-time.

Graduate Enrollment: The total number of matriculated full-time and part-time students in graduate programs in fall 2004 and the percentages of women, men, minority, international, and part-time students are given.

Nursing Student Activities: This section lists organizations open only to nursing students, including nursing clubs, Sigma Theta Tau (the international honor society for nursing), recruiter clubs, and Student Nurses' Association.

Nursing Student Resources: This section lists special learning resources available for nursing students within the nursing school's (or unit's) facilities.

Library Facilities: Figures are provided for the total number of bound volumes held by the college or university, the number of those volumes in health-related subjects, and the number in nursing and the number of periodical subscriptions held and the number of those in health-related subjects.

BACCALAUREATE PROGRAMS

Degree: Baccalaureate degree or degrees awarded are specified.

Available Programs: If, in addition to a generic baccalaureate program in nursing, a school has other baccalaureate nursing programs (e.g., accelerated programs or programs for RNs, LPNs, or college graduates with non-nursing degrees) they are specified here.

Site Options: Locations other than the nursing program's main campus at which baccalaureate programs may be taken, including distance learning, are listed. Off-campus classes generally are held in health-care facilities or other educational facilities that are part of or affiliated with the college or nursing school.

Study Options: Lists full-time and part-time options.

Program Entrance Requirements: Lists special requirements typically required to enter a program of nursing leading to a baccalaureate degree, including completion of a specific program of prerequisite courses, sometimes called prenursing courses. These are specific course credits that must be earned by students who wish to enter the generic baccalaureate program. Students entering into other tracks may be required to prove that they have completed analogous courses. Often the minimum GPA requirement for prerequisite courses differs from that expected for general college courses. Other requirements are generally self-explanatory. This paragraph also indicates if transfer students are accepted into the program and which **Standardized Test** scores the student must have submitted to the institution. These are noted as required, recommended, and required for some. Tests may include American College Testing, Inc.'s ACT; the College Board's SAT or SAT Subject Tests; and the Test of English as a Foreign Language (TOEFL) for nonnative speakers of English. Special tracks will require appropriate proof of experience, diplomas, or other credentials. Finally, application deadlines and fees are given.

Advanced Placement: This entry indicates that program credits may be granted on the basis of examinations or evaluations of earned credits at other facilities by the program's faculty and administrators.

Expenses: In this section, figures are provided for tuition, mandatory and other fees, and room and board, as well as an estimate of costs for books and supplies, based on the 2004–05 academic year. If a school did not return a survey, expenses for the 2003–04 academic year are listed. Unless otherwise indicated, tuition is for one full academic year. If applicable, distinct tuition figures are given for state residents and nonresidents. Part-time, summer, and evening tuition is expressed in terms of the per-unit rate (per credit, per semester hour, etc.) specified by the institution. The tuition structure at some institutions is very complex, with different rates for freshmen and sophomores than for juniors and seniors or with part-time tuition prorated on a sliding scale according to the number of credit hours taken. Mandatory fees include such items as activity fees, health insurance, and malpractice insurance.

Financial Aid: Provides information on college-administered aid for baccalaureate-level nursing students, including the percentage of undergraduate nursing students receiving financial aid, all types of aid offered, and application deadlines. Financial aid programs are organized into four categories: gift aid (need-based), awards based on a student's formally designated inability to pay some or all of the cost of education; gift aid (non-need-based), scholarships given on the basis of a student's special achievements, abilities, or personal characteristics; loans, subsidized low-interest student loans that can be need-based or not; and work-study, a need-based program of part-time work offered to help pay educational expenditures. The application deadline is the deadline by which application forms and need calculations, such as the FAFSA, must be submitted to the institution in order to qualify for need-based and institutional aid.

Contact: This section lists the name, title, mailing address, telephone number, and, if available, fax number and e-mail address of the person to contact for admission information about the baccalaureate program.

GRADUATE PROGRAMS

The first three paragraphs provide information that is common to the college's graduate programs in nursing.

Expenses: In this section, figures are provided for tuition, room and board, and required fees based on the 2004–05 academic year. If a school did not return a survey, expenses for the 2003–04 academic year are listed. Unless otherwise indicated, tuition is for one full academic year. If applicable, distinct tuition figures are given for state residents and nonresidents. Part-time, summer, and evening tuition is expressed in terms of the per-unit rate (per credit, per semester hour, etc.) specified by the institution.

Financial Aid: Provides information on college-administered aid includes the percentage of graduate nursing students receiving financial aid, all types of aid offered, and application deadlines. The major kinds of aid available are listed, including traineeships, low-interest student loans, fellowships, research assistantships, teaching assistantships, and full and partial tuition waivers. If aid is available to part-time students, this is indicated. The application deadline is the deadline by which application forms must be submitted to the college's financial aid office.

Contact: Lists the name, title, mailing address, telephone number, and, if available, fax number and e-mail address of the person to contact for admission information about graduate programs.

MASTER'S DEGREE PROGRAM

Degree(s): Master's degree or degrees awarded are specified. Joint degrees specify which two degrees are given, e.g., M.S.N./M.B.A., M.S./M.H.A., M.S.N./M.P.H., in programs that combine a master's degree (or doctorate) in nursing with a master's degree in another discipline, such as business administration, hospital administration, or public health.

Available Programs: If a college has special tracks that give credit, accelerated programs, or advanced courses designed for students with previous nursing experience or higher education credentials that enable students to complete programs in less time than regularly required, these are specified here in three categories:

For RNs—programs that admit registered nurses with associate degrees or diplomas in nursing and award a master's degree. These include RN-to-master's programs that combine the baccalaureate and master's degrees into one program for nurses who are graduates of associate or hospital diploma programs and programs that admit registered nurses with non-nursing baccalaureate degrees.

For LPNs—programs that admit licensed practical nurses and award a master's degree.
For College Graduates with Non-Nursing Degrees—programs that admit students with baccalaureate or master's degrees in areas other than nursing and award a master's degree in nursing.

Concentrations Available: Specific areas of study and concentrations offered by the school are listed. Areas of specialization in case management, health-care administration, nurse anesthesia, nurse midwifery, nursing administration, nursing education, and nursing informatics are noted. Clinical nurse specialist and nurse practitioner programs and areas of specialization within them are noted.

Site Options: Locations other than the nursing program's main campus at which the master's degree programs are offered, including distance learning, are listed. Off-campus classes generally are held in health-care facilities or other educational facilities that are part of or affiliated with the nursing school.

Study Options: Lists full-time and part-time options.

Program Entrance Requirements: Lists generally self-explanatory requirements.

Advanced Placement: Indicates that program credits may be granted on the basis of examinations or evaluations of earned credits at other facilities by the program's faculty and administrators.

Degree Requirements: Indicates the number of master's program credit hours required to earn the master's degree and the need for a thesis or qualifying score on a comprehensive examination.

POST-MASTER'S PROGRAM

Listed here are the specific areas of clinical nurse specialist programs, nurse practitioner programs, and other specializations offered as post-master's programs.

DOCTORAL DEGREE PROGRAM

Degree: Doctoral degree awarded is specified.

Areas of Study: Lists specific areas of study and concentration offered by the school.

Program Entrance Requirements: Lists generally self-explanatory requirements.

Degree Requirements: Indicates the number of program credit hours required to earn the doctorate and the need for a dissertation, oral examination, written examination, or residency.

POSTDOCTORAL PROGRAM

Areas of Study: Lists areas of study currently reported. These may change, dependent upon the individuals in the program.

Contact: Lists the name, title, mailing address, telephone number, and, if available, fax number and e-mail address of the person to contact for information about postdoctoral programs.

CONTINUING EDUCATION PROGRAM

The appearance of this heading indicates that the nursing school has a program of continuing education. If provided, the name, title, mailing address, telephone number, fax number, and e-mail address of the person to contact regarding the program are given.

Special Messages

Special Messages, which appear within some institutions' profiles, have been written by those colleges or universities that wished to supplement the profile data with timely or important information about their institutions or nursing programs. Some chose to mention degree programs that are not yet accredited.

In-Depth Descriptions of Nursing Programs

The **In-Depth Descriptions of Nursing Programs** section is an open forum for nursing schools to communicate their particular message to prospective students. The absence of any college or university from this section does not constitute an editorial decision on the part of Peterson's. Those who have chosen to write these inclusions are responsible for the accuracy of the content. Statements regarding a school's objectives and accomplishments represent its own beliefs and are not the opinions of the editors. The **In-Depth Descriptions of Nursing Programs** are arranged alphabetically by the official institution name.

Indexes

Indexes at the back of the book provide references to profiles by baccalaureate, master's, doctoral, postdoctoral, distance learning, and continuing education programs offered; for master's-level programs, by area of study or concentration; and by institution name.

Abbreviations Used in This Guide

AACN	American Association of Colleges of Nursing
AACSB	AACSB International—The Association to Advance Collegiate Schools of Business
AAHC	Association of Academic Health Centers
AAS	Associate in Applied Science
ABSN	Accelerated Bachelor of Science in Nursing
ACT	American College Testing, Inc.

ACT ASSET	American College Testing Assessment of Skills for Successful Entry and Transfer
ACT COMP	American College Testing College Outcomes Measures Program
ACT PEP	American College Testing Proficiency Examination Program
AD	Associate Degree
ADN	Associate Degree in Nursing
AHNP	Adult Health Nurse Practitioner
ALE	American Language Exam
AMEDD	Army Medical Department
ANA	American Nurses Association
ANP	Adult Nurse Practitioner
APN	Advanced Practice Nurse
ARNP	Advanced Registered Nurse Practitioner
AS	Associate of Science
ASN	Associate of Science in Nursing
BA	Bachelor of Arts
BAA	Bachelor of Applied Arts
BN	Bachelor of Nursing
BNSc	Bachelor of Nursing Science
BRN	Baccalaureate for the Registered Nurse
BS	Bachelor of Science
BScMH	Bachelor of Science in Mental Health
BScN	Bachelor of Science in Nursing
BSEd	Bachelor of Science in Education
BSN	Bachelor of Science in Nursing
CAI	computer-assisted instruction
CAUSN	Canadian Association of University Schools of Nursing
CCNE	Commission on Collegiate Nursing Education
CCRN	Critical-Care Registered Nurse
CFNP	Certified Family Nurse Practitioner
CGFNS	Commission on Graduates of Foreign Nursing Schools
CINAHL	Cumulative Index to Nursing and Allied Health Literature
CLAST	College-Level Academic Skills Test
CLEP	College-Level Examination Program
CNA	Certified Nurse Assistant, Certified Nursing Assistant, Certified Nurses' Aide
CNAT	Canadian Nurses Association Testing
CNM	Certified Nurse-Midwife
CNS	Clinical Nurse Specialist
CODEC	coder/decoder
CPR	cardiopulmonary resuscitation
CRNA	Certified Registered Nurse Anesthetist
CS	Certified Specialist
CSS	College Scholarship Service
DNS	Doctor of Nursing Science
DNSc	Doctor of Nursing Science
DOE	U.S. Department of Education
DrPH	Doctor of Public Health
DSN	Doctor of Science in Nursing
EdD	Doctor of Education
EFC	expected family contribution
ERIC	Educational Resources Information Center
ESL	English as a second language
ETN	Enterostomal Nurse
FAAN	Fellow in the American Academy of Nursing
FAF	Financial Aid Form
FAFSA	Free Application for Federal Student Aid
FC	family contribution
FNP	Family Nurse Practitioner
FSEOG	Federal Supplemental Educational Opportunity Grants
GED	General Educational Development test
GMAT	Graduate Management Admission Test
GPA	grade point average
GPO	Government Printing Office
GRE	Graduate Record Examinations
Gyn	gynecology
HIV	human immunodeficiency virus
HMO	health maintenance organization
ICEOP	Illinois Consortium for Educational Opportunities Program
ICU	intensive care unit
ISP	Internet service provider
ITV	interactive television
LD	Licensed Dietician
LPN	Licensed Practical Nurse
LVN	Licensed Vocational Nurse
MA	Master of Arts
MAEd	Master of Arts in Education
MAT	Miller Analogies Test
MBA	Master of Business Administration
MCSc	Master of Clinical Science
MDiv	Master of Divinity
MEd	Master of Education
MEDLINE	MEDLARS On-Line
MELAB	Michigan English Language Assessment Battery
MHA	Master of Hospital Administration Master of Health Administration
MHD	Master of Human Development
MHSA	Master of Health Services Administration
MN	Master of Nursing
MNSc	Master of Nursing Science
MOM	Master of Organizational Management
MPA	Master of Public Affairs
MPH	Master of Public Health
MPS	Master of Public Service
MS	Master of Science
MSBA	Master of Science in Business Administration
M Sc	Master of Science
MSc(A)	Master of Science (Applied)
MScN	Master of Science in Nursing
MSEd	Master of Science in Education
MSN	Master of Science in Nursing
MSOB	Master of Science in Organizational Behavior
NCAA	National Collegiate Athletic Association
NCLEX-RN	National Council Licensure Examination for Registered Nurses
ND	Doctor of Nursing
NLN	National League for Nursing
NNP	Neonatal Nurse Practitioner
NP	Nurse Practitioner
NSNA	National Student Nurses' Association
OB	Organizational Behavior
OB/GYN	obstetrics/gynecology
OCLC	Online Computer Library Center
OM	Organizational Management
PEP	Proficiency Examination Program
PhD	Doctor of Philosophy
PHEAA	Pennsylvania Higher Education Assistance Agency
PHS	Public Health Service
PLUS	Parents' Loan for Undergraduate Students
PNNP	Perinatal Nurse Practitioner
PNP	Pediatric Nurse Practitioner

PSAT	Preliminary SAT
RD	Registered Dietician
RN	Registered Nurse
RN, C	Registered Nurse, Certified
RN, CAN	Registered Nurse, Certified in Nursing Administration
RN, CNAA	Registered Nurse, Certified in Nursing Administration, Advanced
RN, CS	Registered Nurse, Certified Specialist
ROTC	Reserve Officers' Training Corps
RPN	Registered Psychiatric Nurse
SAR	Student Aid Report
SAT	SAT and SAT Subject Tests
SLS	Supplemental Loans to Students
SNA	Student Nurses' Association
SNAP	Student Nurses Acting for Progress
SNO	Student Nurses Organization
SUNY	State University of New York
TAP	Tuition Assistance Program
TB	tuberculosis
TOEFL	Test of English as a Foreign Language
TSE	Test of Spoken English
TWE	Test of Written English
USIS	United States Information Service
WHNP	Women's Health Nurse Practitioner

Data Collection Procedures

The data contained in the preponderant number of nursing college profiles, as well as in the indexes to them, were collected through *Thomson Peterson's Survey of Nursing Programs* during winter 2004–05. Questionnaires were posted online for more than 700 colleges and universities with baccalaureate and graduate programs in nursing. With minor exceptions, data for those colleges or schools of nursing that responded to the questionnaires were submitted by officials at the schools themselves. All usable information received in time for publication has been included. For those few schools that failed to respond to Peterson's Web-based survey in time to meet Peterson's deadline, information was drawn from college catalogs and Web sites. The omission of a particular item from a profile means that it is either not applicable to that institution or was not available or usable. In the handful of instances in which no information regarding an eligible nursing program was submitted and research of reliable secondary sources was unable to elicit the desired information, the name, location, and some general information regarding the nursing program appear in the profile section to indicate the existence of the program. Because of the extensive system of checks performed on the data collected by Peterson's, we believe that the information presented in this guide is accurate. Nonetheless, errors and omissions are possible in a data collection and processing endeavor of this scope. Also, facts and figures, such as tuition and fees, can suddenly change. Therefore, students should check with a specific college or university at the time of application to verify all pertinent information.

Criteria for Inclusion in This Book

Peterson's Nursing Programs 2006 covers accredited institutions in the U.S., U.S. territories, and Canada that grant baccalaureate and graduate degrees. The institutions that sponsor the nursing programs must be accredited by accrediting agencies approved by the U.S. Department of Education (USDE) or the Council for Higher Education Accreditation (CHEA) or be candidates for accreditation with an agency recognized by the USDE for its preaccreditation category. Canadian schools may be provincially chartered instead of accredited.

Baccalaureate-level and master's-level nursing programs represented by a profile within the guide are accredited by the National League for Nursing Accrediting Commission (NLNAC) or the Commission on Collegiate Nursing Education (CCNE). Canadian nursing schools are members of the Canadian Association of University Schools of Nursing (CAUSN).

Doctoral, postdoctoral, continuing education, and other nursing programs included in the profiles are offered by nursing schools or departments affiliated with colleges or universities that meet the criteria outlined above.

[illegible]

Criteria for Inclusion in This Book

[illegible]

Data Collection Procedures

[illegible]

QUICK-REFERENCE CHART

Nursing Programs At-a-Glance

	Baccalaureate	Master's	Joint Degree	Post-Master's	Doctoral	Post-doctoral	Continuing Education
U.S. AND U.S. TERRITORIES							
Alabama							
Auburn University	•						
Auburn University Montgomery	•						
Jacksonville State University	•	•					•
Samford University	•	•	•	•			•
Spring Hill College	•						
Troy University	•	•					
Tuskegee University	•						
The University of Alabama	•	•	•	•			•
The University of Alabama at Birmingham	•	•	•	•	•	•	
The University of Alabama in Huntsville	•	•		•			•
University of Mobile	•	•					•
University of North Alabama	•						•
University of South Alabama	•	•		•			
Alaska							
University of Alaska Anchorage	•	•					
Arizona							
Arizona State University	•	•	•	•			•
Grand Canyon University	•	•					•
Northern Arizona University	•	•					
The University of Arizona	•	•		•	•	•	•
University of Phoenix Online Campus	•	•	•	•			
University of Phoenix–Phoenix Campus	•	•	•	•			•
University of Phoenix–Southern Arizona Campus	•	•	•	•			
Arkansas							
Arkansas State University	•	•					
Arkansas Tech University	•						
Harding University	•						
Henderson State University	•						
University of Arkansas	•	•					•
University of Arkansas at Monticello	•						
University of Arkansas at Pine Bluff	•						
University of Arkansas for Medical Sciences	•	•			•		
University of Central Arkansas	•	•		•			
California							
Azusa Pacific University	•	•		•	•		•
Biola University	•						•
California State University, Bakersfield	•	•		•			
California State University, Chico	•	•		•			•
California State University, Dominguez Hills	•	•		•			•
California State University, Fresno	•	•		•			•
California State University, Fullerton	•	•					
California State University, Hayward	•						
California State University, Long Beach	•	•	•	•			
California State University, Los Angeles	•	•		•			
California State University, Northridge	•						
California State University, Sacramento	•	•					•
California State University, San Bernardino	•	•					
California State University, Stanislaus	•						
Dominican University of California	•	•					•

	Baccalaureate	Master's	Joint Degree	Post-Master's	Doctoral	Post-doctoral	Continuing Education
Holy Names University	•	•	•	•			
Humboldt State University	•						
Loma Linda University	•	•	•	•	•		
Mount St. Mary's College	•	•					
National University	•						
Pacific Union College	•						•
Point Loma Nazarene University	•	•					•
Samuel Merritt College	•	•		•			
San Diego State University	•	•		•			•
San Francisco State University	•	•		•			•
San Jose State University	•	•					
Sonoma State University	•	•		•			
University of California, Los Angeles	•	•	•	•	•	•	•
University of California, San Francisco		•			•	•	
University of Phoenix–Northern California Campus	•	•	•	•			
University of Phoenix–Sacramento Campus	•	•	•	•			
University of Phoenix–San Diego Campus	•	•	•	•			
University of Phoenix–Southern California Campus	•	•	•	•			
University of San Diego	•	•	•	•	•		
University of San Francisco	•	•		•			•
Western University of Health Sciences		•		•			
Colorado							
Colorado State University-Pueblo	•	•		•			•
Mesa State College	•						
Metropolitan State College of Denver	•						
Regis University	•	•					
University of Colorado at Colorado Springs	•	•	•	•			•
University of Colorado at Denver and Health Sciences Center—Health Sciences Program	•	•	•	•	•	•	•
University of Northern Colorado	•	•		•	•		
University of Phoenix–Colorado Campus	•	•	•	•			
University of Phoenix–Southern Colorado Campus	•	•	•	•			
Connecticut							
Central Connecticut State University	•						
Fairfield University	•	•		•			
Quinnipiac University	•	•		•			•
Sacred Heart University	•	•	•	•			
Saint Joseph College	•	•		•			
Southern Connecticut State University	•	•		•			
University of Connecticut	•	•	•	•	•		•
University of Hartford	•	•	•				•
Western Connecticut State University	•	•		•			
Yale University		•	•	•	•	•	
Delaware							
Delaware State University	•						
University of Delaware	•	•		•			
Wesley College	•	•		•			•
Wilmington College	•	•	•	•			
District of Columbia							
The Catholic University of America	•	•	•	•	•		
Georgetown University	•	•		•			•
Howard University	•	•		•			
University of the District of Columbia	•						

	Baccalaureate	Master's	Joint Degree	Post-Master's	Doctoral	Post-doctoral	Continuing Education
Florida							
Barry University	•	•	•	•	•		
Bethune-Cookman College	•						
Florida Agricultural and Mechanical University	•	•		•	•		•
Florida Atlantic University	•			•	•		•
Florida Gulf Coast University	•	•		•			•
Florida Hospital College of Health Sciences	•						
Florida International University	•	•		•	•		
Florida Southern College	•						
Florida State University	•	•		•			•
Jacksonville University	•	•	•				
Nova Southeastern University	•						
St. Petersburg College	•						•
University of Central Florida	•	•		•	•		
University of Florida	•	•	•	•	•		
University of Miami	•	•		•	•		•
University of North Florida	•	•		•			
University of Phoenix–Fort Lauderdale Campus	•	•	•	•			
University of Phoenix–Jacksonville Campus	•	•	•	•			
University of Phoenix–Orlando Campus	•	•	•	•			
University of Phoenix–Tampa Campus	•	•	•	•			
University of South Florida	•	•	•	•	•		•
The University of Tampa	•	•		•			
University of West Florida	•						
Georgia							
Albany State University	•	•		•			
Armstrong Atlantic State University	•	•		•			
Brenau University	•	•		•			
Clayton College & State University	•						
Columbus State University	•						
Emory University	•	•	•	•	•	•	
Georgia Baptist College of Nursing of Mercer University	•	•		•			•
Georgia College & State University	•	•	•	•			
Georgia Southern University	•	•		•			
Georgia Southwestern State University	•						•
Georgia State University	•	•		•	•		
Kennesaw State University	•	•					•
LaGrange College	•						
Medical College of Georgia	•	•		•	•		
North Georgia College & State University	•	•		•			
Piedmont College	•						
Thomas University	•						
University of Phoenix–Atlanta Campus	•						
University of West Georgia	•	•		•			
Valdosta State University	•	•					•
Guam							
University of Guam	•						
Hawaii							
Hawai'i Pacific University	•	•	•				
University of Hawaii at Hilo	•						
University of Hawaii at Manoa	•	•		•	•		
University of Phoenix–Hawaii Campus	•	•	•	•			

	Baccalaureate	Master's	Joint Degree	Post-Master's	Doctoral	Post-doctoral	Continuing Education
Idaho							
Boise State University	•						
Idaho State University	•	•		•			
Lewis-Clark State College	•						•
Northwest Nazarene University	•						
Illinois							
Aurora University	•						
Benedictine University	•						
Blessing-Rieman College of Nursing	•						
Bradley University	•	•					
Chicago State University	•						
DePaul University	•	•		•			
Elmhurst College	•						
Governors State University	•	•					
Illinois State University	•	•		•			
Illinois Wesleyan University	•						
Lakeview College of Nursing	•						
Lewis University	•	•	•	•			•
Loyola University Chicago	•	•	•		•		
MacMurray College	•						
McKendree College	•						
Millikin University	•						
Northern Illinois University	•	•	•	•			
North Park University	•	•	•	•			
Olivet Nazarene University	•	•					
Rockford College	•						
Rush University	•	•	•	•	•	•	•
Saint Anthony College of Nursing	•						
Saint Francis Medical Center College of Nursing	•	•					
St. John's College	•						
Saint Xavier University	•	•	•	•			•
Southern Illinois University Edwardsville	•	•					•
Trinity Christian College	•						
University of Illinois at Chicago	•	•	•	•	•	•	•
University of St. Francis	•	•					
West Suburban College of Nursing	•						
Indiana							
Anderson University	•	•	•				
Ball State University	•	•		•			
Bethel College	•	•					
Goshen College	•						
Indiana State University	•	•		•			•
Indiana University Bloomington	•						
Indiana University East	•						
Indiana University Kokomo	•						•
Indiana University Northwest	•						
Indiana University–Purdue University Fort Wayne	•	•					•
Indiana University–Purdue University Indianapolis	•	•	•	•	•	•	•
Indiana University South Bend	•						
Indiana University Southeast	•						
Indiana Wesleyan University	•	•		•			
Marian College	•						
Purdue University	•	•					•
Purdue University Calumet	•	•					
Saint Mary's College	•						

Indiana *(continued)*	Baccalaureate	Master's	Joint Degree	Post-Master's	Doctoral	Post-doctoral	Continuing Education
University of Evansville	•						
University of Indianapolis	•	•	•				
University of Saint Francis	•	•		•			
University of Southern Indiana	•	•		•			•
Valparaiso University	•	•		•			•
Iowa							
Allen College	•	•		•			•
Briar Cliff University		•		•			•
Clarke College	•	•		•			
Coe College	•						
Grand View College	•						•
Iowa Wesleyan College	•						•
Luther College	•						•
Mercy College of Health Sciences	•						
Morningside College	•						
Mount Mercy College	•						•
St. Ambrose University	•						
The University of Iowa	•	•	•	•	•	•	•
Kansas							
Baker University	•						
Bethel College	•						
Emporia State University	•						
Fort Hays State University	•	•		•			
Kansas Wesleyan University	•						
MidAmerica Nazarene University	•						•
Newman University	•						
Pittsburg State University	•	•		•			•
Southwestern College	•						
Tabor College	•						
University of Kansas	•	•	•	•	•		•
Washburn University	•	•		•			•
Wichita State University	•	•	•	•			
Kentucky							
Bellarmine University	•	•	•				•
Berea College	•						•
Eastern Kentucky University	•	•					
Midway College	•						•
Morehead State University	•						
Murray State University	•			•			•
Northern Kentucky University	•	•		•			
Spalding University	•	•		•			•
Thomas More College	•						
University of Kentucky	•	•		•	•		•
University of Louisville	•	•		•			
Western Kentucky University	•	•		•			•
Louisiana							
Dillard University	•						
Grambling State University	•	•		•			
Louisiana College	•						
Louisiana State University Health Sciences Center	•	•			•		•
Loyola University New Orleans	•	•		•			
McNeese State University	•	•		•			•
Nicholls State University	•						•
Northwestern State University of Louisiana	•	•		•			•
Our Lady of Holy Cross College	•						

	Baccalaureate	Master's	Joint Degree	Post-Master's	Doctoral	Post-doctoral	Continuing Education
Our Lady of the Lake College	•						
Southeastern Louisiana University	•	•					
Southern University and Agricultural and Mechanical College	•	•		•	•		
University of Louisiana at Lafayette	•	•		•			•
University of Louisiana at Monroe	•						•
University of Phoenix–Louisiana Campus	•	•	•	•			
Maine							
Husson College	•	•		•			
Saint Joseph's College of Maine	•	•					•
University of Maine	•	•					
University of Maine at Fort Kent	•						
University of New England	•						•
University of Southern Maine	•	•	•	•			•
Maryland							
Bowie State University	•	•					
College of Notre Dame of Maryland	•						
Columbia Union College	•						•
Coppin State University	•	•		•			
The Johns Hopkins University	•	•	•	•	•	•	•
Salisbury University	•	•		•			
Towson University	•	•					
University of Maryland	•	•	•	•	•		•
Villa Julie College	•						
Massachusetts							
American International College	•	•					
Anna Maria College	•						•
Atlantic Union College	•						•
Boston College	•	•	•	•	•		•
Curry College	•						•
Elms College	•						•
Emmanuel College	•						
Endicott College	•						•
Fitchburg State College	•	•					
Framingham State College	•						
MGH Institute of Health Professions		•		•			•
Northeastern University	•	•	•	•			•
Regis College	•	•		•			•
Salem State College	•	•	•				•
Simmons College	•	•		•			•
University of Massachusetts Amherst	•	•	•	•	•		•
University of Massachusetts Boston	•	•		•	•		•
University of Massachusetts Dartmouth	•	•		•			•
University of Massachusetts Lowell	•	•			•		
University of Massachusetts Worcester		•		•	•		•
Worcester State College	•	•					
Michigan							
Andrews University	•	•		•			
Calvin College	•						
Eastern Michigan University	•	•					
Ferris State University	•						
Grand Valley State University	•	•	•	•			•
Hope College	•						
Lake Superior State University	•						
Madonna University	•	•	•	•			•
Michigan State University	•	•		•	•	•	•

Michigan *(continued)*	Baccalaureate	Master's	Joint Degree	Post-Master's	Doctoral	Post-doctoral	Continuing Education
Northern Michigan University	•	•		•			•
Oakland University	•	•		•			•
Saginaw Valley State University	•	•		•			•
Spring Arbor University	•						
University of Detroit Mercy	•	•		•			
University of Michigan	•	•	•	•	•	•	
University of Michigan–Flint	•	•					•
University of Phoenix–Metro Detroit Campus	•	•	•	•			
University of Phoenix–West Michigan Campus	•	•	•	•			
Wayne State University	•	•		•	•	•	
Western Michigan University	•						
Minnesota							
Augsburg College	•	•					
Bemidji State University	•						•
Bethel University	•	•					•
College of Saint Benedict	•						
College of St. Catherine	•	•		•			
The College of St. Scholastica	•	•		•			
Concordia College	•	•					
Gustavus Adolphus College	•						
Metropolitan State University	•	•		•			
Minnesota Intercollegiate Nursing Consortium	•						
Minnesota State University Mankato	•	•		•			•
Minnesota State University Moorhead	•	•					
St. Cloud State University	•						
St. Olaf College	•						
University of Minnesota, Twin Cities Campus	•	•	•		•		•
Winona State University	•	•		•			
Mississippi							
Alcorn State University	•	•		•			
Delta State University	•	•		•			
Mississippi College	•						
Mississippi University for Women	•	•		•			
University of Mississippi Medical Center	•	•		•	•		•
University of Southern Mississippi	•	•		•	•		
William Carey College	•	•					
Missouri							
Avila University	•						
Central Missouri State University	•	•					
Deaconess College of Nursing	•						
Graceland University	•	•		•			
Jewish Hospital College of Nursing and Allied Health	•	•		•			
Lester L. Cox College of Nursing and Health Sciences	•						
Maryville University of Saint Louis	•	•					
Missouri Southern State University	•						
Missouri Western State College	•						•
Research College of Nursing	•	•					
Saint Louis University	•	•	•	•	•		•
Saint Luke's College	•						
Southeast Missouri State University	•	•		•			
Southwest Baptist University	•						
Southwest Missouri State University	•	•		•			•

	Baccalaureate	Master's	Joint Degree	Post-Master's	Doctoral	Post-doctoral	Continuing Education
Truman State University	•						
University of Missouri–Columbia	•	•		•	•		•
University of Missouri–Kansas City	•	•		•	•		
University of Missouri–St. Louis	•	•			•		
Webster University	•	•					
William Jewell College	•						
Montana							
Carroll College	•						•
Montana State University–Bozeman	•	•		•			
Montana State University–Northern	•						•
Nebraska							
Clarkson College	•	•		•			•
College of Saint Mary	•						
Creighton University	•	•		•			
Midland Lutheran College	•						•
Nebraska Methodist College	•	•		•			•
Nebraska Wesleyan University	•	•					
Union College	•						
University of Nebraska Medical Center	•	•		•	•	•	•
Nevada							
University of Nevada, Las Vegas	•	•		•	•		•
University of Nevada, Reno	•	•	•	•			
New Hampshire							
Colby-Sawyer College	•						
Rivier College	•	•	•	•			
Saint Anselm College	•						•
University of New Hampshire	•	•		•			
New Jersey							
Bloomfield College	•						
The College of New Jersey	•	•		•			
College of Saint Elizabeth	•						•
Fairleigh Dickinson University, Metropolitan Campus	•	•		•			
Felician College	•	•		•			
Kean University	•	•	•				•
Monmouth University	•	•		•			•
New Jersey City University	•	•					
The Richard Stockton College of New Jersey	•	•					
Rutgers, The State University of New Jersey, Camden College of Arts and Sciences	•	•					
Rutgers, The State University of New Jersey, College of Nursing	•	•	•	•	•		•
Saint Peter's College	•	•		•			
Seton Hall University	•	•	•	•			•
Thomas Edison State College	•						
University of Medicine and Dentistry of New Jersey	•	•		•			•
William Paterson University of New Jersey	•	•		•			
New Mexico							
Eastern New Mexico University	•						
New Mexico State University	•	•		•			•
University of New Mexico	•	•	•	•	•		
University of Phoenix–New Mexico Campus	•	•	•	•			
New York							
Adelphi University	•	•	•	•			•
College of Mount Saint Vincent	•	•		•			

New York *(continued)*	Baccalaureate	Master's	Joint Degree	Post-Master's	Doctoral	Post-doctoral	Continuing Education
The College of New Rochelle	•	•		•			
College of Staten Island of the City University of New York	•	•		•			
Columbia University	•	•	•	•	•		•
Daemen College	•	•		•			
Dominican College	•	•					
D'Youville College	•	•		•			
Elmira College	•						•
Excelsior College	•	•					
Hartwick College	•						
Hunter College of the City University of New York	•	•	•	•			•
Keuka College	•						
Lehman College of the City University of New York	•	•					
Long Island University, Brooklyn Campus	•	•		•			
Long Island University, C.W. Post Campus	•	•		•			
Medgar Evers College of the City University of New York	•						
Mercy College	•	•		•			•
Molloy College	•	•		•			•
Mount Saint Mary College	•	•		•			
Nazareth College of Rochester	•	•					•
New York University	•	•	•	•	•		•
Pace University	•	•		•			•
Roberts Wesleyan College	•						•
The Sage Colleges	•	•	•	•			
St. John Fisher College	•	•		•			
St. Joseph's College, New York	•						
State University of New York at Binghamton	•	•		•	•		•
State University of New York at New Paltz	•	•					
State University of New York at Plattsburgh	•						•
State University of New York College at Brockport	•						
State University of New York Downstate Medical Center	•	•	•	•			•
State University of New York Institute of Technology	•	•		•			•
State University of New York Upstate Medical University	•	•		•			•
Stony Brook University, State University of New York	•	•		•			•
Teachers College Columbia University					•		
University at Buffalo, The State University of New York	•	•		•	•		
University of Rochester	•	•		•	•	•	•
Utica College	•						•
Wagner College	•	•		•			
York College of the City University of New York	•						
North Carolina							
Barton College	•						
Cabarrus College of Health Sciences	•						
Duke University	•	•	•	•			
East Carolina University	•	•		•	•		
Gardner-Webb University	•	•	•				
Lees-McRae College	•						
Lenoir-Rhyne College	•						
North Carolina Agricultural and Technical State University	•						
North Carolina Central University	•						

	Baccalaureate	Master's	Joint Degree	Post-Master's	Doctoral	Post-doctoral	Continuing Education
Queens University of Charlotte	•	•	•	•			
Southeastern North Carolina Nursing Consortium	•						
The University of North Carolina at Chapel Hill	•	•		•	•	•	•
The University of North Carolina at Charlotte	•	•		•			•
The University of North Carolina at Greensboro	•	•	•	•	•		
The University of North Carolina at Wilmington	•	•					
Western Carolina University	•	•		•			
Winston-Salem State University	•	•					•
North Dakota							
Dickinson State University	•						
Jamestown College	•						
Medcenter One College of Nursing	•						
Minot State University	•						
North Dakota State University	•	•		•			•
University of Mary	•	•					
University of North Dakota	•	•		•	•		
Ohio							
Ashland University	•						
Capital University	•	•					
Case Western Reserve University	•	•	•	•	•	•	•
Cedarville University	•						
Cleveland State University	•	•	•				•
College of Mount St. Joseph	•	•					
Franciscan University of Steubenville	•	•					
Kent State University	•	•	•	•	•		•
Kettering College of Medical Arts	•						
Lourdes College	•						
Malone College	•	•					•
Medical College of Ohio	•	•		•			•
Mercy College of Northwest Ohio	•						
Miami University	•						
Mount Carmel College of Nursing	•	•		•			
The Ohio State University	•	•		•	•		
Ohio University	•	•					
Otterbein College	•	•		•			•
Shawnee State University	•						•
The University of Akron	•	•		•	•		•
University of Cincinnati	•	•	•	•	•		•
University of Phoenix–Cleveland Campus	•	•					
Ursuline College	•	•		•			
Walsh University	•						
Wright State University	•	•	•	•			•
Xavier University	•	•	•				
Youngstown State University	•	•					
Oklahoma							
Bacone College	•						
East Central University	•						
Langston University	•						
Northeastern State University	•						
Northwestern Oklahoma State University	•						
Oklahoma Baptist University	•						
Oklahoma City University	•	•	•				•
Oklahoma Panhandle State University	•						

Oklahoma *(continued)*	Baccalaureate	Master's	Joint Degree	Post-Master's	Doctoral	Post-doctoral	Continuing Education
Oklahoma Wesleyan University	•						
Oral Roberts University	•						
Southern Nazarene University	•	•					
Southwestern Oklahoma State University	•						
University of Central Oklahoma	•						
University of Oklahoma Health Sciences Center	•	•		•			
University of Phoenix–Oklahoma City Campus	•	•	•	•			
University of Phoenix–Tulsa Campus	•	•	•	•			
University of Tulsa	•						
Oregon							
Linfield College	•						•
Oregon Health & Science University	•	•	•	•	•	•	•
University of Portland	•	•		•			
Pennsylvania							
Alvernia College	•						•
Bloomsburg University of Pennsylvania	•	•	•	•			
California University of Pennsylvania	•						
Carlow University	•	•		•			•
Cedar Crest College	•						
Clarion University of Pennsylvania	•	•		•			
College Misericordia	•	•		•			
DeSales University	•	•	•	•			•
Drexel University	•	•		•			•
Duquesne University	•	•	•	•	•		•
Eastern University	•						•
East Stroudsburg University of Pennsylvania	•						
Edinboro University of Pennsylvania	•	•					
Gannon University	•	•		•			
Gwynedd-Mercy College	•	•		•			•
Holy Family University	•	•					•
Immaculata University	•	•					•
Indiana University of Pennsylvania	•	•					
Kutztown University of Pennsylvania	•						•
La Roche College	•	•					•
La Salle University	•	•	•	•			•
Mansfield University of Pennsylvania	•	•					
Marywood University	•	•					
Messiah College	•						
Millersville University of Pennsylvania	•	•		•			•
Moravian College	•						•
Mount Aloysius College	•						•
Neumann College	•	•		•			
Pennsylvania College of Technology	•						
The Pennsylvania State University University Park Campus	•	•		•	•	•	•
Saint Francis University	•						
Slippery Rock University of Pennsylvania	•	•					
Temple University	•	•		•			
Thomas Jefferson University	•	•		•			•
University of Pennsylvania	•	•	•	•	•	•	•
University of Pittsburgh	•	•		•	•	•	•
University of Pittsburgh at Bradford	•						
The University of Scranton	•	•		•			
Villanova University	•	•		•	•		•
Waynesburg College	•	•	•				
West Chester University of Pennsylvania	•	•					

	Baccalaureate	Master's	Joint Degree	Post-Master's	Doctoral	Post-doctoral	Continuing Education
Widener University	•	•		•	•		
Wilkes University	•	•		•			•
York College of Pennsylvania	•	•					
Puerto Rico							
Inter American University of Puerto Rico, Metropolitan Campus	•						
Pontifical Catholic University of Puerto Rico	•						
Universidad Adventista de las Antillas	•						•
Universidad Metropolitana	•						
University of Puerto Rico at Arecibo	•						
University of Puerto Rico at Humacao	•						
University of Puerto Rico, Mayagüez Campus	•						•
University of Puerto Rico, Medical Sciences Campus	•	•					•
University of the Sacred Heart	•	•					
Rhode Island							
Rhode Island College	•						
Salve Regina University	•						•
University of Rhode Island	•	•		•	•		
South Carolina							
Charleston Southern University	•						
Clemson University	•	•		•			•
Lander University	•						
Medical University of South Carolina	•	•		•	•		•
South Carolina State University	•						
University of South Carolina	•	•	•	•	•		
University of South Carolina Aiken	•						
University of South Carolina Upstate	•						
South Dakota							
Augustana College	•	•					
Mount Marty College							
Presentation College	•						
South Dakota State University	•	•		•			•
Tennessee							
Aquinas College	•						
Austin Peay State University	•						
Baptist College of Health Sciences	•						
Belmont University	•	•		•			
Carson-Newman College	•	•		•			
Cumberland University	•						
East Tennessee State University	•	•		•	•		
King College	•						
Lincoln Memorial University	•						
Middle Tennessee State University	•						•
Southern Adventist University	•	•	•				•
Tennessee State University	•	•		•			•
Tennessee Technological University	•	•					
Tennessee Wesleyan College	•						
Union University	•	•					•
The University of Memphis	•	•					
The University of Tennessee	•	•		•	•		•
The University of Tennessee at Chattanooga	•	•		•			•
The University of Tennessee at Martin	•						•
The University of Tennessee Health Science Center	•	•		•	•		•
Vanderbilt University		•	•	•	•	•	•

	Baccalaureate	Master's	Joint Degree	Post-Master's	Doctoral	Post-doctoral	Continuing Education
Texas							
Abilene Intercollegiate School of Nursing	•	•		•			•
Angelo State University	•	•					
Baylor University	•	•		•			
East Texas Baptist University	•						•
Houston Baptist University	•						
Lamar University	•	•					•
Lubbock Christian University	•						
Midwestern State University	•	•		•			•
Prairie View A&M University	•	•					
Southwestern Adventist University	•						•
Stephen F. Austin State University	•						
Tarleton State University	•						•
Texas A&M International University	•	•					•
Texas A&M University–Corpus Christi	•	•		•			•
Texas A&M University–Texarkana	•						
Texas Christian University	•	•					•
Texas Tech University Health Sciences Center	•	•	•	•			•
Texas Woman's University	•	•		•	•		
University of Mary Hardin-Baylor	•						•
The University of Texas at Arlington	•	•	•	•	•		•
The University of Texas at Austin	•	•	•	•	•	•	
The University of Texas at Brownsville	•	•					
The University of Texas at El Paso	•	•		•	•		•
The University of Texas at Tyler	•	•	•	•	•		•
The University of Texas Health Science Center at Houston	•	•	•	•	•		•
The University of Texas Health Science Center at San Antonio	•	•	•	•	•		•
The University of Texas Medical Branch	•	•		•	•		•
The University of Texas–Pan American	•	•		•			
University of the Incarnate Word	•	•	•				
West Texas A&M University	•	•		•			
Utah							
Brigham Young University	•	•		•			
University of Phoenix–Utah Campus	•	•	•	•			
University of Utah	•	•		•	•	•	
Utah Valley State College	•						
Weber State University	•						
Westminster College	•	•		•			
Vermont							
Norwich University	•						
Southern Vermont College	•						
University of Vermont	•	•		•			
Virgin Islands							
University of the Virgin Islands	•						•
Virginia							
Eastern Mennonite University	•						
George Mason University	•	•	•	•	•		•
Hampton University	•	•		•	•		
James Madison University	•	•		•			
Jefferson College of Health Sciences	•	•					•
Liberty University	•	•					
Lynchburg College	•						
Marymount University	•	•		•			

	Baccalaureate	Master's	Joint Degree	Post-Master's	Doctoral	Post-doctoral	Continuing Education
Norfolk State University	•						
Old Dominion University	•	•		•			•
Radford University	•	•					
Shenandoah University	•	•		•			•
University of Virginia	•	•	•	•	•	•	
The University of Virginia's College at Wise	•						
Virginia Commonwealth University	•	•	•	•	•		
Washington							
Gonzaga University	•	•		•			•
Intercollegiate College of Nursing/Washington State University	•	•		•			•
Northwest University	•						
Pacific Lutheran University	•	•					•
Seattle Pacific University	•	•	•	•			
Seattle University	•	•		•			
University of Washington	•	•	•	•	•		•
Walla Walla College	•						
West Virginia							
Alderson-Broaddus College	•						
Bluefield State College	•						
Fairmont State University	•						•
Marshall University	•	•		•			
Mountain State University	•	•		•			•
Shepherd University	•						•
University of Charleston	•						
West Liberty State College	•						
West Virginia University	•	•		•	•		
West Virginia Wesleyan College	•						•
Wheeling Jesuit University	•	•					
Wisconsin							
Alverno College	•						•
Bellin College of Nursing	•	•					
Cardinal Stritch University	•	•					
Columbia College of Nursing/Mount Mary College Nursing Program	•						
Concordia University Wisconsin	•	•					•
Edgewood College	•	•					
Marian College of Fond du Lac	•	•		•			
Marquette University	•	•	•	•	•		•
Milwaukee School of Engineering	•						
University of Wisconsin–Eau Claire	•	•					•
University of Wisconsin–Green Bay	•						
University of Wisconsin–Madison	•	•		•	•	•	•
University of Wisconsin–Milwaukee	•	•	•	•	•		•
University of Wisconsin–Oshkosh	•	•		•			•
Viterbo University	•	•		•			
Wyoming							
University of Wyoming	•	•		•			
CANADA							
Alberta							
Athabasca University	•	•					
University of Alberta	•	•		•	•		•
University of Calgary	•	•		•	•		•
The University of Lethbridge	•	•					

	Baccalaureate	Master's	Joint Degree	Post-Master's	Doctoral	Post-doctoral	Continuing Education
British Columbia							
British Columbia Institute of Technology	•						•
Kwantlen University College	•						
Malaspina University-College	•						
Okanagan University College	•						
Trinity Western University	•						
University College of the Cariboo	•						•
The University of British Columbia	•	•			•	•	•
University of Northern British Columbia	•						
University of Victoria	•	•			•		
Manitoba							
Brandon University	•						
University of Manitoba	•	•					•
New Brunswick							
Université de Moncton	•						•
University of New Brunswick Fredericton	•	•					•
Newfoundland and Labrador							
Memorial University of Newfoundland	•	•					
Nova Scotia							
Dalhousie University	•	•		•	•		
St. Francis Xavier University	•						•
Ontario							
Brock University	•						
Lakehead University	•						
Laurentian University	•						•
McMaster University	•	•			•		
Nipissing University	•						
Queen's University at Kingston	•	•					
Ryerson University	•						•
Trent University	•						
University of Ottawa	•				•		
University of Toronto	•	•	•	•	•		
The University of Western Ontario	•				•		
University of Windsor	•	•					•
York University	•						•
Prince Edward Island							
University of Prince Edward Island	•						
Quebec							
McGill University	•	•			•		
Université de Montréal	•	•			•		
Université de Sherbrooke	•	•			•	•	
Université du Québec à Chicoutimi	•	•					
Université du Québec à Rimouski	•						•
Université du Québec à Trois-Rivières	•	•					
Université du Québec en Abitibi-Témiscamingue	•						
Université du Québec en Outaouais	•						
Université Laval	•	•			•		•
Saskatchewan							
University of Saskatchewan	•	•					•

PROFILES OF NURSING PROGRAMS

U.S. AND U.S. TERRITORIES

ALABAMA

Auburn University

School of Nursing
Auburn University, Alabama

http://www.auburn.edu/academic/nursing/au_nursing.html

Founded in 1856

DEGREE • BSN

Nursing Program Faculty 12 (50% with doctorates).

Baccalaureate Enrollment 152
Women 90% **Men** 10% **Minority** 3%

Nursing Student Activities Nursing Honor Society, Sigma Theta Tau, Student Nurses' Association, nursing club.

Nursing Student Resources Academic advising; academic or career counseling; assistance for students with disabilities; bookstore; campus computer network; career placement assistance; computer lab; computer-assisted instruction; e-mail services; employment services for current students; interactive nursing skills videos; Internet; library services; nursing audiovisuals; placement services for program completers; remedial services; resume preparation assistance; skills, simulation, or other laboratory; tutoring.

Library Facilities 2.6 million volumes; 23,121 periodical subscriptions.

BACCALAUREATE PROGRAMS

Degree BSN

Available Programs Accelerated Baccalaureate for Second Degree; Generic Baccalaureate.

Study Options Full-time.

Program Entrance Requirements Minimum overall college GPA of 2.5, transcript of college record, CPR certification, health exam, health insurance, high school biology, 3 years high school math, 2 years high school science, high school transcript, immunizations, 2 letters of recommendation, minimum high school GPA of 2.0, minimum GPA in nursing prerequisites of 2.5, professional liability insurance/malpractice insurance, prerequisite course work. Transfer students are accepted. **Standardized tests** *Required:* SAT or ACT, TOEFL for international students. **Application** *Deadline:* 8/1 (freshmen), rolling (transfer). *Notification:* continuous (freshmen). *Application fee:* $25.

Expenses (2004–05) *Tuition, state resident:* full-time $5020; part-time $175 per credit hour. *Tuition, nonresident:* full-time $14,240; part-time $525 per credit hour. *International tuition:* $14,240 full-time. *Room and board:* $6686; room only: $5000 per academic year. *Required fees:* full-time $10,040.

Financial Aid 60% of baccalaureate students in nursing programs received some form of financial aid in 2003–04. *Gift aid (need-based):* Federal Pell, FSEOG, state, private, college/university gift aid from institutional funds. *Loans:* FFEL (Subsidized and Unsubsidized Stafford PLUS), Perkins, college/university. *Work-Study:* Federal Work-Study. *Application deadline (priority):* 3/1.

Contact Mrs. Pam Hennessey, Academic Advisor, School of Nursing, Auburn University, 118 Miller Hall, Auburn University, AL 36849-5505. *Telephone:* 334-844-6754. *Fax:* 334-844-4177. *E-mail:* hennepp@auburn.edu.

Auburn University Montgomery

School of Nursing
Montgomery, Alabama

http://www.aum.edu

Founded in 1967

DEGREE • BSN

Nursing Program Faculty 20 (30% with doctorates).

Baccalaureate Enrollment 350
Women 80% **Men** 20% **Minority** 33% **International** 2% **Part-time** 20%

Nursing Student Activities Nursing Honor Society, Sigma Theta Tau, Student Nurses' Association.

Nursing Student Resources Academic advising; academic or career counseling; assistance for students with disabilities; bookstore; campus computer network; career placement assistance; computer lab; computer-assisted instruction; daycare for children of students; e-mail services; housing assistance; interactive nursing skills videos; Internet; learning resource lab; library services; nursing audiovisuals; remedial services; resume preparation assistance; skills, simulation, or other laboratory; tutoring.

Library Facilities 312,110 volumes (9,568 in nursing); 2,044 periodical subscriptions (273 health-care related).

BACCALAUREATE PROGRAMS

Degree BSN

Available Programs Generic Baccalaureate; RN Baccalaureate.

Study Options Full-time and part-time.

Program Entrance Requirements Transcript of college record, CPR certification, health exam, high school transcript, immunizations, minimum GPA in nursing prerequisites of 2.5, professional liability insurance/malpractice insurance, prerequisite course work. Transfer students are accepted. **Standardized tests** *Required:* SAT or ACT, TOEFL for international students. **Application** *Deadline:* rolling (freshmen), rolling (transfer). *Notification:* continuous (freshmen). *Application fee:* $25.

Advanced Placement Credit by examination available.

Expenses (2004–05) *Tuition, state resident:* full-time $3730; part-time $146 per credit hour. *Tuition, nonresident:* full-time $10,780; part-time $428 per credit hour. *International tuition:* $10,780 full-time. *Room and board:* room only: $1730 per academic year.

Financial Aid 75% of baccalaureate students in nursing programs received some form of financial aid in 2003–04. *Gift aid (need-based):* Federal Pell, FSEOG, state, college/university gift aid from institutional funds. *Loans:* FFEL (Subsidized and Unsubsidized Stafford PLUS), Perkins. *Work-Study:* Federal Work-Study. *Application deadline (priority):* 3/1.

Contact Mrs. Lorinda B. Stutheit, Coordinator, Advising and Recruiting, School of Nursing, Auburn University Montgomery, PO Box 244023, Montgomery, AL 36124-4023. *Telephone:* 334-244-3863. *Fax:* 334-244-3243. *E-mail:* lorinda.stutheit@mail.aum.edu.

Jacksonville State University

College of Nursing and Health Sciences
Jacksonville, Alabama

http://www.jsu.edu/depart/nursing

Founded in 1883

DEGREES • BSN • MSN

Nursing Program Faculty 23 (30% with doctorates).

Baccalaureate Enrollment 641
Women 90% **Men** 10% **Minority** 29% **International** 3%

Graduate Enrollment 16
Women 100% **Minority** 6% **Part-time** 55%

Nursing Student Activities Sigma Theta Tau, Student Nurses' Association.

Nursing Student Resources Academic advising; academic or career counseling; campus computer network; computer lab; computer-assisted instruction; e-mail services; Internet; learning resource lab; nursing audiovisuals; remedial services; skills, simulation, or other laboratory; tutoring.

Library Facilities 685,991 volumes (48,347 in health, 1,672 in nursing); 14,376 periodical subscriptions (3,169 health-care related).

BACCALAUREATE PROGRAMS

Degree BSN

Available Programs Generic Baccalaureate; RN Baccalaureate.

Study Options Full-time and part-time.

Program Entrance Requirements Transcript of college record, CPR certification, health exam, health insurance, high school transcript, immunizations, minimum GPA in nursing prerequisites, professional liability insurance/malpractice insurance, prerequisite course work. Transfer students are accepted. **Standardized tests** *Required:* SAT or ACT, TOEFL for international students. **Application** *Deadline:* rolling (freshmen), rolling (transfer). *Notification:* continuous (freshmen). *Application fee:* $20.

Expenses (2003–04) *Tuition, state resident:* full-time $3540; part-time $148 per credit hour. *Tuition, nonresident:* full-time $7080; part-time $296 per credit hour. *International tuition:* $7080 full-time. *Room and board:* $2876; room only: $2063 per academic year.

Financial Aid 70% of baccalaureate students in nursing programs received some form of financial aid in 2002–03.

Contact Dr. Sarah Latham, Student Services Coordinator, College of Nursing and Health Sciences, Jacksonville State University, 700 Pelham Road, North, Jacksonville, AL 36265-1602. *Telephone:* 256-782-5276. *Fax:* 256-782-5406. *E-mail:* slatham@jsucc.jsu.edu.

GRADUATE PROGRAMS

Expenses (2003–04) *Tuition, state resident:* full-time $3540; part-time $177 per credit hour. *Tuition, nonresident:* full-time $7080; part-time $354 per credit hour. *International tuition:* $7080 full-time. *Room and board:* $2876; room only: $2063 per academic year.

Financial Aid 60% of graduate students in nursing programs received some form of financial aid in 2002–03.

Contact Dr. Beth Hembree, Director Graduate Studies, College of Nursing and Health Sciences, Jacksonville State University, 700 Pelham Road, North, Jacksonville, AL 36265-1602. *Telephone:* 256-782-5431. *Fax:* 256-782-5406. *E-mail:* bhembree@jsucc.jsu.edu.

MASTER'S DEGREE PROGRAM

Degree MSN

Available Programs Master's.

Concentrations Available *Clinical nurse specialist programs in:* community health.

Site Options *Distance Learning:* Gadsden, AL; Rainsville, AL; Albertville, AL.

Study Options Full-time and part-time.

Program Entrance Requirements Minimum overall college GPA of 3.0, transcript of college record, written essay, interview, 3 letters of recommendation, nursing research course, physical assessment course, statistics course.

Advanced Placement Credit given for nursing courses completed elsewhere dependent upon specific evaluations.

Degree Requirements 36 total credit hours, thesis or project, comprehensive exam.

CONTINUING EDUCATION PROGRAM

Contact Dr. Sarah Latham, Student Services Coordinator, College of Nursing and Health Sciences, Jacksonville State University, 700 Pelham Road, North, Jacksonville, AL 36265-1602. *Telephone:* 256-782-5276. *Fax:* 256-782-5406. *E-mail:* slatham@jsucc.jsu.edu.

Samford University
Ida V. Moffett School of Nursing
Birmingham, Alabama

http://www.samford.edu
Founded in 1841

DEGREES • BSN • MSN • MSN/MBA

Nursing Program Faculty 30 (54% with doctorates).

Baccalaureate Enrollment 300
Women 97% **Men** 3% **Minority** 5% **International** 2% **Part-time** 10%

Graduate Enrollment 65
Women 88% **Men** 12% **Minority** 32% **Part-time** 5%

Nursing Student Activities Sigma Theta Tau, Student Nurses' Association, nursing club.

Nursing Student Resources Academic advising; academic or career counseling; assistance for students with disabilities; bookstore; campus computer network; career placement assistance; computer lab; computer-assisted instruction; e-mail services; externships; interactive nursing skills videos; Internet; learning resource lab; library services; nursing audiovisuals; paid internships; placement services for program completers; remedial services; resume preparation assistance; skills, simulation, or other laboratory; tutoring; unpaid internships.

Library Facilities 439,760 volumes (7,000 in health, 2,500 in nursing); 3,724 periodical subscriptions (100 health-care related).

BACCALAUREATE PROGRAMS

Degree BSN

Available Programs Baccalaureate for Second Degree; Generic Baccalaureate; RN Baccalaureate.

Study Options Full-time and part-time.

Program Entrance Requirements Minimum overall college GPA of 2.5, transcript of college record, CPR certification, written essay, health exam, health insurance, high school biology, high school chemistry, 2 years high school math, high school transcript, immunizations, minimum high school GPA of 2.5, minimum GPA in nursing prerequisites of 2.0, professional liability insurance/malpractice insurance, prerequisite course work. Transfer students are accepted. **Standardized tests** *Required:* SAT or ACT, TOEFL for international students. **Application** *Deadline:* 8/1 (transfer). *Application fee:* $25.

Advanced Placement Credit given for nursing courses completed elsewhere dependent upon specific evaluations.

Expenses (2004–05) *Tuition:* full-time $13,944; part-time $463 per credit hour. *International tuition:* $13,944 full-time. *Room and board:* $5550; room only: $2726 per academic year. *Required fees:* full-time $1536; part-time $768 per term.

Financial Aid 80% of baccalaureate students in nursing programs received some form of financial aid in 2003–04.

Contact Mrs. Janice G. Paine, Administrative Director of Recruitment and Admissions, Ida V. Moffett School of Nursing, Samford University, 800 Lakeshore Drive, Birmingham, AL 35229. *Telephone:* 205-726-2872 Ext. 2746. *Fax:* 205-726-2219. *E-mail:* jgpaine@samford.edu.

GRADUATE PROGRAMS

Expenses (2004–05) *Tuition:* part-time $457 per credit hour.

Financial Aid 80% of graduate students in nursing programs received some form of financial aid in 2003–04. Career-related internships or fieldwork, Federal Work-Study, and institutionally sponsored loans available. *Financial aid application deadline:* 3/1.

Contact Mrs. Stacy W. Minor, Graduate Admissions and Alumni Relations Administrator, Ida V. Moffett School of Nursing, Samford University, 800 Lakeshore Drive, Birmingham, AL 35229. *Telephone:* 205-726-2047. *Fax:* 205-726-2219. *E-mail:* sewaldre@samford.edu.

MASTER'S DEGREE PROGRAM

Degrees MSN; MSN/MBA

Available Programs Master's; RN to Master's.

Concentrations Available Nurse anesthesia; nursing administration; nursing education. *Clinical nurse specialist programs in:* acute care, adult health, cardiovascular, community health. *Nurse practitioner programs in:* family health, primary care.

Samford University (continued)

Study Options Full-time and part-time.

Program Entrance Requirements Clinical experience, computer literacy, minimum overall college GPA of 3.0, transcript of college record, CPR certification, immunizations, interview, 3 letters of recommendation, nursing research course, physical assessment course, professional liability insurance/malpractice insurance, prerequisite course work, statistics course, GRE General Test or MAT. *Application deadline:* For spring admission, 1/2. Applications are processed on a rolling basis. *Application fee:* $25.

Advanced Placement Credit given for nursing courses completed elsewhere dependent upon specific evaluations.

Degree Requirements 38 total credit hours.

POST-MASTER'S PROGRAM

Areas of Study Nurse anesthesia; nursing administration; nursing education. *Clinical nurse specialist programs in:* acute care, adult health, cardiovascular, community health. *Nurse practitioner programs in:* family health, primary care.

CONTINUING EDUCATION PROGRAM

Contact Dr. Gretchen McDaniel, Coordinator, Ida V. Moffett School of Nursing, Samford University, 800 Lakeshore Drive, Birmingham, AL 35229. *Telephone:* 205-726-2626. *Fax:* 205-726-2219. *E-mail:* gsmcdani@samford.edu.

Spring Hill College
Division of Nursing
Mobile, Alabama

http://faculty.shc.edu/nursing

Founded in 1830

DEGREE • BSN

Nursing Program Faculty 7 (71% with doctorates).

Baccalaureate Enrollment 90
Women 88% **Men** 12% **Minority** 10%

Nursing Student Activities Nursing Honor Society, Student Nurses' Association.

Nursing Student Resources Academic advising; academic or career counseling; assistance for students with disabilities; bookstore; campus computer network; career placement assistance; computer lab; computer-assisted instruction; e-mail services; externships; interactive nursing skills videos; Internet; learning resource lab; library services; nursing audiovisuals; resume preparation assistance; skills, simulation, or other laboratory; tutoring; unpaid internships.

Library Facilities 180,404 volumes (330 in health, 300 in nursing); 2,195 periodical subscriptions (58 health-care related).

BACCALAUREATE PROGRAMS

Degree BSN

Available Programs Generic Baccalaureate.

Study Options Full-time.

Program Entrance Requirements Minimum overall college GPA of 2.5, transcript of college record, CPR certification, written essay, health exam, health insurance, high school transcript, immunizations, 2 letters of recommendation, minimum high school GPA of 2.5, minimum GPA in nursing prerequisites of 2.5, professional liability insurance/malpractice insurance, prerequisite course work. Transfer students are accepted. **Standardized tests** *Required:* SAT or ACT, TOEFL for international students. **Application** *Deadline:* 7/1 (freshmen), 8/10 (transfer). *Notification:* continuous (freshmen). *Application fee:* $25.

Advanced Placement Credit by examination available.

Expenses (2004–05) *Tuition:* full-time $18,722; part-time $701 per credit hour. *Room and board:* $7552; room only: $4000 per academic year. *Required fees:* full-time $1228; part-time $40 per credit.

Financial Aid 80% of baccalaureate students in nursing programs received some form of financial aid in 2003–04.

Contact Dr. Carol Harrison, Chair/Professor, Division of Nursing, Spring Hill College, 4000 Dauphin Street, Mobile, AL 36608. *Telephone:* 334-380-4492. *Fax:* 334-380-4495. *E-mail:* charrison@shc.edu.

Troy University
School of Nursing
Troy, Alabama

Founded in 1887

DEGREES • BSN • MSN

Nursing Program Faculty 40 (47% with doctorates).

Baccalaureate Enrollment 360
Women 88% **Men** 12% **Minority** 35% **International** 4% **Part-time** 17%

Graduate Enrollment 73
Women 97% **Men** 3% **Minority** 23% **Part-time** 29%

Nursing Student Activities Sigma Theta Tau, Student Nurses' Association.

Nursing Student Resources Academic advising; academic or career counseling; assistance for students with disabilities; bookstore; campus computer network; career placement assistance; computer lab; computer-assisted instruction; daycare for children of students; e-mail services; employment services for current students; housing assistance; interactive nursing skills videos; Internet; learning resource lab; library services; nursing audiovisuals; placement services for program completers; remedial services; resume preparation assistance; skills, simulation, or other laboratory; tutoring; unpaid internships.

Library Facilities 389,524 volumes (45,006 in health, 3,843 in nursing); 2,692 periodical subscriptions (703 health-care related).

BACCALAUREATE PROGRAMS

Degree BSN

Available Programs ADN to Baccalaureate; Generic Baccalaureate.

Site Options *Distance Learning:* Phenix City, AL; Montgomery, AL.

Study Options Full-time and part-time.

Program Entrance Requirements Minimum overall college GPA of 2.5, transcript of college record, CPR certification, health exam, health insurance, high school transcript, immunizations, professional liability insurance/malpractice insurance, prerequisite course work. Transfer students are accepted. **Standardized tests** *Required:* SAT or ACT. *Recommended:* TOEFL for international students. **Application** *Deadline:* rolling (freshmen), rolling (transfer). *Application fee:* $20.

Advanced Placement Credit by examination available. Credit given for nursing courses completed elsewhere dependent upon specific evaluations.

Expenses (2004–05) *Tuition, state resident:* full-time $1925; part-time $163 per credit hour. *Tuition, nonresident:* full-time $3850; part-time $326 per credit hour. *International tuition:* $3850 full-time. *Room and board:* $4990; room only: $2650 per academic year. *Required fees:* full-time $502; part-time $13 per credit.

Financial Aid 90% of baccalaureate students in nursing programs received some form of financial aid in 2003–04. *Gift aid (need-based):* Federal Pell, FSEOG, state, private, college/university gift aid from institutional funds. *Loans:* FFEL (Subsidized and Unsubsidized Stafford PLUS), Perkins. *Work-Study:* Federal Work-Study. *Application deadline (priority):* 5/1.

Contact Susan Halley, Chair, Admissions Committee, School of Nursing, Troy University, 400 Pell Avenue, Troy, AL 36082. *Telephone:* 334-670-3428. *Fax:* 334-670-3744. *E-mail:* shalley@troy.edu.

GRADUATE PROGRAMS

Expenses (2004–05) *Tuition, state resident:* part-time $175 per credit hour. *Tuition, nonresident:* part-time $350 per credit hour. *Required fees:* full-time $502; part-time $13 per credit.

Financial Aid 40% of graduate students in nursing programs received some form of financial aid in 2003–04.

Contact Dr. Geraldine Allen, Director, MSN Program, School of Nursing, Troy University, 340 Montgomery Street, Montgomery, AL 36104. *Telephone:* 334-834-2320. *Fax:* 334-241-8627.

MASTER'S DEGREE PROGRAM

Degree MSN

Available Programs Master's; RN to Master's.

Concentrations Available Nursing administration; nursing education; nursing informatics. *Clinical nurse specialist programs in:* adult health, maternity-newborn, pediatric. *Nurse practitioner programs in:* family health.

Site Options *Distance Learning:* Phenix City, AL; Montgomery, AL.

Study Options Full-time and part-time.

Program Entrance Requirements Minimum overall college GPA of 3.0, transcript of college record, CPR certification, immunizations, 3 letters of recommendation, physical assessment course, professional liability insurance/malpractice insurance.

Advanced Placement Credit given for nursing courses completed elsewhere dependent upon specific evaluations.

Degree Requirements 39 total credit hours, thesis or project, comprehensive exam.

Tuskegee University

Program in Nursing
Tuskegee, Alabama

http://www.tusk.edu

Founded in 1881

DEGREE • BSN

Nursing Program Faculty 13 (38% with doctorates).

Baccalaureate Enrollment 176
Women 99.5% **Men** .5% **Minority** 100%

Nursing Student Activities Nursing Honor Society, Student Nurses' Association, nursing club.

Nursing Student Resources Academic advising; academic or career counseling; assistance for students with disabilities; bookstore; campus computer network; career placement assistance; computer lab; computer-assisted instruction; e-mail services; externships; interactive nursing skills videos; Internet; learning resource lab; library services; nursing audiovisuals; placement services for program completers; remedial services; resume preparation assistance; skills, simulation, or other laboratory; tutoring.

Library Facilities 623,824 volumes (1,550 in health, 1,279 in nursing); 81,157 periodical subscriptions (250 health-care related).

BACCALAUREATE PROGRAMS

Degree BSN

Available Programs ADN to Baccalaureate; Generic Baccalaureate; RN Baccalaureate.

Study Options Full-time.

Program Entrance Requirements Minimum overall college GPA of 2.5, transcript of college record, CPR certification, health exam, health insurance, high school biology, high school chemistry, 2 years high school math, 1 year of high school science, high school transcript, immunizations, interview, minimum high school GPA of 3.0, minimum GPA in nursing prerequisites of 2.5, professional liability insurance/malpractice insurance. Transfer students are accepted. **Standardized tests** *Required:* SAT or ACT, TOEFL for international students. **Application** *Deadline:* 4/15 (freshmen), 4/15 (transfer). *Application fee:* $25.

Expenses (2004–05) *Tuition:* full-time $11,990; part-time $1245 per credit hour. *Room and board:* $6150 per academic year. *Required fees:* full-time $600.

Financial Aid 95% of baccalaureate students in nursing programs received some form of financial aid in 2003–04.

Contact Dr. Doris S. Holeman, Associate Dean and Director, Program in Nursing, Tuskegee University, Basil O'Connor Hall, Room 209, Tuskegee, AL 36083. *Telephone:* 334-727-8382. *Fax:* 334-727-5461. *E-mail:* dholeman@tuskegee.edu.

The University of Alabama

Capstone College of Nursing
Tuscaloosa, Alabama

http://nursing.ua.edu

Founded in 1831

DEGREES • BSN • MSN • MSN/MA • MSN/MBA

Nursing Program Faculty 30 (67% with doctorates).

Baccalaureate Enrollment 748
Women 90% **Men** 10% **Minority** 21% **Part-time** 3%

Graduate Enrollment 38
Women 98% **Men** 2% **Minority** 24% **Part-time** 73%

Nursing Student Activities Sigma Theta Tau, Student Nurses' Association.

Nursing Student Resources Academic advising; academic or career counseling; assistance for students with disabilities; bookstore; campus computer network; career placement assistance; computer lab; computer-assisted instruction; e-mail services; employment services for current students; interactive nursing skills videos; Internet; learning resource lab; library services; nursing audiovisuals; paid internships; placement services for program completers; resume preparation assistance; skills, simulation, or other laboratory; tutoring; unpaid internships.

Library Facilities 2.3 million volumes (25,000 in health, 3,500 in nursing); 16,590 periodical subscriptions (1,500 health-care related).

BACCALAUREATE PROGRAMS

Degree BSN

Available Programs Generic Baccalaureate; RN Baccalaureate.

Study Options Full-time and part-time.

Program Entrance Requirements Minimum overall college GPA of 2.5, transcript of college record, CPR certification, health exam, health insurance, 4 years high school math, 4 years high school science, high school transcript, immunizations, minimum high school GPA of 2.5, minimum GPA in nursing prerequisites, professional liability insurance/malpractice insurance, prerequisite course work. Transfer students are accepted. **Standardized tests** *Required:* SAT or ACT, TOEFL for international students. **Application** *Deadline:* 8/1 (freshmen). *Notification:* 9/1 (freshmen). *Application fee:* $25.

Advanced Placement Credit by examination available.

Expenses (2003–04) *Tuition, state resident:* full-time $2067; part-time $519 per credit hour. *Tuition, nonresident:* full-time $5647; part-time $827 per credit hour. *International tuition:* $5647 full-time. *Room and board:* $2129; room only: $1295 per academic year. *Required fees:* full-time $500; part-time $20 per credit.

Financial Aid 50% of baccalaureate students in nursing programs received some form of financial aid in 2002–03.

Contact Mrs. Pat McCullar, Coordinator of Nursing Student Recruitment, Capstone College of Nursing, The University of Alabama, Box 870358, Tuscaloosa, AL 35487-0358. *Telephone:* 205-348-6639. *Fax:* 205-348-5559. *E-mail:* pmcculla@bama.ua.edu.

GRADUATE PROGRAMS

Expenses (2003–04) *Tuition, state resident:* full-time $2067; part-time $529 per credit hour. *Tuition, nonresident:* full-time $5647; part-time $872 per credit hour. *International tuition:* $5647 full-time. *Required fees:* full-time $500; part-time $20 per credit.

Financial Aid 50% of graduate students in nursing programs received some form of financial aid in 2002–03.

Contact Mrs. Pat McCullar, Coordinator of Nursing Student Recruitment, Capstone College of Nursing, The University of Alabama, Box 870358, Tuscaloosa, AL 35487-0358. *Telephone:* 205-348-6640. *Fax:* 205-348-5559. *E-mail:* pmcculla@bama.ua.edu.

MASTER'S DEGREE PROGRAM

Degrees MSN; MSN/MA; MSN/MBA

Available Programs Master's; RN to Master's.

Concentrations Available Nurse case management.

Study Options Full-time and part-time.

The University of Alabama (continued)

Program Entrance Requirements Clinical experience, computer literacy, minimum overall college GPA of 3.0, transcript of college record, CPR certification, written essay, immunizations, 3 letters of recommendation, nursing research course, professional liability insurance/malpractice insurance, statistics course.

Advanced Placement Credit given for nursing courses completed elsewhere dependent upon specific evaluations.

Degree Requirements 35 total credit hours.

POST-MASTER'S PROGRAM

Areas of Study Nurse case management.

CONTINUING EDUCATION PROGRAM

Contact Dr. Carolyn C. Dahl, Dean, College of Continuing Studies, Capstone College of Nursing, The University of Alabama, Box 870388, Tuscaloosa, AL 35487-0388. *Telephone:* 205-348-6331. *Fax:* 205-348-9137. *E-mail:* cdahl@ccs.ua.edu.

The University of Alabama at Birmingham

School of Nursing
Birmingham, Alabama

http://www.uab.edu/son/

Founded in 1969

DEGREES • BSN • MSN • MSN/MPH • PHD

Nursing Program Faculty 48 (100% with doctorates).

Baccalaureate Enrollment 288
Women 89% **Men** 11% **Minority** 21% **International** 2% **Part-time** 16%

Graduate Enrollment 281
Women 93% **Men** 7% **Minority** 27% **International** 4% **Part-time** 73%

Nursing Student Activities Nursing Honor Society, Sigma Theta Tau, Student Nurses' Association, nursing club.

Nursing Student Resources Academic advising; academic or career counseling; assistance for students with disabilities; bookstore; campus computer network; career placement assistance; computer lab; computer-assisted instruction; e-mail services; housing assistance; interactive nursing skills videos; Internet; learning resource lab; library services; nursing audiovisuals; paid internships; placement services for program completers; resume preparation assistance; skills, simulation, or other laboratory.

Library Facilities 853,445 volumes (318,000 in health); 3,934 periodical subscriptions (2,566 health-care related).

BACCALAUREATE PROGRAMS

Degree BSN

Available Programs Accelerated RN Baccalaureate; Baccalaureate for Second Degree; Generic Baccalaureate; RN Baccalaureate.

Study Options Full-time and part-time.

Program Entrance Requirements Minimum overall college GPA of 2.5, transcript of college record, CPR certification, written essay, health exam, health insurance, high school transcript, immunizations, minimum high school GPA of 2.0, minimum GPA in nursing prerequisites of 2.5, prerequisite course work. Transfer students are accepted. **Standardized tests** *Required:* SAT or ACT, TOEFL for international students. **Application** *Deadline:* 7/1 (freshmen), 7/15 (transfer). *Notification:* continuous (freshmen). *Application fee:* $30.

Advanced Placement Credit by examination available. Credit given for nursing courses completed elsewhere dependent upon specific evaluations.

Expenses (2004–05) *Tuition, state resident:* full-time $5396; part-time $142 per credit hour. *Tuition, nonresident:* full-time $13,490; part-time $355 per credit hour. *International tuition:* $13,490 full-time. *Room and board:* $13,115; room only: $7000 per academic year. *Required fees:* full-time $2874; part-time $17 per credit; part-time $391 per term.

Financial Aid 58% of baccalaureate students in nursing programs received some form of financial aid in 2003–04. *Gift aid (need-based):* Federal Pell, FSEOG, state, college/university gift aid from institutional funds. *Loans:* Federal Direct (Subsidized and Unsubsidized Stafford PLUS), Perkins, state, college/university. *Work-Study:* Federal Work-Study. *Application deadline (priority):* 4/1.

Contact Office of Student Affairs, School of Nursing, The University of Alabama at Birmingham, Nursing Building, 1530 3rd Avenue, South, Room 105, Birmingham, AL 35294-1210. *Telephone:* 205-975-7529. *Fax:* 205-975-6142. *E-mail:* studaffr@son.uab.edu.

GRADUATE PROGRAMS

Expenses (2004–05) *Tuition, state resident:* full-time $6501; part-time $197 per credit hour. *Tuition, nonresident:* full-time $16,269; part-time $493 per credit hour. *International tuition:* $16,269 full-time. *Room and board:* $13,115; room only: $7000 per academic year. *Required fees:* full-time $2441; part-time $17 per credit; part-time $391 per term.

Financial Aid 41% of graduate students in nursing programs received some form of financial aid in 2003–04. 3 fellowships (averaging $12,833 per year), 1 research assistantship, teaching assistantships (averaging $6,760 per year) were awarded; Federal Work-Study also available. Aid available to part-time students.

Contact Dr. Elizabeth Stullenbarger, Associate Dean, Graduate Studies, School of Nursing, The University of Alabama at Birmingham, 1530 3rd Avenue South, NB 108, Birmingham, AL 35294-1210. *Telephone:* 205-934-6787. *Fax:* 205-975-6142. *E-mail:* bstullen@uab.edu.

MASTER'S DEGREE PROGRAM

Degrees MSN; MSN/MPH

Available Programs Accelerated RN to Master's; Master's; RN to Master's.

Concentrations Available Health-care administration; nurse case management; nursing administration. *Clinical nurse specialist programs in:* adult health. *Nurse practitioner programs in:* acute care, adult health, family health, neonatal health, occupational health, pediatric, primary care, women's health.

Study Options Full-time and part-time.

Program Entrance Requirements Clinical experience, minimum overall college GPA of 3.0, transcript of college record, CPR certification, written essay, immunizations, interview, 2 letters of recommendation, nursing research course, physical assessment course, prerequisite course work, statistics course, GRE General Test. *Application deadline:* Applications are processed on a rolling basis. *Application fee:* $35 ($60 for international students).

Advanced Placement Credit given for nursing courses completed elsewhere dependent upon specific evaluations.

Degree Requirements 43 total credit hours, thesis or project.

POST-MASTER'S PROGRAM

Areas of Study *Nurse practitioner programs in:* acute care, adult health, family health, neonatal health, pediatric.

DOCTORAL DEGREE PROGRAM

Degree PhD

Available Programs Doctorate; Post-Baccalaureate Doctorate.

Areas of Study Family health, health promotion/disease prevention, nursing research, nursing science.

Program Entrance Requirements Clinical experience, minimum overall college GPA of 3.0, interview by faculty committee, interview, 3 letters of recommendation, MSN or equivalent, scholarly papers, statistics course, vita, writing sample, GRE General Test. *Application deadline:* Applications are processed on a rolling basis. *Application fee:* $35 ($60 for international students).

Degree Requirements 74 total credit hours, dissertation, oral exam, written exam, residency.

POSTDOCTORAL PROGRAM

Areas of Study Community health, family health.

Postdoctoral Program Contact Dr. Carol Dashiff, Chair, Graduate Studies, School of Nursing, The University of Alabama at Birmingham, 1530 3rd Avenue South, NB 302, Birmingham, AL 35294-1210. *Telephone:* 205-934-6852. *Fax:* 205-975-6142. *E-mail:* dashiffc@admin.son.uab.edu.

The University of Alabama in Huntsville

College of Nursing
Huntsville, Alabama

http://www.uah.edu/nursing

Founded in 1950

DEGREES • BSN • MSN

Nursing Program Faculty 40 (30% with doctorates).

Baccalaureate Enrollment 525

Women 90% **Men** 10% **Minority** 20% **International** 1% **Part-time** 18%

Graduate Enrollment 175

Women 88% **Men** 12% **Minority** 18% **International** 1% **Part-time** 58%

Nursing Student Activities Sigma Theta Tau, Student Nurses' Association, nursing club.

Nursing Student Resources Academic advising; academic or career counseling; assistance for students with disabilities; bookstore; campus computer network; career placement assistance; computer lab; computer-assisted instruction; e-mail services; employment services for current students; housing assistance; interactive nursing skills videos; Internet; learning resource lab; library services; nursing audiovisuals; placement services for program completers; remedial services; resume preparation assistance; skills, simulation, or other laboratory; tutoring.

Library Facilities 327,663 volumes (15,000 in health, 11,562 in nursing); 1,051 periodical subscriptions (650 health-care related).

BACCALAUREATE PROGRAMS

Degree BSN

Available Programs Baccalaureate for Second Degree; Generic Baccalaureate; RN Baccalaureate.

Site Options *Distance Learning:* Cullman, AL; Gadsden, AL.

Study Options Full-time and part-time.

Program Entrance Requirements Minimum overall college GPA of 2.0, transcript of college record, CPR certification, health exam, health insurance, immunizations, minimum GPA in nursing prerequisites of 2.0, professional liability insurance/malpractice insurance, prerequisite course work. Transfer students are accepted. **Standardized tests** *Required:* SAT or ACT, TOEFL for international students. **Application** *Deadline:* 8/15 (freshmen). *Notification:* continuous (freshmen). *Application fee:* $30.

Advanced Placement Credit by examination available. Credit given for nursing courses completed elsewhere dependent upon specific evaluations.

Expenses (2004–05) *Tuition, state resident:* full-time $4700; part-time $208 per credit hour. *Tuition, nonresident:* full-time $9900; part-time $443 per credit hour. *International tuition:* $9900 full-time. *Room and board:* $3100; room only: $2800 per academic year. *Required fees:* full-time $650; part-time $325 per term.

Financial Aid 75% of baccalaureate students in nursing programs received some form of financial aid in 2003–04. *Gift aid (need-based):* Federal Pell, FSEOG, state, private, college/university gift aid from institutional funds. *Loans:* Federal Direct (Subsidized and Unsubsidized Stafford PLUS). *Work-Study:* Federal Work-Study. *Application deadline:* 7/31 (priority: 4/1).

Contact Mr. Lavan Wilson, Director of Nursing Student Affairs, College of Nursing, The University of Alabama in Huntsville, Huntsville, AL 35899. *Telephone:* 256-824-6742. *Fax:* 256-824-6026. *E-mail:* wilsonol@uah.edu.

GRADUATE PROGRAMS

Expenses (2004–05) *Tuition, state resident:* full-time $7857; part-time $314 per credit hour. *Tuition, nonresident:* full-time $16,150; part-time $633 per credit hour. *International tuition:* $16,150 full-time. *Room and board:* $3100; room only: $1800 per academic year. *Required fees:* full-time $700; part-time $350 per term.

Financial Aid 65% of graduate students in nursing programs received some form of financial aid in 2003–04. 66 fellowships with full and partial tuition reimbursements available (averaging $1,044 per year), 6 teaching assistantships with full and partial tuition reimbursements available (averaging $7,544 per year) were awarded; research assistantships, career-related internships or fieldwork, Federal Work-Study, institutionally sponsored loans, scholarships, traineeships, tuition waivers (full and partial), and unspecified assistantships also available. Aid available to part-time students. *Financial aid application deadline:* 4/1.

Contact Mr. Lavan Wilson, Director of Nursing Student Affairs, College of Nursing, The University of Alabama in Huntsville, Huntsville, AL 35899. *Telephone:* 256-824-6742. *Fax:* 256-824-6026. *E-mail:* wilsomol@uah.edu.

MASTER'S DEGREE PROGRAM

Degree MSN

Available Programs Master's; RN to Master's.

Concentrations Available Nursing administration. *Clinical nurse specialist programs in:* adult health. *Nurse practitioner programs in:* acute care, family health.

Site Options *Distance Learning:* Gadsden, AL.

Study Options Full-time and part-time.

Program Entrance Requirements Minimum overall college GPA of 3.0, transcript of college record, CPR certification, written essay, immunizations, 3 letters of recommendation, professional liability insurance/malpractice insurance, prerequisite course work, statistics course, MAT (score of 50 preferred) or GRE. *Application deadline:* For fall admission, 5/30 (priority date); for spring admission, 10/10 (priority date). Applications are processed on a rolling basis. *Application fee:* $35.

Advanced Placement Credit given for nursing courses completed elsewhere dependent upon specific evaluations.

Degree Requirements 42 total credit hours, thesis or project, comprehensive exam.

POST-MASTER'S PROGRAM

Areas of Study *Nurse practitioner programs in:* family health.

CONTINUING EDUCATION PROGRAM

Contact Ms. Ina Warboys, Director of Continuing Education, College of Nursing, The University of Alabama in Huntsville, Huntsville, AL 35899. *Telephone:* 256-824-2456. *Fax:* 256-824-6026. *E-mail:* warboysi@uah.edu.

See full description on page 548.

University of Mobile

School of Nursing
Mobile, Alabama

http://www.umobile.edu/main/nursing1.html

Founded in 1961

DEGREES • BSN • MSN

Nursing Program Faculty 18 (25% with doctorates).

Baccalaureate Enrollment 150

Women 80% **Men** 20% **Minority** 25% **Part-time** 5%

Graduate Enrollment 50

Women 85% **Men** 15% **Minority** 30% **Part-time** 50%

Nursing Student Activities Sigma Theta Tau, Student Nurses' Association.

Nursing Student Resources Academic advising; assistance for students with disabilities; bookstore; computer lab; Internet; learning resource lab; library services; nursing audiovisuals; remedial services; skills, simulation, or other laboratory; tutoring; unpaid internships.

Library Facilities 100,250 volumes (7,846 in health, 6,500 in nursing); 1,043 periodical subscriptions (109 health-care related).

BACCALAUREATE PROGRAMS

Degree BSN

Available Programs Generic Baccalaureate; LPN to RN Baccalaureate; RN Baccalaureate.

Study Options Full-time and part-time.

Program Entrance Requirements Minimum overall college GPA of 2.75, transcript of college record, CPR certification, health exam, health insurance, high school transcript, immunizations, prerequisite course work. Transfer students are accepted. **Standardized tests** *Required:* SAT or ACT, TOEFL for international students. **Application** *Deadline:* rolling (freshmen), rolling (transfer). *Notification:* continuous (freshmen). *Application fee:* $30.

University of Mobile (continued)

Advanced Placement Credit given for nursing courses completed elsewhere dependent upon specific evaluations.

Financial Aid 96% of baccalaureate students in nursing programs received some form of financial aid in 2002–03.

Contact Mrs. Mattie Easter, Assistant Professor, School of Nursing, University of Mobile, PO Box 13220, Mobile, AL 36663-0220. *Telephone:* 251-442-2337. *Fax:* 251-442-2520. *E-mail:* mattieeaster@free.mobile.edu.

GRADUATE PROGRAMS

Financial Aid 60% of graduate students in nursing programs received some form of financial aid in 2002–03.

Contact Dr. Elizabeth Flanagan, Dean, School of Nursing, University of Mobile, PO Box 13220, Mobile, AL 36663-0220. *Telephone:* 251-442-2227. *Fax:* 251-442-2520. *E-mail:* elizabethflanagan@free.umobile.edu.

MASTER'S DEGREE PROGRAM

Degree MSN

Available Programs Master's.

Concentrations Available Nursing administration; nursing education. *Nurse practitioner programs in:* family health.

Study Options Full-time and part-time.

Program Entrance Requirements Minimum overall college GPA of 3.0, transcript of college record, CPR certification, immunizations, 3 letters of recommendation, statistics course.

Advanced Placement Credit given for nursing courses completed elsewhere dependent upon specific evaluations.

Degree Requirements 45 total credit hours, thesis or project, comprehensive exam.

CONTINUING EDUCATION PROGRAM

Contact Dr. Elizabeth Flanagan, Dean, School of Nursing, University of Mobile, PO Box 13220, Mobile, AL 36663-0220. *Telephone:* 251-442-2227. *Fax:* 251-442-2520. *E-mail:* elizabethflanagan@free.umobile.edu.

University of North Alabama

College of Nursing and Allied Health
Florence, Alabama

http://www2.una.edu/nursing/

Founded in 1830

DEGREE • BSN

Nursing Program Faculty 22 (29% with doctorates).

Baccalaureate Enrollment 180
Women 90% **Men** 10% **Minority** 10% **International** 2%

Library Facilities 358,393 volumes (343,468 in health, 8,476 in nursing); 3,126 periodical subscriptions (493 health-care related).

BACCALAUREATE PROGRAMS

Degree BSN

Available Programs Generic Baccalaureate; RN Baccalaureate.

Program Entrance Requirements Transfer students are accepted. **Standardized tests** *Required:* SAT or ACT, TOEFL for international students. **Application** *Deadline:* rolling (freshmen), rolling (transfer). *Application fee:* $25.

Expenses (2003–04) *Tuition, state resident:* full-time $3048. *Tuition, nonresident:* full-time $6096. *Room and board:* $4272; room only: $1960 per academic year. *Required fees:* full-time $502.

Financial Aid *Gift aid (need-based):* Federal Pell, FSEOG, state, private, college/university gift aid from institutional funds. *Loans:* FFEL (Subsidized and Unsubsidized Stafford PLUS), Perkins. *Work-Study:* Federal Work-Study. *Application deadline (priority):* 4/1.

Contact Dean. *Telephone:* 256-765-4311. *Fax:* 256-765-4935.

CONTINUING EDUCATION PROGRAM

Contact Director Continuing Education, College of Nursing and Allied Health, University of North Alabama, 210 Stevens Hall, University Box 5054, Florence, AL 35632. *Telephone:* 256-765-4311. *Fax:* 256-765-4935.

University of South Alabama

College of Nursing
Mobile, Alabama

http://www.southalabama.edu/nursing/

Founded in 1963

DEGREES • BSN • MSN

Nursing Program Faculty 57 (30% with doctorates).

Baccalaureate Enrollment 316
Women 82% **Men** 18% **Minority** 24% **International** 3% **Part-time** 11%

Graduate Enrollment 368
Women 86% **Men** 14% **Minority** 19% **Part-time** 22%

Nursing Student Activities Sigma Theta Tau, Student Nurses' Association.

Nursing Student Resources Academic advising; academic or career counseling; assistance for students with disabilities; bookstore; campus computer network; career placement assistance; computer lab; learning resource lab; library services; nursing audiovisuals; resume preparation assistance.

Library Facilities 1 million volumes (2,406 in health, 2,300 in nursing); 5,296 periodical subscriptions (299 health-care related).

BACCALAUREATE PROGRAMS

Degree BSN

Available Programs ADN to Baccalaureate; Accelerated Baccalaureate; Generic Baccalaureate; RN Baccalaureate.

Site Options Fairhope, AL.

Study Options Full-time and part-time.

Program Entrance Requirements Minimum overall college GPA of 2.5, transcript of college record, CPR certification, health exam, health insurance, immunizations, minimum GPA in nursing prerequisites of 2.5, professional liability insurance/malpractice insurance, prerequisite course work. Transfer students are accepted. **Standardized tests** *Required:* SAT or ACT, TOEFL for international students. **Application** *Deadline:* 7/15 (freshmen), 8/10 (transfer). *Notification:* continuous until 8/10 (freshmen). *Application fee:* $25.

Advanced Placement Credit given for nursing courses completed elsewhere dependent upon specific evaluations.

Expenses (2003–04) *Tuition, state resident:* full-time $3390; part-time $113 per credit hour. *Tuition, nonresident:* full-time $3390; part-time $226 per credit hour. *Room and board:* $2065; room only: $1110 per academic year. *Required fees:* full-time $380.

Financial Aid 55% of baccalaureate students in nursing programs received some form of financial aid in 2002–03. *Gift aid (need-based):* Federal Pell, FSEOG, state, college/university gift aid from institutional funds. *Loans:* FFEL (Subsidized and Unsubsidized Stafford PLUS), Perkins. *Work-Study:* Federal Work-Study, part-time campus jobs. *Application deadline:* Continuous.

Contact Dr. Rosemary S. Rhodes, Associate Dean for Academic Affairs, College of Nursing, University of South Alabama, USA Springhill CON 1004, Mobile, AL 36688-0002. *Telephone:* 251-434-3410. *Fax:* 251-434-3413. *E-mail:* rrhodes@usouthal.edu.

GRADUATE PROGRAMS

Expenses (2003–04) *Tuition, state resident:* part-time $149 per credit hour. *Tuition, nonresident:* part-time $298 per credit hour.

Financial Aid 50% of graduate students in nursing programs received some form of financial aid in 2002–03. 1 research assistantship (averaging $5,333 per year) was awarded; traineeships also available. Aid available to part-time students. *Financial aid application deadline:* 4/1.

Contact Dr. Rosemary S. Rhodes, Associate Dean for Academic Affairs, College of Nursing, University of South Alabama, USA Springhill CON 1004, Mobile, AL 36688-0002. *Telephone:* 251-434-3410. *Fax:* 251-434-3413. *E-mail:* rrhodes@usouthal.edu.

MASTER'S DEGREE PROGRAM

Degree MSN

Available Programs Accelerated Master's; Master's; Master's for Nurses with Non-Nursing Degrees.

Concentrations Available Nursing administration; nursing education. *Clinical nurse specialist programs in:* acute care, community health, family health, gerontology, maternity-newborn, pediatric, psychiatric/mental health, women's health. *Nurse practitioner programs in:* acute care, family health, gerontology, neonatal health, pediatric, psychiatric/mental health, women's health.

Study Options Full-time and part-time.

Program Entrance Requirements Computer literacy, minimum overall college GPA of 3.0, transcript of college record, immunizations, nursing research course, physical assessment course, resume. *Application deadline:* For fall admission, 8/1 (priority date); for winter admission, 11/1 (priority date); for spring admission, 5/1 (priority date). Applications are processed on a rolling basis. *Application fee:* $25.

Advanced Placement Credit given for nursing courses completed elsewhere dependent upon specific evaluations.

Degree Requirements 30 total credit hours, thesis or project.

POST-MASTER'S PROGRAM

Areas of Study Nursing administration; nursing education. *Clinical nurse specialist programs in:* acute care, community health, family health, gerontology, maternity-newborn, pediatric, psychiatric/mental health, women's health. *Nurse practitioner programs in:* acute care, family health, gerontology, neonatal health, pediatric, psychiatric/mental health, women's health.

ALASKA

University of Alaska Anchorage

School of Nursing
Anchorage, Alaska

http://www.son.uaa.alaska.edu

Founded in 1954

DEGREES • BS • MS

Nursing Program Faculty 26 (39% with doctorates).

Baccalaureate Enrollment 203

Women 73% **Men** 27% **Minority** 24% **International** 4% **Part-time** 64%

Graduate Enrollment 55

Women 94% **Men** 6% **Minority** 9%

Nursing Student Activities Sigma Theta Tau, Student Nurses' Association.

Nursing Student Resources Academic advising; academic or career counseling; assistance for students with disabilities; bookstore; campus computer network; career placement assistance; computer lab; computer-assisted instruction; daycare for children of students; e-mail services; interactive nursing skills videos; Internet; learning resource lab; library services; nursing audiovisuals; placement services for program completers; remedial services; resume preparation assistance; skills, simulation, or other laboratory; tutoring.

Library Facilities 894,080 volumes (23,000 in health, 150 in nursing); 3,833 periodical subscriptions (780 health-care related).

BACCALAUREATE PROGRAMS

Degree BS

Available Programs Generic Baccalaureate; RN Baccalaureate.

Study Options Full-time and part-time.

Program Entrance Requirements Minimum overall college GPA of 2.7, transcript of college record, CPR certification, written essay, immunizations, 3 letters of recommendation, minimum GPA in nursing prerequisites of 2.7, professional liability insurance/malpractice insurance, prerequisite course work. Transfer students are accepted. **Standardized tests** *Required:* SAT or ACT, TOEFL for international students. **Application** *Deadline:* 7/15 (freshmen). *Application fee:* $40.

Advanced Placement Credit given for nursing courses completed elsewhere dependent upon specific evaluations.

Expenses (2004–05) *Tuition, state resident:* full-time $2376; part-time $112 per credit hour. *Tuition, nonresident:* full-time $7920; part-time $330 per credit hour. *Room and board:* $2815; room only: $1815 per academic year. *Required fees:* full-time $227; part-time $30 per credit; part-time $100 per term.

Financial Aid 90% of baccalaureate students in nursing programs received some form of financial aid in 2003–04. *Gift aid (need-based):* Federal Pell, FSEOG, state, private, college/university gift aid from institutional funds. *Loans:* Federal Direct (Subsidized and Unsubsidized Stafford PLUS), FFEL (Subsidized and Unsubsidized Stafford PLUS), state. *Work-Study:* Federal Work-Study. *Application deadline:* 8/1 (priority: 4/1).

Contact Ms. Marie Samson, Coordinator of Student Affairs, School of Nursing, School of Nursing, University of Alaska Anchorage, 3211 Providence Drive, Anchorage, AK 99508-8030. *Telephone:* 907-786-4550. *Fax:* 907-786-4558. *E-mail:* anms@uaa.alaska.edu.

GRADUATE PROGRAMS

Expenses (2004–05) *Tuition, state resident:* full-time $3996; part-time $222 per credit hour. *Tuition, nonresident:* full-time $6954; part-time $453 per credit hour. *International tuition:* $6954 full-time. *Room and board:* $2815; room only: $1815 per academic year. *Required fees:* full-time $400; part-time $75 per credit; part-time $200 per term.

Financial Aid 30% of graduate students in nursing programs received some form of financial aid in 2003–04. Teaching assistantships, career-related internships or fieldwork and Federal Work-Study available. Aid available to part-time students. *Financial aid application deadline:* 4/1.

Contact Dr. Jacqueline S. Pflaum, Associate Director, School of Nursing, University of Alaska Anchorage, 3211 Providence Drive, Anchorage, AK 99508-8030. *Telephone:* 907-786-4574. *Fax:* 907-786-4558. *E-mail:* afjsp@uaa.alaska.edu.

MASTER'S DEGREE PROGRAM

Degree MS

Available Programs Master's.

Concentrations Available Health-care administration. *Clinical nurse specialist programs in:* community health, psychiatric/mental health. *Nurse practitioner programs in:* family health, psychiatric/mental health.

Study Options Full-time and part-time.

Program Entrance Requirements Clinical experience, minimum overall college GPA of 3.0, transcript of college record, written essay, 3 letters of recommendation, nursing research course, prerequisite course work, statistics course, GRE or MAT. *Application deadline:* For fall admission, 3/1. *Application fee:* $45.

Advanced Placement Credit given for nursing courses completed elsewhere dependent upon specific evaluations.

Degree Requirements 50 total credit hours, thesis or project.

ARIZONA

Arizona State University

College of Nursing
Tempe, Arizona

http://nursing.asu.edu

Founded in 1885

DEGREES • BSN • MS • MS/MPH

Nursing Program Faculty 93 (37% with doctorates).

Baccalaureate Enrollment 1,088 **Women** 93% **Men** 7% **Minority** 28% **International** 1% **Part-time** 17%

Graduate Enrollment 171

Women 90% **Men** 10% **Minority** 18% **International** 1% **Part-time** 50%

Arizona State University (continued)

Nursing Student Activities Nursing Honor Society, Sigma Theta Tau, Student Nurses' Association, nursing club.

Nursing Student Resources Academic advising; academic or career counseling; assistance for students with disabilities; bookstore; campus computer network; career placement assistance; computer lab; computer-assisted instruction; daycare for children of students; e-mail services; employment services for current students; housing assistance; interactive nursing skills videos; Internet; learning resource lab; library services; nursing audiovisuals; paid internships; placement services for program completers; remedial services; resume preparation assistance; skills, simulation, or other laboratory; tutoring; unpaid internships.

Library Facilities 2.4 million volumes (77,814 in health, 7,501 in nursing); 28,159 periodical subscriptions (755 health-care related).

BACCALAUREATE PROGRAMS

Degree BSN

Available Programs Accelerated Baccalaureate; Accelerated Baccalaureate for Second Degree; Accelerated RN Baccalaureate; Baccalaureate for Second Degree; Generic Baccalaureate.

Site Options Phoenix, AZ; Scottsdale, AZ; Chandler/Glendale, AZ.

Study Options Full-time and part-time.

Program Entrance Requirements Minimum overall college GPA of 2.75, transcript of college record, CPR certification, high school chemistry, high school foreign language, 4 years high school math, 3 years high school science, high school transcript, immunizations, minimum high school GPA of 3.0, minimum high school rank 25%, minimum GPA in nursing prerequisites of 2.75, prerequisite course work. Transfer students are accepted. **Standardized tests** *Required:* SAT or ACT, TOEFL for international students. **Application** *Deadline:* rolling (freshmen), rolling (transfer). *Early decision:* 11/1. *Notification:* continuous (freshmen), 12/1 (early action). *Application fee:* $25, $50 for non-residents.

Advanced Placement Credit by examination available. Credit given for nursing courses completed elsewhere dependent upon specific evaluations.

Expenses (2003–04) *Tuition, state resident:* part-time $183 per credit hour. *Tuition, nonresident:* part-time $501 per credit hour. *Room and board:* $5430; room only: $2800 per academic year. *Required fees:* full-time $938; part-time $469 per term.

Financial Aid 70% of baccalaureate students in nursing programs received some form of financial aid in 2002–03. *Gift aid (need-based):* Federal Pell, FSEOG, state, private, college/university gift aid from institutional funds, Federal Nursing. *Loans:* Federal Direct (Subsidized and Unsubsidized Stafford PLUS), FFEL, Perkins. *Work-Study:* Federal Work-Study, part-time campus jobs. *Application deadline (priority):* 2/15.

Contact Ms. Maurine Lee, Office of Student Services, College of Nursing, Arizona State University, Box 872602, Tempe, AZ 85287-2602. *Telephone:* 480-965-2987. *Fax:* 480-965-8468. *E-mail:* maurine.lee@asu.edu.

GRADUATE PROGRAMS

Expenses (2003–04) *Tuition, state resident:* full-time $3708; part-time $194 per credit hour. *Tuition, nonresident:* full-time $12,228; part-time $510 per credit hour. *International tuition:* $12,228 full-time. *Room and board:* $5430; room only: $2800 per academic year. *Required fees:* full-time $87; part-time $22 per term.

Financial Aid 75% of graduate students in nursing programs received some form of financial aid in 2002–03.

Contact Ms. Maurine Lee, Office of Student Services, College of Nursing, Arizona State University, Box 872602, Tempe, AZ 85287-2602. *Telephone:* 480-965-2987. *Fax:* 480-965-8468. *E-mail:* maurine.lee@asu.edu.

MASTER'S DEGREE PROGRAM

Degrees MS; MS/MPH

Available Programs Master's.

Concentrations Available *Clinical nurse specialist programs in:* acute care, adult health, community health, pediatric, psychiatric/mental health. *Nurse practitioner programs in:* acute care, adult health, family health, neonatal health, pediatric, psychiatric/mental health, women's health.

Site Options Phoenix, AZ.

Study Options Full-time and part-time.

Program Entrance Requirements Clinical experience, minimum overall college GPA of 3.0, transcript of college record, immunizations, interview, 3 letters of recommendation, physical assessment course, prerequisite course work, resume, statistics course, GRE. *Application fee:* $45.

Advanced Placement Credit given for nursing courses completed elsewhere dependent upon specific evaluations.

Degree Requirements 40 total credit hours, thesis or project.

POST-MASTER'S PROGRAM

Areas of Study *Clinical nurse specialist programs in:* acute care, adult health, community health, pediatric, psychiatric/mental health. *Nurse practitioner programs in:* acute care, adult health, family health, neonatal health, pediatric, psychiatric/mental health, women's health.

CONTINUING EDUCATION PROGRAM

Contact Dr. David Hrabe, Director of Continuing and Extended Education, College of Nursing, Arizona State University, Box 872602, Tempe, AZ 85287-2602. *Telephone:* 480-965-7431. *Fax:* 480-965-0619. *E-mail:* david.hrabe@asu.edu.

Grand Canyon University
Samaritan College of Nursing
Phoenix, Arizona

Founded in 1949

DEGREES • BSN • MS

Nursing Program Faculty 38 (8% with doctorates).

Baccalaureate Enrollment 237

Women 94% **Men** 6% **Minority** 16% **International** 1%

Graduate Enrollment 8

Nursing Student Activities Sigma Theta Tau, Student Nurses' Association.

Nursing Student Resources Academic advising; academic or career counseling; assistance for students with disabilities; bookstore; campus computer network; career placement assistance; computer lab; computer-assisted instruction; e-mail services; employment services for current students; housing assistance; Internet; learning resource lab; library services; nursing audiovisuals; other; remedial services; resume preparation assistance; skills, simulation, or other laboratory; tutoring.

Library Facilities 75,905 volumes (9,663 in health); 1,174 periodical subscriptions (177 health-care related).

BACCALAUREATE PROGRAMS

Degree BSN

Available Programs Accelerated Baccalaureate; Accelerated RN Baccalaureate; Generic Baccalaureate.

Site Options *Distance Learning:* Phoenix, AZ.

Study Options Full-time.

Program Entrance Requirements Minimum overall college GPA of 2.8, transcript of college record, CPR certification, written essay, health exam, health insurance, immunizations, minimum GPA in nursing prerequisites of 3.0, prerequisite course work. Transfer students are accepted. **Standardized tests** *Required:* SAT or ACT, TOEFL for international students. **Application** *Deadline:* rolling (freshmen), rolling (transfer). *Notification:* continuous until 9/1 (freshmen). *Application fee:* $50.

Expenses (2003–04) *Tuition:* full-time $7250; part-time $605 per credit hour. *Room and board:* $3628 per academic year.

Financial Aid 80% of baccalaureate students in nursing programs received some form of financial aid in 2002–03.

Contact Dr. Cynthia Russell, RN, Dean, Samaritan College of Nursing, Grand Canyon University, 3300 West Camelback Road, Phoenix, AZ 85017. *Telephone:* 602-589-2431. *Fax:* 602-589-2098. *E-mail:* crussell@grand-canyon.edu.

GRADUATE PROGRAMS

Expenses (2003–04) *Tuition:* part-time $605 per credit hour. *Room and board:* $3628 per academic year.

Contact Prof. Elizabeth Gilbert, Associate Dean, Samaritan College of Nursing, Grand Canyon University, Samaritan College of Nursing, 3300 West Camelback Road, Phoenix, AZ 85017. *Telephone:* 602-589-2516. *Fax:* 602-589-2098. *E-mail:* bgilbert@grand-canyon.edu.

MASTER'S DEGREE PROGRAM

Degree MS

Available Programs Master's.

Concentrations Available Health-care administration. *Nurse practitioner programs in:* family health.

Site Options *Distance Learning:* Phoenix, AZ.

Study Options Full-time and part-time.

Program Entrance Requirements Computer literacy, minimum overall college GPA of 3.0, transcript of college record, CPR certification, written essay, immunizations, 2 letters of recommendation, nursing research course, physical assessment course, professional liability insurance/malpractice insurance, resume, statistics course.

Advanced Placement Credit given for nursing courses completed elsewhere dependent upon specific evaluations.

Degree Requirements 49 total credit hours, thesis or project.

CONTINUING EDUCATION PROGRAM

Contact Mrs. Sharon Rayman, RN, Director of RN to BSN Track, Samaritan College of Nursing, Grand Canyon University, 3300 West Camelback Road, Phoenix, AZ 85017. *Telephone:* 602-589-2826. *Fax:* 602-589-2098. *E-mail:* srayman@grand-canyon.edu.

Northern Arizona University

Department of Nursing
Flagstaff, Arizona

http://www.nau.edu/hp/dept/nurse

Founded in 1899

DEGREES • BSN • MS

Nursing Program Faculty 38 (50% with doctorates).

Baccalaureate Enrollment 245

Women 87% **Men** 13% **Minority** 22% **Part-time** 21%

Graduate Enrollment 43

Women 87% **Men** 13% **Minority** 7% **International** 1% **Part-time** 50%

Nursing Student Activities Nursing Honor Society, Sigma Theta Tau, Student Nurses' Association.

Nursing Student Resources Academic advising; academic or career counseling; bookstore; campus computer network; computer lab; computer-assisted instruction; e-mail services; externships; interactive nursing skills videos; Internet; learning resource lab; library services; nursing audiovisuals; paid internships; remedial services; skills, simulation, or other laboratory; tutoring.

Library Facilities 633,417 volumes; 2,595 periodical subscriptions.

BACCALAUREATE PROGRAMS

Degree BSN

Available Programs ADN to Baccalaureate; Accelerated Baccalaureate; Accelerated Baccalaureate for Second Degree; Generic Baccalaureate; RN Baccalaureate.

Site Options *Distance Learning:* Tucson, AZ; Yuma, AZ; Ganado/Chinle, AZ.

Study Options Full-time and part-time.

Program Entrance Requirements Transcript of college record, CPR certification, written essay, health exam, health insurance, high school transcript, immunizations, 2 letters of recommendation, minimum GPA in nursing prerequisites of 2.75, professional liability insurance/malpractice insurance, prerequisite course work. Transfer students are accepted. **Standardized tests** *Required:* TOEFL for international students. *Required for some:* SAT, ACT, SAT or ACT. **Application** *Deadline:* 8/1 (freshmen), rolling (transfer). *Notification:* continuous (freshmen). *Application fee:* $25.

Advanced Placement Credit given for nursing courses completed elsewhere dependent upon specific evaluations.

Expenses (2004–05) *Tuition, state resident:* full-time $3594; part-time $205 per credit hour. *Tuition, nonresident:* full-time $12,114; part-time $523 per credit hour. *International tuition:* $12,114 full-time. *Room and board:* $8502; room only: $3352 per academic year. *Required fees:* part-time $201 per credit.

Financial Aid 75% of baccalaureate students in nursing programs received some form of financial aid in 2003–04. *Gift aid (need-based):* Federal Pell, FSEOG, state, private, college/university gift aid from institutional funds, Federal Nursing. *Loans:* Federal Nursing Student Loans, Federal Direct (Subsidized and Unsubsidized Stafford PLUS), Perkins, college/university. *Work-Study:* Federal Work-Study, part-time campus jobs. *Application deadline (priority):* 2/14.

Contact Coordinator of Student Services, Department of Nursing, Northern Arizona University, Box 15035, Flagstaff, AZ 86011. *Telephone:* 928-523-6717. *Fax:* 928-523-7171.

GRADUATE PROGRAMS

Expenses (2004–05) *Tuition, state resident:* full-time $3794; part-time $216 per credit hour. *Tuition, nonresident:* full-time $12,314; part-time $518 per credit hour. *International tuition:* $12,314 full-time. *Room and board:* $8502; room only: $3352 per academic year.

Financial Aid 75% of graduate students in nursing programs received some form of financial aid in 2003–04. 1 research assistantship was awarded.

Contact Coordinator of Student Services, Department of Nursing, Northern Arizona University, Box 15035, Flagstaff, AZ 86011. *Telephone:* 928-523-6717. *Fax:* 928-523-7171.

MASTER'S DEGREE PROGRAM

Degree MS

Available Programs Master's.

Concentrations Available Nurse case management; nursing education. *Clinical nurse specialist programs in:* public health. *Nurse practitioner programs in:* family health.

Site Options *Distance Learning:* Yuma, AZ.

Study Options Full-time and part-time.

Program Entrance Requirements Clinical experience, minimum overall college GPA of 3.0, transcript of college record, CPR certification, written essay, immunizations, interview, 3 letters of recommendation, nursing research course, physical assessment course, professional liability insurance/malpractice insurance, prerequisite course work, resume, statistics course, GRE General Test. *Application deadline:* For fall admission, 2/15 (priority date). *Application fee:* $45.

Degree Requirements 37 total credit hours, thesis or project.

The University of Arizona

College of Nursing
Tucson, Arizona

http://www.nursing.arizona.edu

Founded in 1885

DEGREES • BSN • MS • PHD

Nursing Program Faculty 57 (58% with doctorates).

Baccalaureate Enrollment 294

Women 92% **Men** 8% **Minority** 30% **International** 1% **Part-time** 14%

Graduate Enrollment 129

Women 94% **Men** 6% **Minority** 17% **International** 12% **Part-time** 54%

Nursing Student Activities Nursing Honor Society, Sigma Theta Tau, Student Nurses' Association.

Nursing Student Resources Academic advising; academic or career counseling; assistance for students with disabilities; bookstore; campus computer network; career placement assistance; computer lab; computer-assisted instruction; e-mail services; externships; housing assistance; interactive nursing skills videos; Internet; learning resource lab; library services; nursing audiovisuals; other; placement services for program completers; skills, simulation, or other laboratory; tutoring.

Library Facilities 4.4 million volumes (215,000 in health, 30,000 in nursing); 23,790 periodical subscriptions (2,000 health-care related).

BACCALAUREATE PROGRAMS

Degree BSN

The University of Arizona (continued)

Available Programs Accelerated Baccalaureate for Second Degree; Generic Baccalaureate.

Study Options Full-time.

Program Entrance Requirements Minimum overall college GPA of 2.75, transcript of college record, CPR certification, written essay, high school foreign language, 4 years high school math, 3 years high school science, immunizations, 2 letters of recommendation, minimum high school GPA of 2.5, minimum GPA in nursing prerequisites of 2.75, prerequisite course work. Transfer students are accepted. **Standardized tests** *Required:* SAT or ACT, TOEFL for international students. **Application** *Deadline:* 4/1 (freshmen), 6/1 (transfer). *Notification:* continuous until 8/1 (freshmen).

Advanced Placement Credit by examination available. Credit given for nursing courses completed elsewhere dependent upon specific evaluations.

Expenses (2004–05) *Tuition, state resident:* full-time $4067. *Tuition, nonresident:* full-time $13,047. *International tuition:* $13,047 full-time. *Room and board:* room only: $6157 per academic year. *Required fees:* full-time $30; part-time $15 per term.

Financial Aid 60% of baccalaureate students in nursing programs received some form of financial aid in 2003–04.

Contact Ms. Vickie Radoye, Assistant Dean for Student Affairs, College of Nursing, The University of Arizona, 1305 North Martin, PO Box 210203, Tucson, AZ 85721-0203. *Telephone:* 520-626-3808. *Fax:* 520-626-6424. *E-mail:* vradoye@nursing.arizona.edu.

GRADUATE PROGRAMS

Expenses (2004–05) *Tuition, state resident:* full-time $8317. *Tuition, nonresident:* full-time $17,297. *International tuition:* $17,297 full-time. *Required fees:* full-time $30; part-time $15 per term.

Financial Aid 52% of graduate students in nursing programs received some form of financial aid in 2003–04. 22 fellowships (averaging $1,136 per year), 16 research assistantships with partial tuition reimbursements available (averaging $15,000 per year), 2 teaching assistantships with partial tuition reimbursements available (averaging $15,000 per year) were awarded; career-related internships or fieldwork, institutionally sponsored loans, scholarships, traineeships, and tuition waivers (full) also available. *Financial aid application deadline:* 6/1.

Contact Mr. Alan Beaudrie, Senior Academic Advisor, College of Nursing, The University of Arizona, 1305 North Martin, PO Box 210203, Tucson, AZ 85721-0203. *Telephone:* 520-626-3808. *Fax:* 520-626-6424. *E-mail:* abeaudrie@nursing.arizona.edu.

MASTER'S DEGREE PROGRAM

Degree MS

Available Programs Master's.

Concentrations Available Nursing informatics. *Nurse practitioner programs in:* adult health, family health, psychiatric/mental health.

Study Options Full-time and part-time.

Program Entrance Requirements Computer literacy, minimum overall college GPA of 3.0, transcript of college record, CPR certification, written essay, immunizations, 3 letters of recommendation, nursing research course, physical assessment course, resume, statistics course, GRE General Test. *Application deadline:* For fall admission, 1/14. *Application fee:* $50.

Advanced Placement Credit given for nursing courses completed elsewhere dependent upon specific evaluations.

Degree Requirements 44 total credit hours, thesis or project.

POST-MASTER'S PROGRAM

Areas of Study Nursing informatics. *Nurse practitioner programs in:* adult health, family health, gerontology, psychiatric/mental health.

DOCTORAL DEGREE PROGRAM

Degree PhD

Available Programs Doctorate; Post-Baccalaureate Doctorate.

Areas of Study Aging, bio-behavioral research, biology of health and illness, gerontology, health-care systems, information systems, nursing research, nursing science.

Site Options *Distance Learning:* Phoenix, AZ.

Program Entrance Requirements Minimum overall college GPA of 3.0, interview by faculty committee, interview, 3 letters of recommendation, scholarly papers, statistics course, vita, writing sample, GRE General Test (not required for applicants with a master's degree). *Application deadline:* For fall admission, 1/14. *Application fee:* $50.

Degree Requirements 75 total credit hours, dissertation, oral exam, written exam, residency.

POSTDOCTORAL PROGRAM

Areas of Study Nursing research.

Postdoctoral Program Contact Ms. Vickie Radoye, Assistant Dean for Student Affairs, College of Nursing, The University of Arizona, 1305 North Martin, PO Box 210203, Tucson, AZ 85721-0203. *Telephone:* 520-626-3808. *Fax:* 520-626-6424. *E-mail:* vradoye@nursing.arizona.edu.

CONTINUING EDUCATION PROGRAM

Contact Ms. Mary Doyle, Administrator for Continuing Education, College of Nursing, The University of Arizona, PO Box 210203, Tucson, AZ 85721. *Telephone:* 520-626-0562. *E-mail:* mdoyle@nursing.arizona.edu.

See full description on page 550.

University of Phoenix Online Campus

College of Health and Human Services
Phoenix, Arizona

http://www.uopxonline.com/

Founded in 1989

DEGREES • BSN • MSN • MSN/MBA

Nursing Program Faculty 469 (31% with doctorates).

Baccalaureate Enrollment 2,985 **Women** 92% **Men** 8% **Minority** 16%

Graduate Enrollment 2,541 **Women** 92% **Men** 8% **Minority** 23%

Nursing Student Activities Sigma Theta Tau.

Nursing Student Resources Academic advising; academic or career counseling; bookstore; library services.

Library Facilities 27.1 million volumes; 11,648 periodical subscriptions (1,426 health-care related).

BACCALAUREATE PROGRAMS

Degree BSN

Available Programs ADN to Baccalaureate; Accelerated RN Baccalaureate.

Study Options Full-time.

Program Entrance Requirements 1 letter of recommendation. Transfer students are accepted. **Application** *Deadline:* rolling (freshmen), rolling (transfer).

Advanced Placement Credit by examination available.

Expenses (2004–05) *Tuition:* full-time $11,550; part-time $385 per credit hour. *International tuition:* $11,550 full-time. *Required fees:* full-time $110.

Financial Aid 5% of baccalaureate students in nursing programs received some form of financial aid in 2003–04.

Contact Program Chair, Healthcare, College of Health and Human Services, University of Phoenix Online Campus, CF-A101, 3157 East Elwood Street, Phoenix, AZ 85034-7209. *Telephone:* 602-387-7000.

GRADUATE PROGRAMS

Expenses (2004–05) *Tuition:* full-time $10,320; part-time $430 per credit hour. *International tuition:* $10,320 full-time. *Required fees:* full-time $110.

Financial Aid 7% of graduate students in nursing programs received some form of financial aid in 2003–04.

Contact Program Chair, Healthcare. *Telephone:* 602-387-7000.

MASTER'S DEGREE PROGRAM

Degrees MSN; MSN/MBA

Available Programs Master's.

Concentrations Available Health-care administration; nursing administration; nursing education. *Nurse practitioner programs in:* family health.

Study Options Full-time.

Program Entrance Requirements Clinical experience, computer literacy, minimum overall college GPA of 2.5, transcript of college record. *Application deadline:* Applications are processed on a rolling basis. *Application fee:* $110.

Degree Requirements 39 total credit hours, thesis or project.

POST-MASTER'S PROGRAM

Areas of Study *Nurse practitioner programs in:* family health.

See full description on page 570.

University of Phoenix–Phoenix Campus

College of Health and Human Services
Phoenix, Arizona

Founded in 1976

DEGREES • BSN • MSN • MSN/MBA

Nursing Program Faculty 80 (25% with doctorates).

Baccalaureate Enrollment 161
Women 93% **Men** 7% **Minority** 11%

Graduate Enrollment 162
Women 88% **Men** 12% **Minority** 15%

Nursing Student Activities Sigma Theta Tau.

Nursing Student Resources Academic advising; academic or career counseling; assistance for students with disabilities; bookstore; computer lab; library services.

Library Facilities 27.1 million volumes; 11,648 periodical subscriptions (1,426 health-care related).

BACCALAUREATE PROGRAMS

Degree BSN

Available Programs ADN to Baccalaureate; Accelerated Baccalaureate.

Site Options Tempe, AZ; Mesa, AZ; Scottsdale, AZ.

Study Options Full-time.

Program Entrance Requirements 1 letter of recommendation. Transfer students are accepted. **Standardized tests** *Required:* TOEFL for international students. **Application** *Deadline:* rolling (freshmen), rolling (transfer). *Application fee:* $85.

Advanced Placement Credit by examination available.

Expenses (2004–05) *Tuition:* full-time $9090; part-time $303 per credit hour. *International tuition:* $9090 full-time. *Required fees:* full-time $110.

Financial Aid 2% of baccalaureate students in nursing programs received some form of financial aid in 2003–04.

Contact Campus College Chair, Nursing, College of Health and Human Services, University of Phoenix–Phoenix Campus, 4635 East Elwood Street, Phoenix, AZ 85040-1958. *Telephone:* 480-804-7600.

GRADUATE PROGRAMS

Expenses (2004–05) *Tuition:* full-time $9120; part-time $335 per credit hour. *International tuition:* $9120 full-time. *Required fees:* full-time $110.

Financial Aid 3% of graduate students in nursing programs received some form of financial aid in 2003–04.

Contact Campus College Chair, Nursing, College of Health and Human Services, University of Phoenix–Phoenix Campus, 4635 East Elwood Street, Phoenix, AZ 85040-1958. *Telephone:* 480-804-7600.

MASTER'S DEGREE PROGRAM

Degrees MSN; MSN/MBA

Available Programs Master's.

Concentrations Available Health-care administration; nursing administration; nursing education. *Nurse practitioner programs in:* family health.

Site Options Tempe, AZ; Mesa, AZ; Scottsdale, AZ.

Study Options Full-time.

Program Entrance Requirements Clinical experience, computer literacy, minimum overall college GPA of 2.5, transcript of college record, 1 letter of recommendation. *Application deadline:* Applications are processed on a rolling basis. *Application fee:* $110.

Degree Requirements 39 total credit hours, thesis or project.

POST-MASTER'S PROGRAM

Areas of Study *Nurse practitioner programs in:* family health.

CONTINUING EDUCATION PROGRAM

Contact Campus College Chair, Nursing, College of Health and Human Services, University of Phoenix–Phoenix Campus, 4635 East Elwood Street, Phoenix, AZ 85040-1958. *Telephone:* 480-804-7600.

University of Phoenix–Southern Arizona Campus

College of Health and Human Services
Tucson, Arizona

Founded in 1979

DEGREES • BSN • MSN • MSN/MBA

Nursing Program Faculty 36 (25% with doctorates).

Baccalaureate Enrollment 89
Women 84% **Men** 16% **Minority** 25%

Graduate Enrollment 25
Women 92% **Men** 8% **Minority** 17%

Nursing Student Activities Sigma Theta Tau.

Nursing Student Resources Academic advising; academic or career counseling; bookstore; computer lab; library services.

Library Facilities 27.1 million volumes; 11,648 periodical subscriptions (1,426 health-care related).

BACCALAUREATE PROGRAMS

Degree BSN

Available Programs ADN to Baccalaureate; Accelerated Baccalaureate.

Site Options Yuma, AZ; Nogales, AZ; Sierra Vista, AZ.

Study Options Full-time.

Program Entrance Requirements 1 letter of recommendation. Transfer students are accepted. **Standardized tests** *Required:* TOEFL for international students. **Application** *Deadline:* rolling (freshmen), rolling (transfer). *Application fee:* $85.

Advanced Placement Credit by examination available.

Expenses (2004–05) *Tuition:* full-time $8910; part-time $297 per credit hour. *International tuition:* $8910 full-time. *Required fees:* full-time $110.

Financial Aid 5% of baccalaureate students in nursing programs received some form of financial aid in 2003–04. *Loans:* Federal Direct (Unsubsidized Stafford PLUS), Perkins. *Application deadline:* Continuous.

Contact Campus College Chair, Nursing, College of Health and Human Services, University of Phoenix–Southern Arizona Campus, 5099 East Grant Road, #120, Tucson, AZ 85712-2732. *Telephone:* 520-881-6512.

GRADUATE PROGRAMS

Expenses (2004–05) *Tuition:* full-time $7968; part-time $332 per credit hour. *International tuition:* $7968 full-time. *Required fees:* full-time $110.

Financial Aid 1% of graduate students in nursing programs received some form of financial aid in 2003–04.

University of Phoenix–Southern Arizona Campus (continued)

Contact Campus College Chair, Nursing, College of Health and Human Services, University of Phoenix–Southern Arizona Campus, 5099 East Grant Road, Tucson, AZ 85712-2732. *Telephone:* 520-881-6512.

MASTER'S DEGREE PROGRAM

Degrees MSN; MSN/MBA

Available Programs Master's.

Concentrations Available Health-care administration; nursing education. *Nurse practitioner programs in:* family health.

Site Options Yuma, AZ; Nogales, AZ; Sierra Vista, AZ.

Study Options Full-time.

Program Entrance Requirements Clinical experience, computer literacy, minimum overall college GPA of 2.5, transcript of college record. *Application deadline:* Applications are processed on a rolling basis. *Application fee:* $110.

Advanced Placement Credit given for nursing courses completed elsewhere dependent upon specific evaluations.

Degree Requirements 39 total credit hours, thesis or project.

POST-MASTER'S PROGRAM

Areas of Study *Nurse practitioner programs in:* family health.

ARKANSAS

Arkansas State University

Department of Nursing
Jonesboro, State University, Arkansas

http://www.conhp.astate.edu/Nursing/

Founded in 1909

DEGREES • BSN • MSN

Nursing Program Faculty 35 (20% with doctorates).

Baccalaureate Enrollment 245

Graduate Enrollment 91

Nursing Student Activities Nursing Honor Society, Sigma Theta Tau.

Library Facilities 586,176 volumes; 1,675 periodical subscriptions.

BACCALAUREATE PROGRAMS

Degree BSN

Available Programs Generic Baccalaureate; LPN to Baccalaureate; RN Baccalaureate.

Site Options Mountain Home, AR; Melbourne, AR; Beebe, AR.

Study Options Full-time.

Program Entrance Requirements Minimum overall college GPA of 2.5, transcript of college record, CPR certification, health exam, immunizations, minimum GPA in nursing prerequisites of 3.5, prerequisite course work. Transfer students are accepted. **Standardized tests** *Required:* SAT I, ACT, ACT COMPASS, or ACT ASSET, ACT preferred, SAT Reasoning or ACT. ***Placement:*** *Required:* SAT or ACT. **Application** *Deadline:* rolling (freshmen), rolling (transfer). *Notification:* continuous (freshmen). *Application fee:* $15.

Advanced Placement Credit given for nursing courses completed elsewhere dependent upon specific evaluations.

Contact Shirley Basinger, Nursing Advisor, Department of Nursing, Arkansas State University, PO Box 910, State University, AR 72467. *Telephone:* 870-972-3074. *Fax:* 870-972-2954. *E-mail:* sbasinge@astate.edu.

GRADUATE PROGRAMS

Contact Dr. Phyllis Skorga, MSN Program Director, Department of Nursing, Arkansas State University, PO Box 910, State University, AR 72467-0069. *Telephone:* 870-972-3074. *Fax:* 870-972-2954. *E-mail:* pskorga@astate.edu.

MASTER'S DEGREE PROGRAM

Degree MSN

Available Programs Master's.

Concentrations Available Nurse anesthesia; nursing education. *Clinical nurse specialist programs in:* adult health. *Nurse practitioner programs in:* primary care.

Site Options Mountain Home, AR; Melbourne, AR; Beebe, AR.

Study Options Full-time and part-time.

Program Entrance Requirements Clinical experience, minimum overall college GPA of 2.75, transcript of college record, CPR certification, written essay, immunizations, interview, letters of recommendation, physical assessment course, professional liability insurance/malpractice insurance, statistics course.

Degree Requirements 39 total credit hours, thesis or project, comprehensive exam.

Arkansas Tech University

Program in Nursing
Russellville, Arkansas

http://nursing.atu.edu

Founded in 1909

DEGREE • BSN

Nursing Program Faculty 23.

Baccalaureate Enrollment 477

Women 88% **Men** 12% **Minority** 9% **International** 7% **Part-time** 19%

Nursing Student Activities Sigma Theta Tau, Student Nurses' Association.

Nursing Student Resources Academic advising; academic or career counseling; assistance for students with disabilities; bookstore; campus computer network; career placement assistance; computer lab; computer-assisted instruction; e-mail services; employment services for current students; housing assistance; Internet; learning resource lab; library services; nursing audiovisuals; other; paid internships; placement services for program completers; remedial services; resume preparation assistance; skills, simulation, or other laboratory; tutoring.

Library Facilities 259,372 volumes (16,900 in health, 2,100 in nursing); 1,054 periodical subscriptions (130 health-care related).

BACCALAUREATE PROGRAMS

Degree BSN

Available Programs ADN to Baccalaureate; Generic Baccalaureate; LPN to Baccalaureate; RN Baccalaureate.

Site Options *Distance Learning:* Fort Smith, AR.

Study Options Full-time and part-time.

Program Entrance Requirements Minimum overall college GPA of 2.75, transcript of college record, CPR certification, health exam, immunizations, minimum GPA in nursing prerequisites, professional liability insurance/malpractice insurance, prerequisite course work. Transfer students are accepted. **Standardized tests** *Required:* SAT or ACT, TOEFL for international students. **Application** *Notification:* continuous (freshmen).

Advanced Placement Credit by examination available. Credit given for nursing courses completed elsewhere dependent upon specific evaluations.

Expenses (2004–05) *Tuition, state resident:* full-time $4158; part-time $154 per credit hour. *Tuition, nonresident:* full-time $7854; part-time $308 per credit hour. *International tuition:* $7854 full-time. *Room and board:* $4785; room only: $3000 per academic year. *Required fees:* full-time $310; part-time $120 per credit; part-time $140 per term.

Financial Aid 80% of baccalaureate students in nursing programs received some form of financial aid in 2003–04. *Gift aid (need-based):* Federal Pell, FSEOG, state, private, college/university gift aid from institutional funds. *Loans:* FFEL (Subsidized and Unsubsidized Stafford PLUS), Perkins. *Work-Study:* Federal Work-Study, part-time campus jobs. *Application deadline (priority):* 4/15.

Contact Dr. Rebecca Frances Burris, Professor and Department Chair, Program in Nursing, Arkansas Tech University, 402 West O Street, Russellville, AR 72801. *Telephone:* 479-968-0383. *Fax:* 479-968-0219. *E-mail:* rebecca.burris@mail.atu.edu.

Harding University
College of Nursing
Searcy, Arkansas

http://www.harding.edu

Founded in 1924

DEGREE • BSN

Nursing Program Faculty 17 (18% with doctorates).

Baccalaureate Enrollment 92
Women 93% **Men** 7% **International** 2% **Part-time** 2%

Nursing Student Activities Nursing Honor Society, Sigma Theta Tau, Student Nurses' Association.

Nursing Student Resources Academic advising; academic or career counseling; assistance for students with disabilities; bookstore; campus computer network; career placement assistance; computer lab; computer-assisted instruction; e-mail services; employment services for current students; externships; housing assistance; interactive nursing skills videos; Internet; learning resource lab; library services; nursing audiovisuals; placement services for program completers; remedial services; resume preparation assistance; skills, simulation, or other laboratory; tutoring.

Library Facilities 253,436 volumes (5,000 in health, 1,729 in nursing); 16,879 periodical subscriptions (145 health-care related).

BACCALAUREATE PROGRAMS

Degree BSN

Available Programs ADN to Baccalaureate; Generic Baccalaureate; LPN to Baccalaureate; LPN to RN Baccalaureate; RN Baccalaureate.

Site Options Searcy, AR.

Study Options Full-time and part-time.

Program Entrance Requirements Minimum overall college GPA of 2.0, transcript of college record, CPR certification, health exam, immunizations, 2 letters of recommendation, minimum GPA in nursing prerequisites of 2.5, prerequisite course work. Transfer students are accepted. **Standardized tests** *Required:* SAT or ACT, TOEFL for international students. **Application** *Deadline:* 7/1 (freshmen), 7/1 (transfer). *Notification:* continuous (freshmen). *Application fee:* $35.

Advanced Placement Credit given for nursing courses completed elsewhere dependent upon specific evaluations.

Expenses (2004–05) *Tuition:* full-time $10,380; part-time $346 per credit hour. *Room and board:* $5182; room only: $2572 per academic year. *Required fees:* full-time $1128.

Financial Aid 95% of baccalaureate students in nursing programs received some form of financial aid in 2003–04. *Gift aid (need-based):* Federal Pell, FSEOG, state, private, college/university gift aid from institutional funds. *Loans:* Federal Nursing Student Loans, FFEL (Subsidized and Unsubsidized Stafford PLUS), Perkins, state, college/university. *Work-Study:* Federal Work-Study, part-time campus jobs. *Application deadline:* Continuous.

Contact Mrs. Summer S. Mills, Assistant to the Dean, College of Nursing, Harding University, Box 12265, Searcy, AR 72149-0001. *Telephone:* 501-279-4682. *Fax:* 501-305-8902. *E-mail:* nursing@harding.edu.

Henderson State University
Department of Nursing
Arkadelphia, Arkansas

http://www.hsu.edu/dept/nsg/index.html

Founded in 1890

DEGREE • BSN

Nursing Program Faculty 9.

Library Facilities 262,572 volumes; 1,516 periodical subscriptions.

BACCALAUREATE PROGRAMS

Degree BSN

Available Programs Generic Baccalaureate.

Program Entrance Requirements Minimum overall college GPA of 2.5, transcript of college record, CPR certification, written essay, immunizations. Transfer students are accepted. **Standardized tests** *Required:* SAT or ACT, TOEFL for international students. *Recommended:* ACT. **Application** *Deadline:* 7/15 (freshmen), rolling (transfer). *Notification:* continuous (freshmen).

Advanced Placement Credit given for nursing courses completed elsewhere dependent upon specific evaluations.

Contact Dr. Laura Meeks Festa, EdD, Professor and Chairperson, Department of Nursing, Henderson State University, Box 7803, 1100 Henderson Street, Arkadelphia, AR 71999-0001. *Telephone:* 870-230-5015. *Fax:* 870-230-5390.

University of Arkansas
Eleanor Mann School of Nursing
Fayetteville, Arkansas

http://www.uark.edu/coehp

Founded in 1871

DEGREES • BSN • MSN

Nursing Program Faculty 19 (26% with doctorates).

Baccalaureate Enrollment 115
Women 95% **Men** 5% **Minority** 7%

Nursing Student Activities Sigma Theta Tau, Student Nurses' Association.

Nursing Student Resources Academic advising; academic or career counseling; assistance for students with disabilities; bookstore; campus computer network; career placement assistance; computer lab; computer-assisted instruction; e-mail services; employment services for current students; housing assistance; interactive nursing skills videos; Internet; learning resource lab; library services; nursing audiovisuals; other; placement services for program completers; remedial services; resume preparation assistance; skills, simulation, or other laboratory; tutoring.

Library Facilities 1.7 million volumes (60,000 in health, 20,000 in nursing); 22,485 periodical subscriptions (130,000 health-care related).

BACCALAUREATE PROGRAMS

Degree BSN

Available Programs Baccalaureate for Second Degree; Generic Baccalaureate; LPN to Baccalaureate; LPN to RN Baccalaureate; RN Baccalaureate.

Study Options Full-time.

Program Entrance Requirements Minimum overall college GPA of 2.75, transcript of college record, CPR certification, health insurance, immunizations, minimum GPA in nursing prerequisites of 2.75, professional liability insurance/malpractice insurance, prerequisite course work. Transfer students are accepted. **Standardized tests** *Required:* SAT or ACT, TOEFL for international students. **Application** *Deadline:* 8/15 (freshmen), 8/15 (transfer). *Early decision:* 11/15. *Notification:* 11/15 (freshmen), 12/15 (early action). *Application fee:* $30.

Advanced Placement Credit by examination available. Credit given for nursing courses completed elsewhere dependent upon specific evaluations.

Expenses (2004–05) *Tuition, state resident:* full-time $4115; part-time $137 per credit hour. *Tuition, nonresident:* full-time $11,405; part-time $380 per credit hour. *Room and board:* $5514; room only: $3038 per academic year. *Required fees:* full-time $1020; part-time $34 per credit.

Financial Aid 80% of baccalaureate students in nursing programs received some form of financial aid in 2003–04. *Gift aid (need-based):* Federal Pell, FSEOG, state, private, college/university gift aid from institutional funds. *Loans:* FFEL (Subsidized and Unsubsidized Stafford PLUS), Perkins, state, college/university. *Work-Study:* Federal Work-Study. *Application deadline (priority):* 3/15.

University of Arkansas (continued)

Contact Dr. Thomas Kippenbrock, Director, Eleanor Mann School of Nursing, University of Arkansas, 217 Ozark Hall, Fayetteville, AR 72701. *Telephone:* 479-575-3907. *Fax:* 479-575-3218. *E-mail:* tkippen@uark.edu.

GRADUATE PROGRAMS

Expenses (2004–05) *Tuition, state resident:* full-time $4115. *Tuition, nonresident:* full-time $11,405. *Room and board:* $11,028; room only: $3038 per academic year. *Required fees:* full-time $1020.

Financial Aid 80% of graduate students in nursing programs received some form of financial aid in 2003–04.

Contact Dr. Thomas Kippenbrock, Director, Eleanor Mann School of Nursing, University of Arkansas, 217 Ozark Hall, Fayetteville, AR 72701. *Telephone:* 479-575-3907. *Fax:* 479-575-3218. *E-mail:* tkippen@uark.edu.

MASTER'S DEGREE PROGRAM

Degree MSN

Available Programs Master's.

Concentrations Available Nursing education. *Clinical nurse specialist programs in:* acute care, medical-surgical.

Study Options Part-time.

Degree Requirements 42 total credit hours, thesis or project.

CONTINUING EDUCATION PROGRAM

Contact Dr. Thomas Kippenbrock, Director, Eleanor Mann School of Nursing, University of Arkansas, 217 Ozark Hall, Fayetteville, AR 72701. *Telephone:* 479-575-3907. *Fax:* 479-575-3218. *E-mail:* tkippen@uark.edu.

University of Arkansas at Monticello

Division of Nursing
Monticello, Arkansas

http://www.uamont.edu/Nursing/

Founded in 1909

DEGREE • BSN

Nursing Program Faculty 7 (14% with doctorates).

Baccalaureate Enrollment 44
Women 95% **Men** 5% **Minority** 27%

Library Facilities 126,229 volumes (441 in health); 862 periodical subscriptions (44 health-care related).

BACCALAUREATE PROGRAMS

Degree BSN

Available Programs ADN to Baccalaureate; LPN to Baccalaureate; RN Baccalaureate.

Study Options Full-time.

Program Entrance Requirements Transcript of college record, CPR certification, written essay, health exam, immunizations, interview, minimum GPA in nursing prerequisites of 2.5, professional liability insurance/malpractice insurance, prerequisite course work. Transfer students are accepted. **Standardized tests** *Required:* TOEFL for international students. ***Placement:*** *Required:* SAT or ACT. *Recommended:* ACT. **Application** *Deadline:* 8/1 (freshmen), 8/1 (transfer).

Advanced Placement Credit by examination available. Credit given for nursing courses completed elsewhere dependent upon specific evaluations.

Expenses (2003–04) *Tuition, state resident:* part-time $90 per credit hour. *Tuition, nonresident:* part-time $204 per credit hour. *Required fees:* part-time $28 per credit.

Financial Aid 89% of baccalaureate students in nursing programs received some form of financial aid in 2002–03. *Gift aid (need-based):* Federal Pell, FSEOG, state, private, college/university gift aid from institutional funds. *Loans:* FFEL (Subsidized and Unsubsidized Stafford PLUS), Perkins. *Work-Study:* Federal Work-Study, part-time campus jobs. *Application deadline:* Continuous.

Contact Dr. Larry W. Eustace, RN, Chair, Division of Nursing, University of Arkansas at Monticello, PO Box 3606, Monticello, AR 71656. *Telephone:* 870-460-1069. *Fax:* 870-460-1969. *E-mail:* Eustace@uamont.edu.

University of Arkansas at Pine Bluff

Department of Nursing
Pine Bluff, Arkansas

http://www.uapb.com

Founded in 1873

DEGREE • BSN

Nursing Program Faculty 7.

Baccalaureate Enrollment 51
Women 94% **Men** 6% **Minority** 96%

Nursing Student Activities Student Nurses' Association.

Nursing Student Resources Academic advising; academic or career counseling; assistance for students with disabilities; bookstore; campus computer network; career placement assistance; computer lab; computer-assisted instruction; e-mail services; housing assistance; interactive nursing skills videos; Internet; learning resource lab; library services; nursing audiovisuals; remedial services; resume preparation assistance; skills, simulation, or other laboratory; tutoring.

Library Facilities 287,857 volumes (2,600 in health, 1,550 in nursing); 3,041 periodical subscriptions (60 health-care related).

BACCALAUREATE PROGRAMS

Degree BSN

Available Programs Generic Baccalaureate.

Study Options Full-time and part-time.

Program Entrance Requirements Minimum overall college GPA of 2.5, transcript of college record, CPR certification, written essay, health exam, immunizations, 3 letters of recommendation, minimum GPA in nursing prerequisites of 2.5, professional liability insurance/malpractice insurance, prerequisite course work. Transfer students are accepted. **Standardized tests** *Required:* TOEFL for international students. ***Placement:*** *Required:* SAT or ACT. **Application** *Deadline:* rolling (freshmen). *Notification:* continuous (freshmen).

Advanced Placement Credit by examination available. Credit given for nursing courses completed elsewhere dependent upon specific evaluations.

Expenses (2003–04) *Tuition, state resident:* full-time $2256; part-time $94 per credit hour. *Tuition, nonresident:* full-time $5256; part-time $219 per credit hour. *Room and board:* $5300; room only: $2344 per academic year. *Required fees:* full-time $6832; part-time $700 per term.

Financial Aid 88% of baccalaureate students in nursing programs received some form of financial aid in 2002–03. *Gift aid (need-based):* Federal Pell, FSEOG, state. *Loans:* FFEL (Subsidized and Unsubsidized Stafford PLUS), signature loans. *Work-Study:* Federal Work-Study. *Application deadline (priority):* 4/1.

Contact Dr. Irene T. Henderson, Department Chairperson, Department of Nursing, University of Arkansas at Pine Bluff, 1200 University Drive, Mail Slot 4973, Pine Bluff, AR 71601. *Telephone:* 870-575-8220. *Fax:* 870-575-8229. *E-mail:* henderson_i@uapb.edu.

University of Arkansas for Medical Sciences

College of Nursing
Little Rock, Arkansas

http://www.nursing.uams.edu

Founded in 1879

DEGREES • BSN • MN SC • PHD

Nursing Program Faculty 61 (46% with doctorates).

Baccalaureate Enrollment 282

Graduate Enrollment 163

Nursing Student Activities Sigma Theta Tau, Student Nurses' Association.

Nursing Student Resources Academic advising; assistance for students with disabilities; bookstore; campus computer network; computer lab; e-mail services; externships; interactive nursing skills videos; Internet; learning resource lab; library services; nursing audiovisuals; remedial services; skills, simulation, or other laboratory; tutoring.

Library Facilities 183,975 volumes (183,975 in health); 1,567 periodical subscriptions (1,567 health-care related).

BACCALAUREATE PROGRAMS

Degree BSN

Available Programs ADN to Baccalaureate; Accelerated Baccalaureate for Second Degree; Accelerated RN Baccalaureate; Generic Baccalaureate; RN Baccalaureate.

Site Options Hope, AR. *Distance Learning:* Texarkana, TX; Fayetteville, AR.

Study Options Full-time.

Program Entrance Requirements Minimum overall college GPA of 2.5, transcript of college record, CPR certification, health insurance, high school transcript, immunizations, professional liability insurance/malpractice insurance, prerequisite course work. Transfer students are accepted.

Advanced Placement Credit by examination available. Credit given for nursing courses completed elsewhere dependent upon specific evaluations.

Expenses (2003–04) *Tuition, state resident:* part-time $144 per credit hour. *Tuition, nonresident:* part-time $361 per credit hour.

Contact College of Nursing, College of Nursing, University of Arkansas for Medical Sciences, 4301 West Markham, #529, Little Rock, AR 72205-7199. *Telephone:* 501-686-5374. *Fax:* 501-686-8350.

GRADUATE PROGRAMS

Expenses (2003–04) *Tuition, state resident:* part-time $215 per credit hour. *Tuition, nonresident:* part-time $461 per credit hour.

Financial Aid Career-related internships or fieldwork and traineeships available.

Contact College of Nursing, College of Nursing, University of Arkansas for Medical Sciences, 4301 West Markham, #529, Little Rock, AR 72205-7199. *Telephone:* 501-686-5374. *Fax:* 501-686-8350.

MASTER'S DEGREE PROGRAM

Degree MN Sc

Concentrations Available Nursing administration; nursing education. *Clinical nurse specialist programs in:* acute care, adult health, pediatric. *Nurse practitioner programs in:* acute care, family health, gerontology, pediatric, women's health.

Site Options *Distance Learning:* Texarkana, TX; Fayetteville, AR.

Study Options Full-time and part-time.

Program Entrance Requirements Clinical experience, minimum overall college GPA of 2.85, transcript of college record, CPR certification, immunizations, physical assessment course, professional liability insurance/malpractice insurance, statistics course, MAT.

Advanced Placement Credit given for nursing courses completed elsewhere dependent upon specific evaluations.

Degree Requirements 39 total credit hours, thesis or project, comprehensive exam.

DOCTORAL DEGREE PROGRAM

Degree PhD

Available Programs Doctorate; Doctorate for Nurses with Non-Nursing Degrees; Post-Baccalaureate Doctorate.

Areas of Study Clinical practice, nursing administration, nursing education, nursing research, nursing science.

Program Entrance Requirements interview by faculty committee, interview, 4 letters of recommendation, MSN or equivalent, scholarly papers, statistics course, writing sample.

Degree Requirements 60 total credit hours, dissertation, oral exam, written exam, residency.

University of Central Arkansas
Department of Nursing
Conway, Arkansas

http://www.uca.edu/divisions/academic/nursing/

Founded in 1907

DEGREES • BSN • MSN

Nursing Program Faculty 26 (33% with doctorates).

Graduate Enrollment 53

Women 94% **Men** 6% **Minority** 8%

Nursing Student Activities Sigma Theta Tau, Student Nurses' Association.

Nursing Student Resources Academic advising; academic or career counseling; assistance for students with disabilities; bookstore; campus computer network; career placement assistance; computer lab; computer-assisted instruction; e-mail services; employment services for current students; externships; housing assistance; interactive nursing skills videos; Internet; learning resource lab; library services; nursing audiovisuals; paid internships; placement services for program completers; remedial services; resume preparation assistance; skills, simulation, or other laboratory; tutoring; unpaid internships.

Library Facilities 505,000 volumes (11,500 in health, 4,500 in nursing); 2,000 periodical subscriptions (80 health-care related).

BACCALAUREATE PROGRAMS

Degree BSN

Available Programs Generic Baccalaureate; LPN to Baccalaureate; RN Baccalaureate.

Program Entrance Requirements Minimum overall college GPA of 2.5, written essay, minimum GPA in nursing prerequisites, prerequisite course work. **Standardized tests** *Required:* SAT or ACT, TOEFL for international students. **Application** *Deadline:* rolling (freshmen), rolling (transfer). *Notification:* continuous (freshmen).

Financial Aid 85% of baccalaureate students in nursing programs received some form of financial aid in 2002–03.

Contact Ann Mattison, Program Coordinator, Department of Nursing, University of Central Arkansas, Doyne Health Science Center, 201 South Donaghey Avenue, Conway, AR 72035. *Telephone:* 501-450-3119. *Fax:* 501-450-5503. *E-mail:* annm@mail.uca.edu.

GRADUATE PROGRAMS

Financial Aid Fellowships (averaging $1,200 per year), 4 research assistantships (averaging $5,700 per year) were awarded; Federal Work-Study, traineeships, and unspecified assistantships also available.

Contact Director of Graduate Program, Department of Nursing, University of Central Arkansas, Doyne Health Science Center, 201 South Donaghey Avenue, Conway, AR 72035. *Telephone:* 501-450-3119. *Fax:* 501-450-5503.

MASTER'S DEGREE PROGRAM

Degree MSN

Available Programs Master's; RN to Master's.

Concentrations Available *Clinical nurse specialist programs in:* community health, family health, medical-surgical, psychiatric/mental health. *Nurse practitioner programs in:* adult health, family health, primary care.

Site Options *Distance Learning:* Fort Smith, AR; Russelville, AR.

Program Entrance Requirements Clinical experience, minimum overall college GPA of 2.7, CPR certification, written essay, immunizations, interview, letters of recommendation, professional liability insurance/malpractice insurance, resume, statistics course, GRE General Test. *Application deadline:* For fall admission, 3/1 (priority date); for spring admission, 10/1. Applications are processed on a rolling basis. *Application fee:* $25 ($40 for international students).

University of Central Arkansas (continued)

POST-MASTER'S PROGRAM

Areas of Study Nursing education. *Nurse practitioner programs in:* adult health, family health.

CALIFORNIA

Azusa Pacific University

School of Nursing
Azusa, California

http://www.apu.edu/nursing/grad

Founded in 1899

DEGREES • BSN • DSN • MSN

Nursing Program Faculty 52 (17% with doctorates).

Baccalaureate Enrollment 188
Women 91% **Men** 9% **Minority** 40% **Part-time** 5%

Graduate Enrollment 74
Women 96% **Men** 4% **Minority** 37%

Nursing Student Resources Assistance for students with disabilities; computer lab; interactive nursing skills videos; learning resource lab; library services; nursing audiovisuals; tutoring.

Library Facilities 185,708 volumes (14,005 in health, 4,692 in nursing); 14,031 periodical subscriptions (394 health-care related).

BACCALAUREATE PROGRAMS

Degree BSN

Available Programs ADN to Baccalaureate; Accelerated Baccalaureate; Accelerated RN Baccalaureate; Generic Baccalaureate.

Study Options Full-time and part-time.

Program Entrance Requirements Minimum overall college GPA of 3.0, transcript of college record, CPR certification, written essay, health exam, high school biology, high school chemistry, 2 years high school math, high school transcript, immunizations, 3 letters of recommendation, minimum high school GPA of 3.0, minimum GPA in nursing prerequisites of 3.0. Transfer students are accepted. **Standardized tests** *Required:* SAT or ACT, TOEFL for international students. **Application** *Deadline:* 6/1 (freshmen), 6/1 (transfer). *Early decision:* 12/1. *Notification:* continuous (freshmen), 1/15 (early action). *Application fee:* $45.

Advanced Placement Credit by examination available. Credit given for nursing courses completed elsewhere dependent upon specific evaluations.

Financial Aid 75% of baccalaureate students in nursing programs received some form of financial aid in 2003–04. *Gift aid (need-based):* Federal Pell, FSEOG, state, private, college/university gift aid from institutional funds, Federal Nursing. *Loans:* Federal Nursing Student Loans, FFEL (Subsidized and Unsubsidized Stafford PLUS), Perkins. *Work-Study:* Federal Work-Study. *Application deadline:* 7/1 (priority: 3/2).

Contact Mrs. Barbara Wiltsey, Administrative Assistant for Admissions, School of Nursing, Azusa Pacific University, 901 East Alosta Avenue, Azusa, CA 91702-7000. *Telephone:* 626-815-6000 Ext. 5501. *Fax:* 626-815-5414. *E-mail:* bwiltsey@apu.edu.

GRADUATE PROGRAMS

Expenses (2004–05) *Tuition:* full-time $5160; part-time $430 per unit.

Financial Aid 50% of graduate students in nursing programs received some form of financial aid in 2003–04. Teaching assistantships, scholarships, traineeships, and unspecified assistantships available. Aid available to part-time students. *Financial aid application deadline:* 10/15.

Contact Mrs. Barb Barthelmess, Graduate Program Coordinator, School of Nursing, Azusa Pacific University, 901 East Alosta Avenue, Azusa, CA 91702. *Telephone:* 626-815-5386. *Fax:* 626-815-5414. *E-mail:* bbarthelmess@apu.edu.

MASTER'S DEGREE PROGRAM

Degree MSN

Available Programs Accelerated Master's for Non-Nursing College Graduates; Accelerated Master's for Nurses with Non-Nursing Degrees; Master's.

Concentrations Available Nursing administration; nursing education. *Clinical nurse specialist programs in:* adult health, medical-surgical, parent-child, pediatric. *Nurse practitioner programs in:* adult health, family health, pediatric, primary care.

Site Options *Distance Learning:* San Bernardino, CA.

Study Options Full-time and part-time.

Program Entrance Requirements Clinical experience, computer literacy, minimum overall college GPA of 3.0, transcript of college record, CPR certification, written essay, immunizations, 3 letters of recommendation, nursing research course, physical assessment course, professional liability insurance/malpractice insurance, prerequisite course work, resume, statistics course. *Application deadline:* Applications are processed on a rolling basis. *Application fee:* $45 ($65 for international students).

Advanced Placement Credit by examination available. Credit given for nursing courses completed elsewhere dependent upon specific evaluations.

Degree Requirements 42 total credit hours, thesis or project, comprehensive exam.

POST-MASTER'S PROGRAM

Areas of Study Nursing administration; nursing education. *Clinical nurse specialist programs in:* adult health, medical-surgical, parent-child, pediatric, school health. *Nurse practitioner programs in:* adult health, family health, pediatric, primary care.

DOCTORAL DEGREE PROGRAM

Degree DSN

Available Programs Doctorate.

Areas of Study Community health, family health, nursing education.

Program Entrance Requirements Clinical experience, minimum overall college GPA of 3.5, interview by faculty committee, interview, 3 letters of recommendation, MSN or equivalent, scholarly papers, statistics course, vita, writing sample. *Application deadline:* Applications are processed on a rolling basis. *Application fee:* $45 ($65 for international students).

Degree Requirements 64 total credit hours, dissertation, oral exam, written exam.

CONTINUING EDUCATION PROGRAM

Contact Mrs. Kathryn Speck, Projects Coordinator, School of Nursing, Azusa Pacific University, 901 East Alosta Avenue, Azusa, CA 91702. *Telephone:* 626-815-5385. *Fax:* 626-815-5414. *E-mail:* Kspeck@apu.edu.

Biola University

Department of Nursing
La Mirada, California

Founded in 1908

DEGREE • BS

Nursing Program Faculty 14 (25% with doctorates).

Baccalaureate Enrollment 230
Women 96% **Men** 4% **Minority** 15% **International** 5% **Part-time** 1%

Nursing Student Activities Student Nurses' Association.

Nursing Student Resources Academic advising; academic or career counseling; assistance for students with disabilities; bookstore; campus computer network; career placement assistance; computer lab; computer-assisted instruction; e-mail services; employment services for current students; housing assistance; Internet; learning resource lab; library services; nursing audiovisuals; placement services for program completers; remedial services; resume preparation assistance; skills, simulation, or other laboratory; tutoring.

Library Facilities 279,560 volumes (20,000 in health, 10,000 in nursing); 13,123 periodical subscriptions (63 health-care related).

BACCALAUREATE PROGRAMS

Degree BS

Available Programs ADN to Baccalaureate; Baccalaureate for Second Degree; Generic Baccalaureate; LPN to Baccalaureate; RN Baccalaureate.

Study Options Full-time.

Program Entrance Requirements Minimum overall college GPA of 3.0, transcript of college record, CPR certification, written essay, health exam, health insurance, high school biology, high school chemistry, high school foreign language, 2 years high school math, high school transcript, immunizations, interview, 2 letters of recommendation, minimum high school GPA of 3.0, minimum GPA in nursing prerequisites of 2.0, professional liability insurance/malpractice insurance, prerequisite course work. Transfer students are accepted. **Standardized tests** *Required:* SAT or ACT, TOEFL for international students. **Application** *Deadline:* 3/1 (freshmen), 3/1 (transfer). *Early decision:* 12/1. *Notification:* 4/1 (freshmen), 12/24 (early action). *Application fee:* $45.

Advanced Placement Credit by examination available. Credit given for nursing courses completed elsewhere dependent upon specific evaluations.

Expenses (2004–05) *Tuition:* full-time $20,932; part-time $873 per credit hour. *International tuition:* $20,932 full-time. *Room and board:* $6800; room only: $3500 per academic year. *Required fees:* full-time $150.

Financial Aid 95% of baccalaureate students in nursing programs received some form of financial aid in 2003–04. *Gift aid (need-based):* Federal Pell, FSEOG, state, private, college/university gift aid from institutional funds. *Loans:* FFEL (Subsidized and Unsubsidized Stafford PLUS), Perkins, college/university, alternative loans. *Work-Study:* Federal Work-Study. *Application deadline (priority):* 3/2.

Contact Dr. Anne L. Gewe, Associate Chair and Associate Professor, Department of Nursing, Biola University, 13800 Biola Avenue, La Mirada, CA 90639. *Telephone:* 562-903-4850. *Fax:* 562-903-4803. *E-mail:* anne.gewe@biola.edu.

CONTINUING EDUCATION PROGRAM

Contact Dr. Anne L. Gewe, Associate Chair/Associate Professor, Department of Nursing, Biola University, 13800 Biola Avenue, La Mirada, CA 90639. *Telephone:* 562-903-4850. *Fax:* 562-903-4803. *E-mail:* anne.gewe@biola.edu.

California State University, Bakersfield

Program in Nursing
Bakersfield, California

http://www.csubak.edu

Founded in 1970

DEGREES • BSN • MSN

Nursing Program Faculty 20 (45% with doctorates).

Baccalaureate Enrollment 125
Women 90% **Men** 10% **Minority** 60% **International** 2% **Part-time** 5%

Graduate Enrollment 55
Women 87% **Men** 13% **Minority** 28%

Nursing Student Activities Sigma Theta Tau, Student Nurses' Association.

Nursing Student Resources Academic advising; assistance for students with disabilities; bookstore; campus computer network; career placement assistance; computer lab; daycare for children of students; e-mail services; employment services for current students; externships; interactive nursing skills videos; Internet; library services; nursing audiovisuals; paid internships; skills, simulation, or other laboratory.

Library Facilities 354,016 volumes (20,000 in health, 1,850 in nursing); 2,260 periodical subscriptions (90 health-care related).

BACCALAUREATE PROGRAMS

Degree BSN

Available Programs Generic Baccalaureate; RN Baccalaureate.

Site Options *Distance Learning:* Visalia, CA; Lancaster, CA.

Study Options Full-time.

Program Entrance Requirements Minimum overall college GPA of 2.0, transcript of college record, CPR certification, health exam, health insurance, high school transcript, immunizations, minimum high school GPA of 2.0, professional liability insurance/malpractice insurance, prerequisite course work. Transfer students are accepted. **Standardized tests** *Required:* SAT or ACT, TOEFL for international students. *Recommended:* SAT Subject Tests. **Application** *Deadline:* 9/23 (freshmen), 9/23 (transfer). *Notification:* continuous (freshmen). *Application fee:* $55.

Advanced Placement Credit given for nursing courses completed elsewhere dependent upon specific evaluations.

Expenses (2003–04) *Tuition, state resident:* full-time $1797; part-time $399 per quarter. *Tuition, nonresident:* full-time $8460; part-time $188 per unit.

Financial Aid 78% of baccalaureate students in nursing programs received some form of financial aid in 2002–03.

Contact Ms. Nancy Haley, Nursing Department Manager, Program in Nursing, California State University, Bakersfield, Romberg Nursing Education Building, 9001 Stockdale Highway, Bakersfield, CA 93311-1099. *Telephone:* 661-664-3101. *Fax:* 661-665-6903. *E-mail:* nhaley@csub.edu.

GRADUATE PROGRAMS

Expenses (2003–04) *Tuition, state resident:* full-time $1875; part-time $415 per quarter. *Tuition, nonresident:* full-time $8460; part-time $188 per unit. *International tuition:* $8460 full-time.

Financial Aid 80% of graduate students in nursing programs received some form of financial aid in 2002–03. Scholarships and traineeships available.

Contact Dr. Candace Meares, Graduate Coordinator, Program in Nursing, California State University, Bakersfield, 9001 Stockdale Highway, Bakersfield, CA 93311-1099. *Telephone:* 661-664-2093. *Fax:* 661-665-6347. *E-mail:* cmeares@csub.edu.

MASTER'S DEGREE PROGRAM

Degree MSN

Available Programs Accelerated RN to Master's; Master's; Master's for Nurses with Non-Nursing Degrees; RN to Master's.

Concentrations Available Nurse case management; nursing administration. *Clinical nurse specialist programs in:* community health. *Nurse practitioner programs in:* family health.

Study Options Full-time and part-time.

Program Entrance Requirements Clinical experience, minimum overall college GPA of 2.5, transcript of college record, CPR certification, written essay, immunizations, 3 letters of recommendation, nursing research course, physical assessment course, professional liability insurance/malpractice insurance, prerequisite course work, resume, statistics course, MAT. *Application deadline:* Applications are processed on a rolling basis. *Application fee:* $55.

Advanced Placement Credit given for nursing courses completed elsewhere dependent upon specific evaluations.

Degree Requirements 57 total credit hours, thesis or project.

POST-MASTER'S PROGRAM

Areas of Study *Clinical nurse specialist programs in:* school health.

California State University, Chico

School of Nursing
Chico, California

http://www.csuchico.edu/nurs/nurs.html

Founded in 1887

DEGREES • BSN • MSN

California State University, Chico (continued)

Nursing Program Faculty 26 (27% with doctorates).

Baccalaureate Enrollment 164
Women 87% **Men** 13% **Minority** 16% **Part-time** 2%

Graduate Enrollment 20
Women 100% **Part-time** 100%

Nursing Student Activities Sigma Theta Tau, Student Nurses' Association, nursing club.

Nursing Student Resources Academic advising; academic or career counseling; assistance for students with disabilities; bookstore; campus computer network; career placement assistance; computer lab; computer-assisted instruction; daycare for children of students; e-mail services; employment services for current students; externships; housing assistance; interactive nursing skills videos; Internet; learning resource lab; library services; nursing audiovisuals; paid internships; placement services for program completers; remedial services; resume preparation assistance; skills, simulation, or other laboratory; tutoring; unpaid internships.

Library Facilities 957,181 volumes (17,727 in health, 1,467 in nursing); 24,244 periodical subscriptions (133 health-care related).

BACCALAUREATE PROGRAMS

Degree BSN

Available Programs ADN to Baccalaureate; Baccalaureate for Second Degree; Generic Baccalaureate; LPN to Baccalaureate; RN Baccalaureate.

Study Options Full-time.

Program Entrance Requirements Minimum overall college GPA of 2.5, transcript of college record, CPR certification, health insurance, immunizations, minimum GPA in nursing prerequisites of 2.3, professional liability insurance/malpractice insurance, prerequisite course work. Transfer students are accepted. **Standardized tests** *Required:* SAT or ACT, TOEFL for international students. **Application** *Deadline:* 11/30 (freshmen), 11/30 (transfer). *Notification:* 3/1 (freshmen). *Application fee:* $55.

Advanced Placement Credit given for nursing courses completed elsewhere dependent upon specific evaluations.

Expenses (2004–05) *Tuition, state resident:* full-time $3154; part-time $1088 per semester. *Tuition, nonresident:* full-time $11,290; part-time $3611 per semester. *Room and board:* $8107; room only: $4999 per academic year. *Required fees:* full-time $300.

Financial Aid 75% of baccalaureate students in nursing programs received some form of financial aid in 2003–04. *Gift aid (need-based):* Federal Pell, FSEOG, state, private, college/university gift aid from institutional funds, United Negro College Fund. *Loans:* Federal Direct (Subsidized and Unsubsidized Stafford PLUS), Perkins, college/university. *Work-Study:* Federal Work-Study. *Application deadline:* Continuous.

Contact Dr. Sherry D. Fox, Director, School of Nursing, California State University, Chico, Chico, CA 95929-0200. *Telephone:* 530-898-5891. *Fax:* 530-898-4363. *E-mail:* sdfox@csuchico.edu.

GRADUATE PROGRAMS

Expenses (2004–05) *Tuition, state resident:* full-time $3640; part-time $1229 per semester. *Tuition, nonresident:* full-time $11,776; part-time $3263 per semester. *International tuition:* $11,776 full-time. *Room and board:* $8107; room only: $4999 per academic year. *Required fees:* full-time $89.

Financial Aid 75% of graduate students in nursing programs received some form of financial aid in 2003–04. Career-related internships or fieldwork available.

Contact Shelley Young, Graduate Coordinator, School of Nursing, California State University, Chico, Chico, CA 95929-0200. *Telephone:* 530-898-6207. *Fax:* 530-898-4363. *E-mail:* syoung@facultypo.csuchico.edu.

MASTER'S DEGREE PROGRAM

Degree MSN

Available Programs Master's.

Concentrations Available Nursing education. *Clinical nurse specialist programs in:* adult health.

Site Options *Distance Learning:* Chico, CA.

Study Options Part-time.

Program Entrance Requirements Clinical experience, minimum overall college GPA of 3.0, transcript of college record, CPR certification, immunizations, physical assessment course, professional liability insurance/malpractice insurance, statistics course, GRE or MAT. *Application deadline:* For fall admission, 3/1. Applications are processed on a rolling basis. *Application fee:* $55.

Advanced Placement Credit given for nursing courses completed elsewhere dependent upon specific evaluations.

Degree Requirements 30 total credit hours, thesis or project.

POST-MASTER'S PROGRAM

Areas of Study Nursing education.

CONTINUING EDUCATION PROGRAM

Contact Ms. Clare Robe, Continuing Education, School of Nursing, California State University, Chico, Chico, CA 95929-0250. *Telephone:* 530-898-6105. *E-mail:* rce@csuchico.edu.

California State University, Dominguez Hills

Program in Nursing
Carson, California

http://www.csudh.edu/soh/don/index.htm

Founded in 1960

DEGREES • BSN • MSN

Nursing Program Faculty 65 (80% with doctorates).

Baccalaureate Enrollment 700
Women 92% **Men** 8% **Minority** 49% **International** 10% **Part-time** 88%

Graduate Enrollment 275
Women 91% **Men** 9% **Minority** 40% **International** 5% **Part-time** 88%

Nursing Student Activities Nursing Honor Society, Sigma Theta Tau, Student Nurses' Association.

Nursing Student Resources Academic advising; academic or career counseling; assistance for students with disabilities; bookstore; campus computer network; career placement assistance; computer lab; computer-assisted instruction; daycare for children of students; e-mail services; externships; interactive nursing skills videos; Internet; learning resource lab; library services; nursing audiovisuals; remedial services; skills, simulation, or other laboratory; tutoring.

Library Facilities 440,181 volumes (10,000 in nursing).

BACCALAUREATE PROGRAMS

Degree BSN

Available Programs RN Baccalaureate.

Site Options *Distance Learning:* Palm Desert, CA; Riverside, CA; Long Beach, CA.

Study Options Full-time and part-time.

Program Entrance Requirements Minimum overall college GPA of 2.0, transcript of college record, prerequisite course work, RN licensure. Transfer students are accepted. **Standardized tests** *Required:* TOEFL for international students. *Required for some:* SAT or ACT. **Application** *Deadline:* rolling (freshmen), rolling (transfer). *Notification:* continuous (freshmen). *Application fee:* $55.

Expenses (2003–04) *Tuition, state resident:* full-time $2278; part-time $710 per semester. *Tuition, nonresident:* full-time $5000; part-time $2500 per semester. *Required fees:* part-time $100 per term.

Financial Aid 90% of baccalaureate students in nursing programs received some form of financial aid in 2002–03. *Gift aid (need-based):* Federal Pell, FSEOG, state, private, college/university gift aid from institutional funds. *Loans:* Federal Direct (Subsidized and Unsubsidized Stafford), FFEL, Perkins. *Work-Study:* Federal Work-Study. *Application deadline:* 4/15 (priority: 3/2).

Contact Dr. Laura M. Inouye, EdD, BSN Coordinator, Program in Nursing, California State University, Dominguez Hills, CSUDH Division of Nursing, 1000 East Victoria Street, WH A320, Welch Hall, 3rd Floor, Carson, CA 90747. *Telephone:* 310-243-2005. *Fax:* 310-516-3542. *E-mail:* linouye@csudh.edu.

GRADUATE PROGRAMS

Expenses (2003–04) *Tuition, state resident:* full-time $2488; part-time $770 per semester. *Tuition, nonresident:* full-time $6000; part-time $3000 per semester. *Required fees:* part-time $100 per term.

Financial Aid 90% of graduate students in nursing programs received some form of financial aid in 2002–03.

Contact Dr. Rose Aguilar Welch, EdD, MSN Coordinator, Program in Nursing, California State University, Dominguez Hills, CSUDH Division of Nursing, 1000 East Victoria Street, WH A320, Carson, CA 90747. *Telephone:* 310-243-2112. *Fax:* 310-516-3542. *E-mail:* rwelch@csudh.edu.

MASTER'S DEGREE PROGRAM

Degree MSN

Available Programs Master's; Master's for Nurses with Non-Nursing Degrees.

Concentrations Available Nursing administration; nursing education. *Clinical nurse specialist programs in:* gerontology, parent-child. *Nurse practitioner programs in:* family health.

Site Options *Distance Learning:* Long Beach, CA.

Study Options Full-time and part-time.

Program Entrance Requirements Clinical experience, minimum overall college GPA of 3.0, transcript of college record, written essay, nursing research course, physical assessment course, prerequisite course work, resume, statistics course. *Application deadline:* For fall admission, 6/1. *Application fee:* $55.

Degree Requirements 45 total credit hours, comprehensive exam.

POST-MASTER'S PROGRAM

Areas of Study Nursing administration; nursing education. *Clinical nurse specialist programs in:* gerontology, parent-child. *Nurse practitioner programs in:* family health.

CONTINUING EDUCATION PROGRAM

Contact Student Services Center, Program in Nursing, California State University, Dominguez Hills, CSUDH, Student Services Center, 1000 East Victoria Street, Carson, CA 90747. *Telephone:* 800-344-5484. *Fax:* 310-516-3542. *E-mail:* sohadvising@csudh.edu.

California State University, Fresno

Department of Nursing
Fresno, California

http://www.csufresno.edu/nursing/

Founded in 1911

DEGREES • BSN • MSN

Nursing Program Faculty 39 (33% with doctorates).

Baccalaureate Enrollment 360

Women 84% **Men** 16% **Minority** 54% **International** 10%

Graduate Enrollment 113

Women 83% **Men** 17% **Minority** 40% **International** 5% **Part-time** 40%

Nursing Student Activities Sigma Theta Tau, Student Nurses' Association.

Nursing Student Resources Academic advising; academic or career counseling; assistance for students with disabilities; bookstore; campus computer network; career placement assistance; computer lab; computer-assisted instruction; daycare for children of students; e-mail services; externships; housing assistance; interactive nursing skills videos; Internet; learning resource lab; library services; nursing audiovisuals; paid internships; placement services for program completers; remedial services; skills, simulation, or other laboratory; tutoring.

Library Facilities 23,961 volumes in health, 1,287 volumes in nursing; 2,617 periodical subscriptions (1,260 health-care related).

BACCALAUREATE PROGRAMS

Degree BSN

Available Programs ADN to Baccalaureate; Baccalaureate for Second Degree; Generic Baccalaureate; RN Baccalaureate.

Study Options Full-time and part-time.

Program Entrance Requirements Transcript of college record, CPR certification, health exam, immunizations, minimum GPA in nursing prerequisites of 3.0, professional liability insurance/malpractice insurance, prerequisite course work. Transfer students are accepted. **Standardized tests** *Required:* SAT or ACT, TOEFL for international students. **Application** *Deadline:* 2/1 (freshmen), 2/1 (transfer). *Application fee:* $55.

Advanced Placement Credit by examination available. Credit given for nursing courses completed elsewhere dependent upon specific evaluations.

Expenses (2004–05) *Tuition, state resident:* full-time $2414. *Tuition, nonresident:* full-time $6768; part-time $282 per credit hour. *International tuition:* $6768 full-time.

Financial Aid 65% of baccalaureate students in nursing programs received some form of financial aid in 2003–04. *Gift aid (need-based):* Federal Pell, FSEOG, state, private, college/university gift aid from institutional funds. *Loans:* Federal Nursing Student Loans, FFEL (Subsidized and Unsubsidized Stafford PLUS), Perkins, college/university. *Work-Study:* Federal Work-Study. *Application deadline (priority):* 3/1.

Contact Dr. Michael F. Russler, Chair and Professor, Department of Nursing, California State University, Fresno, 2345 East San Ramon Avenue, MH25, Fresno, CA 93740-8031. *Telephone:* 559-278-2041. *Fax:* 559-278-6360. *E-mail:* michaelr@csufresno.edu.

GRADUATE PROGRAMS

Expenses (2004–05) *Tuition, state resident:* full-time $2624. *Tuition, nonresident:* full-time $6768. *International tuition:* $6768 full-time.

Financial Aid 30% of graduate students in nursing programs received some form of financial aid in 2003–04. 2 teaching assistantships were awarded; career-related internships or fieldwork, Federal Work-Study, scholarships, and traineeships also available. Aid available to part-time students. *Financial aid application deadline:* 3/1.

Contact Dr. Kenn Kirksey, Professor, Department of Nursing, California State University, Fresno, 2345 East San Ramon Avenue, Fresno, CA 93740-8031. *Telephone:* 559-278-2041. *Fax:* 559-278-6360. *E-mail:* kkirksey@csufresno.edu.

MASTER'S DEGREE PROGRAM

Degree MSN

Available Programs Master's; Master's for Nurses with Non-Nursing Degrees.

Concentrations Available *Clinical nurse specialist programs in:* acute care, community health, critical care, pediatric, psychiatric/mental health, public health. *Nurse practitioner programs in:* family health, pediatric.

Study Options Full-time and part-time.

Program Entrance Requirements Clinical experience, computer literacy, minimum overall college GPA of 3.0, transcript of college record, CPR certification, written essay, 3 letters of recommendation, nursing research course, physical assessment course, professional liability insurance/malpractice insurance, prerequisite course work, resume, statistics course, GRE General Test. *Application deadline:* For fall admission, 8/1 (priority date); for spring admission, 12/1 (priority date). Applications are processed on a rolling basis. *Application fee:* $55.

Degree Requirements 37 total credit hours, thesis or project, comprehensive exam.

POST-MASTER'S PROGRAM

Areas of Study *Nurse practitioner programs in:* family health, pediatric.

CONTINUING EDUCATION PROGRAM

Contact Dr. Audrey Anderson, Dean, Extended Education, Department of Nursing, California State University, Fresno, 5005 North Maple Avenue, ED76, Fresno, CA 93740-0076. *Telephone:* 559-278-0333. *E-mail:* audrey_anderson@csufresno.edu.

California State University, Fullerton

Department of Nursing
Fullerton, California

http://nursing.fullerton.edu/

Founded in 1957

DEGREES • BSN • MSN

California State University, Fullerton (continued)

Nursing Program Faculty 23 (40% with doctorates).

Baccalaureate Enrollment 365
Women 91.5% **Men** 8.5% **Minority** 66% **Part-time** 88%

Graduate Enrollment 149
Women 71% **Men** 29% **Minority** 60% **Part-time** 45%

Nursing Student Activities Nursing Honor Society, Sigma Theta Tau.

Nursing Student Resources Academic advising; academic or career counseling; assistance for students with disabilities; bookstore; campus computer network; computer lab; daycare for children of students; e-mail services; housing assistance; Internet; library services; resume preparation assistance; skills, simulation, or other laboratory; tutoring.

Library Facilities 1.2 million volumes (16,500 in health, 780 in nursing); 10,827 periodical subscriptions (531 health-care related).

BACCALAUREATE PROGRAMS

Degree BSN

Available Programs ADN to Baccalaureate; Baccalaureate for Second Degree; RN Baccalaureate.

Site Options *Distance Learning:* Riverside, CA; Orange, CA.

Study Options Full-time and part-time.

Program Entrance Requirements Transcript of college record, CPR certification, immunizations, 2 letters of recommendation, minimum GPA in nursing prerequisites of 2.0, professional liability insurance/malpractice insurance, prerequisite course work, RN licensure. Transfer students are accepted. **Standardized tests** *Required:* SAT or ACT, TOEFL for international students. **Application** *Deadline:* 11/30 (freshmen), rolling (transfer). *Notification:* continuous (freshmen). *Application fee:* $55.

Advanced Placement Credit given for nursing courses completed elsewhere dependent upon specific evaluations.

Expenses (2004–05) *Tuition, nonresident:* part-time $339 per unit. *Required fees:* full-time $2804; part-time $913 per term.

Financial Aid *Gift aid (need-based):* Federal Pell, FSEOG, state, private, college/university gift aid from institutional funds. *Loans:* FFEL (Subsidized and Unsubsidized Stafford PLUS), Perkins, college/university. *Work-Study:* Federal Work-Study. *Application deadline (priority):* 3/2.

Contact Department of Nursing, California State University, Fullerton, EC-199, PO Box 6868, Fullerton, CA 92834-6868. *Telephone:* 714-278-3336. *Fax:* 714-278-3338. *E-mail:* nursing@fullerton.edu.

GRADUATE PROGRAMS

Expenses (2004–05) *Tuition, nonresident:* part-time $339 per unit. *Required fees:* full-time $3290; part-time $1054 per term.

Contact Department of Nursing, California State University, Fullerton, EC-199, PO Box 6868, Fullerton, CA 92834-6868. *Telephone:* 714-278-3336. *Fax:* 714-278-3338. *E-mail:* nursing@fullerton.edu.

MASTER'S DEGREE PROGRAM

Degree MSN

Available Programs Accelerated AD/RN to Master's; Master's.

Concentrations Available Nurse anesthesia; nurse-midwifery; nursing administration. *Nurse practitioner programs in:* family health, women's health.

Site Options Pasadena, CA.

Study Options Full-time and part-time.

Program Entrance Requirements Clinical experience, minimum overall college GPA of 3.0, transcript of college record, CPR certification, written essay, immunizations, interview, 3 letters of recommendation, nursing research course, professional liability insurance/malpractice insurance, statistics course.

Advanced Placement Credit given for nursing courses completed elsewhere dependent upon specific evaluations.

Degree Requirements 71 total credit hours, thesis or project.

California State University, Hayward

Department of Nursing and Health Sciences
Hayward, California

Founded in 1957

DEGREE • BS

Nursing Program Faculty 22 (42% with doctorates).

Nursing Student Activities Sigma Theta Tau, Student Nurses' Association.

Nursing Student Resources Academic advising; academic or career counseling; assistance for students with disabilities; bookstore; campus computer network; career placement assistance; computer lab; computer-assisted instruction; daycare for children of students; e-mail services; employment services for current students; Internet; learning resource lab; library services; nursing audiovisuals; remedial services; resume preparation assistance; skills, simulation, or other laboratory; tutoring; unpaid internships.

Library Facilities 908,577 volumes; 2,210 periodical subscriptions.

BACCALAUREATE PROGRAMS

Degree BS

Available Programs Generic Baccalaureate; RN Baccalaureate.

Site Options Concord, CA.

Study Options Full-time and part-time.

Program Entrance Requirements Minimum overall college GPA of 2.0, transcript of college record, health exam, minimum GPA in nursing prerequisites of 2.4, prerequisite course work. Transfer students are accepted. **Standardized tests** *Required:* TOEFL for international students. *Required for some:* SAT or ACT. **Application** *Deadline:* 9/7 (freshmen), 9/7 (transfer). *Notification:* continuous (freshmen). *Application fee:* $55.

Advanced Placement Credit given for nursing courses completed elsewhere dependent upon specific evaluations.

Financial Aid 45% of baccalaureate students in nursing programs received some form of financial aid in 2002–03. *Gift aid (need-based):* Federal Pell, FSEOG, state, private, college/university gift aid from institutional funds. *Loans:* FFEL (Subsidized and Unsubsidized Stafford PLUS), Perkins, college/university. *Work-Study:* Federal Work-Study. *Application deadline (priority):* 3/2.

Contact Lynn Condit, Administrative Assistant, Department of Nursing and Health Sciences, California State University, Hayward, 25800 Carlos Bee Boulevard, Hayward, CA 94542. *Telephone:* 510-885-3481. *Fax:* 510-885-2156. *E-mail:* lcondit@csuhayward.edu.

California State University, Long Beach

Department of Nursing
Long Beach, California

http://www.csulb.edu/depts/nursing/

Founded in 1949

DEGREES • BSN • MS/MHSA • MSN

Nursing Student Activities Nursing Honor Society, Sigma Theta Tau, Student Nurses' Association.

Nursing Student Resources Library services; tutoring.

Library Facilities 1.5 million volumes; 18,749 periodical subscriptions.

BACCALAUREATE PROGRAMS

Degree BSN

Available Programs Accelerated Baccalaureate; Accelerated Baccalaureate for Second Degree; Generic Baccalaureate; RN Baccalaureate.

Study Options Full-time.

Program Entrance Requirements Transcript of college record, CPR certification, health exam, immunizations, interview, minimum GPA in nursing prerequisites of 2.5, professional liability insurance/malpractice insurance, prerequisite course work. **Standardized tests** *Required:* SAT or ACT, TOEFL for international students. **Application** *Deadline:* 11/30 (freshmen), 11/30 (transfer). *Notification:* continuous (freshmen). *Application fee:* $55.

Advanced Placement Credit by examination available.

Expenses (2003–04) *Tuition, area resident:* full-time $1181; part-time $752 per semester.

Financial Aid 65% of baccalaureate students in nursing programs received some form of financial aid in 2002–03. *Gift aid (need-based):* Federal Pell, FSEOG, state, private, college/university gift aid from institutional funds. *Loans:* FFEL (Subsidized and Unsubsidized Stafford PLUS), Perkins. *Work-Study:* Federal Work-Study. *Application deadline (priority):* 3/2.

Contact Dr. Beth Keely, Undergraduate Adviser, Department of Nursing, California State University, Long Beach, 1250 Bellflower Boulevard, Long Beach, CA 90840. *Telephone:* 562-985-4478. *Fax:* 562-985-2382. *E-mail:* bkeely@earthlink.com.

GRADUATE PROGRAMS

Expenses (2003–04) *Tuition, state resident:* full-time $2500; part-time $812 per semester. *Tuition, nonresident:* full-time $4250; part-time $2312 per semester.

Financial Aid 50% of graduate students in nursing programs received some form of financial aid in 2002–03. Federal Work-Study, institutionally sponsored loans, and scholarships available. *Financial aid application deadline:* 3/2.

Contact Alison Kliachko-Trafas, Administrative Assistant, Department of Nursing, California State University, Long Beach, 1250 Bellflower Boulevard, Long Beach, CA 90840-0119. *Telephone:* 562-985-4473. *Fax:* 562-985-2382. *E-mail:* akliachk@csulb.edu.

MASTER'S DEGREE PROGRAM

Degrees MS/MHSA; MSN

Available Programs Master's.

Concentrations Available Health-care administration; nursing education. *Clinical nurse specialist programs in:* adult health. *Nurse practitioner programs in:* adult health, family health, gerontology, pediatric, psychiatric/mental health, women's health.

Study Options Full-time and part-time.

Program Entrance Requirements Clinical experience, minimum overall college GPA of 2.75, transcript of college record, written essay, 3 letters of recommendation, physical assessment course, prerequisite course work, resume, statistics course. *Application deadline:* For fall admission, 7/1; for spring admission, 12/1. Applications are processed on a rolling basis. *Application fee:* $55.

Degree Requirements 37 total credit hours, thesis or project, comprehensive exam.

POST-MASTER'S PROGRAM

Areas of Study *Clinical nurse specialist programs in:* adult health. *Nurse practitioner programs in:* adult health, family health, gerontology, pediatric, school health.

California State University, Los Angeles

School of Nursing
Los Angeles, California

http://www.calstatela.edu/dept/nursing/

Founded in 1947

DEGREES • BS • MS

Nursing Program Faculty 31 (39% with doctorates).

Baccalaureate Enrollment 300

Graduate Enrollment 100

Nursing Student Resources Academic advising.

Library Facilities 1.7 million volumes; 2,724 periodical subscriptions.

BACCALAUREATE PROGRAMS

Degree BS

Available Programs Generic Baccalaureate; RN Baccalaureate.

Program Entrance Requirements **Standardized tests** *Required:* SAT or ACT, TOEFL for international students. **Application** *Deadline:* 6/15 (freshmen), 6/15 (transfer). *Application fee:* $55.

Contact Jane G. Connor, Undergraduate Adviser, School of Nursing, California State University, Los Angeles, 5151 State University Drive, Los Angeles, CA 90032-8171. *Telephone:* 323-343-4703. *Fax:* 323-343-6454. *E-mail:* jconner@calstatela.edu.

GRADUATE PROGRAMS

Financial Aid Federal Work-Study available.

Contact Dr. Judith Papenhausen, RN, Chairperson/Head of Nursing Program, School of Nursing, California State University, Los Angeles, 5151 State University Drive, Los Angeles, CA 90032. *Telephone:* 323-343-4700. *Fax:* 323-343-6454. *E-mail:* jpapen@calstatela.edu.

MASTER'S DEGREE PROGRAM

Degree MS

Available Programs Accelerated Master's for Nurses with Non-Nursing Degrees; Accelerated RN to Master's; Master's.

Concentrations Available Nurse case management; nursing administration; nursing education. *Clinical nurse specialist programs in:* psychiatric/mental health. *Nurse practitioner programs in:* acute care, adult health, family health, pediatric, primary care, women's health.

Program Entrance Requirements Minimum overall college GPA of 3.0, nursing research course, professional liability insurance/malpractice insurance, statistics course. *Application deadline:* For fall admission, 6/30; for spring admission, 2/1. Applications are processed on a rolling basis. *Application fee:* $55.

POST-MASTER'S PROGRAM

Areas of Study *Nurse practitioner programs in:* acute care, adult health, family health, pediatric, primary care.

California State University, Northridge

Nursing Program
Northridge, California

http://www.csun.edu/~nursing/

Founded in 1958

DEGREE • BSN

Nursing Program Faculty 8 (38% with doctorates).

Baccalaureate Enrollment 60

Women 88% **Men** 12% **Minority** 60% **International** 12% **Part-time** 90%

Nursing Student Activities Nursing Honor Society, Student Nurses' Association.

Nursing Student Resources Academic advising; academic or career counseling; assistance for students with disabilities; bookstore; campus computer network; career placement assistance; computer lab; computer-assisted instruction; daycare for children of students; e-mail services; housing assistance; Internet; learning resource lab; library services; nursing audiovisuals; remedial services; resume preparation assistance; skills, simulation, or other laboratory; tutoring.

Library Facilities 1.2 million volumes (61,848 in health, 1,401 in nursing); 2,754 periodical subscriptions (303 health-care related).

California State University, Northridge (continued)

BACCALAUREATE PROGRAMS

Degree BSN

Available Programs RN Baccalaureate.

Study Options Full-time and part-time.

Program Entrance Requirements Minimum overall college GPA of 2.5, transcript of college record, CPR certification, written essay, health exam, health insurance, immunizations, interview, 3 letters of recommendation, minimum GPA in nursing prerequisites of 2.5, professional liability insurance/malpractice insurance, prerequisite course work, RN licensure. Transfer students are accepted. **Standardized tests** *Required:* TOEFL for international students. *Recommended:* SAT or ACT. **Application** *Deadline:* 11/30 (freshmen), rolling (transfer). *Early decision:* 8/30. *Notification:* continuous (freshmen), 9/30 (early action). *Application fee:* $55.

Advanced Placement Credit by examination available. Credit given for nursing courses completed elsewhere dependent upon specific evaluations.

Expenses (2004–05) *Tuition, nonresident:* full-time $339; part-time $339 per credit hour. *International tuition:* $339 full-time. *Required fees:* full-time $2778; part-time $900 per term.

Financial Aid 20% of baccalaureate students in nursing programs received some form of financial aid in 2003–04. *Gift aid (need-based):* Federal Pell, FSEOG, state, private, college/university gift aid from institutional funds. *Loans:* FFEL (Subsidized and Unsubsidized Stafford PLUS), Perkins, college/university. *Work-Study:* Federal Work-Study. *Application deadline (priority):* 3/2.

Contact Dr. Martha Highfield, Acting Program Director and Professor of Nursing, Nursing Program, California State University, Northridge, 18111 Nordhoff Street, Northridge, CA 91330-8285. *Telephone:* 818-677-3649. *Fax:* 818-677-2045. *E-mail:* martha.highfield@csun.edu.

California State University, Sacramento

Division of Nursing
Sacramento, California

http://www.hhs.csus.edu/nrs

Founded in 1947

DEGREES • BSN • MS

Nursing Program Faculty 50 (38% with doctorates).

Baccalaureate Enrollment 300

Graduate Enrollment 180

Nursing Student Activities Sigma Theta Tau, Student Nurses' Association.

Nursing Student Resources Academic advising; academic or career counseling; assistance for students with disabilities; bookstore; campus computer network; computer lab; computer-assisted instruction; daycare for children of students; e-mail services; externships; housing assistance; interactive nursing skills videos; Internet; learning resource lab; library services; nursing audiovisuals; placement services for program completers; remedial services; resume preparation assistance; skills, simulation, or other laboratory; tutoring.

Library Facilities 1.3 million volumes (33,000 in health); 3,761 periodical subscriptions (327 health-care related).

BACCALAUREATE PROGRAMS

Degree BSN

Available Programs ADN to Baccalaureate; Generic Baccalaureate; LPN to RN Baccalaureate; RN Baccalaureate.

Study Options Full-time.

Program Entrance Requirements Minimum overall college GPA of 2.75, transcript of college record, CPR certification, health exam, health insurance, high school biology, high school chemistry, high school foreign language, high school math, immunizations, minimum GPA in nursing prerequisites of 2.75, professional liability insurance/malpractice insurance, prerequisite course work. Transfer students are accepted. **Standardized tests** *Required:* TOEFL for international students. *Required for some:* SAT or ACT. **Application** *Deadline:* 11/30 (freshmen), 4/1 (transfer). *Early decision:* 11/30. *Notification:* 11/1 (freshmen), 11/1 (early action). *Application fee:* $55.

Advanced Placement Credit by examination available.

Expenses (2003–04) *Tuition, state resident:* full-time $2039; part-time $1378 per semester. *Tuition, nonresident:* full-time $5518; part-time $2081 per semester. *Required fees:* full-time $2039; part-time $1378 per term.

Financial Aid 60% of baccalaureate students in nursing programs received some form of financial aid in 2002–03. *Gift aid (need-based):* Federal Pell, FSEOG, state, private, college/university gift aid from institutional funds, Federal Nursing. *Loans:* Federal Nursing Student Loans, Federal Direct (Subsidized and Unsubsidized Stafford), FFEL, Perkins, state, college/university. *Work-Study:* Federal Work-Study, part-time campus jobs. *Application deadline (priority):* 3/2.

Contact Nancy Beers, Administrative Support Coordinator, Division of Nursing, California State University, Sacramento, 6000 J Street, Sacramento, CA 95819-6096. *Telephone:* 916-278-6525. *E-mail:* beersnj@csus.edu.

GRADUATE PROGRAMS

Financial Aid Research assistantships, teaching assistantships, career-related internships or fieldwork and Federal Work-Study available.

Contact Kathleen Jarvis, Graduate Coordinator, Division of Nursing, California State University, Sacramento, 6000 J Street, Sacramento, CA 95819-6096. *Telephone:* 916-278-7298. *Fax:* 916-278-6311. *E-mail:* jarviska@csus.edu.

MASTER'S DEGREE PROGRAM

Degree MS

Available Programs Master's; Master's for Nurses with Non-Nursing Degrees.

Concentrations Available Nursing administration; nursing education. *Clinical nurse specialist programs in:* adult health, community health, family health, gerontology, medical-surgical, parent-child, perinatal, psychiatric/mental health, school health. *Nurse practitioner programs in:* family health, primary care.

Study Options Part-time.

Program Entrance Requirements Clinical experience, minimum overall college GPA of 3.0, transcript of college record, CPR certification, written essay, immunizations, 3 letters of recommendation, nursing research course, professional liability insurance/malpractice insurance, prerequisite course work, statistics course, GRE. *Application deadline:* For fall admission, 5/1; for spring admission, 11/1. *Application fee:* $55.

Advanced Placement Credit by examination available. Credit given for nursing courses completed elsewhere dependent upon specific evaluations.

Degree Requirements 39 total credit hours, thesis or project.

CONTINUING EDUCATION PROGRAM

Contact Dr. Robyn M. Nelson, Chairperson, Division of Nursing, California State University, Sacramento, 6000 J Street, Sacramento, CA 95819-6096. *Telephone:* 916-278-6525. *Fax:* 916-278-6311. *E-mail:* nelsonrm@csus.edu.

California State University, San Bernardino

Department of Nursing
San Bernardino, California

http://nursing.csusb.edu

Founded in 1965

DEGREES • BSN • MSN

Nursing Program Faculty 24 (16% with doctorates).

Baccalaureate Enrollment 203

Women 88% **Men** 12% **Minority** 49%

Graduate Enrollment 36
Women 92% **Men** 8% **Minority** 42%

Nursing Student Activities Nursing Honor Society, Sigma Theta Tau, Student Nurses' Association.

Nursing Student Resources Academic advising; academic or career counseling; campus computer network; computer lab; computer-assisted instruction; externships; Internet; nursing audiovisuals; remedial services; skills, simulation, or other laboratory.

Library Facilities 731,259 volumes (1,500 in health, 1,000 in nursing); 2,028 periodical subscriptions (5,000 health-care related).

BACCALAUREATE PROGRAMS

Degree BSN

Available Programs ADN to Baccalaureate; RN Baccalaureate.

Study Options Full-time.

Program Entrance Requirements Transcript of college record, CPR certification, written essay, health exam, health insurance, immunizations, minimum GPA in nursing prerequisites of 3.0, professional liability insurance/malpractice insurance, prerequisite course work. Transfer students are accepted. **Standardized tests** *Required:* TOEFL for international students. *Required for some:* SAT or ACT. **Application** *Deadline:* rolling (freshmen), rolling (transfer). *Notification:* continuous (freshmen). *Application fee:* $55.

Advanced Placement Credit by examination available. Credit given for nursing courses completed elsewhere dependent upon specific evaluations.

Expenses (2003–04) *Tuition, state resident:* full-time $2681; part-time $900 per quarter. *Required fees:* full-time $300.

Financial Aid 79% of baccalaureate students in nursing programs received some form of financial aid in 2002–03. *Gift aid (need-based):* Federal Pell, FSEOG, state, college/university gift aid from institutional funds. *Loans:* Federal Direct (Subsidized and Unsubsidized Stafford), FFEL, Perkins. *Work-Study:* Federal Work-Study, part-time campus jobs. *Application deadline (priority):* 3/2.

Contact Ms. Anna Wilson, Lecturer, Recruiter, Department of Nursing, California State University, San Bernardino, 5500 University Parkway, San Bernadino, CA 92407. *Telephone:* 909-880-5384. *Fax:* 909-880-7089. *E-mail:* amwilson@csusb.edu.

GRADUATE PROGRAMS

Financial Aid 55% of graduate students in nursing programs received some form of financial aid in 2002–03.

Contact Dr. Susan Lloyd, Director, Masters Program, Department of Nursing, California State University, San Bernardino, 5500 University Parkway, San Bernadino, CA 92407. *Telephone:* 909-880-5380. *Fax:* 909-880-7089. *E-mail:* slloyd@csusb.edu.

MASTER'S DEGREE PROGRAM

Degree MSN

Concentrations Available Nurse case management; nursing education. *Clinical nurse specialist programs in:* community health, home health care, school health.

Study Options Full-time and part-time.

Program Entrance Requirements Clinical experience, minimum overall college GPA of 3.0, transcript of college record, prerequisite course work, statistics course.

Advanced Placement Credit given for nursing courses completed elsewhere dependent upon specific evaluations.

Degree Requirements 65 total credit hours, thesis or project.

California State University, Stanislaus

Department of Nursing
Turlock, California

http://www.csustan.edu/Nursing/index.htm

Founded in 1957

DEGREE • BSN

Nursing Program Faculty 13 (23% with doctorates).

Baccalaureate Enrollment 158
Women 87% **Men** 13% **Minority** 38% **Part-time** 30%

Nursing Student Activities Sigma Theta Tau, Student Nurses' Association.

Nursing Student Resources Academic advising; academic or career counseling; assistance for students with disabilities; bookstore; campus computer network; career placement assistance; computer lab; computer-assisted instruction; daycare for children of students; e-mail services; employment services for current students; externships; interactive nursing skills videos; Internet; learning resource lab; library services; nursing audiovisuals; resume preparation assistance; skills, simulation, or other laboratory; tutoring.

Library Facilities 365,870 volumes (12,642 in health, 1,399 in nursing); 1,693 periodical subscriptions (93 health-care related).

BACCALAUREATE PROGRAMS

Degree BSN

Available Programs ADN to Baccalaureate; Generic Baccalaureate; LPN to Baccalaureate.

Site Options *Distance Learning:* Stockton, CA.

Study Options Full-time.

Program Entrance Requirements Minimum overall college GPA of 2.5, transcript of college record, CPR certification, health exam, immunizations, minimum GPA in nursing prerequisites of 2.5, professional liability insurance/malpractice insurance, prerequisite course work. Transfer students are accepted. **Standardized tests** *Required:* SAT or ACT, TOEFL for international students. **Application** *Deadline:* 5/1 (freshmen), 5/1 (transfer). *Early decision:* 11/30. *Notification:* 3/1 (freshmen), 3/1 (out-of-state freshmen), 3/1 (early decision). *Application fee:* $55.

Advanced Placement Credit given for nursing courses completed elsewhere dependent upon specific evaluations.

Expenses (2004–05) *Tuition, state resident:* full-time $2676; part-time $247 per semester. *Tuition, nonresident:* full-time $11,136; part-time $350 per unit. *Room and board:* $7800; room only: $5700 per academic year. *Required fees:* full-time $550.

Financial Aid 43% of baccalaureate students in nursing programs received some form of financial aid in 2003–04. *Gift aid (need-based):* Federal Pell, FSEOG, state, private, college/university gift aid from institutional funds. *Loans:* FFEL (Subsidized and Unsubsidized Stafford PLUS), Perkins, college/university. *Work-Study:* Federal Work-Study, part-time campus jobs. *Application deadline (priority):* 3/2.

Contact Mrs. Ilene M. Worthington, Administrative Coordinator, Department of Nursing, California State University, Stanislaus, 801 West Monte Vista Avenue, Turlock, CA 95382. *Telephone:* 209-667-3141. *Fax:* 209-667-3690. *E-mail:* iworthington@csustan.edu.

Dominican University of California

Program in Occupational Therapy
San Rafael, California

Founded in 1890

DEGREES • BSN • MSN

Nursing Program Faculty 35 (11% with doctorates).

Baccalaureate Enrollment 361
Women 93% **Men** 7% **Minority** 54% **International** 2% **Part-time** 12%

Graduate Enrollment 19
Women 95% **Men** 5% **Minority** 21% **Part-time** 21%

Nursing Student Activities Nursing Honor Society, Sigma Theta Tau, Student Nurses' Association, nursing club.

Nursing Student Resources Academic advising; academic or career counseling; assistance for students with disabilities; bookstore; campus computer network; career placement assistance; computer lab; computer-assisted instruction; e-mail services; housing assistance; interactive nursing skills videos; Internet; learning resource lab; library services; nursing audiovisuals; resume preparation assistance; skills, simulation, or other laboratory; tutoring.

Dominican University of California (continued)

Library Facilities 95,000 volumes (1,200 in health, 1,000 in nursing); 508 periodical subscriptions (1,300 health-care related).

BACCALAUREATE PROGRAMS

Degree BSN

Available Programs ADN to Baccalaureate; Baccalaureate for Second Degree; Generic Baccalaureate; LPN to Baccalaureate; LPN to RN Baccalaureate; RN Baccalaureate.

Study Options Full-time and part-time.

Program Entrance Requirements Minimum overall college GPA of 2.5, transcript of college record, CPR certification, written essay, health exam, health insurance, high school biology, high school chemistry, 2 years high school math, high school transcript, immunizations, 1 letter of recommendation, minimum high school GPA of 2.7, minimum GPA in nursing prerequisites of 2.7, prerequisite course work. Transfer students are accepted. **Standardized tests** *Required:* SAT or ACT, TOEFL for international students. *Recommended:* SAT Subject Tests. **Application** *Deadline:* 8/1 (freshmen), rolling (transfer). *Notification:* continuous until 9/1 (freshmen). *Application fee:* $40.

Advanced Placement Credit by examination available. Credit given for nursing courses completed elsewhere dependent upon specific evaluations.

Expenses (2004–05) *Tuition:* full-time $24,254; part-time $1011 per credit hour. *International tuition:* $24,254 full-time. *Room and board:* $10,270; room only: $5986 per academic year. *Required fees:* full-time $200; part-time $100 per term.

Financial Aid 97% of baccalaureate students in nursing programs received some form of financial aid in 2003–04. *Gift aid (need-based):* Federal Pell, FSEOG, state, private, college/university gift aid from institutional funds. *Loans:* FFEL (Subsidized and Unsubsidized Stafford PLUS), Perkins. *Work-Study:* Federal Work-Study, part-time campus jobs. *Application deadline (priority):* 3/2.

Contact Art Criss, Director of Admissions, Program in Occupational Therapy, Dominican University of California, 50 Acacia Avenue, San Rafael, CA 94901-2298. *Telephone:* 415-257-1376. *Fax:* 415-485-3214. *E-mail:* acriss@dominican.edu.

GRADUATE PROGRAMS

Expenses (2004–05) *Tuition:* full-time $12,150; part-time $675 per credit hour. *International tuition:* $12,150 full-time. *Room and board:* $10,270; room only: $5986 per academic year. *Required fees:* full-time $200; part-time $100 per term.

Financial Aid 53% of graduate students in nursing programs received some form of financial aid in 2003–04. 3 fellowships (averaging $3,000 per year) were awarded; career-related internships or fieldwork, Federal Work-Study, scholarships, and tuition waivers (partial) also available. Aid available to part-time students.

Contact Lorrie Crivello, Director of Pathways and Graduate Admissions, Program in Occupational Therapy, Dominican University of California, 50 Acacia Avenue, San Rafael, CA 94901-2298. *Telephone:* 415-458-3754. *Fax:* 415-485-3214. *E-mail:* lcrivello@dominican.edu.

MASTER'S DEGREE PROGRAM

Degree MSN

Available Programs Master's; Master's for Nurses with Non-Nursing Degrees.

Concentrations Available Integrated health practice. *Clinical nurse specialist programs in:* gerontology.

Study Options Full-time and part-time.

Program Entrance Requirements Clinical experience, minimum overall college GPA of 3.0, transcript of college record, CPR certification, interview, 2 letters of recommendation, nursing research course, statistics course. *Application deadline:* For fall admission, 5/1; for spring admission, 11/1. Applications are processed on a rolling basis. *Application fee:* $40.

Advanced Placement Credit given for nursing courses completed elsewhere dependent upon specific evaluations.

Degree Requirements 45 total credit hours, thesis or project.

CONTINUING EDUCATION PROGRAM

Contact Ms. Lorrie Crivello, Director of Pathways and Graduate Admissions, Program in Occupational Therapy, Dominican University of California, 50 Acacia Avenue, San Rafael, CA 94901-2298. *Telephone:* 415-458-3754. *Fax:* 415-485-3214. *E-mail:* lcrivello@dominican.edu.

See full description on page 474.

Holy Names University
Department of Nursing
Oakland, California

Founded in 1868

DEGREES • BSN • MSN • MSN/MBA

Nursing Program Faculty 44.

Baccalaureate Enrollment 150

Graduate Enrollment 45

Nursing Student Activities Nursing Honor Society, Sigma Theta Tau.

Library Facilities 116,031 volumes; 200 periodical subscriptions.

BACCALAUREATE PROGRAMS

Degree BSN

Available Programs RN Baccalaureate.

Program Entrance Requirements RN licensure. **Standardized tests** *Required:* SAT or ACT, TOEFL for international students. **Application** *Deadline:* 8/1 (freshmen), 8/1 (transfer). *Notification:* continuous (freshmen). *Application fee:* $35.

Expenses (2003–04) *Tuition:* part-time $395 per credit hour.

Contact Dr. Fay L. Bower, Chair and Professor, Department of Nursing, Holy Names University, 3500 Mountain Boulevard, Oakland, CA 94619-1699. *Telephone:* 510-436-1024. *Fax:* 510-436-1376. *E-mail:* bower@hnc.edu.

GRADUATE PROGRAMS

Expenses (2003–04) *Tuition:* part-time $440 per credit hour.

Financial Aid Scholarships available.

Contact Dr. Fay L. Bower, Chair and Professor, Department of Nursing, Holy Names University, 3500 Mountain Boulevard, Oakland, CA 94619-1699. *Telephone:* 510-436-1024. *Fax:* 510-436-1376. *E-mail:* bower@hnc.edu.

MASTER'S DEGREE PROGRAM

Degrees MSN; MSN/MBA

Available Programs Master's.

Concentrations Available Nursing administration. *Nurse practitioner programs in:* family health.

Program Entrance Requirements *Application deadline:* For fall admission, 8/1 (priority date); for spring admission, 12/1 (priority date). Applications are processed on a rolling basis. *Application fee:* $50.

POST-MASTER'S PROGRAM

Areas of Study Nursing administration. *Nurse practitioner programs in:* family health.

Humboldt State University
Department of Nursing
Arcata, California

http://www.humboldt.edu/~nurs

Founded in 1913

DEGREE • BSN

Nursing Program Faculty 12 (25% with doctorates).

Baccalaureate Enrollment 122

Women 89% **Men** 11% **Minority** 22%

Nursing Student Activities Sigma Theta Tau, Student Nurses' Association.

Nursing Student Resources Academic advising; academic or career counseling; assistance for students with disabilities; bookstore; campus computer network; career placement assistance; computer lab; computer-assisted instruction; daycare for children of students; e-mail services; employment services for current students; housing assistance; interactive nursing skills videos; Internet; learning resource lab; library services;

nursing audiovisuals; placement services for program completers; resume preparation assistance; skills, simulation, or other laboratory; tutoring.

Library Facilities 585,386 volumes (16,000 in health, 750 in nursing); 2,629 periodical subscriptions (152 health-care related).

BACCALAUREATE PROGRAMS

Degree BSN

Available Programs ADN to Baccalaureate; Baccalaureate for Second Degree; Generic Baccalaureate; International Nurse to Baccalaureate; LPN to Baccalaureate; RN Baccalaureate.

Study Options Full-time.

Program Entrance Requirements Minimum overall college GPA of 2.5, transcript of college record, CPR certification, health exam, high school foreign language, 2 years high school math, 1 year of high school science, high school transcript, immunizations, minimum GPA in nursing prerequisites of 2.5, professional liability insurance/malpractice insurance, prerequisite course work. Transfer students are accepted. **Standardized tests** *Required:* TOEFL for international students. *Required for some:* SAT or ACT. **Application** *Deadline:* rolling (freshmen), 11/30 (transfer). *Notification:* continuous (freshmen). *Application fee:* $55.

Advanced Placement Credit given for nursing courses completed elsewhere dependent upon specific evaluations.

Expenses (2003–04) *Tuition, state resident:* full-time $2536; part-time $839 per semester. *Tuition, nonresident:* full-time $9304; part-time $282 per contact hour. *International tuition:* $9304 full-time. *Room and board:* $7499; room only: $4449 per academic year. *Required fees:* full-time $120.

Financial Aid 70% of baccalaureate students in nursing programs received some form of financial aid in 2002–03. *Gift aid (need-based):* Federal Pell, FSEOG, state, private, college/university gift aid from institutional funds. *Loans:* Federal Direct (Subsidized and Unsubsidized Stafford PLUS), Perkins. *Work-Study:* Federal Work-Study. *Application deadline (priority):* 3/2.

Contact Marshelle Thobaben, RN, Chair and Professor, Department of Nursing, Humboldt State University, 1 Harpst Street, Arcata, CA 95521. *Telephone:* 707-826-3215. *Fax:* 707-826-5141. *E-mail:* nurs@humboldt.edu.

Loma Linda University

School of Nursing
Loma Linda, California

http://www.llu.edu/llu/nursing/

Founded in 1905

DEGREES • BS • MS • MS/MA • MS/MPH • PHD

Nursing Program Faculty 40 (50% with doctorates).

Baccalaureate Enrollment 324
Women 78% **Men** 22% **Minority** 68% **International** 19% **Part-time** 22%

Graduate Enrollment 53
Women 96% **Men** 4% **Minority** 40% **International** 8% **Part-time** 82%

Nursing Student Activities Nursing Honor Society, Sigma Theta Tau, nursing club.

Nursing Student Resources Academic advising; academic or career counseling; assistance for students with disabilities; bookstore; campus computer network; computer lab; computer-assisted instruction; e-mail services; employment services for current students; housing assistance; interactive nursing skills videos; Internet; learning resource lab; library services; nursing audiovisuals; paid internships; resume preparation assistance; skills, simulation, or other laboratory; tutoring.

Library Facilities 322,657 volumes (158,000 in health, 3,916 in nursing); 1,394 periodical subscriptions (2,152 health-care related).

BACCALAUREATE PROGRAMS

Degree BS

Available Programs Accelerated Baccalaureate for Second Degree; Accelerated RN Baccalaureate; Generic Baccalaureate; RN Baccalaureate.

Study Options Full-time and part-time.

Program Entrance Requirements Minimum overall college GPA of 3.0, transcript of college record, CPR certification, written essay, health exam, high school transcript, immunizations, interview, 2 letters of recommendation, minimum GPA in nursing prerequisites of 3.0, prerequisite course work. Transfer students are accepted. **Standardized tests** *Required:* TOEFL for international students. **Application** *Deadline:* 4/15 (freshmen). *Application fee:* $60.

Advanced Placement Credit by examination available. Credit given for nursing courses completed elsewhere dependent upon specific evaluations.

Expenses (2004–05) *Tuition:* part-time $465 per credit hour.

Financial Aid 95% of baccalaureate students in nursing programs received some form of financial aid in 2003–04.

Contact Mrs. Stephanie Larsen, Director of Admissions, Marketing, and Recruiting, School of Nursing, Loma Linda University, Loma Linda, CA 92350. *Telephone:* 909-558-4923. *Fax:* 909-558-0175. *E-mail:* sllarsen@sn.llu.edu.

GRADUATE PROGRAMS

Financial Aid 26% of graduate students in nursing programs received some form of financial aid in 2003–04.

Contact Ms. Joyce Bates, Administrative Assistant, School of Nursing, Loma Linda University, Loma Linda, CA 92350. *Telephone:* 909-558-8061. *Fax:* 909-558-4134. *E-mail:* jbates@sn.llu.edu.

MASTER'S DEGREE PROGRAM

Degrees MS; MS/MA; MS/MPH

Available Programs Master's; Master's for Nurses with Non-Nursing Degrees; RN to Master's.

Concentrations Available Nursing administration. *Clinical nurse specialist programs in:* adult health, parent-child, pediatric, school health. *Nurse practitioner programs in:* adult health, family health, neonatal health, pediatric, primary care.

Study Options Full-time and part-time.

Program Entrance Requirements Clinical experience, minimum overall college GPA of 3.0, transcript of college record, immunizations, interview, 3 letters of recommendation, nursing research course, prerequisite course work, statistics course.

Degree Requirements 60 total credit hours, comprehensive exam.

POST-MASTER'S PROGRAM

Areas of Study *Nurse practitioner programs in:* adult health, family health, neonatal health, pediatric.

DOCTORAL DEGREE PROGRAM

Degree PhD

Available Programs Doctorate.

Areas of Study Ethics, faculty preparation, health policy, human health and illness, individualized study, nursing education, nursing research, nursing science.

Program Entrance Requirements Clinical experience, minimum overall college GPA of 3.5, interview by faculty committee, interview, 3 letters of recommendation, MSN or equivalent, scholarly papers, statistics course, vita, writing sample.

Degree Requirements 95 total credit hours, dissertation, oral exam, written exam, residency.

See full description on page 510.

Mount St. Mary's College

Department of Nursing
Los Angeles, California

http://www.msmc.la.edu/nursing/

Founded in 1925

DEGREES • BSN • MSN

Nursing Program Faculty 15 (27% with doctorates).

Mount St. Mary's College (continued)

Nursing Student Activities Student Nurses' Association.

Nursing Student Resources Academic advising; bookstore; library services.

Library Facilities 140,000 volumes (4,000 in health, 1,000 in nursing); 750 periodical subscriptions (150 health-care related).

BACCALAUREATE PROGRAMS

Degree BSN

Available Programs ADN to Baccalaureate; Accelerated Baccalaureate; Generic Baccalaureate.

Program Entrance Requirements Minimum overall college GPA of 2.7, transcript of college record, CPR certification, written essay, health exam, high school chemistry, high school transcript, immunizations, 1 letter of recommendation, minimum GPA in nursing prerequisites of 2.5, professional liability insurance/malpractice insurance, prerequisite course work. Transfer students are accepted. **Standardized tests** *Required:* SAT or ACT, TOEFL for international students. *Recommended:* SAT. **Application** *Deadline:* 2/15 (freshmen), 3/15 (transfer). *Early decision:* 12/1. *Notification:* continuous (freshmen), 1/1 (early action). *Application fee:* $40.

Advanced Placement Credit by examination available. Credit given for nursing courses completed elsewhere dependent upon specific evaluations.

Contact Admissions Officer, Department of Nursing, Mount St. Mary's College, 12001 Chalon Road, Los Angeles, CA 90049-1599. *Telephone:* 800-999-9893. *E-mail:* admissions@msmc.la.edu.

GRADUATE PROGRAMS

Contact Graduate Program. *Telephone:* 213-477-2676.

MASTER'S DEGREE PROGRAM

Degree MSN

Available Programs Master's.

Study Options Part-time.

Program Entrance Requirements Minimum overall college GPA of 3.0, transcript of college record, CPR certification, immunizations, professional liability insurance/malpractice insurance.

Degree Requirements 37 total credit hours.

National University

Department of Nursing
La Jolla, California

http://www.nu.edu/nursing-handbook

Founded in 1971

DEGREE • BSN

Nursing Program Faculty 9 (70% with doctorates).

Baccalaureate Enrollment 20

Women 80% **Men** 20% **Part-time** 75%

Nursing Student Resources Academic advising; academic or career counseling; assistance for students with disabilities; bookstore; campus computer network; computer lab; Internet; library services; nursing audiovisuals; other; remedial services; resume preparation assistance; tutoring.

Library Facilities 226,049 volumes (12,195 in health, 1,447 in nursing); 2,794 periodical subscriptions (446 health-care related).

BACCALAUREATE PROGRAMS

Degree BSN

Available Programs RN Baccalaureate.

Study Options Full-time and part-time.

Program Entrance Requirements Minimum overall college GPA of 2.0, transcript of college record, CPR certification, immunizations, interview, minimum GPA in nursing prerequisites of 2.75, professional liability insurance/malpractice insurance, prerequisite course work. Transfer students are accepted. **Standardized tests** *Required:* TOEFL for international students. **Application** *Deadline:* rolling (freshmen), rolling (transfer). *Notification:* continuous (freshmen). *Application fee:* $60.

Advanced Placement Credit given for nursing courses completed elsewhere dependent upon specific evaluations.

Expenses (2003–04) *Tuition:* full-time $11,400; part-time $950 per course. *Required fees:* full-time $60.

Contact Ms. Holly Nyland, Admissions Counselor, Department of Nursing, National University, 11255 North Torrey Pines Road, La Jolla, CA 92037. *Telephone:* 800-628-8648 Ext. 7221. *Fax:* 858-642-8715. *E-mail:* hnyland@nu.edu.

Pacific Union College

Department of Nursing
Angwin, California

Founded in 1882

DEGREE • BSN

Nursing Program Faculty 9 (33% with doctorates).

Baccalaureate Enrollment 50

Women 94% **Men** 6% **Minority** 39% **Part-time** 56%

Nursing Student Activities Student Nurses' Association.

Nursing Student Resources Academic advising; academic or career counseling; assistance for students with disabilities; bookstore; campus computer network; career placement assistance; computer lab; e-mail services; externships; housing assistance; Internet; learning resource lab; library services; nursing audiovisuals; skills, simulation, or other laboratory; tutoring.

Library Facilities 173,839 volumes; 812 periodical subscriptions (109 health-care related).

BACCALAUREATE PROGRAMS

Degree BSN

Site Options Hanford, CA; Fairfield, CA; Los Angeles, CA.

Study Options Full-time and part-time.

Program Entrance Requirements Transcript of college record, CPR certification, health exam, health insurance, immunizations, interview, 2 letters of recommendation, minimum GPA in nursing prerequisites of 2.0, professional liability insurance/malpractice insurance, prerequisite course work, RN licensure. Transfer students are accepted. **Standardized tests** *Required:* SAT and SAT Subject Tests or ACT, TOEFL for international students. *Recommended:* ACT, SAT or ACT. ***Placement:*** *Required:* SAT and SAT Subject Tests or ACT. **Application** *Deadline:* rolling (freshmen), rolling (transfer). *Application fee:* $30.

Advanced Placement Credit given for nursing courses completed elsewhere dependent upon specific evaluations.

Expenses (2003–04) *Tuition:* full-time $17,115; part-time $495 per credit hour. *Room and board:* $4950 per academic year.

Financial Aid 93% of baccalaureate students in nursing programs received some form of financial aid in 2002–03.

Contact Mrs. Carol Williams, RN, Coordinator, BSN Program, Department of Nursing, Pacific Union College, One Angwin Avenue, Angwin, CA 94508. *Telephone:* 707-965-7619. *Fax:* 707-965-6499. *E-mail:* cwilliams@puc.edu.

CONTINUING EDUCATION PROGRAM

Contact Dr. Nancy L. Tucker, Chair, Department of Nursing, Pacific Union College, One Angwin Avenue, Angwin, CA 94508. *Telephone:* 707-965-7262. *Fax:* 707-965-6499. *E-mail:* ntucker@puc.edu.

Point Loma Nazarene University

School of Nursing
San Diego, California

http://www.ptloma.edu/nursing

Founded in 1902

DEGREES • BSN • MSN

Nursing Program Faculty 20 (25% with doctorates).

Baccalaureate Enrollment 138
Women 92% **Men** 8% **Minority** 22% **Part-time** 2%

Graduate Enrollment 32
Women 97% **Men** 3% **Minority** 22% **Part-time** 44%

Nursing Student Activities Sigma Theta Tau, Student Nurses' Association.

Nursing Student Resources Academic advising; academic or career counseling; bookstore; campus computer network; computer lab; computer-assisted instruction; daycare for children of students; e-mail services; employment services for current students; externships; housing assistance; interactive nursing skills videos; Internet; learning resource lab; library services; nursing audiovisuals; paid internships; resume preparation assistance; skills, simulation, or other laboratory; tutoring; unpaid internships.

Library Facilities 152,377 volumes; 25,505 periodical subscriptions.

BACCALAUREATE PROGRAMS

Degree BSN

Available Programs ADN to Baccalaureate; Baccalaureate for Second Degree; Generic Baccalaureate; LPN to RN Baccalaureate; RN Baccalaureate.

Study Options Full-time.

Program Entrance Requirements Minimum overall college GPA of 2.7, transcript of college record, CPR certification, written essay, health exam, health insurance, high school foreign language, 2 years high school math, 1 year of high school science, high school transcript, immunizations, interview, 3 letters of recommendation, minimum high school GPA, minimum GPA in nursing prerequisites of 2.3, prerequisite course work. Transfer students are accepted. **Standardized tests** *Required:* SAT or ACT, TOEFL for international students. *Recommended:* SAT. **Application** *Deadline:* 3/1 (freshmen), rolling (transfer). *Early decision:* 12/1. *Notification:* continuous (freshmen), 1/15 (early action). *Application fee:* $45.

Advanced Placement Credit by examination available. Credit given for nursing courses completed elsewhere dependent upon specific evaluations.

Expenses (2004–05) *Tuition:* full-time $19,040; part-time $795 per unit. *Room and board:* $6680 per academic year. *Required fees:* full-time $500; part-time $250 per term.

Financial Aid 90% of baccalaureate students in nursing programs received some form of financial aid in 2003–04.

Contact Prof. Dottie E. Crummy, Dean, School of Nursing, Point Loma Nazarene University, 3900 Lomaland Drive, San Diego, CA 92106-2899. *Telephone:* 619-849-2425. *Fax:* 619-849-2672. *E-mail:* dcrummy@ptloma.edu.

GRADUATE PROGRAMS

Expenses (2004–05) *Tuition:* full-time $10,500; part-time $495 per unit.

Financial Aid 80% of graduate students in nursing programs received some form of financial aid in 2003–04.

Contact Prof. Barbara Taylor, MSN Director/Associate Dean, School of Nursing, School of Nursing, Point Loma Nazarene University, 3900 Lomaland Drive, San Diego, CA 92106-2899. *Telephone:* 619-849-2425. *E-mail:* bataylor@ptloma.edu.

MASTER'S DEGREE PROGRAM

Degree MSN

Available Programs Master's.

Concentrations Available Nursing education. *Clinical nurse specialist programs in:* family health, gerontology, medical-surgical, psychiatric/mental health.

Site Options San Diego, CA.

Study Options Full-time.

Program Entrance Requirements Computer literacy, minimum overall college GPA of 3.0, transcript of college record, CPR certification, written essay, immunizations, interview, letters of recommendation, nursing research course, physical assessment course, professional liability insurance/malpractice insurance, statistics course.

Advanced Placement Credit given for nursing courses completed elsewhere dependent upon specific evaluations.

Degree Requirements 43 total credit hours, thesis or project.

CONTINUING EDUCATION PROGRAM

Contact Ms. Marsha Reece, Program Assistant, School of Nursing, Point Loma Nazarene University, 3900 Lomaland Drive, San Diego, CA 92106-2899. *Telephone:* 619-849-7055. *Fax:* 619-849-2672. *E-mail:* mreece@ptloma.edu.

Samuel Merritt College

School of Nursing
Oakland, California

Founded in 1909

DEGREES • BSN • MSN

Nursing Program Faculty 89 (18% with doctorates).

Baccalaureate Enrollment 321
Women 92% **Men** 8% **Minority** 61% **Part-time** 10%

Graduate Enrollment 301
Women 83% **Men** 17% **Minority** 47% **Part-time** 19%

Nursing Student Activities Sigma Theta Tau, Student Nurses' Association.

Nursing Student Resources Academic advising; academic or career counseling; assistance for students with disabilities; campus computer network; computer lab; computer-assisted instruction; e-mail services; employment services for current students; housing assistance; interactive nursing skills videos; Internet; learning resource lab; library services; nursing audiovisuals; resume preparation assistance; skills, simulation, or other laboratory; tutoring; unpaid internships.

Library Facilities 33,000 volumes (15,259 in health, 2,637 in nursing); 60 periodical subscriptions (494 health-care related).

BACCALAUREATE PROGRAMS

Degree BSN

Available Programs Generic Baccalaureate.

Study Options Full-time and part-time.

Program Entrance Requirements Minimum overall college GPA of 2.5, transcript of college record, written essay, health exam, health insurance, high school biology, high school chemistry, high school foreign language, 2 years high school math, 3 years high school science, high school transcript, immunizations, 1 letter of recommendation, minimum high school GPA of 2.5, minimum GPA in nursing prerequisites of 2.5, prerequisite course work. Transfer students are accepted. **Standardized tests** *Required:* SAT or ACT, TOEFL for international students. **Application** *Deadline:* 3/1 (freshmen), 3/1 (transfer). *Notification:* continuous (freshmen). *Application fee:* $35.

Advanced Placement Credit by examination available. Credit given for nursing courses completed elsewhere dependent upon specific evaluations.

Expenses (2004–05) *Tuition:* full-time $23,718; part-time $986 per unit. *International tuition:* $23,718 full-time. *Room and board:* room only: $6507 per academic year. *Required fees:* full-time $160.

Financial Aid 86% of baccalaureate students in nursing programs received some form of financial aid in 2003–04.

Contact Ms. Anne E. Seed, Director of Admissions, School of Nursing, Samuel Merritt College, Office of Admissions, 370 Hawthorne Avenue, Oakland, CA 94609. *Telephone:* 510-869-6610. *Fax:* 510-869-6525. *E-mail:* admission@samuelmerritt.edu.

GRADUATE PROGRAMS

Expenses (2004–05) *Tuition:* part-time $723 per unit. *Room and board:* room only: $8676 per academic year. *Required fees:* full-time $50.

Financial Aid 81% of graduate students in nursing programs received some form of financial aid in 2003–04. Career-related internships or fieldwork, Federal Work-Study, scholarships, and traineeships available. Aid available to part-time students. *Financial aid application deadline:* 3/2.

Contact Ms. Anne E. Seed, Director of Admissions, School of Nursing, Samuel Merritt College, Office of Admissions, 370 Hawthorne Avenue, Oakland, CA 94609. *Telephone:* 510-869-6610. *Fax:* 510-869-6525. *E-mail:* aseed@samuelmerritt.edu.

Samuel Merritt College (continued)

MASTER'S DEGREE PROGRAM

Degree MSN

Available Programs Master's; Master's for Non-Nursing College Graduates; Master's for Nurses with Non-Nursing Degrees.

Concentrations Available Nurse anesthesia; nurse case management. *Nurse practitioner programs in:* family health.

Site Options *Distance Learning:* Sacramento, CA.

Study Options Full-time and part-time.

Program Entrance Requirements Clinical experience, computer literacy, minimum overall college GPA of 3.0, transcript of college record, CPR certification, written essay, immunizations, interview, 2 letters of recommendation, prerequisite course work, statistics course. *Application deadline:* For fall admission, 1/15 (priority date). Applications are processed on a rolling basis. *Application fee:* $50.

Advanced Placement Credit by examination available. Credit given for nursing courses completed elsewhere dependent upon specific evaluations.

Degree Requirements Thesis or project, comprehensive exam.

POST-MASTER'S PROGRAM

Areas of Study Nurse anesthesia; nurse case management. *Nurse practitioner programs in:* family health.

San Diego State University

School of Nursing

San Diego, California

http://nursing.sdsu.edu

Founded in 1897

DEGREES • BSN • MSN

Nursing Program Faculty 57 (47% with doctorates).

Nursing Student Resources Computer lab; library services; skills, simulation, or other laboratory.

Library Facilities 1.3 million volumes (36,000 in health, 14,000 in nursing); 8,245 periodical subscriptions (335 health-care related).

BACCALAUREATE PROGRAMS

Degree BSN

Available Programs Generic Baccalaureate; RN Baccalaureate.

Study Options Full-time and part-time.

Program Entrance Requirements Minimum overall college GPA of 3.0, transcript of college record, CPR certification, written essay, health exam, high school foreign language, high school math, high school transcript, immunizations, minimum high school GPA of 2.5, minimum GPA in nursing prerequisites of 2.5, professional liability insurance/malpractice insurance, prerequisite course work. Transfer students are accepted. **Standardized tests** *Required:* SAT or ACT, TOEFL for international students. **Application** *Deadline:* 11/30 (freshmen), 11/30 (transfer). *Notification:* 3/1 (freshmen). *Application fee:* $55.

Advanced Placement Credit given for nursing courses completed elsewhere dependent upon specific evaluations.

Contact School of Nursing, School of Nursing, San Diego State University, 5500 Campanile Drive, San Diego, CA 92182-0254. *Telephone:* 619-594-5357. *Fax:* 619-594-2765.

GRADUATE PROGRAMS

Financial Aid Career-related internships or fieldwork, scholarships, and traineeships available.

Contact Associate Professor and Graduate Adviser, School of Nursing, San Diego State University, 5500 Campanile Drive, San Diego, CA 92182-0254. *Telephone:* 619-594-2770. *Fax:* 619-594-2765.

MASTER'S DEGREE PROGRAM

Degree MSN

Concentrations Available Nurse-midwifery. *Clinical nurse specialist programs in:* adult health, community health, gerontology, school health. *Nurse practitioner programs in:* acute care, adult health, family health, gerontology, women's health.

Study Options Full-time and part-time.

Program Entrance Requirements Clinical experience, minimum overall college GPA of 3.0, transcript of college record, written essay, interview, 3 letters of recommendation, nursing research course, physical assessment course, professional liability insurance/malpractice insurance, statistics course, GRE General Test. *Application deadline:* For fall admission, 1/15; for spring admission, 11/1. Applications are processed on a rolling basis. *Application fee:* $55.

Advanced Placement Credit by examination available. Credit given for nursing courses completed elsewhere dependent upon specific evaluations.

Degree Requirements 39 total credit hours, thesis or project, comprehensive exam.

POST-MASTER'S PROGRAM

Areas of Study Nurse-midwifery.

CONTINUING EDUCATION PROGRAM

Contact School of Nursing, School of Nursing, San Diego State University, 5500 Campanile Drive, San Diego, CA 92182-0254. *Telephone:* 619-594-5357. *Fax:* 619-594-2765.

See full description on page 540.

San Francisco State University

School of Nursing

San Francisco, California

Founded in 1899

DEGREES • BSN • MSN

Nursing Program Faculty 40 (50% with doctorates).

Baccalaureate Enrollment 250

Women 88% **Men** 12% **Minority** 53% **International** 2% **Part-time** 5%

Graduate Enrollment 180

Women 80% **Men** 20% **Minority** 80% **International** 10% **Part-time** 20%

Nursing Student Activities Sigma Theta Tau, Student Nurses' Association.

Nursing Student Resources Academic advising; academic or career counseling; assistance for students with disabilities; bookstore; campus computer network; career placement assistance; computer lab; computer-assisted instruction; daycare for children of students; e-mail services; employment services for current students; externships; housing assistance; interactive nursing skills videos; Internet; learning resource lab; library services; nursing audiovisuals; other; placement services for program completers; remedial services; resume preparation assistance; skills, simulation, or other laboratory; tutoring.

Library Facilities 780,230 volumes (11,000 in health, 1,500 in nursing); 5,679 periodical subscriptions (200 health-care related).

BACCALAUREATE PROGRAMS

Degree BSN

Available Programs ADN to Baccalaureate; Accelerated LPN to Baccalaureate; Generic Baccalaureate; RN Baccalaureate.

Study Options Full-time.

Program Entrance Requirements Minimum overall college GPA of 2.5, transcript of college record, CPR certification, health exam, health insurance, immunizations, minimum GPA in nursing prerequisites of 2.5, professional liability insurance/malpractice insurance, prerequisite course work. Transfer students are accepted. **Standardized tests** *Required:* TOEFL for international students. *Required for some:* SAT or ACT. **Application** *Deadline:* rolling (freshmen). *Notification:* continuous (freshmen). *Application fee:* $55.

Advanced Placement Credit by examination available. Credit given for nursing courses completed elsewhere dependent upon specific evaluations.

Expenses (2003–04) *Tuition, state resident:* full-time $2500; part-time $210 per credit hour. *Tuition, nonresident:* full-time $6000; part-time $300 per credit hour. *International tuition:* $6000 full-time. *Room and board:* $14,400; room only: $1000 per academic year. *Required fees:* full-time $300; part-time $30 per credit; part-time $65 per term.

Financial Aid 60% of baccalaureate students in nursing programs received some form of financial aid in 2002–03.

Contact Dr. Karen C. Johnson-Brennan, Associate Director of Undergraduate Programs and Professor, School of Nursing, San Francisco State University, 1600 Holloway Avenue, San Francsico, CA 94132. *Telephone:* 415-338-2315 Ext. 1. *Fax:* 415-338-0555. *E-mail:* kcjb@sfsu.edu.

GRADUATE PROGRAMS

Expenses (2003–04) *Tuition, state resident:* full-time $2750; part-time $250 per credit hour. *Tuition, nonresident:* full-time $7000; part-time $350 per credit hour. *International tuition:* $7000 full-time. *Room and board:* $14,400; room only: $10,000 per academic year. *Required fees:* full-time $350.

Financial Aid 80% of graduate students in nursing programs received some form of financial aid in 2002–03. 35 fellowships were awarded; career-related internships or fieldwork also available. *Financial aid application deadline:* 3/1.

Contact Dr. Amy Nichols, Associate Director for Graduate Programs, School of Nursing, San Francisco State University, 1600 Holloway Avenue, 371 Burk Hall, San Francisco, CA 94132-4161. *Telephone:* 415-338-1802. *Fax:* 415-338-0555. *E-mail:* anichols@sfsu.edu.

MASTER'S DEGREE PROGRAM

Degree MSN

Available Programs Accelerated Master's for Non-Nursing College Graduates; Accelerated Master's for Nurses with Non-Nursing Degrees; Master's; Master's for Non-Nursing College Graduates; Master's for Nurses with Non-Nursing Degrees.

Concentrations Available Nurse case management; nursing administration. *Clinical nurse specialist programs in:* adult health, perinatal, public health. *Nurse practitioner programs in:* family health.

Study Options Full-time and part-time.

Program Entrance Requirements Minimum overall college GPA of 3.0, transcript of college record, CPR certification, written essay, immunizations, 3 letters of recommendation, nursing research course, professional liability insurance/malpractice insurance, resume, statistics course. *Application deadline:* For fall admission, 11/30 (priority date); for spring admission, 5/31. Applications are processed on a rolling basis. *Application fee:* $55.

Advanced Placement Credit by examination available. Credit given for nursing courses completed elsewhere dependent upon specific evaluations.

Degree Requirements 36 total credit hours, thesis or project.

POST-MASTER'S PROGRAM

Areas of Study Nursing administration. *Nurse practitioner programs in:* family health.

CONTINUING EDUCATION PROGRAM

Contact Dr. Beatrice Crofts Yorker, Director, School of Nursing, San Francisco State University, 371 Burk Hall, 1600 Holloway Avenue, San Francisco, CA 94129. *Telephone:* 415-405-3660. *Fax:* 415-338-0555. *E-mail:* byorker@sfsu.edu.

San Jose State University

School of Nursing
San Jose, California

Founded in 1857

DEGREES • BS • MS

Nursing Program Faculty 55 (52% with doctorates).

Baccalaureate Enrollment 550
Women 92% **Men** 8% **Minority** 76% **Part-time** 20%

Graduate Enrollment 101
Women 92% **Men** 8% **Minority** 46% **Part-time** 83%

Nursing Student Activities Sigma Theta Tau, Student Nurses' Association, nursing club.

Nursing Student Resources Academic advising; academic or career counseling; assistance for students with disabilities; bookstore; career placement assistance; computer lab; computer-assisted instruction; housing assistance; interactive nursing skills videos; Internet; learning resource lab; library services; nursing audiovisuals; skills, simulation, or other laboratory; tutoring.

Library Facilities 280 volumes in health, 250 volumes in nursing; 80 periodical subscriptions health-care related.

BACCALAUREATE PROGRAMS

Degree BS

Available Programs Generic Baccalaureate; RPN to Baccalaureate.

Site Options Salinas, CA; Gilroy, CA.

Study Options Full-time and part-time.

Program Entrance Requirements Transcript of college record, health insurance, 3 years high school math, minimum high school GPA of 2.0, minimum GPA in nursing prerequisites of 2.0, professional liability insurance/malpractice insurance, prerequisite course work. Transfer students are accepted. **Standardized tests** *Required:* TOEFL for international students. *Required for some:* SAT or ACT. **Application** *Deadline:* 11/30 (freshmen), rolling (transfer). *Notification:* continuous (freshmen). *Application fee:* $55.

Advanced Placement Credit by examination available. Credit given for nursing courses completed elsewhere dependent upon specific evaluations.

Contact Ms. Diane Gerrity, Administrative Support Assistant, School of Nursing, San Jose State University, One Washington Square, San Jose, CA 95192-0057. *Telephone:* 408-924-3131. *Fax:* 408-924-3135. *E-mail:* dgerrity@son.sjsu.edu.

GRADUATE PROGRAMS

Contact Dr. Phyllis Connolly, Graduate Coordinator, School of Nursing, San Jose State University, One Washington Square, San Jose, CA 95192. *Telephone:* 408-924-3144. *Fax:* 408-924-3135. *E-mail:* connollyDR@son.sjsu.edu.

MASTER'S DEGREE PROGRAM

Degree MS

Available Programs Master's.

Concentrations Available Nursing administration; nursing education. *Clinical nurse specialist programs in:* gerontology, school health. *Nurse practitioner programs in:* family health.

Study Options Full-time and part-time.

Program Entrance Requirements Minimum overall college GPA of 3.0, transcript of college record, CPR certification, written essay, immunizations, 3 letters of recommendation, nursing research course, physical assessment course, professional liability insurance/malpractice insurance, resume, statistics course.

Degree Requirements 36 total credit hours, thesis or project.

Sonoma State University

Department of Nursing
Rohnert Park, California

http://www.sonoma.edu/nursing

Founded in 1960

DEGREES • BSN • MSN

Nursing Program Faculty 22 (36% with doctorates).

Sonoma State University (continued)

Baccalaureate Enrollment 139
Women 92% **Men** 8% **Minority** 24% **International** 2% **Part-time** 14%

Graduate Enrollment 48
Women 96% **Men** 4% **Minority** 15% **Part-time** 44%

Nursing Student Activities Nursing Honor Society, Sigma Theta Tau, Student Nurses' Association, nursing club.

Nursing Student Resources Academic advising; academic or career counseling; assistance for students with disabilities; bookstore; campus computer network; career placement assistance; computer lab; computer-assisted instruction; daycare for children of students; e-mail services; employment services for current students; externships; housing assistance; interactive nursing skills videos; Internet; learning resource lab; library services; nursing audiovisuals; remedial services; resume preparation assistance; skills, simulation, or other laboratory; tutoring; unpaid internships.

Library Facilities 636,613 volumes (26,700 in health, 1,400 in nursing); 21,115 periodical subscriptions (64 health-care related).

BACCALAUREATE PROGRAMS

Degree BSN

Available Programs ADN to Baccalaureate; Baccalaureate for Second Degree; Generic Baccalaureate; LPN to Baccalaureate; LPN to RN Baccalaureate; RN Baccalaureate.

Study Options Full-time.

Program Entrance Requirements Minimum overall college GPA of 3.0, transcript of college record, CPR certification, written essay, health exam, health insurance, high school biology, high school chemistry, high school foreign language, 3 years high school math, 2 years high school science, high school transcript, immunizations, 2 letters of recommendation, minimum high school GPA of 3.0, minimum GPA in nursing prerequisites of 3.0, professional liability insurance/malpractice insurance, prerequisite course work. Transfer students are accepted. **Standardized tests** *Required:* SAT or ACT, TOEFL for international students. **Application** *Deadline:* 12/31 (freshmen), 1/31 (transfer). *Notification:* continuous (freshmen). *Application fee:* $55.

Advanced Placement Credit by examination available. Credit given for nursing courses completed elsewhere dependent upon specific evaluations.

Expenses (2004–05) *Tuition, state resident:* full-time $3408; part-time $1215 per semester. *Tuition, nonresident:* full-time $13,578; part-time $3249 per semester. *International tuition:* $13,578 full-time. *Room and board:* $7588; room only: $5912 per academic year.

Financial Aid 53% of baccalaureate students in nursing programs received some form of financial aid in 2003–04. *Gift aid (need-based):* Federal Pell, FSEOG, state, private, college/university gift aid from institutional funds. *Loans:* Federal Direct (Subsidized and Unsubsidized Stafford PLUS), Perkins. *Work-Study:* Federal Work-Study, part-time campus jobs. *Application deadline (priority):* 1/31.

Contact Ms. Becky Schroeder Cohen, Administrative Coordinator, Department of Nursing, Sonoma State University, 1801 East Cotati Avenue, Rohnert Park, CA 94928. *Telephone:* 707-664-2465. *Fax:* 707-664-2653. *E-mail:* becky.cohen@sonoma.edu.

GRADUATE PROGRAMS

Expenses (2004–05) *Tuition, state resident:* full-time $3894; part-time $1356 per semester. *Tuition, nonresident:* full-time $12,030; part-time $3390 per semester. *International tuition:* $12,030 full-time.

Financial Aid 90% of graduate students in nursing programs received some form of financial aid in 2003–04.

Contact Ms. Becky Schroeder Cohen, Administrative Coordinator, Department of Nursing, Sonoma State University, 1801 East Cotati Avenue, Rohnert Park, CA 94928. *Telephone:* 707-664-2465. *Fax:* 707-664-2653. *E-mail:* becky.cohen@sonoma.edu.

MASTER'S DEGREE PROGRAM

Degree MSN

Available Programs Master's.

Concentrations Available Nurse case management; nursing administration; nursing education. *Nurse practitioner programs in:* family health.

Site Options *Distance Learning:* Turlock, CA; Chico, CA.

Study Options Full-time.

Program Entrance Requirements Clinical experience, computer literacy, minimum overall college GPA of 3.0, transcript of college record, CPR certification, written essay, immunizations, 3 letters of recommendation, physical assessment course, professional liability insurance/malpractice insurance, prerequisite course work, statistics course.

Advanced Placement Credit given for nursing courses completed elsewhere dependent upon specific evaluations.

Degree Requirements 40 total credit hours, thesis or project, comprehensive exam.

POST-MASTER'S PROGRAM

Areas of Study *Nurse practitioner programs in:* family health.

University of California, Los Angeles
School of Nursing
Los Angeles, California

http://www.nursing.ucla.edu

Founded in 1919

DEGREES • BS • MSN • MSN/MBA • PHD

Nursing Program Faculty 44 (66% with doctorates).

Baccalaureate Enrollment 33
Women 94% **Men** 6% **Minority** 52%

Graduate Enrollment 284
Women 92% **Men** 8% **Minority** 56% **International** 1%

Nursing Student Activities Nursing Honor Society, Sigma Theta Tau, Student Nurses' Association, nursing club.

Nursing Student Resources Academic advising; assistance for students with disabilities; bookstore; campus computer network; computer lab; daycare for children of students; e-mail services; housing assistance; Internet; library services; nursing audiovisuals.

Library Facilities 7.6 million volumes (760,000 in health, 8,000 in nursing); 94,801 periodical subscriptions (600,000 health-care related).

BACCALAUREATE PROGRAMS

Degree BS

Available Programs ADN to Baccalaureate.

Study Options Full-time.

Program Entrance Requirements Minimum overall college GPA of 3.0, transcript of college record, written essay, 3 letters of recommendation, prerequisite course work. Transfer students are accepted. **Standardized tests** *Required:* SAT or ACT, SAT Subject Tests, SAT II Writing Tests, TOEFL for international students. **Application** *Deadline:* 11/30 (freshmen), 11/30 (transfer). *Notification:* 3/15 (freshmen). *Application fee:* $55.

Expenses (2004–05) *Tuition, nonresident:* full-time $16,476. *International tuition:* $16,476 full-time. *Room and board:* $11,879 per academic year. *Required fees:* full-time $6576.

Financial Aid 100% of baccalaureate students in nursing programs received some form of financial aid in 2003–04. *Gift aid (need-based):* Federal Pell, FSEOG, state, private, college/university gift aid from institutional funds, United Negro College Fund, Federal Nursing, National Merit Scholarships. *Loans:* Federal Nursing Student Loans, FFEL (Subsidized and Unsubsidized Stafford PLUS), Perkins, state, college/university. *Work-Study:* Federal Work-Study, part-time campus jobs. *Application deadline (priority):* 3/2.

Contact Ms. Deborah Kafka-Hirsch, Admissions Coordinator, School of Nursing, University of California, Los Angeles, Box 951702, Los Angeles, CA 90095-1702. *Telephone:* 310-825-7181. *Fax:* 310-206-7433. *E-mail:* sonsaff@sonnet.ucla.edu.

GRADUATE PROGRAMS

Expenses (2004–05) *Room and board:* room only: $10,500 per academic year.

Financial Aid 80% of graduate students in nursing programs received some form of financial aid in 2003–04. 195 fellowships, 4 research assistantships, 2 teaching assistantships were awarded; Federal Work-Study, institutionally sponsored loans, scholarships, and tuition waivers (full and partial) also available. *Financial aid application deadline:* 3/1.

Contact Ms. Kathy Scrivner, Student Affairs Officer, School of Nursing, University of California, Los Angeles, Box 951702, Los Angeles, CA 90095-1702. *Telephone:* 310-825-7181. *Fax:* 310-267-0330. *E-mail:* sonsaff@ucla.edu.

MASTER'S DEGREE PROGRAM

Degrees MSN; MSN/MBA

Available Programs Master's.

Concentrations Available Nursing administration. *Clinical nurse specialist programs in:* acute care, gerontology, oncology, pediatric. *Nurse practitioner programs in:* acute care, family health, gerontology, occupational health, oncology, pediatric.

Study Options Full-time.

Program Entrance Requirements Minimum overall college GPA of 3.0, transcript of college record, written essay, 3 letters of recommendation, nursing research course, physical assessment course, prerequisite course work, statistics course, Commission on Graduates of Foreign Nursing Schools Exam. *Application deadline:* For fall admission, 2/1. *Application fee:* $60.

Degree Requirements 72 total credit hours, comprehensive exam.

POST-MASTER'S PROGRAM

Areas of Study Nursing administration. *Nurse practitioner programs in:* acute care, family health, gerontology, oncology, pediatric.

DOCTORAL DEGREE PROGRAM

Degree PhD

Available Programs Doctorate.

Areas of Study Addiction/substance abuse, advanced practice nursing, aging, bio-behavioral research, biology of health and illness, clinical practice, community health, critical care, family health, gerontology, health policy, health promotion/disease prevention, health-care systems, human health and illness, illness and transition, neuro-behavior, nursing administration, nursing research, nursing science, oncology, women's health.

Program Entrance Requirements Minimum overall college GPA of 3.5, 4 letters of recommendation, MSN or equivalent, scholarly papers, statistics course, vita, writing sample, GRE General Test, Commission on Graduates of Foreign Nursing Schools exam. *Application deadline:* For fall admission, 2/1. *Application fee:* $60.

Degree Requirements 127 total credit hours, dissertation, oral exam, written exam, residency.

POSTDOCTORAL PROGRAM

Areas of Study Addiction/substance abuse, adolescent health, aging, cancer care, gerontology, health promotion/disease prevention, nursing research, vulnerable population, women's health.

Postdoctoral Program Contact Dr. Mary Woo, Associate Dean for Research, School of Nursing, University of California, Los Angeles, Box 951702, Los Angeles, CA 90095-1702. *Telephone:* 310-206-2032. *Fax:* 310-206-7433. *E-mail:* mwoo@sonnet.ucla.edu.

CONTINUING EDUCATION PROGRAM

Contact Ms. Salpy Akaragian, Education Specialist, School of Nursing, University of California, Los Angeles, Box 951701, Los Angeles, CA 90095-1701. *Telephone:* 310-206-9581. *E-mail:* nssa@mednet.ucla.edu.

University of California, San Francisco

School of Nursing
San Francisco, California

http://www.nurseweb.ucsf.edu

Founded in 1864

DEGREES • MS • PHD

Nursing Program Faculty 150 (70% with doctorates).

Graduate Enrollment 602

Women 88% **Men** 12% **Minority** 29% **International** 5% **Part-time** 2%

Nursing Student Activities Sigma Theta Tau, Student Nurses' Association.

Nursing Student Resources Academic advising; academic or career counseling; assistance for students with disabilities; bookstore; campus computer network; career placement assistance; computer lab; computer-assisted instruction; daycare for children of students; e-mail services; employment services for current students; housing assistance; interactive nursing skills videos; Internet; learning resource lab; library services; nursing audiovisuals; other; placement services for program completers; remedial services; resume preparation assistance; skills, simulation, or other laboratory; tutoring; unpaid internships.

Library Facilities 856,169 volumes in health, 131,046 volumes in nursing; 3,270 periodical subscriptions health-care related.

GRADUATE PROGRAMS

Expenses (2004–05) *Tuition, state resident:* full-time $8148. *Tuition, nonresident:* full-time $23,087. *International tuition:* $23,087 full-time.

Financial Aid 61% of graduate students in nursing programs received some form of financial aid in 2003–04. Fellowships, career-related internships or fieldwork and Federal Work-Study available. Aid available to part-time students.

Contact Mr. Terry Linton, Admissions and Progression Officer, School of Nursing, University of California, San Francisco, Room N319X, 2 Koret Way, San Francisco, CA 94143-0602. *Telephone:* 415-476-1435. *Fax:* 415-476-9707. *E-mail:* terry.linton@nursing.ucsf.edu.

MASTER'S DEGREE PROGRAM

Degree MS

Available Programs Master's; Master's for Non-Nursing College Graduates; Master's for Nurses with Non-Nursing Degrees.

Concentrations Available Nurse-midwifery; nursing administration; nursing education; nursing informatics. *Clinical nurse specialist programs in:* cardiovascular, community health, critical care, gerontology, occupational health, oncology, perinatal, psychiatric/mental health. *Nurse practitioner programs in:* acute care, adult health, family health, gerontology, neonatal health, occupational health, oncology, pediatric, psychiatric/mental health.

Study Options Full-time.

Program Entrance Requirements Clinical experience, computer literacy, minimum overall college GPA of 3.0, transcript of college record, CPR certification, written essay, immunizations, 4 letters of recommendation, prerequisite course work, statistics course, GRE General Test. *Application deadline:* For fall admission, 3/1. *Application fee:* $40.

Advanced Placement Credit given for nursing courses completed elsewhere dependent upon specific evaluations.

Degree Requirements 36 total credit hours, comprehensive exam.

DOCTORAL DEGREE PROGRAM

Degree PhD

Available Programs Doctorate.

Areas of Study Addiction/substance abuse, aging, bio-behavioral research, biology of health and illness, community health, critical care, ethics, family health, gerontology, health policy, health promotion/disease prevention, health-care systems, human health and illness, illness and transition, individualized study, information systems, maternity-newborn, neuro-behavior, nursing administration, nursing policy, nursing research, nursing science, oncology, urban health, women's health.

Program Entrance Requirements Minimum overall college GPA of 3.0, interview by faculty committee, 4 letters of recommendation, statistics course, writing sample, GRE General Test. *Application deadline:* For fall admission, 3/1. *Application fee:* $40.

Degree Requirements Dissertation, oral exam, written exam, residency.

POSTDOCTORAL PROGRAM

Areas of Study Individualized study.

Postdoctoral Program Contact Mr. Jeff Kilmer, Director, Office of Student and Curricular Affairs, School of Nursing, University of California, San Francisco, Room N319X, 2 Koret Way, San Francisco, CA 94143-0602. *Telephone:* 415-476-1435. *Fax:* 415-476-9707. *E-mail:* jeff.kilmer@nursing.ucsf.edu.

University of Phoenix–Northern California Campus

College of Health and Human Services
Pleasanton, California

DEGREES • BSN • MSN • MSN/MBA

Nursing Program Faculty 39 (28% with doctorates).

Baccalaureate Enrollment 10
Women 80% **Men** 20% **Minority** 78%

Graduate Enrollment 7
Women 86% **Men** 14% **Minority** 67%

Nursing Student Activities Sigma Theta Tau.

Nursing Student Resources Academic advising; academic or career counseling; bookstore; computer lab; library services.

Library Facilities 27.1 million volumes; 11,648 periodical subscriptions (1,426 health-care related).

BACCALAUREATE PROGRAMS

Degree BSN

Available Programs ADN to Baccalaureate; Accelerated Baccalaureate.

Site Options Bakersfield, CA; Oakland, CA; San Francisco, CA.

Study Options Full-time.

Program Entrance Requirements 1 letter of recommendation. Transfer students are accepted. **Standardized tests** *Required:* TOEFL for international students. **Application** *Deadline:* rolling (freshmen), rolling (transfer). *Application fee:* $85.

Advanced Placement Credit by examination available.

Expenses (2004–05) *Tuition:* full-time $11,670; part-time $389 per credit hour. *International tuition:* $11,670 full-time. *Required fees:* full-time $110.

Contact Campus College Chair, Nursing, College of Health and Human Services, University of Phoenix–Northern California Campus, 7901 Stoneridge Drive, Suite #130, Pleasanton, CA 94588-3677. *Telephone:* 877-416-4100.

GRADUATE PROGRAMS

Expenses (2004–05) *Tuition:* full-time $10,320; part-time $430 per credit hour. *International tuition:* $10,320 full-time. *Required fees:* full-time $110.

Contact Campus College Chair, Nursing, College of Health and Human Services, University of Phoenix–Northern California Campus, 7901 Stoneridge Drive, Suite #130, Pleasanton, CA 94588-3677. *Telephone:* 877-416-4100.

MASTER'S DEGREE PROGRAM

Degrees MSN; MSN/MBA

Available Programs Master's.

Concentrations Available Health-care administration; nursing administration; nursing education. *Nurse practitioner programs in:* family health.

Site Options Bakersfield, CA; Oakland, CA; San Francisco, CA.

Study Options Full-time.

Program Entrance Requirements Clinical experience, computer literacy, minimum overall college GPA of 2.5, transcript of college record. *Application deadline:* Applications are processed on a rolling basis. *Application fee:* $110.

Degree Requirements 39 total credit hours, thesis or project.

POST-MASTER'S PROGRAM

Areas of Study *Nurse practitioner programs in:* family health.

University of Phoenix–Sacramento Campus

College of Health and Human Services
Sacramento, California

Founded in 1993

DEGREES • BSN • MSN • MSN/MBA

Nursing Program Faculty 42 (17% with doctorates).

Baccalaureate Enrollment 45
Women 75.5% **Men** 24.5% **Minority** 34%

Graduate Enrollment 65
Women 88% **Men** 12% **Minority** 26%

Nursing Student Activities Sigma Theta Tau.

Nursing Student Resources Academic advising; academic or career counseling; bookstore; computer lab; library services.

Library Facilities 27.1 million volumes; 11,648 periodical subscriptions (1,426 health-care related).

BACCALAUREATE PROGRAMS

Degree BSN

Available Programs ADN to Baccalaureate; Accelerated Baccalaureate.

Site Options Suisun City, CA; Roseville, CA; Lathrop, CA.

Study Options Full-time.

Program Entrance Requirements 1 letter of recommendation. Transfer students are accepted. **Standardized tests** *Required:* TOEFL for international students. **Application** *Deadline:* rolling (freshmen), rolling (transfer). *Application fee:* $85.

Advanced Placement Credit by examination available.

Expenses (2004–05) *Tuition:* full-time $11,550; part-time $385 per credit hour. *International tuition:* $11,550 full-time. *Required fees:* full-time $110.

Financial Aid 2% of baccalaureate students in nursing programs received some form of financial aid in 2003–04.

Contact Campus College Chair, Nursing, College of Health and Human Services, University of Phoenix–Sacramento Campus, 1760 Creekside Oaks Drive, #100, Sacramento, CA 95833-3632. *Telephone:* 800-266-2107.

GRADUATE PROGRAMS

Expenses (2004–05) *Tuition:* full-time $10,560; part-time $440 per credit hour. *International tuition:* $10,560 full-time. *Required fees:* full-time $110.

Financial Aid 10% of graduate students in nursing programs received some form of financial aid in 2003–04.

Contact Campus College Chair, Nursing, College of Health and Human Services, University of Phoenix–Sacramento Campus, 1760 Creekside Oaks Drive, #100, Sacramento, CA 95833-3632. *Telephone:* 800-266-2107.

MASTER'S DEGREE PROGRAM

Degrees MSN; MSN/MBA

Available Programs Master's.

Concentrations Available Health-care administration; nursing administration; nursing education. *Nurse practitioner programs in:* family health.

Site Options Suisun City, CA; Roseville, CA; Lathrop, CA.

Study Options Full-time and part-time.

Program Entrance Requirements Clinical experience, computer literacy, minimum overall college GPA of 2.5, transcript of college record. *Application deadline:* Applications are processed on a rolling basis. *Application fee:* $110.

Degree Requirements 39 total credit hours, thesis or project.

POST-MASTER'S PROGRAM

Areas of Study *Nurse practitioner programs in:* family health.

University of Phoenix–San Diego Campus

College of Health and Human Services
San Diego, California

Founded in 1988

DEGREES • BSN • MSN • MSN/MBA

Nursing Program Faculty 39 (28% with doctorates).

Baccalaureate Enrollment 155
Women 88% **Men** 12% **Minority** 48%
Graduate Enrollment 39
Women 90% **Men** 10% **Minority** 50%
Nursing Student Activities Sigma Theta Tau.
Nursing Student Resources Academic advising; academic or career counseling; bookstore; computer lab; Internet.
Library Facilities 27.1 million volumes; 11,648 periodical subscriptions (1,426 health-care related).

BACCALAUREATE PROGRAMS

Degree BSN
Available Programs ADN to Baccalaureate; Accelerated Baccalaureate.
Site Options Oceanside, CA; San Marcos, CA; Chula Vista, CA.
Study Options Full-time.
Program Entrance Requirements 1 letter of recommendation. Transfer students are accepted. **Standardized tests** *Required:* TOEFL for international students. **Application** *Deadline:* rolling (freshmen), rolling (transfer). *Application fee:* $85.
Advanced Placement Credit by examination available.
Expenses (2004–05) *Tuition:* full-time $11,370; part-time $379 per credit hour. *International tuition:* $11,370 full-time. *Required fees:* full-time $110.
Financial Aid 4% of baccalaureate students in nursing programs received some form of financial aid in 2003–04.
Contact Campus College Chair, Nursing, College of Health and Human Services, University of Phoenix–San Diego Campus, 3870 Murphy Canyon Road, #100, San Diego, CA 92123-4403. *Telephone:* 888-867-4636.

GRADUATE PROGRAMS

Expenses (2004–05) *Tuition:* full-time $10,680; part-time $445 per credit hour. *International tuition:* $10,680 full-time. *Required fees:* full-time $110.
Financial Aid 7% of graduate students in nursing programs received some form of financial aid in 2003–04.
Contact Campus College Chair, Nursing, College of Health and Human Services, University of Phoenix–San Diego Campus, 3870 Murphy Canyon Road, #100, San Diego, CA 92123-4403. *Telephone:* 888-867-4636.

MASTER'S DEGREE PROGRAM

Degrees MSN; MSN/MBA
Available Programs Master's.
Concentrations Available Health-care administration; nursing administration; nursing education. *Nurse practitioner programs in:* family health.
Site Options Oceanside, CA; San Marcos, CA; Chula Vista, CA.
Study Options Full-time.
Program Entrance Requirements Clinical experience, computer literacy, minimum overall college GPA of 2.5, transcript of college record. *Application deadline:* Applications are processed on a rolling basis. *Application fee:* $110.
Degree Requirements 39 total credit hours, thesis or project.

POST-MASTER'S PROGRAM

Areas of Study *Nurse practitioner programs in:* family health.

University of Phoenix–Southern California Campus

College of Health and Human Services
Costa Mesa, California

Founded in 1980

DEGREES • BSN • MSN • MSN/MBA

Nursing Program Faculty 113 (29% with doctorates).
Baccalaureate Enrollment 389
Women 90% **Men** 10% **Minority** 56%
Graduate Enrollment 191
Women 88% **Men** 12% **Minority** 55%
Nursing Student Activities Sigma Theta Tau.
Nursing Student Resources Academic advising; academic or career counseling; bookstore; computer lab; library services.
Library Facilities 27.1 million volumes; 11,648 periodical subscriptions (1,426 health-care related).

BACCALAUREATE PROGRAMS

Degree BSN
Available Programs ADN to Baccalaureate; Accelerated RN Baccalaureate.
Site Options La Marada, CA; Diamond Bar, CA; Oxnard, CA.
Study Options Full-time.
Program Entrance Requirements 1 letter of recommendation. Transfer students are accepted. **Standardized tests** *Required:* TOEFL for international students. **Application** *Deadline:* rolling (freshmen), rolling (transfer). *Application fee:* $85.
Advanced Placement Credit by examination available.
Expenses (2004–05) *Tuition:* full-time $12,360; part-time $412 per credit hour. *International tuition:* $12,360 full-time. *Required fees:* full-time $110.
Financial Aid 5% of baccalaureate students in nursing programs received some form of financial aid in 2003–04.
Contact Campus College Chair, Nursing, College of Health and Human Services, University of Phoenix–Southern California Campus, 10540 Talbert Avenue, West Tower, Suite 120, Fountain Valley, CA 92708-6027. *Telephone:* 800-697-8223.

GRADUATE PROGRAMS

Expenses (2004–05) *Tuition:* full-time $11,376; part-time $474 per credit hour. *International tuition:* $11,376 full-time. *Required fees:* full-time $110.
Financial Aid 12% of graduate students in nursing programs received some form of financial aid in 2003–04.
Contact Campus College Chair, Nursing, College of Health and Human Services, University of Phoenix–Southern California Campus, 10540 Talbert Avenue, West Tower, Suite 120, Fountain Valley, CA 92708-6027. *Telephone:* 800-697-8223.

MASTER'S DEGREE PROGRAM

Degrees MSN; MSN/MBA
Available Programs Master's.
Concentrations Available Health-care administration; nursing administration; nursing education. *Nurse practitioner programs in:* family health.
Site Options La Marada, CA; Diamond Bar, CA; Oxnard, CA.
Study Options Full-time.
Program Entrance Requirements Clinical experience, computer literacy, minimum overall college GPA of 2.5, transcript of college record, 1 letter of recommendation. *Application deadline:* Applications are processed on a rolling basis. *Application fee:* $110.
Degree Requirements 39 total credit hours, thesis or project.

POST-MASTER'S PROGRAM

Areas of Study *Nurse practitioner programs in:* family health.

University of San Diego

Hahn School of Nursing and Health Sciences
San Diego, California

http://www.sandiego.edu

Founded in 1949

DEGREES • BSN • MSN • MSN/MBA • PHD

Nursing Program Faculty 41 (65% with doctorates).

University of San Diego (continued)

Baccalaureate Enrollment 14
Women 86% **Men** 14% **Minority** 50% **Part-time** 5%

Graduate Enrollment 191
Women 89% **Men** 11% **Minority** 27% **International** 3% **Part-time** 53%

Nursing Student Activities Nursing Honor Society, Sigma Theta Tau, Student Nurses' Association.

Nursing Student Resources Academic advising; academic or career counseling; assistance for students with disabilities; bookstore; campus computer network; career placement assistance; computer lab; computer-assisted instruction; daycare for children of students; e-mail services; employment services for current students; interactive nursing skills videos; Internet; learning resource lab; library services; nursing audiovisuals; resume preparation assistance; skills, simulation, or other laboratory; tutoring.

Library Facilities 714,082 volumes (25,000 in health, 15,000 in nursing); 10,451 periodical subscriptions (200 health-care related).

BACCALAUREATE PROGRAMS

Degree BSN

Available Programs ADN to Baccalaureate; RN Baccalaureate.

Program Entrance Requirements Transfer students are accepted. **Standardized tests** *Required:* SAT or ACT, TOEFL for international students. *Recommended:* SAT and SAT Subject Tests or ACT, SAT II Writing Tests. ***Placement:*** *Recommended:* SAT II Writing Tests. **Application** *Deadline:* 1/5 (freshmen), 3/1 (transfer). *Early decision:* 11/15. *Notification:* 4/15 (freshmen), 1/31 (early action). *Application fee:* $55.

Expenses (2004–05) *Tuition:* full-time $26,600; part-time $920 per credit hour. *International tuition:* $26,600 full-time. *Room and board:* $11,720; room only: $9200 per academic year. *Required fees:* full-time $426; part-time $176 per term.

Financial Aid 100% of baccalaureate students in nursing programs received some form of financial aid in 2003–04. *Gift aid (need-based):* Federal Pell, FSEOG, state, private, college/university gift aid from institutional funds. *Loans:* Federal Nursing Student Loans, FFEL (Subsidized and Unsubsidized Stafford PLUS), Perkins, college/university. *Work-Study:* Federal Work-Study, part-time campus jobs. *Application deadline (priority):* 2/20.

Contact Ms. Cathleen Mumper, Director of Student Services and Admissions Officer, Hahn School of Nursing and Health Sciences, University of San Diego, 5998 Alcala Park, San Diego, CA 92110-2492. *Telephone:* 619-260-4163. *Fax:* 619-260-6814. *E-mail:* cmm@sandiego.edu.

GRADUATE PROGRAMS

Expenses (2004–05) *Tuition:* part-time $905 per credit hour. *Required fees:* full-time $366; part-time $183 per term.

Financial Aid 80% of graduate students in nursing programs received some form of financial aid in 2003–04. Institutionally sponsored loans, scholarships, traineeships, tuition waivers (partial), and graduate work program available. Aid available to part-time students. *Financial aid application deadline:* 5/1.

Contact Ms. Cathleen Mumper, Director of Student Services and Admissions Officer, Hahn School of Nursing and Health Sciences, University of San Diego, 5998 Alcala Park, San Diego, CA 92110-2492. *Telephone:* 619-260-4163. *Fax:* 619-260-6814. *E-mail:* cmm@sandiego.edu.

MASTER'S DEGREE PROGRAM

Degrees MSN; MSN/MBA

Available Programs Accelerated AD/RN to Master's; Accelerated RN to Master's; Master's; Master's for Non-Nursing College Graduates; Master's for Nurses with Non-Nursing Degrees.

Concentrations Available Health-care administration. *Clinical nurse specialist programs in:* adult health. *Nurse practitioner programs in:* adult health, family health, gerontology, pediatric.

Study Options Full-time and part-time.

Program Entrance Requirements Computer literacy, minimum overall college GPA of 3.0, transcript of college record, CPR certification, written essay, immunizations, interview, 3 letters of recommendation, professional liability insurance/malpractice insurance, resume, statistics course, GRE General Test or MAT. *Application deadline:* For fall admission, 5/1 (priority date); for spring admission, 11/1 (priority date). Applications are processed on a rolling basis. *Application fee:* $45.

Advanced Placement Credit by examination available. Credit given for nursing courses completed elsewhere dependent upon specific evaluations.

POST-MASTER'S PROGRAM

Areas of Study Health-care administration. *Clinical nurse specialist programs in:* adult health. *Nurse practitioner programs in:* adult health, family health, gerontology, pediatric.

DOCTORAL DEGREE PROGRAM

Degree PhD

Available Programs Doctorate.

Areas of Study Advanced practice nursing, aging, clinical practice, community health, ethics, faculty preparation, family health, health policy, health promotion/disease prevention, health-care systems, human health and illness, illness and transition, individualized study, maternity-newborn, nursing education, nursing science, oncology, women's health.

Program Entrance Requirements Clinical experience, minimum overall college GPA of 3.5, interview by faculty committee, interview, 3 letters of recommendation, MSN or equivalent, scholarly papers, statistics course, vita, writing sample, GRE General Test or MAT. *Application deadline:* For fall admission, 5/1 (priority date); for spring admission, 11/1 (priority date). Applications are processed on a rolling basis. *Application fee:* $45.

Degree Requirements 54 total credit hours, dissertation, oral exam, residency.

See full description on page 576.

University of San Francisco
School of Nursing
San Francisco, California

http://www.usfca.edu/nursing/

Founded in 1855

DEGREES • BSN • MSN

Nursing Program Faculty 49 (83% with doctorates).

Baccalaureate Enrollment 535
Women 78% **Men** 22% **Minority** 49% **International** 9% **Part-time** 7%

Graduate Enrollment 115
Women 81% **Men** 19% **Minority** 51% **International** 1% **Part-time** 10%

Nursing Student Activities Nursing Honor Society, Sigma Theta Tau, Student Nurses' Association, nursing club.

Nursing Student Resources Academic advising; academic or career counseling; assistance for students with disabilities; bookstore; campus computer network; career placement assistance; computer lab; computer-assisted instruction; e-mail services; employment services for current students; housing assistance; interactive nursing skills videos; Internet; learning resource lab; library services; nursing audiovisuals; placement services for program completers; remedial services; resume preparation assistance; skills, simulation, or other laboratory; tutoring.

Library Facilities 1.1 million volumes; 5,560 periodical subscriptions.

BACCALAUREATE PROGRAMS

Degree BSN

Available Programs Baccalaureate for Second Degree; Generic Baccalaureate.

Study Options Full-time and part-time.

Program Entrance Requirements Minimum overall college GPA of 3.0, transcript of college record, CPR certification, written essay, health exam, health insurance, high school biology, high school chemistry, 3 years high school math, 2 years high school science, high school transcript, immunizations, 2 letters of recommendation, minimum high school GPA of 3.0, professional liability insurance/malpractice insurance, prerequisite course work. Transfer students are accepted. **Standardized tests** *Required:* SAT or ACT, TOEFL for international students. **Application**

Deadline: 2/1 (freshmen), rolling (transfer). *Early decision:* 11/15. *Notification:* continuous until 8/15 (freshmen), 1/1 (early action). *Application fee:* $55.

Advanced Placement Credit given for nursing courses completed elsewhere dependent upon specific evaluations.

Expenses (2004–05) *Tuition:* full-time $24,800; part-time $886 per unit. *International tuition:* $24,800 full-time. *Room and board:* $8990; room only: $5900 per academic year. *Required fees:* full-time $480.

Financial Aid 91% of baccalaureate students in nursing programs received some form of financial aid in 2003–04. *Gift aid (need-based):* Federal Pell, FSEOG, state, private, college/university gift aid from institutional funds. *Loans:* Federal Nursing Student Loans, Federal Direct (Subsidized and Unsubsidized Stafford PLUS), Perkins, college/university. *Work-Study:* Federal Work-Study, part-time campus jobs. *Application deadline (priority):* 2/15.

Contact Mr. Robert J. Reed, Assistant Dean, School of Nursing, University of San Francisco, 2130 Fulton Street, San Francisco, CA 94117-1080. *Telephone:* 415-422-6681. *Fax:* 415-422-6877. *E-mail:* reedr@usfca.edu.

GRADUATE PROGRAMS

Expenses (2004–05) *Tuition:* full-time $14,400; part-time $900 per unit. *International tuition:* $14,400 full-time. *Room and board:* $8990; room only: $5900 per academic year. *Required fees:* full-time $300.

Financial Aid 82% of graduate students in nursing programs received some form of financial aid in 2003–04. Institutionally sponsored loans available. *Financial aid application deadline:* 3/2.

Contact Mr. Robert J. Reed, Assistant Dean, School of Nursing, University of San Francisco, 2130 Fulton Street, Cowell Hall 102, San Francisco, CA 94117-1080. *Telephone:* 415-422-6681. *Fax:* 415-422-6877. *E-mail:* reedr@usfca.edu.

MASTER'S DEGREE PROGRAM

Degree MSN

Available Programs Accelerated Master's; Accelerated Master's for Non-Nursing College Graduates; Accelerated Master's for Nurses with Non-Nursing Degrees; Master's; Master's for Non-Nursing College Graduates; Master's for Nurses with Non-Nursing Degrees.

Concentrations Available Health-care administration; nurse case management; nursing informatics. *Clinical nurse specialist programs in:* adult health, family health, psychiatric/mental health. *Nurse practitioner programs in:* adult health, family health, psychiatric/mental health.

Study Options Full-time and part-time.

Program Entrance Requirements Clinical experience, minimum overall college GPA of 3.25, transcript of college record, written essay, immunizations, 2 letters of recommendation, nursing research course, prerequisite course work, resume, statistics course. *Application deadline:* Applications are processed on a rolling basis. *Application fee:* $40.

Advanced Placement Credit given for nursing courses completed elsewhere dependent upon specific evaluations.

Degree Requirements 53 total credit hours, comprehensive exam.

POST-MASTER'S PROGRAM

Areas of Study *Clinical nurse specialist programs in:* family health, psychiatric/mental health. *Nurse practitioner programs in:* adult health, family health, psychiatric/mental health.

CONTINUING EDUCATION PROGRAM

Contact Mr. Robert J. Reed, Assistant Dean, School of Nursing, University of San Francisco, 2130 Fulton Street, San Francisco, CA 94117-1080. *Telephone:* 415-422-6681. *Fax:* 415-422-6877. *E-mail:* reedr@usfca.edu.

Western University of Health Sciences

College of Graduate Nursing
Pomona, California

http://www.westernu.edu/cogn.html

Founded in 1975

DEGREE • MSN

Nursing Student Resources Library services.

GRADUATE PROGRAMS

Expenses (2003–04) *Tuition:* full-time $28,000.

Financial Aid Institutionally sponsored loans and scholarships available.

Contact College of Graduate Nursing, Western University of Health Sciences, 309 East Second Street, College Plaza, Pomona, CA 91766. *Telephone:* 909-469-5523. *Fax:* 909-469-5521.

MASTER'S DEGREE PROGRAM

Degree MSN

Concentrations Available *Nurse practitioner programs in:* family health.

Study Options Full-time and part-time.

Program Entrance Requirements Computer literacy, minimum overall college GPA of 3.0, transcript of college record, 3 letters of recommendation, prerequisite course work, resume, statistics course, GRE General Test. *Application deadline:* For fall admission, 3/1 (priority date). Applications are processed on a rolling basis. *Application fee:* $60.

POST-MASTER'S PROGRAM

Areas of Study *Nurse practitioner programs in:* family health.

COLORADO

Colorado State University-Pueblo

Department of Nursing
Pueblo, Colorado

Founded in 1933

DEGREES • BSN • MS

Nursing Program Faculty 15 (30% with doctorates).

Baccalaureate Enrollment 300
Women 90% **Men** 10% **Minority** 28% **International** 10% **Part-time** 20%

Graduate Enrollment 27

Nursing Student Activities Nursing Honor Society, Sigma Theta Tau, Student Nurses' Association, nursing club.

Nursing Student Resources Academic advising; academic or career counseling; assistance for students with disabilities; bookstore; campus computer network; career placement assistance; computer lab; computer-assisted instruction; daycare for children of students; e-mail services; employment services for current students; externships; housing assistance; interactive nursing skills videos; Internet; learning resource lab; library services; nursing audiovisuals; paid internships; placement services for program completers; remedial services; resume preparation assistance; skills, simulation, or other laboratory; tutoring; unpaid internships.

Library Facilities 270,761 volumes (2,700 in health, 68 in nursing); 1,327 periodical subscriptions (69 health-care related).

BACCALAUREATE PROGRAMS

Degree BSN

Available Programs ADN to Baccalaureate; Baccalaureate for Second Degree; Generic Baccalaureate; LPN to Baccalaureate; LPN to RN Baccalaureate; RN Baccalaureate.

Study Options Full-time.

Program Entrance Requirements Minimum overall college GPA of 2.75, transcript of college record, CPR certification, health exam, immunizations, minimum GPA in nursing prerequisites of 2.50, professional liability insurance/malpractice insurance, prerequisite course work. Transfer students are accepted. **Standardized tests** *Required:* SAT or ACT, TOEFL for international students. ***Placement:*** *Required:* SAT or ACT. **Application** *Deadline:* 8/1 (freshmen), 8/1 (transfer). *Notification:* continuous until 8/1 (freshmen). *Application fee:* $25.

Colorado State University-Pueblo (continued)

Advanced Placement Credit by examination available. Credit given for nursing courses completed elsewhere dependent upon specific evaluations.

Financial Aid 80% of baccalaureate students in nursing programs received some form of financial aid in 2002–03. *Gift aid (need-based):* Federal Pell, FSEOG, state, private, college/university gift aid from institutional funds. *Loans:* FFEL (Subsidized and Unsubsidized Stafford PLUS), Perkins. *Work-Study:* Federal Work-Study, part-time campus jobs. *Application deadline (priority):* 3/1.

Contact Dr. Rhonda L. Johnston, Director and Chair, Department of Nursing, Colorado State University-Pueblo, 2200 Bonforte Boulevard, Pueblo, CO 81001. *Telephone:* 719-549-2871. *Fax:* 719-549-2113. *E-mail:* Rhonda.Johnston@colostate-pueblo.edu.

GRADUATE PROGRAMS

Contact Dr. Rhonda L. Johnston, Nursing Department Chair, Department of Nursing, Colorado State University-Pueblo, 2200 Bonforte Boulevard, Pueblo, CO 81001. *Telephone:* 719-549-2871. *Fax:* 719-549-2113. *E-mail:* Rhonda.Johnston@colostate-pueblo.edu.

MASTER'S DEGREE PROGRAM

Degree MS

Available Programs Accelerated Master's; Accelerated Master's for Non-Nursing College Graduates; Master's; Master's for Non-Nursing College Graduates.

Concentrations Available Health-care administration; nursing education. *Clinical nurse specialist programs in:* acute care, medical-surgical, psychiatric/mental health, school health, women's health. *Nurse practitioner programs in:* acute care.

Study Options Full-time and part-time.

Program Entrance Requirements Clinical experience, computer literacy, minimum overall college GPA of 3.0, transcript of college record, CPR certification, written essay, immunizations, 3 letters of recommendation, nursing research course, professional liability insurance/malpractice insurance, prerequisite course work, resume, statistics course.

Advanced Placement Credit by examination available. Credit given for nursing courses completed elsewhere dependent upon specific evaluations.

Degree Requirements 45 total credit hours, thesis or project, comprehensive exam.

POST-MASTER'S PROGRAM

Areas of Study *Nurse practitioner programs in:* acute care.

CONTINUING EDUCATION PROGRAM

Contact Dr. Rhonda L. Johnston, Nursing Department Chair, Department of Nursing, Colorado State University-Pueblo, 2200 Bonforte Boulevard, Pueblo, CO 81001. *Telephone:* 719-549-2871. *Fax:* 719-549-2113. *E-mail:* Rhonda.Johnston@colostate-pueblo.edu.

Mesa State College

Department of Nursing and Radiologic Sciences
Grand Junction, Colorado

http://www.mesastate.edu/schools/sbps/nars/nursing.htm

Founded in 1925

DEGREE • BSN

Nursing Program Faculty 19 (11% with doctorates).

Baccalaureate Enrollment 150

Women 89% **Men** 11% **Minority** 8% **International** 2% **Part-time** 7%

Nursing Student Activities Sigma Theta Tau, Student Nurses' Association.

Nursing Student Resources Academic advising; academic or career counseling; assistance for students with disabilities; bookstore; campus computer network; career placement assistance; computer lab; computer-assisted instruction; daycare for children of students; e-mail services; employment services for current students; housing assistance; interactive nursing skills videos; Internet; learning resource lab; library services; nursing audiovisuals; placement services for program completers; resume preparation assistance; skills, simulation, or other laboratory; tutoring; unpaid internships.

Library Facilities 247,338 volumes (200 in health, 150 in nursing); 31,992 periodical subscriptions (25 health-care related).

BACCALAUREATE PROGRAMS

Degree BSN

Available Programs ADN to Baccalaureate; Generic Baccalaureate; LPN to Baccalaureate; LPN to RN Baccalaureate; RN Baccalaureate.

Site Options *Distance Learning:* Montrose, CO; Craig, CO; Cortez, CO.

Study Options Full-time and part-time.

Program Entrance Requirements Minimum overall college GPA of 2.0, transcript of college record, CPR certification, written essay, health exam, immunizations, minimum GPA in nursing prerequisites of 2.0, professional liability insurance/malpractice insurance, prerequisite course work. Transfer students are accepted. **Standardized tests** *Required:* SAT or ACT. *Recommended:* TOEFL for international students. **Application** *Deadline:* 8/15 (freshmen), 8/15 (transfer). *Application fee:* $30.

Advanced Placement Credit by examination available. Credit given for nursing courses completed elsewhere dependent upon specific evaluations.

Expenses (2004–05) *Tuition, state resident:* full-time $2062; part-time $94 per credit hour. *Tuition, nonresident:* full-time $8350; part-time $380 per credit hour. *Room and board:* $6500; room only: $3260 per academic year. *Required fees:* part-time $150 per credit; part-time $860 per term.

Financial Aid 85% of baccalaureate students in nursing programs received some form of financial aid in 2003–04.

Contact Judy Goodhart, Program Director, Department of Nursing and Radiologic Sciences, Mesa State College, 1100 North Avenue, Grand Junction, CO 81501. *Telephone:* 970-248-1774. *Fax:* 970-248-1133. *E-mail:* goodhart@mesastate.edu.

Metropolitan State College of Denver

Department of Health Professions
Denver, Colorado

http://www.mscd.edu/~nursing

Founded in 1963

DEGREE • BS

Nursing Program Faculty 6 (35% with doctorates).

Baccalaureate Enrollment 74

Women 88% **Men** 12% **Minority** 23% **Part-time** 72%

Nursing Student Activities Nursing club.

Nursing Student Resources Academic advising; academic or career counseling; assistance for students with disabilities; bookstore; campus computer network; computer lab; computer-assisted instruction; daycare for children of students; e-mail services; Internet; library services; nursing audiovisuals; remedial services; resume preparation assistance.

Library Facilities 607,971 volumes (21,503 in health); 2,380 periodical subscriptions (204 health-care related).

BACCALAUREATE PROGRAMS

Degree BS

Available Programs ADN to Baccalaureate; RN Baccalaureate.

Study Options Full-time and part-time.

Program Entrance Requirements Transcript of college record, CPR certification, immunizations, professional liability insurance/malpractice insurance, prerequisite course work, RN licensure. Transfer students are accepted. **Standardized tests** *Required:* TOEFL for international students. *Required for some:* SAT or ACT. **Application** *Deadline:* 8/12 (freshmen), rolling (transfer). *Notification:* continuous (freshmen). *Application fee:* $25.

Advanced Placement Credit given for nursing courses completed elsewhere dependent upon specific evaluations.

Financial Aid 35% of baccalaureate students in nursing programs received some form of financial aid in 2002–03. *Gift aid (need-based):* Federal Pell, FSEOG, state, private, college/university gift aid from institutional funds. *Loans:* FFEL (Subsidized and Unsubsidized Stafford PLUS), Perkins. *Work-Study:* Federal Work-Study, part-time campus jobs. *Application deadline:* Continuous.

Contact Roberta Hills, Chair of the Nursing Department. *Telephone:* 303-556-8415. *Fax:* 303-556-3439. *E-mail:* hillsro@mscd.edu.

Regis University

Department of Nursing
Denver, Colorado

Founded in 1877

DEGREES • BSN • MS

Nursing Program Faculty 18 (55% with doctorates).

Nursing Student Activities Nursing Honor Society, Sigma Theta Tau, Student Nurses' Association.

Nursing Student Resources Academic advising; academic or career counseling; assistance for students with disabilities; bookstore; campus computer network; computer lab; computer-assisted instruction; e-mail services; interactive nursing skills videos; Internet; learning resource lab; library services; nursing audiovisuals; resume preparation assistance; skills, simulation, or other laboratory; tutoring; unpaid internships.

Library Facilities 350,000 volumes; 20,800 periodical subscriptions.

BACCALAUREATE PROGRAMS

Degree BSN

Available Programs Accelerated Baccalaureate; Generic Baccalaureate; RN Baccalaureate.

Study Options Full-time.

Program Entrance Requirements Minimum overall college GPA of 2.5, transcript of college record, written essay, 2 letters of recommendation, prerequisite course work. Transfer students are accepted. **Standardized tests** *Required:* SAT or ACT, TOEFL for international students. *Recommended:* SAT Subject Tests. **Application** *Deadline:* rolling (freshmen), rolling (out-of-state freshmen), rolling (transfer). *Notification:* continuous (freshmen), continuous (out-of-state freshmen). *Application fee:* $40.

Advanced Placement Credit by examination available.

Expenses (2003–04) *Tuition:* full-time $20,700. *Room and board:* $3750; room only: $2250 per academic year. *Required fees:* full-time $627.

Contact Sarah Andrews, Admissions Counselor, Department of Nursing, Regis University, 3333 Regis Boulevard G-9, Carroll Hall, Room 108L, Denver, CO 80221-1099. *Telephone:* 303-458-4958. *Fax:* 303-964-5533. *E-mail:* sandrews@regis.edu.

GRADUATE PROGRAMS

Expenses (2003–04) *Tuition:* part-time $296 per credit hour.

Contact Alison Campbell, Admissions Counselor, Department of Nursing, Regis University, 3333 Regis Boulevard G-9, Carroll Hall, Room 108K, Denver, CO 80221-1099. *Telephone:* 303-458-4938. *Fax:* 303-964-5533. *E-mail:* acampbel@regis.edu.

MASTER'S DEGREE PROGRAM

Degree MS

Available Programs Master's.

Concentrations Available Health-care administration; nursing administration; nursing education. *Nurse practitioner programs in:* family health, neonatal health.

Study Options Full-time and part-time.

Program Entrance Requirements Minimum overall college GPA of 2.75, transcript of college record, written essay, 3 letters of recommendation, prerequisite course work, statistics course.

Advanced Placement Credit by examination available.

Degree Requirements 42 total credit hours, thesis or project.

University of Colorado at Colorado Springs

Beth-El College of Nursing and Health Sciences
Colorado Springs, Colorado

http://www.uccs.edu

Founded in 1965

DEGREES • BSN • MSN • MSN/MBA

Nursing Program Faculty 47 (32% with doctorates).

Baccalaureate Enrollment 594
Women 93% **Men** 7% **Minority** 13% **Part-time** 20%

Graduate Enrollment 101
Women 92% **Men** 8% **Minority** 40% **Part-time** 21%

Nursing Student Activities Nursing Honor Society, Sigma Theta Tau, Student Nurses' Association, nursing club.

Nursing Student Resources Academic advising; academic or career counseling; assistance for students with disabilities; bookstore; campus computer network; career placement assistance; computer lab; computer-assisted instruction; daycare for children of students; e-mail services; employment services for current students; externships; housing assistance; interactive nursing skills videos; Internet; learning resource lab; library services; nursing audiovisuals; resume preparation assistance; skills, simulation, or other laboratory.

Library Facilities 391,638 volumes (9,497 in health, 848 in nursing); 2,201 periodical subscriptions (229 health-care related).

BACCALAUREATE PROGRAMS

Degree BSN

Available Programs Accelerated Baccalaureate for Second Degree; Generic Baccalaureate; RN Baccalaureate.

Study Options Full-time.

Program Entrance Requirements Minimum overall college GPA of 3.0, transcript of college record, CPR certification, health exam, high school biology, high school chemistry, high school foreign language, 3 years high school math, 1 year of high school science, high school transcript, immunizations, minimum high school GPA of 3.0, minimum high school rank 30%, minimum GPA in nursing prerequisites of 3.0. Transfer students are accepted. **Standardized tests** *Required:* SAT or ACT, TOEFL for international students. **Application** *Deadline:* 7/1 (freshmen), 7/1 (transfer). *Notification:* continuous (freshmen). *Application fee:* $45.

Advanced Placement Credit given for nursing courses completed elsewhere dependent upon specific evaluations.

Expenses (2004–05) *Tuition, state resident:* full-time $2534; part-time $211 per credit hour. *Tuition, nonresident:* full-time $7871; part-time $633 per credit hour. *International tuition:* $7871 full-time. *Room and board:* $5824 per academic year. *Required fees:* full-time $317; part-time $10 per credit; part-time $175 per term.

Financial Aid 69% of baccalaureate students in nursing programs received some form of financial aid in 2003–04. *Gift aid (need-based):* Federal Pell, FSEOG, state, private, college/university gift aid from institutional funds. *Loans:* FFEL (Subsidized and Unsubsidized Stafford PLUS), Perkins, college/university. *Work-Study:* Federal Work-Study, part-time campus jobs. *Application deadline (priority):* 4/1.

Contact Ms. Bev Kratzer, Advisor, Baccalaureate Nursing and Health Sciences, Beth-El College of Nursing and Health Sciences, University of Colorado at Colorado Springs, 1460 Austin Bluffs Parkway, PO Box 7150, Colorado Springs, CO 80933. *Telephone:* 719-262-3260. *Fax:* 719-262-3316. *E-mail:* success@mail.uccs.edu.

GRADUATE PROGRAMS

Expenses (2004–05) *Tuition, state resident:* full-time $3334; part-time $277 per credit hour. *Tuition, nonresident:* full-time $8478; part-time $694 per credit hour. *International tuition:* $8478 full-time. *Room and board:* $5824 per academic year. *Required fees:* full-time $317; part-time $10 per credit; part-time $175 per term.

University of Colorado at Colorado Springs (continued)

Financial Aid 34% of graduate students in nursing programs received some form of financial aid in 2003–04.

Contact Dr. Kathy LaSala, Chair, Department of Graduate Studies, Beth-El College of Nursing and Health Sciences, University of Colorado at Colorado Springs, 1420 Austin Bluffs Parkway, PO Box 7150, Colorado Springs, CO 80933-7150. *Telephone:* 719-262-4411. *Fax:* 719-262-4416. *E-mail:* klasala@uccs.edu.

MASTER'S DEGREE PROGRAM

Degrees MSN; MSN/MBA

Available Programs Master's.

Concentrations Available Health-care administration; nursing administration. *Clinical nurse specialist programs in:* acute care, adult health, community health, critical care, medical-surgical. *Nurse practitioner programs in:* adult health, family health, gerontology, neonatal health, pediatric, psychiatric/mental health, women's health.

Study Options Full-time and part-time.

Program Entrance Requirements Clinical experience, computer literacy, minimum overall college GPA of 3.0, transcript of college record, CPR certification, immunizations, 4 letters of recommendation, nursing research course, physical assessment course, professional liability insurance/malpractice insurance, resume, statistics course.

Advanced Placement Credit by examination available.

Degree Requirements 51 total credit hours, thesis or project, comprehensive exam.

POST-MASTER'S PROGRAM

Areas of Study Nursing education. *Nurse practitioner programs in:* adult health, gerontology, neonatal health.

CONTINUING EDUCATION PROGRAM

Contact Dr. William Crouch, Director, Extended Studies, Beth-El College of Nursing and Health Sciences, University of Colorado at Colorado Springs, 1460 Austin Bluffs Parkway, Mail Stop UH-1, Colorado Springs, CO 80917. *Telephone:* 719-262-4651. *Fax:* 719-262-4416. *E-mail:* wcrouch@uccs.edu.

University of Colorado at Denver and Health Sciences Center—Health Sciences Program

School of Nursing
Denver, Colorado

http://www.uchsc.edu/nursing

Founded in 1883

DEGREES • BS • MS • MSN/MBA • PHD

Nursing Program Faculty 75 (66% with doctorates).

Baccalaureate Enrollment 267
Women 92% **Men** 8% **Minority** 12% **Part-time** 7%

Graduate Enrollment 262
Women 95% **Men** 5% **Minority** 7% **International** 1% **Part-time** 18%

Nursing Student Activities Sigma Theta Tau, Student Nurses' Association, nursing club.

Nursing Student Resources Academic advising; academic or career counseling; assistance for students with disabilities; bookstore; campus computer network; computer lab; computer-assisted instruction; e-mail services; externships; interactive nursing skills videos; Internet; learning resource lab; library services; nursing audiovisuals; paid internships; remedial services; skills, simulation, or other laboratory; tutoring; unpaid internships.

Library Facilities 250,000 volumes (1,000 in health, 40 in nursing); 1,650 periodical subscriptions (200 health-care related).

BACCALAUREATE PROGRAMS

Degree BS

Available Programs Generic Baccalaureate; RN Baccalaureate.

Site Options *Distance Learning:* Denver, CO.

Study Options Full-time and part-time.

Program Entrance Requirements Minimum overall college GPA of 2.75, transcript of college record, written essay, health exam, health insurance, immunizations, minimum GPA in nursing prerequisites of 2.0, prerequisite course work. Transfer students are accepted. **Standardized tests** *Required:* TOEFL for international students. **Application** *Deadline:* 10/1 (transfer). *Application fee:* $50.

Advanced Placement Credit given for nursing courses completed elsewhere dependent upon specific evaluations.

Expenses (2003–04) *Tuition, state resident:* part-time $191 per credit hour. *Tuition, nonresident:* part-time $667 per credit hour. *Required fees:* full-time $1500; part-time $40 per term.

Financial Aid 60% of baccalaureate students in nursing programs received some form of financial aid in 2002–03. *Gift aid (need-based):* Federal Pell, FSEOG, state, private, college/university gift aid from institutional funds. *Loans:* Federal Nursing Student Loans, Federal Direct (Subsidized and Unsubsidized Stafford PLUS), Perkins, college/university, Loans for Disadvantaged Students program, Health Professions Student Loans (HPSL). *Work-Study:* Federal Work-Study, part-time campus jobs. *Application deadline:* Continuous.

Contact Ruby J. Martinez, Director of Student Services & Diversity, School of Nursing, University of Colorado at Denver and Health Sciences Center—Health Sciences Program, 4200 East Ninth Avenue, Box C288-6, Denver, CO 80262. *Telephone:* 303-315-5592. *Fax:* 303-315-8920. *E-mail:* Ruby.Martinez@UCHSC.edu.

GRADUATE PROGRAMS

Expenses (2003–04) *Tuition, state resident:* part-time $272 per credit hour. *Tuition, nonresident:* part-time $867 per credit hour. *Required fees:* full-time $1500; part-time $10 per term.

Financial Aid 35% of graduate students in nursing programs received some form of financial aid in 2002–03. Fellowships, research assistantships, teaching assistantships, career-related internships or fieldwork, Federal Work-Study, and institutionally sponsored loans available. Aid available to part-time students. *Financial aid application deadline:* 3/15.

Contact Dr. Ruby J. Martinez, Director of Student Services & Diversity, School of Nursing, University of Colorado at Denver and Health Sciences Center—Health Sciences Program, 4200 East Ninth Avenue, Box C288-6, Denver, CO 80262. *Telephone:* 303-315-5592. *Fax:* 303-315-5648. *E-mail:* Ruby.Martinez@UCHSC.edu.

MASTER'S DEGREE PROGRAM

Degrees MS; MSN/MBA

Available Programs Master's; RN to Master's.

Concentrations Available Health-care administration; nurse-midwifery; nursing administration; nursing informatics. *Clinical nurse specialist programs in:* adult health, community health, psychiatric/mental health, public health. *Nurse practitioner programs in:* adult health, family health, gerontology, pediatric, psychiatric/mental health, women's health.

Site Options *Distance Learning:* Denver, CO.

Study Options Full-time and part-time.

Program Entrance Requirements Computer literacy, minimum overall college GPA of 3.0, transcript of college record, written essay, immunizations, 4 letters of recommendation, nursing research course, resume, statistics course. *Application deadline:* For fall admission, 12/1 (priority date). *Application fee:* $50.

Advanced Placement Credit given for nursing courses completed elsewhere dependent upon specific evaluations.

Degree Requirements 35 total credit hours, comprehensive exam.

POST-MASTER'S PROGRAM

Areas of Study Health-care administration; nurse-midwifery; nursing administration; nursing informatics. *Clinical nurse specialist programs in:* adult health, community health, psychiatric/mental health, public health. *Nurse practitioner programs in:* adult health, family health, gerontology, pediatric, psychiatric/mental health, women's health.

DOCTORAL DEGREE PROGRAM

Degree PhD

Available Programs Doctorate; Post-Baccalaureate Doctorate.

Areas of Study Community health, health-care systems, human health and illness, illness and transition, individualized study, nursing research, nursing science.

Site Options *Distance Learning:* Denver, CO.

Program Entrance Requirements Minimum overall college GPA of 3.0, interview by faculty committee, interview, 4 letters of recommendation, MSN or equivalent, statistics course, vita, writing sample. *Application deadline:* For fall admission, 12/1 (priority date). *Application fee:* $50.

Degree Requirements 75 total credit hours, dissertation, oral exam, written exam.

POSTDOCTORAL PROGRAM

Areas of Study Adolescent health, cancer care, community health, gerontology, individualized study, information systems, nursing informatics, nursing interventions, nursing research, nursing science, outcomes, vulnerable population.

Postdoctoral Program Contact Dr. Ruby J. Martinez, Director of Student Services & Diversity, School of Nursing, University of Colorado at Denver and Health Sciences Center—Health Sciences Program, 4200 East Ninth Avenue, Box C288-6, Denver, CO 80262. *Telephone:* 303-315-5592. *Fax:* 303-315-5648. *E-mail:* Ruby.Martinez@UCHSC.edu.

CONTINUING EDUCATION PROGRAM

Contact Dr. Mary McHugh, Director of Professional Development and Extended Studies, School of Nursing, University of Colorado at Denver and Health Sciences Center—Health Sciences Program, 4200 East Ninth Avenue, Box C288-6, Denver, CO 80262. *Telephone:* 303-315-8691. *Fax:* 303-315-0907. *E-mail:* mary.mchugh@uchsc.edu.

University of Northern Colorado
School of Nursing
Greeley, Colorado

http://www.unco.edu/HHS/son/son.htm

Founded in 1890

DEGREES • BS • MS • PHD

Nursing Program Faculty 31 (65% with doctorates).

Baccalaureate Enrollment 162
Women 94% **Men** 6% **Minority** 18%

Graduate Enrollment 42
Women 98% **Men** 2% **Minority** 11% **Part-time** 59%

Nursing Student Activities Sigma Theta Tau, Student Nurses' Association.

Nursing Student Resources Academic advising; academic or career counseling; assistance for students with disabilities; bookstore; campus computer network; career placement assistance; computer lab; computer-assisted instruction; e-mail services; employment services for current students; housing assistance; Internet; learning resource lab; library services; nursing audiovisuals; paid internships; placement services for program completers; resume preparation assistance; skills, simulation, or other laboratory; tutoring.

Library Facilities 1 million volumes (43,602 in health, 25,700 in nursing); 3,417 periodical subscriptions (140 health-care related).

BACCALAUREATE PROGRAMS

Degree BS

Available Programs Accelerated Baccalaureate; Generic Baccalaureate; RN Baccalaureate.

Site Options *Distance Learning:* Greeley, CO.

Study Options Full-time.

Program Entrance Requirements Minimum overall college GPA of 2.5, transcript of college record, CPR certification, written essay, health exam, immunizations, 1 letter of recommendation, minimum GPA in nursing prerequisites of 2.5, professional liability insurance/malpractice insurance, prerequisite course work. Transfer students are accepted. **Standardized tests** *Required:* SAT or ACT, TOEFL for international students. **Application** *Deadline:* 8/1 (freshmen), rolling (transfer). *Application fee:* $40.

Advanced Placement Credit given for nursing courses completed elsewhere dependent upon specific evaluations.

Expenses (2004–05) *Tuition, area resident:* full-time $3370; part-time $143 per credit hour. *Tuition, state resident:* full-time $3370; part-time $143 per summer. *Tuition, nonresident:* full-time $13,040; part-time $1425 per credit hour. *Required fees:* full-time $260; part-time $26 per credit.

Financial Aid 70% of baccalaureate students in nursing programs received some form of financial aid in 2003–04. *Gift aid (need-based):* Federal Pell, FSEOG, state, private, college/university gift aid from institutional funds, Robert C. Byrd Scholarships. *Loans:* FFEL (Subsidized and Unsubsidized Stafford PLUS), Perkins, college/university. *Work-Study:* Federal Work-Study, part-time campus jobs. *Application deadline (priority):* 3/1.

Contact Dr. Diane Peters, Assistant Director, School of Nursing, University of Northern Colorado, Box 125, Greeley, CO 80639. *Telephone:* 970-351-1692. *Fax:* 970-351-1707. *E-mail:* diane.peters@unco.edu.

GRADUATE PROGRAMS

Expenses (2004–05) *Tuition, state resident:* full-time $3880; part-time $168 per credit hour. *Tuition, nonresident:* full-time $13,040; part-time $587 per credit hour. *Required fees:* full-time $260; part-time $26 per credit.

Financial Aid 80% of graduate students in nursing programs received some form of financial aid in 2003–04. 3 fellowships (averaging $2,019 per year), 2 research assistantships (averaging $5,421 per year) were awarded; teaching assistantships, unspecified assistantships also available. *Financial aid application deadline:* 3/1.

Contact Dr. Nancy White, MS Program Coordinator and Professor, School of Nursing, University of Northern Colorado, Box 125, Greeley, CO 80639. *Telephone:* 970-351-2662. *Fax:* 970-351-1707. *E-mail:* nancy.white@unco.edu.

MASTER'S DEGREE PROGRAM

Degree MS

Concentrations Available Nursing education. *Nurse practitioner programs in:* family health.

Site Options *Distance Learning:* Greeley, CO.

Study Options Full-time and part-time.

Program Entrance Requirements Clinical experience, minimum overall college GPA of 3.0, transcript of college record, CPR certification, immunizations, 2 letters of recommendation, nursing research course, physical assessment course. *Application deadline:* Applications are processed on a rolling basis. *Application fee:* $50 ($60 for international students).

Advanced Placement Credit given for nursing courses completed elsewhere dependent upon specific evaluations.

Degree Requirements 45 total credit hours, thesis or project, comprehensive exam.

POST-MASTER'S PROGRAM

Areas of Study *Nurse practitioner programs in:* family health.

DOCTORAL DEGREE PROGRAM

Degree PhD

Available Programs Doctorate.

Areas of Study Nursing education.

Program Entrance Requirements Clinical experience, minimum overall college GPA of 3.0, interview. *Application deadline:* Applications are processed on a rolling basis. *Application fee:* $50 ($60 for international students).

Degree Requirements 30 total credit hours, dissertation.

University of Phoenix–Colorado Campus
College of Health and Human Services
Lone Tree, Colorado

DEGREES • BSN • MSN • MSN/MBA

University of Phoenix–Colorado Campus (continued)

Nursing Program Faculty 16 (19% with doctorates).

Baccalaureate Enrollment 36
Women 90% **Men** 10% **Minority** 10%

Graduate Enrollment 15
Women 93% **Men** 7% **Minority** 20%

Nursing Student Activities Sigma Theta Tau.

Nursing Student Resources Academic advising; academic or career counseling; bookstore; computer lab; library services.

Library Facilities 27.1 million volumes; 1,648 periodical subscriptions (1,426 health-care related).

BACCALAUREATE PROGRAMS

Degree BSN

Available Programs ADN to Baccalaureate; Accelerated RN Baccalaureate.

Study Options Full-time.

Program Entrance Requirements 1 letter of recommendation. Transfer students are accepted. **Standardized tests** *Required:* TOEFL for international students. **Application** *Deadline:* rolling (freshmen), rolling (transfer). *Application fee:* $100.

Advanced Placement Credit by examination available.

Expenses (2004–05) *Tuition:* full-time $9000; part-time $300 per credit hour. *International tuition:* $9000 full-time. *Required fees:* full-time $110.

Financial Aid 2% of baccalaureate students in nursing programs received some form of financial aid in 2003–04.

Contact Campus College Chair, Nursing, College of Health and Human Services, University of Phoenix–Colorado Campus, 10004 Park Meadow Drive, Lone Tree, CO 80124-5453. *Telephone:* 303-694-9093.

GRADUATE PROGRAMS

Expenses (2004–05) *Tuition:* full-time $9360; part-time $390 per credit hour. *International tuition:* $9360 full-time. *Required fees:* full-time $110.

Financial Aid 2% of graduate students in nursing programs received some form of financial aid in 2003–04.

Contact Campus College Chair, Nursing, College of Health and Human Services, University of Phoenix–Colorado Campus, 10004 Park Meadow Drive, Lone Tree, CO 80124-5453. *Telephone:* 303-694-9003.

MASTER'S DEGREE PROGRAM

Degrees MSN; MSN/MBA

Available Programs Master's.

Concentrations Available Health-care administration; nursing administration; nursing education. *Nurse practitioner programs in:* family health.

Study Options Full-time.

Program Entrance Requirements Clinical experience, computer literacy, minimum overall college GPA of 2.5, transcript of college record. *Application deadline:* Applications are processed on a rolling basis. *Application fee:* $110.

Degree Requirements 39 total credit hours, thesis or project.

POST-MASTER'S PROGRAM

Areas of Study *Nurse practitioner programs in:* family health.

University of Phoenix–Southern Colorado Campus

College of Health and Human Services
Colorado Springs, Colorado

Founded in 1999

DEGREES • BSN • MSN • MSN/MBA

Nursing Program Faculty 10 (20% with doctorates).

Baccalaureate Enrollment 17
Women 94% **Men** 6% **Minority** 8%

Graduate Enrollment 1
Women 100%

Nursing Student Activities Sigma Theta Tau.

Nursing Student Resources Academic advising; academic or career counseling; bookstore; computer lab; library services.

Library Facilities 27.1 million volumes; 11,648 periodical subscriptions (1,426 health-care related).

BACCALAUREATE PROGRAMS

Degree BSN

Available Programs ADN to Baccalaureate; Accelerated Baccalaureate.

Study Options Full-time.

Program Entrance Requirements 1 letter of recommendation. Transfer students are accepted. **Standardized tests** *Required:* TOEFL for international students. **Application** *Deadline:* rolling (freshmen), rolling (transfer). *Application fee:* $85.

Advanced Placement Credit by examination available.

Expenses (2004–05) *Tuition:* full-time $9000; part-time $300 per credit hour. *International tuition:* $9000 full-time. *Required fees:* full-time $110.

Financial Aid 3% of baccalaureate students in nursing programs received some form of financial aid in 2003–04.

Contact Campus College Chair, Nursing, College of Health and Human Services, University of Phoenix–Southern Colorado Campus, 5475 Tech Center Drive, #130, Colorado Springs, CO 80919-2335. *Telephone:* 719-599-5282.

GRADUATE PROGRAMS

Expenses (2004–05) *Tuition:* full-time $9360; part-time $390 per credit hour. *International tuition:* $9360 full-time. *Required fees:* full-time $110.

Financial Aid 3% of graduate students in nursing programs received some form of financial aid in 2003–04.

Contact Campus College Chair, Nursing, College of Health and Human Services, University of Phoenix–Southern Colorado Campus, 5475 Tech Center Drive, #130, Colorado Springs, CO 80919-2335. *Telephone:* 719-599-5282.

MASTER'S DEGREE PROGRAM

Degrees MSN; MSN/MBA

Available Programs Master's.

Concentrations Available Health-care administration; nursing administration; nursing education. *Nurse practitioner programs in:* family health.

Study Options Full-time.

Program Entrance Requirements Clinical experience, computer literacy, minimum overall college GPA of 2.5, transcript of college record. *Application deadline:* Applications are processed on a rolling basis. *Application fee:* $110.

Degree Requirements 39 total credit hours, thesis or project.

POST-MASTER'S PROGRAM

Areas of Study *Nurse practitioner programs in:* family health.

CONNECTICUT

Central Connecticut State University

Department of Counseling and Family Therapy
New Britain, Connecticut

http://www.ccsu.edu/nursing/

Founded in 1849

DEGREE • BSN

Nursing Program Faculty 5 (80% with doctorates).

Nursing Student Activities Nursing Honor Society.

Library Facilities 639,257 volumes; 2,762 periodical subscriptions.

BACCALAUREATE PROGRAMS

Degree BSN

Available Programs RN Baccalaureate.

Site Options New London, CT.

Program Entrance Requirements Minimum overall college GPA of 2.7, transcript of college record, CPR certification, health exam, immunizations, minimum GPA in nursing prerequisites of 2.7, professional liability insurance/malpractice insurance, prerequisite course work, RN licensure. Transfer students are accepted. **Standardized tests** *Required:* SAT, TOEFL for international students. **Application** *Deadline:* 6/1 (freshmen), 6/1 (transfer). *Notification:* continuous until 7/1 (freshmen). *Application fee:* $50.

Advanced Placement Credit by examination available. Credit given for nursing courses completed elsewhere dependent upon specific evaluations.

Contact Dr. Carol G. Williams, Associate Professor and Interim Department Chairperson, Department of Counseling and Family Therapy, Central Connecticut State University, 1615 Stanley Street, New Britain, CT 06050-4010. *Telephone:* 860-832-0032. *Fax:* 860-832-2188. *E-mail:* williamsca@ccsu.edu.

Fairfield University

School of Nursing
Fairfield, Connecticut

http://www.fairfield.edu/academic/nursing/

Founded in 1942

DEGREES • BS • MSN

Nursing Program Faculty 26 (83% with doctorates).

Baccalaureate Enrollment 281
Women 94% **Men** 6% **Minority** 9% **Part-time** 15%

Graduate Enrollment 46
Women 100% **Minority** 9% **Part-time** 98%

Nursing Student Activities Nursing Honor Society, Sigma Theta Tau, Student Nurses' Association.

Nursing Student Resources Academic advising; academic or career counseling; bookstore; career placement assistance; computer lab; e-mail services; Internet; library services; skills, simulation, or other laboratory.

Library Facilities 325,166 volumes (8,900 in health); 1,793 periodical subscriptions (130 health-care related).

BACCALAUREATE PROGRAMS

Degree BS

Available Programs Accelerated Baccalaureate for Second Degree; Baccalaureate for Second Degree; Generic Baccalaureate; RN Baccalaureate.

Study Options Full-time and part-time.

Program Entrance Requirements Written essay, health exam, high school biology, high school chemistry, high school foreign language, 3 years high school math, 3 years high school science, high school transcript, letters of recommendation, minimum high school GPA of 3.0, minimum high school rank 40%. Transfer students are accepted. **Standardized tests** *Required:* SAT or ACT, TOEFL for international students. **Application** *Deadline:* 1/15 (freshmen), 6/1 (transfer). *Early decision:* 11/15. *Notification:* 4/1 (freshmen), 12/15 (out-of-state freshmen), 12/15 (early decision). *Application fee:* $55.

Expenses (2004–05) *Tuition:* full-time $27,930; part-time $375 per degree program. *International tuition:* $27,930 full-time. *Room and board:* $9270; room only: $5470 per academic year. *Required fees:* full-time $485.

Financial Aid 68% of baccalaureate students in nursing programs received some form of financial aid in 2003–04.

Contact Ms. Karen Pellegrino, Director of Admission, School of Nursing, Fairfield University, 1073 North Benson Road, Fairfield, CT 06824-5195. *Telephone:* 203-254-4100. *Fax:* 203-254-4199. *E-mail:* admis@mail.fairfield.edu.

GRADUATE PROGRAMS

Expenses (2004–05) *Tuition:* part-time $435 per credit hour. *Required fees:* full-time $25.

Financial Aid Traineeships available.

Contact Ms. Marianne Gumpper, Graduate Program Director, School of Nursing, Fairfield University, 1073 North Benson Road, CNS 302, Fairfield, CT 06824-5195. *Telephone:* 203-254-4000 Ext. 2908. *Fax:* 203-254-4073. *E-mail:* admis@mail.fairfield.edu.

MASTER'S DEGREE PROGRAM

Degree MSN

Available Programs Master's.

Concentrations Available *Nurse practitioner programs in:* adult health, family health, psychiatric/mental health.

Study Options Full-time and part-time.

Program Entrance Requirements Computer literacy, minimum overall college GPA of 3.0, transcript of college record, written essay, immunizations, interview, 2 letters of recommendation, physical assessment course, prerequisite course work, resume, statistics course, MAT or GRE. *Application deadline:* For fall admission, 4/1 (priority date); for spring admission, 11/1 (priority date). Applications are processed on a rolling basis. *Application fee:* $55.

Degree Requirements 39 total credit hours, thesis or project.

POST-MASTER'S PROGRAM

Areas of Study *Nurse practitioner programs in:* adult health, family health, psychiatric/mental health.

Quinnipiac University

Department of Nursing
Hamden, Connecticut

Founded in 1929

DEGREES • BSN • MSN

Nursing Program Faculty 37 (90% with doctorates).

Baccalaureate Enrollment 297
Women 98% **Men** 2% **Minority** 7% **International** 1% **Part-time** 1%

Graduate Enrollment 72
Women 99% **Men** 1% **Minority** 6% **International** 1% **Part-time** 58%

Nursing Student Activities Nursing club.

Nursing Student Resources Academic advising; academic or career counseling; bookstore; campus computer network; career placement assistance; e-mail services; employment services for current students; externships; housing assistance; Internet; learning resource lab; library services; paid internships; placement services for program completers; resume preparation assistance; skills, simulation, or other laboratory; tutoring; unpaid internships.

Library Facilities 285,000 volumes (1,000 in nursing); 4,400 periodical subscriptions.

BACCALAUREATE PROGRAMS

Degree BSN

Available Programs Accelerated Baccalaureate for Second Degree; Generic Baccalaureate; RN Baccalaureate.

Study Options Full-time and part-time.

Program Entrance Requirements Minimum overall college GPA of 3.0, transcript of college record, CPR certification, written essay, health exam, high school biology, high school chemistry, 4 years high school math, 3 years high school science, high school transcript, immunizations, 1 letter of recommendation, minimum high school GPA of 3.0, minimum high school rank 50%, minimum GPA in nursing prerequisites of 3.0. Transfer students are accepted. **Standardized tests** *Required:* SAT or ACT,

Quinnipiac University (continued)
TOEFL for international students. **Application** *Deadline:* 2/1 (freshmen), 5/1 (transfer). *Notification:* continuous until 3/1 (freshmen). *Application fee:* $45.

Advanced Placement Credit given for nursing courses completed elsewhere dependent upon specific evaluations.

Expenses (2004–05) *Tuition:* full-time $21,540; part-time $530 per credit hour. *International tuition:* $21,540 full-time. *Room and board:* $9900 per academic year. *Required fees:* full-time $960; part-time $30 per credit.

Financial Aid 69% of baccalaureate students in nursing programs received some form of financial aid in 2003–04.

Contact Ms. Carla Knowlton, Director of Undergraduate Admissions, Department of Nursing, Quinnipiac University, 275 Mount Carmel Avenue, Hamden, CT 06518. *Telephone:* 203-582-8600. *Fax:* 203-582-8906. *E-mail:* admissions@quinnipiac.edu.

GRADUATE PROGRAMS

Expenses (2004–05) *Tuition:* part-time $530 per credit hour. *Required fees:* part-time $30 per credit.

Financial Aid 30% of graduate students in nursing programs received some form of financial aid in 2003–04.

Contact Scott Farber, Director of Graduate Admissions, Department of Nursing, Quinnipiac University, 275 Mount Carmel Avenue, Hamden, CT 06518. *Telephone:* 203-582-8672. *Fax:* 203-582-3443. *E-mail:* graduate@quinnipiac.edu.

MASTER'S DEGREE PROGRAM

Degree MSN

Available Programs Master's.

Concentrations Available Forensic nursing (clinical specialist program); health-care administration. *Nurse practitioner programs in:* adult health, family health.

Study Options Full-time and part-time.

Program Entrance Requirements Clinical experience, minimum overall college GPA of 3.0, transcript of college record, CPR certification, written essay, immunizations, interview, 3 letters of recommendation, professional liability insurance/malpractice insurance, prerequisite course work, resume.

Advanced Placement Credit given for nursing courses completed elsewhere dependent upon specific evaluations.

Degree Requirements 55 total credit hours, thesis or project.

POST-MASTER'S PROGRAM

Areas of Study *Nurse practitioner programs in:* adult health, family health.

CONTINUING EDUCATION PROGRAM

Contact Ms. Mary Wargo, Director of Transfer and Part-Time Admissions, Department of Nursing, Quinnipiac University, 275 Mount Carmel Avenue, Hamden, CT 06518. *Telephone:* 203-582-8612. *Fax:* 203-582-8906. *E-mail:* mary.wargo@quinnipiac.edu.

See full description on page 532.

Sacred Heart University

Program in Nursing
Fairfield, Connecticut

http://nursing.sacredheart.edu/

Founded in 1963

DEGREES • BS • MSN • MSN/MBA

Nursing Program Faculty 23 (30% with doctorates).

Baccalaureate Enrollment 254
Women 93% **Men** 7% **Minority** 22% **Part-time** 51%

Graduate Enrollment 59
Women 91% **Men** 9% **Minority** 14% **Part-time** 94%

Nursing Student Activities Nursing Honor Society, Sigma Theta Tau, Student Nurses' Association, nursing club.

Nursing Student Resources Academic advising; academic or career counseling; assistance for students with disabilities; bookstore; campus computer network; career placement assistance; computer lab; computer-assisted instruction; e-mail services; Internet; learning resource lab; library services; nursing audiovisuals; placement services for program completers; resume preparation assistance; skills, simulation, or other laboratory; tutoring.

Library Facilities 3,729 volumes in health, 1,900 volumes in nursing; 4,100 periodical subscriptions (135 health-care related).

BACCALAUREATE PROGRAMS

Degree BS

Available Programs ADN to Baccalaureate; Generic Baccalaureate; RN Baccalaureate.

Site Options *Distance Learning:* Fairfield, CT.

Study Options Full-time and part-time.

Program Entrance Requirements Minimum overall college GPA of 2.5, transcript of college record, CPR certification, written essay, health exam, health insurance, high school biology, 3 years high school math, 3 years high school science, high school transcript, immunizations, interview, 2 letters of recommendation, minimum high school GPA of 3.0, minimum high school rank 50%, minimum GPA in nursing prerequisites of 2.5, prerequisite course work. Transfer students are accepted. **Standardized tests** *Required:* SAT or ACT, TOEFL for international students. **Application** *Early decision:* 10/1 (for plan 1), 12/1 (for plan 2). *Notification:* continuous (freshmen), 10/15 (out-of-state freshmen), 10/15 (early decision plan 1), 12/15 (early decision plan 2). *Application fee:* $50.

Advanced Placement Credit given for nursing courses completed elsewhere dependent upon specific evaluations.

Expenses (2004–05) *Tuition:* full-time $10,995; part-time $370 per credit hour.

Financial Aid 72% of baccalaureate students in nursing programs received some form of financial aid in 2003–04. *Gift aid (need-based):* Federal Pell, FSEOG, state, private, college/university gift aid from institutional funds, Federal Nursing. *Loans:* FFEL (Subsidized and Unsubsidized Stafford PLUS), Perkins, state, alternative loans. *Work-Study:* Federal Work-Study, part-time campus jobs. *Application deadline (priority):* 2/15.

Contact Ms. Alma C. Haluch, Departmental Assistant, Program in Nursing, Sacred Heart University, 5151 Park Avenue, Fairfield, CT 06825-1000. *Telephone:* 203-371-7715. *Fax:* 203-365-7662. *E-mail:* halucha@sacredheart.edu.

GRADUATE PROGRAMS

Expenses (2004–05) *Tuition:* part-time $430 per credit hour.

Contact Dr. Dori Taylor Sullivan, Chair and Director, Program in Nursing, Sacred Heart University, 5151 Park Avenue, Fairfield, CT 06825-1000. *Telephone:* 203-371-7715. *Fax:* 203-365-7662. *E-mail:* sullivand@sacredheart.edu.

MASTER'S DEGREE PROGRAM

Degrees MSN; MSN/MBA

Available Programs Accelerated AD/RN to Master's; Accelerated Master's for Nurses with Non-Nursing Degrees; Accelerated RN to Master's; Master's; Master's for Nurses with Non-Nursing Degrees; RN to Master's.

Concentrations Available Nursing administration. *Nurse practitioner programs in:* family health.

Site Options *Distance Learning:* Fairfield, CT.

Study Options Full-time and part-time.

Program Entrance Requirements Clinical experience, minimum overall college GPA of 3.0, transcript of college record, written essay, interview, 2 letters of recommendation, physical assessment course, professional liability insurance/malpractice insurance, prerequisite course work, resume, statistics course.

Advanced Placement Credit given for nursing courses completed elsewhere dependent upon specific evaluations.

Degree Requirements 40 total credit hours, thesis or project.

POST-MASTER'S PROGRAM

Areas of Study Nursing administration. *Nurse practitioner programs in:* family health.

See full description on page 536.

Saint Joseph College
Department of Nursing
West Hartford, Connecticut

Founded in 1932

DEGREES • BS • MS

Nursing Program Faculty 19 (34% with doctorates).

Baccalaureate Enrollment 130
Women 100% **Minority** 30% **International** 5% **Part-time** 40%

Graduate Enrollment 55
Women 90% **Men** 10% **Minority** 10% **Part-time** 95%

Nursing Student Activities Sigma Theta Tau, Student Nurses' Association, nursing club.

Nursing Student Resources Academic advising; academic or career counseling; assistance for students with disabilities; bookstore; campus computer network; career placement assistance; computer lab; computer-assisted instruction; daycare for children of students; e-mail services; employment services for current students; externships; housing assistance; interactive nursing skills videos; Internet; learning resource lab; library services; nursing audiovisuals; paid internships; remedial services; resume preparation assistance; skills, simulation, or other laboratory; tutoring; unpaid internships.

Library Facilities 120,094 volumes; 479 periodical subscriptions.

BACCALAUREATE PROGRAMS

Degree BS

Available Programs Accelerated Baccalaureate for Second Degree; Accelerated RN Baccalaureate; Baccalaureate for Second Degree; Generic Baccalaureate; RN Baccalaureate.

Study Options Full-time and part-time.

Program Entrance Requirements Minimum overall college GPA of 2.8, transcript of college record, written essay, health exam, health insurance, high school biology, high school chemistry, 3 years high school math, 3 years high school science, high school transcript, immunizations, 1 letter of recommendation, minimum high school GPA of 2.0, minimum GPA in nursing prerequisites of 2.8. Transfer students are accepted. **Standardized tests** *Required:* SAT or ACT, TOEFL for international students. **Application** *Deadline:* rolling (freshmen), 7/1 (transfer). *Early decision:* 11/15. *Notification:* continuous until 6/14 (freshmen), 12/15 (early action). *Application fee:* $35.

Advanced Placement Credit by examination available. Credit given for nursing courses completed elsewhere dependent upon specific evaluations.

Expenses (2003–04) *Tuition:* full-time $20,350; part-time $515 per credit hour. *Room and board:* $8785; room only: $4140 per academic year. *Required fees:* full-time $550; part-time $55 per credit.

Financial Aid 61% of baccalaureate students in nursing programs received some form of financial aid in 2002–03. *Gift aid (need-based):* Federal Pell, FSEOG, state, private, college/university gift aid from institutional funds. *Loans:* FFEL (Subsidized and Unsubsidized Stafford PLUS), Perkins, state, Connecticut Family Education Loan Program. *Work-Study:* Federal Work-Study, part-time campus jobs. *Application deadline (priority):* 3/15.

Contact Terry L. Bosworth, Chairperson, Department of Nursing, Saint Joseph College, 1678 Asylum Avenue, West Hartford, CT 06117. *Telephone:* 860-231-5304. *E-mail:* tbosworth@sjc.edu.

GRADUATE PROGRAMS

Expenses (2003–04) *Tuition:* part-time $540 per credit hour. *Required fees:* part-time $55 per credit.

Financial Aid 50% of graduate students in nursing programs received some form of financial aid in 2002–03.

Contact Dr. Nancy Drew, Director, Department of Nursing, Saint Joseph College, 1678 Asylum Avenue, West Hartford, CT 06117-2700. *Telephone:* 860-231-5316. *Fax:* 860-231-8396. *E-mail:* ndrew@sjc.edu.

MASTER'S DEGREE PROGRAM

Degree MS

Available Programs Accelerated AD/RN to Master's; Accelerated RN to Master's; Master's; Master's for Nurses with Non-Nursing Degrees; RN to Master's.

Concentrations Available *Clinical nurse specialist programs in:* family health, psychiatric/mental health. *Nurse practitioner programs in:* adult health, family health.

Study Options Full-time and part-time.

Program Entrance Requirements Clinical experience, minimum overall college GPA of 3.0, transcript of college record, written essay, immunizations, 2 letters of recommendation, nursing research course, physical assessment course, professional liability insurance/malpractice insurance, statistics course.

Advanced Placement Credit given for nursing courses completed elsewhere dependent upon specific evaluations.

Degree Requirements 36 total credit hours, thesis or project.

POST-MASTER'S PROGRAM

Areas of Study *Clinical nurse specialist programs in:* family health, psychiatric/mental health. *Nurse practitioner programs in:* family health.

Southern Connecticut State University
Department of Nursing
New Haven, Connecticut

http://www.southernct.edu/departments/nursing

Founded in 1893

DEGREES • BSN • MSN

Nursing Program Faculty 13 (55% with doctorates).

Nursing Student Activities Nursing Honor Society, Sigma Theta Tau, Student Nurses' Association.

Library Facilities 495,660 volumes (35,540 in health, 2,279 in nursing); 3,549 periodical subscriptions (318 health-care related).

BACCALAUREATE PROGRAMS

Degree BSN

Available Programs ADN to Baccalaureate; Generic Baccalaureate; RN Baccalaureate.

Study Options Full-time and part-time.

Program Entrance Requirements Minimum overall college GPA of 2.4, transcript of college record, high school math, high school transcript, prerequisite course work. Transfer students are accepted. **Standardized tests** *Required:* SAT or ACT, TOEFL for international students. **Application** *Deadline:* 7/1 (freshmen), 8/1 (transfer). *Notification:* continuous (freshmen). *Application fee:* $50.

Advanced Placement Credit given for nursing courses completed elsewhere dependent upon specific evaluations.

Contact Dr. Shelley Bochain, Coordinator, BSN Program in Nursing, Department of Nursing, Southern Connecticut State University, 501 Crescent Street, New Haven, CT 06515-1355. *Telephone:* 203-392-6483. *Fax:* 203-392-6493. *E-mail:* bochains@southernct.edu.

GRADUATE PROGRAMS

Contact Dr. Olive Santavenere, Coordinator, Graduate Programs in Nursing, Department of Nursing, Southern Connecticut State University, 501 Crescent Street, New Haven, CT 06515. *Telephone:* 203-392-6486. *Fax:* 203-392-6493. *E-mail:* santavenero1@southernct.edu.

MASTER'S DEGREE PROGRAM

Degree MSN

Concentrations Available Nursing administration; nursing education. *Nurse practitioner programs in:* family health.

Study Options Full-time and part-time.

Southern Connecticut State University (continued)

Program Entrance Requirements Clinical experience, minimum overall college GPA of 2.8, transcript of college record, interview, 2 letters of recommendation, nursing research course, professional liability insurance/malpractice insurance, prerequisite course work, resume, statistics course, GRE, MAT. *Application deadline:* For fall admission, 7/15 (priority date). Applications are processed on a rolling basis. *Application fee:* $40.

Advanced Placement Credit given for nursing courses completed elsewhere dependent upon specific evaluations.

Degree Requirements 42 total credit hours, thesis or project.

POST-MASTER'S PROGRAM

Areas of Study *Nurse practitioner programs in:* family health.

University of Connecticut

School of Nursing
Storrs, Connecticut

http://www.nursing.uconn.edu

Founded in 1881

DEGREES • BS • MS • MSN/MBA • MSN/MPH • PHD

Nursing Program Faculty 47 (50% with doctorates).

Baccalaureate Enrollment 400
Women 90% **Men** 10% **Minority** 23% **Part-time** 5%

Graduate Enrollment 150
Women 89% **Men** 11% **Minority** 5% **International** 2% **Part-time** 70%

Nursing Student Activities Sigma Theta Tau, Student Nurses' Association.

Nursing Student Resources Academic advising; academic or career counseling; assistance for students with disabilities; bookstore; campus computer network; career placement assistance; computer lab; daycare for children of students; e-mail services; externships; housing assistance; interactive nursing skills videos; Internet; library services; paid internships; placement services for program completers; resume preparation assistance; skills, simulation, or other laboratory; tutoring.

Library Facilities 3 million volumes (34,240 in nursing); 17,378 periodical subscriptions (219 health-care related).

BACCALAUREATE PROGRAMS

Degree BS

Available Programs RN Baccalaureate.

Site Options Farmington, CT. *Distance Learning:* Torrington, CT; West Hartford, CT.

Study Options Full-time and part-time.

Program Entrance Requirements Minimum overall college GPA of 2.5, transcript of college record, written essay, health exam, health insurance, high school foreign language, 3 years high school math, 2 years high school science, high school transcript, immunizations, minimum high school GPA of 3.0, minimum GPA in nursing prerequisites of 2.0. Transfer students are accepted. **Standardized tests** *Required:* SAT or ACT, TOEFL for international students. **Application** *Deadline:* 2/1 (freshmen), 4/1 (transfer). *Early decision:* 12/1. *Notification:* 1/1 (early action). *Application fee:* $70.

Advanced Placement Credit by examination available. Credit given for nursing courses completed elsewhere dependent upon specific evaluations.

Expenses (2003–04) *Tuition, state resident:* full-time $7338. *Tuition, nonresident:* full-time $19,066. *International tuition:* $19,066 full-time. *Room and board:* $7300; room only: $3872 per academic year. *Required fees:* full-time $7300.

Financial Aid 31% of baccalaureate students in nursing programs received some form of financial aid in 2002–03.

Contact Office of Academic Advising Services, School of Nursing, University of Connecticut, 231 Glenbrook Road, Unit 2026, Storrs, CT 06269-2026. *Telephone:* 860-486-1968. *Fax:* 860-486-0906. *E-mail:* nuradm11@uconnvm.uconn.edu.

GRADUATE PROGRAMS

Expenses (2003–04) *Tuition, area resident:* full-time $3239; part-time $360 per course. *Tuition, state resident:* full-time $3239; part-time $360 per quarter. *Tuition, nonresident:* full-time $8415; part-time $935 per course. *Room and board:* $3696; room only: $2087 per academic year. *Required fees:* full-time $3840; part-time $213 per credit.

Financial Aid 9 research assistantships, 5 teaching assistantships were awarded; fellowships, Federal Work-Study, scholarships, and unspecified assistantships also available.

Contact Office of Academic Advising Services, School of Nursing, University of Connecticut, 231 Glenbrook Road, Unit 2026, Storrs, CT 06269-2026. *Telephone:* 860-486-1968. *Fax:* 860-486-0906. *E-mail:* nuradm11@uconnvm.uconn.edu.

MASTER'S DEGREE PROGRAM

Degrees MS; MSN/MBA; MSN/MPH

Available Programs Master's; RN to Master's.

Concentrations Available Nursing administration. *Clinical nurse specialist programs in:* acute care, adult health, community health, critical care. *Nurse practitioner programs in:* acute care, adult health, neonatal health, primary care.

Site Options Farmington, CT. *Distance Learning:* Torrington, CT; West Hartford, CT.

Study Options Full-time and part-time.

Program Entrance Requirements Minimum overall college GPA of 3.0, transcript of college record, CPR certification, written essay, immunizations, interview, 3 letters of recommendation, nursing research course, professional liability insurance/malpractice insurance, resume, statistics course. *Application deadline:* For fall admission, 2/1 (priority date); for spring admission, 11/1. Applications are processed on a rolling basis. *Application fee:* $55.

Advanced Placement Credit given for nursing courses completed elsewhere dependent upon specific evaluations.

Degree Requirements 24 total credit hours, comprehensive exam.

POST-MASTER'S PROGRAM

Areas of Study Nursing administration. *Clinical nurse specialist programs in:* acute care, adult health, community health, critical care. *Nurse practitioner programs in:* acute care, adult health, neonatal health, primary care.

DOCTORAL DEGREE PROGRAM

Degree PhD

Available Programs Doctorate.

Areas of Study Nursing research, nursing science.

Program Entrance Requirements Minimum overall college GPA of 3.25, interview by faculty committee, interview, 3 letters of recommendation, MSN or equivalent, statistics course, vita, writing sample. *Application deadline:* For fall admission, 2/1 (priority date); for spring admission, 11/1. Applications are processed on a rolling basis. *Application fee:* $55.

Degree Requirements 48 total credit hours, dissertation, oral exam, written exam, residency.

CONTINUING EDUCATION PROGRAM

Contact Center for Academic Advising Services, School of Nursing, University of Connecticut, 231 Glenbrook Road, Unit 2026, Storrs, CT 06269-2026. *Telephone:* 860-486-1968. *Fax:* 860-486-0906. *E-mail:* nuradm11@uconnvm.uconn.edu.

See full description on page 554.

University of Hartford

College of Education, Nursing, and Health Professions
West Hartford, Connecticut

http://www.hartford.edu/enhp

Founded in 1877

DEGREES • BSN • MSN • MSN/MSOB

Nursing Program Faculty 8 (70% with doctorates).
Baccalaureate Enrollment 108
Women 98% **Men** 2% **Minority** 30% **Part-time** 100%
Graduate Enrollment 140
Women 96% **Men** 4% **Minority** 8% **Part-time** 100%
Nursing Student Activities Sigma Theta Tau.
Library Facilities 468,780 volumes; 2,425 periodical subscriptions.

BACCALAUREATE PROGRAMS

Degree BSN

Available Programs ADN to Baccalaureate; RN Baccalaureate.

Study Options Part-time.

Program Entrance Requirements RN licensure. Transfer students are accepted. **Standardized tests** *Required:* SAT or ACT, TOEFL for international students. **Application** *Deadline:* rolling (freshmen), rolling (transfer). *Notification:* continuous (freshmen). *Application fee:* $35.

Advanced Placement Credit by examination available. Credit given for nursing courses completed elsewhere dependent upon specific evaluations.

Expenses (2004–05) *Tuition:* part-time $320 per credit hour. *Required fees:* part-time $55 per term.

Financial Aid 60% of baccalaureate students in nursing programs received some form of financial aid in 2003–04. *Gift aid (need-based):* Federal Pell, FSEOG, state, private, college/university gift aid from institutional funds. *Loans:* FFEL (Subsidized and Unsubsidized Stafford PLUS), Perkins. *Work-Study:* Federal Work-Study, part-time campus jobs. *Application deadline (priority):* 2/1.

Contact Marlene J. Hall, Assistant Dean, College of Education, Nursing, and Health Professions, College of Education, Nursing, and Health Professions, University of Hartford, 200 Bloomfield Avenue, West Hartford, CT 06117-1599. *Telephone:* 860-768-5116. *Fax:* 860-768-5346. *E-mail:* mhall@hartford.edu.

GRADUATE PROGRAMS

Expenses (2004–05) *Tuition:* part-time $320 per credit hour. *Required fees:* part-time $55 per term.

Financial Aid 60% of graduate students in nursing programs received some form of financial aid in 2003–04. 2 teaching assistantships (averaging $9,580 per year) were awarded; institutionally sponsored loans and unspecified assistantships also available. *Financial aid application deadline:* 6/1.

Contact Marlene J. Hall, Assistant Dean, College of Education, Nursing and Health Professions, College of Education, Nursing, and Health Professions, University of Hartford, 200 Bloomfield Avenue, West Hartford, CT 06117-1599. *Telephone:* 860-768-5116. *Fax:* 860-768-5346. *E-mail:* mhall@hartford.edu.

MASTER'S DEGREE PROGRAM

Degrees MSN; MSN/MSOB

Available Programs Master's; Master's for Nurses with Non-Nursing Degrees.

Concentrations Available Nursing administration; nursing education.

Study Options Part-time.

Program Entrance Requirements Clinical experience, minimum overall college GPA of 3.0, transcript of college record, written essay, 2 letters of recommendation, professional liability insurance/malpractice insurance, resume. *Application deadline:* Applications are processed on a rolling basis. *Application fee:* $40 ($55 for international students).

Advanced Placement Credit given for nursing courses completed elsewhere dependent upon specific evaluations.

Degree Requirements 34 total credit hours, thesis or project.

DOCTORAL DEGREE PROGRAM

Program Entrance Requirements MAT. *Application deadline:* Applications are processed on a rolling basis. *Application fee:* $40 ($55 for international students).

CONTINUING EDUCATION PROGRAM

Contact Ms. Mary Beth Mathews, Chair, Department of Nursing, College of Education, Nursing, and Health Professions, University of Hartford, 200 Bloomfield Avenue, West Hartford, CT 06117-1599. *Telephone:* 860-768-4213. *Fax:* 860-768-5346. *E-mail:* mbmathews@hartford.edu.

Western Connecticut State University

Department of Nursing
Danbury, Connecticut

Founded in 1903

DEGREES • BS • MS

Nursing Program Faculty 18 (56% with doctorates).
Baccalaureate Enrollment 247
Women 95% **Men** 5% **Minority** 20% **Part-time** 30%
Graduate Enrollment 30
Women 100% **Minority** 2% **Part-time** 100%
Nursing Student Activities Sigma Theta Tau, Student Nurses' Association.

Nursing Student Resources Academic advising; academic or career counseling; assistance for students with disabilities; bookstore; campus computer network; career placement assistance; computer lab; computer-assisted instruction; daycare for children of students; e-mail services; employment services for current students; externships; interactive nursing skills videos; Internet; learning resource lab; library services; nursing audiovisuals; remedial services; resume preparation assistance; skills, simulation, or other laboratory; tutoring.

Library Facilities 182,915 volumes; 1,273 periodical subscriptions.

BACCALAUREATE PROGRAMS

Degree BS

Available Programs Generic Baccalaureate; RN Baccalaureate.

Site Options Waterbury, CT.

Study Options Full-time.

Program Entrance Requirements Transcript of college record, CPR certification, health exam, high school biology, high school chemistry, high school foreign language, 3 years high school math, 2 years high school science, high school transcript, immunizations, minimum high school GPA of 2.67, minimum GPA in nursing prerequisites of 2.0, prerequisite course work. Transfer students are accepted. **Standardized tests** *Required:* SAT or ACT, TOEFL for international students. **Application** *Deadline:* 5/1 (freshmen), 7/1 (transfer). *Notification:* continuous (freshmen). *Application fee:* $40.

Advanced Placement Credit by examination available. Credit given for nursing courses completed elsewhere dependent upon specific evaluations.

Expenses (2004–05) *Tuition, state resident:* full-time $3010; part-time $287 per credit hour. *Tuition, nonresident:* full-time $9744; part-time $287 per credit hour. *Room and board:* $6890; room only: $3950 per academic year. *Required fees:* full-time $3765.

Financial Aid *Gift aid (need-based):* Federal Pell, FSEOG, state, private, college/university gift aid from institutional funds. *Loans:* FFEL (Subsidized and Unsubsidized Stafford PLUS), Perkins. *Work-Study:* Federal Work-Study, part-time campus jobs. *Application deadline:* 4/15 (priority: 3/15).

Contact Dr. Barbara Piscopo, BSN Program Coordinator, Department of Nursing, Western Connecticut State University, 181 White Street, Danbury, CT 06810. *Telephone:* 203-837-8557. *Fax:* 203-837-8550. *E-mail:* piscopob@wcsu.edu.

GRADUATE PROGRAMS

Contact Dr. Laurel Halloren, Graduate Program Coordinator, Department of Nursing, Western Connecticut State University, 181 White Street, Danbury, CT 06810. *Telephone:* 203-837-8564. *Fax:* 203-837-8526. *E-mail:* halloran@wcsu.edu.

MASTER'S DEGREE PROGRAM

Degree MS

Available Programs Master's.

Concentrations Available *Clinical nurse specialist programs in:* adult health. *Nurse practitioner programs in:* adult health.

Study Options Full-time and part-time.

Program Entrance Requirements Clinical experience, minimum overall college GPA of 3.3, transcript of college record, CPR certification, immunizations, interview, 2 letters of recommendation, nursing research course, professional liability insurance/malpractice insurance, resume, statistics course.

Western Connecticut State University (continued)

Advanced Placement Credit given for nursing courses completed elsewhere dependent upon specific evaluations.

Degree Requirements 36 total credit hours, thesis or project.

POST-MASTER'S PROGRAM

Areas of Study *Clinical nurse specialist programs in:* adult health. *Nurse practitioner programs in:* adult health.

Yale University
School of Nursing
New Haven, Connecticut

http://www.nursing.yale.edu

Founded in 1701

DEGREES • DN SC • MSN • MSN/MBA • MSN/MPH

Nursing Program Faculty 75 (41% with doctorates).

Graduate Enrollment 280

Women 93% **Men** 7% **Minority** 7% **International** 9% **Part-time** 18%

Nursing Student Activities Sigma Theta Tau.

Nursing Student Resources Academic advising; academic or career counseling; assistance for students with disabilities; bookstore; campus computer network; career placement assistance; computer lab; computer-assisted instruction; e-mail services; employment services for current students; housing assistance; interactive nursing skills videos; Internet; learning resource lab; library services; nursing audiovisuals; placement services for program completers; skills, simulation, or other laboratory.

Library Facilities 11.1 million volumes (400,000 in health); 61,649 periodical subscriptions (2,900 health-care related).

GRADUATE PROGRAMS

Expenses (2004–05) *Tuition:* full-time $25,000. *Room and board:* $12,500 per academic year. *Required fees:* full-time $1100.

Financial Aid 80% of graduate students in nursing programs received some form of financial aid in 2003–04. 63 fellowships (averaging $2,004 per year), 11 research assistantships with tuition reimbursements available (averaging $29,895 per year) were awarded; Federal Work-Study, institutionally sponsored loans, scholarships, and traineeships also available. Aid available to part-time students.

Contact Ms. Sharon E. Sanderson, Office of Student Recruitment, School of Nursing, Yale University, 100 Church Street South, PO Box 9740, New Haven, CT 06536-0740. *Telephone:* 203-737-2557. *Fax:* 203-737-5409. *E-mail:* sharon.sanderson@yale.edu.

MASTER'S DEGREE PROGRAM

Degrees MSN; MSN/MBA; MSN/MPH

Available Programs Master's; Master's for Non-Nursing College Graduates; RN to Master's.

Concentrations Available Nurse-midwifery. *Clinical nurse specialist programs in:* acute care, cardiovascular, critical care, oncology. *Nurse practitioner programs in:* acute care, adult health, family health, gerontology, oncology, pediatric, psychiatric/mental health, women's health.

Study Options Full-time.

Program Entrance Requirements Transcript of college record, CPR certification, written essay, immunizations, interview, 3 letters of recommendation, statistics course, GRE General Test. *Application deadline:* For fall admission, 11/15 (priority date); for spring admission, 1/15 (priority date). Applications are processed on a rolling basis. *Application fee:* $50.

Degree Requirements 40 total credit hours, thesis or project.

POST-MASTER'S PROGRAM

Areas of Study *Nurse practitioner programs in:* acute care, adult health, gerontology, oncology, pediatric.

DOCTORAL DEGREE PROGRAM

Degree DN Sc

Available Programs Doctorate.

Areas of Study Family health, health policy, health-care systems, human health and illness, nursing policy, nursing research.

Program Entrance Requirements Minimum overall college GPA of 3.2, interview by faculty committee, interview, 3 letters of recommendation, MSN or equivalent, statistics course, writing sample, GRE General Test. *Application deadline:* For fall admission, 11/15 (priority date); for spring admission, 1/15 (priority date). Applications are processed on a rolling basis. *Application fee:* $50.

Degree Requirements 60 total credit hours, dissertation, oral exam, written exam.

POSTDOCTORAL PROGRAM

Areas of Study Adolescent health, chronic illness.

Postdoctoral Program Contact Ms. Sharon E. Sanderson, Director, Student Recruitment and Placement, School of Nursing, Yale University, 100 Church Street South, PO Box 9740, New Haven, CT 06536-0740. *Telephone:* 203-737-2258. *Fax:* 203-737-5409. *E-mail:* sharon.sanderson@yale.edu.

DELAWARE

Delaware State University
Department of Nursing
Dover, Delaware

http://www.dsc.edu/schools/professional_studies/nursing

Founded in 1891

DEGREE • BSN

Nursing Program Faculty 11.

Nursing Student Activities Sigma Theta Tau, Student Nurses' Association.

Library Facilities 204,127 volumes; 3,094 periodical subscriptions.

BACCALAUREATE PROGRAMS

Degree BSN

Available Programs Generic Baccalaureate; LPN to Baccalaureate.

Study Options Full-time and part-time.

Program Entrance Requirements High school biology, high school chemistry, high school transcript, minimum high school GPA of 2.0, prerequisite course work. Transfer students are accepted. **Standardized tests** *Required:* SAT or ACT, TOEFL for international students. **Application** *Deadline:* 4/1 (freshmen), 4/1 (transfer). *Application fee:* $15.

Advanced Placement Credit by examination available. Credit given for nursing courses completed elsewhere dependent upon specific evaluations.

Contact Dr. Mary P. Watkins, RN, Chairperson/Professor, Department of Nursing, Delaware State University, 1200 North DuPont Highway, Dover, DE 19901-2277. *Telephone:* 302-857-6750. *Fax:* 302-857-6755. *E-mail:* mwatkins@dsc.edu.

University of Delaware
Department of Nursing
Newark, Delaware

http://www.udel.edu/nursing/udnursing.html

Founded in 1743

DEGREES • BSN • MSN

Nursing Program Faculty 35 (64% with doctorates).

Baccalaureate Enrollment 711
Women 94% **Men** 6% **Minority** 11% **International** 17% **Part-time** 23%
Graduate Enrollment 55
Women 87% **Men** 13% **Minority** 11% **Part-time** 82%

Nursing Student Activities Sigma Theta Tau, Student Nurses' Association.

Nursing Student Resources Academic advising; academic or career counseling; assistance for students with disabilities; bookstore; campus computer network; career placement assistance; computer lab; computer-assisted instruction; e-mail services; employment services for current students; housing assistance; interactive nursing skills videos; Internet; learning resource lab; library services; nursing audiovisuals; resume preparation assistance; skills, simulation, or other laboratory; tutoring.

Library Facilities 2.6 million volumes; 12,476 periodical subscriptions.

BACCALAUREATE PROGRAMS

Degree BSN

Available Programs Accelerated Baccalaureate for Second Degree; Generic Baccalaureate; RN Baccalaureate.

Study Options Full-time.

Program Entrance Requirements Written essay, high school biology, high school chemistry, high school foreign language, 3 years high school math, 4 years high school science, high school transcript, 1 letter of recommendation, minimum high school GPA of 3.0. Transfer students are accepted. **Standardized tests** *Required:* SAT or ACT, TOEFL for international students. *Recommended:* SAT Subject Tests, SAT II Writing Tests. **Application** *Deadline:* 1/15 (freshmen), 5/1 (transfer). *Early decision:* 11/1. *Notification:* 3/15 (freshmen), 12/15 (out-of-state freshmen), 12/15 (early decision). *Application fee:* $60.

Advanced Placement Credit given for nursing courses completed elsewhere dependent upon specific evaluations.

Expenses (2004–05) *Tuition, state resident:* full-time $6304; part-time $263 per credit hour. *Tuition, nonresident:* full-time $15,990; part-time $667 per credit hour. *International tuition:* $15,990 full-time. *Required fees:* full-time $650; part-time $25 per term.

Contact Patricia Drake, Faculty/Recruiter, Department of Nursing, University of Delaware, 391 McDowell Hall, Newark, DE 19716. *Telephone:* 302-831-2193. *Fax:* 302-831-2382. *E-mail:* ud-nursing@udel.edu.

GRADUATE PROGRAMS

Expenses (2004–05) *Tuition, state resident:* full-time $6304; part-time $351 per credit hour. *Tuition, nonresident:* full-time $15,990; part-time $889 per credit hour. *International tuition:* $15,990 full-time. *Required fees:* full-time $522; part-time $25 per term.

Financial Aid 5 fellowships, 1 research assistantship (averaging $11,500 per year), 1 teaching assistantship (averaging $11,500 per year) were awarded; institutionally sponsored loans, scholarships, traineeships, tuition waivers (full), and unspecified assistantships also available.

Contact Ms. Joanne Marra, Senior Secretary, Department of Nursing, University of Delaware, 349 McDowell Hall, Newark, DE 19716. *Telephone:* 302-831-8386. *Fax:* 302-831-2382. *E-mail:* ud-gradnursing@udel.edu.

MASTER'S DEGREE PROGRAM

Degree MSN

Available Programs Master's; RN to Master's.

Concentrations Available Health-care administration. *Clinical nurse specialist programs in:* adult health, pediatric, psychiatric/mental health. *Nurse practitioner programs in:* adult health, family health.

Study Options Full-time and part-time.

Program Entrance Requirements Clinical experience, minimum overall college GPA of 2.5, transcript of college record, immunizations, interview, 3 letters of recommendation. *Application deadline:* For fall admission, 7/1; for spring admission, 12/1. Applications are processed on a rolling basis. *Application fee:* $60.

Advanced Placement Credit given for nursing courses completed elsewhere dependent upon specific evaluations.

Degree Requirements 34 total credit hours.

POST-MASTER'S PROGRAM

Areas of Study Health-care administration. *Clinical nurse specialist programs in:* adult health, pediatric, psychiatric/mental health. *Nurse practitioner programs in:* adult health, family health.

See full description on page 556.

Wesley College
Graduate Nursing Program
Dover, Delaware

http://www.wesley.edu
Founded in 1873

DEGREES • BSN • MSN

Nursing Program Faculty 8 (60% with doctorates).

Baccalaureate Enrollment 100
Women 85% **Men** 15% **Minority** 35% **Part-time** 2%
Graduate Enrollment 54
Women 90% **Men** 10% **Minority** 25% **Part-time** 25%

Nursing Student Activities Sigma Theta Tau, Student Nurses' Association.

Nursing Student Resources Academic advising; academic or career counseling; assistance for students with disabilities; bookstore; campus computer network; career placement assistance; computer lab; computer-assisted instruction; e-mail services; employment services for current students; externships; housing assistance; interactive nursing skills videos; Internet; learning resource lab; library services; nursing audiovisuals; paid internships; placement services for program completers; remedial services; resume preparation assistance; skills, simulation, or other laboratory; tutoring; unpaid internships.

Library Facilities 95,719 volumes (15,000 in health, 1,500 in nursing); 232 periodical subscriptions (30 health-care related).

BACCALAUREATE PROGRAMS

Degree BSN

Available Programs Generic Baccalaureate; LPN to Baccalaureate.

Study Options Full-time and part-time.

Program Entrance Requirements CPR certification, written essay, health exam, high school biology, high school chemistry, 2 years high school math, 2 years high school science, high school transcript, immunizations, minimum high school GPA of 2.5, minimum GPA in nursing prerequisites of 3.0, professional liability insurance/malpractice insurance. Transfer students are accepted. **Standardized tests** *Required:* TOEFL for international students. *Recommended:* SAT. **Application** *Deadline:* rolling (freshmen), rolling (transfer). *Early decision:* 11/15. *Notification:* 12/1 (out-of-state freshmen), 12/1 (early decision). *Application fee:* $20.

Advanced Placement Credit by examination available. Credit given for nursing courses completed elsewhere dependent upon specific evaluations.

Expenses (2004–05) *Tuition:* full-time $12,000; part-time $495 per credit hour. *International tuition:* $12,000 full-time. *Room and board:* $5500; room only: $4500 per academic year. *Required fees:* full-time $450.

Financial Aid 90% of baccalaureate students in nursing programs received some form of financial aid in 2003–04. *Gift aid (need-based):* Federal Pell, FSEOG, state, private, college/university gift aid from institutional funds. *Loans:* Federal Direct (Subsidized and Unsubsidized Stafford PLUS), FFEL (Subsidized and Unsubsidized Stafford PLUS), Perkins, state, college/university. *Work-Study:* Federal Work-Study, part-time campus jobs. *Application deadline (priority):* 4/15.

Contact Dr. Nancy D. Rubino, Program Director, Graduate Nursing Program, Wesley College, 120 North State Street, Dulany Hall, Dover, DE 19901. *Telephone:* 302-736-2550. *Fax:* 302-736-2548. *E-mail:* rubinona@wesley.edu.

GRADUATE PROGRAMS

Expenses (2004–05) *Tuition:* full-time $3990; part-time $285 per credit hour. *International tuition:* $3990 full-time. *Required fees:* full-time $150.

Financial Aid 100% of graduate students in nursing programs received some form of financial aid in 2003–04. 4 teaching assistantships with full tuition reimbursements available were awarded; traineeships also available.

Contact Dr. Lucille C. Gambardella, Chairperson, Graduate Nursing Program, Wesley College, 120 North State Street, Dulany Hall, Dover, DE 19901. *Telephone:* 302-736-2512. *Fax:* 302-736-2548. *E-mail:* gambarlu@wesley.edu.

Wesley College (continued)

MASTER'S DEGREE PROGRAM

Degree MSN

Available Programs Accelerated AD/RN to Master's; Accelerated RN to Master's; Master's.

Concentrations Available *Clinical nurse specialist programs in:* community health.

Site Options New Castle, DE.

Study Options Full-time and part-time.

Program Entrance Requirements Clinical experience, computer literacy, minimum overall college GPA of 3.0, transcript of college record, written essay, interview, 3 letters of recommendation, professional liability insurance/malpractice insurance, resume, GRE or MAT. *Application deadline:* Applications are processed on a rolling basis. *Application fee:* $25.

Advanced Placement Credit by examination available. Credit given for nursing courses completed elsewhere dependent upon specific evaluations.

Degree Requirements 36 total credit hours, thesis or project.

POST-MASTER'S PROGRAM

Areas of Study Nursing education.

CONTINUING EDUCATION PROGRAM

Contact Dr. Lucille C. Gambardella, Chairperson, Graduate Nursing Program, Wesley College, 120 North State Street, Dulany Hall, Dover, DE 19901. *Telephone:* 302-736-2512. *Fax:* 302-736-2548. *E-mail:* gambarlu@wesley.edu.

Wilmington College

Division of Nursing
New Castle, Delaware

Founded in 1967

DEGREES • BSN • MSN • MSN/MBA • MSN/MS

Nursing Program Faculty 10 (40% with doctorates).

Baccalaureate Enrollment 150
Women 96% **Men** 4% **Minority** 8% **Part-time** 90%

Graduate Enrollment 170
Women 92% **Men** 8% **Minority** 17%

Nursing Student Activities Sigma Theta Tau.

Nursing Student Resources Academic advising; academic or career counseling; assistance for students with disabilities; bookstore; computer lab; employment services for current students; interactive nursing skills videos; learning resource lab; library services; nursing audiovisuals; remedial services; resume preparation assistance; tutoring.

Library Facilities 98,713 volumes (5,800 in health, 3,500 in nursing); 425 periodical subscriptions (60 health-care related).

BACCALAUREATE PROGRAMS

Degree BSN

Available Programs Accelerated RN Baccalaureate; RN Baccalaureate.

Site Options Dover, DE; Georgetown, DE.

Study Options Full-time and part-time.

Program Entrance Requirements Transcript of college record, CPR certification, health exam, immunizations, prerequisite course work, RN licensure. Transfer students are accepted. **Standardized tests** *Required:* TOEFL for international students. ***Placement:*** *Recommended:* SAT or ACT. **Application** *Deadline:* rolling (freshmen), rolling (transfer). *Notification:* continuous (freshmen). *Application fee:* $25.

Advanced Placement Credit by examination available. Credit given for nursing courses completed elsewhere dependent upon specific evaluations.

Expenses (2003–04) *Tuition:* part-time $231 per credit hour. *Required fees:* full-time $150; part-time $50 per term.

Financial Aid 85% of baccalaureate students in nursing programs received some form of financial aid in 2002–03. *Gift aid (need-based):* Federal Pell, FSEOG, state, college/university gift aid from institutional funds. *Loans:* FFEL (Subsidized and Unsubsidized Stafford PLUS), alternative loans. *Work-Study:* Federal Work-Study. *Application deadline:* Continuous.

Contact Ms. Johanna Adams, BSN Program Coordinator, Division of Nursing, Wilmington College, 320 DuPont Highway, New Castle, DE 19720. *Telephone:* 302-328-9401 Ext. 172. *Fax:* 302-322-7081. *E-mail:* jadam@wilmcoll.edu.

GRADUATE PROGRAMS

Expenses (2003–04) *Tuition:* part-time $284 per credit hour. *Required fees:* full-time $200; part-time $50 per term.

Financial Aid 65% of graduate students in nursing programs received some form of financial aid in 2002–03. 28 fellowships with tuition reimbursements available (averaging $2,200 per year) were awarded; traineeships also available.

Contact Ms. Kim Christensen, Admissions Associate, Division of Nursing, Wilmington College, 320 DuPont Highway, New Castle, DE 19720. *Telephone:* 302-328-9401 Ext. 188. *Fax:* 302-328-1147. *E-mail:* kchri@wilmcoll.edu.

MASTER'S DEGREE PROGRAM

Degrees MSN; MSN/MBA; MSN/MS

Available Programs Master's.

Concentrations Available Nursing administration; nursing education. *Nurse practitioner programs in:* adult health, family health, gerontology, women's health.

Site Options Georgetown, DE.

Study Options Full-time and part-time.

Program Entrance Requirements Clinical experience, computer literacy, minimum overall college GPA of 3.0, transcript of college record, CPR certification, written essay, immunizations, interview, 2 letters of recommendation, nursing research course, physical assessment course, professional liability insurance/malpractice insurance, prerequisite course work, resume, statistics course. *Application deadline:* For fall admission, 3/31 (priority date). Applications are processed on a rolling basis. *Application fee:* $25.

Advanced Placement Credit given for nursing courses completed elsewhere dependent upon specific evaluations.

Degree Requirements 42 total credit hours, thesis or project.

POST-MASTER'S PROGRAM

Areas of Study Nursing administration; nursing education. *Nurse practitioner programs in:* adult health, family health, gerontology.

DISTRICT OF COLUMBIA

The Catholic University of America

School of Nursing
Washington, District of Columbia

http://www.nursing.cua.edu

Founded in 1887

DEGREES • BSN • DN SC • MA/MSM • MSN

Nursing Program Faculty 27 (74% with doctorates).

Baccalaureate Enrollment 183
Women 91% **Men** 9% **Minority** 18% **International** 2% **Part-time** 3%

Graduate Enrollment 110
Women 98% **Men** 2% **Minority** 22% **International** 9% **Part-time** 69%

Nursing Student Activities Nursing Honor Society, Sigma Theta Tau, Student Nurses' Association.

Nursing Student Resources Academic advising; academic or career counseling; assistance for students with disabilities; bookstore; computer lab; computer-assisted instruction; e-mail services; interactive nursing skills videos; Internet; learning resource lab; library services; nursing audiovisuals.

Library Facilities 1.6 million volumes (39,000 in health, 17,500 in nursing); 5,907 periodical subscriptions (250 health-care related).

BACCALAUREATE PROGRAMS

Degree BSN

Available Programs Accelerated Baccalaureate; Baccalaureate for Second Degree; Generic Baccalaureate.

Site Options California, MD.

Study Options Full-time and part-time.

Program Entrance Requirements Transcript of college record, written essay, health exam, health insurance, high school biology, high school chemistry, 3 years high school math, 2 years high school science, high school transcript, immunizations, 1 letter of recommendation, minimum high school GPA of 3.0, minimum GPA in nursing prerequisites of 2.75, professional liability insurance/malpractice insurance. Transfer students are accepted. **Standardized tests** *Required:* SAT or ACT, TOEFL for international students. *Recommended:* SAT Subject Tests, SAT II Writing Tests. **Application** *Deadline:* 2/1 (freshmen), 8/1 (transfer). *Early decision:* 11/15. *Notification:* continuous until 3/1 (freshmen), 12/20 (out-of-state freshmen), 12/20 (early decision). *Application fee:* $55.

Advanced Placement Credit given for nursing courses completed elsewhere dependent upon specific evaluations.

Expenses (2004–05) *Tuition:* full-time $23,800; part-time $895 per credit hour. *Room and board:* $9000; room only: $5000 per academic year. *Required fees:* full-time $1000; part-time $500 per term.

Financial Aid 50% of baccalaureate students in nursing programs received some form of financial aid in 2003–04. *Gift aid (need-based):* Federal Pell, FSEOG, state, private, college/university gift aid from institutional funds, Federal Nursing. *Loans:* Federal Nursing Student Loans, FFEL (Subsidized and Unsubsidized Stafford PLUS), Perkins. *Work-Study:* Federal Work-Study, part-time campus jobs. *Application deadline:* 2/1 (priority: 1/15).

Contact Rose Queen, Program Contact, School of Nursing, The Catholic University of America, 124 Gowan Hall, Washington, DC 20064. *Telephone:* 202-319-6457. *E-mail:* queenr@cua.edu.

GRADUATE PROGRAMS

Expenses (2004–05) *Tuition:* full-time $23,800; part-time $895 per credit hour. *Room and board:* $5000; room only: $4000 per academic year. *Required fees:* full-time $1000; part-time $500 per term.

Financial Aid 60% of graduate students in nursing programs received some form of financial aid in 2003–04. Research assistantships, teaching assistantships, career-related internships or fieldwork, Federal Work-Study, institutionally sponsored loans, and tuition waivers (full and partial) available. Aid available to part-time students. *Financial aid application deadline:* 2/1.

Contact Rita Rooney, Coordinator of Graduate Recruitment, School of Nursing, The Catholic University of America, 122 Gowan Hall, Washington, DC 20064. *Telephone:* 202-319-6290. *Fax:* 202-238-2060. *E-mail:* rooneyr@cua.edu.

MASTER'S DEGREE PROGRAM

Degrees MA/MSM; MSN

Available Programs Master's.

Concentrations Available Nursing administration; nursing education. *Clinical nurse specialist programs in:* adult health, community health, pediatric, psychiatric/mental health. *Nurse practitioner programs in:* family health, gerontology, pediatric, school health.

Site Options Silver Spring, MD.

Study Options Full-time and part-time.

Program Entrance Requirements Clinical experience, minimum overall college GPA of 3.0, transcript of college record, written essay, immunizations, 3 letters of recommendation, professional liability insurance/malpractice insurance, statistics course, GRE General Test. *Application deadline:* For fall admission, 2/1 (priority date); for spring admission, 11/15 (priority date). Applications are processed on a rolling basis. *Application fee:* $55.

Advanced Placement Credit given for nursing courses completed elsewhere dependent upon specific evaluations.

Degree Requirements 40 total credit hours, comprehensive exam.

POST-MASTER'S PROGRAM

Areas of Study *Clinical nurse specialist programs in:* adult health, community health, pediatric, psychiatric/mental health. *Nurse practitioner programs in:* gerontology, pediatric, school health.

DOCTORAL DEGREE PROGRAM

Degree DN Sc

Available Programs Doctorate.

Areas of Study Clinical practice, nursing research, nursing science.

Program Entrance Requirements Clinical experience, minimum overall college GPA of 3.5, interview by faculty committee, interview, 3 letters of recommendation, MSN or equivalent, scholarly papers, statistics course, writing sample, GRE General Test. *Application deadline:* For fall admission, 2/1 (priority date); for spring admission, 11/15 (priority date). Applications are processed on a rolling basis. *Application fee:* $55.

Degree Requirements 66 total credit hours, dissertation, written exam, residency.

Georgetown University

School of Nursing and Health Studies
Washington, District of Columbia

http://snhs.georgetown.edu

Founded in 1789

DEGREES • BSN • MS

Nursing Program Faculty 51 (50% with doctorates).

Baccalaureate Enrollment 480

Women 85% **Men** 15% **Minority** 26% **International** 1% **Part-time** 2%

Graduate Enrollment 235

Women 73% **Men** 27% **Minority** 24% **International** 1% **Part-time** 20%

Nursing Student Activities Sigma Theta Tau, Student Nurses' Association.

Nursing Student Resources Academic advising; academic or career counseling; assistance for students with disabilities; bookstore; campus computer network; career placement assistance; computer lab; computer-assisted instruction; e-mail services; housing assistance; interactive nursing skills videos; Internet; learning resource lab; library services; nursing audiovisuals; resume preparation assistance; skills, simulation, or other laboratory; tutoring; unpaid internships.

Library Facilities 2.4 million volumes (36,000 in health, 20,000 in nursing); 23,241 periodical subscriptions (92 health-care related).

BACCALAUREATE PROGRAMS

Degree BSN

Available Programs ADN to Baccalaureate; Accelerated Baccalaureate for Second Degree; Generic Baccalaureate; RN Baccalaureate.

Study Options Full-time.

Program Entrance Requirements Minimum overall college GPA of 3.0, transcript of college record, CPR certification, written essay, health exam, health insurance, high school biology, high school chemistry, high school math, 4 years high school science, high school transcript, immunizations, interview, 2 letters of recommendation. Transfer students are accepted. **Standardized tests** *Required:* SAT or ACT, TOEFL for international students. *Recommended:* SAT Subject Tests, SAT II Writing Tests. **Application** *Deadline:* 1/10 (freshmen), 3/1 (transfer). *Early decision:* 11/1. *Notification:* 4/1 (freshmen), 12/15 (early action). *Application fee:* $60.

Advanced Placement Credit by examination available.

Georgetown University (continued)

Expenses (2004–05) *Tuition:* full-time $30,000; part-time $1242 per credit hour. *Room and board:* $9280; room only: $6280 per academic year. *Required fees:* full-time $154.

Financial Aid 55% of baccalaureate students in nursing programs received some form of financial aid in 2003–04.

Contact Mr. Matthew Smith, Associate Director of Admissions and Outreach, School of Nursing and Health Studies, Georgetown University, 3700 Reservoir Road, NW, Washington, DC 20007. *Telephone:* 202-687-2781. *Fax:* 202-687-5553. *E-mail:* gms7@georgetown.edu.

GRADUATE PROGRAMS

Expenses (2004–05) *Tuition:* part-time $1183 per credit hour.

Financial Aid 95% of graduate students in nursing programs received some form of financial aid in 2003–04. Scholarships and traineeships available.

Contact Mr. David Lewis, Coordinator of Graduate Admissions and Outreach, School of Nursing and Health Studies, Georgetown University, 3700 Reservoir Road, NW, Washington, DC 20007. *Telephone:* 202-687-8439. *Fax:* 202-687-5553. *E-mail:* ADL6@georgetown.edu.

MASTER'S DEGREE PROGRAM

Degree MS

Available Programs Master's; Master's for Non-Nursing College Graduates; RN to Master's.

Concentrations Available Health-care administration; nurse anesthesia; nurse-midwifery. *Clinical nurse specialist programs in:* critical care. *Nurse practitioner programs in:* acute care, family health.

Study Options Full-time and part-time.

Program Entrance Requirements Clinical experience, minimum overall college GPA of 3.0, transcript of college record, written essay, interview, 3 letters of recommendation, resume, statistics course, GRE General Test or MAT. *Application fee:* $50 ($55 for international students).

Advanced Placement Credit given for nursing courses completed elsewhere dependent upon specific evaluations.

Degree Requirements 40 total credit hours, thesis or project.

POST-MASTER'S PROGRAM

Areas of Study Nurse-midwifery. *Clinical nurse specialist programs in:* critical care. *Nurse practitioner programs in:* acute care, family health, gerontology.

CONTINUING EDUCATION PROGRAM

Contact Ms. Marianne Lyons, Director of Continuing Education, School of Nursing and Health Studies, Georgetown University, 3700 Reservoir Road, NW, Washington, DC 20007. *Telephone:* 202-687-1561. *Fax:* 202-687-5553. *E-mail:* lyonsm@georgetown.edu.

See full description on page 492.

Howard University

Division of Nursing
Washington, District of Columbia

http://www.howard.edu

Founded in 1867

DEGREES • BSN • MSN

Nursing Program Faculty 30 (50% with doctorates).

Baccalaureate Enrollment 270
Women 90% **Men** 10% **Minority** 88% **International** 12% **Part-time** 20%

Graduate Enrollment 20
Women 92% **Men** 8% **Minority** 84% **International** 11% **Part-time** 50%

Nursing Student Activities Sigma Theta Tau, Student Nurses' Association.

Nursing Student Resources Academic advising; academic or career counseling; assistance for students with disabilities; bookstore; campus computer network; career placement assistance; computer lab; computer-assisted instruction; e-mail services; externships; housing assistance; interactive nursing skills videos; Internet; learning resource lab; library services; nursing audiovisuals; paid internships; placement services for program completers; remedial services; resume preparation assistance; skills, simulation, or other laboratory.

Library Facilities 2.5 million volumes (219,448 in health, 4,500 in nursing); 12,795 periodical subscriptions (5,247 health-care related).

BACCALAUREATE PROGRAMS

Degree BSN

Available Programs ADN to Baccalaureate; Accelerated Baccalaureate; Accelerated Baccalaureate for Second Degree; Accelerated LPN to Baccalaureate; Accelerated RN Baccalaureate; Baccalaureate for Second Degree; Generic Baccalaureate; LPN to Baccalaureate; LPN to RN Baccalaureate; RN Baccalaureate.

Study Options Full-time and part-time.

Program Entrance Requirements Minimum overall college GPA of 2.8, transcript of college record, written essay, health exam, high school biology, high school chemistry, 2 years high school math, 2 years high school science, high school transcript, immunizations, 2 letters of recommendation, minimum high school GPA of 2.5, minimum high school rank 50%, minimum GPA in nursing prerequisites of 2.5. Transfer students are accepted. **Standardized tests** *Required:* SAT or ACT, SAT II Writing Tests, TOEFL for international students. **Application** *Deadline:* 2/15 (freshmen), 4/1 (transfer). *Early decision:* 11/1. *Notification:* continuous (freshmen), 12/24 (early action). *Application fee:* $45.

Advanced Placement Credit by examination available. Credit given for nursing courses completed elsewhere dependent upon specific evaluations.

Expenses (2003–04) *Tuition:* full-time $10,130; part-time $422 per credit hour. *International tuition:* $10,130 full-time. *Room and board:* $5070; room only: $3500 per academic year. *Required fees:* part-time $403 per term.

Financial Aid 92% of baccalaureate students in nursing programs received some form of financial aid in 2002–03. *Gift aid (need-based):* Federal Pell, FSEOG, state, private, college/university gift aid from institutional funds, Federal Nursing. *Loans:* Federal Nursing Student Loans, Federal Direct (Subsidized and Unsubsidized Stafford PLUS), FFEL (Subsidized and Unsubsidized Stafford PLUS), Perkins, state, college/university. *Work-Study:* Federal Work-Study, part-time campus jobs. *Application deadline (priority):* 2/15.

Contact Dr. Sheryl Nichols, Acting Assistant Dean, Student Affairs, Division of Nursing, Howard University, 501 Bryant Street, NW, Room 119, Washington, DC 20059. *Telephone:* 202-806-6509. *Fax:* 202-806-5958. *E-mail:* snichols@howard.edu.

GRADUATE PROGRAMS

Expenses (2003–04) *Tuition:* full-time $12,400; part-time $689 per credit hour. *International tuition:* $12,400 full-time. *Room and board:* $5070; room only: $2500 per academic year. *Required fees:* part-time $403 per term.

Financial Aid 52% of graduate students in nursing programs received some form of financial aid in 2002–03. Teaching assistantships, career-related internships or fieldwork, institutionally sponsored loans, and scholarships available. *Financial aid application deadline:* 4/1.

Contact Dr. Ruth Johnson, Assistant Dean, Graduate Program, Division of Nursing, Howard University, 501 Bryant Street, NW, Washington, DC 20059. *Telephone:* 202-806-7460. *Fax:* 202-806-5978. *E-mail:* rjohnson@howard.edu.

MASTER'S DEGREE PROGRAM

Degree MSN

Available Programs Master's.

Concentrations Available *Nurse practitioner programs in:* family health.

Study Options Full-time and part-time.

Program Entrance Requirements Minimum overall college GPA of 3.0, transcript of college record, written essay, immunizations, interview, 3 letters of recommendation, physical assessment course, professional liability insurance/malpractice insurance, statistics course. *Application deadline:* For fall admission, 4/1 (priority date); for spring admission, 11/1. Applications are processed on a rolling basis. *Application fee:* $45.

Advanced Placement Credit given for nursing courses completed elsewhere dependent upon specific evaluations.

Degree Requirements 42 total credit hours, thesis or project, comprehensive exam.

POST-MASTER'S PROGRAM

Areas of Study *Nurse practitioner programs in:* family health.

University of the District of Columbia

Nursing Education Program
Washington, District of Columbia

Founded in 1976

DEGREE • BSN

Nursing Program Faculty 11 (1% with doctorates).

Nursing Student Activities Student Nurses' Association.

Nursing Student Resources Learning resource lab; library services; skills, simulation, or other laboratory.

Library Facilities 544,412 volumes (100 in health, 20 in nursing); 594 periodical subscriptions (35 health-care related).

BACCALAUREATE PROGRAMS

Degree BSN

Available Programs ADN to Baccalaureate.

Site Options Washington, DC.

Program Entrance Requirements CPR certification, professional liability insurance/malpractice insurance, prerequisite course work. Transfer students are accepted. **Standardized tests** *Required:* TOEFL for international students. *Recommended:* SAT. **Application** *Deadline:* 8/1 (freshmen), 8/1 (transfer). *Notification:* continuous until 8/15 (freshmen). *Application fee:* $20.

Expenses (2003–04) *Tuition, state resident:* full-time $2070; part-time $75 per credit hour. *Tuition, nonresident:* full-time $4710; part-time $185 per credit hour. *International tuition:* $4710 full-time. *Required fees:* full-time $270.

Contact Dr. Connie M. Webster, RN, Chairperson, Nursing Education Program, University of the District of Columbia, 4200 Connecticut Avenue Northwest, Washington, DC 20008. *Telephone:* 202-274-5899. *Fax:* 202-274-5952. *E-mail:* Cwebster@udc.edu.

FLORIDA

Barry University

School of Nursing
Miami Shores, Florida

http://www.barry.edu/nursing

Founded in 1940

DEGREES • BSN • MSN • MSN/MBA • PHD

Nursing Program Faculty 30 (46% with doctorates).

Baccalaureate Enrollment 250

Women 90% **Men** 10% **Minority** 51% **International** 3% **Part-time** 49%

Graduate Enrollment 150

Nursing Student Activities Sigma Theta Tau, Student Nurses' Association.

Nursing Student Resources Academic advising; academic or career counseling; assistance for students with disabilities; bookstore; campus computer network; career placement assistance; computer lab; computer-assisted instruction; e-mail services; employment services for current students; housing assistance; interactive nursing skills videos; Internet; learning resource lab; library services; nursing audiovisuals; paid internships; remedial services; resume preparation assistance; skills, simulation, or other laboratory; tutoring.

Library Facilities 233,938 volumes (15,000 in health, 8,500 in nursing); 2,880 periodical subscriptions (400 health-care related).

BACCALAUREATE PROGRAMS

Degree BSN

Available Programs ADN to Baccalaureate; Accelerated Baccalaureate; Accelerated Baccalaureate for Second Degree; Baccalaureate for Second Degree; Generic Baccalaureate; LPN to Baccalaureate; LPN to RN Baccalaureate; RN Baccalaureate.

Study Options Full-time and part-time.

Program Entrance Requirements Minimum overall college GPA of 2.7, transcript of college record, CPR certification, health exam, health insurance, high school biology, high school chemistry, high school math, high school science, high school transcript, immunizations, 2 letters of recommendation, minimum high school GPA of 2.7, minimum GPA in nursing prerequisites of 2.7, professional liability insurance/malpractice insurance. Transfer students are accepted. **Standardized tests** *Required:* SAT or ACT, TOEFL for international students. **Application** *Deadline:* rolling (freshmen), rolling (transfer). *Notification:* continuous (freshmen). *Application fee:* $30.

Advanced Placement Credit given for nursing courses completed elsewhere dependent upon specific evaluations.

Expenses (2004–05) *Tuition:* full-time $21,500; part-time $630 per credit hour. *International tuition:* $21,500 full-time.

Financial Aid 90% of baccalaureate students in nursing programs received some form of financial aid in 2003–04. *Gift aid (need-based):* Federal Pell, FSEOG, state, private, college/university gift aid from institutional funds, Federal Nursing. *Loans:* Federal Nursing Student Loans, FFEL (Subsidized and Unsubsidized Stafford PLUS), Perkins, college/university, alternative loans. *Work-Study:* Federal Work-Study, part-time campus jobs. *Application deadline:* Continuous.

Contact Ms. Jennifer Morejon, Administrative Assistant, School of Nursing, Barry University, 11300 NE Second Avenue, Miami Shores, FL 33161-6695. *Telephone:* 305-899-3837. *Fax:* 305-899-3831. *E-mail:* jmorejon@mail.barry.edu.

GRADUATE PROGRAMS

Expenses (2004–05) *Tuition:* part-time $650 per credit hour. *Required fees:* full-time $245.

Financial Aid 100% of graduate students in nursing programs received some form of financial aid in 2003–04. 3 research assistantships (averaging $5,000 per year), 3 teaching assistantships (averaging $5,000 per year) were awarded; tuition waivers (full) also available. *Financial aid application deadline:* 5/1.

Contact Dr. Claudette Spalding, Associate Dean, School of Nursing, Barry University, 11300 NE Second Avenue, Miami Shores, FL 33161-6695. *Telephone:* 305-899-3849. *Fax:* 305-899-3831. *E-mail:* cspalding@mail.barry.edu.

MASTER'S DEGREE PROGRAM

Degrees MSN; MSN/MBA

Available Programs Master's.

Concentrations Available Nursing administration; nursing education. *Nurse practitioner programs in:* acute care, family health.

Study Options Part-time.

Program Entrance Requirements Clinical experience, computer literacy, minimum overall college GPA of 3.0, transcript of college record, written essay, 2 letters of recommendation, nursing research course, professional liability insurance/malpractice insurance, statistics course, GRE General Test or MAT. *Application deadline:* For fall admission, 5/1 (priority date). Applications are processed on a rolling basis. *Application fee:* $30.

Advanced Placement Credit given for nursing courses completed elsewhere dependent upon specific evaluations.

Degree Requirements 45 total credit hours.

POST-MASTER'S PROGRAM

Areas of Study Nursing administration; nursing education. *Nurse practitioner programs in:* acute care, family health.

Barry University (continued)

DOCTORAL DEGREE PROGRAM

Degree PhD

Available Programs Doctorate.

Areas of Study Nursing research, nursing science.

Program Entrance Requirements Clinical experience, minimum overall college GPA of 3.0, interview, 2 letters of recommendation, MSN or equivalent, statistics course, writing sample, GRE General Test or MAT. *Application deadline:* For fall admission, 5/1 (priority date). Applications are processed on a rolling basis. *Application fee:* $30.

Degree Requirements 45 total credit hours, dissertation, written exam, residency.

Bethune-Cookman College

School of Nursing
Daytona Beach, Florida

http://www.cookman.edu/Nursing

Founded in 1904

DEGREE • BSN

Nursing Program Faculty 9 (11% with doctorates).

Nursing Student Activities Student Nurses' Association.

Nursing Student Resources Library services.

Library Facilities 173,193 volumes; 770 periodical subscriptions.

BACCALAUREATE PROGRAMS

Degree BSN

Available Programs Generic Baccalaureate; RN Baccalaureate.

Study Options Full-time.

Program Entrance Requirements Minimum overall college GPA of 2.8, transcript of college record, CPR certification, written essay, health exam, high school transcript, immunizations, interview, 2 letters of recommendation, minimum GPA in nursing prerequisites of 2.8, professional liability insurance/malpractice insurance, prerequisite course work. Transfer students are accepted. **Standardized tests** *Required:* SAT or ACT, TOEFL for international students. **Application** *Deadline:* 6/30 (freshmen), 6/30 (transfer). *Notification:* continuous (freshmen). *Application fee:* $25.

Advanced Placement Credit by examination available. Credit given for nursing courses completed elsewhere dependent upon specific evaluations.

Contact Dr. Alma Dixon, RN, Chair and Associate Professor, School of Nursing, Bethune-Cookman College, 640 Dr. Mary McLeod Bethune Boulevard, Daytona Beach, FL 32114-3099. *Telephone:* 386-481-2000. *E-mail:* dixonal@cookman.edu.

Florida Agricultural and Mechanical University

School of Nursing
Tallahassee, Florida

http://www.famu.edu/acad/colleges/son

Founded in 1887

DEGREES • BSN • MSN • PHD

Nursing Program Faculty 28 (18% with doctorates).

Baccalaureate Enrollment 161
Women 90% **Men** 10% **Minority** 98%

Graduate Enrollment 17
Women 83% **Men** 17% **Minority** 76% **Part-time** 12%

Nursing Student Activities Sigma Theta Tau, Student Nurses' Association.

Nursing Student Resources Academic advising; academic or career counseling; bookstore; campus computer network; career placement assistance; computer lab; computer-assisted instruction; daycare for children of students; e-mail services; employment services for current students; externships; interactive nursing skills videos; Internet; library services; nursing audiovisuals; placement services for program completers; remedial services; resume preparation assistance; skills, simulation, or other laboratory; tutoring.

Library Facilities 484,801 volumes (5,000 in health, 4,091 in nursing); 7,672 periodical subscriptions (385 health-care related).

BACCALAUREATE PROGRAMS

Degree BSN

Available Programs Generic Baccalaureate.

Study Options Part-time.

Program Entrance Requirements CPR certification, health exam, immunizations, 3 letters of recommendation, minimum high school GPA of 2.5, prerequisite course work. Transfer students are accepted. **Standardized tests** *Required:* SAT or ACT, TOEFL for international students. **Application** *Deadline:* 5/9 (freshmen), 5/1 (transfer). *Notification:* continuous until 8/1 (freshmen). *Application fee:* $20.

Expenses (2003–04) *Tuition, area resident:* part-time $85 per credit hour. *Tuition, state resident:* full-time $1273; part-time $85 per credit hour. *Tuition, nonresident:* full-time $6045; part-time $403 per credit hour. *Room and board:* $4626; room only: $2760 per academic year. *Required fees:* full-time $1704.

Financial Aid 80% of baccalaureate students in nursing programs received some form of financial aid in 2002–03. *Gift aid (need-based):* Federal Pell, FSEOG, state, private, college/university gift aid from institutional funds, United Negro College Fund, Federal Nursing. *Loans:* Federal Direct (Subsidized and Unsubsidized Stafford PLUS), Perkins. *Work-Study:* Federal Work-Study. *Application deadline:* 6/30 (priority: 3/1).

Contact Miss Kimberly R. Davis, Director of Student Affairs, School of Nursing, Florida Agricultural and Mechanical University, Florida Agricultural & Mechanical University, School of Nursing 118 Ware-Rhaney Building, Tallahassee, FL 32307. *Telephone:* 850-599-3458. *Fax:* 850-599-3508. *E-mail:* kimberly.davis@famu.edu.

GRADUATE PROGRAMS

Expenses (2003–04) *Tuition, state resident:* part-time $179 per credit hour. *Tuition, nonresident:* part-time $671 per credit hour.

Financial Aid 60% of graduate students in nursing programs received some form of financial aid in 2002–03.

Contact Dr. Cornelia P. Porter, Dean & Professor, School of Nursing, Florida Agricultural and Mechanical University, Florida Agricultural & Mechanical University, School of Nursing 103 Ware-Rhaney Building, Tallahassee, FL 32307. *Telephone:* 850-599-3017. *Fax:* 850-599-3508. *E-mail:* cornelia.porter@famu.edu.

MASTER'S DEGREE PROGRAM

Degree MSN

Available Programs Master's.

Concentrations Available *Nurse practitioner programs in:* adult health, gerontology, women's health.

Study Options Full-time and part-time.

Program Entrance Requirements Clinical experience, minimum overall college GPA of 3.0, CPR certification, immunizations, interview, nursing research course, physical assessment course, professional liability insurance/malpractice insurance, statistics course.

Degree Requirements 42 total credit hours, thesis or project.

POST-MASTER'S PROGRAM

Areas of Study *Nurse practitioner programs in:* adult health, gerontology, women's health.

DOCTORAL DEGREE PROGRAM

Degree PhD

Program Entrance Requirements Minimum overall college GPA of 3.5, 3 letters of recommendation, MSN or equivalent.

Degree Requirements 90 total credit hours, dissertation, oral exam, written exam.

CONTINUING EDUCATION PROGRAM

Contact Dr. Cornelia P. Porter, Dean & Professor, School of Nursing, Florida Agricultural and Mechanical University, Florida Agricultural & Mechanical University, School of Nursing 103 Ware-Rhaney Building, Tallahassee, FL 32307. *Telephone:* 850-599-3017. *Fax:* 850-599-3508. *E-mail:* cornelia.porter@famu.edu.

Florida Atlantic University

College of Nursing
Boca Raton, Florida

http://www.fau.edu/nursing

Founded in 1961

DEGREES • BSN • DNS • M SC N

Nursing Program Faculty 63 (50% with doctorates).

Baccalaureate Enrollment 600

Women 85% **Men** 15% **Minority** 30% **International** 10% **Part-time** 30%

Graduate Enrollment 229

Nursing Student Activities Sigma Theta Tau, Student Nurses' Association.

Nursing Student Resources Academic advising; assistance for students with disabilities; bookstore; campus computer network; computer lab; computer-assisted instruction; e-mail services; housing assistance; Internet; learning resource lab; library services; nursing audiovisuals; skills, simulation, or other laboratory; tutoring.

Library Facilities 1.4 million volumes (18,735 in health, 4,713 in nursing); 10,572 periodical subscriptions (333 health-care related).

BACCALAUREATE PROGRAMS

Degree BSN

Available Programs Accelerated Baccalaureate for Second Degree; Generic Baccalaureate; RN Baccalaureate.

Site Options *Distance Learning:* Davie, FL; Port St. Lucie, FL.

Study Options Full-time.

Program Entrance Requirements Minimum overall college GPA of 3.0, transcript of college record, CPR certification, written essay, health exam, health insurance, high school transcript, immunizations, minimum GPA in nursing prerequisites of 2.0, professional liability insurance/malpractice insurance, prerequisite course work, RN licensure. Transfer students are accepted. **Standardized tests** *Required:* SAT and SAT Subject Tests or ACT, TOEFL for international students. **Application** *Deadline:* 6/1 (freshmen), 6/1 (transfer). *Notification:* continuous (freshmen). *Application fee:* $30.

Advanced Placement Credit by examination available. Credit given for nursing courses completed elsewhere dependent upon specific evaluations.

Expenses (2004–05) *Tuition, state resident:* full-time $3710; part-time $103 per contact hour. *Tuition, nonresident:* full-time $18,720; part-time $520 per contact hour. *Room and board:* $2300 per academic year. *Required fees:* full-time $140; part-time $70 per term.

Financial Aid 75% of baccalaureate students in nursing programs received some form of financial aid in 2003–04.

Contact Dr. Theris Touhy, Assistant Dean for Undergraduate Programs, College of Nursing, Florida Atlantic University, 777 Glades Road, Boca Raton, FL 33431. *Telephone:* 561-297-2535. *Fax:* 561-297-3652. *E-mail:* ttouhy@fau.edu.

GRADUATE PROGRAMS

Expenses (2004–05) *Tuition, state resident:* full-time $3777; part-time $210 per credit hour. *Tuition, nonresident:* full-time $13,953; part-time $775 per credit hour.

Financial Aid 11 research assistantships, 6 teaching assistantships were awarded; career-related internships or fieldwork, Federal Work-Study, institutionally sponsored loans, scholarships, and traineeships also available.

Contact Dr. Lynne M. Dunphy, Assistant Dean for Graduate Programs (Master's), College of Nursing, Florida Atlantic University, 777 Glades Road, Boca Raton, FL 33431. *Telephone:* 561-297-3384. *Fax:* 561-297-0088. *E-mail:* ldunphy@fau.edu.

MASTER'S DEGREE PROGRAM

Degree M Sc N

Available Programs Master's; Master's for Nurses with Non-Nursing Degrees; RN to Master's.

Concentrations Available Nursing administration; nursing education. *Clinical nurse specialist programs in:* gerontology. *Nurse practitioner programs in:* adult health, family health, gerontology.

Site Options *Distance Learning:* Davie, FL; Port St. Lucie, FL.

Study Options Full-time and part-time.

Program Entrance Requirements Minimum overall college GPA of 3.0, transcript of college record, CPR certification, written essay, immunizations, 2 letters of recommendation, nursing research course, physical assessment course, professional liability insurance/malpractice insurance, prerequisite course work, resume, statistics course, GRE General Test. *Application deadline:* For fall admission, 6/2; for spring admission, 10/20. Applications are processed on a rolling basis. *Application fee:* $30.

Degree Requirements Thesis or project.

POST-MASTER'S PROGRAM

Areas of Study Nursing administration; nursing education. *Clinical nurse specialist programs in:* gerontology. *Nurse practitioner programs in:* adult health, family health, gerontology.

DOCTORAL DEGREE PROGRAM

Degree DNS

Available Programs Doctorate.

Areas of Study Advanced practice nursing, aging, clinical practice, community health, faculty preparation, family health, gerontology, health policy, health promotion/disease prevention, individualized study, nursing administration, nursing education, nursing policy, nursing research, nursing science.

Program Entrance Requirements Minimum overall college GPA of 3.0, interview by faculty committee, 3 letters of recommendation, MSN or equivalent, statistics course, vita, writing sample, GRE General Test. *Application deadline:* For fall admission, 6/2; for spring admission, 10/20. Applications are processed on a rolling basis. *Application fee:* $30.

Degree Requirements 62 total credit hours, dissertation, written exam, residency.

CONTINUING EDUCATION PROGRAM

Contact Dr. Beth King, Director, College of Nursing, Florida Atlantic University, 777 Glades Road, Boca Raton, FL 33431. *Telephone:* 561-297-3887. *Fax:* 561-297-3652. *E-mail:* bking@fau.edu.

Florida Gulf Coast University

School of Nursing
Fort Myers, Florida

Founded in 1991

DEGREES • BSN • MSN

Nursing Program Faculty 17 (47% with doctorates).

Baccalaureate Enrollment 192

Women 89% **Men** 11% **Minority** 11% **International** 15% **Part-time** 13%

Graduate Enrollment 140

Women 54% **Men** 46% **Minority** 20% **Part-time** 15%

Nursing Student Activities Sigma Theta Tau, Student Nurses' Association.

Nursing Student Resources Academic advising; academic or career counseling; assistance for students with disabilities; bookstore; campus computer network; career placement assistance; computer lab; computer-assisted instruction; daycare for children of students; e-mail services; employment services for current students; housing assistance; Internet; library services; nursing audiovisuals; remedial services; tutoring.

Florida Gulf Coast University (continued)
Library Facilities 282,557 volumes (12,768 in health, 6,742 in nursing); 1,429 periodical subscriptions (471 health-care related).

BACCALAUREATE PROGRAMS

Degree BSN

Available Programs Accelerated RN Baccalaureate; Generic Baccalaureate.

Site Options Port Charlotte, FL.

Study Options Full-time and part-time.

Program Entrance Requirements Minimum overall college GPA of 2.75, transcript of college record, CPR certification, written essay, health insurance, high school foreign language, immunizations, minimum GPA in nursing prerequisites of 2.75, professional liability insurance/malpractice insurance, prerequisite course work. Transfer students are accepted. **Standardized tests** *Required:* SAT or ACT, TOEFL for international students. **Application** *Deadline:* 6/1 (freshmen), rolling (transfer). *Notification:* continuous (freshmen). *Application fee:* $30.

Advanced Placement Credit by examination available. Credit given for nursing courses completed elsewhere dependent upon specific evaluations.

Expenses (2004–05) *Tuition, state resident:* part-time $102 per credit hour. *Tuition, nonresident:* part-time $505 per credit hour. *Required fees:* part-time $48 per term.

Contact Dr. Anne Nolan, Associate Director, School of Nursing, Florida Gulf Coast University, 10501 FGCU Boulevard South, Fort Myers, FL 33931. *Telephone:* 239-590-7513. *Fax:* 239-590-7474. *E-mail:* anolan@fgcu.edu.

GRADUATE PROGRAMS

Expenses (2004–05) *Tuition, state resident:* part-time $220 per credit hour. *Tuition, nonresident:* part-time $841 per credit hour. *Required fees:* part-time $48 per term.

Contact Dr. Karen Miles, Director, School of Nursing, Florida Gulf Coast University, 10501 FGCU Boulevard South, Fort Myers, FL 33931. *Telephone:* 239-590-7454. *Fax:* 239-590-7474. *E-mail:* kmiles@fgcu.edu.

MASTER'S DEGREE PROGRAM

Degree MSN

Available Programs Master's.

Concentrations Available Nurse anesthesia; nursing education. *Nurse practitioner programs in:* family health.

Site Options *Distance Learning:* Tampa, FL.

Study Options Full-time and part-time.

Program Entrance Requirements Clinical experience, minimum overall college GPA of 3.0, transcript of college record, CPR certification, written essay, immunizations, interview, 1 letter of recommendation, nursing research course, physical assessment course, professional liability insurance/malpractice insurance, prerequisite course work, resume, statistics course.

Advanced Placement Credit given for nursing courses completed elsewhere dependent upon specific evaluations.

Degree Requirements 40 total credit hours.

POST-MASTER'S PROGRAM

Areas of Study *Nurse practitioner programs in:* family health.

CONTINUING EDUCATION PROGRAM

Contact Dr. Anne Nolan, Associate Director, School of Nursing, Florida Gulf Coast University, 10501 FGCU Boulevard South, Fort Myers, FL 33931. *Telephone:* 239-590-7513. *Fax:* 239-590-7474. *E-mail:* anolan@fgcu.edu.

Florida Hospital College of Health Sciences

Department of Nursing
Orlando, Florida

http://www.fhchs.edu/

DEGREE • BS

Nursing Program Faculty 12 (16% with doctorates).

Nursing Student Resources Campus computer network; computer lab; computer-assisted instruction; Internet; learning resource lab; library services; nursing audiovisuals; skills, simulation, or other laboratory.

Library Facilities 74,581 volumes; 158 periodical subscriptions.

BACCALAUREATE PROGRAMS

Degree BS

Available Programs Generic Baccalaureate; RN Baccalaureate.

Study Options Full-time and part-time.

Program Entrance Requirements Minimum overall college GPA of 2.5, transcript of college record, health exam, 1 letter of recommendation, prerequisite course work, RN licensure. Transfer students are accepted. **Standardized tests** *Required for some:* SAT or ACT. **Application** *Deadline:* 7/18 (freshmen), 7/18 (out-of-state freshmen), 7/18 (transfer). *Notification:* continuous until 8/30 (freshmen), continuous until 8/30 (out-of-state freshmen). *Application fee:* $20.

Advanced Placement Credit by examination available. Credit given for nursing courses completed elsewhere dependent upon specific evaluations.

Contact Department of Nursing, Department of Nursing, Florida Hospital College of Health Sciences, 800 Lake Estelle Drive, Orlando, FL 32803. *Telephone:* 407-303-9798. *Fax:* 407-303-9408. *E-mail:* fhcinfo@fhchs.edu.

Florida International University

School of Nursing
Miami, Florida

http://www.fiu.edu

Founded in 1965

DEGREES • BSN • MSN • PHD

Nursing Program Faculty 74 (32% with doctorates).

Baccalaureate Enrollment 484
Women 72% **Men** 28% **Minority** 82% **International** 1% **Part-time** 21%

Graduate Enrollment 232
Women 76% **Men** 24% **Minority** 59% **International** 1% **Part-time** 28%

Nursing Student Activities Sigma Theta Tau, Student Nurses' Association.

Nursing Student Resources Academic advising; academic or career counseling; assistance for students with disabilities; bookstore; campus computer network; career placement assistance; computer lab; computer-assisted instruction; e-mail services; externships; housing assistance; interactive nursing skills videos; Internet; learning resource lab; library services; nursing audiovisuals; paid internships; remedial services; resume preparation assistance; skills, simulation, or other laboratory; tutoring.

Library Facilities 1.8 million volumes (200,500 in health, 9,600 in nursing); 16,920 periodical subscriptions (1,500 health-care related).

BACCALAUREATE PROGRAMS

Degree BSN

Available Programs Accelerated Baccalaureate for Second Degree; Generic Baccalaureate; RN Baccalaureate.

Site Options *Distance Learning:* Pembroke Pines, FL.

Study Options Full-time.

Program Entrance Requirements Minimum overall college GPA of 3.0, transcript of college record, CPR certification, written essay, health exam, health insurance, high school foreign language, high school transcript, immunizations, minimum GPA in nursing prerequisites of 3.0, prerequisite course work. Transfer students are accepted. **Standardized tests** *Required:* SAT or ACT, TOEFL for international students. **Application** *Deadline:* rolling (freshmen), rolling (transfer). *Notification:* continuous until 8/1 (freshmen). *Application fee:* $25.

Advanced Placement Credit by examination available. Credit given for nursing courses completed elsewhere dependent upon specific evaluations.

Expenses (2004–05) *Tuition, state resident:* full-time $2854; part-time $95 per credit hour. *Tuition, nonresident:* full-time $15,260; part-time $509 per credit hour. *International tuition:* $15,260 full-time. *Room and board:* $9000; room only: $7500 per academic year. *Required fees:* full-time $336; part-time $112 per term.

Financial Aid 75% of baccalaureate students in nursing programs received some form of financial aid in 2003–04.

Contact Mrs. Paula Delpech, RN, Assistant Director, Student Services, School of Nursing, Florida International University, 3000 Northeast 151st Street, ACII 230, North Miami, FL 33181. *Telephone:* 305-919-5915. *Fax:* 305-919-5395. *E-mail:* jeany@fiu.edu.

GRADUATE PROGRAMS

Expenses (2004–05) *Tuition, state resident:* full-time $8823; part-time $225 per credit hour. *Tuition, nonresident:* full-time $25,966; part-time $866 per credit hour. *International tuition:* $25,966 full-time. *Room and board:* $9000; room only: $7500 per academic year. *Required fees:* full-time $336; part-time $112 per term.

Financial Aid 60% of graduate students in nursing programs received some form of financial aid in 2003–04.

Contact Mrs. Paula Delpech, RN, Assistant Director, Student Services, School of Nursing, Florida International University, 3000 Northeast 151st Street, ACII 230, North Miami, FL 33181. *Telephone:* 305-919-5915. *Fax:* 305-919-5395. *E-mail:* jeany@fiu.edu.

MASTER'S DEGREE PROGRAM

Degree MSN

Available Programs Master's; Master's for Nurses with Non-Nursing Degrees.

Concentrations Available Nurse anesthesia; nursing administration. *Clinical nurse specialist programs in:* adult health, family health, pediatric, psychiatric/mental health. *Nurse practitioner programs in:* adult health, family health, pediatric, psychiatric/mental health.

Site Options *Distance Learning:* Pembroke Pines, FL.

Study Options Full-time and part-time.

Program Entrance Requirements Clinical experience, computer literacy, minimum overall college GPA of 3.0, transcript of college record, CPR certification, written essay, immunizations, interview, 3 letters of recommendation, nursing research course, physical assessment course, professional liability insurance/malpractice insurance, prerequisite course work, statistics course, GRE General Test. *Application deadline:* For fall admission, 4/1 (priority date); for spring admission, 10/1. Applications are processed on a rolling basis. *Application fee:* $20.

Advanced Placement Credit given for nursing courses completed elsewhere dependent upon specific evaluations.

Degree Requirements 42 total credit hours.

POST-MASTER'S PROGRAM

Areas of Study Nursing administration. *Clinical nurse specialist programs in:* adult health, family health, pediatric, psychiatric/mental health. *Nurse practitioner programs in:* adult health, family health, pediatric, psychiatric/mental health.

DOCTORAL DEGREE PROGRAM

Degree PhD

Available Programs Doctorate.

Areas of Study Faculty preparation, health policy, health-care systems, individualized study, information systems, nursing administration, nursing education, nursing policy, nursing research, nursing science.

Program Entrance Requirements Clinical experience, minimum overall college GPA of 3.0, interview by faculty committee, 3 letters of recommendation, MSN or equivalent, statistics course. *Application deadline:* For fall admission, 4/1 (priority date); for spring admission, 10/1. Applications are processed on a rolling basis. *Application fee:* $20.

Degree Requirements 84 total credit hours, dissertation, oral exam, written exam.

Florida Southern College

Department of Nursing
Lakeland, Florida

http://www.flsouthern.edu/nursing/

Founded in 1885

DEGREE • BSN

Nursing Program Faculty 3 (67% with doctorates).

Baccalaureate Enrollment 74

Nursing Student Resources Academic advising; academic or career counseling; bookstore; campus computer network; computer lab; computer-assisted instruction; e-mail services; Internet; library services; nursing audiovisuals; resume preparation assistance; tutoring.

Library Facilities 172,803 volumes; 939 periodical subscriptions.

BACCALAUREATE PROGRAMS

Degree BSN

Available Programs ADN to Baccalaureate.

Site Options Orlando, FL.

Program Entrance Requirements Transcript of college record, health exam, professional liability insurance/malpractice insurance, RN licensure. Transfer students are accepted. **Standardized tests** *Required:* SAT or ACT, TOEFL for international students. **Application** *Deadline:* 4/1 (freshmen), rolling (transfer). *Early decision:* 12/1. *Notification:* continuous (freshmen), 12/15 (out-of-state freshmen), 12/15 (early decision). *Application fee:* $30.

Advanced Placement Credit given for nursing courses completed elsewhere dependent upon specific evaluations.

Expenses (2003–04) *Tuition:* part-time $185 per credit hour.

Contact Sheila F. Marks, DNS, Associate Professor & Chairperson, Department of Nursing, Florida Southern College, 111 Lake Hollingsworth Drive, Lakeland, FL 33801. *Telephone:* 863-680-4315. *Fax:* 863-680-4120. *E-mail:* smarks@flsouthern.edu.

Florida State University

School of Nursing
Tallahassee, Florida

Founded in 1851

DEGREES • BSN • MSN • MSN/MS

Nursing Program Faculty 43 (12% with doctorates).

Baccalaureate Enrollment 351
Women 94% **Men** 6% **Minority** 22% **International** 1% **Part-time** 12%

Graduate Enrollment 93
Women 91% **Men** 9% **Minority** 91% **Part-time** 87%

Nursing Student Activities Nursing Honor Society, Sigma Theta Tau, Student Nurses' Association, nursing club.

Nursing Student Resources Academic advising; academic or career counseling; assistance for students with disabilities; bookstore; campus computer network; career placement assistance; computer lab; computer-assisted instruction; daycare for children of students; e-mail services; externships; housing assistance; interactive nursing skills videos; Internet; learning resource lab; library services; nursing audiovisuals; resume preparation assistance; skills, simulation, or other laboratory; unpaid internships.

Library Facilities 2.7 million volumes (220,248 in nursing); 38,271 periodical subscriptions.

BACCALAUREATE PROGRAMS

Degree BSN

Available Programs Generic Baccalaureate; RN Baccalaureate.

Site Options Panama City, FL. *Distance Learning:* Marianna, FL; Lake City, FL.

Study Options Full-time.

Program Entrance Requirements Minimum overall college GPA of 3.0, transcript of college record, CPR certification, health exam, high school foreign language, high school transcript, immunizations, minimum GPA in nursing prerequisites of 3.0, professional liability insurance/malpractice insurance, prerequisite course work. Transfer students are accepted. **Standardized tests** *Required:* SAT or ACT, TOEFL for international students. **Application** *Deadline:* 3/1 (freshmen), 7/1 (transfer). *Notification:* continuous until 3/15 (freshmen). *Application fee:* $30.

Florida State University (continued)

Expenses (2003–04) *Tuition, state resident:* full-time $2500; part-time $90 per credit hour. *Tuition, nonresident:* full-time $12,824; part-time $458 per credit hour. *International tuition:* $12,824 full-time. *Room and board:* $5000; room only: $3280 per academic year. *Required fees:* full-time $5760; part-time $1260 per term.

Financial Aid 92% of baccalaureate students in nursing programs received some form of financial aid in 2002–03. *Gift aid (need-based):* Federal Pell, FSEOG, state, private, college/university gift aid from institutional funds. *Loans:* FFEL (Subsidized and Unsubsidized Stafford PLUS), Perkins, college/university. *Work-Study:* Federal Work-Study, part-time campus jobs. *Application deadline (priority):* 2/15.

Contact Ms. Brenda Arosemena, Academic Coordinator, School of Nursing, Florida State University, 104H Vivian M. Duxbury Hall, Tallahassee, FL 32306-4310. *Telephone:* 850-644-5107. *Fax:* 850-644-7660. *E-mail:* barosemena@nursing.fsu.edu.

GRADUATE PROGRAMS

Expenses (2003–04) *Tuition, state resident:* full-time $7066; part-time $5300 per semester. *Tuition, nonresident:* full-time $26,309; part-time $19,732 per semester. *International tuition:* $26,309 full-time. *Required fees:* full-time $1330; part-time $333 per credit; part-time $998 per term.

Financial Aid 60% of graduate students in nursing programs received some form of financial aid in 2002–03. 20 fellowships, 5 research assistantships with partial tuition reimbursements available (averaging $3,000 per year), 12 teaching assistantships with partial tuition reimbursements available (averaging $3,000 per year) were awarded; career-related internships or fieldwork, Federal Work-Study, institutionally sponsored loans, traineeships, and tuition waivers (partial) also available. *Financial aid application deadline:* 4/15.

Contact Mr. Eddie Page, Graduate Program Advisor, School of Nursing, Florida State University, 461C Vivian M. Duxbury Hall, Tallahassee, FL 32306-4310. *Telephone:* 850-644-5638. *Fax:* 850-644-7660. *E-mail:* epage@nursing.fsu.edu.

MASTER'S DEGREE PROGRAM

Degrees MSN; MSN/MS

Available Programs Master's.

Concentrations Available Nurse case management; nursing education. *Clinical nurse specialist programs in:* adult health, family health. *Nurse practitioner programs in:* adult health, family health.

Study Options Full-time and part-time.

Program Entrance Requirements Minimum overall college GPA of 3.0, transcript of college record, CPR certification, immunizations, 3 letters of recommendation, nursing research course, physical assessment course, professional liability insurance/malpractice insurance, prerequisite course work, resume, statistics course, GRE General Test. *Application deadline:* For fall admission, 6/15 (priority date); for spring admission, 10/15 (priority date). Applications are processed on a rolling basis. *Application fee:* $20.

Advanced Placement Credit given for nursing courses completed elsewhere dependent upon specific evaluations.

Degree Requirements 64 total credit hours, thesis or project.

POST-MASTER'S PROGRAM

Areas of Study *Clinical nurse specialist programs in:* adult health, family health. *Nurse practitioner programs in:* adult health, family health.

CONTINUING EDUCATION PROGRAM

Contact Dr. Katherine P. Mason, Dean and Professor, School of Nursing, Florida State University, 102 Vivian M. Duxbury Hall, Tallahassee, FL 32306-4310. *Telephone:* 850-644-3299. *Fax:* 850-644-7660. *E-mail:* kmason@nursing.fsu.edu.

Jacksonville University

School of Nursing
Jacksonville, Florida

http://www.jacksonville.edu

Founded in 1934

DEGREES • BSN • MSN • MSN/MBA

Nursing Program Faculty 28 (25% with doctorates).

Baccalaureate Enrollment 648

Women 89% **Men** 11% **Minority** 22% **Part-time** 77%

Graduate Enrollment 35

Women 97% **Men** 3% **Minority** 32% **Part-time** 89%

Nursing Student Activities Nursing Honor Society, Sigma Theta Tau, Student Nurses' Association, nursing club.

Nursing Student Resources Academic advising; academic or career counseling; assistance for students with disabilities; bookstore; campus computer network; career placement assistance; computer lab; computer-assisted instruction; e-mail services; interactive nursing skills videos; Internet; learning resource lab; library services; nursing audiovisuals; remedial services; resume preparation assistance; skills, simulation, or other laboratory; tutoring; unpaid internships.

Library Facilities 374,016 volumes (2,661 in health, 447 in nursing); 686 periodical subscriptions (71 health-care related).

BACCALAUREATE PROGRAMS

Degree BSN

Available Programs ADN to Baccalaureate; Accelerated Baccalaureate for Second Degree; Baccalaureate for Second Degree; Generic Baccalaureate; RN Baccalaureate.

Site Options St. Augustine, FL.

Study Options Full-time and part-time.

Program Entrance Requirements Minimum overall college GPA of 2.5, transcript of college record, CPR certification, written essay, health exam, 3 years high school math, 2 years high school science, high school transcript, immunizations, interview, 3 letters of recommendation, minimum high school GPA of 2.0, minimum GPA in nursing prerequisites of 2.5, prerequisite course work. Transfer students are accepted. **Standardized tests** *Required:* SAT or ACT, TOEFL for international students. **Application** *Deadline:* rolling (freshmen), rolling (transfer). *Application fee:* $30.

Advanced Placement Credit given for nursing courses completed elsewhere dependent upon specific evaluations.

Financial Aid 92% of baccalaureate students in nursing programs received some form of financial aid in 2003–04. *Gift aid (need-based):* Federal Pell, FSEOG, state, private, college/university gift aid from institutional funds. *Loans:* FFEL (Subsidized and Unsubsidized Stafford PLUS), Perkins, college/university. *Work-Study:* Federal Work-Study. *Application deadline (priority):* 2/1.

Contact Becky Cromwell, Coordinator of Nursing, School of Nursing, Jacksonville University, 2800 University Boulevard North, Jacksonville, FL 32211. *Telephone:* 904-256-7286. *Fax:* 904-256-7287. *E-mail:* bcromwe@ju.edu.

GRADUATE PROGRAMS

Contact Ms. Laura Winn, Coordinator, RN-BSN Program and MSN Program, School of Nursing, Jacksonville University, 2800 University Boulevard North, Jacksonville, FL 32211. *Telephone:* 904-256-7034. *Fax:* 904-256-7287. *E-mail:* lwinn@ju.edu.

MASTER'S DEGREE PROGRAM

Degrees MSN; MSN/MBA

Available Programs Accelerated RN to Master's; Master's; RN to Master's.

Concentrations Available Nursing administration; nursing education.

Study Options Full-time and part-time.

Program Entrance Requirements Clinical experience, minimum overall college GPA of 3.0, transcript of college record, CPR certification, written essay, immunizations, interview, 2 letters of recommendation, prerequisite course work, resume.

Advanced Placement Credit given for nursing courses completed elsewhere dependent upon specific evaluations.

Degree Requirements 32 total credit hours, thesis or project.

Nova Southeastern University

College of Allied Health and Nursing
Fort Lauderdale, Florida

Founded in 1964

DEGREE • BSN

Library Facilities 668,738 volumes; 22,837 periodical subscriptions.

BACCALAUREATE PROGRAMS

Degree BSN

Available Programs Generic Baccalaureate; RN Baccalaureate.

Program Entrance Requirements **Standardized tests** *Required:* SAT or ACT, TOEFL for international students. **Application** *Deadline:* rolling (freshmen), rolling (transfer). *Notification:* continuous (freshmen). *Application fee:* $50.

Contact Nursing Department, College of Allied Health and Nursing, Nova Southeastern University, 3200 South University Drive, Fort Lauderdale, FL 33328. *Telephone:* 800-541-6682 Ext. 1983. *E-mail:* nursinginfo@nsu.nova.edu.

St. Petersburg College

Department of Nursing
St. Petersburg, Florida

http://www.spcollege.edu

Founded in 1927

DEGREE • BSN

Nursing Program Faculty 70 (10% with doctorates).

Baccalaureate Enrollment 201
Women 91% **Men** 9% **Minority** 20%

Nursing Student Activities Student Nurses' Association, nursing club.

Nursing Student Resources Academic advising; academic or career counseling; assistance for students with disabilities; bookstore; campus computer network; career placement assistance; computer lab; computer-assisted instruction; e-mail services; employment services for current students; interactive nursing skills videos; Internet; learning resource lab; library services; nursing audiovisuals; paid internships; placement services for program completers; remedial services; skills, simulation, or other laboratory; unpaid internships.

Library Facilities 222,990 volumes (1,000 in health, 1,000 in nursing); 1,393 periodical subscriptions (50 health-care related).

BACCALAUREATE PROGRAMS

Degree BSN

Available Programs ADN to Baccalaureate; RN Baccalaureate.

Site Options Oakhill, FL; Clearwater, FL.

Study Options Full-time and part-time.

Program Entrance Requirements Minimum overall college GPA of 2.0, RN licensure. Transfer students are accepted. **Standardized tests** *Required:* TOEFL for international students. ***Placement:*** *Required for some:* SAT and SAT Subject Tests or ACT, SAT II Writing Tests, CPT. **Application** *Deadline:* rolling (freshmen). *Notification:* continuous (freshmen). *Application fee:* $35.

Advanced Placement Credit given for nursing courses completed elsewhere dependent upon specific evaluations.

Expenses (2004–05) *Tuition, state resident:* full-time $3879; part-time $73 per credit hour. *Tuition, nonresident:* part-time $272 per credit hour.

Financial Aid 80% of baccalaureate students in nursing programs received some form of financial aid in 2003–04. *Gift aid (need-based):* Federal Pell, FSEOG, state, private, college/university gift aid from institutional funds. *Loans:* FFEL (Subsidized and Unsubsidized Stafford PLUS), college/university. *Work-Study:* Federal Work-Study. *Application deadline (priority):* 4/15.

Contact Dr. Jean M. Wortock, Dean, Department of Nursing, St. Petersburg College, PO Box 13489, St. Petersburg, FL 33733. *Telephone:* 727-341-3640. *Fax:* 727-341-3546. *E-mail:* wortock.jean@spcollege.edu.

CONTINUING EDUCATION PROGRAM

Contact Denise Kerwin, Program Director, Department of Nursing, St. Petersburg College, 7200 66th Street North, Pinellas Park, FL 33781. *Telephone:* 727-341-4549. *Fax:* 727-341-3494. *E-mail:* kerwin.denise@spcollege.edu.

University of Central Florida

School of Nursing
Orlando, Florida

http://www.cohpa.ucf.edu/nursing

Founded in 1963

DEGREES • BSN • MSN • PHD

Nursing Program Faculty 56 (43% with doctorates).

Baccalaureate Enrollment 379
Women 91% **Men** 9% **Minority** 25% **Part-time** 32%

Graduate Enrollment 136
Women 87% **Men** 13% **Minority** 10% **Part-time** 75%

Nursing Student Activities Sigma Theta Tau, Student Nurses' Association.

Nursing Student Resources Academic advising; academic or career counseling; assistance for students with disabilities; bookstore; campus computer network; computer lab; computer-assisted instruction; daycare for children of students; e-mail services; employment services for current students; externships; housing assistance; interactive nursing skills videos; Internet; learning resource lab; library services; nursing audiovisuals; skills, simulation, or other laboratory; tutoring.

Library Facilities 1.2 million volumes (38,944 in health, 2,848 in nursing); 9,866 periodical subscriptions (360 health-care related).

BACCALAUREATE PROGRAMS

Degree BSN

Available Programs Accelerated Baccalaureate for Second Degree; Generic Baccalaureate; RN Baccalaureate.

Site Options *Distance Learning:* Cocoa Beach, FL; Daytona Beach, FL; Leesburg, FL.

Study Options Full-time and part-time.

Program Entrance Requirements Minimum overall college GPA of 2.5, transcript of college record, CPR certification, health exam, health insurance, high school foreign language, high school math, high school transcript, immunizations, minimum high school GPA of 2.5, prerequisite course work. Transfer students are accepted. **Standardized tests** *Required:* SAT or ACT, TOEFL for international students. **Application** *Deadline:* 5/1 (freshmen), 5/1 (transfer). *Notification:* continuous until 10/1 (freshmen). *Application fee:* $30.

Advanced Placement Credit given for nursing courses completed elsewhere dependent upon specific evaluations.

Expenses (2003–04) *Tuition, state resident:* part-time $94 per credit hour. *Tuition, nonresident:* part-time $482 per credit hour. *Required fees:* part-time $94 per credit.

Financial Aid 30% of baccalaureate students in nursing programs received some form of financial aid in 2002–03. *Gift aid (need-based):* Federal Pell, FSEOG, state, private, college/university gift aid from institutional funds. *Loans:* FFEL (Subsidized and Unsubsidized Stafford PLUS), Perkins. *Work-Study:* Federal Work-Study, part-time campus jobs. *Application deadline:* 6/30 (priority: 3/1).

Contact Ms. Patricia Leli, Undergraduate Program Coordinator, School of Nursing, University of Central Florida, PO Box 162210, Orlando, FL 32816-2210. *Telephone:* 407-823-2744. *Fax:* 407-823-5675. *E-mail:* ucfnurse@mail.ucf.edu.

GRADUATE PROGRAMS

Expenses (2003–04) *Tuition, state resident:* part-time $207 per credit hour. *Tuition, nonresident:* part-time $776 per credit hour. *Required fees:* part-time $207 per credit.

Financial Aid 70% of graduate students in nursing programs received some form of financial aid in 2002–03.

Contact Dr. Jean Kijek, Graduate Program Coordinator, School of Nursing, University of Central Florida, PO Box 162210, Orlando, FL 32816-2210. *Telephone:* 407-823-2744. *Fax:* 407-823-5675. *E-mail:* gradnurs@mail.ucf.edu.

MASTER'S DEGREE PROGRAM

Degree MSN

Available Programs Master's; RN to Master's.

University of Central Florida (continued)

Concentrations Available Nurse case management; nursing administration; nursing education. *Clinical nurse specialist programs in:* acute care, critical care. *Nurse practitioner programs in:* adult health, family health, pediatric.

Study Options Full-time and part-time.

Program Entrance Requirements Clinical experience, minimum overall college GPA of 3.0, transcript of college record, CPR certification, written essay, immunizations, 3 letters of recommendation, physical assessment course, resume, statistics course.

Advanced Placement Credit given for nursing courses completed elsewhere dependent upon specific evaluations.

Degree Requirements 47 total credit hours, thesis or project.

POST-MASTER'S PROGRAM

Areas of Study *Nurse practitioner programs in:* adult health, family health, pediatric.

DOCTORAL DEGREE PROGRAM

Degree PhD

Available Programs Doctorate.

Areas of Study Health policy, health-care systems, individualized study, information systems, nursing research.

Program Entrance Requirements Minimum overall college GPA of 3.5, interview by faculty committee, 3 letters of recommendation, MSN or equivalent, statistics course, vita.

Degree Requirements 57 total credit hours, dissertation.

University of Florida

College of Nursing
Gainesville, Florida

http://www.nursing.ufl.edu

Founded in 1853

DEGREES • BSN • MSN • MSN/MBA • MSN/MPH • MSN/PHD

Library Facilities 5 million volumes (260,000 in health, 3,000 in nursing); 28,103 periodical subscriptions (200 health-care related).

BACCALAUREATE PROGRAMS

Degree BSN

Available Programs Generic Baccalaureate; RN Baccalaureate.

Study Options Full-time.

Program Entrance Requirements CPR certification, health exam, immunizations, minimum GPA in nursing prerequisites of 2.8, professional liability insurance/malpractice insurance, prerequisite course work. Transfer students are accepted. **Standardized tests** *Required:* SAT or ACT, TOEFL for international students. **Application** *Deadline:* 1/12 (freshmen). *Early decision:* 10/1. *Notification:* continuous (freshmen), 12/1 (out-of-state freshmen), 12/1 (early decision). *Application fee:* $30.

Expenses (2003–04) *Tuition, state resident:* full-time $2770; part-time $93 per credit hour. *Tuition, nonresident:* full-time $13,800; part-time $460 per credit hour. *Room and board:* $5800 per academic year.

Financial Aid 85% of baccalaureate students in nursing programs received some form of financial aid in 2002–03. *Gift aid (need-based):* Federal Pell, FSEOG, state, private, college/university gift aid from institutional funds. *Loans:* Federal Direct (Subsidized and Unsubsidized Stafford PLUS), Perkins, college/university. *Work-Study:* Federal Work-Study, part-time campus jobs. *Application deadline (priority):* 3/15.

Contact Mr. Kenneth Foote, Program Assistant to the Admissions Coordinator, College of Nursing, University of Florida, PO Box 100197, HPNT Building, Gainesville, FL 32610-0197. *Telephone:* 352-273-6383. *Fax:* 352-273-6440. *E-mail:* Kfoote@nursing.ufl.edu.

GRADUATE PROGRAMS

Expenses (2003–04) *Tuition, state resident:* part-time $205 per credit hour. *Tuition, nonresident:* part-time $775 per credit hour.

Financial Aid 1 fellowship (averaging $15,000 per year), 4 research assistantships, 2 teaching assistantships were awarded; career-related internships or fieldwork and Federal Work-Study also available.

Contact Dr. Karin Polisko-Harris, Associate Dean for Academic and Student Affairs, College of Nursing, University of Florida, PO Box 100197, HPNT Building, Gainesville, FL 32610-0197. *Telephone:* 352-273-6331. *Fax:* 352-273-6440. *E-mail:* kpolisko@nursing.ufl.edu.

MASTER'S DEGREE PROGRAM

Degrees MSN; MSN/MBA; MSN/MPH; MSN/PhD

Concentrations Available Nurse-midwifery. *Clinical nurse specialist programs in:* psychiatric/mental health. *Nurse practitioner programs in:* acute care, adult health, family health, neonatal health, oncology, pediatric, psychiatric/mental health.

Study Options Full-time and part-time.

Program Entrance Requirements Computer literacy, minimum overall college GPA of 3.0, transcript of college record, CPR certification, written essay, immunizations, 2 letters of recommendation, resume, statistics course, GRE General Test. *Application deadline:* For fall admission, 3/1 (priority date). Applications are processed on a rolling basis. *Application fee:* $30.

Advanced Placement Credit given for nursing courses completed elsewhere dependent upon specific evaluations.

Degree Requirements 48 total credit hours, comprehensive exam.

POST-MASTER'S PROGRAM

Areas of Study Nurse-midwifery. *Clinical nurse specialist programs in:* psychiatric/mental health. *Nurse practitioner programs in:* acute care, adult health, family health, neonatal health, oncology, pediatric, psychiatric/mental health.

DOCTORAL DEGREE PROGRAM

Degree PhD

Areas of Study Aging, bio-behavioral research, health policy, illness and transition, nursing science, oncology, women's health.

Program Entrance Requirements Minimum overall college GPA of 3.5, interview by faculty committee, interview, 3 letters of recommendation, MSN or equivalent, statistics course, vita, writing sample, GRE General Test. *Application deadline:* For fall admission, 3/1 (priority date). Applications are processed on a rolling basis. *Application fee:* $30.

Degree Requirements 92 total credit hours, residency.

University of Miami

School of Nursing
Coral Gables, Florida

http://www.miami.edu/nur

Founded in 1925

DEGREES • BSN • MSN • PHD

Nursing Program Faculty 37 (47% with doctorates).

Baccalaureate Enrollment 354
Women 80% **Men** 20% **Minority** 65% **International** 1% **Part-time** 17%

Graduate Enrollment 54
Women 97% **Men** 3% **Minority** 55% **International** 1% **Part-time** 50%

Nursing Student Activities Sigma Theta Tau, Student Nurses' Association.

Nursing Student Resources Academic advising; academic or career counseling; assistance for students with disabilities; bookstore; campus computer network; career placement assistance; computer lab; computer-assisted instruction; daycare for children of students; e-mail services; employment services for current students; externships; housing assistance; interactive nursing skills videos; Internet; learning resource lab; library services; nursing audiovisuals; placement services for program completers; remedial services; resume preparation assistance; skills, simulation, or other laboratory; tutoring; unpaid internships.

Library Facilities 1.4 million volumes (2,000 in nursing); 16,305 periodical subscriptions (89 health-care related).

BACCALAUREATE PROGRAMS

Degree BSN

Available Programs Accelerated Baccalaureate; Accelerated Baccalaureate for Second Degree; Baccalaureate for Second Degree; Generic Baccalaureate; RN Baccalaureate.

Study Options Full-time and part-time.

Program Entrance Requirements Transcript of college record, written essay, 1 letter of recommendation, minimum high school GPA of 2.8, prerequisite course work. Transfer students are accepted. **Standardized tests** *Required:* SAT or ACT, TOEFL for international students. *Required for some:* SAT Subject Tests. **Application** *Deadline:* 2/1 (freshmen), 3/1 (transfer). *Early decision:* 11/1, 11/1. *Notification:* 4/15 (freshmen), 12/20 (out-of-state freshmen), 12/20 (early decision), 2/1 (early action). *Application fee:* $65.

Advanced Placement Credit given for nursing courses completed elsewhere dependent upon specific evaluations.

Expenses (2004–05) *Tuition:* full-time $27,384; part-time $1149 per credit hour. *International tuition:* $27,384 full-time. *Room and board:* $8858; room only: $3500 per academic year. *Required fees:* full-time $500; part-time $228 per term.

Financial Aid 85% of baccalaureate students in nursing programs received some form of financial aid in 2003–04. *Gift aid (need-based):* Federal Pell, FSEOG, state, private, college/university gift aid from institutional funds, Federal Nursing. *Loans:* Federal Nursing Student Loans, FFEL (Subsidized and Unsubsidized Stafford PLUS), Perkins, Signature Loans, alternative loans. *Work-Study:* Federal Work-Study, part-time campus jobs. *Application deadline (priority):* 2/15.

Contact Dr. Valerie Ann Browne-Krimsley, RN, Associate Dean for Student Services, School of Nursing, University of Miami, 5801 Red Road, Coral Gables, FL 33143. *Telephone:* 305-284-4325. *Fax:* 305-284-4827. *E-mail:* vbkrimsley@miami.edu.

GRADUATE PROGRAMS

Expenses (2004–05) *Tuition:* full-time $10,260; part-time $1140 per credit hour. *International tuition:* $10,260 full-time. *Room and board:* $8330; room only: $5000 per academic year. *Required fees:* full-time $200; part-time $100 per term.

Financial Aid 95% of graduate students in nursing programs received some form of financial aid in 2003–04. 1 research assistantship with tuition reimbursement available (averaging $9,000 per year), 8 teaching assistantships with tuition reimbursements available (averaging $9,000 per year) were awarded; fellowships, Federal Work-Study, institutionally sponsored loans, scholarships, and unspecified assistantships also available. Aid available to part-time students. *Financial aid application deadline:* 3/1.

Contact Dr. Valerie Ann Browne-Krimsley, RN, Associate Dean for Student Services, School of Nursing, University of Miami, 5801 Red Road, Coral Gables, FL 33143-2343. *Telephone:* 305-284-4325. *Fax:* 305-284-4827.

MASTER'S DEGREE PROGRAM

Degree MSN

Available Programs Accelerated Master's; Master's.

Concentrations Available Nurse anesthesia; nurse-midwifery. *Clinical nurse specialist programs in:* acute care, adult health, community health, family health, psychiatric/mental health, women's health. *Nurse practitioner programs in:* acute care, adult health, community health, family health, primary care, psychiatric/mental health, women's health.

Study Options Full-time and part-time.

Program Entrance Requirements Clinical experience, minimum overall college GPA of 3.0, transcript of college record, written essay, interview, 3 letters of recommendation, resume, statistics course, GRE General Test. *Application deadline:* For fall admission, 3/1 (priority date); for spring admission, 10/1 (priority date). Applications are processed on a rolling basis. *Application fee:* $50.

Degree Requirements 39 total credit hours.

POST-MASTER'S PROGRAM

Areas of Study Nursing administration; nursing education. *Clinical nurse specialist programs in:* adult health, family health, psychiatric/mental health, women's health. *Nurse practitioner programs in:* adult health, family health, psychiatric/mental health, women's health.

DOCTORAL DEGREE PROGRAM

Degree PhD

Available Programs Doctorate.

Areas of Study Faculty preparation, nursing education, nursing research, nursing science.

Program Entrance Requirements Minimum overall college GPA of 3.0, interview by faculty committee, interview, 3 letters of recommendation, MSN or equivalent, vita, writing sample, GRE General Test. *Application deadline:* For fall admission, 3/1 (priority date); for spring admission, 10/1 (priority date). Applications are processed on a rolling basis. *Application fee:* $50.

Degree Requirements 60 total credit hours, dissertation, written exam.

CONTINUING EDUCATION PROGRAM

Contact Dr. Valerie Ann Browne-Krimsley, RN, Associate Dean for Student Services, School of Nursing, University of Miami, 5801 Red Road, Coral Gables, FL 33124. *Telephone:* 305-284-4325. *Fax:* 305-284-4827. *E-mail:* vbkrimsley@miami.edu.

University of North Florida
School of Nursing
Jacksonville, Florida

http://www.unf.edu/coh/cohnursi.htm

Founded in 1965

DEGREES • BSN • MSN

Nursing Program Faculty 19 (50% with doctorates).

Baccalaureate Enrollment 279

Women 85% **Men** 15% **Minority** 20% **International** 1% **Part-time** 27%

Graduate Enrollment 35

Women 86% **Men** 14% **Minority** 6% **Part-time** 70%

Nursing Student Activities Sigma Theta Tau, Student Nurses' Association.

Nursing Student Resources Academic advising; academic or career counseling; assistance for students with disabilities; bookstore; campus computer network; career placement assistance; computer lab; computer-assisted instruction; e-mail services; interactive nursing skills videos; Internet; learning resource lab; library services; nursing audiovisuals; resume preparation assistance; skills, simulation, or other laboratory.

Library Facilities 746,604 volumes (30,466 in health, 3,000 in nursing); 3,466 periodical subscriptions (200 health-care related).

BACCALAUREATE PROGRAMS

Degree BSN

Available Programs Accelerated Baccalaureate for Second Degree; Generic Baccalaureate; RN Baccalaureate.

Study Options Full-time.

Program Entrance Requirements Minimum overall college GPA of 2.7, CPR certification, written essay, health exam, immunizations, interview, minimum high school GPA, minimum GPA in nursing prerequisites of 3.0, professional liability insurance/malpractice insurance, prerequisite course work. Transfer students are accepted. **Standardized tests** *Required:* SAT or ACT, TOEFL for international students. **Application** *Deadline:* 7/2 (freshmen), 7/2 (transfer). *Early decision:* 11/15. *Notification:* continuous (freshmen), 12/2 (early action). *Application fee:* $30.

Advanced Placement Credit given for nursing courses completed elsewhere dependent upon specific evaluations.

Expenses (2004–05) *Tuition, state resident:* full-time $3101; part-time $103 per credit hour. *Tuition, nonresident:* full-time $14,851; part-time $495 per credit hour. *Room and board:* room only: $2900 per academic year. *Required fees:* full-time $650.

Financial Aid 20% of baccalaureate students in nursing programs received some form of financial aid in 2003–04.

Contact Ms. Bethany Dibble, Admissions Coordinator, School of Nursing, University of North Florida, 4567 St. Johns Bluff Road, South, Building 39, Jacksonville, FL 32224-2673. *Telephone:* 904-620-2418. *E-mail:* bdibble@unf.edu.

GRADUATE PROGRAMS

Expenses (2004–05) *Tuition, state resident:* part-time $232 per credit hour. *Tuition, nonresident:* part-time $833 per credit hour. *Required fees:* full-time $500.

University of North Florida (continued)

Financial Aid 5% of graduate students in nursing programs received some form of financial aid in 2003–04.

Contact Dr. Li Loriz, NP, Director, School of Nursing and MSN Coordinator, School of Nursing, University of North Florida, 4567 St. Johns Bluff Road, South, Building 39, Room 2036, Jacksonville, FL 32224-2673. *Telephone:* 904-620-2684. *Fax:* 904-620-2848. *E-mail:* lloriz@unf.edu.

MASTER'S DEGREE PROGRAM

Degree MSN

Available Programs Master's; RN to Master's.

Concentrations Available *Clinical nurse specialist programs in:* adult health, cardiovascular, community health, critical care, gerontology, maternity-newborn, medical-surgical, pediatric, psychiatric/mental health, women's health. *Nurse practitioner programs in:* family health, primary care.

Study Options Full-time and part-time.

Program Entrance Requirements Clinical experience, computer literacy, minimum overall college GPA of 3.0, transcript of college record, CPR certification, written essay, immunizations, 2 letters of recommendation, nursing research course, physical assessment course, professional liability insurance/malpractice insurance, resume, statistics course.

Advanced Placement Credit given for nursing courses completed elsewhere dependent upon specific evaluations.

Degree Requirements 43 total credit hours, thesis or project.

POST-MASTER'S PROGRAM

Areas of Study *Nurse practitioner programs in:* family health, primary care.

University of Phoenix–Fort Lauderdale Campus

College of Health and Human Services
Fort Lauderdale, Florida

DEGREES • BSN • MSN • MSN/MBA

Nursing Program Faculty 43 (26% with doctorates).

Baccalaureate Enrollment 113
Women 92% **Men** 8% **Minority** 70%

Graduate Enrollment 99
Women 94% **Men** 6% **Minority** 75%

Nursing Student Activities Sigma Theta Tau.

Nursing Student Resources Academic advising; academic or career counseling; bookstore; computer lab; library services.

Library Facilities 27.1 million volumes; 11,648 periodical subscriptions (1,426 health-care related).

BACCALAUREATE PROGRAMS

Degree BSN

Available Programs ADN to Baccalaureate; Accelerated RN Baccalaureate.

Study Options Full-time.

Program Entrance Requirements 1 letter of recommendation. Transfer students are accepted. **Standardized tests** *Required:* TOEFL for international students. **Application** *Deadline:* rolling (freshmen), rolling (transfer). *Application fee:* $100.

Advanced Placement Credit by examination available.

Expenses (2004–05) *Tuition:* full-time $10,170; part-time $339 per credit hour. *International tuition:* $10,170 full-time. *Required fees:* full-time $110.

Financial Aid 6% of baccalaureate students in nursing programs received some form of financial aid in 2003–04.

Contact Campus College Chair, Nursing, College of Health and Human Services, University of Phoenix–Fort Lauderdale Campus, 600 North Pine Island Road, Suite #500, Plantation, FL 33324-1393. *Telephone:* 954-382-5303.

GRADUATE PROGRAMS

Expenses (2004–05) *Tuition:* full-time $9504; part-time $396 per credit hour. *International tuition:* $9504 full-time. *Required fees:* full-time $110.

Financial Aid 10% of graduate students in nursing programs received some form of financial aid in 2003–04.

Contact Campus College Chair, Nursing, College of Health and Human Services, University of Phoenix–Fort Lauderdale Campus, 600 North Pine Island Road, Suite #500, Plantation, FL 33324-1393. *Telephone:* 954-382-5303.

MASTER'S DEGREE PROGRAM

Degrees MSN; MSN/MBA

Available Programs Master's.

Concentrations Available Health-care administration; nursing administration; nursing education. *Nurse practitioner programs in:* family health.

Study Options Full-time.

Program Entrance Requirements Clinical experience, computer literacy, minimum overall college GPA of 2.5, transcript of college record. *Application deadline:* Applications are processed on a rolling basis. *Application fee:* $110.

Advanced Placement Credit by examination available.

Degree Requirements 39 total credit hours, thesis or project.

POST-MASTER'S PROGRAM

Areas of Study *Nurse practitioner programs in:* family health.

University of Phoenix–Jacksonville Campus

College of Health and Human Services
Jacksonville, Florida

Founded in 1976

DEGREES • BSN • MSN • MSN/MBA

Nursing Program Faculty 22 (32% with doctorates).

Baccalaureate Enrollment 27
Women 93% **Men** 7% **Minority** 48%

Graduate Enrollment 21
Women 100% **Minority** 59%

Nursing Student Activities Sigma Theta Tau.

Nursing Student Resources Academic advising; academic or career counseling; assistance for students with disabilities; bookstore; computer lab; library services.

Library Facilities 27.1 million volumes; 11,648 periodical subscriptions (1,426 health-care related).

BACCALAUREATE PROGRAMS

Degree BSN

Available Programs ADN to Baccalaureate; Accelerated RN Baccalaureate.

Site Options Jacksonville, FL; Orange Park, FL.

Study Options Full-time.

Program Entrance Requirements 1 letter of recommendation. Transfer students are accepted. **Standardized tests** *Required:* TOEFL for international students. **Application** *Deadline:* rolling (freshmen), rolling (transfer). *Application fee:* $100.

Advanced Placement Credit by examination available.

Expenses (2004–05) *Tuition:* full-time $10,170; part-time $339 per credit hour. *International tuition:* $10,170 full-time. *Required fees:* full-time $110.

Financial Aid 4% of baccalaureate students in nursing programs received some form of financial aid in 2003–04.

Contact Campus College Chair, Nursing, College of Health and Human Services, University of Phoenix–Jacksonville Campus, 4500 Salisbury Road, Suite 200, Jacksonville, FL 32216-0959. *Telephone:* 904-636-6645.

GRADUATE PROGRAMS

Expenses (2004–05) *Tuition:* full-time $9504; part-time $396 per credit hour. *International tuition:* $9504 full-time. *Required fees:* full-time $110.

Financial Aid 6% of graduate students in nursing programs received some form of financial aid in 2003–04.

Contact Campus College Chair, Nursing, College of Health and Human Services, University of Phoenix–Jacksonville Campus, 4500 Salisbury Road, Suite 200, Jacksonville, FL 32216-0959. *Telephone:* 904-636-6645.

MASTER'S DEGREE PROGRAM

Degrees MSN; MSN/MBA

Available Programs Master's.

Concentrations Available Health-care administration; nursing administration; nursing education. *Nurse practitioner programs in:* family health.

Site Options Jacksonville, FL; Orange Park, FL.

Program Entrance Requirements Clinical experience, computer literacy, minimum overall college GPA of 2.5, transcript of college record. *Application deadline:* Applications are processed on a rolling basis. *Application fee:* $110.

Degree Requirements 39 total credit hours, thesis or project.

POST-MASTER'S PROGRAM

Areas of Study *Nurse practitioner programs in:* family health.

University of Phoenix–Orlando Campus

College of Health and Human Services
Maitland, Florida

Founded in 1996

DEGREES • BSN • MSN • MSN/MBA

Nursing Program Faculty 25 (24% with doctorates).

Baccalaureate Enrollment 63
Women 92% **Men** 8% **Minority** 24%

Graduate Enrollment 60
Women 90% **Men** 10% **Minority** 57%

Nursing Student Activities Sigma Theta Tau.

Nursing Student Resources Academic advising; academic or career counseling; bookstore; computer lab; library services.

Library Facilities 27.1 million volumes; 11,648 periodical subscriptions (1,426 health-care related).

BACCALAUREATE PROGRAMS

Degree BSN

Available Programs ADN to Baccalaureate; Accelerated Baccalaureate.

Site Options Orlando, FL.

Study Options Full-time.

Program Entrance Requirements 1 letter of recommendation. Transfer students are accepted. **Standardized tests** *Required:* TOEFL for international students. **Application** *Deadline:* rolling (freshmen), rolling (transfer). *Application fee:* $85.

Advanced Placement Credit by examination available.

Expenses (2004–05) *Tuition:* full-time $10,170; part-time $339 per credit hour. *International tuition:* $10,170 full-time. *Required fees:* full-time $110.

Financial Aid 6% of baccalaureate students in nursing programs received some form of financial aid in 2003–04.

Contact Campus College Chair, Nursing, College of Health and Human Services, University of Phoenix–Orlando Campus, 2290 Lucien Way, Suite 400, Maitland, FL 32751-7057. *Telephone:* 407-667-0555.

GRADUATE PROGRAMS

Expenses (2004–05) *Tuition:* full-time $9504; part-time $396 per credit hour. *International tuition:* $9504 full-time. *Required fees:* full-time $110.

Financial Aid 9% of graduate students in nursing programs received some form of financial aid in 2003–04.

Contact Campus College Chair, Nursing, College of Health and Human Services, University of Phoenix–Orlando Campus, 2290 Lucien Way, Suite 400, Maitland, FL 32751-7057. *Telephone:* 407-667-0555.

MASTER'S DEGREE PROGRAM

Degrees MSN; MSN/MBA

Available Programs Master's.

Concentrations Available Health-care administration; nursing administration; nursing education. *Nurse practitioner programs in:* family health.

Site Options Orlando, FL.

Study Options Full-time.

Program Entrance Requirements Clinical experience, computer literacy, minimum overall college GPA of 2.5, transcript of college record. *Application deadline:* Applications are processed on a rolling basis. *Application fee:* $110.

Degree Requirements 39 total credit hours, thesis or project.

POST-MASTER'S PROGRAM

Areas of Study *Nurse practitioner programs in:* family health.

University of Phoenix–Tampa Campus

College of Health and Human Services
Tampa, Florida

DEGREES • BSN • MSN • MSN/MBA

Nursing Program Faculty 27 (30% with doctorates).

Baccalaureate Enrollment 46
Women 85% **Men** 15% **Minority** 22%

Graduate Enrollment 40
Women 95% **Men** 5% **Minority** 38%

Nursing Student Activities Sigma Theta Tau.

Nursing Student Resources Academic advising; academic or career counseling; bookstore; computer lab; library services.

Library Facilities 27.1 million volumes; 11,648 periodical subscriptions (1,426 health-care related).

BACCALAUREATE PROGRAMS

Degree BSN

Available Programs ADN to Baccalaureate; Accelerated Baccalaureate.

Site Options Clearwater, FL.

Study Options Full-time.

Program Entrance Requirements 1 letter of recommendation. Transfer students are accepted. **Standardized tests** *Required:* TOEFL for international students. **Application** *Deadline:* rolling (freshmen), rolling (transfer). *Application fee:* $85.

Advanced Placement Credit by examination available.

Expenses (2004–05) *Tuition:* full-time $10,170; part-time $339 per credit hour. *International tuition:* $10,170 full-time. *Required fees:* full-time $110.

Financial Aid 6% of baccalaureate students in nursing programs received some form of financial aid in 2003–04.

Contact Campus College Chair, Nursing, College of Health and Human Services, University of Phoenix–Tampa Campus, 100 Tampa Oaks Boulevard, Suite #200, Temple Terrace, FL 33637-1920. *Telephone:* 813-626-7911.

GRADUATE PROGRAMS

Expenses (2004–05) *Tuition:* full-time $9504; part-time $396 per credit hour. *International tuition:* $9504 full-time. *Required fees:* full-time $110.

Financial Aid 5% of graduate students in nursing programs received some form of financial aid in 2003–04.

University of Phoenix–Tampa Campus (continued)

Contact Campus College Chair, Nursing, College of Health and Human Services, University of Phoenix–Tampa Campus, 100 Tampa Oaks Boulevard, Suite #200, Temple Terrace, FL 33637-1920. *Telephone:* 813-626-7911.

MASTER'S DEGREE PROGRAM

Degrees MSN; MSN/MBA

Available Programs Master's.

Concentrations Available Health-care administration; nursing administration; nursing education. *Nurse practitioner programs in:* family health.

Site Options Clearwater, FL.

Study Options Full-time.

Program Entrance Requirements Clinical experience, computer literacy, minimum overall college GPA of 2.5, transcript of college record. *Application deadline:* Applications are processed on a rolling basis. *Application fee:* $110.

Degree Requirements 39 total credit hours, thesis or project.

POST-MASTER'S PROGRAM

Areas of Study *Nurse practitioner programs in:* family health.

University of South Florida
College of Nursing
Tampa, Florida

http://hsc.usf.edu/nursing

Founded in 1956

DEGREES • BS • MS • MSN/MPH • PHD

Nursing Program Faculty 51 (51% with doctorates).

Baccalaureate Enrollment 481
Women 91% **Men** 9% **Minority** 25% **International** 1% **Part-time** 40%

Graduate Enrollment 191
Women 88% **Men** 12% **Minority** 20% **International** .5% **Part-time** 64%

Nursing Student Activities Nursing Honor Society, Sigma Theta Tau, Student Nurses' Association.

Nursing Student Resources Academic advising; academic or career counseling; assistance for students with disabilities; bookstore; campus computer network; career placement assistance; computer lab; computer-assisted instruction; daycare for children of students; e-mail services; employment services for current students; housing assistance; Internet; learning resource lab; library services; nursing audiovisuals; remedial services; resume preparation assistance; skills, simulation, or other laboratory; tutoring.

Library Facilities 2 million volumes (106,028 in health, 3,898 in nursing); 20,571 periodical subscriptions (1,581 health-care related).

BACCALAUREATE PROGRAMS

Degree BS

Available Programs ADN to Baccalaureate; Accelerated Baccalaureate; Baccalaureate for Second Degree; Generic Baccalaureate; RN Baccalaureate.

Site Options Sarasota/Bradenton, FL; Winterhaven, FL.

Study Options Full-time.

Program Entrance Requirements Minimum overall college GPA of 3.0, transcript of college record, health insurance, high school foreign language, immunizations, prerequisite course work. Transfer students are accepted. **Standardized tests** *Required:* SAT or ACT, TOEFL for international students. **Application** *Deadline:* 4/15 (freshmen), 4/15 (transfer). *Notification:* continuous (freshmen). *Application fee:* $30.

Advanced Placement Credit by examination available. Credit given for nursing courses completed elsewhere dependent upon specific evaluations.

Expenses (2004–05) *Tuition, state resident:* full-time $1237; part-time $103 per credit hour. *Tuition, nonresident:* full-time $6387; part-time $532 per credit hour. *International tuition:* $6387 full-time. *Room and board:* $6355; room only: $4750 per academic year.

Financial Aid 40% of baccalaureate students in nursing programs received some form of financial aid in 2003–04. *Gift aid (need-based):* Federal Pell, FSEOG, state, private, college/university gift aid from institutional funds. *Loans:* FFEL (Subsidized and Unsubsidized Stafford PLUS), Perkins, college/university. *Work-Study:* Federal Work-Study. *Application deadline (priority):* 3/1.

Contact Mr. Carl Storck, Director of Student Affairs, College of Nursing, University of South Florida, 12901 Bruce B. Downs Boulevard, MDC Box 22, Tampa, FL 33612-4766. *Telephone:* 813-974-7513. *Fax:* 813-974-5418. *E-mail:* cstorck@hsc.usf.edu.

GRADUATE PROGRAMS

Expenses (2004–05) *Tuition, state resident:* full-time $2797; part-time $233 per credit hour. *Tuition, nonresident:* full-time $10,734; part-time $895 per credit hour. *International tuition:* $10,734 full-time. *Room and board:* $6355; room only: $4750 per academic year.

Financial Aid 40% of graduate students in nursing programs received some form of financial aid in 2003–04. 4 fellowships with partial tuition reimbursements available (averaging $11,250 per year), 4 research assistantships with partial tuition reimbursements available (averaging $16,500 per year), 18 teaching assistantships with partial tuition reimbursements available (averaging $8,000 per year) were awarded; Federal Work-Study, institutionally sponsored loans, scholarships, traineeships, tuition waivers (partial), and unspecified assistantships also available. *Financial aid application deadline:* 1/15.

Contact Mr. Carl Storck, Director of Student Affairs, College of Nursing, University of South Florida, 12901 Bruce B. Downs Boulevard, MDC Box 22, Tampa, FL 33612-4766. *Telephone:* 813-974-7513. *Fax:* 813-974-5418. *E-mail:* cstorck@hsc.usf.edu.

MASTER'S DEGREE PROGRAM

Degrees MS; MSN/MPH

Available Programs Master's; Master's for Nurses with Non-Nursing Degrees; RN to Master's.

Concentrations Available Nursing education; nursing informatics. *Clinical nurse specialist programs in:* gerontology, oncology, psychiatric/mental health. *Nurse practitioner programs in:* acute care, adult health, family health, gerontology, occupational health, oncology, pediatric, psychiatric/mental health.

Site Options Sarasota/Bradenton, FL.

Study Options Full-time and part-time.

Program Entrance Requirements Computer literacy, minimum overall college GPA of 3.0, transcript of college record, written essay, immunizations, interview, 3 letters of recommendation, resume. *Application deadline:* For fall admission, 6/1 (priority date); for spring admission, 10/15 (priority date). Applications are processed on a rolling basis. *Application fee:* $30.

Advanced Placement Credit given for nursing courses completed elsewhere dependent upon specific evaluations.

Degree Requirements 44 total credit hours, thesis or project, comprehensive exam.

POST-MASTER'S PROGRAM

Areas of Study Nursing education; nursing informatics. *Nurse practitioner programs in:* adult health, family health, oncology, pediatric, psychiatric/mental health.

DOCTORAL DEGREE PROGRAM

Degree PhD

Available Programs Doctorate.

Areas of Study Addiction/substance abuse, advanced practice nursing, aging, faculty preparation, family health, gerontology, health policy, health promotion/disease prevention, health-care systems, human health and illness, information systems, nurse case management, nursing administration, nursing education, nursing policy, nursing research, oncology.

Program Entrance Requirements Minimum overall college GPA of 3.5, interview by faculty committee, interview, 3 letters of recommendation, scholarly papers, vita, writing sample. *Application deadline:* For fall admission, 6/1 (priority date); for spring admission, 10/15 (priority date). Applications are processed on a rolling basis. *Application fee:* $30.

Degree Requirements 94 total credit hours, dissertation.

CONTINUING EDUCATION PROGRAM

Contact Dr. Patricia Gorzka, Coordinator of Continuing Medical Education, College of Nursing, University of South Florida, 12901 Bruce B. Downs Boulevard, MDC Box 22, Tampa, FL 33612-4766. *Telephone:* 813-974-4392. *Fax:* 813-974-5418. *E-mail:* pgorzka@hsc.usf.edu.

The University of Tampa

Department of Nursing
Tampa, Florida

http://www.utampa.edu/academics/liberalarts/departments/nursingbsn.html

Founded in 1931

DEGREES • BSN • MSN

Nursing Program Faculty 12.

Nursing Student Activities Nursing Honor Society, Sigma Theta Tau, Student Nurses' Association.

Library Facilities 252,147 volumes; 10,854 periodical subscriptions.

BACCALAUREATE PROGRAMS

Degree BSN

Available Programs ADN to Baccalaureate; Generic Baccalaureate; RN Baccalaureate.

Program Entrance Requirements Minimum overall college GPA of 2.0, transcript of college record, CPR certification, health exam, high school transcript, immunizations, professional liability insurance/malpractice insurance. Transfer students are accepted. **Standardized tests** *Required:* SAT or ACT, TOEFL for international students. **Application** *Deadline:* rolling (freshmen), rolling (transfer). *Application fee:* $35.

Advanced Placement Credit by examination available. Credit given for nursing courses completed elsewhere dependent upon specific evaluations.

Expenses (2003–04) *Tuition:* part-time $356 per credit hour. *Required fees:* full-time $451.

Contact Dr. Nancy Ross, Director, Department of Nursing, The University of Tampa, 401 West Kennedy Boulevard, Tampa, FL 33606-1490. *Telephone:* 813-253-3333. *Fax:* 813-258-7214. *E-mail:* nross@ut.edu.

GRADUATE PROGRAMS

Contact Dr. Nancy Ross, Director, Department of Nursing, The University of Tampa, 401 West Kennedy Boulevard, Tampa, FL 33606-1490. *Telephone:* 813-253-3333. *Fax:* 813-258-7214. *E-mail:* nross@ut.edu.

MASTER'S DEGREE PROGRAM

Degree MSN

Available Programs Accelerated RN to Master's; Master's.

Concentrations Available Nursing education. *Nurse practitioner programs in:* adult health, family health.

Study Options Full-time and part-time.

Program Entrance Requirements Computer literacy, minimum overall college GPA of 3.0, transcript of college record, CPR certification, written essay, immunizations, interview, 2 letters of recommendation, physical assessment course, professional liability insurance/malpractice insurance, resume, statistics course.

Advanced Placement Credit by examination available.

Degree Requirements Comprehensive exam.

POST-MASTER'S PROGRAM

Areas of Study Nursing education. *Nurse practitioner programs in:* adult health, family health.

See full description on page 580.

University of West Florida

Department of Nursing
Pensacola, Florida

http://uwf.edu/nursing

Founded in 1963

DEGREE • BSN

Nursing Program Faculty 4.

Baccalaureate Enrollment 103

Women 98% **Men** 2% **Minority** 20% **International** 2% **Part-time** 90%

Library Facilities 414,418 volumes (3,500 in health, 1,950 in nursing); 3,236 periodical subscriptions (54 health-care related).

BACCALAUREATE PROGRAMS

Degree BSN

Available Programs ADN to Baccalaureate; Generic Baccalaureate; RN Baccalaureate.

Study Options Full-time and part-time.

Program Entrance Requirements Transcript of college record, health insurance, immunizations, professional liability insurance/malpractice insurance, prerequisite course work. Transfer students are accepted. **Standardized tests** *Required:* SAT or ACT, TOEFL for international students. **Application** *Deadline:* 6/30 (freshmen), 6/30 (transfer). *Notification:* continuous (freshmen). *Application fee:* $30.

Advanced Placement Credit given for nursing courses completed elsewhere dependent upon specific evaluations.

Financial Aid 60% of baccalaureate students in nursing programs received some form of financial aid in 2002–03.

Contact The University of West Florida Nursing Department, Department of Nursing, University of West Florida, 11000 University Parkway, Pensacola, FL 32514. *Telephone:* 850-494-3802. *E-mail:* nursing@uwf.edu.

GEORGIA

Albany State University

College of Health Professions
Albany, Georgia

http://asuweb.asurams.edu

Founded in 1903

DEGREES • BSN • MSN

Nursing Program Faculty 14 (43% with doctorates).

Baccalaureate Enrollment 151

Women 93% **Men** 7% **Minority** 91% **Part-time** 20%

Graduate Enrollment 27

Women 93% **Men** 7% **Minority** 48% **International** 7% **Part-time** 59%

Nursing Student Activities Nursing Honor Society, Student Nurses' Association, nursing club.

Nursing Student Resources Academic advising; academic or career counseling; assistance for students with disabilities; bookstore; campus computer network; career placement assistance; computer lab; computer-assisted instruction; e-mail services; interactive nursing skills videos; Internet; learning resource lab; library services; nursing audiovisuals; paid internships; placement services for program completers; remedial services; resume preparation assistance; skills, simulation, or other laboratory; tutoring; unpaid internships.

Library Facilities 338,744 volumes (9,000 in health, 6,800 in nursing); 1,066 periodical subscriptions (75 health-care related).

Albany State University (continued)

BACCALAUREATE PROGRAMS

Degree BSN

Available Programs ADN to Baccalaureate; Accelerated RN Baccalaureate; Generic Baccalaureate; RN Baccalaureate.

Site Options Bainbridge, GA.

Study Options Full-time.

Program Entrance Requirements Minimum overall college GPA of 2.75, transcript of college record, written essay, health exam, health insurance, high school biology, high school foreign language, high school math, high school transcript, immunizations, interview, minimum GPA in nursing prerequisites of 2.75, professional liability insurance/malpractice insurance, prerequisite course work. Transfer students are accepted. **Standardized tests** *Required:* SAT or ACT, TOEFL for international students. **Application** *Deadline:* 7/1 (freshmen), 7/1 (transfer). *Application fee:* $20.

Advanced Placement Credit given for nursing courses completed elsewhere dependent upon specific evaluations.

Expenses (2004–05) *Tuition, state resident:* full-time $2896; part-time $97 per contact hour. *Tuition, nonresident:* full-time $9290; part-time $388 per contact hour. *Room and board:* $3648; room only: $1644 per academic year. *Required fees:* full-time $574.

Financial Aid 80% of baccalaureate students in nursing programs received some form of financial aid in 2003–04. *Gift aid (need-based):* Federal Pell, FSEOG, state, private, college/university gift aid from institutional funds, Federal Nursing, Thurgood Marshall Scholarship Fund. *Loans:* Federal Direct (Subsidized and Unsubsidized Stafford PLUS), Perkins, state. *Work-Study:* Federal Work-Study, part-time campus jobs. *Application deadline (priority):* 4/15.

Contact Dr. Linda P. Grimsley, RN, Chair, College of Health Professions, Albany State University, 504 College Drive, Albany, GA 31705. *Telephone:* 229-430-4724. *Fax:* 229-430-3937. *E-mail:* linda.grimsley@asurams.edu.

GRADUATE PROGRAMS

Expenses (2004–05) *Tuition, state resident:* full-time $2680; part-time $117 per contact hour. *Tuition, nonresident:* full-time $8370; part-time $465 per contact hour.

Financial Aid 70% of graduate students in nursing programs received some form of financial aid in 2003–04. Scholarships and traineeships available.

Contact Dr. Linda P. Grimsley, RN, Chair, College of Health Professions, Albany State University, 504 College Drive, Albany, GA 31705. *Telephone:* 229-430-4727. *Fax:* 229-430-3937. *E-mail:* linda.grimsley@asurams.edu.

MASTER'S DEGREE PROGRAM

Degree MSN

Available Programs Accelerated Master's; Master's.

Concentrations Available Nursing administration; nursing education. *Clinical nurse specialist programs in:* community health. *Nurse practitioner programs in:* family health.

Study Options Full-time and part-time.

Program Entrance Requirements Clinical experience, computer literacy, minimum overall college GPA of 3.0, transcript of college record, CPR certification, immunizations, interview, 2 letters of recommendation, nursing research course, physical assessment course, professional liability insurance/malpractice insurance, prerequisite course work, resume, statistics course, GRE General Test or MAT. *Application deadline:* For fall admission, 4/15; for spring admission, 11/15. Applications are processed on a rolling basis. *Application fee:* $20.

Advanced Placement Credit given for nursing courses completed elsewhere dependent upon specific evaluations.

Degree Requirements 36 total credit hours, thesis or project, comprehensive exam.

POST-MASTER'S PROGRAM

Areas of Study Nursing education. *Clinical nurse specialist programs in:* psychiatric/mental health. *Nurse practitioner programs in:* family health.

Armstrong Atlantic State University
Program in Nursing
Savannah, Georgia

http://www.don.armstrong.edu/

Founded in 1935

DEGREES • BSN • MN/MHSA • MSN

Nursing Program Faculty 29 (38% with doctorates).

Baccalaureate Enrollment 200
Women 87% **Men** 13% **Minority** 31% **Part-time** 5%

Graduate Enrollment 59
Women 97% **Men** 3% **Minority** 24% **Part-time** 68%

Nursing Student Activities Nursing Honor Society, Sigma Theta Tau, Student Nurses' Association.

Nursing Student Resources Academic advising; assistance for students with disabilities; bookstore; campus computer network; career placement assistance; computer lab; computer-assisted instruction; e-mail services; employment services for current students; housing assistance; interactive nursing skills videos; Internet; learning resource lab; library services; nursing audiovisuals; placement services for program completers; remedial services; resume preparation assistance; skills, simulation, or other laboratory; tutoring.

Library Facilities 223,412 volumes (8,000 in nursing); 1,166 periodical subscriptions (96 health-care related).

BACCALAUREATE PROGRAMS

Degree BSN

Available Programs ADN to Baccalaureate; Baccalaureate for Second Degree; Generic Baccalaureate; LPN to Baccalaureate; RN Baccalaureate.

Site Options *Distance Learning:* Brunswick, GA.

Study Options Full-time and part-time.

Program Entrance Requirements Transcript of college record, CPR certification, health exam, health insurance, immunizations, minimum GPA in nursing prerequisites of 2.5, professional liability insurance/malpractice insurance. Transfer students are accepted. **Standardized tests** *Required:* SAT or ACT, TOEFL for international students. *Required for some:* SAT Subject Tests. **Application** *Deadline:* 7/1 (freshmen), 7/1 (transfer). *Notification:* continuous (freshmen). *Application fee:* $20.

Expenses (2004–05) *Tuition, state resident:* full-time $1161; part-time $97 per credit hour. *Tuition, nonresident:* full-time $4645; part-time $388 per credit hour. *Required fees:* full-time $206.

Financial Aid 95% of baccalaureate students in nursing programs received some form of financial aid in 2003–04.

Contact Dr. Helen Taggart, Student Services Coordinator, Program in Nursing, Armstrong Atlantic State University, 11935 Abercorn Street, Savannah, GA 31419-1997. *Telephone:* 912-927-5302. *Fax:* 912-920-6579. *E-mail:* taggarhe@mail.armstrong.edu.

GRADUATE PROGRAMS

Expenses (2004–05) *Tuition, state resident:* full-time $1599; part-time $133 per credit hour. *Tuition, nonresident:* full-time $5779; part-time $443 per credit hour. *Required fees:* full-time $195.

Financial Aid Research assistantships (averaging $2,500 per year); Federal Work-Study, scholarships, and unspecified assistantships also available.

Contact Dr. Camille Stern, Department Head, Program in Nursing, Armstrong Atlantic State University, 11935 Abercorn Street, Savannah, GA 31419-1997. *Telephone:* 912-927-5311. *Fax:* 912-920-6579. *E-mail:* sterncam@mail.armstrong.edu.

MASTER'S DEGREE PROGRAM

Degrees MN/MHSA; MSN

Available Programs Master's.

Concentrations Available Nursing administration. *Clinical nurse specialist programs in:* adult health. *Nurse practitioner programs in:* adult health.

Study Options Full-time and part-time.

Program Entrance Requirements Clinical experience, minimum overall college GPA of 3.0, transcript of college record, CPR certification, written essay, immunizations, interview, 3 letters of recommendation, nursing research course, physical assessment course, professional liability insurance/malpractice insurance, prerequisite course work, statistics course, GRE General Test or MAT. *Application deadline:* For fall admission, 7/1 (priority date); for spring admission, 11/15 (priority date). Applications are processed on a rolling basis. *Application fee:* $25.

Advanced Placement Credit by examination available.

Degree Requirements 37 total credit hours, thesis or project.

POST-MASTER'S PROGRAM

Areas of Study Nursing administration. *Clinical nurse specialist programs in:* adult health. *Nurse practitioner programs in:* adult health.

Brenau University

School of Health and Science
Gainesville, Georgia

Founded in 1878

DEGREES • BSN • MSN

Nursing Program Faculty 14 (65% with doctorates).

Baccalaureate Enrollment 60
Women 97% **Men** 3% **Minority** 20% **Part-time** 5%

Graduate Enrollment 20
Women 100% **Minority** 10% **Part-time** 100%

Nursing Student Activities Sigma Theta Tau, Student Nurses' Association.

Nursing Student Resources Academic advising; academic or career counseling; assistance for students with disabilities; bookstore; campus computer network; computer lab; computer-assisted instruction; e-mail services; employment services for current students; housing assistance; interactive nursing skills videos; Internet; learning resource lab; library services; nursing audiovisuals; remedial services; resume preparation assistance; skills, simulation, or other laboratory; tutoring.

Library Facilities 61,059 volumes (6,000 in health, 5,000 in nursing); 205 periodical subscriptions (75 health-care related).

BACCALAUREATE PROGRAMS

Degree BSN

Available Programs ADN to Baccalaureate; Generic Baccalaureate.

Site Options Atlanta, GA.

Study Options Full-time and part-time.

Program Entrance Requirements Minimum overall college GPA of 2.5, transcript of college record, health exam, 2 years high school math, 1 year of high school science, high school transcript, immunizations, minimum high school GPA of 2.0, minimum GPA in nursing prerequisites of 2.5, professional liability insurance/malpractice insurance, prerequisite course work. Transfer students are accepted. **Standardized tests** *Required:* SAT or ACT, TOEFL for international students. **Application** *Deadline:* rolling (freshmen), rolling (transfer). *Notification:* continuous (freshmen). *Application fee:* $35.

Financial Aid 65% of baccalaureate students in nursing programs received some form of financial aid in 2002–03. *Gift aid (need-based):* Federal Pell, FSEOG, state, private, college/university gift aid from institutional funds. *Loans:* FFEL (Subsidized and Unsubsidized Stafford PLUS), Perkins, state. *Work-Study:* Federal Work-Study, part-time campus jobs. *Application deadline (priority):* 3/15.

Contact Ms. Teresa Chastain, Undergraduate Admissions Coordinator for Women's College, School of Health and Science, Brenau University, One Centennial Circle, Gainesville, GA 30501. *Telephone:* 770-534-6100. *Fax:* 770-538-4306. *E-mail:* tchastain@lib.brenau.edu.

GRADUATE PROGRAMS

Financial Aid 30% of graduate students in nursing programs received some form of financial aid in 2002–03. Scholarships available. Aid available to part-time students. *Financial aid application deadline:* 7/15.

Contact Dr. Lynn Minish, Graduate Admissions Coordinator, School of Health and Science, Brenau University, One Centennial Circle, Gainesville, GA 30501. *Telephone:* 770-534-6162. *E-mail:* lminish@lib.brenau.edu.

MASTER'S DEGREE PROGRAM

Degree MSN

Available Programs Master's.

Concentrations Available *Nurse practitioner programs in:* family health.

Site Options Atlanta, GA.

Study Options Part-time.

Program Entrance Requirements Clinical experience, minimum overall college GPA of 3.0, transcript of college record, written essay, 3 letters of recommendation, nursing research course, physical assessment course, statistics course, GRE General Test or MAT. *Application deadline:* Applications are processed on a rolling basis. *Application fee:* $30.

Degree Requirements 42 total credit hours.

POST-MASTER'S PROGRAM

Areas of Study *Nurse practitioner programs in:* family health.

Clayton College & State University

Department of Nursing
Morrow, Georgia

http://www.healthsci.clayton.edu

Founded in 1969

DEGREE • BSN

Nursing Program Faculty 30 (45% with doctorates).

Baccalaureate Enrollment 135
Women 88% **Men** 12% **Minority** 50% **International** 10%

Nursing Student Activities Sigma Theta Tau, Student Nurses' Association.

Nursing Student Resources Academic advising; academic or career counseling; assistance for students with disabilities; bookstore; campus computer network; career placement assistance; computer lab; computer-assisted instruction; e-mail services; employment services for current students; externships; housing assistance; interactive nursing skills videos; Internet; learning resource lab; library services; nursing audiovisuals; paid internships; placement services for program completers; remedial services; resume preparation assistance; skills, simulation, or other laboratory; tutoring.

Library Facilities 77,043 volumes (3,450 in health, 1,800 in nursing); 4,250 periodical subscriptions (151 health-care related).

BACCALAUREATE PROGRAMS

Degree BSN

Available Programs Generic Baccalaureate; RN Baccalaureate.

Study Options Full-time.

Program Entrance Requirements Minimum overall college GPA of 2.5, transcript of college record, CPR certification, health exam, health insurance, immunizations, interview, minimum GPA in nursing prerequisites of 2.5, professional liability insurance/malpractice insurance, prerequisite course work. Transfer students are accepted. **Standardized tests** *Required:* SAT or ACT, TOEFL for international students. *Required for some:* SAT Subject Tests. **Application** *Deadline:* 7/17 (freshmen). *Notification:* continuous (freshmen). *Application fee:* $40.

Advanced Placement Credit by examination available.

Expenses (2004–05) *Tuition, state resident:* full-time $2802; part-time $337 per credit hour. *Tuition, nonresident:* full-time $9300; part-time $628 per credit hour. *International tuition:* $9300 full-time.

Financial Aid 25% of baccalaureate students in nursing programs received some form of financial aid in 2003–04.

Clayton College & State University (continued)
Contact Dr. Deborah J. Clark, Associate Dean for Nursing, Department of Nursing, Clayton College & State University, 5900 North Lee Street, Business and Health Sciences Building, Morrow, GA 30260. *Telephone:* 770-961-3484. *Fax:* 770-961-3639. *E-mail:* deborahclark@mail.clayton.edu.

Columbus State University
Nursing Program
Columbus, Georgia

http://nursing.colstate.edu
Founded in 1958

DEGREE • BSN

Nursing Program Faculty 28 (7% with doctorates).

Baccalaureate Enrollment 134
Women 91% **Men** 9% **Minority** 34% **International** 1%

Nursing Student Activities Sigma Theta Tau, Student Nurses' Association.

Nursing Student Resources Academic advising; academic or career counseling; assistance for students with disabilities; bookstore; campus computer network; career placement assistance; computer lab; computer-assisted instruction; e-mail services; interactive nursing skills videos; Internet; learning resource lab; library services; nursing audiovisuals; remedial services; resume preparation assistance; skills, simulation, or other laboratory; tutoring.

Library Facilities 250,000 volumes; 1,400 periodical subscriptions (475 health-care related).

BACCALAUREATE PROGRAMS

Degree BSN

Available Programs Accelerated RN Baccalaureate; Generic Baccalaureate.

Study Options Full-time.

Program Entrance Requirements Minimum overall college GPA of 2.5, transcript of college record, CPR certification, health exam, immunizations, 3 letters of recommendation, minimum GPA in nursing prerequisites of 2.5, professional liability insurance/malpractice insurance, prerequisite course work. Transfer students are accepted. **Standardized tests** *Required:* SAT or ACT, TOEFL for international students. *Required for some:* SAT Subject Tests. **Application** *Deadline:* 7/28 (freshmen), 7/28 (transfer). *Application fee:* $25.

Expenses (2004–05) *Tuition, state resident:* full-time $2212; part-time $97 per credit hour. *Tuition, nonresident:* full-time $9290; part-time $388 per credit hour. *International tuition:* $9290 full-time. *Room and board:* $5880; room only: $2350 per academic year. *Required fees:* full-time $486; part-time $179 per credit.

Financial Aid 95% of baccalaureate students in nursing programs received some form of financial aid in 2003–04.

Contact Dr. June S. Goyne, Department Chair and Director of BSN Program, Nursing Program, Columbus State University, 4225 University Avenue, Columbus, GA 31907. *Telephone:* 706-565-3649. *Fax:* 706-569-3101. *E-mail:* goyne_june@colstate.edu.

Emory University
Nell Hodgson Woodruff School of Nursing
Atlanta, Georgia

http://www.nursing.emory.edu
Founded in 1836

DEGREES • BSN • MSN • MSN/MPH • PHD

Nursing Program Faculty 62 (37% with doctorates).

Baccalaureate Enrollment 182
Women 95% **Men** 5% **Minority** 31% **International** 1%

Graduate Enrollment 173
Women 95% **Men** 5% **Minority** 37% **International** 1% **Part-time** 54%

Nursing Student Activities Sigma Theta Tau, Student Nurses' Association.

Nursing Student Resources Academic advising; academic or career counseling; assistance for students with disabilities; bookstore; campus computer network; career placement assistance; computer lab; daycare for children of students; e-mail services; housing assistance; interactive nursing skills videos; Internet; learning resource lab; library services; nursing audiovisuals; skills, simulation, or other laboratory; tutoring; unpaid internships.

Library Facilities 2.5 million volumes (206,000 in health); 51,500 periodical subscriptions (2,300 health-care related).

BACCALAUREATE PROGRAMS

Degree BSN

Available Programs Accelerated Baccalaureate for Second Degree; Generic Baccalaureate; RN Baccalaureate.

Study Options Full-time.

Program Entrance Requirements Minimum overall college GPA of 2.5, transcript of college record, CPR certification, written essay, health exam, health insurance, immunizations, 3 letters of recommendation, minimum GPA in nursing prerequisites of 2.5, prerequisite course work. Transfer students are accepted. **Standardized tests** *Required:* SAT or ACT. *Recommended:* SAT Subject Tests, TOEFL for international students. **Application** *Deadline:* 1/15 (freshmen), 6/1 (transfer). *Early decision:* 11/1 (for plan 1), 1/1 (for plan 2). *Notification:* 4/1 (freshmen), 12/15 (out-of-state freshmen), 12/15 (early decision plan 1), 2/1 (early decision plan 2). *Application fee:* $40.

Advanced Placement Credit given for nursing courses completed elsewhere dependent upon specific evaluations.

Expenses (2004–05) *Tuition:* full-time $26,218; part-time $1092 per credit hour. *International tuition:* $26,218 full-time. *Room and board:* $8992; room only: $5612 per academic year. *Required fees:* full-time $352; part-time $5 per credit; part-time $176 per term.

Financial Aid 94% of baccalaureate students in nursing programs received some form of financial aid in 2003–04.

Contact Ms. Beth Taylor, Associate Director of Admissions and Student Services, Nell Hodgson Woodruff School of Nursing, Emory University, 1520 Clifton Road, NE, Atlanta, GA 30322. *Telephone:* 404-727-7980. *Fax:* 404-727-8509. *E-mail:* admit@nurse.emory.edu.

GRADUATE PROGRAMS

Expenses (2004–05) *Tuition:* full-time $26,218; part-time $1092 per credit hour. *International tuition:* $26,218 full-time. *Room and board:* $8992; room only: $5612 per academic year. *Required fees:* full-time $295; part-time $5 per credit; part-time $292 per term.

Financial Aid 96% of graduate students in nursing programs received some form of financial aid in 2003–04. Fellowships, career-related internships or fieldwork, Federal Work-Study, institutionally sponsored loans, scholarships, traineeships, and tuition waivers (full and partial) available. Aid available to part-time students. *Financial aid application deadline:* 3/15.

Contact Ms. Beth Taylor, Associate Director of Admissions and Student Services, Nell Hodgson Woodruff School of Nursing, Emory University, 1520 Clifton Road, NE, Atlanta, GA 30322. *Telephone:* 404-727-7980. *Fax:* 404-727-8509. *E-mail:* admit@nurse.emory.edu.

MASTER'S DEGREE PROGRAM

Degrees MSN; MSN/MPH

Available Programs Master's; RN to Master's.

Concentrations Available Health-care administration; nurse-midwifery; nursing administration. *Clinical nurse specialist programs in:* acute care, adult health, community health, critical care, gerontology, medical-surgical, oncology, pediatric, public health. *Nurse practitioner programs in:* acute care, adult health, community health, family health, gerontology, oncology, pediatric, women's health.

Study Options Full-time and part-time.

Program Entrance Requirements Clinical experience, minimum overall college GPA of 3.0, transcript of college record, CPR certification, written essay, immunizations, interview, 3 letters of recommendation, physical assessment course, professional liability insurance/malpractice insurance, prerequisite course work, statistics course, GRE General Test or MAT. *Application deadline:* For fall admission, 2/15 (priority date); for spring admission, 10/1 (priority date). Applications are processed on a rolling basis. *Application fee:* $50.

Advanced Placement Credit given for nursing courses completed elsewhere dependent upon specific evaluations.

Degree Requirements 36 total credit hours.

POST-MASTER'S PROGRAM

Areas of Study Health-care administration; nurse-midwifery; nursing administration. *Clinical nurse specialist programs in:* acute care, adult health, community health, critical care, gerontology, medical-surgical, oncology, pediatric, public health. *Nurse practitioner programs in:* acute care, adult health, community health, family health, gerontology, oncology, pediatric, women's health.

DOCTORAL DEGREE PROGRAM

Degree PhD

Available Programs Doctorate.

Areas of Study Ethics, health policy, nursing research.

Program Entrance Requirements Minimum overall college GPA of 3.0, interview by faculty committee, interview, 3 letters of recommendation, MSN or equivalent, statistics course, vita, writing sample. *Application deadline:* For fall admission, 2/15 (priority date); for spring admission, 10/1 (priority date). Applications are processed on a rolling basis. *Application fee:* $50.

Degree Requirements 49 total credit hours, dissertation, written exam.

POSTDOCTORAL PROGRAM

Areas of Study Adolescent health, aging, cancer care, chronic illness, community health, family health, gerontology, individualized study, nursing interventions, nursing research, outcomes, vulnerable population.

Postdoctoral Program Contact Jane B. Clark, Assistant Director of Academic Affairs Services, Nell Hodgson Woodruff School of Nursing, Emory University, 1520 Clifton Road, NE, Atlanta, GA 30322. *Telephone:* 404-727-7977. *Fax:* 404-727-4645. *E-mail:* jbclark@emory.edu.

See full description on page 484.

Georgia Baptist College of Nursing of Mercer University

Department of Nursing
Atlanta, Georgia

http://nursing.mercer.edu

Founded in 1988

DEGREES • BSN • MSN

Nursing Program Faculty 47 (30% with doctorates).

Baccalaureate Enrollment 411
Women 96% **Men** 4% **Minority** 36% **Part-time** 13%

Graduate Enrollment 16
Women 100% **Minority** 36% **Part-time** 56%

Nursing Student Activities Nursing Honor Society, Sigma Theta Tau, Student Nurses' Association, nursing club.

Nursing Student Resources Academic advising; academic or career counseling; assistance for students with disabilities; bookstore; campus computer network; computer lab; computer-assisted instruction; e-mail services; employment services for current students; housing assistance; interactive nursing skills videos; Internet; learning resource lab; library services; nursing audiovisuals; skills, simulation, or other laboratory; tutoring.

Library Facilities 12,836 volumes (10,551 in health, 5,487 in nursing); 182 periodical subscriptions (98 health-care related).

BACCALAUREATE PROGRAMS

Degree BSN

Available Programs Generic Baccalaureate; RN Baccalaureate.

Study Options Full-time and part-time.

Program Entrance Requirements Transcript of college record, written essay, health exam, health insurance, high school biology, high school foreign language, 3 years high school math, 3 years high school science, high school transcript, immunizations, 1 letter of recommendation. Transfer students are accepted. **Standardized tests** *Required:* SAT or ACT, TOEFL for international students. **Application** *Deadline:* 5/15 (freshmen), 5/15 (transfer). *Notification:* continuous until 6/1 (freshmen). *Application fee:* $35.

Advanced Placement Credit by examination available. Credit given for nursing courses completed elsewhere dependent upon specific evaluations.

Expenses (2004–05) *Tuition:* full-time $13,944; part-time $581 per semester. *International tuition:* $13,944 full-time. *Room and board:* $8550; room only: $571 per academic year.

Financial Aid 79% of baccalaureate students in nursing programs received some form of financial aid in 2003–04.

Contact Ms. Lynn Vines, Associate Director of Admissions, Department of Nursing, Georgia Baptist College of Nursing of Mercer University, 3001 Mercer University Drive, Atlanta, GA 30341. *Telephone:* 678-547-6700. *Fax:* 678-547-6794. *E-mail:* vines_ml@mercer.edu.

GRADUATE PROGRAMS

Expenses (2004–05) *Tuition:* full-time $12,376; part-time $688 per contact hour.

Financial Aid 69% of graduate students in nursing programs received some form of financial aid in 2003–04.

Contact Dr. Linda Streit, Associate Dean for the Graduate Program, Department of Nursing, Georgia Baptist College of Nursing of Mercer University, 3001 Mercer University Drive, Atlanta, GA 30341. *Telephone:* 678-547-6774. *Fax:* 678-547-6777. *E-mail:* streit_la@mercer.edu.

MASTER'S DEGREE PROGRAM

Degree MSN

Available Programs Master's.

Concentrations Available Nursing education. *Clinical nurse specialist programs in:* acute care.

Study Options Full-time and part-time.

Program Entrance Requirements Clinical experience, computer literacy, minimum overall college GPA of 3.0, transcript of college record, CPR certification, immunizations, interview, letters of recommendation, nursing research course, physical assessment course, statistics course.

Advanced Placement Credit given for nursing courses completed elsewhere dependent upon specific evaluations.

Degree Requirements 42 total credit hours, thesis or project.

POST-MASTER'S PROGRAM

Areas of Study Nursing education.

CONTINUING EDUCATION PROGRAM

Contact Dr. Susan S. Gunby, RN, Dean, Department of Nursing, Georgia Baptist College of Nursing of Mercer University, 3001 Mercer University Drive, Atlanta, GA 30341. *Telephone:* 678-547-6798. *Fax:* 678-547-6796. *E-mail:* gunby_ss@mercer.edu.

Georgia College & State University

School of Health Sciences
Milledgeville, Georgia

http://www.gcsu.edu/acad_affairs/school_healthsci/healthsci

Founded in 1889

DEGREES • BSN • MSN • MSN/MBA

Nursing Program Faculty 35.

Georgia College & State University (continued)
Baccalaureate Enrollment 267
Women 85% **Men** 15% **Minority** 12% **International** 1% **Part-time** 30%
Graduate Enrollment 73
Women 80% **Men** 20% **Minority** 16% **International** 1% **Part-time** 100%
Nursing Student Activities Sigma Theta Tau, Student Nurses' Association.

Nursing Student Resources Academic advising; academic or career counseling; assistance for students with disabilities; bookstore; campus computer network; computer lab; computer-assisted instruction; e-mail services; employment services for current students; housing assistance; interactive nursing skills videos; Internet; learning resource lab; library services; nursing audiovisuals; remedial services; skills, simulation, or other laboratory.

Library Facilities 169,735 volumes (3,086 in health, 1,464 in nursing); 13,165 periodical subscriptions (313 health-care related).

BACCALAUREATE PROGRAMS

Degree BSN
Available Programs Generic Baccalaureate; RN Baccalaureate.
Site Options Macon, GA.
Study Options Full-time and part-time.
Program Entrance Requirements Minimum overall college GPA, transcript of college record, CPR certification, written essay, health exam, health insurance, high school biology, high school foreign language, 4 years high school math, 3 years high school science, high school transcript, immunizations, interview, minimum GPA in nursing prerequisites of 2.75, professional liability insurance/malpractice insurance, prerequisite course work. Transfer students are accepted. **Standardized tests** *Required:* SAT or ACT, TOEFL for international students. *Required for some:* SAT Subject Tests. **Application** *Deadline:* 4/1 (freshmen), 7/1 (transfer). *Early decision:* 11/1. *Notification:* continuous (freshmen), 12/1 (early action). *Application fee:* $25.

Advanced Placement Credit by examination available. Credit given for nursing courses completed elsewhere dependent upon specific evaluations.

Expenses (2004–05) *Tuition, state resident:* full-time $1501; part-time $126 per credit hour. *Tuition, nonresident:* full-time $6004; part-time $501 per credit hour. *International tuition:* $6004 full-time. *Room and board:* $3000; room only: $1600 per academic year. *Required fees:* full-time $379; part-time $337 per term.

Financial Aid 80% of baccalaureate students in nursing programs received some form of financial aid in 2003–04. *Gift aid (need-based):* Federal Pell, FSEOG, state, college/university gift aid from institutional funds. *Loans:* Federal Direct PLUS), FFEL (Subsidized and Unsubsidized Stafford PLUS), Perkins, state, college/university. *Work-Study:* Federal Work-Study. *Application deadline:* Continuous.

Contact Dr. Cheryl Pope Kish, Associate Dean for Health Sciences/ Director of Nursing Programs, School of Health Sciences, Georgia College & State University, Milledgeville, GA 31061. *Telephone:* 478-445-2633. *Fax:* 478-445-1913. *E-mail:* cheryl.kish@gcsu.edu.

GRADUATE PROGRAMS

Expenses (2004–05) *Tuition, state resident:* part-time $151 per credit hour. *Tuition, nonresident:* part-time $601 per credit hour. *Required fees:* part-time $38 per term.

Financial Aid 80% of graduate students in nursing programs received some form of financial aid in 2003–04. 17 research assistantships with tuition reimbursements available were awarded; career-related internships or fieldwork, Federal Work-Study, and unspecified assistantships also available. Aid available to part-time students. *Financial aid application deadline:* 3/1.

Contact Dr. Karen Frith, Graduate Coordinator, School of Health Sciences, Georgia College & State University, CBX 64, 231 West Hancock Street, Milledgeville, GA 31061. *Telephone:* 478-445-1795. *Fax:* 478-445-1913. *E-mail:* kfrith@gcsu.edu.

MASTER'S DEGREE PROGRAM

Degrees MSN; MSN/MBA
Available Programs Master's; RN to Master's.
Concentrations Available Nursing administration; nursing education; nursing informatics. *Clinical nurse specialist programs in:* adult health. *Nurse practitioner programs in:* family health.
Site Options Macon, GA.
Study Options Part-time.
Program Entrance Requirements Clinical experience, computer literacy, transcript of college record, CPR certification, immunizations, interview, nursing research course, professional liability insurance/ malpractice insurance, resume, statistics course, GRE, GMAT or MAT. *Application deadline:* For fall admission, 7/15 (priority date). Applications are processed on a rolling basis. *Application fee:* $25.

Advanced Placement Credit given for nursing courses completed elsewhere dependent upon specific evaluations.

Degree Requirements 36 total credit hours.

POST-MASTER'S PROGRAM

Areas of Study Nursing education; nursing informatics. *Nurse practitioner programs in:* family health.

Georgia Southern University
School of Nursing
Statesboro, Georgia

http://www.georgiasouthern.edu
Founded in 1906

DEGREES • BSN • MSN

Nursing Program Faculty 27 (56% with doctorates).
Baccalaureate Enrollment 225
Women 91% **Men** 9% **Minority** 19% **Part-time** 26%
Graduate Enrollment 39
Women 95% **Men** 5% **Minority** 10% **Part-time** 3%
Nursing Student Activities Sigma Theta Tau, Student Nurses' Association.

Nursing Student Resources Academic advising; academic or career counseling; assistance for students with disabilities; bookstore; campus computer network; career placement assistance; computer lab; computer-assisted instruction; e-mail services; housing assistance; interactive nursing skills videos; Internet; learning resource lab; library services; nursing audiovisuals; placement services for program completers; resume preparation assistance; skills, simulation, or other laboratory; tutoring.

Library Facilities 568,551 volumes (25,000 in health, 12,000 in nursing); 2,697 periodical subscriptions (20,000 health-care related).

BACCALAUREATE PROGRAMS

Degree BSN
Available Programs ADN to Baccalaureate; Accelerated RN Baccalaureate; Generic Baccalaureate; LPN to Baccalaureate.
Study Options Full-time and part-time.
Program Entrance Requirements Minimum overall college GPA of 2.7, transcript of college record, CPR certification, written essay, health exam, health insurance, high school biology, high school chemistry, high school foreign language, 2 years high school math, 4 years high school science, high school transcript, immunizations, interview, minimum GPA in nursing prerequisites of 2.7, professional liability insurance/malpractice insurance, prerequisite course work. Transfer students are accepted. **Standardized tests** *Required:* SAT or ACT, TOEFL for international students. *Required for some:* SAT II Writing Tests. **Application** *Deadline:* 8/1 (freshmen), 7/1 (transfer). *Notification:* continuous (freshmen). *Application fee:* $20.

Advanced Placement Credit by examination available. Credit given for nursing courses completed elsewhere dependent upon specific evaluations.

Expenses (2004–05) *Tuition, state resident:* full-time $2322; part-time $97 per credit hour. *Tuition, nonresident:* full-time $9290; part-time $388 per credit hour. *International tuition:* $9290 full-time. *Room and board:* $6266; room only: $4000 per academic year. *Required fees:* full-time $830; part-time $415 per term.

Financial Aid 89% of baccalaureate students in nursing programs received some form of financial aid in 2003–04. *Gift aid (need-based):* Federal Pell, FSEOG, state, private, college/university gift aid from institutional funds, Georgia HOPE Scholarships. *Loans:* Federal Direct (Subsidized and Unsubsidized Stafford PLUS), Perkins, Service-Cancelable State Direct Student Loans, alternative loans. *Work-Study:* Federal Work-Study. *Application deadline (priority):* 3/31.

Contact Dr. Danette Wood, BSN Program Director, School of Nursing, Georgia Southern University, PO Box 8158, Statesboro, GA 30460-8158. *Telephone:* 912-681-5242. *Fax:* 912-681-0536. *E-mail:* danette_wood@georgiasouthern.edu.

GRADUATE PROGRAMS

Expenses (2004–05) *Tuition, state resident:* full-time $2786; part-time $117 per credit hour. *Tuition, nonresident:* full-time $11,146; part-time $465 per credit hour. *International tuition:* $11,146 full-time. *Room and board:* $6266; room only: $4000 per academic year. *Required fees:* full-time $830; part-time $415 per term.

Financial Aid 66% of graduate students in nursing programs received some form of financial aid in 2003–04. Research assistantships with partial tuition reimbursements available (averaging $5,500 per year), teaching assistantships with partial tuition reimbursements available (averaging $5,500 per year) were awarded; career-related internships or fieldwork, Federal Work-Study, scholarships, traineeships, and unspecified assistantships also available. Aid available to part-time students. *Financial aid application deadline:* 4/15.

Contact Dr. Donna Hodnicki, Director, MSN Program, School of Nursing, Georgia Southern University, PO Box 8158, Statesboro, GA 30460-8158. *Telephone:* 912-681-5056. *Fax:* 912-681-0536. *E-mail:* dhodnicki@georgiasouthern.edu.

MASTER'S DEGREE PROGRAM

Degree MSN

Available Programs Accelerated RN to Master's; Master's; Master's for Nurses with Non-Nursing Degrees; RN to Master's.

Concentrations Available *Clinical nurse specialist programs in:* community health. *Nurse practitioner programs in:* family health, women's health.

Study Options Full-time and part-time.

Program Entrance Requirements Clinical experience, computer literacy, minimum overall college GPA of 3.0, transcript of college record, CPR certification, immunizations, interview, 3 letters of recommendation, professional liability insurance/malpractice insurance, statistics course, GRE General Test or MAT. *Application deadline:* For fall admission, 3/1 (priority date); for spring admission, 10/1 (priority date). Applications are processed on a rolling basis. *Application fee:* $30.

Advanced Placement Credit given for nursing courses completed elsewhere dependent upon specific evaluations.

Degree Requirements 48 total credit hours, thesis or project, comprehensive exam.

POST-MASTER'S PROGRAM

Areas of Study *Clinical nurse specialist programs in:* community health. *Nurse practitioner programs in:* family health, women's health.

Georgia Southwestern State University

School of Nursing
Americus, Georgia

http://www.gsw.edu

Founded in 1906

DEGREE • BSN

Nursing Program Faculty 10 (33% with doctorates).

Baccalaureate Enrollment 38

Women 83% **Men** 17% **Minority** 18% **International** 3% **Part-time** 29%

Nursing Student Activities Sigma Theta Tau, Student Nurses' Association.

Nursing Student Resources Academic advising; academic or career counseling; assistance for students with disabilities; bookstore; campus computer network; career placement assistance; computer lab; computer-assisted instruction; e-mail services; employment services for current students; interactive nursing skills videos; Internet; learning resource lab; library services; nursing audiovisuals; placement services for program completers; remedial services; resume preparation assistance; skills, simulation, or other laboratory; tutoring.

Library Facilities 428,197 volumes (627 in health, 528 in nursing); 516 periodical subscriptions (141 health-care related).

BACCALAUREATE PROGRAMS

Degree BSN

Available Programs Baccalaureate for Second Degree; Generic Baccalaureate; RN Baccalaureate.

Study Options Full-time and part-time.

Program Entrance Requirements Minimum overall college GPA of 2.5, transcript of college record, CPR certification, written essay, health exam, health insurance, high school foreign language, 4 years high school math, 4 years high school science, high school transcript, immunizations, 2 letters of recommendation, minimum GPA in nursing prerequisites of 2.5, professional liability insurance/malpractice insurance, prerequisite course work. Transfer students are accepted. **Standardized tests** *Required:* SAT or ACT, TOEFL for international students. **Application** *Deadline:* rolling (freshmen), rolling (transfer). *Early decision:* 12/15. *Notification:* continuous until 8/1 (freshmen), 1/15 (out-of-state freshmen), 1/15 (early decision). *Application fee:* $20.

Advanced Placement Credit given for nursing courses completed elsewhere dependent upon specific evaluations.

Expenses (2003–04) *Tuition, state resident:* full-time $2212; part-time $93 per credit hour. *Tuition, nonresident:* full-time $8848. *International tuition:* $10,639 full-time.

Financial Aid 82% of baccalaureate students in nursing programs received some form of financial aid in 2002–03.

Contact Dr. Judith M. Malachowski, Chair, BSN Program, School of Nursing, Georgia Southwestern State University, 800 Wheatley Street, Americus, GA 31709. *Telephone:* 229-931-2662. *Fax:* 229-931-2288. *E-mail:* jmm@canes.gsw.edu.

CONTINUING EDUCATION PROGRAM

Contact Dr. Judith M. Malachowski, Chair, BSN Program, School of Nursing, Georgia Southwestern State University, 800 Wheatley Street, Americus, GA 31709. *Telephone:* 229-931-2662. *Fax:* 229-931-2288. *E-mail:* jmm@canes.gsw.edu.

Georgia State University

School of Nursing
Atlanta, Georgia

http://chhs.gsu.edu/nursing/

Founded in 1913

DEGREES • BS • MS • PHD

Nursing Program Faculty 52 (32% with doctorates).

Baccalaureate Enrollment 250

Graduate Enrollment 195

Nursing Student Activities Sigma Theta Tau, Student Nurses' Association.

Nursing Student Resources Academic advising; academic or career counseling; assistance for students with disabilities; bookstore; campus computer network; career placement assistance; computer lab; computer-assisted instruction; daycare for children of students; e-mail services; externships; interactive nursing skills videos; Internet; learning resource lab; library services; nursing audiovisuals; skills, simulation, or other laboratory.

Library Facilities 2.2 million volumes (52,835 in health, 20,856 in nursing); 4,788 periodical subscriptions (725 health-care related).

BACCALAUREATE PROGRAMS

Degree BS

Available Programs Accelerated Baccalaureate; Accelerated RN Baccalaureate; Generic Baccalaureate; RN Baccalaureate.

Study Options Full-time and part-time.

Georgia State University (continued)

Program Entrance Requirements Minimum overall college GPA of 2.5, transcript of college record, CPR certification, written essay, health exam, immunizations, interview, 2 letters of recommendation, minimum GPA in nursing prerequisites of 2.5, professional liability insurance/malpractice insurance, prerequisite course work. Transfer students are accepted. **Standardized tests** *Required:* SAT or ACT, TOEFL for international students. *Required for some:* SAT Subject Tests. **Application** *Deadline:* 3/1 (freshmen), 6/1 (transfer). *Notification:* continuous (freshmen). *Application fee:* $50.

Advanced Placement Credit given for nursing courses completed elsewhere dependent upon specific evaluations.

Expenses (2004–05) *Tuition, state resident:* full-time $1684; part-time $141 per credit hour. *Tuition, nonresident:* full-time $6737; part-time $562 per semester. *International tuition:* $6737 full-time. *Room and board:* $3215; room only: $2565 per academic year.

Contact Office of Academic Assistance, School of Nursing, Georgia State University, College of Health and Human Sciences, Atlanta, GA 30303-3083. *Telephone:* 404-651-3083. *Fax:* 404-651-4871. *E-mail:* schoolofnursing@gsu.edu.

GRADUATE PROGRAMS

Expenses (2004–05) *Tuition, state resident:* full-time $2162; part-time $181 per credit hour. *Tuition, nonresident:* full-time $8648; part-time $721 per credit hour. *International tuition:* $8648 full-time. *Room and board:* $3215; room only: $2565 per academic year. *Required fees:* full-time $1086; part-time $393 per term.

Financial Aid 80 fellowships, 34 research assistantships were awarded; teaching assistantships, Federal Work-Study, institutionally sponsored loans, scholarships, traineeships, and tuition waivers (partial) also available.

Contact Office of Academic Assistance, School of Nursing, Georgia State University, College of Health and Human Sciences, Atlanta, GA 30303-3083. *Telephone:* 404-651-3064. *Fax:* 404-651-4871. *E-mail:* schoolofnursing@gsu.edu.

MASTER'S DEGREE PROGRAM

Degree MS

Available Programs Master's; RN to Master's.

Concentrations Available *Clinical nurse specialist programs in:* adult health, pediatric, perinatal, psychiatric/mental health. *Nurse practitioner programs in:* family health, pediatric, women's health.

Study Options Full-time and part-time.

Program Entrance Requirements Clinical experience, minimum overall college GPA of 2.75, transcript of college record, CPR certification, interview, 2 letters of recommendation, professional liability insurance/malpractice insurance. *Application deadline:* For fall admission, 3/1; for spring admission, 10/1. Applications are processed on a rolling basis. *Application fee:* $50.

Advanced Placement Credit given for nursing courses completed elsewhere dependent upon specific evaluations.

Degree Requirements 48 total credit hours, thesis or project.

POST-MASTER'S PROGRAM

Areas of Study *Clinical nurse specialist programs in:* adult health, pediatric, perinatal, psychiatric/mental health. *Nurse practitioner programs in:* family health, pediatric, women's health.

DOCTORAL DEGREE PROGRAM

Degree PhD

Available Programs Doctorate.

Areas of Study Faculty preparation, family health, health promotion/disease prevention, individualized study, nursing research, nursing science.

Program Entrance Requirements Minimum overall college GPA of 3.0, interview by faculty committee, interview, 3 letters of recommendation, MSN or equivalent, scholarly papers, vita, GRE General Test. *Application deadline:* For fall admission, 3/1; for spring admission, 10/1. Applications are processed on a rolling basis. *Application fee:* $50.

Degree Requirements 60 total credit hours, dissertation, written exam, residency.

Kennesaw State University
School of Nursing
Kennesaw, Georgia

http://www.kennesaw.edu/chhs/schoolofnursing

Founded in 1963

DEGREES • BSN • MSN

Nursing Program Faculty 38 (52% with doctorates).

Baccalaureate Enrollment 325

Women 90% **Men** 10% **Minority** 21% **International** 11% **Part-time** 60%

Graduate Enrollment 73

Women 94% **Men** 6% **Minority** 18% **International** 7%

Nursing Student Activities Sigma Theta Tau, Student Nurses' Association.

Nursing Student Resources Academic advising; academic or career counseling; assistance for students with disabilities; bookstore; campus computer network; career placement assistance; computer lab; computer-assisted instruction; e-mail services; employment services for current students; externships; housing assistance; interactive nursing skills videos; Internet; learning resource lab; library services; nursing audiovisuals; paid internships; placement services for program completers; resume preparation assistance; skills, simulation, or other laboratory.

Library Facilities 608,342 volumes (20,000 in health, 10,000 in nursing); 4,580 periodical subscriptions (178 health-care related).

BACCALAUREATE PROGRAMS

Degree BSN

Available Programs ADN to Baccalaureate; Accelerated Baccalaureate; Accelerated Baccalaureate for Second Degree; Generic Baccalaureate; RN Baccalaureate.

Site Options Rome, GA.

Study Options Full-time and part-time.

Program Entrance Requirements Minimum overall college GPA of 2.7, transcript of college record, CPR certification, health exam, health insurance, 2 years high school math, 2 years high school science, high school transcript, immunizations, 1 letter of recommendation, minimum high school GPA of 2.0, minimum GPA in nursing prerequisites of 2.7, professional liability insurance/malpractice insurance, prerequisite course work. Transfer students are accepted. **Standardized tests** *Required:* SAT or ACT, TOEFL for international students. *Required for some:* SAT Subject Tests. **Application** *Deadline:* 5/27 (freshmen), 6/28 (transfer). *Notification:* continuous (freshmen). *Application fee:* $40.

Advanced Placement Credit by examination available. Credit given for nursing courses completed elsewhere dependent upon specific evaluations.

Expenses (2004–05) *Tuition, state resident:* full-time $2321; part-time $97 per credit hour. *Tuition, nonresident:* full-time $11,611; part-time $485 per credit hour. *International tuition:* $11,611 full-time. *Room and board:* room only: $5130 per academic year. *Required fees:* full-time $661; part-time $331 per term.

Financial Aid 50% of baccalaureate students in nursing programs received some form of financial aid in 2003–04. *Gift aid (need-based):* Federal Pell, FSEOG, state, private, college/university gift aid from institutional funds. *Loans:* FFEL (Subsidized and Unsubsidized Stafford PLUS), Perkins, state, college/university. *Work-Study:* Federal Work-Study. *Application deadline:* Continuous.

Contact Fran Paul, Admissions Coordinator, School of Nursing, Kennesaw State University, 1000 Chastain Road, Kennesaw, GA 30144. *Telephone:* 770-499-3211. *Fax:* 770-423-6627. *E-mail:* fpaul@kennesaw.edu.

GRADUATE PROGRAMS

Financial Aid 50% of graduate students in nursing programs received some form of financial aid in 2003–04.

Contact Dr. Regina Dorman, Coordinator, School of Nursing, Kennesaw State University, 1000 Chastain Road, Kennesaw, GA 30144. *Telephone:* 770-423-6061. *Fax:* 770-423-6627. *E-mail:* gdorman@ksumail.kennesaw.edu.

MASTER'S DEGREE PROGRAM

Degree MSN

Available Programs Master's.

Concentrations Available *Clinical nurse specialist programs in:* adult health. *Nurse practitioner programs in:* adult health, family health, primary care.

Study Options Full-time.

Program Entrance Requirements Clinical experience, minimum overall college GPA of 3.0, transcript of college record, CPR certification, written essay, immunizations, 2 letters of recommendation, nursing research course, physical assessment course, professional liability insurance/malpractice insurance, prerequisite course work, resume.

Advanced Placement Credit given for nursing courses completed elsewhere dependent upon specific evaluations.

Degree Requirements 40 total credit hours, thesis or project.

CONTINUING EDUCATION PROGRAM

Contact Dr. Vanice Wise Roberts, Associate Dean, School of Nursing, Kennesaw State University, 1000 Chastain Road #1601, Kennesaw, GA 30144. *Telephone:* 770-423-6064. *Fax:* 770-423-6627. *E-mail:* vroberts@kennesaw.edu.

See full description on page 506.

LaGrange College
Department of Nursing
LaGrange, Georgia

http://www.lagrange.edu

Founded in 1831

DEGREE • BSN

Nursing Program Faculty 6 (20% with doctorates).

Baccalaureate Enrollment 60
Women 90% **Men** 10% **Minority** 20% **International** 5% **Part-time** 5%

Nursing Student Activities Nursing Honor Society, Student Nurses' Association.

Nursing Student Resources Academic advising; academic or career counseling; assistance for students with disabilities; bookstore; campus computer network; career placement assistance; computer lab; computer-assisted instruction; e-mail services; employment services for current students; externships; interactive nursing skills videos; Internet; learning resource lab; library services; nursing audiovisuals; paid internships; placement services for program completers; remedial services; resume preparation assistance; skills, simulation, or other laboratory; tutoring; unpaid internships.

Library Facilities 108,389 volumes (19,000 in health, 10,000 in nursing); 512 periodical subscriptions (100 health-care related).

BACCALAUREATE PROGRAMS

Degree BSN

Available Programs RN Baccalaureate.

Study Options Full-time.

Program Entrance Requirements Minimum overall college GPA of 2.5, transcript of college record, CPR certification, written essay, health exam, health insurance, immunizations, minimum GPA in nursing prerequisites of 2.5, professional liability insurance/malpractice insurance, prerequisite course work. Transfer students are accepted. **Standardized tests** *Required:* SAT or ACT, TOEFL for international students. **Application** *Deadline:* 8/30 (freshmen), 8/15 (transfer). *Notification:* continuous (freshmen). *Application fee:* $20.

Advanced Placement Credit given for nursing courses completed elsewhere dependent upon specific evaluations.

Expenses (2003–04) *Tuition:* full-time $7241; part-time $597 per credit hour. *International tuition:* $7241 full-time. *Room and board:* $6018 per academic year. *Required fees:* full-time $100; part-time $25 per term.

Financial Aid 100% of baccalaureate students in nursing programs received some form of financial aid in 2002–03. *Gift aid (need-based):* Federal Pell, FSEOG, state, private, college/university gift aid from institutional funds. *Loans:* FFEL (Subsidized and Unsubsidized Stafford PLUS), Perkins. *Work-Study:* Federal Work-Study, part-time campus jobs. *Application deadline:* 3/1.

Contact Dr. Maranah A. Sauter, RN, Chair, Department of Nursing, LaGrange College, 601 Broad Street, LaGrange, GA 30240-2999. *Telephone:* 706-880-8220. *Fax:* 706-880-8029. *E-mail:* msauter@lagrange.edu.

Medical College of Georgia
School of Nursing
Augusta, Georgia

http://www.mcg.edu/son

Founded in 1828

DEGREES • BSN • MSN • PHD

Nursing Program Faculty 51 (25% with doctorates).

Baccalaureate Enrollment 355
Women 91% **Men** 9% **Minority** 12% **International** 1% **Part-time** 12%

Graduate Enrollment 86
Women 77% **Men** 23% **Minority** 14% **Part-time** 41%

Nursing Student Activities Sigma Theta Tau, Student Nurses' Association, nursing club.

Nursing Student Resources Academic advising; academic or career counseling; assistance for students with disabilities; bookstore; campus computer network; career placement assistance; computer lab; computer-assisted instruction; daycare for children of students; e-mail services; employment services for current students; externships; housing assistance; interactive nursing skills videos; Internet; learning resource lab; library services; nursing audiovisuals; paid internships; remedial services; skills, simulation, or other laboratory; tutoring.

Library Facilities 164,154 volumes (178,650 in health, 14,650 in nursing); 2,458 periodical subscriptions (1,307 health-care related).

BACCALAUREATE PROGRAMS

Degree BSN

Available Programs ADN to Baccalaureate; Generic Baccalaureate; RN Baccalaureate.

Site Options *Distance Learning:* Barnesville, GA; Columbus, GA; Athens, GA.

Study Options Full-time.

Program Entrance Requirements Minimum overall college GPA of 2.5, transcript of college record, CPR certification, written essay, immunizations, 3 letters of recommendation, prerequisite course work. Transfer students are accepted. **Standardized tests** *Required:* TOEFL for international students.

Expenses (2004–05) *Tuition, state resident:* full-time $3368; part-time $141 per credit hour. *Tuition, nonresident:* full-time $13,474; part-time $562 per credit hour. *Room and board:* room only: $2711 per academic year. *Required fees:* full-time $800; part-time $400 per term.

Financial Aid 93% of baccalaureate students in nursing programs received some form of financial aid in 2003–04.

Contact Office of Academic Admissions, School of Nursing, Medical College of Georgia, AA-170 Kelly Building, Augusta, GA 30912. *Telephone:* 706-721-2725. *Fax:* 706-721-0186. *E-mail:* underadm@mail.mcg.edu.

GRADUATE PROGRAMS

Expenses (2004–05) *Tuition, state resident:* full-time $4044; part-time $169 per credit hour. *Tuition, nonresident:* full-time $16,170; part-time $674 per credit hour. *Room and board:* room only: $2711 per academic year.

Financial Aid 84% of graduate students in nursing programs received some form of financial aid in 2003–04.

Contact Director, Academic Admissions, School of Nursing, Medical College of Georgia, AA-170 Kelly Building, Augusta, GA 30912. *Telephone:* 706-721-2725. *Fax:* 706-721-0186. *E-mail:* gradadm@mail.mcg.edu.

MASTER'S DEGREE PROGRAM

Degree MSN

Available Programs Master's; RN to Master's.

Concentrations Available Nurse anesthesia. *Clinical nurse specialist programs in:* acute care, adult health, community health, critical care, parent-child, psychiatric/mental health. *Nurse practitioner programs in:* family health, pediatric.

Medical College of Georgia (continued)

Site Options *Distance Learning:* Columbus, GA; Athens, GA.

Study Options Full-time and part-time.

Program Entrance Requirements Clinical experience, minimum overall college GPA of 3.0, transcript of college record, written essay, interview, 3 letters of recommendation, physical assessment course, professional liability insurance/malpractice insurance, statistics course.

Degree Requirements 36 total credit hours.

POST-MASTER'S PROGRAM

Areas of Study Nurse anesthesia. *Nurse practitioner programs in:* family health.

DOCTORAL DEGREE PROGRAM

Degree PhD

Available Programs Doctorate.

Areas of Study Bio-behavioral research, nursing research.

Program Entrance Requirements Clinical experience, minimum overall college GPA of 3.2, interview by faculty committee, interview, 3 letters of recommendation, MSN or equivalent, scholarly papers, statistics course, vita, writing sample.

Degree Requirements 60 total credit hours, dissertation, oral exam, written exam.

See full description on page 518.

North Georgia College & State University

Department of Nursing
Dahlonega, Georgia

Founded in 1873

DEGREES • BSN • MS

Nursing Program Faculty 31 (23% with doctorates).

Baccalaureate Enrollment 58
Women 96% **Men** 4% **Minority** 9% **Part-time** 66%

Graduate Enrollment 32
Women 84% **Men** 16% **Minority** 13% **Part-time** 9%

Nursing Student Activities Nursing Honor Society, Student Nurses' Association.

Nursing Student Resources Academic advising; academic or career counseling; assistance for students with disabilities; bookstore; campus computer network; career placement assistance; computer lab; computer-assisted instruction; e-mail services; interactive nursing skills videos; Internet; learning resource lab; library services; nursing audiovisuals; remedial services; resume preparation assistance; skills, simulation, or other laboratory; tutoring.

Library Facilities 146,888 volumes (8,616 in health, 2,500 in nursing); 2,548 periodical subscriptions (70 health-care related).

BACCALAUREATE PROGRAMS

Degree BSN

Available Programs RN Baccalaureate.

Study Options Full-time and part-time.

Program Entrance Requirements Minimum overall college GPA of 2.5, transcript of college record, CPR certification, health exam, health insurance, high school biology, high school chemistry, high school foreign language, 3 years high school math, 2 years high school science, high school transcript, immunizations, 2 letters of recommendation, professional liability insurance/malpractice insurance. Transfer students are accepted. **Standardized tests** *Required:* SAT or ACT, TOEFL for international students. **Application** *Deadline:* 7/1 (freshmen), rolling (transfer). *Notification:* continuous (freshmen). *Application fee:* $25.

Expenses (2004–05) *Tuition, state resident:* full-time $2322; part-time $97 per credit hour. *Tuition, nonresident:* full-time $9290; part-time $388 per credit hour. *International tuition:* $9290 full-time. *Room and board:* $4408; room only: $2204 per academic year. *Required fees:* full-time $1212; part-time $606 per term.

Financial Aid 75% of baccalaureate students in nursing programs received some form of financial aid in 2003–04.

Contact Dr. Donna Waddell, RN, Coordinator, BSN Program, Department of Nursing, North Georgia College & State University, Campus Circle, Dahlonega, GA 30597. *Telephone:* 706-864-1652. *Fax:* 706-864-1845. *E-mail:* dwaddell@ngcsu.edu.

GRADUATE PROGRAMS

Expenses (2004–05) *Tuition, state resident:* full-time $2786; part-time $117 per credit hour. *Tuition, nonresident:* full-time $11,146; part-time $465 per credit hour. *International tuition:* $11,146 full-time. *Room and board:* $4408; room only: $2204 per academic year.

Financial Aid 60% of graduate students in nursing programs received some form of financial aid in 2003–04.

Contact Dr. Toni Barnett, Coordinator, FNP Program, Department of Nursing, North Georgia College & State University, Sunset Boulevard, Dahlonega, GA 30597. *Telephone:* 706-867-2800. *Fax:* 706-864-1845. *E-mail:* tbarnett@ngsu.edu.

MASTER'S DEGREE PROGRAM

Degree MS

Available Programs Master's.

Concentrations Available *Nurse practitioner programs in:* family health.

Study Options Full-time and part-time.

Program Entrance Requirements Clinical experience, computer literacy, minimum overall college GPA of 2.75, transcript of college record, CPR certification, written essay, immunizations, interview, 3 letters of recommendation, nursing research course, physical assessment course, professional liability insurance/malpractice insurance, prerequisite course work, statistics course.

Degree Requirements 46 total credit hours, thesis or project.

POST-MASTER'S PROGRAM

Areas of Study *Nurse practitioner programs in:* family health.

Piedmont College

School of Nursing
Demorest, Georgia

http://www.piedmont.edu/schools/index.html#nursing

Founded in 1897

DEGREE • BSN

Nursing Program Faculty 9 (10% with doctorates).

Baccalaureate Enrollment 125
Women 98% **Men** 2% **Minority** 12% **International** 1% **Part-time** 20%

Nursing Student Activities Nursing Honor Society, Student Nurses' Association.

Nursing Student Resources Academic advising; academic or career counseling; assistance for students with disabilities; bookstore; campus computer network; career placement assistance; computer lab; computer-assisted instruction; e-mail services; externships; housing assistance; interactive nursing skills videos; Internet; learning resource lab; library services; nursing audiovisuals; other; paid internships; resume preparation assistance; skills, simulation, or other laboratory; tutoring.

Library Facilities 118,750 volumes (2,040 in health, 400 in nursing); 366 periodical subscriptions (40 health-care related).

BACCALAUREATE PROGRAMS

Degree BSN

Available Programs Accelerated RN Baccalaureate; RN Baccalaureate.

Study Options Full-time.

Program Entrance Requirements Transcript of college record, CPR certification, health exam, health insurance, high school foreign language, 2 years high school math, 3 years high school science, high school transcript, immunizations, minimum GPA in nursing prerequisites of 2.8, professional liability insurance/malpractice insurance, prerequisite course work. Transfer students are accepted. **Standardized tests** *Required:* SAT or ACT, TOEFL for international students. **Application** *Deadline:* rolling (freshmen), rolling (transfer).

Advanced Placement Credit given for nursing courses completed elsewhere dependent upon specific evaluations.

Expenses (2003–04) *Tuition:* full-time $12,550; part-time $521 per credit hour. *Room and board:* $4400; room only: $2250 per academic year.

Financial Aid 90% of baccalaureate students in nursing programs received some form of financial aid in 2002–03. *Gift aid (need-based):* Federal Pell, FSEOG, state, private, college/university gift aid from institutional funds. *Loans:* Federal Direct (Subsidized and Unsubsidized Stafford PLUS), state. *Work-Study:* Federal Work-Study, part-time campus jobs. *Application deadline (priority):* 5/1.

Contact Dr. Barbara Crosson, Dean, School of Nursing. *Telephone:* 706-776-0116. *E-mail:* bcrosson@piedmont.edu.

Thomas University

Division of Nursing
Thomasville, Georgia

http://www.thomasu.edu/nursing.htm

Founded in 1950

DEGREE • BSN

Nursing Program Faculty 5 (40% with doctorates).

Baccalaureate Enrollment 26
Women 70% **Men** 30% **Minority** 30%

Nursing Student Resources Academic advising; academic or career counseling; assistance for students with disabilities; bookstore; campus computer network; career placement assistance; computer lab; computer-assisted instruction; e-mail services; interactive nursing skills videos; Internet; library services; nursing audiovisuals; skills, simulation, or other laboratory; tutoring.

Library Facilities 61,096 volumes (200 in health, 100 in nursing); 408 periodical subscriptions (30 health-care related).

BACCALAUREATE PROGRAMS

Degree BSN

Available Programs RN Baccalaureate.

Study Options Full-time.

Program Entrance Requirements Minimum overall college GPA of 2.5, transcript of college record, CPR certification, health exam, immunizations, professional liability insurance/malpractice insurance, prerequisite course work, RN licensure. Transfer students are accepted. **Standardized tests** *Required:* TOEFL for international students. ***Placement:*** *Required:* MAPS. *Recommended:* SAT or ACT. **Application** *Deadline:* rolling (freshmen), rolling (transfer). *Application fee:* $25.

Advanced Placement Credit given for nursing courses completed elsewhere dependent upon specific evaluations.

Contact Dr. Deanna Epley, PhD, Program Contact, Division of Nursing, Thomas University, 1501 Millpond Road, Thomasville, GA 31792-7490. *Telephone:* 800-538-9784. *Fax:* 229-226-1653. *E-mail:* depley@thomasu.edu.

University of Phoenix–Atlanta Campus

College of Health and Human Services
Atlanta, Georgia

DEGREE • BSN

Nursing Program Faculty 17 (18% with doctorates).

Baccalaureate Enrollment 18
Women 89% **Men** 11% **Minority** 30%

Nursing Student Resources Academic advising; academic or career counseling; bookstore; library services.

Library Facilities 27.1 million volumes; 11,648 periodical subscriptions (1,426 health-care related).

BACCALAUREATE PROGRAMS

Degree BSN

Available Programs ADN to Baccalaureate; RN Baccalaureate.

Program Entrance Requirements RN licensure. **Standardized tests** *Required:* TOEFL for international students. **Application** *Deadline:* rolling (freshmen), rolling (transfer). *Application fee:* $100.

Expenses (2004–05) *Tuition:* full-time $10,830; part-time $361 per credit hour. *International tuition:* $10,830 full-time. *Required fees:* full-time $110.

Contact Campus College Chair, Nursing. *Telephone:* 678-731-0555. *Fax:* 678-731-9666.

University of West Georgia

Department of Nursing
Carrollton, Georgia

http://www.westga.edu/~nurs/

Founded in 1933

DEGREES • BSN • MSN

Nursing Program Faculty 19 (42% with doctorates).

Baccalaureate Enrollment 138
Women 88% **Men** 12% **Minority** 11% **Part-time** 49%

Graduate Enrollment 14
Women 100% **Minority** 7% **Part-time** 21%

Nursing Student Activities Sigma Theta Tau, Student Nurses' Association.

Nursing Student Resources Academic advising; academic or career counseling; assistance for students with disabilities; bookstore; campus computer network; career placement assistance; computer lab; computer-assisted instruction; e-mail services; employment services for current students; externships; housing assistance; interactive nursing skills videos; Internet; learning resource lab; library services; nursing audiovisuals; placement services for program completers; remedial services; resume preparation assistance; skills, simulation, or other laboratory; tutoring.

Library Facilities 391,330 volumes (8,605 in health, 554 in nursing); 1,194 periodical subscriptions (92 health-care related).

BACCALAUREATE PROGRAMS

Degree BSN

Available Programs Generic Baccalaureate; RN Baccalaureate.

Site Options *Distance Learning:* Dalton, GA; Rome, GA.

Study Options Full-time.

Program Entrance Requirements Minimum overall college GPA of 2.75, transcript of college record, CPR certification, health exam, health insurance, immunizations, minimum GPA in nursing prerequisites of 2.75, professional liability insurance/malpractice insurance, prerequisite course work. Transfer students are accepted. **Standardized tests** *Required:* SAT or ACT, TOEFL for international students. **Application** *Deadline:* 7/1 (freshmen), 6/1 (transfer). *Notification:* continuous until 8/1 (freshmen). *Application fee:* $20.

Advanced Placement Credit given for nursing courses completed elsewhere dependent upon specific evaluations.

Expenses (2004–05) *Tuition, state resident:* full-time $2906; part-time $779 per semester. *Tuition, nonresident:* full-time $9874; part-time $2525 per semester. *International tuition:* $9874 full-time. *Room and board:* $3585; room only: $2610 per academic year. *Required fees:* full-time $343; part-time $172 per term.

Financial Aid 65% of baccalaureate students in nursing programs received some form of financial aid in 2003–04.

University of West Georgia (continued)

Contact Dr. Kathryn Mary Grams, RN, Chair and Professor, Department of Nursing, University of West Georgia, 1601 Maple Street, Carrollton, GA 30118. *Telephone:* 678-839-5624. *Fax:* 678-839-6553. *E-mail:* kgrams@westga.edu.

GRADUATE PROGRAMS

Expenses (2004–05) *Tuition, state resident:* full-time $2595; part-time $569 per semester. *Tuition, nonresident:* full-time $8859; part-time $1961 per semester. *International tuition:* $8859 full-time. *Room and board:* $3585; room only: $2610 per academic year.

Financial Aid 43% of graduate students in nursing programs received some form of financial aid in 2003–04.

Contact Dr. Laurie Taylor, RN, Coordinator of Graduate Program and Professor, Department of Nursing, University of West Georgia, 1601 Maple Street, Carrollton, GA 30118. *Telephone:* 678-839-5631. *Fax:* 678-839-6553. *E-mail:* ltaylor@westga.edu.

MASTER'S DEGREE PROGRAM

Degree MSN

Available Programs Master's.

Concentrations Available Nursing administration; nursing education.

Study Options Full-time and part-time.

Program Entrance Requirements Clinical experience, computer literacy, minimum overall college GPA of 3.0, transcript of college record, CPR certification, written essay, immunizations, interview, 3 letters of recommendation, nursing research course, professional liability insurance/malpractice insurance, prerequisite course work, resume, statistics course.

Degree Requirements 36 total credit hours, thesis or project, comprehensive exam.

POST-MASTER'S PROGRAM

Areas of Study Nursing administration; nursing education.

Valdosta State University

College of Nursing
Valdosta, Georgia

http://www.valdosta.edu/nursing/

Founded in 1906

DEGREES • BSN • MSN

Nursing Program Faculty 23 (52% with doctorates).

Baccalaureate Enrollment 183

Women 87% **Men** 13% **Minority** 21% **International** 1% **Part-time** 7%

Graduate Enrollment 25

Women 99% **Men** 1% **Minority** 15% **International** 1% **Part-time** 49%

Nursing Student Activities Sigma Theta Tau, Student Nurses' Association.

Nursing Student Resources Academic advising; academic or career counseling; assistance for students with disabilities; bookstore; campus computer network; career placement assistance; computer lab; computer-assisted instruction; e-mail services; employment services for current students; externships; housing assistance; Internet; learning resource lab; library services; nursing audiovisuals; placement services for program completers; resume preparation assistance; skills, simulation, or other laboratory; tutoring; unpaid internships.

Library Facilities 467,560 volumes (21,688 in health); 2,815 periodical subscriptions (75 health-care related).

BACCALAUREATE PROGRAMS

Degree BSN

Available Programs Generic Baccalaureate; RN Baccalaureate.

Site Options *Distance Learning:* Kings Bay, GA; Tifton, GA; Waycross, GA.

Study Options Full-time.

Program Entrance Requirements Minimum overall college GPA of 2.8, transcript of college record, CPR certification, health exam, health insurance, immunizations, minimum GPA in nursing prerequisites of 2.8, professional liability insurance/malpractice insurance, prerequisite course work. Transfer students are accepted. **Standardized tests** *Required:* SAT or ACT, TOEFL for international students. **Application** *Deadline:* 7/1 (freshmen), 8/1 (transfer). *Notification:* continuous (freshmen). *Application fee:* $20.

Advanced Placement Credit given for nursing courses completed elsewhere dependent upon specific evaluations.

Expenses (2003–04) *Tuition, state resident:* full-time $2434; part-time $122 per credit hour. *Tuition, nonresident:* full-time $8664; part-time $373 per credit hour. *International tuition:* $8664 full-time. *Room and board:* $4680; room only: $2328 per academic year. *Required fees:* full-time $3951; part-time $1236 per term.

Financial Aid 80% of baccalaureate students in nursing programs received some form of financial aid in 2002–03. *Gift aid (need-based):* Federal Pell, FSEOG, state, private, college/university gift aid from institutional funds. *Loans:* Federal Direct (Subsidized and Unsubsidized Stafford PLUS), college/university. *Work-Study:* Federal Work-Study. *Application deadline (priority):* 5/1.

Contact Dr. Joan W. Futch, Acting Dean, College of Nursing, Valdosta State University, 1300 North Patterson Street, Valdosta, GA 31698-0130. *Telephone:* 229-333-5959. *Fax:* 229-333-7300. *E-mail:* jwfutch@valdosta.edu.

GRADUATE PROGRAMS

Expenses (2003–04) *Tuition, state resident:* full-time $3036; part-time $139 per credit hour. *Tuition, nonresident:* full-time $10,272; part-time $440 per credit hour. *International tuition:* $10,272 full-time. *Room and board:* $4680; room only: $2328 per academic year. *Required fees:* full-time $1518; part-time $30 per credit; part-time $274 per term.

Financial Aid 26% of graduate students in nursing programs received some form of financial aid in 2002–03. 2 research assistantships with full tuition reimbursements available (averaging $2,452 per year) were awarded; institutionally sponsored loans, scholarships, and unspecified assistantships also available. Aid available to part-time students. *Financial aid application deadline:* 7/1.

Contact Dr. Joan W. Futch, Acting Dean, College of Nursing, Valdosta State University, 1300 North Patterson Street, Valdosta, GA 31698-0130. *Telephone:* 229-333-5959. *Fax:* 229-333-7300. *E-mail:* jwfutch@valdosta.edu.

MASTER'S DEGREE PROGRAM

Degree MSN

Available Programs Master's; RN to Master's.

Concentrations Available Nurse case management; nursing administration; nursing education. *Clinical nurse specialist programs in:* adult health, family health, psychiatric/mental health.

Site Options *Distance Learning:* Kings Bay, GA; Tifton, GA; Waycross, GA.

Study Options Full-time and part-time.

Program Entrance Requirements Minimum overall college GPA of 2.8, transcript of college record, CPR certification, immunizations, 3 letters of recommendation, physical assessment course, professional liability insurance/malpractice insurance, statistics course, GRE General Test. *Application deadline:* For fall admission, 7/1; for spring admission, 11/15. Applications are processed on a rolling basis. *Application fee:* $20.

Advanced Placement Credit given for nursing courses completed elsewhere dependent upon specific evaluations.

Degree Requirements 36 total credit hours, thesis or project, comprehensive exam.

CONTINUING EDUCATION PROGRAM

Contact Dr. M. M. Richardson, Assistant Dean, College of Nursing, Valdosta State University, 1300 North Patterson Street, Valdosta, GA 31698. *Telephone:* 229-333-5960.

GUAM

University of Guam
College of Nursing and Health Sciences
Mangilao, Guam

http://www.uog.edu/cnhs/index.html
Founded in 1952

DEGREE • BSN

Nursing Program Faculty 10 (30% with doctorates).

Baccalaureate Enrollment 175
Women 97% **Men** 3% **International** 2%

Nursing Student Activities Student Nurses' Association.

Nursing Student Resources Academic advising; academic or career counseling; assistance for students with disabilities; bookstore; campus computer network; career placement assistance; computer lab; daycare for children of students; e-mail services; employment services for current students; interactive nursing skills videos; Internet; learning resource lab; library services; nursing audiovisuals; remedial services; skills, simulation, or other laboratory; tutoring.

Library Facilities 327,925 volumes (5,246 in health, 982 in nursing); 3,060 periodical subscriptions (53 health-care related).

BACCALAUREATE PROGRAMS

Degree BSN

Available Programs ADN to Baccalaureate; Generic Baccalaureate; RN Baccalaureate.

Study Options Full-time and part-time.

Program Entrance Requirements Transcript of college record, CPR certification, written essay, health exam, high school biology, high school chemistry, 1 year of high school math, 1 year of high school science, high school transcript, immunizations, interview, minimum high school GPA of 2.5, minimum GPA in nursing prerequisites of 2.7, prerequisite course work. Transfer students are accepted. **Application** *Deadline:* 7/8 (freshmen), 7/8 (transfer). *Notification:* continuous (freshmen).

Advanced Placement Credit by examination available. Credit given for nursing courses completed elsewhere dependent upon specific evaluations.

Expenses (2003–04) *Tuition, state resident:* part-time $118 per credit hour. *Tuition, nonresident:* part-time $351 per credit hour. *International tuition:* $351 full-time.

Financial Aid 73% of baccalaureate students in nursing programs received some form of financial aid in 2002–03. *Gift aid (need-based):* Federal Pell, FSEOG, state, private. *Loans:* Federal Direct (Subsidized and Unsubsidized Stafford), FFEL (Subsidized and Unsubsidized Stafford), state. *Work-Study:* Federal Work-Study. *Application deadline (priority):* 6/30.

Contact Dr. Deborah Leon Guerrero, Registrar, College of Nursing and Health Sciences, University of Guam, Admissions and Records Office, UOG Station, Mangilao, GU 96923. *Telephone:* 671-735-2210. *Fax:* 671-734-4245. *E-mail:* admitme@uog9.uog.edu.

HAWAII

Hawai'i Pacific University
School of Nursing
Honolulu, Hawaii

http://www.hpu.edu
Founded in 1965

DEGREES • BSN • MSN • MSN/MBA

Nursing Program Faculty 85 (11% with doctorates).

Baccalaureate Enrollment 1,040 **Women** 88% **Men** 12% **Minority** 75% **International** 1% **Part-time** 33%

Graduate Enrollment 46
Women 95% **Men** 5% **Minority** 44% **International** 1% **Part-time** 57%

Nursing Student Activities Sigma Theta Tau.

Nursing Student Resources Academic advising; academic or career counseling; assistance for students with disabilities; bookstore; campus computer network; career placement assistance; computer lab; computer-assisted instruction; e-mail services; employment services for current students; externships; housing assistance; Internet; learning resource lab; library services; paid internships; placement services for program completers; resume preparation assistance; tutoring.

Library Facilities 162,000 volumes (5,587 in health, 1,950 in nursing); 12,000 periodical subscriptions (1,033 health-care related).

■ Hawai'i Pacific University's BSN program offers hands-on experiences in both classroom and clinical settings in which multicultural nursing is an everyday opportunity. Students are accepted directly into the nursing major when they apply to the University but must achieve a minimum 2.75 GPA in courses required for the major before progressing into nursing courses. In the sophomore year, HPU students begin their clinical experiences. Small clinical laboratories (8–10 students) utilize health-care facilities all over the island of Oahu for clinical experiences. The MSN is available to registered nurses and offers 2 concentrations: community clinical nurse specialist (CNS) studies and family nurse practitioner (FNP) studies. Hawai'i Pacific's BSN and MSN programs are accredited by the National League for Nursing Accrediting Commission and approved by the State of Hawai'i Board of Nursing.

BACCALAUREATE PROGRAMS

Degree BSN

Available Programs Accelerated Baccalaureate; Generic Baccalaureate; International Nurse to Baccalaureate; LPN to Baccalaureate; RN Baccalaureate.

Study Options Full-time and part-time.

Program Entrance Requirements Minimum overall college GPA of 2.5, transcript of college record, 3 years high school math, 2 years high school science, high school transcript, minimum high school GPA of 2.5. Transfer students are accepted. **Standardized tests** *Required:* SAT or ACT. *Recommended:* TOEFL for international students. **Application** *Deadline:* rolling (freshmen), rolling (transfer). *Application fee:* $50.

Advanced Placement Credit given for nursing courses completed elsewhere dependent upon specific evaluations.

Expenses (2004–05) *Tuition:* full-time $15,632; part-time $651 per credit hour. *Room and board:* $9020 per academic year. *Required fees:* full-time $80.

Financial Aid 60% of baccalaureate students in nursing programs received some form of financial aid in 2003–04.

Contact Mrs. Cherie Andrade, Director of Admissions, School of Nursing, Hawai'i Pacific University, 1164 Bishop Street, Honolulu, HI 96813. *Telephone:* 808-544-0238. *Fax:* 808-544-1136. *E-mail:* candrade@hpu.edu.

GRADUATE PROGRAMS

Expenses (2004–05) *Tuition:* full-time $15,632; part-time $651 per credit hour. *Room and board:* $9020 per academic year. *Required fees:* full-time $80.

Financial Aid 50% of graduate students in nursing programs received some form of financial aid in 2003–04. Career-related internships or fieldwork, Federal Work-Study, scholarships, and unspecified assistantships available. Aid available to part-time students. *Financial aid application deadline:* 3/1.

Contact Patricia Lange-Otsuka, Coordinator for Nursing Graduate Program, School of Nursing, Hawai'i Pacific University, 45-045 Kamehameha Highway, Kaneohe, HI 96744-5297. *Telephone:* 808-236-3552. *Fax:* 808-236-5818. *E-mail:* plangeot@hpu.edu.

Hawai'i Pacific University (continued)

MASTER'S DEGREE PROGRAM

Degrees MSN; MSN/MBA

Available Programs Master's.

Concentrations Available *Clinical nurse specialist programs in:* community health. *Nurse practitioner programs in:* community health, family health.

Study Options Full-time and part-time.

Program Entrance Requirements Clinical experience, minimum overall college GPA of 3.0, transcript of college record, CPR certification, written essay, immunizations, 2 letters of recommendation, nursing research course, physical assessment course, professional liability insurance/malpractice insurance, resume, statistics course. *Application deadline:* Applications are processed on a rolling basis. *Application fee:* $50.

Advanced Placement Credit given for nursing courses completed elsewhere dependent upon specific evaluations.

Degree Requirements 42 total credit hours.

See full description on page 496.

University of Hawaii at Hilo

Department in Nursing
Hilo, Hawaii

http://www.uhh.hawaii.edu

Founded in 1970

DEGREE • BSN

Nursing Program Faculty 11 (27% with doctorates).

Baccalaureate Enrollment 47

Women 98% **Men** 2% **Minority** 75% **International** 2% **Part-time** 6%

Nursing Student Activities Student Nurses' Association, nursing club.

Nursing Student Resources Academic advising; academic or career counseling; assistance for students with disabilities; bookstore; campus computer network; career placement assistance; computer lab; computer-assisted instruction; daycare for children of students; e-mail services; employment services for current students; externships; housing assistance; Internet; learning resource lab; library services; nursing audiovisuals; remedial services; resume preparation assistance; skills, simulation, or other laboratory; tutoring; unpaid internships.

Library Facilities 250,000 volumes; 2,500 periodical subscriptions (15,000 health-care related).

BACCALAUREATE PROGRAMS

Degree BSN

Available Programs ADN to Baccalaureate; Generic Baccalaureate; RN Baccalaureate.

Site Options *Distance Learning:* Lihue, HI; Kona, HI; Kahalui, HI.

Study Options Full-time.

Program Entrance Requirements Minimum overall college GPA of 2.7, transcript of college record, CPR certification, written essay, health exam, health insurance, 4 years high school math, 3 years high school science, high school transcript, immunizations, interview, 2 letters of recommendation, minimum high school GPA of 3.0, minimum GPA in nursing prerequisites of 3.0, professional liability insurance/malpractice insurance, prerequisite course work. **Standardized tests** *Required:* SAT or ACT. *Recommended:* TOEFL for international students. **Application** *Deadline:* 7/1 (freshmen), 7/1 (transfer). *Notification:* 7/31 (freshmen). *Application fee:* $40.

Expenses (2004–05) *Tuition, state resident:* full-time $1212; part-time $101 per credit hour. *Tuition, nonresident:* full-time $3996; part-time $333 per credit hour. *International tuition:* $3996 full-time. *Room and board:* $3700; room only: $2500 per academic year. *Required fees:* full-time $126; part-time $35 per term.

Financial Aid 65% of baccalaureate students in nursing programs received some form of financial aid in 2003–04.

Contact Dr. Cecilia Mukai, Chair and Program Director, Department in Nursing, University of Hawaii at Hilo, 200 West Kawili Street, UCB 239, Hilo, HI 96720. *Telephone:* 808-974-7760. *Fax:* 808-974-7665. *E-mail:* cmukai@hawaii.edu.

University of Hawaii at Manoa

School of Nursing and Dental Hygiene
Honolulu, Hawaii

http://www.nursing.hawaii.edu

Founded in 1907

DEGREES • BS • MS • PHD

Nursing Program Faculty 53 (38% with doctorates).

Baccalaureate Enrollment 258

Women 81% **Men** 19% **Minority** 86% **International** 1% **Part-time** 15%

Graduate Enrollment 85

Women 87% **Men** 13% **Minority** 43% **International** 5%

Nursing Student Activities Nursing Honor Society, Sigma Theta Tau, Student Nurses' Association, nursing club.

Nursing Student Resources Academic advising; academic or career counseling; assistance for students with disabilities; bookstore; computer lab; computer-assisted instruction; e-mail services; employment services for current students; housing assistance; Internet; learning resource lab; library services; nursing audiovisuals; resume preparation assistance; skills, simulation, or other laboratory.

Library Facilities 3.2 million volumes (98,176 in health, 3,205 in nursing); 27,328 periodical subscriptions (1,680 health-care related).

■ The School of Nursing and Dental Hygiene's vision is to be the leader in nursing education and research in Hawaii, with outreach to Asia and the Pacific Basin. Hawaii's unique multicultural population provides the richness of the learning environment that facilitates the cultural competence and commitment to underserved people. The School offers programs leading to the Bachelor of Science, Master of Science, post-master's certificate, and PhD. The undergraduate curriculum provides 3 curricular options: the generic BS option, the RN/BS option, and the accelerated program for second degree candidates. The MS degree prepares nurses to function as advanced practice nurses in psychiatric–mental health nursing and primary care or as managers of clinical systems. Graduates of the PhD program are prepared for culturally appropriate clinical scholarship and to teach in nursing programs.

BACCALAUREATE PROGRAMS

Degree BS

Available Programs ADN to Baccalaureate; Generic Baccalaureate; RN Baccalaureate.

Site Options *Distance Learning:* Lihue, HI; Kailua Kona, HI; Kahului—Maui, HI.

Study Options Full-time and part-time.

Program Entrance Requirements Minimum overall college GPA of 2.5, transcript of college record, CPR certification, health exam, health insurance, immunizations, minimum GPA in nursing prerequisites of 2.5, professional liability insurance/malpractice insurance, prerequisite course work. Transfer students are accepted. **Standardized tests** *Required:* SAT or ACT, TOEFL for international students. **Application** *Deadline:* 5/1 (freshmen), 5/1 (transfer). *Notification:* continuous (freshmen). *Application fee:* $50.

Advanced Placement Credit by examination available. Credit given for nursing courses completed elsewhere dependent upon specific evaluations.

Expenses (2003–04) *Tuition, state resident:* full-time $3312. *Tuition, nonresident:* full-time $9792. *Room and board:* $6101 per academic year.

Financial Aid 50% of baccalaureate students in nursing programs received some form of financial aid in 2002–03.

Contact Katherine Thompson, Academic Advisor, School of Nursing and Dental Hygiene, University of Hawaii at Manoa, 2528 McCarthy Mall, Honolulu, HI 96822. *Telephone:* 808-956-8939. *Fax:* 808-956-5977. *E-mail:* nursing@hawaii.edu.

GRADUATE PROGRAMS

Expenses (2003–04) *Tuition, state resident:* full-time $4464. *Tuition, nonresident:* full-time $10,608.

Financial Aid 10% of graduate students in nursing programs received some form of financial aid in 2002–03. 1 research assistantship (averaging $15,552 per year) was awarded.

Contact Dr. Jillian Inouye, Graduate Chair, School of Nursing and Dental Hygiene, University of Hawaii at Manoa, 2528 McCarthy Mall, Honolulu, HI 96822. *Telephone:* 808-956-5326. *Fax:* 808-956-5296. *E-mail:* jinouye@hawaii.edu.

MASTER'S DEGREE PROGRAM

Degree MS

Available Programs Master's.

Concentrations Available Health-care administration. *Clinical nurse specialist programs in:* psychiatric/mental health. *Nurse practitioner programs in:* adult health, family health, gerontology, primary care.

Site Options *Distance Learning:* Kailua Kona, HI; Kahului—Maui, HI.

Study Options Full-time and part-time.

Program Entrance Requirements Minimum overall college GPA of 3.0, transcript of college record, CPR certification, written essay, immunizations, interview, 2 letters of recommendation, nursing research course, professional liability insurance/malpractice insurance, resume, statistics course. *Application deadline:* For fall admission, 3/1; for spring admission, 10/1. *Application fee:* $50.

Advanced Placement Credit given for nursing courses completed elsewhere dependent upon specific evaluations.

Degree Requirements 52 total credit hours.

POST-MASTER'S PROGRAM

Areas of Study Health-care administration. *Clinical nurse specialist programs in:* psychiatric/mental health. *Nurse practitioner programs in:* adult health, family health, gerontology, pediatric, women's health.

DOCTORAL DEGREE PROGRAM

Degree PhD

Areas of Study Faculty preparation, nursing education, nursing research, nursing science.

Program Entrance Requirements Clinical experience, minimum overall college GPA of 3.0, interview by faculty committee, interview, 3 letters of recommendation, MSN or equivalent, scholarly papers, statistics course, vita, writing sample. *Application deadline:* For fall admission, 3/1; for spring admission, 10/1. *Application fee:* $50.

Degree Requirements 46 total credit hours, dissertation, oral exam, residency.

University of Phoenix–Hawaii Campus

College of Health and Human Services
Honolulu, Hawaii

DEGREES • BSN • MSN • MSN/MBA

Nursing Program Faculty 35 (14% with doctorates).

Baccalaureate Enrollment 23
Women 91% **Men** 9% **Minority** 33%

Nursing Student Activities Sigma Theta Tau.

Nursing Student Resources Academic advising; academic or career counseling; bookstore; computer lab; library services.

Library Facilities 27.1 million volumes; 11,648 periodical subscriptions (1,426 health-care related).

BACCALAUREATE PROGRAMS

Degree BSN

Available Programs ADN to Baccalaureate; Accelerated RN Baccalaureate.

Site Options Kapolei, HI; Mililani, HI; Maui, HI.

Study Options Full-time.

Program Entrance Requirements 1 letter of recommendation. Transfer students are accepted. **Standardized tests** *Required:* TOEFL for international students. **Application** *Deadline:* rolling (freshmen), rolling (transfer). *Application fee:* $100.

Advanced Placement Credit by examination available.

Expenses (2004–05) *Tuition:* full-time $10,650; part-time $355 per credit hour. *International tuition:* $10,650 full-time. *Required fees:* full-time $110.

Financial Aid 2% of baccalaureate students in nursing programs received some form of financial aid in 2003–04.

Contact Campus College Chair, Nursing, College of Health and Human Services, University of Phoenix–Hawaii Campus, 827 Fort Street, Hololulu, HI 96813-4317. *Telephone:* 808-536-2686.

GRADUATE PROGRAMS

Expenses (2004–05) *Tuition:* full-time $10,200; part-time $425 per credit hour. *International tuition:* $10,200 full-time. *Required fees:* full-time $110.

Contact Campus College Chair, Nursing, College of Health and Human Services, University of Phoenix–Hawaii Campus, 827 Fort Street, Hololulu, HI 96813-4317. *Telephone:* 808-536-2686.

MASTER'S DEGREE PROGRAM

Degrees MSN; MSN/MBA

Available Programs Master's.

Concentrations Available Health-care administration; nursing administration; nursing education. *Nurse practitioner programs in:* family health.

Site Options Kapolei, HI; Mililani, HI; Maui, HI.

Study Options Full-time.

Program Entrance Requirements Clinical experience, computer literacy, minimum overall college GPA of 2.5, transcript of college record. *Application deadline:* Applications are processed on a rolling basis. *Application fee:* $110.

Degree Requirements 39 total credit hours, thesis or project.

POST-MASTER'S PROGRAM

Areas of Study *Nurse practitioner programs in:* family health.

IDAHO

Boise State University

Department of Nursing
Boise, Idaho

http://nursing.boisestate.edu

Founded in 1932

DEGREE • BS

Nursing Program Faculty 40 (8% with doctorates).

Baccalaureate Enrollment 535
Women 90% **Men** 10% **International** 1%

Nursing Student Activities Nursing Honor Society, Sigma Theta Tau, Student Nurses' Association.

Boise State University (continued)

Nursing Student Resources Academic advising; academic or career counseling; assistance for students with disabilities; bookstore; campus computer network; career placement assistance; computer lab; computer-assisted instruction; daycare for children of students; e-mail services; employment services for current students; housing assistance; interactive nursing skills videos; Internet; learning resource lab; library services; nursing audiovisuals; placement services for program completers; remedial services; resume preparation assistance; skills, simulation, or other laboratory; tutoring.

Library Facilities 675,000 volumes; 5,000 periodical subscriptions.

BACCALAUREATE PROGRAMS

Degree BS

Available Programs Accelerated Baccalaureate; Generic Baccalaureate; LPN to Baccalaureate; RN Baccalaureate.

Site Options *Distance Learning:* Nampa, ID.

Study Options Full-time.

Program Entrance Requirements Transfer students are accepted. **Standardized tests** *Required:* TOEFL for international students. *Required for some:* SAT or ACT. **Application** *Deadline:* 7/14 (freshmen), 7/14 (transfer). *Notification:* continuous (freshmen). *Application fee:* $30.

Advanced Placement Credit by examination available. Credit given for nursing courses completed elsewhere dependent upon specific evaluations.

Financial Aid *Gift aid (need-based):* Federal Pell, FSEOG, state, private, college/university gift aid from institutional funds, Leveraged Educational Assistance Program (LEAP). *Loans:* Federal Direct (Subsidized and Unsubsidized Stafford PLUS), Perkins, state, college/university, Alaska Loans. *Work-Study:* Federal Work-Study, part-time campus jobs. *Application deadline:* 6/1 (priority: 2/15).

Contact Pat Taylor, Program Director, Department of Nursing, Boise State University, 1910 University Drive, Boise, ID 83725-0399. *Telephone:* 208-426-3783. *Fax:* 208-426-1370. *E-mail:* ptaylor@boisestate.edu.

Idaho State University

Department of Nursing
Pocatello, Idaho

Founded in 1901

DEGREES • BSN • MS

Nursing Program Faculty 25 (60% with doctorates).

Baccalaureate Enrollment 130
Women 89% **Men** 11%

Graduate Enrollment 37
Women 99% **Men** 1% **Part-time** 40%

Nursing Student Activities Sigma Theta Tau, Student Nurses' Association.

Nursing Student Resources Academic advising; bookstore; campus computer network; computer lab; computer-assisted instruction; e-mail services; interactive nursing skills videos; Internet; learning resource lab; library services; nursing audiovisuals; skills, simulation, or other laboratory.

Library Facilities 712,041 volumes (500 in health, 35 in nursing); 6,672 periodical subscriptions (3,391 health-care related).

BACCALAUREATE PROGRAMS

Degree BSN

Available Programs ADN to Baccalaureate; Accelerated Baccalaureate for Second Degree; Generic Baccalaureate; LPN to Baccalaureate.

Site Options *Distance Learning:* Boise, ID; Twin Falls, ID.

Study Options Full-time.

Program Entrance Requirements Minimum overall college GPA of 2.5, transcript of college record, CPR certification, health exam, health insurance, high school transcript, immunizations, minimum high school GPA of 2.0, minimum GPA in nursing prerequisites of 2.8, prerequisite course work. Transfer students are accepted. **Standardized tests** *Required:* SAT or ACT, TOEFL for international students. **Application** *Deadline:* 8/1 (freshmen), 8/1 (transfer). *Application fee:* $35.

Advanced Placement Credit given for nursing courses completed elsewhere dependent upon specific evaluations.

Expenses (2003–04) *Tuition, state resident:* full-time $1724; part-time $172 per credit hour. *Tuition, nonresident:* full-time $5024; part-time $267 per credit hour. *International tuition:* $5024 full-time. *Room and board:* $2100; room only: $1500 per academic year. *Required fees:* full-time $250.

Financial Aid 75% of baccalaureate students in nursing programs received some form of financial aid in 2002–03. *Gift aid (need-based):* Federal Pell, FSEOG, state, private. *Loans:* Federal Direct (Subsidized and Unsubsidized Stafford PLUS), Perkins. *Work-Study:* Federal Work-Study, part-time campus jobs. *Application deadline:* Continuous.

Contact Dr. Diana McLaughlin, RN, Associate Chair Undergraduate Studies, Department of Nursing, Idaho State University, Campus Box 8101, Pocatello, ID 83209. *Telephone:* 208-236-2152. *Fax:* 208-236-4476. *E-mail:* mcladian@isu.edu.

GRADUATE PROGRAMS

Expenses (2003–04) *Tuition, state resident:* full-time $2054; part-time $267 per credit hour. *Tuition, nonresident:* full-time $5354; part-time $300 per credit hour. *International tuition:* $5354 full-time. *Room and board:* $2100; room only: $1500 per academic year. *Required fees:* full-time $1000; part-time $500 per term.

Financial Aid 35% of graduate students in nursing programs received some form of financial aid in 2002–03. Research assistantships, teaching assistantships with full and partial tuition reimbursements available, career-related internships or fieldwork, Federal Work-Study, scholarships, and traineeships available. Aid available to part-time students. *Financial aid application deadline:* 1/1.

Contact Dr. Carol Ashton, RN, Associate Chairperson, Graduate Studies, Department of Nursing, Idaho State University, Campus Box 8101, Pocatello, ID 83209-8101. *Telephone:* 208-282-2443. *Fax:* 208-282-4476. *E-mail:* ashtcaro@isu.edu.

MASTER'S DEGREE PROGRAM

Degree MS

Available Programs Master's.

Concentrations Available Nursing administration; nursing education. *Nurse practitioner programs in:* community health, family health.

Site Options *Distance Learning:* Boise, ID; Twin Falls, ID; Lewiston, ID.

Study Options Full-time and part-time.

Program Entrance Requirements Clinical experience, minimum overall college GPA of 3.0, transcript of college record, interview, 3 letters of recommendation, nursing research course, physical assessment course, professional liability insurance/malpractice insurance, prerequisite course work, statistics course, GRE General Test. *Application deadline:* For fall admission, 7/1 (priority date); for spring admission, 12/1 (priority date). Applications are processed on a rolling basis. *Application fee:* $35.

Advanced Placement Credit given for nursing courses completed elsewhere dependent upon specific evaluations.

Degree Requirements 36 total credit hours, thesis or project.

POST-MASTER'S PROGRAM

Areas of Study Nursing administration; nursing education. *Nurse practitioner programs in:* community health, family health.

Lewis-Clark State College

Division of Nursing and Health Sciences
Lewiston, Idaho

http://www.lcsc.edu/Nurdiv/

Founded in 1893

DEGREE • BSN

Nursing Program Faculty 22 (36% with doctorates).

Baccalaureate Enrollment 203
Women 86% **Men** 14% **Minority** 3% **International** .4% **Part-time** 41%

Nursing Student Activities Student Nurses' Association, nursing club.

Nursing Student Resources Academic advising; academic or career counseling; assistance for students with disabilities; bookstore; campus computer network; career placement assistance; computer lab; computer-assisted instruction; daycare for children of students; e-mail services; employment services for current students; housing assistance; interactive nursing skills videos; Internet; learning resource lab; library services; nursing audiovisuals; remedial services; resume preparation assistance; skills, simulation, or other laboratory; tutoring; unpaid internships.

Library Facilities 139,499 volumes (19,920 in health, 5,101 in nursing); 1,612 periodical subscriptions (12,058 health-care related).

BACCALAUREATE PROGRAMS

Degree BSN

Available Programs ADN to Baccalaureate; Generic Baccalaureate; LPN to Baccalaureate; RN Baccalaureate.

Site Options *Distance Learning:* Coeur d'Alene, ID.

Study Options Full-time.

Program Entrance Requirements Minimum overall college GPA of 2.5, transcript of college record, CPR certification, health exam, health insurance, high school biology, high school chemistry, high school transcript, immunizations, 2 letters of recommendation, minimum high school GPA of 2.0, minimum GPA in nursing prerequisites of 2.0, professional liability insurance/malpractice insurance, prerequisite course work. Transfer students are accepted. **Standardized tests** *Required:* TOEFL for international students. *Required for some:* SAT or ACT, ACT COMPASS. **Application** *Deadline:* rolling (freshmen), rolling (transfer). *Notification:* continuous (freshmen). *Application fee:* $35.

Advanced Placement Credit by examination available. Credit given for nursing courses completed elsewhere dependent upon specific evaluations.

Expenses (2004–05) *Tuition, area resident:* full-time $3392; part-time $171 per credit hour. *Tuition, state resident:* full-time $6560; part-time $171 per credit hour. *Tuition, nonresident:* full-time $9632; part-time $171 per credit hour. *Room and board:* $2000 per academic year. *Required fees:* full-time $200; part-time $171 per credit.

Financial Aid 70% of baccalaureate students in nursing programs received some form of financial aid in 2003–04. *Gift aid (need-based):* Federal Pell, FSEOG, state, private, college/university gift aid from institutional funds. *Loans:* Federal Nursing Student Loans, FFEL (Subsidized and Unsubsidized Stafford PLUS), Perkins. *Work-Study:* Federal Work-Study, part-time campus jobs. *Application deadline (priority):* 3/1.

Contact Mrs. Dianne Blum, Office Specialist I, Division of Nursing and Health Sciences, Lewis-Clark State College, Division of Nursing and Health Sciences, Lewis-Clark State College, 500 8th Avenue, Lewiston, ID 83501. *Telephone:* 208-792-2250. *Fax:* 208-792-2062. *E-mail:* dblum@lcsc.edu.

CONTINUING EDUCATION PROGRAM

Contact Ms. Dianne Blum, Office Specialist I, Division of Nursing and Health Sciences, Lewis-Clark State College, Division of Nursing and Health Sciences, Lewis-Clark State College, 500 8th Avenue, Lewiston, ID 83501. *Telephone:* 208-792-2250. *Fax:* 208-792-2062. *E-mail:* dblum@lcsc.edu.

Northwest Nazarene University
School of Health and Science
Nampa, Idaho

Founded in 1913

DEGREE • BSN

Nursing Program Faculty 7 (40% with doctorates).

Baccalaureate Enrollment 50
Women 95% **Men** 5% **Minority** 5%

Nursing Student Activities Student Nurses' Association, nursing club.

Nursing Student Resources Academic advising; academic or career counseling; assistance for students with disabilities; bookstore; campus computer network; computer lab; computer-assisted instruction; e-mail services; housing assistance; interactive nursing skills videos; Internet; learning resource lab; library services; nursing audiovisuals; remedial services; resume preparation assistance; skills, simulation, or other laboratory; tutoring; unpaid internships.

Library Facilities 100,966 volumes; 821 periodical subscriptions.

BACCALAUREATE PROGRAMS

Degree BSN

Available Programs Generic Baccalaureate.

Study Options Full-time.

Program Entrance Requirements Minimum overall college GPA of 2.5, high school chemistry, minimum GPA in nursing prerequisites of 2.5. Transfer students are accepted. **Standardized tests** *Required:* ACT, TOEFL for international students. **Application** *Deadline:* 8/8 (freshmen), 8/8 (transfer). *Early decision:* 12/1. *Notification:* continuous (freshmen), 1/15 (early action). *Application fee:* $25.

Advanced Placement Credit given for nursing courses completed elsewhere dependent upon specific evaluations.

Expenses (2003–04) *Tuition:* full-time $15,330; part-time $665 per credit hour. *Room and board:* $4440 per academic year. *Required fees:* full-time $590.

Financial Aid 90% of baccalaureate students in nursing programs received some form of financial aid in 2002–03.

Contact Chair, School of Health and Science, Northwest Nazarene University, 623 Holly Street, Nampa, ID 83686. *Telephone:* 208-467-8650. *Fax:* 208-467-8651. *E-mail:* nursing@nnu.edu.

ILLINOIS

Aurora University
School of Nursing
Aurora, Illinois

http://www.aurora.edu

Founded in 1893

DEGREE • BSN

Nursing Program Faculty 6 (33% with doctorates).

Baccalaureate Enrollment 132
Women 94% **Men** 6% **Minority** 40% **Part-time** 6%

Nursing Student Activities Sigma Theta Tau, Student Nurses' Association, nursing club.

Nursing Student Resources Academic advising; academic or career counseling; assistance for students with disabilities; bookstore; campus computer network; career placement assistance; computer lab; computer-assisted instruction; e-mail services; externships; interactive nursing skills videos; Internet; learning resource lab; library services; nursing audiovisuals; resume preparation assistance; skills, simulation, or other laboratory; tutoring.

Library Facilities 115,642 volumes (5,285 in health, 86 in nursing); 748 periodical subscriptions (698 health-care related).

BACCALAUREATE PROGRAMS

Degree BSN

Available Programs Generic Baccalaureate; RN Baccalaureate.

Site Options Aurora, IL.

Study Options Full-time and part-time.

Program Entrance Requirements Minimum overall college GPA of 2.75, transcript of college record, CPR certification, written essay, health exam, health insurance, 3 years high school math, 3 years high school science, high school transcript, immunizations, interview, minimum high school GPA of 2.75, minimum high school rank 50%, minimum GPA in nursing prerequisites of 2.75, prerequisite course work. Transfer students are accepted. **Standardized tests** *Required:* TOEFL for international

Aurora University (continued)

students. *Recommended:* SAT or ACT, SAT Subject Tests. **Application** *Deadline:* rolling (freshmen), rolling (transfer). *Notification:* continuous (freshmen). *Application fee:* $25.

Advanced Placement Credit given for nursing courses completed elsewhere dependent upon specific evaluations.

Expenses (2004–05) *Tuition:* full-time $14,750; part-time $475 per credit hour. *Room and board:* $3046; room only: $1480 per academic year. *Required fees:* part-time $7375 per term.

Financial Aid 85% of baccalaureate students in nursing programs received some form of financial aid in 2003–04.

Contact Dr. Maryanne Phyllis Locklin, Director and Associate Professor, School of Nursing, Aurora University, 347 South Gladstone Avenue, Aurora, IL 60506-4892. *Telephone:* 630-844-5130. *Fax:* 630-844-7822. *E-mail:* mlocklin@aurora.edu.

Benedictine University
Department of Nursing
Lisle, Illinois

Founded in 1887

DEGREE • BSN

Nursing Program Faculty 3 (3% with doctorates).

Baccalaureate Enrollment 32
Women 99% **Men** 1% **Minority** 47% **Part-time** 100%

Nursing Student Activities Nursing Honor Society, Sigma Theta Tau.

Nursing Student Resources Academic advising; academic or career counseling; assistance for students with disabilities; bookstore; campus computer network; computer lab; computer-assisted instruction; e-mail services; interactive nursing skills videos; Internet; learning resource lab; library services; nursing audiovisuals; resume preparation assistance; skills, simulation, or other laboratory.

Library Facilities 1,350 volumes in health, 850 volumes in nursing; 291 periodical subscriptions health-care related.

BACCALAUREATE PROGRAMS

Degree BSN

Available Programs Accelerated RN Baccalaureate.

Site Options Rockford, IL.

Study Options Full-time and part-time.

Program Entrance Requirements Transcript of college record. Transfer students are accepted. **Standardized tests** *Required:* ACT, TOEFL for international students. **Application** *Deadline:* rolling (freshmen), rolling (transfer). *Notification:* continuous (freshmen). *Application fee:* $40.

Advanced Placement Credit given for nursing courses completed elsewhere dependent upon specific evaluations.

Expenses (2003–04) *Tuition:* part-time $380 per credit hour.

Financial Aid 20% of baccalaureate students in nursing programs received some form of financial aid in 2002–03. *Gift aid (need-based):* Federal Pell, FSEOG, state, private, college/university gift aid from institutional funds. *Loans:* FFEL (Subsidized and Unsubsidized Stafford PLUS), Perkins, alternative loans. *Work-Study:* Federal Work-Study. *Application deadline:* 4/15 (priority: 4/15).

Contact Dr. Shirley A. Moore, Department Chair, Department of Nursing, Benedictine University, 5700 College Road, Lisle, IL 60532. *Telephone:* 630-829-6567. *Fax:* 630-829-6551. *E-mail:* smoore@ben.edu.

Blessing–Rieman College of Nursing
Blessing–Rieman College of Nursing
Quincy, Illinois

DEGREE • BSN

Nursing Program Faculty 14 (27% with doctorates).

Baccalaureate Enrollment 248
Women 95% **Men** 5% **Minority** 3% **Part-time** 9%

Nursing Student Activities Sigma Theta Tau, Student Nurses' Association.

Nursing Student Resources Academic advising; academic or career counseling; bookstore; campus computer network; computer lab; computer-assisted instruction; daycare for children of students; e-mail services; employment services for current students; externships; interactive nursing skills videos; Internet; learning resource lab; library services; nursing audiovisuals; paid internships; resume preparation assistance; skills, simulation, or other laboratory; tutoring.

Library Facilities 4,282 volumes in health, 3,962 volumes in nursing; 123 periodical subscriptions health-care related.

BACCALAUREATE PROGRAMS

Degree BSN

Available Programs Accelerated Baccalaureate for Second Degree; Generic Baccalaureate; LPN to Baccalaureate; RN Baccalaureate.

Study Options Full-time and part-time.

Program Entrance Requirements Minimum overall college GPA of 2.0, transcript of college record, CPR certification, health insurance, high school biology, high school chemistry, 2 years high school math, 2 years high school science, high school transcript, immunizations, minimum high school GPA of 3.0, minimum high school rank 50%, minimum GPA in nursing prerequisites of 2.0, prerequisite course work. Transfer students are accepted.

Advanced Placement Credit by examination available. Credit given for nursing courses completed elsewhere dependent upon specific evaluations.

Expenses (2004–05) *Tuition:* full-time $13,200; part-time $289 per credit hour. *International tuition:* $13,200 full-time. *Room and board:* $5865; room only: $2765 per academic year. *Required fees:* full-time $500; part-time $250 per term.

Financial Aid 98% of baccalaureate students in nursing programs received some form of financial aid in 2003–04.

Contact Miss Erin Flesner, Admission Counselor, Blessing–Rieman College of Nursing, Broadway at 11th Street, Quincy, IL 62305-7005. *Telephone:* 217-228-5520 Ext. 6961. *Fax:* 217-223-4661. *E-mail:* admissions@brcn.edu.

See full description on page 460.

Bradley University
Department of Nursing
Peoria, Illinois

http://www.bradley.edu/academics/ehs/nur/nur_index.html

Founded in 1897

DEGREES • BSN • MSN

Nursing Program Faculty 27 (22% with doctorates).

Baccalaureate Enrollment 187
Women 93% **Men** 7% **Minority** 15% **Part-time** 5%

Graduate Enrollment 57
Women 65% **Men** 35% **Minority** 14% **Part-time** 72%

Nursing Student Activities Sigma Theta Tau, Student Nurses' Association.

Nursing Student Resources Academic advising; bookstore; campus computer network; career placement assistance; computer lab; computer-assisted instruction; e-mail services; housing assistance; Internet; learning resource lab; library services; nursing audiovisuals; placement services for program completers; resume preparation assistance; skills, simulation, or other laboratory; tutoring.

Library Facilities 435,394 volumes (9,869 in health, 2,097 in nursing); 1,724 periodical subscriptions (122 health-care related).

BACCALAUREATE PROGRAMS

Degree BSN

Available Programs Accelerated LPN to Baccalaureate; Accelerated RN Baccalaureate; Generic Baccalaureate.

Study Options Full-time and part-time.

Program Entrance Requirements Minimum overall college GPA of 2.5, transcript of college record, health exam, high school biology, high school chemistry, 3 years high school math, 3 years high school science, high school transcript, immunizations, minimum high school GPA of 2.5, minimum GPA in nursing prerequisites of 2.0, professional liability insurance/malpractice insurance. Transfer students are accepted. **Standardized tests** *Required:* SAT or ACT, TOEFL for international students. **Application** *Deadline:* rolling (freshmen). *Notification:* continuous (freshmen). *Application fee:* $35.

Advanced Placement Credit by examination available. Credit given for nursing courses completed elsewhere dependent upon specific evaluations.

Expenses (2004–05) *Tuition:* full-time $17,600; part-time $590 per credit hour. *International tuition:* $17,600 full-time. *Room and board:* $6040; room only: $3400 per academic year. *Required fees:* full-time $250; part-time $125 per term.

Financial Aid 96% of baccalaureate students in nursing programs received some form of financial aid in 2003–04. *Gift aid (need-based):* Federal Pell, FSEOG, state, private, college/university gift aid from institutional funds. *Loans:* Federal Nursing Student Loans, Federal Direct (Subsidized and Unsubsidized Stafford PLUS), FFEL, Perkins. *Work-Study:* Federal Work-Study. *Application deadline (priority):* 3/1.

Contact Ms. Marilyn Miller, Student Records Coordinator, Department of Nursing, Bradley University, Peoria, IL 61625. *Telephone:* 309-677-2530. *Fax:* 309-677-2566. *E-mail:* mmiller@bradley.edu.

GRADUATE PROGRAMS

Expenses (2004–05) *Tuition:* full-time $10,170; part-time $480 per credit hour. *International tuition:* $10,170 full-time. *Room and board:* $6040; room only: $3400 per academic year. *Required fees:* full-time $110; part-time $85 per term.

Financial Aid 83% of graduate students in nursing programs received some form of financial aid in 2003–04. 3 research assistantships with full and partial tuition reimbursements available (averaging $5,060 per year) were awarded; scholarships and tuition waivers (partial) also available. *Financial aid application deadline:* 3/1.

Contact Ms. Marilyn Miller, Student Records Coordinator, Department of Nursing, Bradley University, Peoria, IL 61625. *Telephone:* 309-677-2530. *Fax:* 309-677-2527. *E-mail:* mmiller@bradley.edu.

MASTER'S DEGREE PROGRAM

Degree MSN

Available Programs Accelerated Master's for Nurses with Non-Nursing Degrees; Master's.

Concentrations Available Nurse anesthesia; nursing administration.

Site Options Decatur, IL.

Study Options Full-time and part-time.

Program Entrance Requirements Clinical experience, minimum overall college GPA of 3.0, transcript of college record, interview, 3 letters of recommendation, nursing research course, physical assessment course, prerequisite course work, resume, statistics course, GRE General Test or MAT. *Application deadline:* For fall admission, 7/1 (priority date); for spring admission, 11/1. Applications are processed on a rolling basis. *Application fee:* $40 ($50 for international students).

Advanced Placement Credit given for nursing courses completed elsewhere dependent upon specific evaluations.

Degree Requirements Thesis or project, comprehensive exam.

Chicago State University

College of Nursing and Allied Health Professions
Chicago, Illinois

http://www.csu.edu

Founded in 1867

DEGREE • BSN

Nursing Program Faculty 23 (60% with doctorates).

Baccalaureate Enrollment 372

Women 90% **Men** 10% **Minority** 97% **International** 15% **Part-time** 24%

Nursing Student Activities Nursing Honor Society, Student Nurses' Association.

Nursing Student Resources Academic advising; academic or career counseling; assistance for students with disabilities; bookstore; campus computer network; computer lab; computer-assisted instruction; daycare for children of students; e-mail services; employment services for current students; externships; interactive nursing skills videos; Internet; learning resource lab; library services; nursing audiovisuals; remedial services; resume preparation assistance; skills, simulation, or other laboratory; tutoring; unpaid internships.

Library Facilities 320,000 volumes; 1,539 periodical subscriptions.

BACCALAUREATE PROGRAMS

Degree BSN

Available Programs Generic Baccalaureate; LPN to Baccalaureate; RN Baccalaureate.

Site Options *Distance Learning:* Chicago, IL.

Study Options Full-time.

Program Entrance Requirements Minimum overall college GPA of 2.5, transcript of college record, written essay, health exam, health insurance, 3 years high school math, 3 years high school science, high school transcript, immunizations, interview, 3 letters of recommendation, minimum GPA in nursing prerequisites of 2.5, professional liability insurance/malpractice insurance, prerequisite course work. Transfer students are accepted. **Standardized tests** *Required:* SAT or ACT, TOEFL for international students. **Application** *Deadline:* 7/15 (freshmen), 7/15 (transfer). *Notification:* continuous (freshmen). *Application fee:* $25.

Advanced Placement Credit by examination available.

Expenses (2003–04) *Tuition, state resident:* full-time $1584; part-time $132 per credit hour. *Tuition, nonresident:* full-time $4776; part-time $398 per credit hour. *Required fees:* part-time $204 per credit; part-time $608 per term.

Financial Aid 95% of baccalaureate students in nursing programs received some form of financial aid in 2002–03.

Contact Dr. Linda B. Hureston, RN, Acting Chairperson, College of Nursing and Allied Health Professions, Chicago State University, 9501 South Martin Luther King Drive, Chicago, IL 60628. *Telephone:* 773-995-3992. *Fax:* 773-821-2438. *E-mail:* Nursing@csu.edu.

DePaul University

Department of Nursing
Chicago, Illinois

http://www.depaul.edu/~nursing

Founded in 1898

DEGREES • BS • MS

Nursing Program Faculty 19 (89% with doctorates).

Baccalaureate Enrollment 5

Graduate Enrollment 131

Women 87% **Men** 13% **Minority** 23% **Part-time** 35%

Nursing Student Activities Sigma Theta Tau, Student Nurses' Association.

Nursing Student Resources Academic advising; academic or career counseling; assistance for students with disabilities; bookstore; campus computer network; computer lab; computer-assisted instruction; e-mail services; employment services for current students; externships; housing assistance; interactive nursing skills videos; Internet; learning resource lab; library services; nursing audiovisuals; resume preparation assistance; skills, simulation, or other laboratory; tutoring.

Library Facilities 896,864 volumes; 26,822 periodical subscriptions (193 health-care related).

BACCALAUREATE PROGRAMS

Degree BS

DePaul University (continued)

Available Programs Accelerated RN Baccalaureate.

Study Options Full-time and part-time.

Program Entrance Requirements Minimum overall college GPA of 2.5, transcript of college record, CPR certification, health exam, immunizations, professional liability insurance/malpractice insurance, RN licensure. Transfer students are accepted. **Standardized tests** *Required:* SAT or ACT, TOEFL for international students. **Application** *Deadline:* rolling (freshmen), rolling (transfer). *Early decision:* 11/15, 11/15. *Notification:* 10/15 (freshmen), 1/15 (early action). *Application fee:* $40.

Advanced Placement Credit given for nursing courses completed elsewhere dependent upon specific evaluations.

Financial Aid *Gift aid (need-based):* Federal Pell, FSEOG, state, private, college/university gift aid from institutional funds, United Negro College Fund. *Loans:* Federal Direct (Subsidized and Unsubsidized Stafford PLUS), Perkins. *Work-Study:* Federal Work-Study, part-time campus jobs. *Application deadline:* 4/1 (priority: 3/1).

Contact Ms. Christine Werdrick, Coordinator of Student Academic Services, Department of Nursing, DePaul University, 990 West Fullerton Avenue, Suite 3000, Chicago, IL 60614. *Telephone:* 773-325-7280. *Fax:* 773-325-7282. *E-mail:* cwerdric@depaul.edu.

GRADUATE PROGRAMS

Expenses (2003–04) *Tuition:* part-time $395 per quarter.

Financial Aid 20% of graduate students in nursing programs received some form of financial aid in 2002–03. 5 fellowships (averaging $2,000 per year) were awarded; traineeships also available.

Contact Ms. Christine Werdrick, Coordinator of Student Academic Services, Department of Nursing, DePaul University, 990 West Fullerton Avenue, Suite 3000, Chicago, IL 60614. *Telephone:* 773-325-7280. *Fax:* 773-325-7282. *E-mail:* cwerdric@depaul.edu.

MASTER'S DEGREE PROGRAM

Degree MS

Available Programs Master's; Master's for Non-Nursing College Graduates; Master's for Nurses with Non-Nursing Degrees; RN to Master's.

Concentrations Available Nurse anesthesia; nurse case management; nursing administration; nursing education. *Clinical nurse specialist programs in:* community health, medical-surgical. *Nurse practitioner programs in:* adult health, community health, family health, pediatric, women's health.

Study Options Full-time and part-time.

Program Entrance Requirements Computer literacy, minimum overall college GPA of 2.75, transcript of college record, CPR certification, physical assessment course, professional liability insurance/malpractice insurance, prerequisite course work, statistics course, GRE. *Application fee:* $25.

Advanced Placement Credit given for nursing courses completed elsewhere dependent upon specific evaluations.

Degree Requirements 52 total credit hours, thesis or project.

POST-MASTER'S PROGRAM

Areas of Study Nurse anesthesia. *Nurse practitioner programs in:* adult health, community health, family health, pediatric, women's health.

Elmhurst College

Deicke Center for Nursing Education
Elmhurst, Illinois

Founded in 1871

DEGREE • BSN

Nursing Program Faculty 8 (50% with doctorates).

Library Facilities 222,441 volumes (6,000 in health); 2,010 periodical subscriptions (80 health-care related).

BACCALAUREATE PROGRAMS

Degree BSN

Available Programs Generic Baccalaureate; RN Baccalaureate.

Study Options Full-time.

Program Entrance Requirements Minimum overall college GPA of 2.75, transcript of college record, CPR certification, immunizations, minimum GPA in nursing prerequisites of 2.0, prerequisite course work. Transfer students are accepted. **Standardized tests** *Required:* SAT or ACT, TOEFL for international students. **Application** *Deadline:* 7/15 (freshmen). *Notification:* continuous (freshmen). *Application fee:* $25.

Advanced Placement Credit given for nursing courses completed elsewhere dependent upon specific evaluations.

Contact Dr. Linda K. Niedringhaus, Director, Deicke Center for Nursing Education, Elmhurst College, 190 Prospect Avenue, Elmhurst, IL 60126. *Telephone:* 630-617-3344. *Fax:* 630-617-3237. *E-mail:* lindan@elmhurst.edu.

Governors State University

Division of Nursing, Communication Disorders, Occupational Therapy, and Physical Therapy
University Park, Illinois

http://www.govst.edu/nursing/index.html

Founded in 1969

DEGREES • BS • MS

Nursing Program Faculty 7 (85% with doctorates).

Nursing Student Activities Sigma Theta Tau.

Nursing Student Resources Academic advising; assistance for students with disabilities; bookstore; campus computer network; computer lab; daycare for children of students; e-mail services; Internet; learning resource lab; library services; nursing audiovisuals; tutoring.

Library Facilities 260,000 volumes; 2,200 periodical subscriptions.

BACCALAUREATE PROGRAMS

Degree BS

Available Programs RN Baccalaureate.

Study Options Part-time.

Program Entrance Requirements Transcript of college record, CPR certification, health exam, health insurance, immunizations, minimum GPA in nursing prerequisites of 2.0, professional liability insurance/malpractice insurance, prerequisite course work, RN licensure. Transfer students are accepted. **Standardized tests** *Required:* TOEFL for international students. **Application** *Deadline:* 7/15 (transfer).

Contact Linda McCann, Program Advisor, Division of Nursing, Communication Disorders, Occupational Therapy, and Physical Therapy, Governors State University, University Park, IL 60466-0975. *Telephone:* 708-534-4053. *Fax:* 708-534-2197. *E-mail:* l-mccann@govst.edu.

GRADUATE PROGRAMS

Financial Aid Research assistantships, career-related internships or fieldwork, Federal Work-Study, institutionally sponsored loans, scholarships, and tuition waivers (full and partial) available.

Contact Linda McCann, Program Advisor, Division of Nursing, Communication Disorders, Occupational Therapy, and Physical Therapy, Governors State University, University Park, IL 60466-0975. *Telephone:* 708-534-4053. *Fax:* 708-534-2197. *E-mail:* l-mccann@govst.edu.

MASTER'S DEGREE PROGRAM

Degree MS

Concentrations Available *Clinical nurse specialist programs in:* adult health.

Study Options Part-time.

Program Entrance Requirements Clinical experience, computer literacy, minimum overall college GPA of 3.0, transcript of college record, CPR certification, written essay, immunizations, nursing research course, physical assessment course, professional liability insurance/malpractice insurance, prerequisite course work, statistics course. *Application deadline:* Applications are processed on a rolling basis.

Degree Requirements 41 total credit hours, comprehensive exam.

Illinois State University
Mennonite College of Nursing
Normal, Illinois

http://www.mcn.ilstu.edu

Founded in 1857

DEGREES • BSN • MSN

Nursing Program Faculty 36 (33% with doctorates).

Baccalaureate Enrollment 237
Women 96% **Men** 4% **Minority** 7% **Part-time** 8%

Graduate Enrollment 32
Women 97% **Men** 3% **Part-time** 22%

Nursing Student Activities Nursing Honor Society, Sigma Theta Tau, Student Nurses' Association.

Nursing Student Resources Academic advising; academic or career counseling; assistance for students with disabilities; bookstore; campus computer network; career placement assistance; computer lab; computer-assisted instruction; daycare for children of students; e-mail services; employment services for current students; externships; interactive nursing skills videos; Internet; learning resource lab; library services; nursing audiovisuals; placement services for program completers; resume preparation assistance; skills, simulation, or other laboratory; tutoring.

Library Facilities 1.6 million volumes (18,000 in health, 4,000 in nursing); 14,166 periodical subscriptions (700 health-care related).

BACCALAUREATE PROGRAMS

Degree BSN

Available Programs ADN to Baccalaureate; Generic Baccalaureate; RN Baccalaureate.

Study Options Full-time.

Program Entrance Requirements Minimum overall college GPA of 2.7, transcript of college record, CPR certification, health exam, health insurance, immunizations, minimum GPA in nursing prerequisites of 2.0, prerequisite course work. Transfer students are accepted. **Standardized tests** *Required:* SAT or ACT, TOEFL for international students. *Recommended:* ACT. **Application** *Deadline:* 3/1 (freshmen), rolling (transfer). *Notification:* continuous (freshmen). *Application fee:* $30.

Advanced Placement Credit given for nursing courses completed elsewhere dependent upon specific evaluations.

Expenses (2004–05) *Tuition, state resident:* full-time $4800; part-time $160 per credit hour. *Tuition, nonresident:* full-time $10,020; part-time $334 per credit hour. *Room and board:* $5212; room only: $2682 per academic year. *Required fees:* full-time $1382; part-time $43 per credit; part-time $691 per term.

Financial Aid 70% of baccalaureate students in nursing programs received some form of financial aid in 2003–04.

Contact Mrs. Tenna Webb, Academic Advising Secretary, Mennonite College of Nursing, Illinois State University, 5810 Edwards Hall, Normal, IL 61790-5810. *Telephone:* 309-438-2252. *Fax:* 309-438-2620. *E-mail:* tlwebb@ilstu.edu.

GRADUATE PROGRAMS

Expenses (2004–05) *Tuition, state resident:* full-time $4350; part-time $145 per credit hour. *Tuition, nonresident:* full-time $9090; part-time $303 per credit hour. *Room and board:* $5212; room only: $2682 per academic year. *Required fees:* full-time $1382; part-time $43 per credit; part-time $691 per term.

Financial Aid 56% of graduate students in nursing programs received some form of financial aid in 2003–04. 3 research assistantships (averaging $6,375 per year) were awarded; teaching assistantships.

Contact Dr. Brenda R. Jeffers, Director of Graduate Program and Research, Mennonite College of Nursing, Illinois State University, 5810 Edwards Hall, Normal, IL 61790-5810. *Telephone:* 309-438-2349. *Fax:* 309-438-2280. *E-mail:* brjeffe@ilstu.edu.

MASTER'S DEGREE PROGRAM

Degree MSN

Available Programs Master's.

Concentrations Available Nursing administration. *Nurse practitioner programs in:* family health.

Study Options Full-time and part-time.

Program Entrance Requirements Clinical experience, minimum overall college GPA of 3.0, transcript of college record, CPR certification, written essay, immunizations, 3 letters of recommendation, prerequisite course work, resume, statistics course. *Application fee:* $30.

Advanced Placement Credit given for nursing courses completed elsewhere dependent upon specific evaluations.

Degree Requirements 44 total credit hours.

POST-MASTER'S PROGRAM

Areas of Study Nursing education. *Nurse practitioner programs in:* family health.

See full description on page 500.

Illinois Wesleyan University
School of Nursing
Bloomington, Illinois

http://titan.iwu.edu/~nursing

Founded in 1850

DEGREE • BSN

Nursing Program Faculty 17 (53% with doctorates).

Baccalaureate Enrollment 92
Women 92% **Men** 8% **Minority** 10%

Nursing Student Activities Nursing Honor Society, Sigma Theta Tau, Student Nurses' Association.

Nursing Student Resources Academic advising; academic or career counseling; assistance for students with disabilities; bookstore; campus computer network; career placement assistance; computer lab; computer-assisted instruction; e-mail services; employment services for current students; externships; housing assistance; interactive nursing skills videos; Internet; learning resource lab; library services; nursing audiovisuals; paid internships; placement services for program completers; resume preparation assistance; skills, simulation, or other laboratory; tutoring; unpaid internships.

Library Facilities 314,894 volumes (314,894 in health, 15,780 in nursing); 15,226 periodical subscriptions (83 health-care related).

BACCALAUREATE PROGRAMS

Degree BSN

Available Programs Generic Baccalaureate; RN Baccalaureate.

Study Options Full-time and part-time.

Program Entrance Requirements Minimum overall college GPA of 3.0, transcript of college record, written essay, health exam, health insurance, high school biology, high school chemistry, 2 years high school math, 2 years high school science, high school transcript, immunizations, interview, minimum high school GPA of 3.0, minimum high school rank 25%. Transfer students are accepted. **Standardized tests** *Required:* SAT or ACT, TOEFL for international students. **Application** *Deadline:* 2/15 (freshmen). *Notification:* 4/15 (freshmen).

Advanced Placement Credit by examination available. Credit given for nursing courses completed elsewhere dependent upon specific evaluations.

Expenses (2004–05) *Tuition:* full-time $25,980; part-time $12,990 per semester. *International tuition:* $25,980 full-time. *Room and board:* $6140; room only: $3680 per academic year.

Financial Aid 89% of baccalaureate students in nursing programs received some form of financial aid in 2003–04. *Gift aid (need-based):* Federal Pell, FSEOG, state, private, college/university gift aid from institutional funds. *Loans:* Federal Nursing Student Loans, FFEL (Subsidized and Unsubsidized Stafford PLUS), Perkins, college/university. *Work-Study:* Federal Work-Study, part-time campus jobs. *Application deadline:* 3/1.

Illinois Wesleyan University (continued)

Contact Dr. Donna L. Hartweg, Caroline F. Rupert Professor of Nursing and Director, School of Nursing, Illinois Wesleyan University, PO Box 2900, Bloomington, IL 61701-2900. *Telephone:* 309-556-3051. *Fax:* 309-556-3043. *E-mail:* dhartweg@titan.iwu.edu.

Lakeview College of Nursing

Lakeview College of Nursing
Danville, Illinois

http://www.lakeviewcol.edu

Founded in 1987

DEGREE • BSN

Nursing Program Faculty 13.

Baccalaureate Enrollment 147
Women 89% **Men** 11% **Minority** 4% **Part-time** 15%

Nursing Student Activities Nursing Honor Society, Sigma Theta Tau, Student Nurses' Association.

Nursing Student Resources Academic advising; academic or career counseling; assistance for students with disabilities; bookstore; campus computer network; career placement assistance; computer lab; Internet; library services; nursing audiovisuals; resume preparation assistance; skills, simulation, or other laboratory; tutoring.

Library Facilities 1,500 volumes; 60 periodical subscriptions.

BACCALAUREATE PROGRAMS

Degree BSN

Available Programs Accelerated RN Baccalaureate; Generic Baccalaureate; RN Baccalaureate.

Site Options *Distance Learning:* Charleston, IL.

Study Options Full-time and part-time.

Program Entrance Requirements Minimum overall college GPA of 2.5, CPR certification, written essay, health exam, immunizations, 2 letters of recommendation, prerequisite course work. Transfer students are accepted. **Application** *Deadline:* rolling (transfer). *Application fee:* $50.

Advanced Placement Credit given for nursing courses completed elsewhere dependent upon specific evaluations.

Expenses (2004–05) *Tuition:* full-time $300; part-time $300 per credit hour.

Financial Aid 55% of baccalaureate students in nursing programs received some form of financial aid in 2003–04.

Contact Ms. Errin Davis, Director of Admissions and Records/Registrar, Lakeview College of Nursing, 903 North Logan Avenue, Danville, IL 61832. *Telephone:* 217-554-6899. *Fax:* 217-442-2279. *E-mail:* edavis@lakeviewcol.edu.

Lewis University

Program in Nursing
Romeoville, Illinois

http://www.lewisu.edu/academics/nursing/index.htm

Founded in 1932

DEGREES • BSN • MSN • MSN/MBA

Nursing Program Faculty 25 (29% with doctorates).

Baccalaureate Enrollment 632
Women 95% **Men** 5% **Minority** 31% **International** 8% **Part-time** 69%

Graduate Enrollment 185
Women 90% **Men** 10% **Minority** 16% **International** 2%

Nursing Student Activities Sigma Theta Tau, Student Nurses' Association.

Nursing Student Resources Academic advising; academic or career counseling; assistance for students with disabilities; bookstore; campus computer network; career placement assistance; computer lab; computer-assisted instruction; e-mail services; employment services for current students; Internet; learning resource lab; library services; nursing audiovisuals; remedial services; resume preparation assistance; skills, simulation, or other laboratory; tutoring.

Library Facilities 149,870 volumes (3,100 in health, 2,038 in nursing); 1,990 periodical subscriptions (85 health-care related).

BACCALAUREATE PROGRAMS

Degree BSN

Available Programs Accelerated Baccalaureate for Second Degree; Accelerated RN Baccalaureate; Generic Baccalaureate.

Site Options Hickory Hills, IL; Oak Brook, IL; Tinley Park, IL.

Study Options Full-time.

Program Entrance Requirements Minimum overall college GPA of 2.5, transcript of college record, CPR certification, health exam, health insurance, high school transcript, immunizations, minimum high school GPA of 2.5, minimum GPA in nursing prerequisites of 2.0, prerequisite course work. Transfer students are accepted. **Standardized tests** *Required:* SAT or ACT, TOEFL for international students. **Application** *Deadline:* 8/1 (freshmen), rolling (transfer). *Application fee:* $35.

Advanced Placement Credit given for nursing courses completed elsewhere dependent upon specific evaluations.

Expenses (2003–04) *Tuition:* full-time $15,950; part-time $515 per credit hour. *International tuition:* $15,950 full-time. *Room and board:* $6500; room only: $4000 per academic year. *Required fees:* full-time $1000.

Financial Aid 80% of baccalaureate students in nursing programs received some form of financial aid in 2002–03. *Gift aid (need-based):* Federal Pell, FSEOG, state, private, college/university gift aid from institutional funds, Federal Nursing. *Loans:* FFEL (Subsidized and Unsubsidized Stafford PLUS), Perkins. *Work-Study:* Federal Work-Study, part-time campus jobs. *Application deadline (priority):* 5/1.

Contact Dr. Peggy Rice, Undergraduate Nursing Program Director, Program in Nursing, Lewis University, One University Parkway, Romeoville, IL 60446. *Telephone:* 815-836-5245. *Fax:* 815-838-8306. *E-mail:* Ricepe@lewisu.edu.

GRADUATE PROGRAMS

Expenses (2003–04) *Tuition:* full-time $9720; part-time $540 per credit hour. *International tuition:* $9720 full-time. *Room and board:* $6500; room only: $4000 per academic year. *Required fees:* full-time $1000.

Financial Aid 40% of graduate students in nursing programs received some form of financial aid in 2002–03. Federal Work-Study, scholarships, tuition waivers (full and partial), and unspecified assistantships available. *Financial aid application deadline:* 5/1.

Contact Lois Stephens, Director, Graduate Program, Program in Nursing, Lewis University, One University Parkway, Romeoville, IL 60446-2298. *Telephone:* 815-836-5355 Ext. 5363. *Fax:* 815-838-8306. *E-mail:* stephelo@lewisu.edu.

MASTER'S DEGREE PROGRAM

Degrees MSN; MSN/MBA

Available Programs Accelerated Master's; RN to Master's.

Concentrations Available Health-care administration; nurse case management; nursing administration; nursing education. *Clinical nurse specialist programs in:* community health.

Site Options Hickory Hills, IL; Oak Brook, IL.

Study Options Full-time and part-time.

Program Entrance Requirements Clinical experience, minimum overall college GPA of 2.75, transcript of college record, CPR certification, immunizations, 3 letters of recommendation, nursing research course, professional liability insurance/malpractice insurance, prerequisite course work, resume, statistics course, GRE General Test, GRE Subject Test. *Application deadline:* Applications are processed on a rolling basis. *Application fee:* $40.

Degree Requirements 45 total credit hours, thesis or project.

POST-MASTER'S PROGRAM

Areas of Study *Clinical nurse specialist programs in:* community health.

CONTINUING EDUCATION PROGRAM

Contact Ms. Linda Elsik, RN, Director of RN/BSN and Allied Health Program, Program in Nursing, Lewis University, One University Parkway, Box 404, Romeoville, IL 60446. *Telephone:* 815-836-5798. *Fax:* 815-838-8306. *E-mail:* elsikli@lewisu.edu.

Loyola University Chicago

Marcella Niehoff School of Nursing
Chicago, Illinois

http://www.luc.edu/schools/nursing/

Founded in 1870

DEGREES • BSN • MSN • MSN/MBA • MSN/MDIV • PHD

Nursing Program Faculty 40 (90% with doctorates).

Nursing Student Activities Nursing Honor Society, Sigma Theta Tau, Student Nurses' Association.

Library Facilities 1.1 million volumes (51,674 in health, 4,966 in nursing); 68,886 periodical subscriptions (2,630 health-care related).

BACCALAUREATE PROGRAMS

Degree BSN

Available Programs Accelerated Baccalaureate; Generic Baccalaureate; RN Baccalaureate.

Site Options Maywood, IL; Chicago, IL.

Study Options Full-time and part-time.

Program Entrance Requirements Transcript of college record, CPR certification, written essay, health exam, health insurance, high school biology, high school chemistry, 2 years high school math, high school transcript, immunizations, 2 letters of recommendation, minimum high school GPA of 3.0, minimum high school rank 25%, prerequisite course work. Transfer students are accepted. **Standardized tests** *Required:* SAT or ACT, TOEFL for international students. **Application** *Deadline:* 4/1 (freshmen), 8/1 (transfer). *Notification:* continuous (freshmen). *Application fee:* $25.

Advanced Placement Credit given for nursing courses completed elsewhere dependent upon specific evaluations.

Contact Eileen Lynch, Assistant Dean of Students, Undergraduate Programs, Marcella Niehoff School of Nursing, Loyola University Chicago, 6525 North Sheridan Road, DH 507, Chicago, IL 60626. *Telephone:* 773-508-3249. *Fax:* 773-508-3241. *E-mail:* elynch1@luc.edu.

GRADUATE PROGRAMS

Financial Aid 1 fellowship, 7 research assistantships, 1 teaching assistantship were awarded; career-related internships or fieldwork, Federal Work-Study, institutionally sponsored loans, traineeships, and unspecified assistantships also available.

Contact Lauren Groves, Assistant Dean of Students, Graduate Programs, Marcella Niehoff School of Nursing, Loyola University Chicago, 6525 North Sheridan Road, Chicago, IL 60626. *Telephone:* 773-508-3249. *Fax:* 773-508-3241. *E-mail:* lgroves@luc.edu.

MASTER'S DEGREE PROGRAM

Degrees MSN; MSN/MBA; MSN/MDIV

Available Programs Master's; RN to Master's.

Concentrations Available Nurse-midwifery; nursing administration. *Clinical nurse specialist programs in:* acute care, cardiovascular, oncology. *Nurse practitioner programs in:* acute care, adult health, family health, pediatric, women's health.

Site Options Maywood, IL; Chicago, IL.

Study Options Full-time and part-time.

Program Entrance Requirements Clinical experience, minimum overall college GPA of 3.0, transcript of college record, CPR certification, written essay, immunizations, interview, 3 letters of recommendation, physical assessment course, professional liability insurance/malpractice insurance, statistics course. *Application deadline:* Applications are processed on a rolling basis. *Application fee:* $40.

Advanced Placement Credit given for nursing courses completed elsewhere dependent upon specific evaluations.

Degree Requirements 48 total credit hours, comprehensive exam.

DOCTORAL DEGREE PROGRAM

Degree PhD

Available Programs Post-Baccalaureate Doctorate.

Areas of Study Ethics, nursing education, nursing research, nursing science.

Site Options Maywood, IL; Chicago, IL.

Program Entrance Requirements interview by faculty committee, interview, 3 letters of recommendation, scholarly papers, statistics course, vita, writing sample, GRE General Test. *Application deadline:* Applications are processed on a rolling basis. *Application fee:* $40.

Degree Requirements 64 total credit hours, dissertation, oral exam, written exam.

MacMurray College

Department of Nursing
Jacksonville, Illinois

http://www.mac.edu/academics/nursing.html

Founded in 1846

DEGREE • BSN

Nursing Program Faculty 7 (43% with doctorates).

Baccalaureate Enrollment 85

Women 89% **Men** 11% **Minority** 10% **International** 3% **Part-time** 15%

Nursing Student Activities Student Nurses' Association.

Nursing Student Resources Academic advising; academic or career counseling; assistance for students with disabilities; bookstore; campus computer network; career placement assistance; computer lab; computer-assisted instruction; e-mail services; employment services for current students; externships; interactive nursing skills videos; Internet; learning resource lab; library services; nursing audiovisuals; paid internships; placement services for program completers; remedial services; resume preparation assistance; skills, simulation, or other laboratory; tutoring; unpaid internships.

Library Facilities 1.8 million volumes (1,800 in health, 1,000 in nursing); 185 periodical subscriptions (40 health-care related).

BACCALAUREATE PROGRAMS

Degree BSN

Available Programs ADN to Baccalaureate; Accelerated LPN to Baccalaureate; Generic Baccalaureate; LPN to Baccalaureate; LPN to RN Baccalaureate; RN Baccalaureate.

Study Options Full-time and part-time.

Program Entrance Requirements Minimum overall college GPA of 2.5, transcript of college record, 2 years high school math, high school transcript, immunizations, minimum high school GPA of 2.5, minimum high school rank 50%, minimum GPA in nursing prerequisites of 2.5. Transfer students are accepted. **Standardized tests** *Required:* SAT or ACT, TOEFL for international students. **Application** *Deadline:* rolling (freshmen), rolling (transfer). *Notification:* continuous (freshmen).

Advanced Placement Credit given for nursing courses completed elsewhere dependent upon specific evaluations.

Expenses (2004–05) *Tuition:* full-time $14,500. *Room and board:* $5625; room only: $2575 per academic year. *Required fees:* full-time $200.

Financial Aid 95% of baccalaureate students in nursing programs received some form of financial aid in 2003–04.

Contact Devonna L. Dugan, Administrative Assistant, Department of Nursing, MacMurray College, 447 East College Avenue, Jacksonville, IL 62650. *Telephone:* 217-479-7083. *Fax:* 217-479-7078. *E-mail:* nursing.dept@mac.edu.

McKendree College
Department of Nursing
Lebanon, Illinois

Founded in 1828

DEGREE • BSN

Nursing Program Faculty 12 (60% with doctorates).

Baccalaureate Enrollment 195
Women 94% **Men** 6% **Minority** 9% **Part-time** 94%

Nursing Student Activities Nursing Honor Society.

Nursing Student Resources Academic advising; academic or career counseling; bookstore; campus computer network; career placement assistance; computer lab; computer-assisted instruction; e-mail services; Internet; learning resource lab; library services; nursing audiovisuals; resume preparation assistance; tutoring.

Library Facilities 105,000 volumes (1,921 in health, 732 in nursing); 450 periodical subscriptions (67 health-care related).

BACCALAUREATE PROGRAMS

Degree BSN

Available Programs ADN to Baccalaureate.

Site Options Marion, IL; Louisville, KY; Paducah, KY.

Program Entrance Requirements Minimum overall college GPA of 2.0, transcript of college record, CPR certification, health exam, high school transcript, immunizations, prerequisite course work, RN licensure. Transfer students are accepted. **Standardized tests** *Required:* SAT or ACT, TOEFL for international students. **Application** *Deadline:* rolling (freshmen), rolling (transfer). *Notification:* continuous (freshmen). *Application fee:* $40.

Advanced Placement Credit given for nursing courses completed elsewhere dependent upon specific evaluations.

Expenses (2004–05) *Tuition:* part-time $250 per credit hour.

Financial Aid 90% of baccalaureate students in nursing programs received some form of financial aid in 2003–04. *Gift aid (need-based):* Federal Pell, FSEOG, state, private, college/university gift aid from institutional funds. *Loans:* FFEL (Subsidized and Unsubsidized Stafford PLUS), Perkins. *Work-Study:* Federal Work-Study. *Application deadline (priority):* 5/31.

Contact Kim Niebling, Associate Director of Nursing Admissions, Department of Nursing, McKendree College, 701 College Road, Lebanon, IL 62254. *Telephone:* 800-232-7228 Ext. 6411. *Fax:* 618-537-6259.

Millikin University
School of Nursing
Decatur, Illinois

Founded in 1901

DEGREE • BSN

Nursing Program Faculty 9 (67% with doctorates).

Baccalaureate Enrollment 151
Women 92% **Men** 8% **Minority** 15% **Part-time** 2%

Nursing Student Activities Nursing Honor Society, Student Nurses' Association.

Nursing Student Resources Academic advising; academic or career counseling; assistance for students with disabilities; bookstore; campus computer network; career placement assistance; computer lab; computer-assisted instruction; e-mail services; employment services for current students; housing assistance; interactive nursing skills videos; Internet; learning resource lab; library services; nursing audiovisuals; other; remedial services; resume preparation assistance; skills, simulation, or other laboratory; tutoring; unpaid internships.

Library Facilities 199,660 volumes (10,000 in health, 6,000 in nursing); 927 periodical subscriptions (64 health-care related).

BACCALAUREATE PROGRAMS

Degree BSN

Available Programs Accelerated RN Baccalaureate; Generic Baccalaureate.

Study Options Full-time and part-time.

Program Entrance Requirements Minimum overall college GPA of 2.3, transcript of college record, CPR certification, health exam, high school biology, high school chemistry, 2 years high school math, 2 years high school science, high school transcript, immunizations, minimum high school GPA of 3.0, minimum high school rank 25%, minimum GPA in nursing prerequisites of 2.3. Transfer students are accepted. **Standardized tests** *Required:* SAT or ACT, TOEFL for international students. **Application** *Deadline:* rolling (freshmen). *Notification:* continuous (freshmen).

Advanced Placement Credit given for nursing courses completed elsewhere dependent upon specific evaluations.

Expenses (2003–04) *Tuition:* full-time $18,834; part-time $535 per credit hour. *Room and board:* $6321; room only: $3513 per academic year. *Required fees:* full-time $400.

Financial Aid 95% of baccalaureate students in nursing programs received some form of financial aid in 2002–03.

Contact Dr. Kathy J. Booker, RN, Dean, School of Nursing, Millikin University, 1184 West Main Street, Decatur, IL 62522. *Telephone:* 217-424-6393. *Fax:* 217-420-6731. *E-mail:* kbooker@mail.millikin.edu.

Northern Illinois University
School of Nursing
De Kalb, Illinois

http://www.nursing.niu.edu

Founded in 1895

DEGREES • BS • MS • MSN/MPH

Nursing Program Faculty 40 (52% with doctorates).

Baccalaureate Enrollment 364
Women 96% **Men** 4% **Minority** 25% **Part-time** 31%

Graduate Enrollment 122
Women 97% **Men** 3% **Minority** 21% **Part-time** 86%

Nursing Student Activities Nursing Honor Society, Sigma Theta Tau, Student Nurses' Association, nursing club.

Nursing Student Resources Academic advising; academic or career counseling; assistance for students with disabilities; bookstore; campus computer network; career placement assistance; computer lab; computer-assisted instruction; daycare for children of students; e-mail services; employment services for current students; externships; housing assistance; interactive nursing skills videos; Internet; learning resource lab; library services; nursing audiovisuals; paid internships; placement services for program completers; remedial services; resume preparation assistance; skills, simulation, or other laboratory; tutoring; unpaid internships.

Library Facilities 3.1 million volumes (39,869 in health, 7,600 in nursing); 24,696 periodical subscriptions (676 health-care related).

BACCALAUREATE PROGRAMS

Degree BS

Available Programs Generic Baccalaureate; RN Baccalaureate.

Site Options *Distance Learning:* Highland , IL; Rockford, IL; Hoffman Estates, IL.

Study Options Full-time and part-time.

Program Entrance Requirements Transcript of college record, CPR certification, health exam, health insurance, high school transcript, immunizations, minimum high school rank 50%, professional liability insurance/malpractice insurance. Transfer students are accepted. **Standardized tests** *Required:* SAT or ACT, TOEFL for international students. **Application** *Deadline:* 8/1 (freshmen), 8/1 (transfer). *Notification:* continuous (freshmen).

Advanced Placement Credit given for nursing courses completed elsewhere dependent upon specific evaluations.

Expenses (2003–04) *Tuition, state resident:* full-time $3106; part-time $133 per contact hour. *Tuition, nonresident:* full-time $6212; part-time $264 per contact hour. *International tuition:* $6212 full-time. *Room and board:* $7780; room only: $4352 per academic year. *Required fees:* full-time $1230; part-time $48 per credit; part-time $571 per term.

Financial Aid 76% of baccalaureate students in nursing programs received some form of financial aid in 2002–03. *Gift aid (need-based):* Federal Pell, FSEOG, state, private, college/university gift aid from institutional funds, Federal Nursing. *Loans:* FFEL (Subsidized and Unsubsidized Stafford PLUS), Perkins, college/university. *Work-Study:* Federal Work-Study, part-time campus jobs. *Application deadline (priority):* 3/1.

Contact Ms. Constance Uhlken, RN, Undergraduate Academic Adviser, School of Nursing, Northern Illinois University, 1240 Normal Road, De Kalb, IL 60115. *Telephone:* 815-753-6557. *Fax:* 815-753-0814. *E-mail:* cuhlken@niu.edu.

GRADUATE PROGRAMS

Expenses (2003–04) *Tuition, state resident:* full-time $3968; part-time $165 per contact hour. *Tuition, nonresident:* full-time $7937; part-time $331 per contact hour. *Room and board:* $7780; room only: $4352 per academic year. *Required fees:* full-time $1680; part-time $52 per credit; part-time $840 per term.

Financial Aid 72% of graduate students in nursing programs received some form of financial aid in 2002–03. 9 research assistantships with full tuition reimbursements available, 1 teaching assistantship with full tuition reimbursement available were awarded; fellowships with full tuition reimbursements available, career-related internships or fieldwork, Federal Work-Study, scholarships, tuition waivers (full), and unspecified assistantships also available. Aid available to part-time students.

Contact Dr. Marilyn Frank Stromberg, Chair, School of Nursing, Northern Illinois University, 1240 Normal Road, De Kalb, IL 60115-2864. *Telephone:* 815-753-6557. *Fax:* 815-753-0814. *E-mail:* gradadvisor@niu.edu.

MASTER'S DEGREE PROGRAM

Degrees MS; MSN/MPH

Available Programs Master's.

Concentrations Available *Clinical nurse specialist programs in:* adult health, community health. *Nurse practitioner programs in:* adult health, family health.

Site Options *Distance Learning:* Rockford, IL; Hoffman Estates, IL.

Study Options Full-time and part-time.

Program Entrance Requirements Minimum overall college GPA of 3.0, transcript of college record, CPR certification, written essay, immunizations, 2 letters of recommendation, nursing research course, physical assessment course, professional liability insurance/malpractice insurance, statistics course. *Application deadline:* For fall admission, 6/1; for spring admission, 11/1. Applications are processed on a rolling basis. *Application fee:* $30.

Degree Requirements 48 total credit hours.

POST-MASTER'S PROGRAM

Areas of Study *Nurse practitioner programs in:* family health.

North Park University

School of Nursing
Chicago, Illinois

http://www.northpark.edu

Founded in 1891

DEGREES • BS • MS • MSN/MA • MSN/MBA

Nursing Program Faculty 23 (65% with doctorates).

Baccalaureate Enrollment 71
Women 86% **Men** 14% **Minority** 42% **International** 4% **Part-time** 27%

Graduate Enrollment 128
Women 95% **Men** 5% **Minority** 27% **Part-time** 73%

Nursing Student Activities Sigma Theta Tau, Student Nurses' Association.

Nursing Student Resources Academic advising; academic or career counseling; bookstore; campus computer network; career placement assistance; computer lab; computer-assisted instruction; e-mail services; employment services for current students; interactive nursing skills videos; Internet; learning resource lab; library services; nursing audiovisuals; remedial services; skills, simulation, or other laboratory; tutoring.

Library Facilities 260,685 volumes (3,959 in health, 1,791 in nursing); 1,178 periodical subscriptions (239 health-care related).

BACCALAUREATE PROGRAMS

Degree BS

Available Programs Generic Baccalaureate.

Site Options Arlington Heights, IL.

Study Options Full-time.

Program Entrance Requirements Minimum overall college GPA of 2.75, transcript of college record, CPR certification, health exam, health insurance, immunizations, minimum GPA in nursing prerequisites of 2.75, prerequisite course work. Transfer students are accepted. **Standardized tests** *Required:* SAT or ACT, TOEFL for international students. **Application** *Deadline:* rolling (freshmen), rolling (transfer). *Notification:* continuous (freshmen). *Application fee:* $20.

Expenses (2003–04) *Tuition:* full-time $19,470; part-time $650 per credit hour. *International tuition:* $19,470 full-time. *Room and board:* $6260; room only: $3510 per academic year. *Required fees:* part-time $90 per credit.

Financial Aid 92% of baccalaureate students in nursing programs received some form of financial aid in 2002–03.

Contact Mr. Trevor James, Senior Admissions Counselor, School of Nursing, North Park University, 3225 West Foster Avenue, Chicago, IL 60625. *Telephone:* 773-244-5508. *Fax:* 773-244-4953. *E-mail:* tjames@northpark.edu.

GRADUATE PROGRAMS

Expenses (2003–04) *Tuition:* part-time $490 per credit hour.

Financial Aid 95% of graduate students in nursing programs received some form of financial aid in 2002–03.

Contact Mr. Trevor James, Graduate and Continuing Studies Admission, School of Nursing, North Park University, 3225 West Foster Avenue, Chicago, IL 60625. *Telephone:* 773-244-5508. *Fax:* 773-279-7994. *E-mail:* tjames@northpark.edu.

MASTER'S DEGREE PROGRAM

Degrees MS; MSN/MA; MSN/MBA

Available Programs Master's.

Concentrations Available Health-care administration. *Clinical nurse specialist programs in:* community health. *Nurse practitioner programs in:* adult health.

Site Options Arlington Heights, IL.

Study Options Full-time and part-time.

Program Entrance Requirements Clinical experience, minimum overall college GPA of 3.0, transcript of college record, CPR certification, immunizations, 2 letters of recommendation, nursing research course, physical assessment course, professional liability insurance/malpractice insurance, prerequisite course work, resume, statistics course.

Degree Requirements 37 total credit hours, thesis or project.

POST-MASTER'S PROGRAM

Areas of Study *Nurse practitioner programs in:* adult health.

Olivet Nazarene University

Division of Nursing
Bourbonnais, Illinois

http://www.olivet.edu/academics/divisions/nursing

Founded in 1907

DEGREES • BSN • MSN

Nursing Program Faculty 9 (44% with doctorates).

Baccalaureate Enrollment 266
Women 98% **Men** 2% **Minority** 21% **International** 1% **Part-time** 1%

Graduate Enrollment 6
Women 100% **Minority** 50%

Olivet Nazarene University (continued)

Nursing Student Activities Sigma Theta Tau, nursing club.

Nursing Student Resources Academic advising; academic or career counseling; assistance for students with disabilities; bookstore; campus computer network; career placement assistance; computer lab; computer-assisted instruction; e-mail services; employment services for current students; externships; housing assistance; interactive nursing skills videos; Internet; learning resource lab; library services; nursing audiovisuals; placement services for program completers; remedial services; resume preparation assistance; skills, simulation, or other laboratory; tutoring.

Library Facilities 160,039 volumes (8,847 in health, 5,489 in nursing); 925 periodical subscriptions (722 health-care related).

BACCALAUREATE PROGRAMS

Degree BSN

Available Programs Accelerated RN Baccalaureate; Generic Baccalaureate.

Site Options Chicago, IL; Libertyville, IL; Chicago Heights, IL.

Study Options Full-time and part-time.

Program Entrance Requirements Transcript of college record, CPR certification, health exam, health insurance, high school biology, high school chemistry, 2 years high school science, high school transcript, immunizations, 2 letters of recommendation. Transfer students are accepted. **Standardized tests** *Required:* ACT, TOEFL for international students. **Application** *Deadline:* rolling (freshmen), rolling (transfer). *Notification:* continuous (freshmen).

Advanced Placement Credit by examination available. Credit given for nursing courses completed elsewhere dependent upon specific evaluations.

Expenses (2004–05) *Tuition:* full-time $14,900; part-time $414 per credit hour. *International tuition:* $14,900 full-time. *Room and board:* $5800 per academic year. *Required fees:* full-time $1070.

Financial Aid 98% of baccalaureate students in nursing programs received some form of financial aid in 2003–04. *Gift aid (need-based):* Federal Pell, FSEOG, state, private, college/university gift aid from institutional funds. *Loans:* FFEL (Subsidized and Unsubsidized Stafford PLUS), Perkins, alternative loans. *Work-Study:* Federal Work-Study, part-time campus jobs. *Application deadline (priority):* 3/1.

Contact Mr. Brian Parker, Director of Admissions, Division of Nursing, Olivet Nazarene University, One University Avenue, Bourbonnais, IL 60914-2345. *Telephone:* 815-939-5203. *Fax:* 815-939-5203. *E-mail:* bparker@olivet.edu.

GRADUATE PROGRAMS

Expenses (2004–05) *Tuition:* full-time $8064; part-time $448 per credit hour. *International tuition:* $8064 full-time. *Required fees:* full-time $363.

Financial Aid 84% of graduate students in nursing programs received some form of financial aid in 2003–04.

Contact Mr. Spencer Barnard, Director of Enrollment Development, Division of Nursing, Olivet Nazarene University, One University Avenue, Bourbonnais, IL 60914-2345. *Telephone:* 815-939-5003. *Fax:* 815-935-4991. *E-mail:* sbarnard@olivet.edu.

MASTER'S DEGREE PROGRAM

Degree MSN

Available Programs Master's.

Concentrations Available Health-care administration; nursing education. *Clinical nurse specialist programs in:* community health, family health.

Study Options Full-time.

Program Entrance Requirements Minimum overall college GPA of 2.5, transcript of college record, CPR certification, immunizations, professional liability insurance/malpractice insurance, statistics course.

Degree Requirements 36 total credit hours, thesis or project.

Quincy University

Blessing–Rieman College of Nursing
Quincy, Illinois

http://www.quincy.edu/

See description of programs under Blessing–Rieman College of Nursing (Quincy, Illinois).

Rockford College

Department of Nursing
Rockford, Illinois

http://www.rockford.edu

Founded in 1847

DEGREE • BSN

Nursing Program Faculty 5.

Baccalaureate Enrollment 122

Women 89% **Men** 11% **Minority** 16% **Part-time** 14%

Nursing Student Activities Student Nurses' Association.

Nursing Student Resources Academic advising; academic or career counseling; assistance for students with disabilities; bookstore; campus computer network; career placement assistance; computer lab; computer-assisted instruction; e-mail services; employment services for current students; externships; housing assistance; interactive nursing skills videos; Internet; learning resource lab; library services; nursing audiovisuals; paid internships; placement services for program completers; remedial services; resume preparation assistance; skills, simulation, or other laboratory; tutoring.

Library Facilities 140,000 volumes (655 in health, 600 in nursing); 831 periodical subscriptions (55 health-care related).

BACCALAUREATE PROGRAMS

Degree BSN

Available Programs ADN to Baccalaureate; Generic Baccalaureate; RN Baccalaureate.

Site Options Rockford, IL.

Study Options Full-time and part-time.

Program Entrance Requirements Minimum overall college GPA of 2.75, transcript of college record, CPR certification, health exam, health insurance, high school biology, high school chemistry, 2 years high school math, 2 years high school science, high school transcript, immunizations, interview, minimum high school GPA of 2.75, minimum high school rank 50%, minimum GPA in nursing prerequisites of 2.75, prerequisite course work. Transfer students are accepted. **Standardized tests** *Required:* SAT or ACT, TOEFL for international students. **Application** *Deadline:* rolling (freshmen), rolling (transfer). *Application fee:* $35.

Advanced Placement Credit given for nursing courses completed elsewhere dependent upon specific evaluations.

Expenses (2004–05) *Tuition:* full-time $21. *Room and board:* $6780 per academic year.

Financial Aid 90% of baccalaureate students in nursing programs received some form of financial aid in 2003–04. *Gift aid (need-based):* Federal Pell, FSEOG, state, private, college/university gift aid from institutional funds. *Loans:* FFEL (Subsidized and Unsubsidized Stafford PLUS), Perkins, college/university, alternative loans. *Work-Study:* Federal Work-Study, part-time campus jobs. *Application deadline (priority):* 3/15.

Contact Mr. Michael Plocinski, Director of Admissions, Department of Nursing, Rockford College, 5050 East State Street, Rockford, IL 61108-2393. *Telephone:* 815-226-4050. *Fax:* 815-226-2822. *E-mail:* mplocinski@rockford.edu.

Rush University
College of Nursing
Chicago, Illinois

http://www.rushu.rush.edu/nursing

Founded in 1969

DEGREES • BSN • DN SC • MSN • MSN/MBA

Nursing Program Faculty 85 (75% with doctorates).

Baccalaureate Enrollment 160
Women 90% **Men** 10% **Minority** 22% **International** 1% **Part-time** 7%

Graduate Enrollment 263
Women 90% **Men** 10% **Minority** 15% **International** 1% **Part-time** 76%

Nursing Student Activities Nursing Honor Society, Sigma Theta Tau, Student Nurses' Association.

Nursing Student Resources Academic advising; academic or career counseling; assistance for students with disabilities; bookstore; campus computer network; computer lab; computer-assisted instruction; daycare for children of students; e-mail services; employment services for current students; housing assistance; interactive nursing skills videos; Internet; learning resource lab; library services; nursing audiovisuals; other; resume preparation assistance; skills, simulation, or other laboratory; tutoring.

Library Facilities 120,042 volumes (120,000 in health); 1,100 periodical subscriptions (2,000 health-care related).

BACCALAUREATE PROGRAMS

Degree BSN

Available Programs ADN to Baccalaureate; Accelerated Baccalaureate for Second Degree; Generic Baccalaureate; RN Baccalaureate.

Study Options Full-time.

Program Entrance Requirements Minimum overall college GPA of 2.75, transcript of college record, written essay, health exam, immunizations, 3 letters of recommendation, minimum GPA in nursing prerequisites of 2.75, prerequisite course work. Transfer students are accepted. **Standardized tests** *Required:* TOEFL for international students. **Application** *Deadline:* rolling (transfer). *Application fee:* $40.

Advanced Placement Credit by examination available. Credit given for nursing courses completed elsewhere dependent upon specific evaluations.

Expenses (2004–05) *Tuition:* full-time $19,656; part-time $486 per credit hour. *Room and board:* room only: $9600 per academic year.

Financial Aid 82% of baccalaureate students in nursing programs received some form of financial aid in 2003–04. *Gift aid (need-based):* Federal Pell, FSEOG, state, private, college/university gift aid from institutional funds. *Loans:* Federal Nursing Student Loans, FFEL (Subsidized and Unsubsidized Stafford PLUS), Perkins, state, college/university, credit-based loans. *Work-Study:* Federal Work-Study, part-time campus jobs. *Application deadline:* 5/1 (priority: 3/1).

Contact Ms. Hicela Castruita-Woods, College Admissions Services, College of Nursing, Rush University, 600 South Paulina Street, Armour Academic Center, Room 440, Chicago, IL 60612. *Telephone:* 312-942-7100. *Fax:* 312-942-2219. *E-mail:* Rush_Admissions@rush.edu.

GRADUATE PROGRAMS

Expenses (2004–05) *Tuition:* full-time $24,052; part-time $529 per credit hour. *Room and board:* room only: $9600 per academic year.

Financial Aid 60% of graduate students in nursing programs received some form of financial aid in 2003–04. 8 research assistantships (averaging $3,500 per year), 8 teaching assistantships with tuition reimbursements available (averaging $20,000 per year) were awarded; fellowships, Federal Work-Study, institutionally sponsored loans, scholarships, and traineeships also available. Aid available to part-time students.

Contact Ms. Hicela Castruita-Woods, College Admissions Services, College of Nursing, Rush University, 600 South Paulina Street, Armour Academic Center, Room 440, Chicago, IL 60612. *Telephone:* 312-942-7100. *Fax:* 312-942-2219. *E-mail:* Rush_Admissions@rush.edu.

MASTER'S DEGREE PROGRAM

Degrees MSN; MSN/MBA

Available Programs Master's; Master's for Nurses with Non-Nursing Degrees; RN to Master's.

Concentrations Available Nurse anesthesia. *Clinical nurse specialist programs in:* critical care, gerontology, medical-surgical, parent-child, pediatric, psychiatric/mental health, public health. *Nurse practitioner programs in:* acute care, adult health, family health, gerontology, neonatal health, pediatric, psychiatric/mental health.

Study Options Full-time and part-time.

Program Entrance Requirements Minimum overall college GPA of 3.0, transcript of college record, CPR certification, written essay, immunizations, interview, 3 letters of recommendation, resume, GRE General Test. *Application deadline:* For fall admission, 7/1; for winter admission, 11/1; for spring admission, 1/15. Applications are processed on a rolling basis. *Application fee:* $40.

Advanced Placement Credit by examination available. Credit given for nursing courses completed elsewhere dependent upon specific evaluations.

Degree Requirements 55 total credit hours, thesis or project.

POST-MASTER'S PROGRAM

Areas of Study Nurse anesthesia. *Clinical nurse specialist programs in:* critical care, gerontology, medical-surgical, parent-child, pediatric, psychiatric/mental health, public health. *Nurse practitioner programs in:* acute care, adult health, family health, gerontology, neonatal health, pediatric, psychiatric/mental health.

DOCTORAL DEGREE PROGRAM

Degree DN Sc

Available Programs Doctorate; Post-Baccalaureate Doctorate.

Areas of Study Addiction/substance abuse, advanced practice nursing, aging, bio-behavioral research, biology of health and illness, clinical practice, community health, critical care, ethics, family health, gerontology, health policy, health promotion/disease prevention, health-care systems, human health and illness, illness and transition, individualized study, maternity-newborn, neuro-behavior, nursing policy, nursing research, oncology, urban health, women's health.

Program Entrance Requirements Minimum overall college GPA of 3.25, interview, 3 letters of recommendation, MSN or equivalent, statistics course, vita, writing sample, GRE General Test. *Application deadline:* For fall admission, 7/1; for winter admission, 11/1; for spring admission, 1/15. Applications are processed on a rolling basis. *Application fee:* $40.

Degree Requirements 70 total credit hours, dissertation, oral exam.

POSTDOCTORAL PROGRAM

Areas of Study Aging, cancer care, chronic illness, community health, family health, gerontology, health promotion/disease prevention, individualized study, neuro-behavior, nursing interventions, nursing research, outcomes, vulnerable population, women's health.

Postdoctoral Program Contact Dr. Ann Minnick, Associate Dean for Research, College of Nursing, Rush University, 600 South Paulina Street, 1062A AR, Chicago, IL 60612. *Telephone:* 312-942-6990. *Fax:* 312-942-3038. *E-mail:* Ann_F_Minnick@rush.edu.

CONTINUING EDUCATION PROGRAM

Contact Dr. Ruth Kleinpell, College of Nursing, Rush University, 600 South Paulina Street, Suite 1080 AR, Chicago, IL 60612-3832. *Telephone:* 312-942-7117. *Fax:* 312-942-3043. *E-mail:* Ruth_Kleinpell@rush.edu.

Saint Anthony College of Nursing
Saint Anthony College of Nursing
Rockford, Illinois

http://www.sacn.edu

Founded in 1915

DEGREE • BSN

Nursing Program Faculty 13 (8% with doctorates).

Baccalaureate Enrollment 113
Women 89% **Men** 11% **Minority** 12% **Part-time** 17%

Saint Anthony College of Nursing (continued)

Nursing Student Activities Student Nurses' Association.

Nursing Student Resources Academic advising; academic or career counseling; campus computer network; computer lab; computer-assisted instruction; e-mail services; interactive nursing skills videos; Internet; learning resource lab; library services; paid internships; skills, simulation, or other laboratory; tutoring.

Library Facilities 1,394 volumes (1,280 in health, 980 in nursing); 3,136 periodical subscriptions (5,160 health-care related).

BACCALAUREATE PROGRAMS

Degree BSN

Available Programs Baccalaureate for Second Degree; Generic Baccalaureate; RN Baccalaureate.

Site Options Woodstock, IL.

Study Options Full-time and part-time.

Program Entrance Requirements Minimum overall college GPA of 2.5, transcript of college record, CPR certification, written essay, health exam, health insurance, immunizations, interview, 3 letters of recommendation, prerequisite course work. Transfer students are accepted. **Application** *Deadline:* 8/15 (transfer). *Application fee:* $50.

Advanced Placement Credit by examination available. Credit given for nursing courses completed elsewhere dependent upon specific evaluations.

Expenses (2004–05) *Tuition:* full-time $14,700; part-time $460 per credit hour. *Required fees:* full-time $112; part-time $50 per term.

Financial Aid 87% of baccalaureate students in nursing programs received some form of financial aid in 2003–04.

Contact Ms. Cheryl Delgado, Admissions Representative, Saint Anthony College of Nursing, 5658 East State Street, Rockford, IL 61108-2468. *Telephone:* 815-227-2141. *Fax:* 815-227-2730. *E-mail:* cheryldelgado@sacn.edu.

See full description on page 538.

Saint Francis Medical Center College of Nursing

Baccalaureate Nursing Program
Peoria, Illinois

http://www.sfmccon.edu

Founded in 1986

DEGREES • BSN • MSN

Nursing Program Faculty 27 (26% with doctorates).

Baccalaureate Enrollment 223

Women 91% **Men** 9% **Minority** 3% **Part-time** 17%

Graduate Enrollment 47

Women 89% **Men** 11% **Minority** 1% **Part-time** 94%

Nursing Student Activities Nursing Honor Society, Student Nurses' Association.

Nursing Student Resources Academic advising; academic or career counseling; campus computer network; computer lab; computer-assisted instruction; e-mail services; housing assistance; interactive nursing skills videos; Internet; learning resource lab; library services; nursing audiovisuals; skills, simulation, or other laboratory; tutoring.

Library Facilities 6,215 volumes (2,228 in nursing); 125 periodical subscriptions (130 health-care related).

BACCALAUREATE PROGRAMS

Degree BSN

Available Programs ADN to Baccalaureate; Generic Baccalaureate.

Study Options Full-time and part-time.

Program Entrance Requirements Transcript of college record, CPR certification, written essay, health exam, high school transcript, immunizations, minimum GPA in nursing prerequisites of 2.5, professional liability insurance/malpractice insurance, prerequisite course work. Transfer students are accepted. **Application** *Deadline:* rolling (transfer). *Application fee:* $50.

Advanced Placement Credit given for nursing courses completed elsewhere dependent upon specific evaluations.

Expenses (2004–05) *Tuition:* full-time $9888; part-time $412 per credit hour. *International tuition:* $9888 full-time. *Room and board:* room only: $1880 per academic year. *Required fees:* full-time $440; part-time $220 per term.

Financial Aid 94% of baccalaureate students in nursing programs received some form of financial aid in 2003–04.

Contact Ms. Janice E. Farquharson, Director of Admissions/Registrar, Baccalaureate Nursing Program, Saint Francis Medical Center College of Nursing, 511 NE Greenleaf Street, Peoria, IL 61603-3783. *Telephone:* 309-624-8980. *Fax:* 309-624-8973. *E-mail:* janice.farquharson@osfhealthcare.org.

GRADUATE PROGRAMS

Expenses (2004–05) *Tuition:* part-time $412 per credit hour. *Room and board:* room only: $1880 per academic year.

Financial Aid 67% of graduate students in nursing programs received some form of financial aid in 2003–04.

Contact Dr. Janice F. Boundy, Associate Dean of Graduate Program, Baccalaureate Nursing Program, Saint Francis Medical Center College of Nursing, 511 NE Greenleaf Street, Peoria, IL 61603. *Telephone:* 309-655-2230. *Fax:* 309-655-3648. *E-mail:* jan.f.boundy@osfhealthcare.org.

MASTER'S DEGREE PROGRAM

Degree MSN

Available Programs Master's; Master's for Nurses with Non-Nursing Degrees; RN to Master's.

Concentrations Available Nursing education. *Clinical nurse specialist programs in:* medical-surgical.

Study Options Full-time and part-time.

Program Entrance Requirements Clinical experience, computer literacy, minimum overall college GPA of 2.8, transcript of college record, CPR certification, written essay, immunizations, interview, 3 letters of recommendation, nursing research course, physical assessment course, professional liability insurance/malpractice insurance, prerequisite course work, statistics course.

Advanced Placement Credit given for nursing courses completed elsewhere dependent upon specific evaluations.

Degree Requirements 45 total credit hours, thesis or project.

St. John's College

Department of Nursing
Springfield, Illinois

http://www.st-johns.org/collegeofnursing

Founded in 1886

DEGREE • BSN

Nursing Program Faculty 15 (13% with doctorates).

Baccalaureate Enrollment 81

Women 93% **Men** 7% **Minority** 4% **International** 1% **Part-time** 5%

Nursing Student Activities Student Nurses' Association.

Nursing Student Resources Academic advising; computer lab; daycare for children of students; interactive nursing skills videos; Internet; library services; resume preparation assistance; skills, simulation, or other laboratory.

Library Facilities 7,715 volumes; 349 periodical subscriptions.

BACCALAUREATE PROGRAMS

Degree BSN

Available Programs Generic Baccalaureate.

Study Options Full-time and part-time.

Program Entrance Requirements Transcript of college record, CPR certification, health exam, high school transcript, immunizations, 2 letters of recommendation, minimum GPA in nursing prerequisites of 2.4, professional liability insurance/malpractice insurance, prerequisite course work. Transfer students are accepted. **Application** *Application fee:* $25.

Advanced Placement Credit given for nursing courses completed elsewhere dependent upon specific evaluations.

Expenses (2004–05) *Tuition:* full-time $9504; part-time $396 per credit hour. *Required fees:* full-time $366; part-time $183 per credit.

Financial Aid 63% of baccalaureate students in nursing programs received some form of financial aid in 2003–04.

Contact Beth Beasley, Student Development Office, Department of Nursing, St. John's College, 421 North Ninth Street, Springfield, IL 62702. *Telephone:* 217-525-5628. *Fax:* 217-757-6870. *E-mail:* bbeasley@st-johns.org.

Saint Xavier University

School of Nursing
Chicago, Illinois

http://www.sxu.edu/son

Founded in 1847

DEGREES • BSN • MSN • MSN/MBA

Nursing Program Faculty 31 (61% with doctorates).

Baccalaureate Enrollment 529

Women 94% **Men** 6% **Minority** 43% **Part-time** 24%

Graduate Enrollment 95

Women 97% **Men** 3% **Minority** 35% **Part-time** 94%

Nursing Student Activities Sigma Theta Tau, Student Nurses' Association.

Nursing Student Resources Academic advising; academic or career counseling; assistance for students with disabilities; bookstore; campus computer network; career placement assistance; computer lab; computer-assisted instruction; daycare for children of students; e-mail services; employment services for current students; externships; interactive nursing skills videos; Internet; learning resource lab; library services; nursing audiovisuals; placement services for program completers; remedial services; resume preparation assistance; skills, simulation, or other laboratory; tutoring.

Library Facilities 170,753 volumes (7,600 in health, 4,400 in nursing); 717 periodical subscriptions (1,029 health-care related).

BACCALAUREATE PROGRAMS

Degree BSN

Available Programs ADN to Baccalaureate; Generic Baccalaureate; LPN to Baccalaureate.

Site Options Orland Park, IL; Chicago, IL; Elk Grove Village, IL.

Study Options Full-time and part-time.

Program Entrance Requirements Minimum overall college GPA of 2.5, transcript of college record, CPR certification, health exam, health insurance, high school biology, high school chemistry, high school foreign language, 3 years high school math, 3 years high school science, high school transcript, minimum high school GPA of 2.5, minimum GPA in nursing prerequisites of 2.75, prerequisite course work. Transfer students are accepted. **Standardized tests** *Required:* SAT or ACT, TOEFL for international students. **Application** *Deadline:* rolling (freshmen), rolling (transfer). *Notification:* continuous (freshmen). *Application fee:* $25.

Advanced Placement Credit by examination available. Credit given for nursing courses completed elsewhere dependent upon specific evaluations.

Expenses (2004–05) *Tuition:* full-time $17,150; part-time $575 per credit hour. *International tuition:* $17,150 full-time. *Room and board:* $6724 per academic year. *Required fees:* full-time $430; part-time $215 per term.

Financial Aid 83% of baccalaureate students in nursing programs received some form of financial aid in 2003–04. *Gift aid (need-based):* Federal Pell, FSEOG, state, private, college/university gift aid from institutional funds. *Loans:* FFEL (Subsidized and Unsubsidized Stafford PLUS), Perkins. *Work-Study:* Federal Work-Study, part-time campus jobs. *Application deadline (priority):* 3/1.

Contact Dr. Phyllis Baker, Assistant Dean, Undergraduate Nursing Program, School of Nursing, Saint Xavier University, 3700 West 103rd Street, Chicago, IL 60655. *Telephone:* 773-298-3707. *Fax:* 773-298-3704. *E-mail:* baker@sxu.edu.

GRADUATE PROGRAMS

Expenses (2004–05) *Tuition:* full-time $13,200; part-time $550 per credit hour. *International tuition:* $13,200 full-time. *Room and board:* $6724 per academic year. *Required fees:* full-time $320; part-time $160 per term.

Financial Aid 18% of graduate students in nursing programs received some form of financial aid in 2003–04. Available to part-time students.

Contact Dr. Ann Filipski, Assistant Dean, Graduate Program, School of Nursing, Saint Xavier University, 3700 West 103rd Street, Chicago, IL 60655. *Telephone:* 773-298-3708. *Fax:* 773-298-3704. *E-mail:* filipski@sxu.edu.

MASTER'S DEGREE PROGRAM

Degrees MSN; MSN/MBA

Available Programs Master's; Master's for Nurses with Non-Nursing Degrees; RN to Master's.

Concentrations Available Nursing administration. *Clinical nurse specialist programs in:* adult health, community health, psychiatric/mental health. *Nurse practitioner programs in:* family health.

Site Options Chicago, IL; Elk Grove Village, IL.

Study Options Full-time and part-time.

Program Entrance Requirements Minimum overall college GPA of 3.0, transcript of college record, written essay, interview, 2 letters of recommendation, prerequisite course work, GRE General Test or MAT. *Application deadline:* For fall admission, 2/15; for spring admission, 9/15. Applications are processed on a rolling basis. *Application fee:* $35.

Advanced Placement Credit given for nursing courses completed elsewhere dependent upon specific evaluations.

Degree Requirements 46 total credit hours.

POST-MASTER'S PROGRAM

Areas of Study *Nurse practitioner programs in:* family health.

CONTINUING EDUCATION PROGRAM

Contact Dr. Michelle Poradzisz, Continuing Education Director, School of Nursing, Saint Xavier University, 3700 West 103rd Street, Chicago, IL 60655. *Telephone:* 773-298-3730. *Fax:* 773-298-3704. *E-mail:* poradzisz@sxu.edu.

Southern Illinois University Edwardsville

School of Nursing
Edwardsville, Illinois

http://www.siue.edu/NURSING

Founded in 1957

DEGREES • BS • MS

Nursing Program Faculty 57 (38% with doctorates).

Baccalaureate Enrollment 285

Women 79% **Men** 21% **Minority** 19% **International** 2% **Part-time** 16%

Graduate Enrollment 200

Women 63% **Men** 37% **Minority** 21% **International** 4% **Part-time** 48%

Nursing Student Activities Nursing Honor Society, Sigma Theta Tau, Student Nurses' Association, nursing club.

Nursing Student Resources Academic advising; academic or career counseling; assistance for students with disabilities; bookstore; campus computer network; career placement assistance; computer lab; computer-assisted instruction; daycare for children of students; e-mail services; employment services for current students; housing assistance; interactive nursing skills videos; Internet; learning resource lab; library services; nursing audiovisuals; placement services for program completers; remedial services; skills, simulation, or other laboratory; tutoring.

Library Facilities 788,003 volumes; 14,371 periodical subscriptions (281 health-care related).

BACCALAUREATE PROGRAMS

Degree BS

Southern Illinois University Edwardsville (continued)

Available Programs Accelerated Baccalaureate; Generic Baccalaureate; RN Baccalaureate.

Site Options *Distance Learning:* Springfield, IL.

Study Options Full-time.

Program Entrance Requirements Minimum overall college GPA of 2.5, transcript of college record, CPR certification, written essay, health exam, health insurance, high school transcript, immunizations, minimum GPA in nursing prerequisites of 2.7, prerequisite course work. Transfer students are accepted. **Standardized tests** *Required:* SAT or ACT, TOEFL for international students. **Application** *Deadline:* 5/1 (freshmen), 7/22 (transfer). *Notification:* continuous (freshmen). *Application fee:* $30.

Expenses (2004–05) *Tuition, state resident:* full-time $4700; part-time $120 per credit hour. *Tuition, nonresident:* full-time $8500; part-time $240 per credit hour. *International tuition:* $8500 full-time. *Room and board:* $5600; room only: $3250 per academic year. *Required fees:* full-time $750.

Financial Aid 85% of baccalaureate students in nursing programs received some form of financial aid in 2003–04. *Gift aid (need-based):* Federal Pell, FSEOG, state, private, college/university gift aid from institutional funds, Federal Nursing. *Loans:* Federal Nursing Student Loans, Federal Direct (Subsidized and Unsubsidized Stafford PLUS), FFEL, Perkins, college/university, alternative loans. *Work-Study:* Federal Work-Study, part-time campus jobs. *Application deadline (priority):* 3/1.

Contact Mr. Stephen Wayne Held, Director of Student Recruitment, Admissions, Progression, and Retention, School of Nursing, Southern Illinois University Edwardsville, Alumni Hall, Room 2119, Edwardsville, IL 62026. *Telephone:* 618-650-5612. *Fax:* 618-650-3854. *E-mail:* sheld@siue.edu.

GRADUATE PROGRAMS

Expenses (2004–05) *Tuition, state resident:* full-time $4062; part-time $190 per credit hour. *Tuition, nonresident:* full-time $7490; part-time $380 per credit hour. *Room and board:* $3150; room only: $3150 per academic year. *Required fees:* full-time $850.

Financial Aid 70% of graduate students in nursing programs received some form of financial aid in 2003–04. 2 fellowships with full tuition reimbursements available were awarded; research assistantships, teaching assistantships, career-related internships or fieldwork, Federal Work-Study, institutionally sponsored loans, scholarships, traineeships, and unspecified assistantships also available. Aid available to part-time students. *Financial aid application deadline:* 3/1.

Contact Ms. Angela White, Academic Advisor, School of Nursing, Southern Illinois University Edwardsville, Alumni Hall, Room 2107, Edwardsville, IL 62026-1066. *Telephone:* 618-650-3956. *Fax:* 618-650-2522. *E-mail:* angewhi@siue.edu.

MASTER'S DEGREE PROGRAM

Degree MS

Available Programs Master's.

Concentrations Available Health-care administration; nurse anesthesia; nursing education. *Clinical nurse specialist programs in:* community health, medical-surgical, psychiatric/mental health. *Nurse practitioner programs in:* adult health, family health.

Site Options *Distance Learning:* Springfield, IL.

Study Options Full-time and part-time.

Program Entrance Requirements Clinical experience, minimum overall college GPA of 3.0, transcript of college record, CPR certification, immunizations, interview, 3 letters of recommendation, nursing research course, physical assessment course, professional liability insurance/malpractice insurance, prerequisite course work, statistics course. *Application deadline:* For fall admission, 7/20; for spring admission, 12/7. *Application fee:* $25.

Advanced Placement Credit by examination available. Credit given for nursing courses completed elsewhere dependent upon specific evaluations.

Degree Requirements 33 total credit hours, thesis or project, comprehensive exam.

CONTINUING EDUCATION PROGRAM

Contact Dr. Karen Kelly, Coordinator of Continuing Education, School of Nursing, Southern Illinois University Edwardsville, Box 1066, School of Nursing, Edwardsville, IL 62026-1066. *Telephone:* 618-650-3908. *Fax:* 618-650-3854. *E-mail:* kkelly@siue.edu.

Trinity Christian College
Department of Nursing
Palos Heights, Illinois

http://www.trnty/depts/nursing/

Founded in 1959

DEGREE • BSN

Nursing Program Faculty 9 (33% with doctorates).

Baccalaureate Enrollment 111
Women 92% **Men** 8% **Minority** 7% **International** 1% **Part-time** 1%

Nursing Student Activities Student Nurses' Association.

Nursing Student Resources Academic advising; academic or career counseling; assistance for students with disabilities; bookstore; campus computer network; career placement assistance; computer lab; computer-assisted instruction; e-mail services; Internet; learning resource lab; library services; nursing audiovisuals; resume preparation assistance; skills, simulation, or other laboratory; tutoring; unpaid internships.

Library Facilities 77,833 volumes (2,500 in health, 500 in nursing); 437 periodical subscriptions (100 health-care related).

BACCALAUREATE PROGRAMS

Degree BSN

Available Programs Generic Baccalaureate; RN Baccalaureate.

Study Options Full-time.

Program Entrance Requirements Minimum overall college GPA of 2.5, transcript of college record, CPR certification, health exam, health insurance, high school biology, high school chemistry, high school foreign language, 3 years high school math, 2 years high school science, high school transcript, immunizations, minimum high school GPA of 2.2, minimum GPA in nursing prerequisites of 2.5, prerequisite course work. Transfer students are accepted. **Standardized tests** *Required:* SAT or ACT, TOEFL for international students. **Application** *Deadline:* rolling (freshmen). *Notification:* continuous (freshmen). *Application fee:* $20.

Advanced Placement Credit given for nursing courses completed elsewhere dependent upon specific evaluations.

Expenses (2004–05) *Tuition:* full-time $16,250; part-time $545 per credit hour. *International tuition:* $16,250 full-time. *Room and board:* $6044; room only: $3224 per academic year. *Required fees:* full-time $190.

Financial Aid 90% of baccalaureate students in nursing programs received some form of financial aid in 2003–04.

Contact Admissions Office, Department of Nursing, Trinity Christian College, 6601 West College Drive, Palos Heights, IL 60463. *Telephone:* 866-874-6463. *Fax:* 708-385-5665. *E-mail:* admissions@trnty.edu.

University of Illinois at Chicago
College of Nursing
Chicago, Illinois

http://www.uic.edu/nursing

Founded in 1946

DEGREES • BSN • MS • MS/MBA • PHD

Nursing Program Faculty 111 (68% with doctorates).

Baccalaureate Enrollment 200
Women 90% **Men** 10% **Minority** 23% **International** 3% **Part-time** 20%

Graduate Enrollment 480
Women 95% **Men** 5% **Minority** 10% **International** 6%

Nursing Student Activities Sigma Theta Tau, Student Nurses' Association.

Nursing Student Resources Academic advising; assistance for students with disabilities; campus computer network; computer lab; e-mail services; Internet; tutoring.

Library Facilities 2.2 million volumes (500,000 in health); 21,571 periodical subscriptions.

■ The University of Illinois at Chicago College of Nursing, consistently rated among the top 10 colleges of nursing in the United States, continues at the forefront of nursing education and research. In 2003, the College was 3rd in the nation in total NIH research and research training dollars. Graduates guide the nursing practice of tomorrow, create and maintain high-quality health-care delivery systems, and ensure that excellent nursing services are available to the public. Diversity is a characteristic of both the specializations available for study and the students, whose backgrounds and clinical experiences enrich the broad range of topics that are the focus of study and investigation.

BACCALAUREATE PROGRAMS

Degree BSN

Available Programs Generic Baccalaureate; RPN to Baccalaureate.

Site Options *Distance Learning:* Urbana, IL.

Study Options Full-time and part-time.

Program Entrance Requirements Minimum overall college GPA of 2.5, transcript of college record, written essay, 2 letters of recommendation, minimum GPA in nursing prerequisites of 2.5, prerequisite course work. Transfer students are accepted. **Standardized tests** *Required:* SAT or ACT, TOEFL for international students. **Application** *Deadline:* 1/15 (freshmen), 3/1 (transfer). *Notification:* continuous (freshmen). *Application fee:* $40.

Expenses (2004–05) *Tuition, state resident:* full-time $4042; part-time $3023 per semester. *Tuition, nonresident:* full-time $9666; part-time $6772 per semester. *International tuition:* $9666 full-time. *Room and board:* $3500 per academic year.

Financial Aid 65% of baccalaureate students in nursing programs received some form of financial aid in 2003–04. *Gift aid (need-based):* Federal Pell, FSEOG, state, private, college/university gift aid from institutional funds. *Loans:* Federal Nursing Student Loans, Federal Direct (Subsidized and Unsubsidized Stafford PLUS), Perkins, college/university. *Work-Study:* Federal Work-Study, part-time campus jobs. *Application deadline (priority):* 3/1.

Contact Ms. Andrea Schmoyer, Undergraduate Program Coordinator, College of Nursing, University of Illinois at Chicago, 845 South Damen Avenue, Chicago, IL 60612-7350. *Telephone:* 312-996-5786. *Fax:* 312-996-8066. *E-mail:* schmoyer@uic.edu.

GRADUATE PROGRAMS

Expenses (2004–05) *Tuition, state resident:* full-time $6195; part-time $4458 per semester. *Tuition, nonresident:* full-time $11,802; part-time $8196 per semester. *International tuition:* $11,802 full-time. *Room and board:* $3500 per academic year.

Financial Aid 75% of graduate students in nursing programs received some form of financial aid in 2003–04. Fellowships with full tuition reimbursements available, research assistantships with full tuition reimbursements available, teaching assistantships with full tuition reimbursements available, career-related internships or fieldwork, Federal Work-Study, institutionally sponsored loans, scholarships, traineeships, tuition waivers (full and partial), and unspecified assistantships available. Aid available to part-time students. *Financial aid application deadline:* 3/1.

Contact Ms. Kate D. DiAna, Graduate Program Coordinator, College of Nursing, University of Illinois at Chicago, 845 South Damen Avenue, Chicago, IL 60612-7350. *Telephone:* 312-996-2184. *Fax:* 312-996-8066. *E-mail:* kdiana@uic.edu.

MASTER'S DEGREE PROGRAM

Degrees MS; MS/MBA

Available Programs Master's; Master's for Non-Nursing College Graduates.

Concentrations Available Health-care administration; nurse-midwifery; nursing administration; nursing informatics. *Clinical nurse specialist programs in:* acute care, adult health, cardiovascular, community health, family health, gerontology, maternity-newborn, medical-surgical, occupational health, pediatric, perinatal, psychiatric/mental health, public health, school health, women's health. *Nurse practitioner programs in:* acute care, adult health, family health, gerontology, occupational health, pediatric, psychiatric/mental health, school health, women's health.

Site Options *Distance Learning:* Urbana, IL; Peoria, IL; Rockford, IL.

Study Options Full-time and part-time.

Program Entrance Requirements Clinical experience, computer literacy, minimum overall college GPA of 3.0, transcript of college record, CPR certification, written essay, immunizations, interview, 3 letters of recommendation, nursing research course, physical assessment course, prerequisite course work, resume, statistics course, GRE General Test. *Application deadline:* For fall admission, 5/15; for spring admission, 10/15. Applications are processed on a rolling basis. *Application fee:* $40 ($50 for international students).

Advanced Placement Credit given for nursing courses completed elsewhere dependent upon specific evaluations.

Degree Requirements Thesis or project.

POST-MASTER'S PROGRAM

Areas of Study Health-care administration; nurse-midwifery; nursing administration; nursing education; nursing informatics. *Clinical nurse specialist programs in:* acute care, adult health, cardiovascular, family health, gerontology, medical-surgical, occupational health, pediatric, psychiatric/mental health, public health, school health, women's health. *Nurse practitioner programs in:* acute care, adult health, family health, gerontology, occupational health, pediatric, psychiatric/mental health, school health, women's health.

DOCTORAL DEGREE PROGRAM

Degree PhD

Available Programs Doctorate; Post-Baccalaureate Doctorate.

Areas of Study Bio-behavioral research, clinical practice, community health, faculty preparation, family health, gerontology, health policy, health-care systems, individualized study, maternity-newborn, nursing administration, nursing policy, nursing research, nursing science, women's health.

Program Entrance Requirements Minimum overall college GPA of 3.0, interview by faculty committee, interview, 3 letters of recommendation, MSN or equivalent, statistics course, vita, writing sample, GRE General Test. *Application deadline:* For fall admission, 5/15; for spring admission, 10/15. Applications are processed on a rolling basis. *Application fee:* $40 ($50 for international students).

Degree Requirements 96 total credit hours, dissertation.

POSTDOCTORAL PROGRAM

Areas of Study Individualized study, nursing interventions, nursing research, nursing science.

Postdoctoral Program Contact Jan Larson, Department Head, Medical-Surgical Nursing, College of Nursing, University of Illinois at Chicago, 845 South Damen Avenue, Chicago, IL 60612-7350. *Telephone:* 312-996-7900. *E-mail:* jllarson@uic.edu.

CONTINUING EDUCATION PROGRAM

Contact Dr. Beth Brooks, Director, Nursing Institute, College of Nursing, University of Illinois at Chicago, 845 South Damen Avenue, Chicago, IL 60612-7350. *Telephone:* 312-355-3092. *E-mail:* brooksbe@uic.edu.

See full description on page 558.

University of St. Francis

College of Nursing and Allied Health
Joliet, Illinois

http://www.stfrancis.edu/conah/

Founded in 1920

DEGREES • BSN • MSN

Nursing Program Faculty 29 (21% with doctorates).

Baccalaureate Enrollment 366
Women 91% **Men** 9% **Minority** 25% **International** 1% **Part-time** 37%

Graduate Enrollment 40
Women 95% **Men** 5% **Minority** 35% **Part-time** 95%

University of St. Francis (continued)

Nursing Student Activities Nursing Honor Society, Student Nurses' Association.

Nursing Student Resources Academic advising; academic or career counseling; assistance for students with disabilities; bookstore; campus computer network; career placement assistance; computer lab; computer-assisted instruction; e-mail services; employment services for current students; externships; housing assistance; interactive nursing skills videos; Internet; learning resource lab; library services; nursing audiovisuals; remedial services; skills, simulation, or other laboratory; tutoring.

Library Facilities 106,346 volumes (2,689 in health, 824 in nursing); 776 periodical subscriptions (151 health-care related).

BACCALAUREATE PROGRAMS

Degree BSN

Available Programs Accelerated RN Baccalaureate; Generic Baccalaureate.

Study Options Full-time and part-time.

Program Entrance Requirements Minimum overall college GPA of 2.5, transcript of college record, CPR certification, health exam, 2 years high school math, 2 years high school science, high school transcript, immunizations, minimum high school GPA of 2.0, minimum high school rank 50%, minimum GPA in nursing prerequisites of 2.0, prerequisite course work. Transfer students are accepted. **Standardized tests** *Required:* SAT or ACT, TOEFL for international students. **Application** *Deadline:* 8/1 (freshmen). *Notification:* continuous (freshmen). *Application fee:* $20.

Advanced Placement Credit by examination available. Credit given for nursing courses completed elsewhere dependent upon specific evaluations.

Expenses (2004–05) *Tuition:* full-time $17,310; part-time $500 per credit hour. *Room and board:* $6180; room only: $2996 per academic year. *Required fees:* full-time $360; part-time $20 per term.

Financial Aid 87% of baccalaureate students in nursing programs received some form of financial aid in 2003–04. *Gift aid (need-based):* Federal Pell, FSEOG, state, private, college/university gift aid from institutional funds. *Loans:* Federal Direct (Subsidized and Unsubsidized Stafford PLUS), Perkins, alternative loans. *Work-Study:* Federal Work-Study, part-time campus jobs. *Application deadline (priority):* 5/1.

Contact Ms. Caryn Jakielski, Associate Director Graduate/Off-Campus Admissions, College of Nursing and Allied Health, University of St. Francis, 500 Wilcox Street, Joliet, IL 60435. *Telephone:* 866-890-8329. *Fax:* 815-740-3431. *E-mail:* cjakielski@stfrancis.edu.

GRADUATE PROGRAMS

Expenses (2004–05) *Tuition:* part-time $485 per credit hour.

Financial Aid 43% of graduate students in nursing programs received some form of financial aid in 2003–04.

Contact Ms. Caryn Jakielski, Associate Director, Graduate/Off-Campus Admissions, College of Nursing and Allied Health, University of St. Francis, 500 Wilcox Street, Joliet, IL 60435. *Telephone:* 866-890-8329. *Fax:* 815-740-3431. *E-mail:* cjakielski@stfrancis.edu.

MASTER'S DEGREE PROGRAM

Degree MSN

Available Programs Master's for Nurses with Non-Nursing Degrees; RN to Master's.

Concentrations Available Nursing education. *Clinical nurse specialist programs in:* adult health, gerontology, medical-surgical. *Nurse practitioner programs in:* adult health, family health, gerontology.

Site Options Albuquerque, NM.

Study Options Part-time.

Program Entrance Requirements Clinical experience, computer literacy, minimum overall college GPA of 3.0, transcript of college record, CPR certification, written essay, immunizations, interview, 3 letters of recommendation, nursing research course, physical assessment course, professional liability insurance/malpractice insurance, prerequisite course work, resume, statistics course.

Advanced Placement Credit by examination available. Credit given for nursing courses completed elsewhere dependent upon specific evaluations.

Degree Requirements 44 total credit hours, thesis or project.

See full description on page 574.

West Suburban College of Nursing

West Suburban College of Nursing
Oak Park, Illinois

Founded in 1982

DEGREE • BSN

Nursing Program Faculty 12 (15% with doctorates).

Baccalaureate Enrollment 101
Women 92% **Men** 8% **Minority** 30% **Part-time** 15%

Nursing Student Activities Student Nurses' Association, nursing club.

Nursing Student Resources Academic advising; academic or career counseling; bookstore; campus computer network; career placement assistance; computer lab; computer-assisted instruction; e-mail services; employment services for current students; externships; Internet; learning resource lab; library services; nursing audiovisuals; skills, simulation, or other laboratory; tutoring.

Library Facilities 2,400 volumes in health, 1,100 volumes in nursing; 300 periodical subscriptions health-care related.

BACCALAUREATE PROGRAMS

Degree BSN

Available Programs ADN to Baccalaureate; Accelerated Baccalaureate for Second Degree; Baccalaureate for Second Degree; Generic Baccalaureate; RN Baccalaureate.

Study Options Full-time and part-time.

Program Entrance Requirements Minimum overall college GPA of 2.75, transcript of college record, CPR certification, written essay, health exam, health insurance, immunizations, 1 letter of recommendation, minimum GPA in nursing prerequisites of 2.75, prerequisite course work. Transfer students are accepted. **Standardized tests** *Required:* TOEFL for international students. **Application** *Deadline:* rolling (freshmen), rolling (transfer). *Notification:* continuous until 8/21 (freshmen).

Advanced Placement Credit by examination available. Credit given for nursing courses completed elsewhere dependent upon specific evaluations.

Expenses (2004–05) *Tuition:* full-time $18,100; part-time $612 per credit hour. *Required fees:* full-time $340; part-time $170 per term.

Financial Aid 95% of baccalaureate students in nursing programs received some form of financial aid in 2003–04.

Contact Mr. J.C. Crane, Assistant Director of Enrollment Management, West Suburban College of Nursing, Office of Enrollment Management, 3 Erie Court, Oak Park, IL 60302. *Telephone:* 708-763-6507. *Fax:* 708-763-1531. *E-mail:* jc.crane@wscn.edu.

INDIANA

Anderson University

Department of Nursing
Anderson, Indiana

http://www.anderson.edu/academics/nurs/

Founded in 1917

DEGREES • BSN • MSN • MSN/MBA

Nursing Program Faculty 9 (33% with doctorates).

Library Facilities 245,019 volumes (7,500 in health, 6,218 in nursing); 937 periodical subscriptions (892 health-care related).

BACCALAUREATE PROGRAMS

Degree BSN

Available Programs Generic Baccalaureate.

Study Options Full-time and part-time.

Program Entrance Requirements Minimum overall college GPA of 2.5, transcript of college record, CPR certification, health exam, high school chemistry, 2 years high school science, high school transcript, immunizations, 3 letters of recommendation, minimum high school GPA of 3.0, minimum high school rank 33%, minimum GPA in nursing prerequisites of 2.0, professional liability insurance/malpractice insurance, prerequisite course work. Transfer students are accepted. **Standardized tests** *Required:* SAT or ACT. *Recommended:* TOEFL for international students. **Application** *Deadline:* 7/1 (freshmen), 8/25 (transfer). *Notification:* continuous until 9/1 (freshmen). *Application fee:* $20.

Advanced Placement Credit given for nursing courses completed elsewhere dependent upon specific evaluations.

Expenses (2004–05) *Tuition:* full-time $17,995; part-time $750 per credit hour. *International tuition:* $17,995 full-time. *Room and board:* $5820; room only: $3500 per academic year.

Financial Aid 97% of baccalaureate students in nursing programs received some form of financial aid in 2003–04. *Gift aid (need-based):* Federal Pell, FSEOG, state, private, college/university gift aid from institutional funds. *Loans:* FFEL (Subsidized and Unsubsidized Stafford PLUS), Perkins, GATE Loans. *Work-Study:* Federal Work-Study, part-time campus jobs. *Application deadline (priority):* 3/1.

Contact Ms. Kelly Noel, Office Manager and Admissions Counselor, Department of Nursing, Anderson University, 1100 East 5th Street, Anderson, IN 46012. *Telephone:* 765-641-4390. *Fax:* 765-641-3095. *E-mail:* sdailey@anderson.edu.

GRADUATE PROGRAMS

Expenses (2004–05) *Tuition:* full-time $4176; part-time $350 per credit hour. *International tuition:* $4176 full-time.

Financial Aid 100% of graduate students in nursing programs received some form of financial aid in 2003–04.

Contact Paula Boley, Director of MSN/MBA Program, Department of Nursing, Anderson University, 1100 East 5th Street, Anderson, IL 46012. *Telephone:* 765-641-4387. *Fax:* 765-641-3095. *E-mail:* pboley@anderson.edu.

MASTER'S DEGREE PROGRAM

Degrees MSN; MSN/MBA

Available Programs Master's.

Concentrations Available Nursing administration.

Study Options Full-time.

Program Entrance Requirements Clinical experience, minimum overall college GPA of 3.0, transcript of college record, CPR certification, written essay, immunizations, letters of recommendation, prerequisite course work, statistics course.

Advanced Placement Credit given for nursing courses completed elsewhere dependent upon specific evaluations.

Degree Requirements 52 total credit hours, thesis or project.

Ball State University
School of Nursing
Muncie, Indiana

http://www.bsu.edu/nursing

Founded in 1918

DEGREES • BS • MS

Nursing Program Faculty 37 (11% with doctorates).

Baccalaureate Enrollment 215
Women 95% **Men** 5% **Minority** 7%

Graduate Enrollment 234
Women 95% **Men** 5% **Minority** 10% **Part-time** 100%

Nursing Student Activities Nursing Honor Society, Sigma Theta Tau, Student Nurses' Association, nursing club.

Nursing Student Resources Academic advising; academic or career counseling; assistance for students with disabilities; bookstore; campus computer network; career placement assistance; computer lab; computer-assisted instruction; e-mail services; employment services for current students; housing assistance; interactive nursing skills videos; Internet; learning resource lab; library services; nursing audiovisuals; remedial services; resume preparation assistance; skills, simulation, or other laboratory; tutoring.

Library Facilities 1.1 million volumes; 2,937 periodical subscriptions.

BACCALAUREATE PROGRAMS

Degree BS

Available Programs Accelerated Baccalaureate for Second Degree; Generic Baccalaureate; LPN to Baccalaureate; RN Baccalaureate.

Study Options Full-time and part-time.

Program Entrance Requirements Minimum overall college GPA of 2.75, CPR certification, health exam, immunizations, minimum GPA in nursing prerequisites, prerequisite course work. Transfer students are accepted. **Standardized tests** *Required:* TOEFL for international students. *Required for some:* SAT or ACT. **Application** *Deadline:* 5/1 (freshmen), rolling (transfer). *Notification:* continuous (freshmen). *Application fee:* $25.

Expenses (2004–05) *Tuition, state resident:* full-time $5752. *Tuition, nonresident:* full-time $14,928. *Room and board:* $6228 per academic year. *Required fees:* full-time $408.

Financial Aid 90% of baccalaureate students in nursing programs received some form of financial aid in 2003–04. *Gift aid (need-based):* Federal Pell, FSEOG, state, private, college/university gift aid from institutional funds. *Loans:* Federal Direct (Subsidized and Unsubsidized Stafford PLUS), Perkins. *Work-Study:* Federal Work-Study, part-time campus jobs. *Application deadline (priority):* 3/1.

Contact Dr. Nancy Dillard, RN, Associate Director, School of Nursing, Ball State University, Muncie, IN 47306. *Telephone:* 765-285-5570. *Fax:* 765-285-2169. *E-mail:* ndillard@bsu.edu.

GRADUATE PROGRAMS

Expenses (2004–05) *Tuition, state resident:* part-time $192 per credit hour. *Tuition, nonresident:* part-time $325 per credit hour. *Required fees:* full-time $230.

Financial Aid 1 research assistantship (averaging $8,546 per year), 2 teaching assistantships (averaging $8,546 per year) were awarded; career-related internships or fieldwork also available.

Contact Dr. Marilyn Ryan, RN, Associate Director, Graduate Program, School of Nursing, Ball State University, Muncie, IN 47306. *Telephone:* 765-285-5764. *Fax:* 765-285-2169. *E-mail:* mryan@bsu.edu.

MASTER'S DEGREE PROGRAM

Degree MS

Available Programs Master's; RN to Master's.

Concentrations Available Nursing administration; nursing education. *Nurse practitioner programs in:* adult health, family health.

Study Options Part-time.

Program Entrance Requirements Clinical experience, computer literacy, minimum overall college GPA of 2.8, transcript of college record, interview, 2 letters of recommendation, nursing research course, physical assessment course, professional liability insurance/malpractice insurance. *Application fee:* $25 ($35 for international students).

Degree Requirements Thesis or project.

POST-MASTER'S PROGRAM

Areas of Study Nursing administration; nursing education. *Nurse practitioner programs in:* adult health, family health.

Bethel College
Department of Nursing
Mishawaka, Indiana

http://www.bethelcollege.edu

Founded in 1947

DEGREES • BSN • MSN

Bethel College (continued)

Nursing Program Faculty 25 (8% with doctorates).

Baccalaureate Enrollment 125
Women 90% **Men** 10% **Minority** 5% **Part-time** 40%

Graduate Enrollment 15

Nursing Student Activities Sigma Theta Tau, Student Nurses' Association.

Nursing Student Resources Academic advising; academic or career counseling; assistance for students with disabilities; campus computer network; career placement assistance; computer lab; computer-assisted instruction; e-mail services; employment services for current students; housing assistance; Internet; learning resource lab; library services; nursing audiovisuals; placement services for program completers; remedial services; resume preparation assistance; skills, simulation, or other laboratory; tutoring.

Library Facilities 106,584 volumes (3,000 in health, 2,000 in nursing); 450 periodical subscriptions (150 health-care related).

BACCALAUREATE PROGRAMS

Degree BSN

Available Programs ADN to Baccalaureate; Generic Baccalaureate; LPN to Baccalaureate; RN Baccalaureate.

Site Options Winona Lake, IN.

Study Options Full-time and part-time.

Program Entrance Requirements Minimum overall college GPA of 2.5, transcript of college record, CPR certification, written essay, health exam, high school chemistry, high school transcript, immunizations, 1 letter of recommendation, minimum high school GPA of 2.5, minimum high school rank 35%, minimum GPA in nursing prerequisites of 2.5. Transfer students are accepted. **Standardized tests** *Required:* SAT or ACT, TOEFL for international students. **Application** *Deadline:* 8/6 (freshmen), 8/6 (transfer). *Notification:* continuous (freshmen). *Application fee:* $25.

Advanced Placement Credit by examination available. Credit given for nursing courses completed elsewhere dependent upon specific evaluations.

Expenses (2004–05) *Tuition:* full-time $15,000; part-time $250 per credit hour. *International tuition:* $15,000 full-time. *Room and board:* $4500; room only: $2500 per academic year. *Required fees:* full-time $600.

Financial Aid 90% of baccalaureate students in nursing programs received some form of financial aid in 2003–04. *Gift aid (need-based):* Federal Pell, FSEOG, state, private, college/university gift aid from institutional funds, Federal Nursing. *Loans:* FFEL (Subsidized and Unsubsidized Stafford PLUS), Perkins, college/university, GATE Loans. *Work-Study:* Federal Work-Study, part-time campus jobs. *Application deadline (priority):* 3/1.

Contact Dr. Ruth Elaine Davidhizar, Dean of Nursing, Department of Nursing, Bethel College, 1001 West McKinley Street, Mishawaka, IN 46545. *Telephone:* 574-257-2594 Ext. 2594. *Fax:* 574-257-3326. *E-mail:* davidhr@bethelcollege.edu.

GRADUATE PROGRAMS

Expenses (2004–05) *Tuition:* full-time $4950; part-time $330 per credit hour. *International tuition:* $4950 full-time. *Room and board:* $4500; room only: $2500 per academic year. *Required fees:* full-time $120.

Financial Aid 90% of graduate students in nursing programs received some form of financial aid in 2003–04.

Contact Dr. Ruth Elaine Davidhizar, Dean of Nursing, Department of Nursing, Bethel College, 1001 West McKinley Street, Mishawaka, IN 46545. *Telephone:* 574-257-2594 Ext. 2594. *Fax:* 574-257-2683. *E-mail:* davidhr@bethelcollege.edu.

MASTER'S DEGREE PROGRAM

Degree MSN

Available Programs Master's.

Concentrations Available Nursing education.

Study Options Part-time.

Program Entrance Requirements Clinical experience, minimum overall college GPA of 3.0, transcript of college record, CPR certification, immunizations, 3 letters of recommendation, nursing research course, physical assessment course, statistics course.

Advanced Placement Credit given for nursing courses completed elsewhere dependent upon specific evaluations.

Degree Requirements 36 total credit hours, thesis or project.

Goshen College
Department of Nursing
Goshen, Indiana

http://www.goshen.edu

Founded in 1894

DEGREE • BSN

Nursing Program Faculty 7 (29% with doctorates).

Baccalaureate Enrollment 137
Women 91% **Men** 9% **Minority** 8% **International** 9%

Nursing Student Activities Sigma Theta Tau, Student Nurses' Association.

Nursing Student Resources Academic advising; academic or career counseling; bookstore; campus computer network; career placement assistance; computer lab; e-mail services; employment services for current students; externships; library services; nursing audiovisuals; placement services for program completers; resume preparation assistance.

Library Facilities 127,028 volumes (80 in health, 75 in nursing); 750 periodical subscriptions (67 health-care related).

BACCALAUREATE PROGRAMS

Degree BSN

Available Programs Generic Baccalaureate; RN Baccalaureate.

Study Options Full-time and part-time.

Program Entrance Requirements Minimum overall college GPA of 2.5, transcript of college record, CPR certification, health exam, high school chemistry, high school foreign language, 2 years high school math, high school science, high school transcript, immunizations, 2 letters of recommendation, minimum high school GPA of 2.5, minimum high school rank 50%. Transfer students are accepted. **Standardized tests** *Required:* SAT or ACT, TOEFL for international students. **Application** *Deadline:* 8/15 (freshmen), 8/15 (transfer). *Early decision:* 12/1. *Notification:* continuous (freshmen), 12/15 (early action). *Application fee:* $25.

Advanced Placement Credit by examination available. Credit given for nursing courses completed elsewhere dependent upon specific evaluations.

Expenses (2004–05) *Tuition:* full-time $18,200. *International tuition:* $18,200 full-time. *Room and board:* $6200; room only: $3300 per academic year. *Required fees:* full-time $200.

Financial Aid 98% of baccalaureate students in nursing programs received some form of financial aid in 2003–04. *Gift aid (need-based):* Federal Pell, FSEOG, state, private, college/university gift aid from institutional funds. *Loans:* Federal Nursing Student Loans, Federal Direct (Subsidized and Unsubsidized Stafford PLUS), Perkins, college/university. *Work-Study:* Federal Work-Study, part-time campus jobs. *Application deadline (priority):* 2/15.

Contact Admissions, Department of Nursing, Goshen College, 1700 South Main Street, Goshen, IN 46526. *Telephone:* 219-535-7535. *Fax:* 219-535-7609. *E-mail:* admissions@goshen.edu.

See full description on page 494.

Indiana State University
School of Nursing
Terre Haute, Indiana

http://www.indstate.edu/nurs/

Founded in 1865

DEGREES • BS • MS

Nursing Program Faculty 35 (24% with doctorates).

Baccalaureate Enrollment 199
Women 93% **Men** 7% **Minority** 6.5% **International** .05% **Part-time** 14%

Graduate Enrollment 26
Women 92% **Men** 8% **Part-time** 23%

Nursing Student Activities Sigma Theta Tau, Student Nurses' Association.

Nursing Student Resources Academic advising; academic or career counseling; assistance for students with disabilities; bookstore; campus computer network; career placement assistance; computer lab; computer-assisted instruction; daycare for children of students; e-mail services; employment services for current students; externships; housing assistance; interactive nursing skills videos; Internet; learning resource lab; library services; nursing audiovisuals; paid internships; placement services for program completers; remedial services; resume preparation assistance; skills, simulation, or other laboratory; tutoring; unpaid internships.

Library Facilities 2.5 million volumes (33,560 in nursing); 2,827 periodical subscriptions (104 health-care related).

BACCALAUREATE PROGRAMS

Degree BS

Available Programs Generic Baccalaureate; LPN to Baccalaureate; RN Baccalaureate.

Site Options *Distance Learning:* Terre Haute, IN.

Study Options Full-time and part-time.

Program Entrance Requirements Minimum overall college GPA of 2.0, transcript of college record, CPR certification, health exam, high school chemistry, high school foreign language, 2 years high school math, 1 year of high school science, high school transcript, immunizations, minimum high school GPA of 3.0, minimum GPA in nursing prerequisites of 2.25, prerequisite course work. Transfer students are accepted. **Standardized tests** *Required:* SAT or ACT, TOEFL for international students. **Application** *Deadline:* 8/1 (freshmen). *Notification:* continuous (freshmen). *Application fee:* $25.

Advanced Placement Credit given for nursing courses completed elsewhere dependent upon specific evaluations.

Expenses (2003–04) *Tuition, area resident:* full-time $5322; part-time $192 per credit hour. *Tuition, state resident:* full-time $6358; part-time $237 per credit hour. *Tuition, nonresident:* full-time $11,790; part-time $416 per credit hour. *International tuition:* $11,790 full-time. *Room and board:* $5297; room only: $5297 per academic year. *Required fees:* full-time $5442; part-time $2721 per term.

Financial Aid 50% of baccalaureate students in nursing programs received some form of financial aid in 2002–03. *Gift aid (need-based):* Federal Pell, FSEOG, state, private, college/university gift aid from institutional funds. *Loans:* FFEL (Subsidized and Unsubsidized Stafford PLUS), Perkins. *Work-Study:* Federal Work-Study, part-time campus jobs. *Application deadline:* 3/1 (priority: 3/1).

Contact Lynn C. Foster, Director of Student Affairs, School of Nursing, Indiana State University, 749 Chestnut Street, Terre Haute, IN 47809. *Telephone:* 812-237-2317. *Fax:* 812-237-4300. *E-mail:* nufoster@isugw.indstate.edu.

GRADUATE PROGRAMS

Expenses (2003–04) *Tuition, area resident:* part-time $242 per credit hour. *Tuition, state resident:* full-time $4326; part-time $242 per credit hour. *Tuition, nonresident:* full-time $8658; part-time $481 per credit hour. *International tuition:* $8658 full-time. *Room and board:* $5297; room only: $5297 per academic year. *Required fees:* full-time $6782; part-time $3416 per term.

Financial Aid 19% of graduate students in nursing programs received some form of financial aid in 2002–03. 2 research assistantships with partial tuition reimbursements available, 1 teaching assistantship with partial tuition reimbursement available were awarded; career-related internships or fieldwork and Federal Work-Study also available. Aid available to part-time students. *Financial aid application deadline:* 3/1.

Contact Lynn C. Foster, Director of Student Affairs, School of Nursing, Indiana State University, 749 Chestnut Street, Terre Haute, IN 47809. *Telephone:* 812-237-2317. *Fax:* 812-237-4300. *E-mail:* nufoster@isugw.indstate.edu.

MASTER'S DEGREE PROGRAM

Degree MS

Available Programs Master's.

Concentrations Available *Clinical nurse specialist programs in:* adult health, community health. *Nurse practitioner programs in:* family health.

Site Options *Distance Learning:* Terre Haute, IN.

Study Options Full-time and part-time.

Program Entrance Requirements Clinical experience, minimum overall college GPA of 3.0, transcript of college record, CPR certification, written essay, immunizations, 3 letters of recommendation, nursing research course, prerequisite course work, statistics course. *Application deadline:* For fall admission, 7/1 (priority date); for spring admission, 11/1 (priority date). Applications are processed on a rolling basis. *Application fee:* $35.

Advanced Placement Credit given for nursing courses completed elsewhere dependent upon specific evaluations.

Degree Requirements 36 total credit hours, thesis or project.

POST-MASTER'S PROGRAM

Areas of Study *Nurse practitioner programs in:* family health.

CONTINUING EDUCATION PROGRAM

Contact Ms. Michelle Pantle, RN, Director of Continuing Education, School of Nursing, Indiana State University, Landsbaum Center LCHE 111, 1433 North 61/2 Street, Terre Haute, IN 47807. *Telephone:* 812-237-3696. *Fax:* 812-237-8248. *E-mail:* nupantle@isugw.indstate.edu.

Indiana University Bloomington

Department of Nursing–Bloomington Division
Bloomington, Indiana

Founded in 1820

DEGREE • BSN

Nursing Program Faculty 14 (2% with doctorates).

Baccalaureate Enrollment 100
Women 95% **Men** 5% **Minority** 1% **Part-time** 1%

Nursing Student Activities Nursing Honor Society, Sigma Theta Tau, Student Nurses' Association, nursing club.

Nursing Student Resources Academic advising; academic or career counseling; campus computer network; computer lab; interactive nursing skills videos; learning resource lab; nursing audiovisuals; resume preparation assistance; skills, simulation, or other laboratory; tutoring.

Library Facilities 6.5 million volumes (2,000 in nursing); 60,019 periodical subscriptions (12 health-care related).

BACCALAUREATE PROGRAMS

Degree BSN

Available Programs Generic Baccalaureate.

Site Options Bloomington, IN; Nashville, IN; Columbus, IN.

Study Options Full-time.

Program Entrance Requirements Minimum overall college GPA of 2.3, CPR certification, health exam, health insurance, high school biology, high school chemistry, high school foreign language, 3 years high school math, 1 year of high school science, high school transcript, immunizations, prerequisite course work. Transfer students are accepted. **Standardized tests** *Required:* SAT or ACT. *Recommended:* SAT Subject Tests, TOEFL for international students. **Application** *Deadline:* 4/1 (freshmen), rolling (transfer). *Notification:* continuous (freshmen). *Application fee:* $50.

Advanced Placement Credit given for nursing courses completed elsewhere dependent upon specific evaluations.

Expenses (2003–04) *Tuition, state resident:* full-time $4756; part-time $48 per credit hour. *Tuition, nonresident:* full-time $15,790; part-time $180 per credit hour. *Room and board:* $5400 per academic year. *Required fees:* full-time $598; part-time $148 per credit.

Financial Aid 50% of baccalaureate students in nursing programs received some form of financial aid in 2002–03. *Gift aid (need-based):* Federal Pell, FSEOG, state, private, college/university gift aid from institutional funds. *Loans:* Federal Nursing Student Loans, Federal Direct (Subsidized and Unsubsidized Stafford PLUS), Perkins, college/university. *Work-Study:* Federal Work-Study. *Application deadline:* Continuous.

Indiana University Bloomington (continued)

Contact Mrs. Lisa Wrasse, Academic Advisor, Department of Nursing–Bloomington Division, Indiana University Bloomington, Sycamore Hall, Room 401, Bloomington, IN 47405. *Telephone:* 812-855-2592. *Fax:* 812-855-6986. *E-mail:* lwrasse@indiana.edu.

Indiana University East

Division of Nursing
Richmond, Indiana

http://www.indiana.edu/nursing

Founded in 1971

DEGREE • BSN

Nursing Program Faculty 15.

Baccalaureate Enrollment 115
Women 90% **Men** 10% **Minority** 1%

Nursing Student Activities Sigma Theta Tau, Student Nurses' Association.

Nursing Student Resources Academic advising; academic or career counseling; assistance for students with disabilities; bookstore; campus computer network; career placement assistance; computer lab; computer-assisted instruction; daycare for children of students; e-mail services; interactive nursing skills videos; Internet; learning resource lab; library services; nursing audiovisuals; placement services for program completers; remedial services; resume preparation assistance; skills, simulation, or other laboratory; tutoring.

Library Facilities 67,036 volumes (5,039 in health, 3,418 in nursing); 435 periodical subscriptions (70 health-care related).

BACCALAUREATE PROGRAMS

Degree BSN

Available Programs ADN to Baccalaureate; Generic Baccalaureate; RN Baccalaureate.

Study Options Full-time.

Program Entrance Requirements Minimum overall college GPA of 2.5, transcript of college record, CPR certification, high school biology, high school chemistry, 3 years high school math, 2 years high school science, high school transcript, immunizations, minimum high school GPA of 2.0, minimum high school rank 50%, minimum GPA in nursing prerequisites of 2.0, prerequisite course work. Transfer students are accepted. **Standardized tests** *Recommended:* SAT or ACT. **Application** *Deadline:* rolling (freshmen), rolling (transfer). *Notification:* continuous (freshmen). *Application fee:* $25.

Advanced Placement Credit by examination available. Credit given for nursing courses completed elsewhere dependent upon specific evaluations.

Expenses (2004–05) *Tuition, state resident:* full-time $3762; part-time $125 per credit hour. *Tuition, nonresident:* full-time $10,143; part-time $338 per credit hour. *Required fees:* full-time $752; part-time $375 per credit.

Financial Aid 65% of baccalaureate students in nursing programs received some form of financial aid in 2003–04. *Gift aid (need-based):* Federal Pell, FSEOG, state, private, college/university gift aid from institutional funds. *Loans:* Federal Nursing Student Loans, FFEL (Subsidized and Unsubsidized Stafford PLUS), Perkins, college/university. *Work-Study:* Federal Work-Study. *Application deadline (priority):* 3/1.

Contact Dr. Karen R. Clark, Dean of Nursing, Division of Nursing, Indiana University East, 2325 Chester Boulevard, Richmond, IN 47374-1289. *Telephone:* 765-973-8242. *Fax:* 765-973-8220. *E-mail:* krclark@indiana.edu.

Indiana University Kokomo

Indiana University School Of Nursing
Kokomo, Indiana

Founded in 1945

DEGREE • BSN

Nursing Program Faculty 14 (43% with doctorates).

Baccalaureate Enrollment 198
Women 95% **Men** 5% **Minority** 1% **International** 1% **Part-time** 32%

Nursing Student Activities Student Nurses' Association.

Nursing Student Resources Academic advising; academic or career counseling; assistance for students with disabilities; bookstore; campus computer network; career placement assistance; computer lab; computer-assisted instruction; daycare for children of students; e-mail services; employment services for current students; externships; interactive nursing skills videos; Internet; learning resource lab; library services; nursing audiovisuals; paid internships; remedial services; resume preparation assistance; skills, simulation, or other laboratory; tutoring.

Library Facilities 132,424 volumes (2,881 in health, 1,513 in nursing); 1,513 periodical subscriptions (75 health-care related).

BACCALAUREATE PROGRAMS

Degree BSN

Available Programs Accelerated RN Baccalaureate; Generic Baccalaureate.

Site Options Logansport, IN; Marion, IN; Peru, IN.

Study Options Full-time.

Program Entrance Requirements Minimum overall college GPA of 2.5, transcript of college record, CPR certification, high school biology, high school chemistry, 4 years high school math, high school transcript, immunizations, minimum high school GPA of 2.0, minimum high school rank 50%, minimum GPA in nursing prerequisites of 2.7, prerequisite course work. Transfer students are accepted. **Standardized tests** *Required:* SAT or ACT, TOEFL for international students. **Application** *Deadline:* 8/3 (freshmen). *Notification:* continuous (freshmen). *Application fee:* $30.

Expenses (2004–05) *Tuition, state resident:* full-time $4800. *Tuition, nonresident:* part-time $338 per semester. *International tuition:* $4800 full-time. *Required fees:* full-time $600.

Financial Aid 75% of baccalaureate students in nursing programs received some form of financial aid in 2003–04. *Gift aid (need-based):* Federal Pell, FSEOG, state, private, college/university gift aid from institutional funds. *Loans:* Federal Nursing Student Loans, FFEL (Subsidized and Unsubsidized Stafford PLUS), Perkins, college/university. *Work-Study:* Federal Work-Study. *Application deadline (priority):* 3/1.

Contact Mr. Morris S. Starkey, Coordinator of Nursing Student Services, Indiana University School Of Nursing, Indiana University Kokomo, 2300 South Washington Street, PO Box 9003, Kokomo, IN 46904-9003. *Telephone:* 765-455-9384. *Fax:* 765-455-9421. *E-mail:* mstarke@iuk.edu.

CONTINUING EDUCATION PROGRAM

Contact Coordinator, Indiana University School Of Nursing, Indiana University Kokomo, 2300 South Washington Street, PO Box 9003, Kokomo, IN 46904-9003. *Telephone:* 765-455-9264. *Fax:* 765-455-9421.

Indiana University Northwest

School of Nursing and Health Professions
Gary, Indiana

http://www.iun.edu/~nurse

Founded in 1959

DEGREE • BSN

Nursing Program Faculty 14 (15% with doctorates).

Baccalaureate Enrollment 100
Women 95% **Men** 5% **Minority** 25%

Nursing Student Activities Sigma Theta Tau, Student Nurses' Association.

Nursing Student Resources Academic advising; academic or career counseling; assistance for students with disabilities; bookstore; campus computer network; career placement assistance; computer lab; computer-assisted instruction; daycare for children of students; e-mail services; externships; interactive nursing skills videos; Internet; learning resource lab; library services; nursing audiovisuals; placement services for program completers; skills, simulation, or other laboratory; tutoring.

Library Facilities 251,508 volumes (42,000 in health, 15,000 in nursing); 1,541 periodical subscriptions (200 health-care related).

BACCALAUREATE PROGRAMS

Degree BSN

Available Programs Generic Baccalaureate; RN Baccalaureate.

Study Options Full-time.

Program Entrance Requirements Minimum overall college GPA of 2.5, transcript of college record, CPR certification, health exam, health insurance, high school biology, high school chemistry, high school foreign language, 4 years high school science, high school transcript, immunizations, minimum high school rank 25%, prerequisite course work. Transfer students are accepted. **Standardized tests** *Required:* SAT or ACT. *Recommended:* TOEFL for international students. **Application** *Deadline:* 8/1 (freshmen), rolling (transfer). *Notification:* continuous (freshmen). *Application fee:* $35.

Advanced Placement Credit given for nursing courses completed elsewhere dependent upon specific evaluations.

Expenses (2003–04) *Tuition, state resident:* full-time $2894; part-time $121 per credit hour. *Tuition, nonresident:* full-time $7655; part-time $319 per credit hour. *International tuition:* $7655 full-time. *Required fees:* full-time $1125; part-time $562 per term.

Financial Aid 54% of baccalaureate students in nursing programs received some form of financial aid in 2002–03. *Gift aid (need-based):* Federal Pell, FSEOG, state, private, college/university gift aid from institutional funds, Federal Nursing. *Loans:* FFEL (Subsidized and Unsubsidized Stafford PLUS), Perkins, college/university. *Work-Study:* Federal Work-Study. *Application deadline (priority):* 3/1.

Contact Ms. Anne Mitchell, Nursing Student Services Coordinator, School of Nursing and Health Professions, Indiana University Northwest, 3400 Broadway, Gary, IN 46408. *Telephone:* 219-980-6611. *Fax:* 219-980-6578. *E-mail:* amitchel@iun.edu.

Indiana University–Purdue University Fort Wayne

Department of Nursing
Fort Wayne, Indiana

http://www.ipfw.edu/nursing

Founded in 1917

DEGREES • BS • MS

Nursing Program Faculty 42 (10% with doctorates).

Baccalaureate Enrollment 32
Women 94% **Men** 6% **Minority** 13% **Part-time** 75%

Graduate Enrollment 8
Women 100% **Part-time** 100%

Nursing Student Activities Sigma Theta Tau, nursing club.

Nursing Student Resources Academic advising; academic or career counseling; assistance for students with disabilities; bookstore; campus computer network; career placement assistance; computer lab; computer-assisted instruction; daycare for children of students; e-mail services; employment services for current students; housing assistance; interactive nursing skills videos; Internet; learning resource lab; library services; nursing audiovisuals; placement services for program completers; remedial services; resume preparation assistance; skills, simulation, or other laboratory; tutoring.

Library Facilities 479,992 volumes (1,100 in health, 500 in nursing); 10,964 periodical subscriptions (120 health-care related).

BACCALAUREATE PROGRAMS

Degree BS

Available Programs RN Baccalaureate.

Study Options Full-time and part-time.

Program Entrance Requirements Minimum overall college GPA, transcript of college record, health exam, high school transcript, immunizations, professional liability insurance/malpractice insurance, prerequisite course work, RN licensure. Transfer students are accepted. **Standardized tests** *Required:* SAT or ACT, TOEFL for international students. **Application** *Deadline:* 8/1 (freshmen). *Notification:* continuous (freshmen). *Application fee:* $30.

Advanced Placement Credit by examination available. Credit given for nursing courses completed elsewhere dependent upon specific evaluations.

Expenses (2004–05) *Tuition, state resident:* part-time $177 per credit hour. *Tuition, nonresident:* part-time $408 per credit hour.

Financial Aid 50% of baccalaureate students in nursing programs received some form of financial aid in 2003–04.

Contact Dr. Linda H. Meyer, Director of Undergraduate Programs/Associate Professor in Nursing, Department of Nursing, Indiana University–Purdue University Fort Wayne, 2101 East Coliseum Boulevard, Fort Wayne, IN 46805. *Telephone:* 260-481-6276. *Fax:* 260-481-5767. *E-mail:* meyer@ipfw.edu.

GRADUATE PROGRAMS

Expenses (2004–05) *Tuition, state resident:* part-time $219 per credit hour. *Tuition, nonresident:* part-time $475 per credit hour.

Contact Dr. Carol Sternberger, Chair/Professor of Nursing, Department of Nursing, Indiana University–Purdue University Fort Wayne, 2101 East Coliseum Boulevard, Fort Wayne, IN 46805-1499. *Telephone:* 260-481-6284. *Fax:* 260-481-5767. *E-mail:* leverman@ipfw.edu.

MASTER'S DEGREE PROGRAM

Degree MS

Available Programs Master's.

Concentrations Available Nursing administration. *Clinical nurse specialist programs in:* adult health, critical care, psychiatric/mental health. *Nurse practitioner programs in:* family health.

Site Options *Distance Learning:* Hammond, IN.

Study Options Full-time and part-time.

Program Entrance Requirements Clinical experience, minimum overall college GPA of 3.0, transcript of college record, interview, prerequisite course work, statistics course.

Advanced Placement Credit by examination available. Credit given for nursing courses completed elsewhere dependent upon specific evaluations.

Degree Requirements 45 total credit hours, thesis or project.

CONTINUING EDUCATION PROGRAM

Contact Roberta Barnes, Registrar, Continuing Studies, Department of Nursing, Indiana University–Purdue University Fort Wayne, 2101 East Coliseum Boulevard, Fort Wayne, IN 46805. *Telephone:* 260-481-6626. *E-mail:* barnes@ipfw.edu.

Indiana University–Purdue University Indianapolis

School of Nursing
Indianapolis, Indiana

http://www.nursing.iupui.edu

Founded in 1969

DEGREES • BSN • MSN • MSN/MPH • PHD

Nursing Program Faculty 185 (30% with doctorates).

Baccalaureate Enrollment 774
Women 94% **Men** 6% **Minority** 7% **International** 2% **Part-time** 11%

Graduate Enrollment 488
Women 94% **Men** 6% **Minority** 11% **International** 4% **Part-time** 85%

Nursing Student Activities Sigma Theta Tau, Student Nurses' Association.

Nursing Student Resources Academic advising; academic or career counseling; assistance for students with disabilities; bookstore; campus computer network; career placement assistance; computer lab; computer-assisted instruction; daycare for children of students; e-mail services; employment services for current students; externships; housing assistance;

Indiana University–Purdue University Indianapolis (continued)
interactive nursing skills videos; Internet; learning resource lab; library services; nursing audiovisuals; other; paid internships; remedial services; resume preparation assistance; skills, simulation, or other laboratory; tutoring; unpaid internships.

Library Facilities 1.5 million volumes (209,344 in health, 3,002 in nursing); 14,673 periodical subscriptions (2,717 health-care related).

BACCALAUREATE PROGRAMS

Degree BSN

Available Programs ADN to Baccalaureate; Accelerated Baccalaureate for Second Degree; Generic Baccalaureate; RN Baccalaureate.

Site Options Bloomington, IN.

Study Options Full-time and part-time.

Program Entrance Requirements Minimum overall college GPA of 2.5, transcript of college record, CPR certification, health insurance, high school chemistry, 2 years high school math, 1 year of high school science, high school transcript, immunizations, minimum high school rank 50%, minimum GPA in nursing prerequisites of 2.7, prerequisite course work. Transfer students are accepted. **Standardized tests** *Required:* SAT or ACT, TOEFL for international students. **Application** *Deadline:* rolling (freshmen), rolling (transfer). *Notification:* continuous (freshmen). *Application fee:* $50.

Advanced Placement Credit by examination available. Credit given for nursing courses completed elsewhere dependent upon specific evaluations.

Expenses (2004–05) *Tuition, state resident:* full-time $4526; part-time $151 per credit hour. *Tuition, nonresident:* full-time $14,346; part-time $478 per credit hour. *International tuition:* $14,346 full-time. *Room and board:* room only: $5500 per academic year. *Required fees:* full-time $550.

Financial Aid 75% of baccalaureate students in nursing programs received some form of financial aid in 2003–04. *Gift aid (need-based):* Federal Pell, FSEOG, state, private, college/university gift aid from institutional funds. *Loans:* Federal Nursing Student Loans, FFEL (Subsidized and Unsubsidized Stafford PLUS), Perkins, college/university. *Work-Study:* Federal Work-Study. *Application deadline (priority):* 3/1.

Contact Dr. Donna Boland, Associate Dean for Undergraduate Programs, School of Nursing, Indiana University–Purdue University Indianapolis, 1111 Middle Drive, NU 140, Indianapolis, IN 46202-5107. *Telephone:* 317-274-8010. *Fax:* 317-274-2996. *E-mail:* dboland@iupui.edu.

GRADUATE PROGRAMS

Expenses (2004–05) *Tuition, state resident:* full-time $6858; part-time $229 per credit hour. *Tuition, nonresident:* full-time $20,730; part-time $691 per credit hour. *International tuition:* $20,730 full-time. *Room and board:* room only: $5500 per academic year. *Required fees:* full-time $534.

Financial Aid 25% of graduate students in nursing programs received some form of financial aid in 2003–04. Fellowships with full tuition reimbursements available (averaging $10,000 per year), 50 research assistantships with full tuition reimbursements available (averaging $3,000 per year), 10 teaching assistantships with full tuition reimbursements available (averaging $3,500 per year) were awarded; Federal Work-Study, scholarships, traineeships, and tuition waivers (full) also available. Aid available to part-time students. *Financial aid application deadline:* 5/1.

Contact Dr. Joanne R. Warner, Associate Dean for Graduate Programs, School of Nursing, Indiana University–Purdue University Indianapolis, 1111 Middle Drive, NU 136, Indianapolis, IN 46202-5107. *Telephone:* 317-274-3115. *Fax:* 317-274-2996. *E-mail:* warnerjr@iupui.edu.

MASTER'S DEGREE PROGRAM

Degrees MSN; MSN/MPH

Available Programs Master's; RN to Master's.

Concentrations Available Nursing administration. *Clinical nurse specialist programs in:* adult health, community health, pediatric, psychiatric/mental health. *Nurse practitioner programs in:* acute care, adult health, family health, neonatal health, pediatric, women's health.

Site Options Bloomington, IN; Kokomo, IN.

Study Options Full-time and part-time.

Program Entrance Requirements Clinical experience, computer literacy, minimum overall college GPA of 3.0, transcript of college record, immunizations, 3 letters of recommendation, physical assessment course, resume, statistics course, GRE General Test. *Application fee:* $45 ($55 for international students).

Advanced Placement Credit given for nursing courses completed elsewhere dependent upon specific evaluations.

Degree Requirements 42 total credit hours, thesis or project.

POST-MASTER'S PROGRAM

Areas of Study Nursing administration. *Clinical nurse specialist programs in:* adult health, community health, pediatric, psychiatric/mental health. *Nurse practitioner programs in:* acute care, adult health, family health, neonatal health, pediatric, women's health.

DOCTORAL DEGREE PROGRAM

Degree PhD

Available Programs Doctorate; Post-Baccalaureate Doctorate.

Areas of Study Family health, health policy, health promotion/disease prevention, information systems, nursing administration, nursing education, nursing research, nursing science.

Program Entrance Requirements Minimum overall college GPA of 3.0, interview by faculty committee, interview, 3 letters of recommendation, statistics course, vita, writing sample, GRE General Test. *Application fee:* $45 ($55 for international students).

Degree Requirements 90 total credit hours, dissertation, oral exam, written exam, residency.

POSTDOCTORAL PROGRAM

Areas of Study Adolescent health, cancer care, chronic illness, family health, health promotion/disease prevention, nursing informatics, nursing science.

Postdoctoral Program Contact Dr. Joan K. Austin, Distinguished Professor, School of Nursing, Indiana University–Purdue University Indianapolis, 1111 Middle Drive, Indianapolis, IN 46202-5107. *Telephone:* 317-274-8254. *Fax:* 317-278-1811. *E-mail:* joausti@iupui.edu.

CONTINUING EDUCATION PROGRAM

Contact Janice Ward, Director, Lifelong Learning, School of Nursing, Indiana University–Purdue University Indianapolis, 1111 Middle Drive, NU 347, Indianapolis, IN 46202-5107. *Telephone:* 317-274-7779. *Fax:* 317-274-0012. *E-mail:* jaward@iupui.edu.

See full description on page 502.

Indiana University South Bend

Division of Nursing and Health Professions
South Bend, Indiana

http://www.iusb.edu/~health/

Founded in 1922

DEGREE • BSN

Nursing Program Faculty 22 (33% with doctorates).

Baccalaureate Enrollment 188

Women 94% **Men** 6% **Minority** 11% **International** 1% **Part-time** 36%

Nursing Student Activities Sigma Theta Tau, Student Nurses' Association.

Nursing Student Resources Academic advising; academic or career counseling; assistance for students with disabilities; bookstore; campus computer network; career placement assistance; computer lab; computer-assisted instruction; daycare for children of students; e-mail services; employment services for current students; interactive nursing skills videos; Internet; learning resource lab; library services; nursing audiovisuals; placement services for program completers; resume preparation assistance; skills, simulation, or other laboratory; tutoring.

Library Facilities 300,202 volumes (4,300 in health, 2,300 in nursing); 1,937 periodical subscriptions (145 health-care related).

BACCALAUREATE PROGRAMS

Degree BSN

Available Programs Accelerated Baccalaureate for Second Degree; Generic Baccalaureate; RN Baccalaureate.

Study Options Full-time and part-time.

Program Entrance Requirements Minimum overall college GPA of 2.3, transcript of college record, CPR certification, health exam, health insurance, high school biology, high school chemistry, high school transcript, immunizations, minimum high school GPA of 2.0, minimum high school rank 50%, minimum GPA in nursing prerequisites of 2.5, prerequisite course work. Transfer students are accepted. **Standardized tests** *Required:* SAT or ACT. *Recommended:* TOEFL for international students. **Application** *Deadline:* 7/1 (freshmen), 6/1 (transfer). *Notification:* continuous (freshmen). *Application fee:* $42.

Advanced Placement Credit given for nursing courses completed elsewhere dependent upon specific evaluations.

Expenses (2003–04) *Tuition, state resident:* full-time $4500; part-time $139 per credit hour. *Tuition, nonresident:* part-time $359 per credit hour. *International tuition:* $11,500 full-time. *Required fees:* full-time $600; part-time $400 per term.

Financial Aid 65% of baccalaureate students in nursing programs received some form of financial aid in 2002–03. *Gift aid (need-based):* Federal Pell, FSEOG, state, private, college/university gift aid from institutional funds. *Loans:* Federal Nursing Student Loans, Federal Direct (Subsidized and Unsubsidized Stafford PLUS), Perkins, college/university. *Work-Study:* Federal Work-Study. *Application deadline (priority):* 3/1.

Contact Office of Student Serices, School of Nursing, Division of Nursing and Health Professions, Indiana University South Bend, 1700 Mishawaka Avenue, PO Box 7111, South Bend, IN 46634-7111. *Telephone:* 574-237-4571. *Fax:* 574-237-4461. *E-mail:* nursing@iusb.edu.

Indiana University Southeast

Division of Nursing
New Albany, Indiana

http://www.ius.edu/Nursing/homepage1.htm

Founded in 1941

DEGREE • BSN

Nursing Program Faculty 14 (35% with doctorates).

Baccalaureate Enrollment 124
Women 97% **Men** 3% **Minority** 3% **International** 2%

Nursing Student Activities Sigma Theta Tau, Student Nurses' Association.

Nursing Student Resources Academic advising; assistance for students with disabilities; Internet; library services; skills, simulation, or other laboratory; tutoring.

Library Facilities 215,429 volumes; 962 periodical subscriptions.

BACCALAUREATE PROGRAMS

Degree BSN

Available Programs Generic Baccalaureate; RN Baccalaureate.

Study Options Full-time.

Program Entrance Requirements Transcript of college record, CPR certification, immunizations, prerequisite course work. Transfer students are accepted. **Standardized tests** *Required:* SAT or ACT, TOEFL for international students. **Application** *Deadline:* 7/15 (freshmen), 7/1 (transfer). *Notification:* continuous (freshmen). *Application fee:* $30.

Advanced Placement Credit given for nursing courses completed elsewhere dependent upon specific evaluations.

Expenses (2004–05) *Tuition, state resident:* full-time $4709; part-time $143 per credit hour. *Tuition, nonresident:* full-time $11,027; part-time $356 per credit hour. *International tuition:* $11,027 full-time. *Required fees:* full-time $150.

Financial Aid 90% of baccalaureate students in nursing programs received some form of financial aid in 2003–04. *Gift aid (need-based):* Federal Pell, FSEOG, state, private, college/university gift aid from institutional funds. *Loans:* Federal Nursing Student Loans, FFEL (Subsidized and Unsubsidized Stafford PLUS), Perkins, college/university. *Work-Study:* Federal Work-Study. *Application deadline (priority):* 3/1.

Contact Division of Nursing, Indiana University Southeast, 4201 Grant Line Road, Life Sciences Building, Room 276, New Albany, IN 47150-6405. *Telephone:* 812-941-2340. *Fax:* 812-941-2687.

Indiana Wesleyan University

Division of Nursing
Marion, Indiana

http://www.indwes.edu/academics/Nursing

Founded in 1920

DEGREES • BS • MS

Nursing Program Faculty 121 (20% with doctorates).

Baccalaureate Enrollment 703
Women 95% **Men** 5% **Minority** 14% **Part-time** 5%

Graduate Enrollment 171
Women 93% **Men** 7% **Minority** 19% **Part-time** 4%

Nursing Student Activities Nursing Honor Society, Sigma Theta Tau, Student Nurses' Association.

Nursing Student Resources Academic advising; academic or career counseling; assistance for students with disabilities; bookstore; campus computer network; career placement assistance; computer lab; computer-assisted instruction; e-mail services; housing assistance; Internet; learning resource lab; library services; nursing audiovisuals; remedial services; resume preparation assistance; skills, simulation, or other laboratory; tutoring.

Library Facilities 110,000 volumes (12,394 in health, 9,619 in nursing); 154 periodical subscriptions health-care related.

BACCALAUREATE PROGRAMS

Degree BS

Available Programs ADN to Baccalaureate; Generic Baccalaureate.

Site Options Terre Haute, IN; Indianapolis, IN; Fort Wayne, IN.

Study Options Full-time and part-time.

Program Entrance Requirements Minimum overall college GPA of 2.75, transcript of college record, CPR certification, health exam, high school biology, high school chemistry, high school transcript, immunizations, minimum high school GPA of 2.3, minimum GPA in nursing prerequisites of 2.75, prerequisite course work. Transfer students are accepted. **Standardized tests** *Required:* SAT or ACT, TOEFL for international students. **Application** *Deadline:* rolling (freshmen), rolling (transfer). *Notification:* continuous (freshmen). *Application fee:* $25.

Advanced Placement Credit by examination available. Credit given for nursing courses completed elsewhere dependent upon specific evaluations.

Expenses (2004–05) *Tuition:* full-time $15,204.

Financial Aid 90% of baccalaureate students in nursing programs received some form of financial aid in 2003–04. *Gift aid (need-based):* Federal Pell, FSEOG, state, private, college/university gift aid from institutional funds. *Loans:* FFEL (Subsidized and Unsubsidized Stafford PLUS), Perkins, college/university. *Work-Study:* Federal Work-Study, part-time campus jobs. *Application deadline (priority):* 3/1.

Contact Mrs. Sandra Mindach, Office Manager, Division of Nursing, Indiana Wesleyan University, 4201 South Washington Street, Marion, IN 46953. *Telephone:* 765-677-2130. *Fax:* 765-677-2333. *E-mail:* smindach@indwes.edu.

GRADUATE PROGRAMS

Expenses (2004–05) *Tuition:* part-time $385 per credit hour.

Financial Aid 62% of graduate students in nursing programs received some form of financial aid in 2003–04. 15 fellowships were awarded; career-related internships or fieldwork, scholarships, and traineeships also available. Aid available to part-time students. *Financial aid application deadline:* 3/15.

Contact Mrs. Pam Giles, Chair, Department of Graduate Nursing Studies, Division of Nursing, Indiana Wesleyan University, 4201 South Washington Street, Marion, IN 46953. *Telephone:* 765-677-1716 Ext. 2357. *Fax:* 765-677-2380. *E-mail:* pam.giles@indwes.edu.

MASTER'S DEGREE PROGRAM

Degree MS

Available Programs Master's.

Indiana Wesleyan University (continued)

Concentrations Available *Clinical nurse specialist programs in:* community health. *Nurse practitioner programs in:* adult health, family health, gerontology.

Site Options Indianapolis, IN; Fort Wayne, IN.

Study Options Full-time and part-time.

Program Entrance Requirements Clinical experience, minimum overall college GPA of 3.0, transcript of college record, immunizations, interview, 3 letters of recommendation, nursing research course, physical assessment course, resume, statistics course, GRE. *Application deadline:* For fall admission, 7/31 (priority date); for winter admission, 11/15 (priority date); for spring admission, 4/15 (priority date).

Advanced Placement Credit given for nursing courses completed elsewhere dependent upon specific evaluations.

Degree Requirements 36 total credit hours, thesis or project.

POST-MASTER'S PROGRAM

Areas of Study *Nurse practitioner programs in:* adult health, family health, gerontology.

Marian College

Department of Nursing and Nutritional Science
Indianapolis, Indiana

http://www.sonak.marian.edu/academ/nursing/index.html

Founded in 1851

DEGREE • BSN

Nursing Program Faculty 16 (1% with doctorates).

Nursing Student Activities Nursing Honor Society, Sigma Theta Tau, Student Nurses' Association.

Nursing Student Resources Academic advising; academic or career counseling; assistance for students with disabilities; bookstore; campus computer network; career placement assistance; computer lab; computer-assisted instruction; e-mail services; employment services for current students; interactive nursing skills videos; Internet; learning resource lab; library services; nursing audiovisuals; resume preparation assistance; skills, simulation, or other laboratory; tutoring.

Library Facilities 132,000 volumes (3,250 in health, 2,000 in nursing); 300 periodical subscriptions (116 health-care related).

BACCALAUREATE PROGRAMS

Degree BSN

Available Programs Accelerated Baccalaureate for Second Degree; Generic Baccalaureate; LPN to Baccalaureate; RN Baccalaureate.

Study Options Full-time and part-time.

Program Entrance Requirements Minimum overall college GPA of 2.5, transcript of college record, CPR certification, high school biology, high school chemistry, high school transcript, immunizations, minimum high school GPA of 2.7, minimum GPA in nursing prerequisites of 2.67, prerequisite course work. Transfer students are accepted. **Standardized tests** *Required:* SAT or ACT, TOEFL for international students. **Application** *Deadline:* 8/15 (freshmen), 8/1 (transfer). *Notification:* continuous until 8/24 (freshmen). *Application fee:* $20.

Advanced Placement Credit by examination available. Credit given for nursing courses completed elsewhere dependent upon specific evaluations.

Expenses (2003–04) *Tuition:* full-time $8400; part-time $735 per credit hour. *International tuition:* $8400 full-time. *Room and board:* $5800; room only: $5600 per academic year. *Required fees:* full-time $660; part-time $330 per term.

Financial Aid 92% of baccalaureate students in nursing programs received some form of financial aid in 2002–03. *Gift aid (need-based):* Federal Pell, FSEOG, state, private, college/university gift aid from institutional funds. *Loans:* FFEL (Subsidized and Unsubsidized Stafford PLUS), Perkins, college/university. *Work-Study:* Federal Work-Study, part-time campus jobs. *Application deadline (priority):* 3/1.

Contact Ms. Barbara Hart, RN, BSN Academic Advisor, Department of Nursing and Nutritional Science, Marian College, 3200 Cold Spring Road, Indianapolis, IN 46222-1997. *Telephone:* 317-955-6157. *Fax:* 317-955-6135. *E-mail:* bhart@marian.edu.

Purdue University

School of Nursing
West Lafayette, Indiana

http://www.nursing.purdue.edu

Founded in 1869

DEGREES • BS • MS

Nursing Program Faculty 48.

Baccalaureate Enrollment 519
Women 95% **Men** 5% **Minority** 2%

Graduate Enrollment 8
Women 99% **Men** 1%

Nursing Student Activities Sigma Theta Tau, Student Nurses' Association.

Nursing Student Resources Academic advising; academic or career counseling; assistance for students with disabilities; bookstore; campus computer network; career placement assistance; computer lab; computer-assisted instruction; e-mail services; interactive nursing skills videos; Internet; learning resource lab; library services; nursing audiovisuals; placement services for program completers; resume preparation assistance; skills, simulation, or other laboratory; tutoring.

Library Facilities 2.4 million volumes (200,000 in health, 10,000 in nursing); 19,957 periodical subscriptions (1,000 health-care related).

BACCALAUREATE PROGRAMS

Degree BS

Available Programs Accelerated Baccalaureate for Second Degree; Generic Baccalaureate; RN Baccalaureate.

Study Options Full-time and part-time.

Program Entrance Requirements High school biology, high school chemistry, high school foreign language, 3 years high school math, 3 years high school science, high school transcript, minimum high school GPA of 2.5. Transfer students are accepted. **Standardized tests** *Required:* SAT or ACT, TOEFL for international students. **Application** *Deadline:* 3/1 (freshmen), rolling (transfer). *Notification:* continuous (freshmen). *Application fee:* $30.

Advanced Placement Credit by examination available. Credit given for nursing courses completed elsewhere dependent upon specific evaluations.

Expenses (2004–05) *Tuition, state resident:* full-time $6092; part-time $218 per credit hour. *Tuition, nonresident:* full-time $18,700; part-time $621 per credit hour. *Room and board:* $7020 per academic year. *Required fees:* full-time $125.

Contact Office of Admissions, School of Nursing, Purdue University, Schleman Hall of Student Services, West Lafayette, IN 47907-2069. *Telephone:* 765-494-1776. *Fax:* 765-494-0544. *E-mail:* admissions@purdue.edu.

GRADUATE PROGRAMS

Expenses (2004–05) *Tuition, state resident:* full-time $6092; part-time $218 per credit hour. *Tuition, nonresident:* full-time $18,700; part-time $621 per credit hour. *Room and board:* $7020 per academic year. *Required fees:* full-time $125.

Contact Barb Wall, Interim Program Director, School of Nursing, Purdue University, 206 Johnson Hall of Nursing, West Lafayette, IN 47907-2069. *Telephone:* 765-494-4023. *Fax:* 765-494-6339. *E-mail:* bwall@nursing.purdue.edu.

MASTER'S DEGREE PROGRAM

Degree MS

Available Programs Master's.

Concentrations Available *Nurse practitioner programs in:* adult health.

Program Entrance Requirements Computer literacy, minimum overall college GPA of 3.0, transcript of college record, written essay, interview, 3 letters of recommendation, prerequisite course work, resume, statistics course.

Advanced Placement Credit given for nursing courses completed elsewhere dependent upon specific evaluations.

Degree Requirements 46 total credit hours, thesis or project.

CONTINUING EDUCATION PROGRAM

Contact Dr. Patricia Coyle-Rogers, Director of Continuing Education, School of Nursing, Purdue University, 502 North University Street, Office 220, West Lafayette, IN 47907-2069. *Telephone:* 765-494-4030. *Fax:* 765-494-6339. *E-mail:* pcrogers@nursing.purdue.edu.

Purdue University Calumet
School of Nursing
Hammond, Indiana

Founded in 1951

DEGREES • BS • MS

Nursing Program Faculty 30 (45% with doctorates).

Baccalaureate Enrollment 107
Women 96% **Men** 4% **Minority** 39% **Part-time** 43%

Graduate Enrollment 83
Women 95% **Men** 5% **Minority** 19% **Part-time** 86%

Nursing Student Activities Sigma Theta Tau, Student Nurses' Association.

Nursing Student Resources Academic advising; academic or career counseling; assistance for students with disabilities; bookstore; campus computer network; career placement assistance; computer lab; computer-assisted instruction; daycare for children of students; e-mail services; employment services for current students; externships; interactive nursing skills videos; Internet; learning resource lab; library services; nursing audiovisuals; paid internships; placement services for program completers; remedial services; resume preparation assistance; skills, simulation, or other laboratory; tutoring; unpaid internships.

Library Facilities 269,648 volumes (400 in health, 300 in nursing); 1,228 periodical subscriptions (110 health-care related).

BACCALAUREATE PROGRAMS

Degree BS

Available Programs Baccalaureate for Second Degree; Generic Baccalaureate; RN Baccalaureate.

Study Options Full-time and part-time.

Program Entrance Requirements Minimum overall college GPA of 2.5, transcript of college record, CPR certification, health exam, high school biology, high school chemistry, 2 years high school math, high school transcript, immunizations, minimum high school rank 65%. Transfer students are accepted. **Standardized tests** *Required for some:* SAT or ACT.
Application *Deadline:* rolling (freshmen), rolling (transfer).

Advanced Placement Credit by examination available. Credit given for nursing courses completed elsewhere dependent upon specific evaluations.

Expenses (2004–05) *Tuition, state resident:* full-time $4564; part-time $147 per credit hour. *Tuition, nonresident:* full-time $10,337; part-time $346 per credit hour. *Required fees:* full-time $462; part-time $50 per credit; part-time $231 per term.

Financial Aid 35% of baccalaureate students in nursing programs received some form of financial aid in 2003–04. *Gift aid (need-based):* Federal Pell, FSEOG, state, private, college/university gift aid from institutional funds. *Loans:* Federal Direct (Subsidized and Unsubsidized Stafford PLUS), Perkins. *Work-Study:* Federal Work-Study, part-time campus jobs. *Application deadline (priority):* 3/10.

Contact Ms. Kathleen M. Nix, RN, Undergraduate Program Coordinator, School of Nursing, Purdue University Calumet, 2200 169th Street, Hammond, IN 46323-2094. *Telephone:* 219-989-2814. *Fax:* 219-989-2848. *E-mail:* nix@calumet.purdue.edu.

GRADUATE PROGRAMS

Expenses (2004–05) *Tuition, state resident:* full-time $4192; part-time $186 per credit hour. *Tuition, nonresident:* full-time $9064; part-time $403 per credit hour. *Required fees:* full-time $297; part-time $10 per credit; part-time $22 per term.

Financial Aid 30% of graduate students in nursing programs received some form of financial aid in 2003–04.

Contact Dr. Jane Walker, Graduate Program Coordinator, School of Nursing, Purdue University Calumet, 2200 169th Street, Hammond, IN 46323-2094. *Telephone:* 219-989-2815. *Fax:* 219-989-2848. *E-mail:* walkerj@calumet.purdue.edu.

MASTER'S DEGREE PROGRAM

Degree MS

Available Programs Accelerated RN to Master's; Master's.

Concentrations Available *Clinical nurse specialist programs in:* adult health, critical care. *Nurse practitioner programs in:* family health.

Site Options Crown Point, IN. *Distance Learning:* Fort Wayne, IN; West Lafayette, IN.

Study Options Full-time and part-time.

Program Entrance Requirements Clinical experience, minimum overall college GPA of 3.0, transcript of college record, written essay, interview, 3 letters of recommendation, physical assessment course, resume, statistics course.

Advanced Placement Credit given for nursing courses completed elsewhere dependent upon specific evaluations.

Degree Requirements 45 total credit hours.

Saint Mary's College
Department of Nursing
Notre Dame, Indiana

http://www.saintmarys.edu

Founded in 1844

DEGREE • BS

Nursing Program Faculty 11 (13% with doctorates).

Baccalaureate Enrollment 136
Women 100% **Minority** 4%

Nursing Student Activities Nursing Honor Society, Sigma Theta Tau, Student Nurses' Association.

Nursing Student Resources Academic advising; academic or career counseling; assistance for students with disabilities; bookstore; campus computer network; career placement assistance; computer lab; computer-assisted instruction; daycare for children of students; e-mail services; employment services for current students; externships; interactive nursing skills videos; Internet; learning resource lab; library services; nursing audiovisuals; paid internships; remedial services; resume preparation assistance; skills, simulation, or other laboratory; tutoring; unpaid internships.

Library Facilities 215,616 volumes (9,787 in health, 5,149 in nursing); 759 periodical subscriptions (70 health-care related).

BACCALAUREATE PROGRAMS

Degree BS

Available Programs Accelerated Baccalaureate; Generic Baccalaureate.

Site Options Goshen, IN; South Bend, IN.

Study Options Full-time.

Program Entrance Requirements Minimum overall college GPA of 3.0, transcript of college record, CPR certification, written essay, health exam, high school foreign language, 3 years high school math, 2 years high school science, high school transcript, immunizations, interview, 2 letters of recommendation, minimum GPA in nursing prerequisites of 2.5. Transfer students are accepted. **Standardized tests** *Required:* SAT or ACT, TOEFL

Saint Mary's College (continued)
for international students. ***Placement:*** *Required:* SAT Subject Tests. **Application** *Deadline:* 3/1 (freshmen), rolling (transfer). *Early decision:* 11/15. *Notification:* continuous (freshmen), 12/15 (out-of-state freshmen), 12/15 (early decision). *Application fee:* $30.

Advanced Placement Credit given for nursing courses completed elsewhere dependent upon specific evaluations.

Expenses (2004–05) *Tuition:* full-time $23,600. *Room and board:* $6000 per academic year. *Required fees:* full-time $200.

Financial Aid 75% of baccalaureate students in nursing programs received some form of financial aid in 2003–04. *Gift aid (need-based):* Federal Pell, FSEOG, state, private, college/university gift aid from institutional funds. *Loans:* FFEL (Subsidized and Unsubsidized Stafford PLUS), Perkins, college/university. *Work-Study:* Federal Work-Study, part-time campus jobs. *Application deadline (priority):* 3/1.

Contact Maria C. Bowe, Associate Director, Admissions Office, Department of Nursing, Saint Mary's College, 124 LeMans, Notre Dame, IN 46556. *Telephone:* 574-284-4587. *Fax:* 574-284-4716. *E-mail:* mbowe@saintmarys.edu.

University of Evansville
Department of Nursing
Evansville, Indiana

http://nursing.evansville.edu
Founded in 1854

DEGREE • BSN

Nursing Program Faculty 8 (12% with doctorates).

Baccalaureate Enrollment 67
Women 99% **Men** 1% **Minority** 2%

Nursing Student Activities Sigma Theta Tau, Student Nurses' Association.

Nursing Student Resources Academic advising; academic or career counseling; assistance for students with disabilities; bookstore; campus computer network; career placement assistance; computer lab; computer-assisted instruction; e-mail services; employment services for current students; externships; housing assistance; Internet; learning resource lab; library services; nursing audiovisuals; paid internships; placement services for program completers; remedial services; resume preparation assistance; skills, simulation, or other laboratory; tutoring; unpaid internships.

Library Facilities 281,729 volumes (11,000 in nursing); 1,200 periodical subscriptions (155 health-care related).

BACCALAUREATE PROGRAMS

Degree BSN

Available Programs Generic Baccalaureate.

Study Options Full-time.

Program Entrance Requirements Health exam, health insurance, high school biology, high school chemistry, 4 years high school math, 4 years high school science, high school transcript, immunizations, minimum high school rank 67%, professional liability insurance/malpractice insurance. Transfer students are accepted. **Standardized tests** *Required:* SAT or ACT, TOEFL for international students. **Application** *Deadline:* rolling (freshmen), 7/1 (transfer). *Early decision:* 12/1. *Notification:* continuous until 3/1 (freshmen), 12/15 (early action). *Application fee:* $35.

Expenses (2003–04) *Tuition:* full-time $18,900; part-time $525 per contact hour. *International tuition:* $18,900 full-time. *Room and board:* $5960; room only: $2930 per academic year. *Required fees:* full-time $300.

Financial Aid 100% of baccalaureate students in nursing programs received some form of financial aid in 2002–03.

Contact Mrs. Jane P. Allen, Chair, Department of Nursing, University of Evansville, 1800 Lincoln Avenue, Evansville, IN 47722. *Telephone:* 812-479-2584. *Fax:* 812-479-2717. *E-mail:* ja2@evansville.edu.

University of Indianapolis
School of Nursing
Indianapolis, Indiana

http://www.uindy.edu
Founded in 1902

DEGREES • BSN • MSN • MSN/MBA

Nursing Program Faculty 43 (45% with doctorates).

Baccalaureate Enrollment 121
Women 96% **Men** 4% **Minority** 3% **International** 2% **Part-time** 2%

Graduate Enrollment 65
Women 98% **Men** 2% **Minority** 2% **Part-time** 80%

Nursing Student Activities Nursing Honor Society, Sigma Theta Tau, Student Nurses' Association.

Nursing Student Resources Academic advising; academic or career counseling; assistance for students with disabilities; bookstore; campus computer network; career placement assistance; computer lab; computer-assisted instruction; e-mail services; employment services for current students; housing assistance; interactive nursing skills videos; Internet; learning resource lab; library services; nursing audiovisuals; remedial services; resume preparation assistance; skills, simulation, or other laboratory; tutoring.

Library Facilities 173,363 volumes (14,800 in health, 915 in nursing); 1,015 periodical subscriptions (190 health-care related).

BACCALAUREATE PROGRAMS

Degree BSN

Available Programs Accelerated RN Baccalaureate; Generic Baccalaureate.

Site Options Indianapolis, IN.

Study Options Full-time and part-time.

Program Entrance Requirements Minimum overall college GPA of 2.82, transcript of college record, CPR certification, health exam, health insurance, high school biology, high school chemistry, high school foreign language, 2 years high school math, 2 years high school science, high school transcript, immunizations, minimum high school GPA of 2.82, minimum GPA in nursing prerequisites of 2.75, prerequisite course work. Transfer students are accepted. **Standardized tests** *Required:* SAT or ACT, TOEFL for international students. **Application** *Deadline:* rolling (freshmen), rolling (transfer). *Notification:* continuous (freshmen). *Application fee:* $20.

Advanced Placement Credit by examination available. Credit given for nursing courses completed elsewhere dependent upon specific evaluations.

Expenses (2004–05) *Tuition:* full-time $17,200; part-time $718 per credit hour. *International tuition:* $17,200 full-time. *Room and board:* $3075; room only: $3075 per academic year. *Required fees:* full-time $200; part-time $100 per term.

Financial Aid 88% of baccalaureate students in nursing programs received some form of financial aid in 2003–04. *Gift aid (need-based):* Federal Pell, FSEOG, state, private, college/university gift aid from institutional funds. *Loans:* Federal Nursing Student Loans, FFEL (Subsidized and Unsubsidized Stafford PLUS), Perkins. *Work-Study:* Federal Work-Study. *Application deadline (priority):* 3/1.

Contact Erna Karla Backer, BSN Program Coordinator, School of Nursing, University of Indianapolis, 1400 East Hanna Avenue, Indianapolis, IN 46227-3697. *Telephone:* 317-788-3324. *Fax:* 317-788-3542. *E-mail:* backer@uindy.edu.

GRADUATE PROGRAMS

Expenses (2004–05) *Tuition:* full-time $8176; part-time $511 per credit hour. *International tuition:* $8176 full-time. *Required fees:* full-time $220; part-time $110 per term.

Financial Aid 75% of graduate students in nursing programs received some form of financial aid in 2003–04.

Contact Anita Siccardi, MSN Program Coordinator, School of Nursing, University of Indianapolis, 1400 East Hanna Avenue, Indianapolis, IN 46227-3697. *Telephone:* 317-788-3471. *Fax:* 317-788-3542. *E-mail:* siccardi@uindy.edu.

MASTER'S DEGREE PROGRAM

Degrees MSN; MSN/MBA

Available Programs Master's.

Concentrations Available Nurse-midwifery; nursing administration; nursing education. *Nurse practitioner programs in:* family health, gerontology.

Site Options Indianapolis, IN.

Study Options Full-time and part-time.

Program Entrance Requirements Clinical experience, minimum overall college GPA of 3.0, transcript of college record, CPR certification, written essay, immunizations, interview, 3 letters of recommendation.

Advanced Placement Credit given for nursing courses completed elsewhere dependent upon specific evaluations.

Degree Requirements 46 total credit hours, thesis or project.

University of Saint Francis

Department of Nursing
Fort Wayne, Indiana

http://www.sf.edu

Founded in 1890

DEGREES • BSN • MSN

Nursing Program Faculty 51 (6% with doctorates).

Baccalaureate Enrollment 216

Women 94% **Men** 6% **Minority** 5% **Part-time** 8%

Graduate Enrollment 29

Women 100% **Minority** 1% **Part-time** 100%

Nursing Student Activities Sigma Theta Tau, Student Nurses' Association.

Nursing Student Resources Academic advising; academic or career counseling; assistance for students with disabilities; bookstore; campus computer network; career placement assistance; computer lab; computer-assisted instruction; e-mail services; employment services for current students; externships; housing assistance; interactive nursing skills videos; Internet; learning resource lab; library services; nursing audiovisuals; paid internships; remedial services; resume preparation assistance; skills, simulation, or other laboratory; tutoring; unpaid internships.

Library Facilities 50,186 volumes (4,500 in health, 1,750 in nursing); 449 periodical subscriptions (182 health-care related).

BACCALAUREATE PROGRAMS

Degree BSN

Available Programs Generic Baccalaureate; RN Baccalaureate.

Site Options *Distance Learning:* Fort Wayne, IN.

Study Options Full-time and part-time.

Program Entrance Requirements Minimum overall college GPA of 2.7, transcript of college record, CPR certification, health exam, high school biology, high school chemistry, 1 year of high school math, high school transcript, immunizations, minimum high school GPA of 2.7, minimum high school rank 50%, minimum GPA in nursing prerequisites of 2.7, prerequisite course work. Transfer students are accepted. **Standardized tests** *Required:* TOEFL for international students. *Required for some:* SAT or ACT. **Application** *Deadline:* rolling (freshmen), rolling (transfer). *Notification:* continuous until 8/15 (freshmen). *Application fee:* $20.

Advanced Placement Credit given for nursing courses completed elsewhere dependent upon specific evaluations.

Expenses (2004–05) *Tuition:* full-time $15,800; part-time $500 per credit hour. *International tuition:* $15,800 full-time. *Room and board:* $5450 per academic year. *Required fees:* full-time $710.

Financial Aid 97% of baccalaureate students in nursing programs received some form of financial aid in 2003–04.

Contact Lorene Arnold, BSN/MSN Program Director, Department of Nursing, University of Saint Francis, 2701 Spring Street, Fort Wayne, IN 46808. *Telephone:* 260-434-7644. *Fax:* 260-434-7404. *E-mail:* larnold@sf.edu.

GRADUATE PROGRAMS

Expenses (2004–05) *Tuition:* part-time $530 per credit hour. *Room and board:* $5450 per academic year. *Required fees:* full-time $710.

Financial Aid 70% of graduate students in nursing programs received some form of financial aid in 2003–04. Federal Work-Study and unspecified assistantships available.

Contact Lorene Arnold, BSN/MSN Program Director, Department of Nursing, University of Saint Francis, 2701 Spring Street, Fort Wayne, IN 46808. *Telephone:* 260-434-7644. *Fax:* 260-434-7404. *E-mail:* larnold@sf.edu.

MASTER'S DEGREE PROGRAM

Degree MSN

Available Programs Accelerated RN to Master's; Master's; Master's for Nurses with Non-Nursing Degrees.

Concentrations Available Nurse case management; nursing administration; nursing education. *Nurse practitioner programs in:* family health.

Study Options Full-time and part-time.

Program Entrance Requirements Computer literacy, minimum overall college GPA of 3.2, transcript of college record, CPR certification, written essay, immunizations, interview, 3 letters of recommendation, nursing research course, physical assessment course, resume, statistics course, GRE. *Application deadline:* For fall admission, 7/1 (priority date); for spring admission, 11/1 (priority date). Applications are processed on a rolling basis. *Application fee:* $20.

Advanced Placement Credit given for nursing courses completed elsewhere dependent upon specific evaluations.

Degree Requirements 48 total credit hours, thesis or project.

POST-MASTER'S PROGRAM

Areas of Study *Nurse practitioner programs in:* family health.

University of Southern Indiana

School of Nursing and Health Professions
Evansville, Indiana

http://health.usi.edu

Founded in 1965

DEGREES • BSN • MSN

Nursing Program Faculty 25 (36% with doctorates).

Baccalaureate Enrollment 280

Women 93% **Men** 7% **Minority** 3% **Part-time** 40%

Graduate Enrollment 210

Women 95% **Men** 5% **Minority** 5% **International** 2% **Part-time** 98%

Nursing Student Activities Sigma Theta Tau, Student Nurses' Association.

Nursing Student Resources Academic advising; academic or career counseling; assistance for students with disabilities; bookstore; campus computer network; career placement assistance; computer lab; computer-assisted instruction; daycare for children of students; e-mail services; employment services for current students; housing assistance; interactive nursing skills videos; Internet; learning resource lab; library services; nursing audiovisuals; placement services for program completers; remedial services; resume preparation assistance; skills, simulation, or other laboratory; tutoring; unpaid internships.

Library Facilities 247,329 volumes (9,000 in health, 1,175 in nursing); 14,276 periodical subscriptions (1,175 health-care related).

BACCALAUREATE PROGRAMS

Degree BSN

Available Programs Accelerated Baccalaureate for Second Degree; Generic Baccalaureate; RN Baccalaureate.

Study Options Full-time and part-time.

Program Entrance Requirements Minimum overall college GPA of 2.7, transcript of college record, CPR certification, written essay, health exam, high school transcript, immunizations, minimum high school GPA of 3.0, minimum GPA in nursing prerequisites of 2.0, professional liability

University of Southern Indiana (continued)
insurance/malpractice insurance. Transfer students are accepted. **Standardized tests** *Required:* SAT or ACT, TOEFL for international students. **Application** *Deadline:* 8/15 (freshmen). *Notification:* continuous until 8/27 (freshmen). *Application fee:* $25.

Advanced Placement Credit by examination available. Credit given for nursing courses completed elsewhere dependent upon specific evaluations.

Expenses (2004–05) *Tuition, state resident:* full-time $3200; part-time $134 per credit hour. *Tuition, nonresident:* full-time $7680; part-time $320 per credit hour. *Room and board:* $6000; room only: $3000 per academic year. *Required fees:* full-time $500; part-time $20 per credit; part-time $200 per term.

Financial Aid 56% of baccalaureate students in nursing programs received some form of financial aid in 2003–04. *Gift aid (need-based):* Federal Pell, FSEOG, state, private, college/university gift aid from institutional funds. *Loans:* FFEL (Subsidized and Unsubsidized Stafford PLUS), Perkins. *Work-Study:* Federal Work-Study. *Application deadline:* 3/1.

Contact Dr. Ann H. White, Assistant Dean for Nursing, School of Nursing and Health Professions, University of Southern Indiana, 8600 University Boulevard, Evansville, IN 47712. *Telephone:* 812-465-1173. *Fax:* 812-465-7092. *E-mail:* awhite@usi.edu.

GRADUATE PROGRAMS

Expenses (2004–05) *Tuition, state resident:* full-time $4100; part-time $195 per credit hour. *Tuition, nonresident:* full-time $4100; part-time $195 per credit hour. *Room and board:* $6000; room only: $3000 per academic year. *Required fees:* full-time $400; part-time $20 per credit; part-time $150 per term.

Financial Aid 45% of graduate students in nursing programs received some form of financial aid in 2003–04. Federal Work-Study, scholarships, tuition waivers (full and partial), and unspecified assistantships available. *Financial aid application deadline:* 3/1.

Contact Dr. Ann H. White, Assistant Dean for Nursing, School of Nursing and Health Professions, University of Southern Indiana, 8600 University Boulevard, Evansville, IN 47712. *Telephone:* 812-465-1173. *Fax:* 812-465-7092. *E-mail:* awhite@usi.edu.

MASTER'S DEGREE PROGRAM

Degree MSN

Available Programs Master's; RN to Master's.

Concentrations Available Nursing administration; nursing education. *Clinical nurse specialist programs in:* adult health, medical-surgical. *Nurse practitioner programs in:* acute care, family health.

Study Options Full-time and part-time.

Program Entrance Requirements Clinical experience, computer literacy, minimum overall college GPA of 3.0, transcript of college record, CPR certification, written essay, immunizations, 2 letters of recommendation, professional liability insurance/malpractice insurance, resume, statistics course. *Application deadline:* Applications are processed on a rolling basis. *Application fee:* $25.

Advanced Placement Credit given for nursing courses completed elsewhere dependent upon specific evaluations.

Degree Requirements 42 total credit hours, thesis or project.

POST-MASTER'S PROGRAM

Areas of Study Nursing administration; nursing education. *Clinical nurse specialist programs in:* adult health, medical-surgical. *Nurse practitioner programs in:* acute care, family health.

CONTINUING EDUCATION PROGRAM

Contact Peggy Graul, Coordinator of Continuing Education for Nursing and Health Professions, School of Nursing and Health Professions, University of Southern Indiana, 8600 University Boulevard, Evansville, IN 47712. *Telephone:* 812-465-1161. *Fax:* 812-465-7092. *E-mail:* pgraul@usi.edu.

See full description on page 578.

Valparaiso University
College of Nursing
Valparaiso, Indiana

http://www.valpo.edu/nursing

Founded in 1859

DEGREES • BSN • MSN

Nursing Program Faculty 12 (33% with doctorates).

Baccalaureate Enrollment 225
Women 83% **Men** 17% **Minority** 18% **Part-time** 14%

Graduate Enrollment 43
Women 91% **Men** 9% **Minority** 18% **Part-time** 74%

Nursing Student Activities Sigma Theta Tau, Student Nurses' Association.

Nursing Student Resources Academic advising; academic or career counseling; assistance for students with disabilities; bookstore; campus computer network; career placement assistance; computer lab; computer-assisted instruction; e-mail services; employment services for current students; externships; housing assistance; interactive nursing skills videos; Internet; learning resource lab; library services; nursing audiovisuals; placement services for program completers; remedial services; resume preparation assistance; skills, simulation, or other laboratory; tutoring; unpaid internships.

Library Facilities 1.1 million volumes (9,600 in health, 950 in nursing); 21,360 periodical subscriptions (1,000 health-care related).

BACCALAUREATE PROGRAMS

Degree BSN

Available Programs Accelerated Baccalaureate; Generic Baccalaureate; RN Baccalaureate.

Study Options Full-time and part-time.

Program Entrance Requirements Minimum overall college GPA of 3.0, transcript of college record, written essay, 2 years high school math, 4 years high school science, high school transcript, immunizations, minimum high school GPA of 2.0, minimum GPA in nursing prerequisites of 2.5. Transfer students are accepted. **Standardized tests** *Required:* SAT or ACT, TOEFL for international students. **Application** *Deadline:* 8/15 (freshmen). *Early decision:* 11/1. *Notification:* 12/1 (early action). *Application fee:* $30.

Advanced Placement Credit by examination available. Credit given for nursing courses completed elsewhere dependent upon specific evaluations.

Expenses (2004–05) *Tuition:* full-time $21,000; part-time $925 per credit hour. *International tuition:* $21,000 full-time. *Room and board:* $5840; room only: $3690 per academic year. *Required fees:* full-time $1124; part-time $120 per term.

Financial Aid 82% of baccalaureate students in nursing programs received some form of financial aid in 2003–04.

Contact Ellen Johnson, Admissions Coordinator, College of Nursing, Valparaiso University, Office of Admission, Kretzmann Hall, Valparaiso, IN 46383. *Telephone:* 219-464-5011. *Fax:* 219-464-6888. *E-mail:* ellen.johnson@valpo.edu.

GRADUATE PROGRAMS

Expenses (2004–05) *Tuition:* full-time $10,200; part-time $425 per credit hour. *International tuition:* $10,200 full-time. *Required fees:* full-time $194; part-time $60 per term.

Financial Aid 39% of graduate students in nursing programs received some form of financial aid in 2003–04. Institutionally sponsored loans available.

Contact Dr. Janet M. Brown, Dean, College of Nursing, Valparaiso University, 836 LaPorte Avenue, Valparaiso, IN 46383-6493. *Telephone:* 219-464-5289. *Fax:* 219-464-5425. *E-mail:* janet.brown@valpo.edu.

MASTER'S DEGREE PROGRAM

Degree MSN

Available Programs Master's; RN to Master's.

Concentrations Available *Clinical nurse specialist programs in:* adult health, parent-child, women's health.

Study Options Full-time and part-time.

Program Entrance Requirements Minimum overall college GPA of 3.0, transcript of college record, CPR certification, written essay, immunizations, 2 letters of recommendation, nursing research course, physical assessment course, prerequisite course work, statistics course. *Application deadline:* Applications are processed on a rolling basis. *Application fee:* $30 ($50 for international students).

Advanced Placement Credit given for nursing courses completed elsewhere dependent upon specific evaluations.

Degree Requirements 36 total credit hours, thesis or project.

POST-MASTER'S PROGRAM

Areas of Study *Nurse practitioner programs in:* family health.

CONTINUING EDUCATION PROGRAM

Contact Mrs. Julie Koch, Assistant Professor, College of Nursing, Valparaiso University, 836 LaPorte Avenue, Valparaiso, IN 46383. *Telephone:* 219-464-5291. *Fax:* 219-464-5425. *E-mail:* julie.koch@valpo.edu.

IOWA

Allen College
Program in Nursing
Waterloo, Iowa

http://www.allencollege.edu

Founded in 1989

DEGREES • BSN • MSN

Nursing Program Faculty 30 (13% with doctorates).

Baccalaureate Enrollment 297
Women 96% **Men** 4% **Minority** 3% **Part-time** 13%

Graduate Enrollment 31
Women 97% **Men** 3% **Part-time** 68%

Nursing Student Activities Sigma Theta Tau, Student Nurses' Association, nursing club.

Nursing Student Resources Academic advising; academic or career counseling; campus computer network; career placement assistance; computer lab; computer-assisted instruction; daycare for children of students; employment services for current students; housing assistance; Internet; library services; nursing audiovisuals; other; placement services for program completers; resume preparation assistance; tutoring.

Library Facilities 2,797 volumes (2,800 in health, 2,600 in nursing); 199 periodical subscriptions (199 health-care related).

BACCALAUREATE PROGRAMS

Degree BSN

Available Programs ADN to Baccalaureate; Accelerated Baccalaureate; Accelerated Baccalaureate for Second Degree; Accelerated RN Baccalaureate; Baccalaureate for Second Degree; Generic Baccalaureate; RN Baccalaureate.

Study Options Full-time and part-time.

Program Entrance Requirements Minimum overall college GPA of 2.0, transcript of college record, written essay, health exam, high school biology, high school chemistry, 3 years high school math, 3 years high school science, high school transcript, immunizations, 1 letter of recommendation, minimum high school rank 50%. Transfer students are accepted. **Standardized tests** *Required:* SAT and SAT Subject Tests or ACT, TOEFL for international students. **Application** *Deadline:* 7/1 (freshmen), 7/1 (transfer). *Notification:* continuous until 8/20 (freshmen). *Application fee:* $50.

Advanced Placement Credit given for nursing courses completed elsewhere dependent upon specific evaluations.

Expenses (2004–05) *Tuition:* full-time $9901; part-time $380 per credit hour. *Room and board:* $5164; room only: $3000 per academic year. *Required fees:* part-time $688 per term.

Financial Aid 95% of baccalaureate students in nursing programs received some form of financial aid in 2003–04. *Gift aid (need-based):* Federal Pell, FSEOG, state, private, college/university gift aid from institutional funds, Federal Nursing, Federal Scholarships for Disadvantaged Students. *Loans:* Federal Nursing Student Loans, Federal Direct (Subsidized and Unsubsidized Stafford PLUS), Perkins, college/university. *Work-Study:* Federal Work-Study, part-time campus jobs. *Application deadline:* Continuous.

Contact Cindy Heyerhoff, Enrollment Management Assistant, Program in Nursing, Allen College, 1825 Logan Avenue, Waterloo, IA 50703. *Telephone:* 319-226-2000. *Fax:* 319-226-2051. *E-mail:* AllenCollegeAdmissions@ihs.org.

GRADUATE PROGRAMS

Expenses (2004–05) *Tuition:* full-time $10,300; part-time $515 per credit hour. *Room and board:* $5164; room only: $3000 per academic year. *Required fees:* part-time $433 per term.

Financial Aid 77% of graduate students in nursing programs received some form of financial aid in 2003–04. Fellowships with partial tuition reimbursements available, research assistantships with partial tuition reimbursements available, teaching assistantships with partial tuition reimbursements available, Federal Work-Study, institutionally sponsored loans, scholarships, and traineeships available. Aid available to part-time students. *Financial aid application deadline:* 8/15.

Contact Cindy Heyerhoff, Enrollment Management Assistant, Program in Nursing, Allen College, 1825 Logan Avenue, Waterloo, IA 50703. *Telephone:* 319-226-2000. *Fax:* 319-226-2051. *E-mail:* AllenCollegeAdmissions@ihs.org.

MASTER'S DEGREE PROGRAM

Degree MSN

Available Programs Master's; Master's for Nurses with Non-Nursing Degrees.

Concentrations Available Nursing administration; nursing education. *Nurse practitioner programs in:* family health.

Study Options Full-time and part-time.

Program Entrance Requirements Clinical experience, minimum overall college GPA of 3.0, transcript of college record, CPR certification, written essay, immunizations, interview, 3 letters of recommendation, nursing research course, professional liability insurance/malpractice insurance, prerequisite course work, resume. *Application deadline:* For fall admission, 8/1 (priority date); for spring admission, 12/1 (priority date). Applications are processed on a rolling basis. *Application fee:* $50.

Advanced Placement Credit given for nursing courses completed elsewhere dependent upon specific evaluations.

Degree Requirements 40 total credit hours.

POST-MASTER'S PROGRAM

Areas of Study Nursing administration; nursing education. *Nurse practitioner programs in:* family health.

POSTDOCTORAL PROGRAM

Postdoctoral Program Contact Dr. Diane Young, Department Chair, MSN Program, Program in Nursing, Allen College, 1825 Logan Avenue, Waterloo, IA 50703. *Telephone:* 319-226-2047. *Fax:* 319-226-2070. *E-mail:* YoungDM@ihs.org.

CONTINUING EDUCATION PROGRAM

Contact Mrs. Mary Kay Frost, Continuing Education Coordinator, Program in Nursing, Allen College, 1825 Logan Avenue, Waterloo, IA 50703. *Telephone:* 319-226-2028. *Fax:* 319-226-2051. *E-mail:* FrostMK@ihs.org.

Briar Cliff University
Department of Nursing
Sioux City, Iowa

http://www.briarcliff.edu/nursing

Founded in 1930

DEGREES • BSC PN • MSN

Briar Cliff University (continued)

Nursing Program Faculty 8 (15% with doctorates).

Baccalaureate Enrollment 200
Women 90% **Men** 10% **Minority** 5% **Part-time** 50%

Graduate Enrollment 25

Nursing Student Activities Sigma Theta Tau, Student Nurses' Association.

Nursing Student Resources Academic advising; academic or career counseling; assistance for students with disabilities; bookstore; campus computer network; career placement assistance; computer lab; computer-assisted instruction; e-mail services; employment services for current students; externships; interactive nursing skills videos; Internet; learning resource lab; library services; nursing audiovisuals; placement services for program completers; remedial services; resume preparation assistance; skills, simulation, or other laboratory; tutoring.

Library Facilities 84,411 volumes; 7,786 periodical subscriptions.

BACCALAUREATE PROGRAMS

Degree BSc PN

Available Programs ADN to Baccalaureate; Generic Baccalaureate; LPN to Baccalaureate; RN Baccalaureate.

Site Options Sioux Center, IA; Orange City, IA; Sioux City, IA.

Study Options Full-time and part-time.

Program Entrance Requirements Minimum overall college GPA of 2.5, transcript of college record, CPR certification, written essay, health exam, high school transcript, immunizations, minimum GPA in nursing prerequisites of 2.0, prerequisite course work. Transfer students are accepted. **Standardized tests** *Required:* SAT or ACT. *Recommended:* TOEFL for international students. **Application** *Deadline:* rolling (freshmen), rolling (transfer). *Application fee:* $20.

Advanced Placement Credit by examination available. Credit given for nursing courses completed elsewhere dependent upon specific evaluations.

Expenses (2004–05) *Tuition:* full-time $15,960; part-time $532 per credit hour. *Room and board:* $5200; room only: $3600 per academic year. *Required fees:* full-time $520; part-time $33 per credit; part-time $160 per term.

Financial Aid 90% of baccalaureate students in nursing programs received some form of financial aid in 2003–04.

Contact Dr. Ruth Daumer, Chairperson, Department of Nursing, Briar Cliff University, 3303 Rebecca Street, PO Box 2100, Sioux City, IA 51104. *Telephone:* 712-279-5458. *Fax:* 712-279-5497. *E-mail:* ruth.daumer@briarcliff.edu.

GRADUATE PROGRAMS

Contact Dr. Ruth Daumer, Chairperson, Department of Nursing, Briar Cliff University, 3303 Rebecca Street, Sioux City, IA 51104. *Telephone:* 712-279-5458. *Fax:* 712-279-1698.

MASTER'S DEGREE PROGRAM

Degree MSN

Available Programs Master's.

Concentrations Available Nursing education. *Nurse practitioner programs in:* family health.

Study Options Full-time and part-time.

Program Entrance Requirements Clinical experience, computer literacy, transcript of college record, CPR certification, written essay, immunizations, 2 letters of recommendation, nursing research course, physical assessment course, professional liability insurance/malpractice insurance, resume, statistics course.

Advanced Placement Credit given for nursing courses completed elsewhere dependent upon specific evaluations.

Degree Requirements 40 total credit hours, thesis or project.

POST-MASTER'S PROGRAM

Areas of Study Nursing education. *Nurse practitioner programs in:* family health.

CONTINUING EDUCATION PROGRAM

Contact Judith Scherer Connealy, Director of Continuing Education, Department of Nursing, Briar Cliff University, 3303 Rebecca Street, Sioux City, IA 51104. *Telephone:* 712-279-1774. *Fax:* 712-279-5497. *E-mail:* schererj@briarcliff.edu.

Clarke College

Department of Nursing and Health
Dubuque, Iowa

Founded in 1843

DEGREES • BS • MSN

Nursing Program Faculty 17 (18% with doctorates).

Baccalaureate Enrollment 18
Women 96% **Men** 4% **Minority** 2% **Part-time** 13%

Graduate Enrollment 44
Women 100% **Part-time** 50%

Nursing Student Activities Nursing Honor Society, Sigma Theta Tau, Student Nurses' Association.

Nursing Student Resources Academic advising; academic or career counseling; assistance for students with disabilities; bookstore; campus computer network; career placement assistance; computer lab; computer-assisted instruction; e-mail services; employment services for current students; externships; housing assistance; interactive nursing skills videos; Internet; learning resource lab; library services; nursing audiovisuals; paid internships; placement services for program completers; remedial services; resume preparation assistance; skills, simulation, or other laboratory; tutoring; unpaid internships.

Library Facilities 157,576 volumes (7,000 in health, 2,856 in nursing); 884 periodical subscriptions (124 health-care related).

BACCALAUREATE PROGRAMS

Degree BS

Available Programs Baccalaureate for Second Degree; Generic Baccalaureate; RN Baccalaureate.

Study Options Full-time and part-time.

Program Entrance Requirements Minimum overall college GPA of 2.75, transcript of college record, CPR certification, written essay, health exam, health insurance, high school chemistry, high school foreign language, high school math, high school transcript, immunizations, interview, 2 letters of recommendation, minimum high school GPA of 2.0, minimum high school rank 50%, professional liability insurance/malpractice insurance, prerequisite course work. Transfer students are accepted. **Standardized tests** *Required:* SAT or ACT, TOEFL for international students. **Application** *Deadline:* rolling (freshmen), rolling (transfer). *Notification:* continuous until 7/15 (freshmen). *Application fee:* $25.

Advanced Placement Credit given for nursing courses completed elsewhere dependent upon specific evaluations.

Expenses (2004–05) *Tuition:* full-time $17,410; part-time $443 per credit hour. *Room and board:* $6289; room only: $3059 per academic year. *Required fees:* full-time $630.

Financial Aid 97% of baccalaureate students in nursing programs received some form of financial aid in 2003–04.

Contact Dr. Katherine Helen Frommelt, Chair, Department of Nursing and Health, Clarke College, MS 1727, 1550 Clarke Drive, Dubuque, IA 52001-3198. *Telephone:* 563-588-6361. *Fax:* 563-588-8684. *E-mail:* kay.frommelt@clarke.edu.

GRADUATE PROGRAMS

Expenses (2004–05) *Tuition:* full-time $4140; part-time $460 per credit hour. *Required fees:* full-time $55.

Financial Aid 50% of graduate students in nursing programs received some form of financial aid in 2003–04. Career-related internships or fieldwork available. Aid available to part-time students.

Contact Dr. Katherine Helen Frommelt, Chair, Department of Nursing and Health, Clarke College, 1550 Clarke Drive, Dubuque, IA 52001. *Telephone:* 563-588-6361. *Fax:* 563-588-8684. *E-mail:* kay.frommelt@clarke.edu.

MASTER'S DEGREE PROGRAM

Degree MSN

Available Programs Master's.

Concentrations Available Nursing administration; nursing education. *Nurse practitioner programs in:* family health.

Study Options Full-time and part-time.

Program Entrance Requirements Computer literacy, minimum overall college GPA of 3.0, transcript of college record, CPR certification, written essay, immunizations, interview, 3 letters of recommendation, nursing research course, physical assessment course, prerequisite course work, resume, statistics course, GRE General Test or MAT. *Application deadline:* For fall admission, 2/15 (priority date); for spring admission, 12/15 (priority date). Applications are processed on a rolling basis. *Application fee:* $25.

Advanced Placement Credit given for nursing courses completed elsewhere dependent upon specific evaluations.

Degree Requirements 37 total credit hours, thesis or project.

POST-MASTER'S PROGRAM

Areas of Study *Nurse practitioner programs in:* family health.

Coe College
Department of Nursing
Cedar Rapids, Iowa

Founded in 1851

DEGREE • BSN

Nursing Program Faculty 5 (40% with doctorates).

Baccalaureate Enrollment 43
Women 95% **Men** 5% **Minority** 2%

Nursing Student Activities Student Nurses' Association.

Nursing Student Resources Academic advising; academic or career counseling; assistance for students with disabilities; bookstore; campus computer network; career placement assistance; computer lab; e-mail services; employment services for current students; housing assistance; Internet; learning resource lab; library services; nursing audiovisuals; remedial services; resume preparation assistance; skills, simulation, or other laboratory; tutoring; unpaid internships.

Library Facilities 218,881 volumes (2,929 in health, 492 in nursing); 1,576 periodical subscriptions (34 health-care related).

BACCALAUREATE PROGRAMS

Degree BSN

Available Programs Generic Baccalaureate; RN Baccalaureate.

Study Options Full-time and part-time.

Program Entrance Requirements Minimum overall college GPA of 2.7, transcript of college record, CPR certification, written essay, health exam, health insurance, high school chemistry, high school transcript, immunizations, minimum high school GPA of 2.0, minimum GPA in nursing prerequisites of 2.7, prerequisite course work. Transfer students are accepted. **Standardized tests** *Required:* SAT or ACT, TOEFL for international students. **Application** *Deadline:* 3/1 (freshmen), rolling (transfer). *Early decision:* 12/10. *Notification:* 3/15 (freshmen), 1/20 (early action). *Application fee:* $30.

Advanced Placement Credit given for nursing courses completed elsewhere dependent upon specific evaluations.

Expenses (2004–05) *Tuition:* full-time $21,280; part-time $1030 per course. *Room and board:* $5780; room only: $2720 per academic year. *Required fees:* full-time $325.

Contact Dr. H. Jule Ohrt, Chair, Department of Nursing, Coe College, 1220 First Avenue, NE, Cedar Rapids, IA 52402. *Telephone:* 319-369-8120. *Fax:* 319-369-8121. *E-mail:* johrt@coe.edu.

Grand View College
Division of Nursing
Des Moines, Iowa

http://www.gvc.edu/academics/nursing/

Founded in 1896

DEGREE • BSN

Nursing Program Faculty 16 (25% with doctorates).

Nursing Student Activities Student Nurses' Association.

Library Facilities 104,225 volumes (3,868 in health); 8,141 periodical subscriptions (91 health-care related).

BACCALAUREATE PROGRAMS

Degree BSN

Available Programs Generic Baccalaureate; RN Baccalaureate.

Study Options Full-time and part-time.

Program Entrance Requirements Minimum overall college GPA of 2.2, transcript of college record, CPR certification, health exam, high school chemistry, high school transcript, immunizations, 3 letters of recommendation, minimum GPA in nursing prerequisites of 2.2, prerequisite course work. Transfer students are accepted. **Standardized tests** *Required:* SAT or ACT, TOEFL for international students. **Application** *Deadline:* 8/15 (freshmen), 8/15 (transfer). *Notification:* continuous until 9/15 (freshmen). *Application fee:* $35.

Advanced Placement Credit by examination available. Credit given for nursing courses completed elsewhere dependent upon specific evaluations.

Contact Dr. Jean Logan, RN, Head, Division of Nursing, Division of Nursing, Grand View College, 1200 Grandview Avenue, Des Moines, IA 50316. *Telephone:* 515-263-2866. *Fax:* 515-263-6077. *E-mail:* jlogan@gvc.edu.

CONTINUING EDUCATION PROGRAM

Contact Karen Anderson, Dean of the College for Professional and Adult Learning, Division of Nursing, Grand View College, 1200 Grandview Avenue, Des Moines, IA 50316-1599. *Telephone:* 515-263-2912. *Fax:* 515-263-6190. *E-mail:* kanderson@gvc.edu.

Iowa Wesleyan College
Division of Health and Natural Sciences
Mount Pleasant, Iowa

http://www.iwc.edu

Founded in 1842

DEGREE • BSN

Nursing Program Faculty 8 (12% with doctorates).

Baccalaureate Enrollment 76
Women 89% **Men** 11% **Minority** 13% **Part-time** 18%

Nursing Student Activities Student Nurses' Association.

Nursing Student Resources Academic advising; academic or career counseling; assistance for students with disabilities; bookstore; campus computer network; computer lab; computer-assisted instruction; e-mail services; Internet; learning resource lab; library services; nursing audiovisuals; remedial services; resume preparation assistance; skills, simulation, or other laboratory; tutoring; unpaid internships.

Library Facilities 107,227 volumes (500 in health, 300 in nursing); 431 periodical subscriptions (40 health-care related).

BACCALAUREATE PROGRAMS

Degree BSN

Available Programs ADN to Baccalaureate; Generic Baccalaureate; LPN to RN Baccalaureate; RN Baccalaureate.

Study Options Full-time and part-time.

Program Entrance Requirements Minimum overall college GPA of 2.0, transcript of college record, CPR certification, health exam, health insurance, high school transcript, immunizations, minimum high school GPA of 2.0, minimum high school rank 50%, minimum GPA in nursing prerequisites of 2.0, professional liability insurance/malpractice insurance, prerequisite course work. Transfer students are accepted. **Standardized tests** *Required:* SAT or ACT, TOEFL for international students. ***Placement:*** *Required:* SAT or ACT. **Application** *Deadline:* 8/15 (freshmen), 8/15 (transfer).

Advanced Placement Credit given for nursing courses completed elsewhere dependent upon specific evaluations.

Iowa Wesleyan College (continued)

Expenses (2004–05) *Tuition:* full-time $16,070; part-time $396 per credit hour. *International tuition:* $16,070 full-time. *Room and board:* $4920; room only: $2050 per academic year.

Financial Aid 98% of baccalaureate students in nursing programs received some form of financial aid in 2003–04.

Contact Mr. Cary Owens, Director, Enrollment Management, Division of Health and Natural Sciences, Iowa Wesleyan College, 601 North Main Street, Mount Pleasant, IA 52641. *Telephone:* 800-582-2383 Ext. 6231. *Fax:* 319-385-6296. *E-mail:* cowens@iwc.edu.

CONTINUING EDUCATION PROGRAM

Contact David File, Dean of Extended Learning, Division of Health and Natural Sciences, Iowa Wesleyan College, 601 North Main Street, Mount Pleasant, IA 52641. *Telephone:* 800-582-2383 Ext. 6245. *Fax:* 319-385-6296. *E-mail:* dfile@iwc.edu.

Luther College

Department of Nursing
Decorah, Iowa

http://nursing.luther.edu/

Founded in 1861

DEGREE • BA

Nursing Program Faculty 15 (20% with doctorates).

Baccalaureate Enrollment 100
Women 96% **Men** 4% **Minority** 3% **International** 2% **Part-time** 1%

Nursing Student Activities Sigma Theta Tau, nursing club.

Nursing Student Resources Academic advising; academic or career counseling; assistance for students with disabilities; bookstore; campus computer network; career placement assistance; computer lab; e-mail services; Internet; learning resource lab; library services; nursing audiovisuals; placement services for program completers; remedial services; resume preparation assistance; tutoring; unpaid internships.

Library Facilities 339,173 volumes (4,324 in health, 3,337 in nursing); 1,122 periodical subscriptions (35 health-care related).

BACCALAUREATE PROGRAMS

Degree BA

Site Options Rochester, MN.

Study Options Full-time and part-time.

Program Entrance Requirements Minimum overall college GPA of 2.3, transcript of college record, written essay, health exam, high school foreign language, 3 years high school math, 2 years high school science, high school transcript, immunizations, 1 letter of recommendation, minimum high school rank 50%, minimum GPA in nursing prerequisites of 2.0. Transfer students are accepted. **Standardized tests** *Required:* SAT or ACT, TOEFL for international students. **Application** *Notification:* continuous (freshmen). *Application fee:* $25.

Advanced Placement Credit given for nursing courses completed elsewhere dependent upon specific evaluations.

Expenses (2003–04) *Tuition:* full-time $21,600. *Room and board:* $4100; room only: $2000 per academic year.

Financial Aid 98% of baccalaureate students in nursing programs received some form of financial aid in 2002–03.

Contact Ms. Ruth Green, Secretary, Department of Nursing, Luther College, 700 College Drive, Decorah, IA 52101. *Telephone:* 563-387-1057. *Fax:* 563-387-2149. *E-mail:* greenru@luther.edu.

CONTINUING EDUCATION PROGRAM

Contact Ms. Ruth Green, Secretary, Department of Nursing, Luther College, 700 College Drive, Decorah, IA 52101. *Telephone:* 563-387-1057. *Fax:* 563-387-2149. *E-mail:* greenru@luther.edu.

See full description on page 514.

Mercy College of Health Sciences

Division of Nursing
Des Moines, Iowa

http://www.mchs.edu/divnurs.html

Founded in 1995

DEGREE • BSN

Nursing Program Faculty 22 (2% with doctorates).

Baccalaureate Enrollment 71
Women 98% **Men** 2% **Part-time** 98%

Nursing Student Activities Sigma Theta Tau, Student Nurses' Association.

Nursing Student Resources Academic advising; academic or career counseling; assistance for students with disabilities; campus computer network; career placement assistance; computer lab; computer-assisted instruction; daycare for children of students; e-mail services; employment services for current students; interactive nursing skills videos; Internet; learning resource lab; library services; nursing audiovisuals; placement services for program completers; skills, simulation, or other laboratory.

BACCALAUREATE PROGRAMS

Degree BSN

Available Programs ADN to Baccalaureate; Accelerated Baccalaureate; Accelerated Baccalaureate for Second Degree; RN Baccalaureate.

Study Options Full-time and part-time.

Program Entrance Requirements Minimum overall college GPA of 2.7, transcript of college record, prerequisite course work. Transfer students are accepted. **Standardized tests** *Required:* ACT, TOEFL for international students. **Application** *Deadline:* rolling (freshmen). *Notification:* continuous (freshmen). *Application fee:* $25.

Expenses (2004–05) *Tuition:* full-time $11,300; part-time $375 per credit hour.

Contact General Information, Division of Nursing, Mercy College of Health Sciences, 928 6th Avenue, Des Moines, IA 50309. *Telephone:* 515-643-3180. *Fax:* 515-643-6698. *E-mail:* information@mchs.edu.

Morningside College

Department of Nursing Education
Sioux City, Iowa

http://www.morningside.edu/academicdepartments/nursing.htm

Founded in 1894

DEGREE • BSN

Nursing Program Faculty 7 (14% with doctorates).

Baccalaureate Enrollment 53
Women 97% **Men** 3% **Minority** 11% **International** 6% **Part-time** 2%

Nursing Student Activities Student Nurses' Association, nursing club.

Nursing Student Resources Academic advising; academic or career counseling; assistance for students with disabilities; bookstore; campus computer network; computer lab; computer-assisted instruction; e-mail services; employment services for current students; externships; housing assistance; interactive nursing skills videos; Internet; learning resource lab; library services; nursing audiovisuals; resume preparation assistance; skills, simulation, or other laboratory; tutoring; unpaid internships.

Library Facilities 113,169 volumes (2,464 in health, 2,464 in nursing); 528 periodical subscriptions (43 health-care related).

BACCALAUREATE PROGRAMS

Degree BSN

Available Programs Baccalaureate for Second Degree; Generic Baccalaureate; International Nurse to Baccalaureate; LPN to Baccalaureate; RN Baccalaureate.

Study Options Full-time and part-time.

Program Entrance Requirements Minimum overall college GPA of 2.5, transcript of college record, CPR certification, high school transcript, immunizations, interview, minimum GPA in nursing prerequisites of 2.5, professional liability insurance/malpractice insurance, prerequisite course work. Transfer students are accepted. **Standardized tests** *Required:* SAT or ACT, TOEFL for international students. **Application** *Deadline:* rolling (freshmen), rolling (transfer). *Notification:* continuous (freshmen). *Application fee:* $25.

Advanced Placement Credit given for nursing courses completed elsewhere dependent upon specific evaluations.

Expenses (2004–05) *Tuition:* full-time $17,170; part-time $315 per credit hour. *Room and board:* $5400 per academic year. *Required fees:* full-time $230.

Financial Aid 99% of baccalaureate students in nursing programs received some form of financial aid in 2003–04.

Contact Mary Kovarna, RN, Chair, Associate Professor, Department of Nursing Education, Morningside College, 1501 Morningside Avenue, Sioux City, IA 51106-1751. *Telephone:* 712-274-5154. *Fax:* 712-274-5101. *E-mail:* kovarna@morningside.edu.

Mount Mercy College
Department of Nursing
Cedar Rapids, Iowa

http://www.mtmercy.edu
Founded in 1928

DEGREE • BSN

Nursing Program Faculty 22 (9% with doctorates).

Baccalaureate Enrollment 166
Women 97% **Men** 3% **Minority** 1% **International** 1% **Part-time** 30%

Nursing Student Activities Sigma Theta Tau, Student Nurses' Association, nursing club.

Nursing Student Resources Academic advising; academic or career counseling; assistance for students with disabilities; bookstore; campus computer network; career placement assistance; computer lab; computer-assisted instruction; e-mail services; employment services for current students; externships; housing assistance; interactive nursing skills videos; Internet; learning resource lab; library services; nursing audiovisuals; placement services for program completers; remedial services; resume preparation assistance; skills, simulation, or other laboratory; tutoring; unpaid internships.

Library Facilities 118,000 volumes (4,700 in health, 1,450 in nursing); 1,000 periodical subscriptions (130 health-care related).

BACCALAUREATE PROGRAMS

Degree BSN

Available Programs Accelerated RN Baccalaureate; Generic Baccalaureate.

Study Options Full-time and part-time.

Program Entrance Requirements Minimum overall college GPA of 2.5, transcript of college record, CPR certification, health exam, health insurance, high school chemistry, immunizations, interview, minimum GPA in nursing prerequisites of 2.5, prerequisite course work. Transfer students are accepted. **Standardized tests** *Required:* SAT or ACT, TOEFL for international students. **Application** *Deadline:* 8/30 (freshmen), 8/30 (transfer). *Notification:* continuous (freshmen). *Application fee:* $20.

Advanced Placement Credit by examination available. Credit given for nursing courses completed elsewhere dependent upon specific evaluations.

Expenses (2004–05) *Tuition:* full-time $16,880; part-time $470 per credit hour. *Room and board:* $5400; room only: $1400 per academic year. *Required fees:* full-time $500.

Financial Aid 90% of baccalaureate students in nursing programs received some form of financial aid in 2003–04. *Gift aid (need-based):* Federal Pell, FSEOG, state, college/university gift aid from institutional funds. *Loans:* Federal Direct (Subsidized and Unsubsidized Stafford PLUS), Perkins, state, college/university. *Work-Study:* Federal Work-Study, part-time campus jobs. *Application deadline (priority):* 3/1.

Contact Dr. Mary P. Tarbox, Professor and Chair, Department of Nursing, Mount Mercy College, 1330 Elmhurst Drive, NE, Cedar Rapids, IA 52402-4798. *Telephone:* 800-248-4504 Ext. 6460. *Fax:* 319-368-6479. *E-mail:* mtarbox@mtmercy.edu.

CONTINUING EDUCATION PROGRAM

Contact Dr. Mary P. Tarbox, Professor and Chair, Department of Nursing, Mount Mercy College, 1330 Elmhurst Drive, NE, Cedar Rapids, IA 52402-4797. *Telephone:* 319-368-6471. *Fax:* 319-368-6479. *E-mail:* mtarbox@mtmercy.edu.

St. Ambrose University
Program in Nursing (BSN)
Davenport, Iowa

Founded in 1882

DEGREE • BSN

Library Facilities 143,634 volumes; 739 periodical subscriptions.

BACCALAUREATE PROGRAMS

Degree BSN

Available Programs Generic Baccalaureate; RN Baccalaureate.

Program Entrance Requirements Standardized tests *Required:* SAT or ACT, TOEFL for international students. *Recommended:* ACT. **Application** *Deadline:* rolling (freshmen), rolling (transfer). *Notification:* 10/1 (freshmen). *Application fee:* $25.

Contact Nursing Department, Program in Nursing (BSN), St. Ambrose University, 518 West Locust Street, Davenport, IA 52803. *Telephone:* 563-333-6076. *E-mail:* nursing@sau.edu.

The University of Iowa
College of Nursing
Iowa City, Iowa

http://www.nursing.uiowa.edu
Founded in 1847

DEGREES • BSN • MSN • MSN/MBA • MSN/MPH • PHD

Nursing Program Faculty 69 (60% with doctorates).

Baccalaureate Enrollment 532
Women 95% **Men** 5% **Minority** 4% **Part-time** 25%

Graduate Enrollment 185
Women 94% **Men** 6% **Minority** 3% **International** 8.6% **Part-time** 60.5%

Nursing Student Activities Sigma Theta Tau, Student Nurses' Association.

Nursing Student Resources Academic advising; academic or career counseling; career placement assistance; computer lab; computer-assisted instruction; employment services for current students; learning resource lab; nursing audiovisuals; placement services for program completers; resume preparation assistance; skills, simulation, or other laboratory; tutoring.

Library Facilities 4 million volumes (273,469 in health); 44,644 periodical subscriptions (2,500 health-care related).

BACCALAUREATE PROGRAMS

Degree BSN

Available Programs Generic Baccalaureate; RN Baccalaureate.

Site Options *Distance Learning:* Mason City, IA; Fort Dodge, IA; Emmetsburg, IA.

Study Options Full-time and part-time.

Program Entrance Requirements Minimum overall college GPA of 2.7, transcript of college record, CPR certification, written essay, health exam, health insurance, high school biology, high school chemistry, high school foreign language, 3 years high school math, 3 years high school

The University of Iowa (continued)
science, high school transcript, immunizations, minimum GPA in nursing prerequisites of 2.7, professional liability insurance/malpractice insurance, prerequisite course work. Transfer students are accepted. **Standardized tests** *Required:* SAT or ACT, TOEFL for international students. **Application** *Deadline:* 4/1 (freshmen), 4/1 (transfer). *Notification:* continuous (freshmen). *Application fee:* $40.

Advanced Placement Credit given for nursing courses completed elsewhere dependent upon specific evaluations.

Expenses (2003–04) *Tuition, state resident:* full-time $4342; part-time $181 per credit hour. *Tuition, nonresident:* full-time $14,634; part-time $610 per credit hour. *Room and board:* $5961; room only: $3885 per academic year. *Required fees:* full-time $651; part-time $54 per credit.

Financial Aid 64% of baccalaureate students in nursing programs received some form of financial aid in 2002–03. *Gift aid (need-based):* Federal Pell, FSEOG, state, private, college/university gift aid from institutional funds. *Loans:* Federal Nursing Student Loans, Federal Direct (Subsidized and Unsubsidized Stafford PLUS), Perkins, college/university. *Work-Study:* Federal Work-Study, part-time campus jobs. *Application deadline:* Continuous.

Contact Linda Myers, Student Services, College of Nursing, The University of Iowa, 30 D Nursing Building, Iowa City, IA 52242. *Telephone:* 319-335-7016. *Fax:* 319-335-5590. *E-mail:* linda-myers@uiowa.edu.

GRADUATE PROGRAMS

Expenses (2003–04) *Tuition, state resident:* full-time $3869; part-time $430 per credit hour. *Tuition, nonresident:* full-time $8886. *International tuition:* $8886 full-time.

Financial Aid 17 fellowships, 19 research assistantships, 22 teaching assistantships were awarded.

Contact Program Associate, Nursing Graduate Program, College of Nursing, The University of Iowa, 444 Nursing Building, Iowa City, IA 52242. *Telephone:* 319-335-7021. *Fax:* 319-335-9990. *E-mail:* nursing-graduateprogram@uiowa.edu.

MASTER'S DEGREE PROGRAM

Degrees MSN; MSN/MBA; MSN/MPH

Available Programs Master's.

Concentrations Available Nurse anesthesia; nurse case management; nursing administration; nursing education; nursing informatics. *Clinical nurse specialist programs in:* adult health, community health, gerontology, occupational health, pediatric, psychiatric/mental health. *Nurse practitioner programs in:* adult health, family health, gerontology, pediatric.

Site Options *Distance Learning:* Mason City, IA; Fort Dodge, IA; Emmetsburg, IA.

Study Options Full-time and part-time.

Program Entrance Requirements Computer literacy, minimum overall college GPA of 3.0, transcript of college record, written essay, immunizations, 3 letters of recommendation, nursing research course, physical assessment course, professional liability insurance/malpractice insurance, prerequisite course work, statistics course, GRE General Test. *Application deadline:* For fall admission, 2/1. *Application fee:* $50 ($75 for international students).

Advanced Placement Credit given for nursing courses completed elsewhere dependent upon specific evaluations.

Degree Requirements 33 total credit hours, thesis or project.

POST-MASTER'S PROGRAM

Areas of Study Nursing informatics. *Clinical nurse specialist programs in:* adult health, occupational health, psychiatric/mental health.

DOCTORAL DEGREE PROGRAM

Degree PhD

Available Programs Doctorate; Post-Baccalaureate Doctorate.

Areas of Study Aging, family health, gerontology, individualized study, information systems, nursing administration.

Program Entrance Requirements Minimum overall college GPA of 3.0, interview by faculty committee, interview, 3 letters of recommendation, MSN or equivalent, statistics course, vita, GRE General Test. *Application deadline:* For fall admission, 2/1. *Application fee:* $50 ($75 for international students).

Degree Requirements 60 total credit hours, dissertation, oral exam, written exam, residency.

POSTDOCTORAL PROGRAM

Areas of Study Aging, family health, gerontology, nursing informatics, nursing interventions, outcomes.

Postdoctoral Program Contact Program Associate, College of Nursing, The University of Iowa, Iowa City, IA 52242. *Telephone:* 319-335-7018. *Fax:* 319-335-9990.

CONTINUING EDUCATION PROGRAM

Contact Ms. Nancy Lathrop, Office of Continuing Education, College of Nursing, The University of Iowa, 342 Nursing Building, Iowa City, IA 52242. *Telephone:* 319-335-7075. *Fax:* 319-335-9990. *E-mail:* nancy-lathrop@uiowa.edu.

KANSAS

Baker University
School of Nursing
Topeka, Kansas

http://www.bakeru.edu
Founded in 1858

DEGREE • BSN

Nursing Program Faculty 15 (7% with doctorates).

Baccalaureate Enrollment 132
Women 95% **Men** 5% **Minority** 6% **Part-time** 2%

Nursing Student Activities Nursing Honor Society, Sigma Theta Tau, Student Nurses' Association.

Nursing Student Resources Academic advising; computer lab; e-mail services; Internet; learning resource lab; library services; nursing audiovisuals; resume preparation assistance; skills, simulation, or other laboratory; tutoring.

Library Facilities 98,258 volumes (5,000 in health, 2,716 in nursing); 482 periodical subscriptions (414 health-care related).

BACCALAUREATE PROGRAMS

Degree BSN

Available Programs Generic Baccalaureate; RN Baccalaureate.

Study Options Full-time and part-time.

Program Entrance Requirements Transcript of college record, CPR certification, written essay, health exam, health insurance, high school transcript, immunizations, interview, minimum GPA in nursing prerequisites of 2.7, prerequisite course work. Transfer students are accepted. **Standardized tests** *Required:* SAT or ACT, TOEFL for international students. **Application** *Deadline:* rolling (freshmen), rolling (transfer).

Advanced Placement Credit given for nursing courses completed elsewhere dependent upon specific evaluations.

Expenses (2004–05) *Tuition:* full-time $10,250; part-time $325 per credit hour. *Required fees:* full-time $250; part-time $195 per term.

Financial Aid 87% of baccalaureate students in nursing programs received some form of financial aid in 2003–04. *Gift aid (need-based):* Federal Pell, FSEOG, state, private, college/university gift aid from institutional funds. *Loans:* FFEL (Subsidized and Unsubsidized Stafford PLUS), Perkins, college/university, alternative loans. *Work-Study:* Federal Work-Study, part-time campus jobs. *Application deadline (priority):* 3/1.

Contact Mrs. Debbie Wallace, Student Affairs Specialist, School of Nursing, Baker University, 1500 Southwest 10th Street, Topeka, KS 66604-1353. *Telephone:* 785-354-5850. *Fax:* 785-354-5832. *E-mail:* debbie.wallace@bakeru.edu.

See full description on page 458.

Bethel College
Department of Nursing
North Newton, Kansas

http://www.bethelks.edu
Founded in 1887

DEGREE • BSN

Nursing Program Faculty 6 (16% with doctorates).

Baccalaureate Enrollment 43

Nursing Student Activities Nursing Honor Society, Sigma Theta Tau, Student Nurses' Association.

Nursing Student Resources Academic advising; academic or career counseling; assistance for students with disabilities; bookstore; computer lab; e-mail services; employment services for current students; housing assistance; Internet; learning resource lab; library services; nursing audiovisuals; resume preparation assistance; skills, simulation, or other laboratory; tutoring.

Library Facilities 137,130 volumes (5,690 in health, 3,150 in nursing); 571 periodical subscriptions (445 health-care related).

BACCALAUREATE PROGRAMS

Degree BSN

Available Programs Generic Baccalaureate; LPN to Baccalaureate; RN Baccalaureate.

Study Options Full-time and part-time.

Program Entrance Requirements Minimum overall college GPA of 2.5, transcript of college record, CPR certification, written essay, health exam, health insurance, high school transcript, immunizations, interview, 2 letters of recommendation, minimum high school GPA of 2.5, minimum GPA in nursing prerequisites of 2.0, prerequisite course work. Transfer students are accepted. **Standardized tests** *Required:* SAT or ACT, TOEFL for international students. **Application** *Deadline:* rolling (freshmen), rolling (transfer). *Notification:* continuous (freshmen). *Application fee:* $20.

Advanced Placement Credit given for nursing courses completed elsewhere dependent upon specific evaluations.

Expenses (2003–04) *Tuition:* full-time $13,000.

Financial Aid 97% of baccalaureate students in nursing programs received some form of financial aid in 2002–03. *Gift aid (need-based):* Federal Pell, FSEOG, state, college/university gift aid from institutional funds. *Loans:* FFEL (Subsidized and Unsubsidized Stafford PLUS), Perkins. *Work-Study:* Federal Work-Study, part-time campus jobs. *Application deadline (priority):* 3/15.

Contact Dr. Carol Moore, Chairperson, Department of Nursing, Bethel College, 300 East 27th Street, North Newton, KS 67117. *Telephone:* 316-283-2500 Ext. 308. *Fax:* 316-284-5286. *E-mail:* moore@bethelks.edu.

Emporia State University
Newman Division of Nursing
Emporia, Kansas

http://www.emporia.edu/ndn
Founded in 1863

DEGREE • BSN

Nursing Program Faculty 10 (40% with doctorates).

Baccalaureate Enrollment 101
Women 89% **Men** 11% **International** 6% **Part-time** 3%

Nursing Student Activities Student Nurses' Association.

Nursing Student Resources Academic advising; academic or career counseling; assistance for students with disabilities; bookstore; campus computer network; career placement assistance; computer lab; computer-assisted instruction; daycare for children of students; e-mail services; employment services for current students; housing assistance; interactive nursing skills videos; Internet; learning resource lab; library services; nursing audiovisuals; placement services for program completers; remedial services; resume preparation assistance; skills, simulation, or other laboratory; tutoring.

Library Facilities 2.4 million volumes (50,596 in health, 2,459 in nursing); 815 periodical subscriptions (372 health-care related).

BACCALAUREATE PROGRAMS

Degree BSN

Available Programs ADN to Baccalaureate; Generic Baccalaureate; LPN to Baccalaureate; RN Baccalaureate.

Study Options Full-time and part-time.

Program Entrance Requirements Minimum overall college GPA of 2.0, transcript of college record, written essay, prerequisite course work. Transfer students are accepted. **Standardized tests** *Required:* SAT or ACT, TOEFL for international students. **Application** *Deadline:* rolling (freshmen), rolling (transfer). *Application fee:* $30.

Advanced Placement Credit given for nursing courses completed elsewhere dependent upon specific evaluations.

Expenses (2004–05) *Tuition, state resident:* full-time $2410; part-time $80 per credit hour. *Tuition, nonresident:* full-time $9130; part-time $304 per credit hour. *International tuition:* $9130 full-time. *Room and board:* $4108; room only: $2208 per academic year. *Required fees:* full-time $626; part-time $38 per credit.

Financial Aid 83% of baccalaureate students in nursing programs received some form of financial aid in 2003–04.

Contact Dr. Judith E. Calhoun, Division Chair, Newman Division of Nursing, Emporia State University, 1127 Chestnut Street, Emporia, KS 66801-2523. *Telephone:* 620-343-6800 Ext. 5641. *Fax:* 620-341-7871. *E-mail:* calhounj@emporia.edu.

Fort Hays State University
Department of Nursing
Hays, Kansas

http://www.fhsu.edu/nursing/
Founded in 1902

DEGREES • BSN • MSN

Nursing Program Faculty 17 (29% with doctorates).

Baccalaureate Enrollment 61
Women 95% **Men** 5% **Minority** 8% **Part-time** 3%

Graduate Enrollment 60
Women 97% **Men** 3% **Minority** 5% **Part-time** 83%

Nursing Student Activities Sigma Theta Tau, Student Nurses' Association, nursing club.

Nursing Student Resources Academic advising; academic or career counseling; assistance for students with disabilities; bookstore; campus computer network; career placement assistance; computer lab; computer-assisted instruction; daycare for children of students; e-mail services; employment services for current students; housing assistance; interactive nursing skills videos; Internet; learning resource lab; library services; nursing audiovisuals; paid internships; placement services for program completers; remedial services; resume preparation assistance; skills, simulation, or other laboratory; tutoring.

Library Facilities 624,637 volumes (9,840 in health, 1,393 in nursing); 1,689 periodical subscriptions (177 health-care related).

BACCALAUREATE PROGRAMS

Degree BSN

Available Programs Generic Baccalaureate; RN Baccalaureate.

Study Options Full-time and part-time.

Program Entrance Requirements Minimum overall college GPA of 2.5, transcript of college record, CPR certification, written essay, health exam, health insurance, immunizations, 2 letters of recommendation, minimum GPA in nursing prerequisites of 2.0, professional liability insurance/malpractice insurance, prerequisite course work. Transfer students are accepted. **Standardized tests** *Required:* ACT, SAT or ACT, TOEFL for international students. **Application** *Deadline:* rolling (freshmen), rolling (transfer). *Notification:* continuous (freshmen). *Application fee:* $30.

Fort Hays State University (continued)

Advanced Placement Credit by examination available. Credit given for nursing courses completed elsewhere dependent upon specific evaluations.

Expenses (2004–05) *Tuition, area resident:* full-time $2901; part-time $97 per credit hour. *Tuition, state resident:* full-time $3660; part-time $122 per credit hour. *Tuition, nonresident:* full-time $9025; part-time $301 per credit hour. *International tuition:* $9025 full-time. *Room and board:* $5061 per academic year.

Financial Aid 92% of baccalaureate students in nursing programs received some form of financial aid in 2003–04.

Contact Dr. Liane Connelly, Interim Chair, Department of Nursing, Fort Hays State University, 600 Park Street, Stroup Hall, 122D, Hays, KS 67601-4099. *Telephone:* 785-628-4511. *Fax:* 785-628-4080. *E-mail:* lconnell@fhsu.edu.

GRADUATE PROGRAMS

Expenses (2004–05) *Tuition, area resident:* full-time $2396; part-time $133 per credit hour. *Tuition, state resident:* full-time $2952; part-time $164 per credit hour. *Tuition, nonresident:* full-time $6293; part-time $350 per credit hour. *International tuition:* $6293 full-time. *Room and board:* $5896 per academic year.

Financial Aid 90% of graduate students in nursing programs received some form of financial aid in 2003–04. 1 teaching assistantship (averaging $5,000 per year) was awarded; research assistantships.

Contact Dr. Liane Connelly, Interim Chair, Department of Nursing, Fort Hays State University, 600 Park Street, Stroup Hall, 122D, Hays, KS 67601-4099. *Telephone:* 785-628-4511. *Fax:* 785-628-4080. *E-mail:* lconnell@fhsu.edu.

MASTER'S DEGREE PROGRAM

Degree MSN

Available Programs Master's.

Concentrations Available Nursing administration; nursing education. *Nurse practitioner programs in:* family health.

Study Options Full-time and part-time.

Program Entrance Requirements Clinical experience, minimum overall college GPA of 3.0, transcript of college record, CPR certification, written essay, immunizations, 2 letters of recommendation, physical assessment course, professional liability insurance/malpractice insurance, statistics course, GRE General Test or MAT. *Application deadline:* For fall admission, 7/1 (priority date). Applications are processed on a rolling basis. *Application fee:* $30 ($35 for international students).

Advanced Placement Credit given for nursing courses completed elsewhere dependent upon specific evaluations.

Degree Requirements 34 total credit hours, thesis or project, comprehensive exam.

POST-MASTER'S PROGRAM

Areas of Study Nursing administration; nursing education. *Nurse practitioner programs in:* family health.

Kansas Wesleyan University

Department of Nursing Education
Salina, Kansas

http://www.kwu.edu/nursing

Founded in 1886

DEGREE • BSN

Nursing Program Faculty 9 (22% with doctorates).

Baccalaureate Enrollment 26

Women 92% **Men** 8% **Minority** 4% **Part-time** 54%

Nursing Student Activities Nursing club.

Nursing Student Resources Academic advising; academic or career counseling; assistance for students with disabilities; bookstore; campus computer network; career placement assistance; computer lab; computer-assisted instruction; e-mail services; employment services for current students; housing assistance; Internet; learning resource lab; library services; nursing audiovisuals; resume preparation assistance; skills, simulation, or other laboratory; tutoring.

Library Facilities 1,091 volumes in health, 1,008 volumes in nursing; 370 periodical subscriptions (1,123 health-care related).

BACCALAUREATE PROGRAMS

Degree BSN

Available Programs ADN to Baccalaureate; Generic Baccalaureate; RN Baccalaureate.

Study Options Full-time and part-time.

Program Entrance Requirements Minimum overall college GPA of 2.6, transcript of college record, high school transcript, minimum GPA in nursing prerequisites of 2.6, prerequisite course work. Transfer students are accepted. **Standardized tests** *Required:* SAT or ACT, TOEFL for international students. *Recommended:* SAT, ACT. **Application** *Deadline:* rolling (freshmen), rolling (transfer). *Notification:* continuous (freshmen). *Application fee:* $20.

Advanced Placement Credit by examination available. Credit given for nursing courses completed elsewhere dependent upon specific evaluations.

Expenses (2004–05) *Tuition:* full-time $15,000; part-time $200 per credit hour. *Room and board:* $5400; room only: $2400 per academic year. *Required fees:* full-time $240.

Financial Aid 57% of baccalaureate students in nursing programs received some form of financial aid in 2003–04.

Contact Dr. Patricia L. Brown, RN, Professor and Chair for the Division of Nursing Education, Department of Nursing Education, Kansas Wesleyan University, 100 East Claflin Avenue, Box 39, Salina, KS 67401-6196. *Telephone:* 785-827-5541 Ext. 2311. *Fax:* 785-827-0927. *E-mail:* pbrown@kwu.edu.

MidAmerica Nazarene University

Division of Nursing
Olathe, Kansas

http://www.mnu.edu

Founded in 1966

DEGREE • BSN

Nursing Program Faculty 10 (40% with doctorates).

Baccalaureate Enrollment 28

Women 96.5% **Men** 3.5% **International** 3.5%

Nursing Student Activities Nursing club.

Nursing Student Resources Academic advising; academic or career counseling; assistance for students with disabilities; bookstore; campus computer network; career placement assistance; computer lab; computer-assisted instruction; e-mail services; interactive nursing skills videos; Internet; learning resource lab; library services; nursing audiovisuals; resume preparation assistance; skills, simulation, or other laboratory; tutoring; unpaid internships.

Library Facilities 132,991 volumes (2,579 in nursing); 1,250 periodical subscriptions (45 health-care related).

BACCALAUREATE PROGRAMS

Degree BSN

Available Programs ADN to Baccalaureate; Accelerated Baccalaureate; Accelerated Baccalaureate for Second Degree; Accelerated LPN to Baccalaureate; Accelerated RN Baccalaureate; Generic Baccalaureate; RN Baccalaureate.

Study Options Full-time.

Program Entrance Requirements Minimum overall college GPA of 2.6, transcript of college record, CPR certification, written essay, health exam, health insurance, high school transcript, immunizations, 2 letters of recommendation, minimum GPA in nursing prerequisites of 2.6, prerequisite course work. Transfer students are accepted. **Standardized tests**

Required: SAT or ACT, TOEFL for international students. **Application** *Deadline:* 8/1 (freshmen), 8/1 (transfer). *Notification:* continuous (freshmen). *Application fee:* $15.

Advanced Placement Credit by examination available. Credit given for nursing courses completed elsewhere dependent upon specific evaluations.

Expenses (2003–04) *Tuition:* full-time $11,910; part-time $397 per credit hour. *International tuition:* $11,910 full-time. *Room and board:* $5828 per academic year. *Required fees:* full-time $1862; part-time $365 per term.

Financial Aid 95% of baccalaureate students in nursing programs received some form of financial aid in 2002–03. *Gift aid (need-based):* Federal Pell, FSEOG, state, private, college/university gift aid from institutional funds. *Loans:* FFEL (Subsidized and Unsubsidized Stafford PLUS), Perkins. *Work-Study:* Federal Work-Study. *Application deadline (priority):* 3/1.

Contact Dr. Palma Lenn Smith, Chair, Division of Nursing, MidAmerica Nazarene University, 2030 East College Way, Olathe, KS 66062. *Telephone:* 913-782-3750 Ext. 298. *Fax:* 913-791-3408. *E-mail:* psmith@mnu.edu.

CONTINUING EDUCATION PROGRAM

Contact Dr. Susan G. Larson, Continuing Education Coordinator, Division of Nursing, MidAmerica Nazarene University, 2030 East College Way, Olathe, KS 66062-1899. *Telephone:* 913-782-3750 Ext. 291. *Fax:* 913-791-3408. *E-mail:* slarson@mnu.edu.

Newman University
Division of Nursing
Wichita, Kansas

http://www.newmanu.edu

Founded in 1933

DEGREES • BSN • M SC N

Nursing Program Faculty 13 (31% with doctorates).

Baccalaureate Enrollment 122
Women 87% **Men** 13% **Minority** 29% **International** 10% **Part-time** 1%

Graduate Enrollment 31
Women 81% **Men** 19% **Minority** 3% **Part-time** 23%

Nursing Student Activities Sigma Theta Tau, nursing club.

Nursing Student Resources Academic advising; academic or career counseling; assistance for students with disabilities; bookstore; campus computer network; computer lab; computer-assisted instruction; daycare for children of students; e-mail services; employment services for current students; housing assistance; Internet; learning resource lab; library services; nursing audiovisuals; placement services for program completers; remedial services; resume preparation assistance; skills, simulation, or other laboratory; tutoring.

Library Facilities 107,057 volumes (8,900 in health, 6,500 in nursing); 327 periodical subscriptions (85 health-care related).

BACCALAUREATE PROGRAMS

Degree BSN

Available Programs Generic Baccalaureate; LPN to Baccalaureate; RN Baccalaureate.

Study Options Full-time and part-time.

Program Entrance Requirements Minimum overall college GPA of 2.0, transcript of college record, CPR certification, written essay, health exam, health insurance, immunizations, interview, 2 letters of recommendation, minimum GPA in nursing prerequisites, professional liability insurance/malpractice insurance, prerequisite course work. Transfer students are accepted. **Standardized tests** *Required:* SAT or ACT, TOEFL for international students. **Application** *Deadline:* rolling (freshmen), rolling (transfer). *Notification:* continuous (freshmen). *Application fee:* $20.

Advanced Placement Credit given for nursing courses completed elsewhere dependent upon specific evaluations.

Expenses (2004–05) *Tuition:* full-time $14,650; part-time $488 per credit hour. *Room and board:* $6452 per academic year. *Required fees:* full-time $426; part-time $6 per credit.

Financial Aid 98% of baccalaureate students in nursing programs received some form of financial aid in 2003–04.

Contact Dr. Joan Felts, RN, Dean, School of Science, Nursing, and Allied Health, Division of Nursing, Newman University, 3100 McCormick Avenue, Wichita, KS 67213. *Telephone:* 316-942-4291 Ext. 2244. *Fax:* 316-942-4483. *E-mail:* feltsj@newmanu.edu.

GRADUATE PROGRAMS

Expenses (2004–05) *Tuition:* full-time $23,000. *Required fees:* full-time $200; part-time $6 per credit.

Contact Ms. Sharon Niemann, Interim Director, Master of Science in Nurse Anesthesia Program, Division of Nursing, Newman University, 3100 McCormick Avenue, Wichita, KS 67213. *Telephone:* 316-942-4291 Ext. 2272. *Fax:* 316-942-4483. *E-mail:* niemanns@newmanu.edu.

MASTER'S DEGREE PROGRAM

Degree M Sc N

Available Programs RN to Master's.

Concentrations Available Nurse anesthesia.

Study Options Full-time.

Program Entrance Requirements Clinical experience, minimum overall college GPA of 3.0, transcript of college record, CPR certification, written essay, immunizations, interview, 3 letters of recommendation, professional liability insurance/malpractice insurance, prerequisite course work, resume, statistics course, MAT. *Application deadline:* For fall admission, 8/15. Applications are processed on a rolling basis. *Application fee:* $25.

Advanced Placement Credit given for nursing courses completed elsewhere dependent upon specific evaluations.

Degree Requirements 54 total credit hours, thesis or project.

Pittsburg State University
Department of Nursing
Pittsburg, Kansas

http://www.pittstate.edu/nurs

Founded in 1903

DEGREES • BSN • MSN

Nursing Program Faculty 29 (34% with doctorates).

Baccalaureate Enrollment 130

Graduate Enrollment 15

Nursing Student Activities Nursing Honor Society, Sigma Theta Tau, Student Nurses' Association.

Nursing Student Resources Academic advising; academic or career counseling; assistance for students with disabilities; bookstore; career placement assistance; computer lab; computer-assisted instruction; e-mail services; employment services for current students; externships; housing assistance; interactive nursing skills videos; Internet; learning resource lab; library services; nursing audiovisuals; placement services for program completers; resume preparation assistance; skills, simulation, or other laboratory; tutoring; unpaid internships.

Library Facilities 639,136 volumes (2,717 in nursing); 7,038 periodical subscriptions.

BACCALAUREATE PROGRAMS

Degree BSN

Available Programs Generic Baccalaureate; RN Baccalaureate.

Study Options Full-time and part-time.

Program Entrance Requirements Minimum overall college GPA of 2.5, transcript of college record, CPR certification, health exam, immunizations, 3 letters of recommendation, professional liability insurance/malpractice insurance, prerequisite course work. Transfer students are accepted. **Standardized tests** *Required:* ACT, TOEFL for international students. **Application** *Deadline:* rolling (freshmen), rolling (transfer). *Application fee:* $30.

Pittsburg State University (continued)

Advanced Placement Credit by examination available. Credit given for nursing courses completed elsewhere dependent upon specific evaluations.

Expenses (2003–04) *Tuition, state resident:* full-time $2962; part-time $105 per credit hour. *Tuition, nonresident:* full-time $8784; part-time $299 per credit hour.

Contact Dr. Barbara Ruth McClaskey, Coordinator of Bachelor of Science in Nursing Program, Department of Nursing, Pittsburg State University, 1701 South Broadway, Pittsburg, KS 66762. *Telephone:* 620-235-4437. *Fax:* 620-235-4449. *E-mail:* bmcclask@pittstate.edu.

GRADUATE PROGRAMS

Expenses (2003–04) *Tuition, state resident:* full-time $3350; part-time $141 per credit hour. *Tuition, nonresident:* full-time $8334; part-time $349 per credit hour.

Contact Dr. Sharon Bowling, Master of Science Coordinator, Department of Nursing, Pittsburg State University, 1701 South Broadway, Pittsburg, KS 66762. *Telephone:* 316-235-4435. *Fax:* 316-235-4449. *E-mail:* sbowling@pittstate.edu.

MASTER'S DEGREE PROGRAM

Degree MSN

Available Programs RN to Master's.

Concentrations Available *Clinical nurse specialist programs in:* family health, gerontology. *Nurse practitioner programs in:* family health.

Study Options Full-time and part-time.

Program Entrance Requirements Clinical experience, minimum overall college GPA of 3.0, transcript of college record, CPR certification, written essay, immunizations, 3 letters of recommendation, nursing research course, physical assessment course, professional liability insurance/malpractice insurance, statistics course, GRE General Test. *Application fee:* $40 for international students).

Advanced Placement Credit given for nursing courses completed elsewhere dependent upon specific evaluations.

Degree Requirements 45 total credit hours, thesis or project, comprehensive exam.

POST-MASTER'S PROGRAM

Areas of Study *Nurse practitioner programs in:* family health.

CONTINUING EDUCATION PROGRAM

Contact Dr. A. Ruthellyn H. Hinton, Coordinator of Continuing Nursing Education, Department of Nursing, Pittsburg State University, 1701 South Broadway, Pittsburg, KS 66762. *Telephone:* 620-235-4440. *Fax:* 620-235-4449. *E-mail:* arhinton@pittstate.edu.

Southwestern College
Nursing Program
Winfield, Kansas

Founded in 1885

DEGREE • BSN

Nursing Program Faculty 6 (33% with doctorates).

Baccalaureate Enrollment 79

Nursing Student Activities Nursing Honor Society, Sigma Theta Tau, Student Nurses' Association, nursing club.

Nursing Student Resources Academic advising; academic or career counseling; assistance for students with disabilities; bookstore; campus computer network; career placement assistance; computer lab; computer-assisted instruction; e-mail services; externships; housing assistance; interactive nursing skills videos; Internet; learning resource lab; library services; nursing audiovisuals; paid internships; placement services for program completers; remedial services; resume preparation assistance; skills, simulation, or other laboratory; tutoring; unpaid internships.

Library Facilities 77,000 volumes; 320 periodical subscriptions.

BACCALAUREATE PROGRAMS

Degree BSN

Available Programs Generic Baccalaureate; RN Baccalaureate.

Site Options Wichita, KS.

Study Options Full-time and part-time.

Program Entrance Requirements Transcript of college record, minimum high school GPA of 2.5. Transfer students are accepted. **Standardized tests** *Required:* SAT or ACT, TOEFL for international students. **Application** *Deadline:* 3/1 (freshmen), 8/15 (transfer). *Notification:* continuous (freshmen). *Application fee:* $20.

Advanced Placement Credit given for nursing courses completed elsewhere dependent upon specific evaluations.

Financial Aid 45% of baccalaureate students in nursing programs received some form of financial aid in 2002–03. *Gift aid (need-based):* Federal Pell, FSEOG, state, private, college/university gift aid from institutional funds. *Loans:* Federal Direct (Subsidized and Unsubsidized Stafford PLUS), FFEL (Subsidized and Unsubsidized Stafford PLUS), Perkins. *Work-Study:* Federal Work-Study, part-time campus jobs. *Application deadline (priority):* 4/1.

Contact Dr. Martha R. Butler, RN, Professor of Nursing, Nursing Program, Southwestern College, 100 College Street, Winfield, KS 67156. *Telephone:* 620-229-6306. *E-mail:* mbutler@sckans.edu.

Tabor College
Department of Nursing
Hillsboro, Kansas

http://www.tabor.edu/

Founded in 1908

DEGREE • BSN

Nursing Program Faculty 8.

Baccalaureate Enrollment 42

Women 93% **Men** 7% **Minority** 5% **Part-time** 100%

Nursing Student Activities Nursing Honor Society.

Nursing Student Resources Academic advising; bookstore; campus computer network; computer lab; e-mail services; Internet; library services; nursing audiovisuals; skills, simulation, or other laboratory; tutoring.

Library Facilities 80,099 volumes (150 in health, 60 in nursing); 265 periodical subscriptions.

BACCALAUREATE PROGRAMS

Degree BSN

Available Programs Accelerated RN Baccalaureate.

Site Options Wichita, KS.

Study Options Part-time.

Program Entrance Requirements Minimum overall college GPA of 2.5, transcript of college record, CPR certification, written essay, health exam, health insurance, immunizations, interview, professional liability insurance/malpractice insurance, prerequisite course work, RN licensure. Transfer students are accepted. **Standardized tests** *Required:* SAT or ACT, TOEFL for international students. ***Placement:*** *Required:* SAT or ACT. **Application** *Deadline:* 8/1 (freshmen), 8/1 (transfer). *Early decision:* 1/1 (for plan 1), 4/1 (for plan 2). *Notification:* continuous (freshmen). *Application fee:* $20.

Advanced Placement Credit by examination available. Credit given for nursing courses completed elsewhere dependent upon specific evaluations.

Expenses (2004–05) *Tuition:* part-time $289 per credit hour. *Required fees:* part-time $40 per credit.

Financial Aid 100% of baccalaureate students in nursing programs received some form of financial aid in 2003–04.

Contact Mrs. Tona L. Leiker, Chairperson, Nursing Department, Department of Nursing, Tabor College, 7348 West 21st Street, Suite 117, Wichita, KS 67205. *Telephone:* 316-729-6333 Ext. 207. *Fax:* 316-773-5436. *E-mail:* tleiker@tabor.edu.

University of Kansas
School of Nursing
Kansas City, Kansas

http://www2.kumc.edu/son

Founded in 1866

DEGREES • BSN • MS • MS/MHSA • MS/MPH • PHD

Nursing Program Faculty 81 (60% with doctorates).

Baccalaureate Enrollment 301
Women 92% **Men** 8% **Minority** 13% **International** 1% **Part-time** 7%

Graduate Enrollment 161
Women 96% **Men** 4% **Minority** 4% **International** 3% **Part-time** 77%

Nursing Student Activities Nursing Honor Society, Sigma Theta Tau, Student Nurses' Association, nursing club.

Nursing Student Resources Academic advising; academic or career counseling; assistance for students with disabilities; bookstore; campus computer network; computer lab; computer-assisted instruction; e-mail services; employment services for current students; interactive nursing skills videos; Internet; learning resource lab; library services; nursing audiovisuals; remedial services; resume preparation assistance; skills, simulation, or other laboratory.

Library Facilities 4.8 million volumes (1,554 in health, 1,554 in nursing); 41,830 periodical subscriptions (96 health-care related).

BACCALAUREATE PROGRAMS

Degree BSN

Available Programs ADN to Baccalaureate; Generic Baccalaureate; RN Baccalaureate.

Study Options Full-time and part-time.

Program Entrance Requirements Minimum overall college GPA of 2.5, transcript of college record, CPR certification, written essay, health exam, health insurance, immunizations, 3 letters of recommendation, minimum GPA in nursing prerequisites of 2.5, prerequisite course work. Transfer students are accepted. **Standardized tests** *Required:* SAT or ACT. *Recommended:* TOEFL for international students. **Application** *Deadline:* 4/1 (freshmen), 5/1 (transfer). *Notification:* continuous (freshmen). *Application fee:* $30.

Advanced Placement Credit given for nursing courses completed elsewhere dependent upon specific evaluations.

Expenses (2003–04) *Tuition, state resident:* full-time $3527; part-time $118 per credit hour. *Tuition, nonresident:* full-time $11,003; part-time $367 per credit hour. *Required fees:* part-time $189 per term.

Financial Aid 71% of baccalaureate students in nursing programs received some form of financial aid in 2002–03.

Contact Office of Student Affairs, School of Nursing, University of Kansas, 3901 Rainbow Boulevard, Mail Stop 2029, Kansas City, KS 66160. *Telephone:* 913-588-1619. *Fax:* 913-588-1615. *E-mail:* soninfo@kumc.edu.

GRADUATE PROGRAMS

Expenses (2003–04) *Tuition, state resident:* full-time $3745; part-time $156 per credit hour. *Tuition, nonresident:* full-time $10,075; part-time $420 per credit hour. *International tuition:* $10,075 full-time. *Required fees:* part-time $84 per term.

Financial Aid 26% of graduate students in nursing programs received some form of financial aid in 2002–03. 6 research assistantships, 12 teaching assistantships with full and partial tuition reimbursements available were awarded; traineeships also available.

Contact Dr. Rita Clifford, RN, Associate Dean, Student Affairs, School of Nursing, University of Kansas, 3901 Rainbow Boulevard, Mail Stop 2029, Kansas City, KS 66160. *Telephone:* 913-588-1619. *Fax:* 913-588-1615. *E-mail:* soninfo@kumc.edu.

MASTER'S DEGREE PROGRAM

Degrees MS; MS/MHSA; MS/MPH

Concentrations Available Health-care administration; nurse-midwifery; nursing administration; nursing education; nursing informatics. *Clinical nurse specialist programs in:* adult health, gerontology. *Nurse practitioner programs in:* adult health, family health, gerontology, psychiatric/mental health.

Site Options *Distance Learning:* Garden City, KS.

Study Options Full-time and part-time.

Program Entrance Requirements Clinical experience, minimum overall college GPA of 3.0, transcript of college record, interview, 3 letters of recommendation, physical assessment course, resume, statistics course, GRE General Test. *Application deadline:* For fall admission, 4/1; for winter admission, 7/1; for spring admission, 9/1. *Application fee:* $35.

Advanced Placement Credit given for nursing courses completed elsewhere dependent upon specific evaluations.

Degree Requirements 43 total credit hours, thesis or project, comprehensive exam.

POST-MASTER'S PROGRAM

Areas of Study Health-care administration; nurse-midwifery; nursing administration; nursing education. *Clinical nurse specialist programs in:* adult health, gerontology. *Nurse practitioner programs in:* adult health, family health, gerontology, psychiatric/mental health.

DOCTORAL DEGREE PROGRAM

Degree PhD

Available Programs Doctorate; Post-Baccalaureate Doctorate.

Areas of Study Nursing research.

Program Entrance Requirements Minimum overall college GPA of 3.5, interview by faculty committee, interview, 3 letters of recommendation, statistics course, vita, writing sample, GRE General Test. *Application deadline:* For fall admission, 4/1; for winter admission, 7/1; for spring admission, 9/1. *Application fee:* $35.

Degree Requirements 65 total credit hours, dissertation, oral exam, written exam, residency.

CONTINUING EDUCATION PROGRAM

Contact Ilene Brawner, Director, School of Nursing, University of Kansas, 3901 Rainbow Boulevard, Mail Stop 4001, Kansas City, KS 66160. *Telephone:* 913-588-4488. *Fax:* 913-588-4486. *E-mail:* ceinfo@kumc.edu.

Washburn University
School of Nursing
Topeka, Kansas

http://www.washburn.edu/sonu/index.html

Founded in 1865

DEGREES • BSN • MSN

Nursing Program Faculty 29 (24% with doctorates).

Baccalaureate Enrollment 201
Women 89% **Men** 11% **Minority** 10% **International** 1% **Part-time** 1%

Nursing Student Activities Sigma Theta Tau, Student Nurses' Association, nursing club.

Nursing Student Resources Academic advising; academic or career counseling; assistance for students with disabilities; bookstore; campus computer network; career placement assistance; computer lab; computer-assisted instruction; e-mail services; employment services for current students; interactive nursing skills videos; Internet; learning resource lab; library services; nursing audiovisuals; remedial services; resume preparation assistance; skills, simulation, or other laboratory; tutoring; unpaid internships.

Library Facilities 1.5 million volumes (12,880 in health, 1,612 in nursing); 14,000 periodical subscriptions (84 health-care related).

BACCALAUREATE PROGRAMS

Degree BSN

Available Programs ADN to Baccalaureate; Baccalaureate for Second Degree; Generic Baccalaureate; LPN to Baccalaureate; RN Baccalaureate.

Study Options Full-time.

Program Entrance Requirements Minimum overall college GPA of 2.7, transcript of college record, CPR certification, written essay, health exam, health insurance, immunizations, interview, 2 letters of recommendation, minimum GPA in nursing prerequisites of 2.0, professional

Washburn University (continued)
liability insurance/malpractice insurance, prerequisite course work. Transfer students are accepted. **Standardized tests** *Required:* ACT, TOEFL for international students. **Application** *Deadline:* rolling (freshmen), 8/1 (transfer). *Notification:* continuous (freshmen). *Application fee:* $20.

Advanced Placement Credit by examination available. Credit given for nursing courses completed elsewhere dependent upon specific evaluations.

Expenses (2004–05) *Tuition, state resident:* full-time $4500. *Tuition, nonresident:* full-time $10,170. *International tuition:* $10,170 full-time. *Required fees:* full-time $62; part-time $15 per term.

Financial Aid 60% of baccalaureate students in nursing programs received some form of financial aid in 2003–04.

Contact Mary V. Allen, Nursing Advisor, School of Nursing, Washburn University, 1700 Southwest College Avenue, Topeka, KS 66621. *Telephone:* 785-231-1032 Ext. 1525. *Fax:* 785-231-1032. *E-mail:* mary.allen@washburn.edu.

GRADUATE PROGRAMS

Expenses (2004–05) *Tuition, state resident:* full-time $5500; part-time $275 per contact hour. *Tuition, nonresident:* full-time $9900; part-time $495 per contact hour. *International tuition:* $9900 full-time. *Required fees:* full-time $62; part-time $15 per term.

Contact Ms. Mary V. Allen, Nursing Advisor, School of Nursing, Washburn University, 1700 College, Topeka, KS 66621-1117. *Telephone:* 785-231-1010 Ext. 1533. *Fax:* 785-213-1032. *E-mail:* mary.allen@washburn.edu.

MASTER'S DEGREE PROGRAM

Degree MSN

Available Programs Master's.

Concentrations Available Nursing administration. *Clinical nurse specialist programs in:* gerontology. *Nurse practitioner programs in:* adult health, community health.

Study Options Full-time and part-time.

Program Entrance Requirements Computer literacy, transcript of college record, CPR certification, written essay, immunizations, 2 letters of recommendation, nursing research course, physical assessment course, professional liability insurance/malpractice insurance, prerequisite course work, resume, statistics course.

Degree Requirements 42 total credit hours, thesis or project.

POST-MASTER'S PROGRAM

Areas of Study Nursing education.

CONTINUING EDUCATION PROGRAM

Contact Dr. Cynthia Ann Hornberger, Dean, School of Nursing, Washburn University, 1700 Southwest College Avenue, Topeka, KS 66621. *Telephone:* 785-231-1010 Ext. 1526. *Fax:* 785-231-1032. *E-mail:* cynthia.hornberger@washburn.edu.

See full description on page 594.

Wichita State University

School of Nursing
Wichita, Kansas

http://www.wichita.edu/nurs

Founded in 1895

DEGREES • BSN • MSN • MSN/MBA

Nursing Program Faculty 36 (25% with doctorates).

Baccalaureate Enrollment 204
Women 88% **Men** 12% **Minority** 10% **International** 1% **Part-time** 1%

Graduate Enrollment 150
Women 94% **Men** 6% **Minority** 6% **International** 1% **Part-time** 60%

Nursing Student Activities Sigma Theta Tau, Student Nurses' Association.

Nursing Student Resources Academic advising; academic or career counseling; assistance for students with disabilities; bookstore; campus computer network; computer lab; computer-assisted instruction; daycare for children of students; e-mail services; employment services for current students; housing assistance; interactive nursing skills videos; Internet; learning resource lab; library services; nursing audiovisuals; skills, simulation, or other laboratory.

Library Facilities 1.6 million volumes (31,320 in health, 2,746 in nursing); 15,169 periodical subscriptions (406 health-care related).

■ Wichita State University School of Nursing, located in the major medical referral center for south-central Kansas, provides high-quality and diverse clinical learning experiences in urban and rural agencies throughout the state. Progression to the baccalaureate degree is facilitated for traditional and nontraditional students through both fall and spring admissions and includes an LPN to RN option. Internet courses provide RN to BSN, RN to MSN, and continuing education students with convenience and flexibility in scheduling. The graduate program prepares advanced practice nurses as clinical nurse specialists, nurse practitioners, nurse midwives, administrators, and educators. An MSN/MBA dual degree and graduate (post-master's) certificate options are offered.

BACCALAUREATE PROGRAMS

Degree BSN

Available Programs Generic Baccalaureate; LPN to RN Baccalaureate; RN Baccalaureate.

Study Options Full-time.

Program Entrance Requirements Minimum overall college GPA of 2.5, transcript of college record, CPR certification, health exam, health insurance, immunizations, minimum GPA in nursing prerequisites of 2.0, professional liability insurance/malpractice insurance, prerequisite course work. Transfer students are accepted. **Standardized tests** *Required:* TOEFL for international students. *Required for some:* ACT. **Application** *Deadline:* rolling (freshmen), rolling (transfer). *Notification:* continuous (freshmen). *Application fee:* $30.

Advanced Placement Credit given for nursing courses completed elsewhere dependent upon specific evaluations.

Expenses (2004–05) *Tuition, state resident:* full-time $3892; part-time $129 per credit hour. *Tuition, nonresident:* full-time $11,328; part-time $378 per credit hour. *International tuition:* $11,328 full-time. *Room and board:* $4810 per academic year. *Required fees:* full-time $166.

Financial Aid 80% of baccalaureate students in nursing programs received some form of financial aid in 2003–04.

Contact Mrs. Treva Lichti, RN, Academic Advisor, School of Nursing, Wichita State University, 1845 Fairmount Street, Wichita, KS 67260-0041. *Telephone:* 316-978-5732. *Fax:* 316-978-3094. *E-mail:* treva.lichti@wichita.edu.

GRADUATE PROGRAMS

Expenses (2004–05) *Tuition, state resident:* part-time $174 per credit hour. *Tuition, nonresident:* part-time $474 per credit hour. *Room and board:* $4810 per academic year. *Required fees:* full-time $150.

Financial Aid 60% of graduate students in nursing programs received some form of financial aid in 2003–04. 3 teaching assistantships with full tuition reimbursements available (averaging $8,243 per year) were awarded; fellowships, research assistantships, Federal Work-Study, institutionally sponsored loans, scholarships, traineeships, and unspecified assistantships also available. Aid available to part-time students. *Financial aid application deadline:* 4/1.

Contact Dr. Alicia Huckstadt, Director, Graduate Program, School of Nursing, Wichita State University, 1845 Fairmount Street, Wichita, KS 67260-0041. *Telephone:* 316-978-3610. *Fax:* 316-978-3094. *E-mail:* alicia.huckstadt@wichita.edu.

MASTER'S DEGREE PROGRAM

Degrees MSN; MSN/MBA

Available Programs Master's; RN to Master's.

Concentrations Available Nursing administration. *Clinical nurse specialist programs in:* acute care, pediatric. *Nurse practitioner programs in:* acute care, family health, pediatric, psychiatric/mental health.

Study Options Full-time and part-time.

Program Entrance Requirements Clinical experience, computer literacy, minimum overall college GPA of 3.0, transcript of college record, CPR certification, immunizations, professional liability insurance/malpractice insurance, resume, statistics course, GRE. *Application deadline:* For fall admission, 6/30 (priority date); for spring admission, 1/1. Applications are processed on a rolling basis. *Application fee:* $35 ($50 for international students).

Advanced Placement Credit given for nursing courses completed elsewhere dependent upon specific evaluations.

Degree Requirements 39 total credit hours, comprehensive exam.

POST-MASTER'S PROGRAM

Areas of Study *Clinical nurse specialist programs in:* acute care, pediatric. *Nurse practitioner programs in:* acute care, family health, pediatric, psychiatric/mental health.

KENTUCKY

Bellarmine University

Donna and Allan Lansing School of Nursing and Health Sciences
Louisville, Kentucky

http://www.bellarmine.edu

Founded in 1950

DEGREES • BSN • MSN • MSN/MBA

Nursing Program Faculty 76 (6% with doctorates).

Baccalaureate Enrollment 139
Women 90% **Men** 10% **Minority** 9% **Part-time** 15%

Graduate Enrollment 118
Women 94% **Men** 6% **Minority** 8% **Part-time** 100%

Nursing Student Activities Sigma Theta Tau, Student Nurses' Association.

Nursing Student Resources Academic advising; academic or career counseling; assistance for students with disabilities; bookstore; campus computer network; career placement assistance; computer lab; computer-assisted instruction; e-mail services; employment services for current students; externships; housing assistance; interactive nursing skills videos; Internet; learning resource lab; library services; nursing audiovisuals; paid internships; placement services for program completers; remedial services; resume preparation assistance; skills, simulation, or other laboratory; tutoring; unpaid internships.

Library Facilities 97,737 volumes (100 in health, 60 in nursing); 401 periodical subscriptions (125 health-care related).

BACCALAUREATE PROGRAMS

Degree BSN

Available Programs ADN to Baccalaureate; Accelerated Baccalaureate for Second Degree; Generic Baccalaureate; RN Baccalaureate.

Site Options Ashland, KY.

Study Options Full-time and part-time.

Program Entrance Requirements Minimum overall college GPA of 2.5, transcript of college record, CPR certification, health exam, high school transcript, immunizations, minimum GPA in nursing prerequisites of 2.5, prerequisite course work. Transfer students are accepted. **Standardized tests** *Required:* SAT or ACT, TOEFL for international students. **Application** *Deadline:* 2/1 (freshmen), 8/15 (transfer). *Early decision:* 11/1. *Notification:* 12/1 (early action). *Application fee:* $25.

Advanced Placement Credit by examination available. Credit given for nursing courses completed elsewhere dependent upon specific evaluations.

Expenses (2004–05) *Tuition:* full-time $19,250; part-time $440 per credit hour. *International tuition:* $19,250 full-time. *Room and board:* $3250; room only: $2000 per academic year. *Required fees:* full-time $820; part-time $130 per term.

Financial Aid 90% of baccalaureate students in nursing programs received some form of financial aid in 2003–04.

Contact Ms. Julie Armstrong-Binnix, Lansing School Marketing/Recruiter, Donna and Allan Lansing School of Nursing and Health Sciences, Bellarmine University, Miles Hall, #201, 2001 Newburg Road, Louisville, KY 40205-0671. *Telephone:* 502-452-8364. *Fax:* 502-452-8058. *E-mail:* jarmstrong-binnix@bellarmine.edu.

GRADUATE PROGRAMS

Expenses (2004–05) *Tuition:* part-time $450 per credit hour. *Room and board:* $3250; room only: $2000 per academic year. *Required fees:* part-time $90 per term.

Financial Aid 20% of graduate students in nursing programs received some form of financial aid in 2003–04.

Contact Mrs. Julie Armstrong-Binnix, Lansing School Marketing/Recruiter, Donna and Allan Lansing School of Nursing and Health Sciences, Bellarmine University, Miles Hall, #201, 2001 Newburg Road, Louisville, KY 40205-0671. *Telephone:* 502-452-8364. *Fax:* 502-452-8058. *E-mail:* jarmstrong-binnix@bellarmine.edu.

MASTER'S DEGREE PROGRAM

Degrees MSN; MSN/MBA

Available Programs Master's; Master's for Nurses with Non-Nursing Degrees; RN to Master's.

Concentrations Available Nursing administration; nursing education.

Site Options Ashland, KY.

Study Options Part-time.

Program Entrance Requirements Minimum overall college GPA of 2.75, transcript of college record, professional liability insurance/malpractice insurance, GRE General Test. *Application deadline:* For fall admission, 8/1 (priority date). Applications are processed on a rolling basis. *Application fee:* $25.

Advanced Placement Credit given for nursing courses completed elsewhere dependent upon specific evaluations.

Degree Requirements 38 total credit hours, thesis or project.

CONTINUING EDUCATION PROGRAM

Contact Ms. Linda Bailey, Director, Continuing Education, Donna and Allan Lansing School of Nursing and Health Sciences, Bellarmine University, Continuing Education Office, 2001 Newburg Road, Louisville, KY 40205-0671. *Telephone:* 502-452-8161. *Fax:* 502-452-8203. *E-mail:* lbailey@bellarmine.edu.

Berea College

Department of Nursing
Berea, Kentucky

http://www.berea.edu

Founded in 1855

DEGREE • BS

Nursing Program Faculty 8 (25% with doctorates).

Baccalaureate Enrollment 66
Women 90% **Men** 10% **Minority** 20% **International** 10%

Nursing Student Activities Student Nurses' Association.

Nursing Student Resources Academic advising; academic or career counseling; assistance for students with disabilities; bookstore; campus computer network; career placement assistance; computer lab; computer-assisted instruction; daycare for children of students; e-mail services; employment services for current students; externships; housing assistance; interactive nursing skills videos; Internet; learning resource lab; library

Berea College (continued)

services; nursing audiovisuals; paid internships; placement services for program completers; remedial services; resume preparation assistance; skills, simulation, or other laboratory; tutoring; unpaid internships.

Library Facilities 358,556 volumes (5,760 in health, 4,871 in nursing); 1,918 periodical subscriptions (95 health-care related).

BACCALAUREATE PROGRAMS

Degree BS

Available Programs Generic Baccalaureate.

Study Options Full-time.

Program Entrance Requirements Transcript of college record, written essay, high school transcript, immunizations, 3 letters of recommendation, minimum high school rank 20%. Transfer students are accepted. **Standardized tests** *Required:* SAT or ACT, TOEFL for international students. **Application** *Deadline:* rolling (freshmen), rolling (transfer). *Notification:* 4/30 (freshmen).

Advanced Placement Credit given for nursing courses completed elsewhere dependent upon specific evaluations.

Financial Aid 100% of baccalaureate students in nursing programs received some form of financial aid in 2002–03.

Contact Dr. Pam Farley, Chairperson and Professor, Department of Nursing, Berea College, CPO 1794, Berea, KY 40404. *Telephone:* 859-985-3384. *Fax:* 859-985-3917. *E-mail:* pam_farley@berea.edu.

CONTINUING EDUCATION PROGRAM

Contact Dr. Pam Farley, Chairperson and Associate Professor, Department of Nursing, Berea College, CPO 1794, Berea, KY 40404. *Telephone:* 859-985-3384. *Fax:* 859-985-3917. *E-mail:* pam_farley@berea.edu.

Eastern Kentucky University

Department of Baccalaureate and Graduate Nursing

Richmond, Kentucky

http://www.bsn-gn.eku.edu

Founded in 1906

DEGREES • BSN • MSN

Nursing Program Faculty 22.

Nursing Student Activities Sigma Theta Tau.

Library Facilities 768,300 volumes; 3,128 periodical subscriptions.

BACCALAUREATE PROGRAMS

Degree BSN

Available Programs Generic Baccalaureate; RN Baccalaureate.

Site Options *Distance Learning:* Corbin, KY; Hazard, KY; Somerset, KY.

Study Options Full-time and part-time.

Program Entrance Requirements Minimum high school GPA of 2.5, prerequisite course work. Transfer students are accepted. **Standardized tests** *Required:* ACT, TOEFL for international students. **Application** *Deadline:* 8/1 (freshmen), rolling (transfer). *Notification:* continuous (freshmen). *Application fee:* $30.

Advanced Placement Credit by examination available. Credit given for nursing courses completed elsewhere dependent upon specific evaluations.

Contact Department of Baccalaureate and Graduate Nursing, Department of Baccalaureate and Graduate Nursing, Eastern Kentucky University, 223 Rowlett Building, 521 Lancaster Avenue, Richmond, KY 40475-3102. *Telephone:* 859-622-1956. *Fax:* 859-622-1972.

GRADUATE PROGRAMS

Contact Outreach and Graduate Coordinator, Department of Baccalaureate and Graduate Nursing, Eastern Kentucky University, 223 Rowlett Building, 521 Lancaster Avenue, Richmond, KY 40475. *Telephone:* 859-622-1827. *Fax:* 859-622-1972.

MASTER'S DEGREE PROGRAM

Degree MSN

Available Programs Master's.

Concentrations Available *Nurse practitioner programs in:* community health, family health.

Site Options *Distance Learning:* Corbin, KY.

Study Options Full-time and part-time.

Program Entrance Requirements Minimum overall college GPA of 2.75, transcript of college record, written essay, 3 letters of recommendation, physical assessment course, prerequisite course work.

Midway College

Program in Nursing (Baccalaureate)

Midway, Kentucky

http://www.midway.edu/degreeprograms/nursing.html

Founded in 1847

DEGREE • BSN

Nursing Program Faculty 2.

Nursing Student Resources Academic advising; campus computer network; computer-assisted instruction; e-mail services; interactive nursing skills videos; Internet; learning resource lab; library services; nursing audiovisuals; remedial services; skills, simulation, or other laboratory.

Library Facilities 96,236 volumes (1,200 in health, 800 in nursing); 250 periodical subscriptions (102 health-care related).

BACCALAUREATE PROGRAMS

Degree BSN

Available Programs ADN to Baccalaureate; Accelerated RN Baccalaureate; Generic Baccalaureate; RN Baccalaureate.

Site Options Danville, KY.

Study Options Full-time and part-time.

Program Entrance Requirements Minimum overall college GPA of 2.3, transcript of college record, high school transcript, interview, 1 letter of recommendation, minimum GPA in nursing prerequisites of 2.0, prerequisite course work, RN licensure. Transfer students are accepted. **Standardized tests** *Required:* SAT or ACT, TOEFL for international students. **Application** *Deadline:* rolling (freshmen), rolling (transfer). *Notification:* continuous (freshmen). *Application fee:* $25.

Advanced Placement Credit given for nursing courses completed elsewhere dependent upon specific evaluations.

Financial Aid 95% of baccalaureate students in nursing programs received some form of financial aid in 2002–03. *Gift aid (need-based):* Federal Pell, FSEOG, state, private, college/university gift aid from institutional funds. *Loans:* FFEL (Subsidized and Unsubsidized Stafford PLUS), Perkins, college/university. *Work-Study:* Federal Work-Study, part-time campus jobs. *Application deadline (priority):* 3/15.

Contact Ms. Barbara Kitchen, RN, Coordinator, Baccalaureate Nursing Program, Program in Nursing (Baccalaureate), Midway College, 512 East Stephens Street, Midway, KY 40347. *Telephone:* 859-846-5725. *E-mail:* bkitchen@midway.edu.

CONTINUING EDUCATION PROGRAM

Contact Mrs. Barbara Kitchen, Coordinator, Baccalaureate Nursing Program, Program in Nursing (Baccalaureate), Midway College, 512 East Stephens Street, Midway, KY 40347. *Telephone:* 859-846-5735. *E-mail:* bkitchen@midway.edu.

Morehead State University

Department of Nursing and Allied Health Sciences

Morehead, Kentucky

http://www.moreheadstate.edu/colleges/science/nahs/

Founded in 1922

DEGREE • BSN

Nursing Program Faculty 9 (11% with doctorates).

Baccalaureate Enrollment 94
Women 89% **Men** 11% **Minority** 4% **Part-time** 8%

Nursing Student Activities Student Nurses' Association.

Nursing Student Resources Academic advising; academic or career counseling; assistance for students with disabilities; bookstore; campus computer network; career placement assistance; computer lab; computer-assisted instruction; daycare for children of students; e-mail services; interactive nursing skills videos; Internet; learning resource lab; library services; nursing audiovisuals; remedial services; resume preparation assistance; skills, simulation, or other laboratory; tutoring.

Library Facilities 333,518 volumes (2,000 in health, 850 in nursing); 2,627 periodical subscriptions (45 health-care related).

BACCALAUREATE PROGRAMS

Degree BSN

Available Programs Generic Baccalaureate; RN Baccalaureate.

Site Options *Distance Learning:* Prestonsburg, KY; Ashland, KY; Maysville, KY.

Study Options Full-time and part-time.

Program Entrance Requirements Minimum overall college GPA of 2.0, transcript of college record, CPR certification, health exam, immunizations, minimum GPA in nursing prerequisites of 2.5, prerequisite course work. Transfer students are accepted. **Standardized tests** *Required:* SAT or ACT, TOEFL for international students. *Recommended:* ACT. **Application** *Deadline:* rolling (freshmen), rolling (transfer). *Notification:* continuous (freshmen).

Advanced Placement Credit by examination available. Credit given for nursing courses completed elsewhere dependent upon specific evaluations.

Expenses (2004–05) *Tuition, state resident:* full-time $7680; part-time $240 per credit hour. *Tuition, nonresident:* full-time $20,400; part-time $360 per credit hour. *International tuition:* $20,400 full-time. *Room and board:* $8820; room only: $4200 per academic year. *Required fees:* full-time $220; part-time $85 per credit; part-time $105 per term.

Financial Aid 75% of baccalaureate students in nursing programs received some form of financial aid in 2003–04. *Gift aid (need-based):* Federal Pell, FSEOG, state, private, college/university gift aid from institutional funds. *Loans:* Federal Direct (Subsidized and Unsubsidized Stafford PLUS), Perkins, college/university. *Work-Study:* Federal Work-Study, part-time campus jobs. *Application deadline (priority):* 3/15.

Contact Shannon Harr, Student Services Officer, Department of Nursing and Allied Health Sciences, Morehead State University, Reed Hall 234, Morehead, KY 40351. *Telephone:* 606-783-2772. *Fax:* 606-783-9104. *E-mail:* s.harr@moreheadstate.edu.

Murray State University

Department of Nursing
Murray, Kentucky

http://www.murraystate.edu/

Founded in 1922

DEGREES • BSN • M SC N

Nursing Program Faculty 17 (47% with doctorates).

Baccalaureate Enrollment 248
Women 94% **Men** 6% **Minority** 3%

Graduate Enrollment 50
Women 85% **Men** 15%

Nursing Student Activities Sigma Theta Tau, Student Nurses' Association.

Nursing Student Resources Academic advising; academic or career counseling; assistance for students with disabilities; bookstore; campus computer network; career placement assistance; computer lab; computer-assisted instruction; daycare for children of students; e-mail services; employment services for current students; externships; housing assistance; interactive nursing skills videos; Internet; learning resource lab; library services; nursing audiovisuals; placement services for program completers; remedial services; resume preparation assistance; skills, simulation, or other laboratory; tutoring; unpaid internships.

Library Facilities 400,000 volumes (4,060 in health, 2,160 in nursing); 2,500 periodical subscriptions (124 health-care related).

BACCALAUREATE PROGRAMS

Degree BSN

Available Programs Generic Baccalaureate; RN Baccalaureate.

Site Options *Distance Learning:* Madisonville, KY; Paducah, KY; Hopkinsville, KY.

Study Options Full-time.

Program Entrance Requirements Transcript of college record, CPR certification, immunizations, minimum GPA in nursing prerequisites of 2.5, professional liability insurance/malpractice insurance, prerequisite course work. Transfer students are accepted. **Standardized tests** *Required:* ACT, TOEFL for international students. **Application** *Notification:* continuous until 8/1 (freshmen). *Application fee:* $25.

Advanced Placement Credit by examination available. Credit given for nursing courses completed elsewhere dependent upon specific evaluations.

Expenses (2004–05) *Tuition, state resident:* full-time $3984; part-time $166 per credit hour. *Tuition, nonresident:* full-time $10,836; part-time $452 per credit hour. *International tuition:* $10,836 full-time. *Room and board:* $2406; room only: $1128 per academic year.

Financial Aid 70% of baccalaureate students in nursing programs received some form of financial aid in 2003–04. *Gift aid (need-based):* Federal Pell, FSEOG, state, private, college/university gift aid from institutional funds. *Loans:* Federal Nursing Student Loans, FFEL (Subsidized and Unsubsidized Stafford PLUS), Perkins, college/university. *Work-Study:* Federal Work-Study, part-time campus jobs. *Application deadline (priority):* 4/1.

Contact Dr. Marcia B. Hobbs, Chair, Department of Nursing, Murray State University, 120 Mason Hall, Murray, KY 42071-0009. *Telephone:* 270-762-2193. *Fax:* 270-762-6662. *E-mail:* marcia.hobbs@murraystate.edu.

GRADUATE PROGRAMS

Expenses (2004–05) *Tuition, state resident:* full-time $4185; part-time $233 per credit hour. *Tuition, nonresident:* full-time $11,700; part-time $650 per credit hour. *International tuition:* $11,700 full-time. *Room and board:* $4662; room only: $2256 per academic year.

Financial Aid 70% of graduate students in nursing programs received some form of financial aid in 2003–04. Research assistantships, teaching assistantships, Federal Work-Study available. *Financial aid application deadline:* 4/1.

Contact Dr. Nancey E. M. France, RN, Graduate Coordinator, Department of Nursing, Murray State University, 120 Mason Hall, Murray, KY 42071-0009. *Telephone:* 270-762-6671. *Fax:* 270-762-6662. *E-mail:* nancey.france@murraystate.edu.

MASTER'S DEGREE PROGRAM

Degree M Sc N

Available Programs Master's.

Concentrations Available Nurse anesthesia. *Clinical nurse specialist programs in:* adult health, critical care, medical-surgical. *Nurse practitioner programs in:* family health.

Site Options *Distance Learning:* Madisonville, KY; Paducah, KY; Hopkinsville, KY.

Study Options Full-time and part-time.

Program Entrance Requirements Clinical experience, minimum overall college GPA of 3.0, transcript of college record, CPR certification, immunizations, interview, 3 letters of recommendation, nursing research course, physical assessment course, professional liability insurance/malpractice insurance, prerequisite course work, statistics course, GRE General Test. *Application deadline:* Applications are processed on a rolling basis. *Application fee:* $25.

Advanced Placement Credit given for nursing courses completed elsewhere dependent upon specific evaluations.

Degree Requirements 64 total credit hours.

Murray State University (continued)

POST-MASTER'S PROGRAM

Areas of Study Nurse anesthesia. *Nurse practitioner programs in:* family health.

CONTINUING EDUCATION PROGRAM

Contact Sandy Minor, Department of Nursing, Murray State University, 120 Mason Hall, Murray, KY 42071-0009. *Telephone:* 270-762-6674. *Fax:* 270-762-6662. *E-mail:* ann.minor@murraystate.edu.

Northern Kentucky University

Department of Nursing
Highland Heights, Kentucky

Founded in 1968

DEGREES • BSN • MSN

Nursing Program Faculty 42 (50% with doctorates).

Baccalaureate Enrollment 53
Women 95% **Men** 5% **Minority** 2% **International** 1% **Part-time** 50%

Graduate Enrollment 99
Women 95% **Men** 5% **Minority** 1%

Nursing Student Activities Sigma Theta Tau, Student Nurses' Association.

Nursing Student Resources Academic advising; academic or career counseling; assistance for students with disabilities; bookstore; campus computer network; career placement assistance; computer lab; computer-assisted instruction; daycare for children of students; e-mail services; interactive nursing skills videos; Internet; learning resource lab; library services; nursing audiovisuals; tutoring.

Library Facilities 325,721 volumes (6,380 in health, 3,500 in nursing); 2,217 periodical subscriptions (100 health-care related).

BACCALAUREATE PROGRAMS

Degree BSN

Available Programs Accelerated Baccalaureate for Second Degree; Generic Baccalaureate; RN Baccalaureate.

Site Options *Distance Learning:* Highland Heights, KY.

Study Options Full-time and part-time.

Program Entrance Requirements Minimum overall college GPA of 2.5, transcript of college record, CPR certification, health exam, health insurance, high school biology, high school chemistry, 1 year of high school math, high school transcript, immunizations, prerequisite course work. Transfer students are accepted. **Standardized tests** *Required:* SAT or ACT, TOEFL for international students. *Recommended:* ACT. **Application** *Deadline:* 8/1 (freshmen), 8/1 (transfer). *Early decision:* 2/1. *Notification:* continuous (freshmen), 2/15 (early action). *Application fee:* $25.

Advanced Placement Credit by examination available. Credit given for nursing courses completed elsewhere dependent upon specific evaluations.

Expenses (2003–04) *Tuition, area resident:* full-time $1872; part-time $156 per credit hour. *Tuition, nonresident:* full-time $3996; part-time $333 per credit hour. *International tuition:* $3996 full-time. *Room and board:* $2000 per academic year.

Financial Aid 10% of baccalaureate students in nursing programs received some form of financial aid in 2002–03.

Contact Dr. Ann Keller, Director, BSN Program, Department of Nursing, Northern Kentucky University, Nunn Drive, AHC 303, Highland Heights, KY 41099. *Telephone:* 859-572-5248. *Fax:* 859-572-6098. *E-mail:* kelleran@nku.edu.

GRADUATE PROGRAMS

Expenses (2003–04) *Tuition, state resident:* part-time $210 per credit hour. *Tuition, nonresident:* part-time $483 per credit hour. *Room and board:* $2000 per academic year. *Required fees:* full-time $3780.

Financial Aid 15% of graduate students in nursing programs received some form of financial aid in 2002–03.

Contact Dr. Denise Robinson, Director of Graduate Nursing Program, Department of Nursing, Northern Kentucky University, Highland Heights, KY 41099. *Telephone:* 859-572-5178. *Fax:* 859-572-6098. *E-mail:* robinson@nku.edu.

MASTER'S DEGREE PROGRAM

Degree MSN

Concentrations Available Nursing administration; nursing education. *Nurse practitioner programs in:* adult health, family health, gerontology, pediatric.

Site Options *Distance Learning:* Highland Heights, KY.

Study Options Full-time and part-time.

Program Entrance Requirements Clinical experience, minimum overall college GPA of 3.0, transcript of college record, CPR certification, immunizations, nursing research course, physical assessment course, professional liability insurance/malpractice insurance, statistics course.

Advanced Placement Credit by examination available. Credit given for nursing courses completed elsewhere dependent upon specific evaluations.

Degree Requirements 36 total credit hours, thesis or project.

POST-MASTER'S PROGRAM

Areas of Study Nursing administration; nursing education. *Nurse practitioner programs in:* adult health, family health, gerontology, pediatric.

Spalding University

School of Nursing
Louisville, Kentucky

http://www.spalding.edu/nursing

Founded in 1814

DEGREES • BSN • MSN

Nursing Program Faculty 33 (18% with doctorates).

Baccalaureate Enrollment 159
Women 94% **Men** 6% **Minority** 24%

Graduate Enrollment 41
Women 100% **Minority** 2% **Part-time** 50%

Nursing Student Activities Sigma Theta Tau, Student Nurses' Association.

Nursing Student Resources Academic advising; academic or career counseling; assistance for students with disabilities; bookstore; campus computer network; career placement assistance; computer lab; computer-assisted instruction; e-mail services; employment services for current students; externships; interactive nursing skills videos; Internet; learning resource lab; library services; nursing audiovisuals; remedial services; resume preparation assistance; skills, simulation, or other laboratory; tutoring; unpaid internships.

Library Facilities 185,498 volumes (2,875 in health, 1,125 in nursing); 592 periodical subscriptions (367 health-care related).

BACCALAUREATE PROGRAMS

Degree BSN

Available Programs Accelerated Baccalaureate for Second Degree; Accelerated RN Baccalaureate; Generic Baccalaureate.

Study Options Full-time and part-time.

Program Entrance Requirements Minimum overall college GPA of 2.5, transcript of college record, CPR certification, health exam, health insurance, high school transcript, immunizations, interview, minimum GPA in nursing prerequisites of 2.5, professional liability insurance/malpractice insurance, prerequisite course work. Transfer students are accepted. **Standardized tests** *Required:* SAT or ACT, TOEFL for international students. **Application** *Deadline:* 8/1 (freshmen), 8/1 (transfer). *Notification:* continuous (freshmen). *Application fee:* $20.

Advanced Placement Credit given for nursing courses completed elsewhere dependent upon specific evaluations.

Expenses (2004–05) *Tuition:* full-time $18,900; part-time $450 per credit hour. *International tuition:* $18,900 full-time. *Room and board:* $6575; room only: $3710 per academic year. *Required fees:* full-time $1050; part-time $25 per credit.

Financial Aid 80% of baccalaureate students in nursing programs received some form of financial aid in 2003–04. *Gift aid (need-based):* Federal Pell, FSEOG, state, private, college/university gift aid from institutional funds. *Loans:* Federal Nursing Student Loans, FFEL (Subsidized and Unsubsidized Stafford PLUS), Perkins, college/university. *Work-Study:* Federal Work-Study, part-time campus jobs. *Application deadline (priority):* 3/1.

Contact Dr. Veronica Abdur-Rahman, PhD, Director Baccalaureate Program in Nursing, School of Nursing, Spalding University, 851 South Fourth Street, Louisville, KY 40203. *Telephone:* 502-585-7125. *Fax:* 502-588-7175. *E-mail:* vrahman@spalding.edu.

GRADUATE PROGRAMS

Expenses (2004–05) *Tuition:* full-time $9900; part-time $495 per credit hour. *International tuition:* $9900 full-time. *Required fees:* full-time $500; part-time $25 per credit; part-time $225 per term.

Financial Aid 85% of graduate students in nursing programs received some form of financial aid in 2003–04. 1 research assistantship (averaging $2,800 per year) was awarded; career-related internships or fieldwork, scholarships, and traineeships also available. Aid available to part-time students. *Financial aid application deadline:* 3/15.

Contact Dr. Michael L. Huggins, RN, EdD, Director, Graduate Programs, School of Nursing, Spalding University, 851 South Fourth Street, Louisville, KY 40203-2188. *Telephone:* 502-585-7125. *Fax:* 502-588-7175. *E-mail:* mhuggins@spalding.edu.

MASTER'S DEGREE PROGRAM

Degree MSN

Available Programs Accelerated Master's for Non-Nursing College Graduates; Accelerated RN to Master's; Master's.

Concentrations Available Nursing administration; nursing education. *Nurse practitioner programs in:* adult health, family health, pediatric.

Site Options Louisville, KY.

Study Options Full-time and part-time.

Program Entrance Requirements Minimum overall college GPA of 2.7, transcript of college record, CPR certification, written essay, immunizations, interview, 2 letters of recommendation, physical assessment course, professional liability insurance/malpractice insurance, prerequisite course work, resume, statistics course, GRE General Test. *Application deadline:* For fall admission, 8/15 (priority date); for spring admission, 12/15 (priority date). Applications are processed on a rolling basis. *Application fee:* $30.

Advanced Placement Credit by examination available. Credit given for nursing courses completed elsewhere dependent upon specific evaluations.

Degree Requirements 40 total credit hours, thesis or project.

POST-MASTER'S PROGRAM

Areas of Study Nursing administration; nursing education. *Nurse practitioner programs in:* adult health, family health, pediatric.

CONTINUING EDUCATION PROGRAM

Contact Dr. Ignatius Perkins, OP, DNS, Continuing Education Administrator, School of Nursing, Spalding University, 851 South Fourth Street, Louisville, KY 40203-2188. *Telephone:* 502-585-7125. *Fax:* 502-588-7175. *E-mail:* iperkins@spalding.edu.

Thomas More College

Program in Nursing
Crestview Hills, Kentucky

http://www.thomasmore.edu

Founded in 1921

DEGREE • BSN

Nursing Program Faculty 6 (33% with doctorates).

Baccalaureate Enrollment 70

Women 98% **Men** 2% **Minority** 1% **International** 1% **Part-time** 5%

Nursing Student Activities Student Nurses' Association, nursing club.

Nursing Student Resources Academic advising; academic or career counseling; assistance for students with disabilities; bookstore; campus computer network; career placement assistance; computer lab; computer-assisted instruction; e-mail services; employment services for current students; externships; interactive nursing skills videos; Internet; learning resource lab; library services; nursing audiovisuals; other; placement services for program completers; remedial services; resume preparation assistance; skills, simulation, or other laboratory; tutoring.

Library Facilities 127,429 volumes (350 in health, 200 in nursing); 609 periodical subscriptions (50 health-care related).

BACCALAUREATE PROGRAMS

Degree BSN

Available Programs Generic Baccalaureate.

Study Options Full-time.

Program Entrance Requirements CPR certification, health exam, health insurance, 1 year of high school math, immunizations, minimum GPA in nursing prerequisites of 2.5, professional liability insurance/malpractice insurance, prerequisite course work. Transfer students are accepted. **Standardized tests** *Required:* SAT or ACT, TOEFL for international students. **Application** *Deadline:* 8/15 (freshmen), 8/15 (transfer). *Notification:* continuous (freshmen). *Application fee:* $25.

Advanced Placement Credit given for nursing courses completed elsewhere dependent upon specific evaluations.

Expenses (2003–04) *Tuition:* full-time $16,200; part-time $375 per credit hour. *International tuition:* $16,200 full-time. *Room and board:* $2500 per academic year. *Required fees:* full-time $200; part-time $30 per credit.

Financial Aid 80% of baccalaureate students in nursing programs received some form of financial aid in 2002–03.

Contact Dr. Lisa Spangler Torok, Chair, Program in Nursing, Thomas More College, 333 Thomas More Parkway, Crestview Hills, KY 41017. *Telephone:* 859-344-3413. *Fax:* 859-344-3537. *E-mail:* Lisa.spangler-torok@thomasmore.edu.

University of Kentucky

Graduate School Programs in the College of Nursing
Lexington, Kentucky

http://www.mc.uky.edu/nursing

Founded in 1865

DEGREES • BSN • MSN • PHD

Nursing Program Faculty 65 (54% with doctorates).

Baccalaureate Enrollment 223

Women 94% **Men** 6% **Minority** 4% **Part-time** 14%

Graduate Enrollment 205

Women 91% **Men** 9% **Minority** 9% **International** 5% **Part-time** 64%

Nursing Student Activities Sigma Theta Tau, Student Nurses' Association.

Nursing Student Resources Academic advising; academic or career counseling; assistance for students with disabilities; bookstore; campus computer network; career placement assistance; computer lab; computer-assisted instruction; e-mail services; interactive nursing skills videos; Internet; learning resource lab; library services; nursing audiovisuals; skills, simulation, or other laboratory.

Library Facilities 3.1 million volumes (105,793 in health); 29,633 periodical subscriptions (3,347 health-care related).

BACCALAUREATE PROGRAMS

Degree BSN

Available Programs Generic Baccalaureate; RN Baccalaureate.

University of Kentucky (continued)

Study Options Full-time and part-time.

Program Entrance Requirements Minimum overall college GPA of 2.5, transcript of college record, CPR certification, written essay, high school transcript, immunizations, 1 letter of recommendation, minimum GPA in nursing prerequisites of 2.5, prerequisite course work. Transfer students are accepted. **Standardized tests** *Required:* SAT or ACT, TOEFL for international students. **Application** *Deadline:* 2/15 (freshmen), 8/1 (transfer). *Notification:* continuous (freshmen). *Application fee:* $30.

Advanced Placement Credit by examination available. Credit given for nursing courses completed elsewhere dependent upon specific evaluations.

Expenses (2003–04) *Tuition, state resident:* full-time $4002; part-time $167 per credit hour. *Tuition, nonresident:* full-time $10,682; part-time $167 per credit hour. *International tuition:* $10,682 full-time. *Room and board:* $4335; room only: $2784 per academic year. *Required fees:* full-time $545; part-time $14 per credit.

Financial Aid 60% of baccalaureate students in nursing programs received some form of financial aid in 2002–03. *Gift aid (need-based):* Federal Pell, FSEOG, state, private, college/university gift aid from institutional funds. *Loans:* Federal Nursing Student Loans, Federal Direct (Subsidized and Unsubsidized Stafford PLUS), Perkins, college/university. *Work-Study:* Federal Work-Study, part-time campus jobs. *Application deadline (priority):* 2/15.

Contact Office of Student Services, Graduate School Programs in the College of Nursing, University of Kentucky, Room 309 College of Nursing Building, University of Kentucky, Lexington, KY 40536-0232. *Telephone:* 859-323-5108. *Fax:* 859-323-1057. *E-mail:* conss@uky.edu.

GRADUATE PROGRAMS

Expenses (2003–04) *Tuition, state resident:* full-time $4430; part-time $247 per credit hour. *Tuition, nonresident:* full-time $11,770; part-time $654 per credit hour. *International tuition:* $11,770 full-time. *Room and board:* $5700; room only: $4200 per academic year. *Required fees:* full-time $545; part-time $14 per credit.

Financial Aid 40% of graduate students in nursing programs received some form of financial aid in 2002–03. 3 fellowships, 24 research assistantships, 8 teaching assistantships were awarded; Federal Work-Study and institutionally sponsored loans also available. Aid available to part-time students. *Financial aid application deadline:* 3/1.

Contact Office of Student Services, Graduate School Programs in the College of Nursing, University of Kentucky, Room 309 College of Nursing Building, University of Kentucky, Lexington, KY 40536-0232. *Telephone:* 859-323-5108. *Fax:* 859-323-1057. *E-mail:* conss@uky.edu.

MASTER'S DEGREE PROGRAM

Degree MSN

Available Programs Master's; RN to Master's.

Concentrations Available Nurse case management. *Clinical nurse specialist programs in:* acute care, adult health, community health, critical care, gerontology, medical-surgical, oncology, parent-child, pediatric, perinatal, psychiatric/mental health, public health, women's health. *Nurse practitioner programs in:* acute care, adult health, family health, gerontology, pediatric, psychiatric/mental health.

Study Options Full-time and part-time.

Program Entrance Requirements Clinical experience, minimum overall college GPA of 2.75, transcript of college record, written essay, interview, 3 letters of recommendation, physical assessment course, statistics course, GRE General Test. *Application deadline:* For fall admission, 3/1. Applications are processed on a rolling basis. *Application fee:* $35 ($45 for international students).

Advanced Placement Credit given for nursing courses completed elsewhere dependent upon specific evaluations.

Degree Requirements 40 total credit hours, comprehensive exam.

POST-MASTER'S PROGRAM

Areas of Study Nurse case management. *Nurse practitioner programs in:* acute care, adult health, family health, gerontology, pediatric, psychiatric/mental health.

DOCTORAL DEGREE PROGRAM

Degree PhD

Available Programs Doctorate.

Areas of Study Nursing research.

Program Entrance Requirements Minimum overall college GPA of 3.3, interview, 3 letters of recommendation, MSN or equivalent, statistics course, writing sample, GRE General Test. *Application deadline:* For fall admission, 3/1. Applications are processed on a rolling basis. *Application fee:* $35 ($45 for international students).

Degree Requirements 63 total credit hours, dissertation, oral exam, written exam, residency.

CONTINUING EDUCATION PROGRAM

Contact Dr. Marcia Stanhope, Coordinator, Graduate School Programs in the College of Nursing, University of Kentucky, Room 315 College of Nursing Building, University of Kentucky, Lexington, KY 40536-0232. *Telephone:* 859-257-9335. *Fax:* 859-323-1057. *E-mail:* mkstan00@uky.edu.

University of Louisville
School of Nursing
Louisville, Kentucky

http://www.louisville.edu/nursing

Founded in 1798

DEGREES • BSN • MSN

Nursing Program Faculty 53 (40% with doctorates).

Baccalaureate Enrollment 256

Women 93% **Men** 7% **Minority** 17% **International** 1% **Part-time** 2%

Graduate Enrollment 100

Women 95% **Men** 5% **Minority** 10% **Part-time** 71%

Nursing Student Activities Nursing Honor Society, Sigma Theta Tau, Student Nurses' Association.

Nursing Student Resources Academic advising; assistance for students with disabilities; bookstore; campus computer network; career placement assistance; computer lab; computer-assisted instruction; e-mail services; employment services for current students; housing assistance; interactive nursing skills videos; Internet; learning resource lab; library services; nursing audiovisuals; placement services for program completers; skills, simulation, or other laboratory; tutoring.

Library Facilities 2 million volumes (220,948 in health, 2,852 in nursing); 24,910 periodical subscriptions (3,800 health-care related).

BACCALAUREATE PROGRAMS

Degree BSN

Available Programs Accelerated Baccalaureate for Second Degree; Accelerated RN Baccalaureate; Generic Baccalaureate.

Study Options Full-time.

Program Entrance Requirements Minimum overall college GPA of 2.5, transcript of college record, CPR certification, written essay, health exam, health insurance, high school biology, high school chemistry, high school foreign language, 3 years high school math, 2 years high school science, high school transcript, immunizations, interview, minimum high school GPA of 2.5, minimum GPA in nursing prerequisites of 2.5, professional liability insurance/malpractice insurance, prerequisite course work. Transfer students are accepted. **Standardized tests** *Required:* SAT or ACT, TOEFL for international students. **Application** *Deadline:* rolling (freshmen). *Notification:* continuous (freshmen). *Application fee:* $30.

Advanced Placement Credit by examination available. Credit given for nursing courses completed elsewhere dependent upon specific evaluations.

Expenses (2004–05) *Tuition, state resident:* full-time $5040; part-time $210 per credit hour. *Tuition, nonresident:* full-time $13,752; part-time $573 per credit hour. *Room and board:* room only: $4440 per academic year.

Financial Aid *Gift aid (need-based):* Federal Pell, FSEOG, state, private, college/university gift aid from institutional funds. *Loans:* Federal Nursing Student Loans, FFEL (Subsidized and Unsubsidized Stafford PLUS), Perkins, college/university. *Work-Study:* Federal Work-Study. *Application deadline (priority):* 3/15.

Contact Dianne Foster, Director of Student Services, School of Nursing, University of Louisville, 555 South Floyd Street, Louisville, KY 40202. *Telephone:* 502-852-5366. *Fax:* 502-852-8783. *E-mail:* ddfost01@louisville.edu.

GRADUATE PROGRAMS

Expenses (2004–05) *Tuition, state resident:* full-time $5472; part-time $304 per credit hour. *Tuition, nonresident:* full-time $15,084; part-time $838 per credit hour. *Room and board:* room only: $4440 per academic year.

Financial Aid 1 research assistantship (averaging $10,800 per year) was awarded; institutionally sponsored loans, scholarships, and traineeships also available.

Contact Dr. Cynthia McCurren, Associate Dean for Academic Programs, School of Nursing, University of Louisville, 555 South Floyd Street, Louisville, KY 40202. *Telephone:* 502-852-5366. *Fax:* 502-852-8783. *E-mail:* camccu01@louisville.edu.

MASTER'S DEGREE PROGRAM

Degree MSN

Available Programs Master's.

Concentrations Available *Clinical nurse specialist programs in:* adult health, oncology, psychiatric/mental health. *Nurse practitioner programs in:* adult health, family health, gerontology, neonatal health, psychiatric/mental health, women's health.

Study Options Full-time and part-time.

Program Entrance Requirements Clinical experience, minimum overall college GPA of 3.0, transcript of college record, CPR certification, written essay, immunizations, interview, 2 letters of recommendation, physical assessment course, professional liability insurance/malpractice insurance, GRE General Test. *Application deadline:* For fall admission, 5/1 (priority date); for spring admission, 10/1 (priority date). Applications are processed on a rolling basis. *Application fee:* $50.

Advanced Placement Credit given for nursing courses completed elsewhere dependent upon specific evaluations.

Degree Requirements 45 total credit hours, thesis or project.

POST-MASTER'S PROGRAM

Areas of Study *Clinical nurse specialist programs in:* adult health, oncology, psychiatric/mental health. *Nurse practitioner programs in:* adult health, family health, gerontology, neonatal health, psychiatric/mental health, women's health.

Western Kentucky University

Department of Nursing
Bowling Green, Kentucky

http://www.wku.edu

Founded in 1906

DEGREES • BSN • MSN

Nursing Program Faculty 18 (58% with doctorates).

Baccalaureate Enrollment 163
Women 89% **Men** 11% **Minority** 3% **Part-time** 40%

Graduate Enrollment 34
Women 89% **Men** 11% **Minority** 2%

Nursing Student Activities Nursing Honor Society, Sigma Theta Tau, Student Nurses' Association.

Nursing Student Resources Academic advising; academic or career counseling; assistance for students with disabilities; bookstore; campus computer network; career placement assistance; computer lab; computer-assisted instruction; e-mail services; employment services for current students; externships; housing assistance; interactive nursing skills videos; Internet; learning resource lab; library services; nursing audiovisuals; paid internships; placement services for program completers; remedial services; resume preparation assistance; skills, simulation, or other laboratory; tutoring; unpaid internships.

Library Facilities 17,880 volumes in health, 1,697 volumes in nursing; 217 periodical subscriptions health-care related.

BACCALAUREATE PROGRAMS

Degree BSN

Site Options *Distance Learning:* Elizabethtown, KY; Glasgow, KY; Owensboro, KY.

Study Options Full-time.

Program Entrance Requirements Minimum overall college GPA of 2.75, transcript of college record, CPR certification, health exam, health insurance, high school transcript, immunizations, professional liability insurance/malpractice insurance. Transfer students are accepted. **Standardized tests** *Required:* SAT or ACT, TOEFL for international students. **Application** *Deadline:* 8/1 (freshmen), 6/1 (out-of-state freshmen), 8/1 (transfer). *Notification:* continuous (freshmen), continuous (out-of-state freshmen). *Application fee:* $35.

Advanced Placement Credit given for nursing courses completed elsewhere dependent upon specific evaluations.

Expenses (2003–04) *Tuition, state resident:* full-time $3850; part-time $169 per credit hour. *Tuition, nonresident:* full-time $8698; part-time $371 per credit hour.

Financial Aid 36% of baccalaureate students in nursing programs received some form of financial aid in 2002–03.

Contact Dr. Deborah Williams, Professor, Department of Nursing, Western Kentucky University, 1 Big Red Way, Bowling Green, KY 42101-3576. *Telephone:* 270-745-3391. *Fax:* 270-745-3392. *E-mail:* deborah.williams@wku.edu.

GRADUATE PROGRAMS

Expenses (2003–04) *Tuition, state resident:* full-time $4198; part-time $222 per credit hour. *Tuition, nonresident:* full-time $4558; part-time $242 per credit hour. *International tuition:* $4881 full-time.

Financial Aid 25% of graduate students in nursing programs received some form of financial aid in 2002–03. 1 research assistantship with partial tuition reimbursement available (averaging $7,400 per year), 2 teaching assistantships with partial tuition reimbursements available (averaging $9,000 per year) were awarded; Federal Work-Study, institutionally sponsored loans, traineeships, tuition waivers (partial), and unspecified assistantships also available. Aid available to part-time students. *Financial aid application deadline:* 4/1.

Contact Dr. Beverly C. Siegrist, Professor, Department of Nursing, Western Kentucky University, 1 Big Red Way, Academic Complex 108G, Bowling Green, KY 42101-3576. *Telephone:* 270-745-3490. *Fax:* 270-745-3392. *E-mail:* beverly.siegrist@wku.edu.

MASTER'S DEGREE PROGRAM

Degree MSN

Concentrations Available Nursing administration; nursing education. *Nurse practitioner programs in:* primary care.

Site Options *Distance Learning:* Elizabethtown, KY; Glasgow, KY; Owensboro, KY.

Study Options Full-time and part-time.

Program Entrance Requirements Computer literacy, minimum overall college GPA of 2.75, transcript of college record, CPR certification, written essay, immunizations, interview, 3 letters of recommendation, nursing research course, physical assessment course, professional liability insurance/malpractice insurance, statistics course, GRE General Test. *Application deadline:* For fall admission, 8/1 (priority date); for spring admission, 4/14. Applications are processed on a rolling basis. *Application fee:* $30.

Advanced Placement Credit given for nursing courses completed elsewhere dependent upon specific evaluations.

Degree Requirements 45 total credit hours, thesis or project, comprehensive exam.

POST-MASTER'S PROGRAM

Areas of Study *Nurse practitioner programs in:* primary care.

CONTINUING EDUCATION PROGRAM

Contact Ms. Angela Drexler, Continuing Nursing Education, Department of Nursing, Western Kentucky University, 1 Big Red Way, Academic Complex 119, Bowling Green, KY 42101-3576. *Telephone:* 270-745-3762. *Fax:* 270-745-3392. *E-mail:* angelyn.drexler@wku.edu.

LOUISIANA

Dillard University
Division of Nursing
New Orleans, Louisiana

http://www.dillard.edu/academic/nursing

Founded in 1869

DEGREE • BSN

Nursing Program Faculty 14 (14% with doctorates).

Baccalaureate Enrollment 58
Women 99% **Men** 1% **Minority** 100%

Nursing Student Activities Student Nurses' Association.

Nursing Student Resources Academic advising; academic or career counseling; bookstore; campus computer network; career placement assistance; computer lab; computer-assisted instruction; e-mail services; externships; interactive nursing skills videos; Internet; learning resource lab; library services; nursing audiovisuals; paid internships; placement services for program completers; remedial services; resume preparation assistance; skills, simulation, or other laboratory; tutoring.

BACCALAUREATE PROGRAMS

Degree BSN

Available Programs Generic Baccalaureate; RN Baccalaureate.

Study Options Full-time.

Program Entrance Requirements Minimum overall college GPA of 2.5, transcript of college record, CPR certification, health exam, health insurance, high school transcript, immunizations, letters of recommendation, prerequisite course work. Transfer students are accepted. **Standardized tests** *Required:* SAT or ACT, TOEFL for international students. **Application** *Deadline:* 7/1 (freshmen), 7/1 (transfer). *Notification:* continuous until 8/1 (freshmen). *Application fee:* $20.

Expenses (2003–04) *Tuition:* full-time $5300; part-time $442 per contact hour. *International tuition:* $5350 full-time. *Room and board:* $3220; room only: $2065 per academic year. *Required fees:* full-time $1515.

Financial Aid 80% of baccalaureate students in nursing programs received some form of financial aid in 2002–03. *Gift aid (need-based):* Federal Pell, FSEOG, state, private, college/university gift aid from institutional funds, United Negro College Fund. *Loans:* FFEL (Subsidized and Unsubsidized Stafford PLUS), Perkins, alternative loans. *Work-Study:* Federal Work-Study, part-time campus jobs. *Application deadline (priority):* 3/1.

Contact Division of Nursing, Division of Nursing, Dillard University, 2601 Gentilly Boulevard, New Orleans, LA 70122. *Telephone:* 504-816-4717. *Fax:* 504-816-4861.

Grambling State University
School of Nursing
Grambling, Louisiana

Founded in 1901

DEGREES • BSN • MSN

Nursing Program Faculty 18 (17% with doctorates).

Baccalaureate Enrollment 350
Women 88% **Men** 12% **Minority** 94% **International** 5% **Part-time** 6%

Graduate Enrollment 35
Women 86% **Men** 14% **Minority** 17% **Part-time** 9%

Nursing Student Activities Student Nurses' Association.

Nursing Student Resources Academic advising; academic or career counseling; assistance for students with disabilities; bookstore; campus computer network; career placement assistance; computer lab; computer-assisted instruction; e-mail services; Internet; learning resource lab; library services; nursing audiovisuals; skills, simulation, or other laboratory.

Library Facilities 208,935 volumes (10,000 in health, 5,000 in nursing); 1,253 periodical subscriptions (65 health-care related).

BACCALAUREATE PROGRAMS

Degree BSN

Available Programs Generic Baccalaureate; LPN to Baccalaureate; RN Baccalaureate.

Study Options Full-time.

Program Entrance Requirements Transcript of college record, CPR certification, health exam, immunizations, minimum GPA in nursing prerequisites of 2.75, professional liability insurance/malpractice insurance, prerequisite course work. Transfer students are accepted. **Standardized tests** *Required:* SAT or ACT, TOEFL for international students. **Application** *Deadline:* 7/15 (freshmen), 7/15 (transfer). *Early decision:* 4/15. *Notification:* continuous until 8/1 (freshmen), 4/20 (out-of-state freshmen), 4/20 (early decision). *Application fee:* $20.

Advanced Placement Credit given for nursing courses completed elsewhere dependent upon specific evaluations.

Expenses (2004–05) *Tuition, state resident:* full-time $3554; part-time $150 per credit hour. *Tuition, nonresident:* full-time $8904; part-time $371 per credit hour. *International tuition:* $9024 full-time. *Room and board:* $3642; room only: $1800 per academic year. *Required fees:* full-time $500; part-time $250 per term.

Financial Aid 95% of baccalaureate students in nursing programs received some form of financial aid in 2003–04. *Gift aid (need-based):* Federal Pell, FSEOG, state. *Loans:* FFEL (Subsidized and Unsubsidized Stafford PLUS), alternative loans. *Work-Study:* Federal Work-Study, part-time campus jobs. *Application deadline:* 6/1.

Contact Dr. Anna Karin Jones, RN, Director, BSN Program, School of Nursing, Grambling State University, PO Box 1192, 1 Cole Street, Grambling, LA 71245. *Telephone:* 318-274-2672. *Fax:* 318-274-3491. *E-mail:* jonesak@gram.edu.

GRADUATE PROGRAMS

Expenses (2004–05) *Tuition, state resident:* full-time $3554; part-time $150 per credit hour. *Tuition, nonresident:* full-time $8904; part-time $371 per credit hour. *International tuition:* $9024 full-time. *Room and board:* $3642; room only: $1800 per academic year. *Required fees:* full-time $500; part-time $250 per term.

Financial Aid 35% of graduate students in nursing programs received some form of financial aid in 2003–04. *Application deadline:* 5/31.

Contact Dr. Rhonda Hensley, NP, Director, MSN Program, School of Nursing, Grambling State University, PO Box 1192, 1 Cole Street, Grambling, LA 71245. *Telephone:* 318-274-2897. *Fax:* 318-274-3491. *E-mail:* hensleyr@gram.edu.

MASTER'S DEGREE PROGRAM

Degree MSN

Available Programs Master's.

Concentrations Available Nursing education. *Nurse practitioner programs in:* family health.

Study Options Full-time and part-time.

Program Entrance Requirements Clinical experience, minimum overall college GPA of 3.0, transcript of college record, CPR certification, immunizations, interview, 3 letters of recommendation, physical assessment course, professional liability insurance/malpractice insurance, prerequisite course work, statistics course, GRE. *Application deadline:* For fall admission, 7/1; for spring admission, 12/1. Applications are processed on a rolling basis. *Application fee:* $20 ($30 for international students).

Advanced Placement Credit given for nursing courses completed elsewhere dependent upon specific evaluations.

Degree Requirements 49 total credit hours, thesis or project, comprehensive exam.

POST-MASTER'S PROGRAM

Areas of Study *Nurse practitioner programs in:* family health.

Louisiana College
Department of Nursing
Pineville, Louisiana

http://www.lacollege.edu

Founded in 1906

DEGREE • BSN

Nursing Program Faculty 6 (17% with doctorates).

Baccalaureate Enrollment 100

Nursing Student Activities Sigma Theta Tau, Student Nurses' Association.

Nursing Student Resources Academic advising; academic or career counseling; assistance for students with disabilities; bookstore; campus computer network; career placement assistance; computer lab; computer-assisted instruction; e-mail services; employment services for current students; externships; Internet; learning resource lab; library services; nursing audiovisuals; skills, simulation, or other laboratory; tutoring; unpaid internships.

Library Facilities 135,566 volumes (3,426 in health, 500 in nursing); 380 periodical subscriptions (142 health-care related).

BACCALAUREATE PROGRAMS

Degree BSN

Available Programs Generic Baccalaureate.

Study Options Full-time.

Program Entrance Requirements Minimum overall college GPA of 2.6, transcript of college record, CPR certification, health exam, health insurance, immunizations, interview, minimum high school GPA of 2.0, minimum high school rank 50%, minimum GPA in nursing prerequisites of 2.6, professional liability insurance/malpractice insurance, prerequisite course work. Transfer students are accepted. **Standardized tests** *Required:* SAT or ACT, TOEFL for international students. **Application** *Deadline:* 8/15 (freshmen). *Notification:* continuous (freshmen). *Application fee:* $25.

Advanced Placement Credit given for nursing courses completed elsewhere dependent upon specific evaluations.

Expenses (2003–04) *Tuition:* part-time $295 per credit hour.

Contact Division of Nursing, Department of Nursing, Louisiana College, PO Box 556, Pineville, LA 71359-0556. *Telephone:* 318-487-7127. *Fax:* 318-487-7488.

Louisiana State University Health Sciences Center

School of Nursing
New Orleans, Louisiana

http://nursing.lsuhsc.edu

Founded in 1931

DEGREES • BSN • DNS • MN

Nursing Program Faculty 77 (33% with doctorates).

Nursing Student Activities Nursing Honor Society, Sigma Theta Tau, Student Nurses' Association.

Nursing Student Resources Academic advising; academic or career counseling; bookstore; computer lab; computer-assisted instruction; e-mail services; housing assistance; interactive nursing skills videos; Internet; learning resource lab; library services; nursing audiovisuals; skills, simulation, or other laboratory.

Library Facilities 232,617 volumes (181,235 in health); 2,359 periodical subscriptions (1,964 health-care related).

BACCALAUREATE PROGRAMS

Degree BSN

Available Programs Generic Baccalaureate; RN Baccalaureate.

Study Options Full-time and part-time.

Program Entrance Requirements Minimum overall college GPA of 2.8, transcript of college record, interview, prerequisite course work. Transfer students are accepted. **Application** *Deadline:* 3/1 (transfer). *Application fee:* $50.

Contact Tasha Torrence, BSN Program Contact, School of Nursing, Louisiana State University Health Sciences Center, 1900 Gravier Street, New Orleans, LA 70112. *Telephone:* 504-568-4197. *E-mail:* ttore@lsuhsc.edu.

GRADUATE PROGRAMS

Financial Aid 12 fellowships, 1 research assistantship were awarded; teaching assistantships, Federal Work-Study, institutionally sponsored loans, and unspecified assistantships also available.

Contact Sylvia Toval, School of Nursing, Louisiana State University Health Sciences Center, 1900 Gravier Street, New Orleans, LA 70112. *Telephone:* 504-568-4213. *E-mail:* stoval@lsuhsc.edu.

MASTER'S DEGREE PROGRAM

Degree MN

Available Programs Master's.

Concentrations Available Health-care administration; nurse anesthesia; nursing administration; nursing education. *Clinical nurse specialist programs in:* adult health, community health, parent-child, psychiatric/mental health. *Nurse practitioner programs in:* neonatal health, primary care.

Study Options Full-time and part-time.

Program Entrance Requirements Clinical experience, minimum overall college GPA of 3.0, transcript of college record, CPR certification, interview, 3 letters of recommendation, statistics course, GRE General Test, MAT. *Application deadline:* For spring admission, 6/1. *Application fee:* $50.

Degree Requirements 38 total credit hours.

DOCTORAL DEGREE PROGRAM

Degree DNS

Available Programs Doctorate.

Areas of Study Clinical practice, nursing education.

Program Entrance Requirements Clinical experience, minimum overall college GPA of 3.5, 3 letters of recommendation, MSN or equivalent, scholarly papers, writing sample, GRE General Test. *Application deadline:* For spring admission, 6/1. *Application fee:* $50.

Degree Requirements 54 total credit hours, dissertation, oral exam.

POSTDOCTORAL PROGRAM

Postdoctoral Program Contact Dr. Anita Hufft, Associate Dean, School of Nursing, Louisiana State University Health Sciences Center, 1900 Gravier Street, New Orleans, LA 70112. *Telephone:* 504-568-4107. *Fax:* 504-568-5853. *E-mail:* ahufft@lsuhsc.edu.

CONTINUING EDUCATION PROGRAM

Contact Barbara Y. Kearney, RN, Associate Dean for Professional Services and Community Activities, School of Nursing, Louisiana State University Health Sciences Center, 1900 Gravier Street, New Orleans, LA 70112. *Telephone:* 504-568-4202. *Fax:* 504-568-5859. *E-mail:* nsgconted@lsuhsc.edu.

Loyola University New Orleans

Program in Nursing
New Orleans, Louisiana

http://www.loyno.edu/~nursing

Founded in 1912

DEGREES • BSN • MSN

Nursing Program Faculty 10 (70% with doctorates).

Nursing Student Activities Sigma Theta Tau.

Nursing Student Resources Academic advising; academic or career counseling; assistance for students with disabilities; bookstore; campus computer network; career placement assistance; computer lab; computer-assisted instruction; e-mail services; Internet; library services; tutoring.

Library Facilities 401,548 volumes; 4,948 periodical subscriptions.

BACCALAUREATE PROGRAMS

Degree BSN

Available Programs RN Baccalaureate.

Site Options Baton Rouge, LA.

Study Options Part-time.

Loyola University New Orleans (continued)

Program Entrance Requirements Minimum overall college GPA of 2.5, transcript of college record, written essay, immunizations, professional liability insurance/malpractice insurance. Transfer students are accepted. **Standardized tests** *Required:* SAT or ACT, TOEFL for international students. *Required for some:* PAA. **Application** *Deadline:* 1/15 (freshmen), rolling (transfer). *Notification:* continuous (freshmen). *Application fee:* $20.

Advanced Placement Credit by examination available. Credit given for nursing courses completed elsewhere dependent upon specific evaluations.

Contact Dr. Billie Ann Wilson, RN, Department Chairperson, Program in Nursing, Loyola University New Orleans, 6363 St. Charles Avenue, Campus Box 14, New Orleans, LA 70118. *Telephone:* 504-865-3142. *Fax:* 504-865-3254. *E-mail:* nursing@loyno.edu.

GRADUATE PROGRAMS

Financial Aid Scholarships available.

Contact Dr. Billie Ann Wilson, RN, Director, Program in Nursing, Loyola University New Orleans, 6363 St. Charles Avenue, Campus Box 14, New Orleans, LA 70118. *Telephone:* 504-865-3142. *Fax:* 504-865-3254. *E-mail:* nursing@loyno.edu.

MASTER'S DEGREE PROGRAM

Degree MSN

Available Programs Master's; Master's for Nurses with Non-Nursing Degrees; RN to Master's.

Concentrations Available Health-care administration; nurse case management. *Nurse practitioner programs in:* adult health, family health.

Study Options Full-time and part-time.

Program Entrance Requirements Clinical experience, minimum overall college GPA of 2.8, transcript of college record, written essay, interview, 3 letters of recommendation, nursing research course, professional liability insurance/malpractice insurance, prerequisite course work, statistics course, GRE. *Application deadline:* For fall admission, 3/1 (priority date). *Application fee:* $20.

Advanced Placement Credit given for nursing courses completed elsewhere dependent upon specific evaluations.

Degree Requirements 39 total credit hours, comprehensive exam.

POST-MASTER'S PROGRAM

Areas of Study *Nurse practitioner programs in:* adult health, family health.

McNeese State University
College of Nursing
Lake Charles, Louisiana

http://www.mcneese.edu

Founded in 1939

DEGREES • BSN • MSN

Nursing Program Faculty 29 (14% with doctorates).

Baccalaureate Enrollment 734

Women 80% **Men** 20% **Minority** 21% **International** 2% **Part-time** 16%

Graduate Enrollment 54

Women 82% **Men** 18% **Minority** 3% **International** 1% **Part-time** 66%

Nursing Student Activities Sigma Theta Tau, Student Nurses' Association.

Nursing Student Resources Academic advising; academic or career counseling; assistance for students with disabilities; bookstore; campus computer network; career placement assistance; computer lab; computer-assisted instruction; daycare for children of students; e-mail services; employment services for current students; housing assistance; interactive nursing skills videos; Internet; learning resource lab; library services; nursing audiovisuals; placement services for program completers; resume preparation assistance; skills, simulation, or other laboratory; tutoring.

Library Facilities 351,708 volumes (40,857 in health, 21,513 in nursing); 1,679 periodical subscriptions (110 health-care related).

BACCALAUREATE PROGRAMS

Degree BSN

Available Programs ADN to Baccalaureate; Generic Baccalaureate.

Study Options Full-time and part-time.

Program Entrance Requirements Minimum overall college GPA of 2.7, transcript of college record, CPR certification, health exam, health insurance, high school transcript, immunizations, minimum high school GPA of 2.5, minimum GPA in nursing prerequisites of 2.7, prerequisite course work. Transfer students are accepted. **Standardized tests** *Required:* SAT or ACT, TOEFL for international students. **Application** *Deadline:* rolling (freshmen), rolling (transfer). *Notification:* continuous (freshmen). *Application fee:* $20.

Advanced Placement Credit by examination available. Credit given for nursing courses completed elsewhere dependent upon specific evaluations.

Expenses (2003–04) *Tuition, state resident:* full-time $2050. *Tuition, nonresident:* full-time $8106. *Room and board:* $4118; room only: $2650 per academic year. *Required fees:* full-time $727.

Financial Aid 65% of baccalaureate students in nursing programs received some form of financial aid in 2002–03.

Contact Dr. Peggy L. Wolfe, Dean and Professor, College of Nursing, McNeese State University, PO Box 90415, Lake Charles, LA 70609-0415. *Telephone:* 337-475-5820. *Fax:* 337-475-5924. *E-mail:* pwolfe@mail.mcneese.edu.

GRADUATE PROGRAMS

Expenses (2003–04) *Tuition, state resident:* full-time $2050; part-time $420 per credit hour. *Tuition, nonresident:* full-time $11,670; part-time $430 per credit hour. *Room and board:* $4118; room only: $2650 per academic year. *Required fees:* full-time $300; part-time $5 per credit.

Financial Aid 15% of graduate students in nursing programs received some form of financial aid in 2002–03.

Contact Dr. Ruth Brewer, MSN Co-Coordinator, College of Nursing, McNeese State University, PO Box 90415, Lake Charles, LA 70609-0415. *Telephone:* 337-475-5753. *Fax:* 337-475-5702. *E-mail:* rbrewer@acc.mcneese.edu.

MASTER'S DEGREE PROGRAM

Degree MSN

Available Programs Master's.

Concentrations Available Nursing administration; nursing education. *Clinical nurse specialist programs in:* adult health. *Nurse practitioner programs in:* adult health, family health.

Site Options *Distance Learning:* Lake Charles, LA; Baton Rouge, LA; Lafayette, LA.

Study Options Full-time and part-time.

Program Entrance Requirements Minimum overall college GPA of 2.7, transcript of college record, physical assessment course, statistics course, GRE. *Application deadline:* For fall admission, 7/15 (priority date). Applications are processed on a rolling basis. *Application fee:* $20 ($30 for international students).

Advanced Placement Credit given for nursing courses completed elsewhere dependent upon specific evaluations.

Degree Requirements 42 total credit hours, thesis or project, comprehensive exam.

POST-MASTER'S PROGRAM

Areas of Study *Nurse practitioner programs in:* adult health, family health.

CONTINUING EDUCATION PROGRAM

Contact Mrs. Patsy Trahan, Continuing Education Coordinator, College of Nursing, McNeese State University, PO Box 90415, Lake Charles, LA 70609-0415. *Telephone:* 337-475-5832. *Fax:* 337-475-5924. *E-mail:* ptrahan@acc.mcneese.edu.

Nicholls State University
Department of Nursing
Thibodaux, Louisiana

http://www.nicholls.edu/nursing/

Founded in 1948

DEGREE • BSN

Nursing Program Faculty 19 (21% with doctorates).

Library Facilities 303,962 volumes; 1,341 periodical subscriptions.

BACCALAUREATE PROGRAMS

Degree BSN

Available Programs Generic Baccalaureate; LPN to Baccalaureate; RN Baccalaureate.

Program Entrance Requirements Minimum overall college GPA of 2.75, transcript of college record, minimum GPA in nursing prerequisites of 2.0, prerequisite course work. Transfer students are accepted. **Standardized tests** *Required:* SAT or ACT. **Application** *Deadline:* rolling (transfer). *Notification:* 9/1 (freshmen). *Application fee:* $20.

Contact Dr. Thomas J. Smith, Program Director, Department of Nursing, Nicholls State University, PO Box 2143, 161 Betsy C. Ayo Hall, Thibodaux, LA 70310. *Telephone:* 985-448-4696. *Fax:* 985-448-4932. *E-mail:* nurs-tjs@mail.nich.edu.

CONTINUING EDUCATION PROGRAM

Contact Jeanne M. LeBlanc, RN, Director, Department of Nursing, Nicholls State University, PO Box 2143, Thibodaux, LA 70310. *Telephone:* 985-448-4696. *Fax:* 985-448-4932.

Northwestern State University of Louisiana
College of Nursing
Shreveport, Louisiana

http://www.nsula.edu

Founded in 1884

DEGREES • BSN • MSN

Nursing Program Faculty 37 (22% with doctorates).

Baccalaureate Enrollment 1,151 **Women** 85% **Men** 15% **Minority** 31% **Part-time** 41%

Graduate Enrollment 100
Women 92% **Men** 8% **Minority** 15% **Part-time** 87%

Nursing Student Activities Sigma Theta Tau, Student Nurses' Association.

Nursing Student Resources Academic advising; academic or career counseling; assistance for students with disabilities; bookstore; campus computer network; computer lab; computer-assisted instruction; e-mail services; employment services for current students; interactive nursing skills videos; Internet; learning resource lab; library services; nursing audiovisuals; remedial services; skills, simulation, or other laboratory; tutoring.

Library Facilities 325,829 volumes (11,104 in health, 6,809 in nursing); 7,978 periodical subscriptions (2,106 health-care related).

BACCALAUREATE PROGRAMS

Degree BSN

Available Programs ADN to Baccalaureate; Generic Baccalaureate; LPN to Baccalaureate; RN Baccalaureate.

Site Options *Distance Learning:* Bunkie, LA; Alexandria, LA; Ferriday, LA.

Study Options Full-time and part-time.

Program Entrance Requirements Minimum overall college GPA of 2.0, transcript of college record, health exam, immunizations, minimum GPA in nursing prerequisites of 2.7, prerequisite course work. Transfer students are accepted. **Standardized tests** *Required:* SAT or ACT, TOEFL for international students. **Application** *Deadline:* 7/6 (freshmen), 7/6 (transfer). *Notification:* continuous (freshmen). *Application fee:* $20.

Advanced Placement Credit by examination available. Credit given for nursing courses completed elsewhere dependent upon specific evaluations.

Expenses (2004–05) *Tuition, state resident:* full-time $4176. *Tuition, nonresident:* full-time $9117. *Required fees:* part-time $500 per term.

Financial Aid 75% of baccalaureate students in nursing programs received some form of financial aid in 2003–04. *Gift aid (need-based):* Federal Pell, FSEOG, state, private, college/university gift aid from institutional funds, United Negro College Fund, Federal Nursing, third party scholarships. *Loans:* FFEL (Subsidized and Unsubsidized Stafford PLUS), Perkins. *Work-Study:* Federal Work-Study, part-time campus jobs. *Application deadline (priority):* 5/1.

Contact Mrs. Shirley Cashio, Director, Undergraduate Studies in Nursing, College of Nursing, Northwestern State University of Louisiana, 1800 Line Avenue, Shreveport, LA 71101. *Telephone:* 318-677-3100. *Fax:* 318-677-3127. *E-mail:* cashios@nsula.edu.

GRADUATE PROGRAMS

Expenses (2004–05) *Tuition, state resident:* full-time $4005. *Tuition, nonresident:* full-time $9117. *Required fees:* part-time $400 per term.

Financial Aid 15% of graduate students in nursing programs received some form of financial aid in 2003–04. Career-related internships or fieldwork and Federal Work-Study available. Aid available to part-time students. *Financial aid application deadline:* 7/15.

Contact Dr. Sally Cook, Director, Graduate Studies and Research in Nursing, College of Nursing, Northwestern State University of Louisiana, 1800 Line Avenue, Shreveport, LA 71101. *Telephone:* 318-677-3100. *Fax:* 318-677-3127. *E-mail:* cooks@nsula.edu.

MASTER'S DEGREE PROGRAM

Degree MSN

Available Programs Master's.

Concentrations Available Nursing administration; nursing education. *Clinical nurse specialist programs in:* adult health, critical care, maternity-newborn, psychiatric/mental health. *Nurse practitioner programs in:* acute care, family health, neonatal health, pediatric, women's health.

Site Options *Distance Learning:* Bunkie, LA; Alexandria, LA; Ferriday, LA.

Study Options Full-time and part-time.

Program Entrance Requirements Clinical experience, minimum overall college GPA of 3.0, transcript of college record, written essay, immunizations, 2 letters of recommendation, physical assessment course, professional liability insurance/malpractice insurance, statistics course, GRE General Test. *Application deadline:* For fall admission, 8/1 (priority date); for spring admission, 1/10. Applications are processed on a rolling basis. *Application fee:* $20 ($30 for international students).

Degree Requirements 42 total credit hours, thesis or project, comprehensive exam.

POST-MASTER'S PROGRAM

Areas of Study *Nurse practitioner programs in:* acute care, family health, neonatal health, pediatric, women's health.

CONTINUING EDUCATION PROGRAM

Contact Ms. Diane Graham Webb, Director, Non-Traditional Studies in Nursing, College of Nursing, Northwestern State University of Louisiana, 1800 Line Avenue, Shreveport, LA 71101. *Telephone:* 318-677-3100. *Fax:* 318-677-3127. *E-mail:* grahamd@nsula.edu.

Our Lady of Holy Cross College
Division of Nursing
New Orleans, Louisiana

http://www.olhcc.edu

Founded in 1916

DEGREE • BSN

Nursing Program Faculty 16 (27% with doctorates).

Baccalaureate Enrollment 145
Women 90% **Men** 10% **Minority** 15% **Part-time** 11%

Nursing Student Activities Sigma Theta Tau, Student Nurses' Association.

Our Lady of Holy Cross College (continued)

Nursing Student Resources Academic advising; academic or career counseling; assistance for students with disabilities; bookstore; campus computer network; computer lab; computer-assisted instruction; e-mail services; interactive nursing skills videos; Internet; learning resource lab; library services; nursing audiovisuals; remedial services; resume preparation assistance; skills, simulation, or other laboratory.

Library Facilities 83,631 volumes (5,000 in health, 3,100 in nursing); 1,002 periodical subscriptions (103 health-care related).

BACCALAUREATE PROGRAMS

Degree BSN

Available Programs Generic Baccalaureate.

Study Options Full-time.

Program Entrance Requirements Minimum overall college GPA of 2.5, transcript of college record, CPR certification, written essay, health exam, health insurance, high school transcript, immunizations, 3 letters of recommendation, minimum high school GPA of 2.0, minimum GPA in nursing prerequisites of 2.5, professional liability insurance/malpractice insurance, prerequisite course work. Transfer students are accepted. **Standardized tests** *Required:* TOEFL for international students. ***Placement:*** *Required:* SAT or ACT. *Recommended:* ACT. **Application** *Deadline:* 7/20 (freshmen), rolling (transfer). *Notification:* continuous (freshmen). *Application fee:* $15.

Advanced Placement Credit by examination available. Credit given for nursing courses completed elsewhere dependent upon specific evaluations.

Expenses (2004–05) *Tuition:* full-time $6870. *Required fees:* full-time $600.

Financial Aid 80% of baccalaureate students in nursing programs received some form of financial aid in 2003–04. *Gift aid (need-based):* Federal Pell, FSEOG, state, private, college/university gift aid from institutional funds, Federal Nursing. *Loans:* FFEL (Subsidized and Unsubsidized Stafford PLUS). *Work-Study:* Federal Work-Study. *Application deadline (priority):* 4/15.

Contact Miss Anne Katherine Lene, Director of Admissions and Career Services, Division of Nursing, Our Lady of Holy Cross College, 4123 Woodland Drive, New Orleans, LA 70131. *Telephone:* 504-394-7744 Ext. 110. *Fax:* 504-391-2421. *E-mail:* alene@olhcc.edu.

Our Lady of the Lake College

Division of Nursing
Baton Rouge, Louisiana

http://www.ololcollege.edu

Founded in 1990

DEGREE • BSN

Nursing Program Faculty 24 (13% with doctorates).

Baccalaureate Enrollment 30

Nursing Student Resources Academic advising; campus computer network; computer lab; Internet.

Library Facilities 12,409 volumes; 328 periodical subscriptions.

BACCALAUREATE PROGRAMS

Degree BSN

Program Entrance Requirements Minimum overall college GPA of 2.0, immunizations, minimum high school GPA of 2.0, RN licensure. Transfer students are accepted. **Standardized tests** *Required:* ACT, ACT ASSET. **Application** *Deadline:* rolling (freshmen), rolling (transfer). *Notification:* 8/1 (freshmen). *Application fee:* $35.

Advanced Placement Credit by examination available.

Expenses (2003–04) *Tuition:* full-time $3280; part-time $205 per credit hour. *Required fees:* full-time $300; part-time $150 per term.

Contact Admissions Office, Division of Nursing, Our Lady of the Lake College, 7434 Perkins Road, Baton Rouge, LA 70808. *Telephone:* 225-768-1700. *E-mail:* admission@ololcollege.edu.

Southeastern Louisiana University

College of Nursing and Health Sciences
Hammond, Louisiana

http://www.selu.edu/Academics/Nursing

Founded in 1925

DEGREES • BS • MSN

Nursing Program Faculty 55 (25% with doctorates).

Baccalaureate Enrollment 1,753 **Women** 86% **Men** 14% **Minority** 21% **Part-time** 22%

Graduate Enrollment 55
Women 89% **Men** 11% **Minority** 5% **Part-time** 73%

Nursing Student Activities Nursing Honor Society, Sigma Theta Tau, Student Nurses' Association.

Nursing Student Resources Academic advising; academic or career counseling; assistance for students with disabilities; bookstore; campus computer network; career placement assistance; computer lab; computer-assisted instruction; e-mail services; employment services for current students; housing assistance; interactive nursing skills videos; Internet; learning resource lab; library services; nursing audiovisuals; other; paid internships; placement services for program completers; remedial services; resume preparation assistance; skills, simulation, or other laboratory; tutoring; unpaid internships.

Library Facilities 572,563 volumes; 2,387 periodical subscriptions (307 health-care related).

BACCALAUREATE PROGRAMS

Degree BS

Available Programs Generic Baccalaureate; RN Baccalaureate.

Site Options *Distance Learning:* Baton Rouge, LA.

Study Options Full-time and part-time.

Program Entrance Requirements CPR certification, health exam, minimum GPA in nursing prerequisites of 2.7. Transfer students are accepted. **Standardized tests** *Required:* SAT or ACT, TOEFL for international students. *Recommended:* SAT Subject Tests. **Application** *Deadline:* 8/16 (freshmen), rolling (transfer). *Notification:* continuous (freshmen). *Application fee:* $20.

Advanced Placement Credit by examination available. Credit given for nursing courses completed elsewhere dependent upon specific evaluations.

Expenses (2004–05) *Tuition, state resident:* full-time $3191; part-time $133 per credit hour. *Tuition, nonresident:* full-time $8519; part-time $355 per credit hour. *International tuition:* $8639 full-time. *Room and board:* $4290; room only: $2300 per academic year.

Financial Aid 82% of baccalaureate students in nursing programs received some form of financial aid in 2003–04.

Contact Dr. Barbara Moffett, Director, School of Nursing, College of Nursing and Health Sciences, Southeastern Louisiana University, SLU 10835, Hammond, LA 70402. *Telephone:* 985-549-2156. *Fax:* 985-549-2869. *E-mail:* nursing@selu.edu.

GRADUATE PROGRAMS

Expenses (2004–05) *Tuition, state resident:* full-time $2986; part-time $166 per credit hour. *Tuition, nonresident:* full-time $6982; part-time $388 per credit hour. *International tuition:* $7102 full-time. *Room and board:* $4290; room only: $2300 per academic year.

Financial Aid 38% of graduate students in nursing programs received some form of financial aid in 2003–04. 13 research assistantships with full tuition reimbursements available (averaging $2,200 per year), 1 teaching assistantship with full tuition reimbursement available (averaging $2,200 per year) were awarded; career-related internships or fieldwork, Federal Work-Study, institutionally sponsored loans, scholarships, unspecified assistantships, and administrative assistantship also available. Aid available to part-time students. *Financial aid application deadline:* 5/1.

Contact Dr. Cynthia Prestholdt, Program Contact, College of Nursing and Health Sciences, Southeastern Louisiana University, SLU 10835, Hammond, LA 70402. *Telephone:* 985-549-5045. *Fax:* 985-549-2869. *E-mail:* cprestholdt@selu.edu.

MASTER'S DEGREE PROGRAM

Degree MSN

Available Programs Master's.

Concentrations Available Nursing administration; nursing education. *Clinical nurse specialist programs in:* community health, family health. *Nurse practitioner programs in:* adult health.

Site Options *Distance Learning:* Lafayette, LA; Lake Charles, LA.

Study Options Full-time and part-time.

Program Entrance Requirements Clinical experience, minimum overall college GPA of 2.7, transcript of college record, immunizations, physical assessment course, statistics course, GRE General Test. *Application deadline:* For fall admission, 7/15 (priority date); for spring admission, 12/1 (priority date). Applications are processed on a rolling basis. *Application fee:* $20 ($30 for international students).

Degree Requirements 36 total credit hours, thesis or project, comprehensive exam.

Southern University and Agricultural and Mechanical College

School of Nursing
Baton Rouge, Louisiana

http://www.subr.edu/suson

Founded in 1880

DEGREES • BSN • MSN • PHD

Nursing Program Faculty 36 (3% with doctorates).

Baccalaureate Enrollment 1,020 **Women** 91% **Men** 9% **Minority** 96% **International** 1% **Part-time** 12%

Nursing Student Activities Nursing Honor Society, Student Nurses' Association, nursing club.

Nursing Student Resources Academic advising; academic or career counseling; assistance for students with disabilities; bookstore; campus computer network; computer lab; computer-assisted instruction; e-mail services; interactive nursing skills videos; Internet; learning resource lab; library services; nursing audiovisuals; resume preparation assistance; skills, simulation, or other laboratory; tutoring.

Library Facilities 808,365 volumes (4,220 in health, 716 in nursing); 1,857 periodical subscriptions (114 health-care related).

BACCALAUREATE PROGRAMS

Degree BSN

Available Programs Generic Baccalaureate.

Study Options Full-time and part-time.

Program Entrance Requirements Minimum overall college GPA of 2.6, CPR certification, health exam, immunizations, minimum GPA in nursing prerequisites, prerequisite course work. Transfer students are accepted. **Standardized tests** *Required:* ACT, SAT or ACT, TOEFL for international students. ***Placement:*** *Required:* ACT, SAT or ACT. *Recommended:* SAT, SAT Subject Tests. **Application** *Deadline:* 7/1 (freshmen), 7/1 (transfer). *Notification:* continuous (freshmen). *Application fee:* $5.

Expenses (2003–04) *Tuition, area resident:* full-time $1542; part-time $518 per credit hour. *Tuition, state resident:* full-time $3066; part-time $1311 per credit hour. *Tuition, nonresident:* full-time $8858. *International tuition:* $8918 full-time. *Room and board:* $2175 per academic year. *Required fees:* full-time $160; part-time $40 per credit; part-time $80 per term.

Financial Aid 93% of baccalaureate students in nursing programs received some form of financial aid in 2002–03. *Gift aid (need-based):* Federal Pell, FSEOG, state, private, college/university gift aid from institutional funds. *Loans:* Federal Direct (Subsidized and Unsubsidized Stafford PLUS), FFEL (Subsidized and Unsubsidized Stafford PLUS), college/university. *Work-Study:* Federal Work-Study, part-time campus jobs. *Application deadline (priority):* 5/15.

Contact Ms. Mary L. Abadie, School of Nursing, School of Nursing, Southern University and Agricultural and Mechanical College, PO Box 11784, Baton Rouge, LA 70813. *Telephone:* 225-771-3416. *Fax:* 225-771-2651. *E-mail:* maryabaie@suson.subr.edu.

GRADUATE PROGRAMS

Expenses (2003–04) *Tuition, area resident:* full-time $1339; part-time $317 per credit hour. *Tuition, state resident:* full-time $1062; part-time $317 per credit hour. *Tuition, nonresident:* full-time $3922; part-time $317 per credit hour. *International tuition:* $3943 full-time. *Room and board:* $1789; room only: $907 per academic year. *Required fees:* full-time $160; part-time $40 per credit; part-time $80 per term.

Financial Aid 92% of graduate students in nursing programs received some form of financial aid in 2002–03. 2 fellowships with tuition reimbursements available (averaging $3,480 per year), 4 research assistantships (averaging $7,000 per year), 2 teaching assistantships (averaging $20,000 per year) were awarded; Federal Work-Study, institutionally sponsored loans, scholarships, traineeships, and unspecified assistantships also available.

Contact Ladonna Strauss, Education Program Coordinator, School of Nursing, Southern University and Agricultural and Mechanical College, PO Box 11784, Baton Rouge, LA 70813. *Telephone:* 225-771-2663. *Fax:* 225-771-3547. *E-mail:* ladonnastrauss@suson.subr.edu.

MASTER'S DEGREE PROGRAM

Degree MSN

Available Programs Master's.

Concentrations Available Health-care administration; nursing education. *Clinical nurse specialist programs in:* family health. *Nurse practitioner programs in:* family health.

Study Options Full-time and part-time.

Program Entrance Requirements Minimum overall college GPA of 3.0, transcript of college record, 3 letters of recommendation, physical assessment course, statistics course, GRE General Test. *Application deadline:* For fall admission, 7/1; for spring admission, 11/1. Applications are processed on a rolling basis. *Application fee:* $25.

Degree Requirements 46 total credit hours, thesis or project, comprehensive exam.

POST-MASTER'S PROGRAM

Areas of Study *Nurse practitioner programs in:* family health.

DOCTORAL DEGREE PROGRAM

Degree PhD

Areas of Study Advanced practice nursing, nursing education, nursing research, women's health.

Program Entrance Requirements Clinical experience, minimum overall college GPA of 3.2, interview by faculty committee, 3 letters of recommendation, MSN or equivalent, scholarly papers, statistics course, vita, writing sample, GRE General Test. *Application deadline:* For fall admission, 7/1; for spring admission, 11/1. Applications are processed on a rolling basis. *Application fee:* $25.

Degree Requirements 60 total credit hours, dissertation, written exam.

University of Louisiana at Lafayette

College of Nursing
Lafayette, Louisiana

http://www.nursing.louisiana.edu

Founded in 1898

DEGREES • BSN • MSN

Nursing Program Faculty 38 (16% with doctorates).

Baccalaureate Enrollment 1,551 **Women** 85% **Men** 15% **Minority** 25% **International** 6% **Part-time** 15%

Graduate Enrollment 46
Women 85% **Men** 15% **Minority** 7% **Part-time** 70%

University of Louisiana at Lafayette (continued)

Nursing Student Activities Nursing Honor Society, Sigma Theta Tau, Student Nurses' Association.

Nursing Student Resources Academic advising; academic or career counseling; assistance for students with disabilities; bookstore; campus computer network; career placement assistance; computer lab; computer-assisted instruction; daycare for children of students; e-mail services; employment services for current students; externships; housing assistance; interactive nursing skills videos; Internet; learning resource lab; library services; nursing audiovisuals; other; paid internships; placement services for program completers; remedial services; resume preparation assistance; skills, simulation, or other laboratory; tutoring; unpaid internships.

Library Facilities 986,000 volumes (6,883 in health, 4,593 in nursing); 5,174 periodical subscriptions (184 health-care related).

BACCALAUREATE PROGRAMS

Degree BSN

Available Programs ADN to Baccalaureate; Accelerated Baccalaureate for Second Degree; LPN to RN Baccalaureate; RN Baccalaureate.

Study Options Full-time and part-time.

Program Entrance Requirements Minimum overall college GPA of 2.5, transcript of college record, CPR certification, health exam, health insurance, immunizations, minimum high school GPA, professional liability insurance/malpractice insurance, prerequisite course work. Transfer students are accepted. **Standardized tests** *Required:* SAT or ACT, TOEFL for international students. **Application** *Deadline:* rolling (freshmen), rolling (transfer). *Application fee:* $20.

Advanced Placement Credit by examination available. Credit given for nursing courses completed elsewhere dependent upon specific evaluations.

Expenses (2004–05) *Tuition, state resident:* full-time $1593; part-time $407 per credit hour. *Tuition, nonresident:* full-time $4683; part-time $407 per credit hour. *International tuition:* $4751 full-time. *Room and board:* $1693 per academic year. *Required fees:* full-time $1175; part-time $85 per credit; part-time $1025 per term.

Financial Aid *Gift aid (need-based):* Federal Pell, FSEOG, state, college/university gift aid from institutional funds. *Loans:* Federal Nursing Student Loans, FFEL (Subsidized and Unsubsidized Stafford PLUS), Perkins. *Work-Study:* Federal Work-Study, part-time campus jobs. *Application deadline (priority):* 5/1.

Contact Jan Byrd, Secretary, College of Nursing, University of Louisiana at Lafayette, PO Box 43810, Lafayette, LA 70504-3810. *Telephone:* 337-482-5604. *Fax:* 337-482-5649.

GRADUATE PROGRAMS

Expenses (2004–05) *Tuition, state resident:* full-time $3013; part-time $422 per credit hour. *Tuition, nonresident:* full-time $9193; part-time $422 per credit hour. *International tuition:* $9329 full-time. *Room and board:* $1693 per academic year. *Required fees:* full-time $366; part-time $102 per credit; part-time $183 per term.

Financial Aid 10% of graduate students in nursing programs received some form of financial aid in 2003–04. 1 fellowship with full tuition reimbursement available (averaging $14,500 per year) was awarded.

Contact Dr. Carolyn Delahoussaye, MSN Coordinator, College of Nursing, University of Louisiana at Lafayette, PO Box 43810, Lafayette, LA 70504-3810. *Telephone:* 337-482-5617. *Fax:* 337-482-5650. *E-mail:* carolyn@louisiana.edu.

MASTER'S DEGREE PROGRAM

Degree MSN

Available Programs Master's.

Concentrations Available Nursing education. *Clinical nurse specialist programs in:* adult health. *Nurse practitioner programs in:* adult health.

Site Options *Distance Learning:* Lake Charles, LA; Baton Rouge, LA; Hammond, LA.

Study Options Full-time and part-time.

Program Entrance Requirements Minimum overall college GPA of 2.75, transcript of college record, immunizations, 3 letters of recommendation, physical assessment course, statistics course, GRE General Test. *Application deadline:* For fall admission, 5/15; for spring admission, 10/1. Applications are processed on a rolling basis. *Application fee:* $20 ($30 for international students).

Advanced Placement Credit given for nursing courses completed elsewhere dependent upon specific evaluations.

Degree Requirements 38 total credit hours, thesis or project, comprehensive exam.

POST-MASTER'S PROGRAM

Areas of Study Nursing education. *Clinical nurse specialist programs in:* adult health. *Nurse practitioner programs in:* adult health.

CONTINUING EDUCATION PROGRAM

Contact Patricia Miller, Director of Continuing Education, College of Nursing, University of Louisiana at Lafayette, PO Box 43810, Lafayette, LA 70504-3810. *Telephone:* 337-482-5648. *Fax:* 337-482-5053.

University of Louisiana at Monroe
Nursing
Monroe, Louisiana

http://www.ulm.edu/nursing

Founded in 1931

DEGREE • BS

Nursing Program Faculty 36 (8% with doctorates).

Baccalaureate Enrollment 245

Women 88% **Men** 12% **Minority** 23% **Part-time** 17%

Nursing Student Activities Sigma Theta Tau, Student Nurses' Association.

Nursing Student Resources Academic advising; academic or career counseling; assistance for students with disabilities; bookstore; campus computer network; computer lab; computer-assisted instruction; daycare for children of students; e-mail services; employment services for current students; interactive nursing skills videos; Internet; learning resource lab; library services; nursing audiovisuals; placement services for program completers; remedial services; resume preparation assistance; skills, simulation, or other laboratory; tutoring.

Library Facilities 355,748 volumes (19,924 in health, 2,651 in nursing); 2,912 periodical subscriptions (400 health-care related).

BACCALAUREATE PROGRAMS

Degree BS

Available Programs ADN to Baccalaureate; Accelerated Baccalaureate; LPN to Baccalaureate; RN Baccalaureate.

Study Options Full-time and part-time.

Program Entrance Requirements Transcript of college record, CPR certification, health exam, high school transcript, immunizations, minimum high school GPA of 2.0, minimum high school rank 50%, minimum GPA in nursing prerequisites of 2.5, professional liability insurance/malpractice insurance, prerequisite course work. Transfer students are accepted. **Standardized tests** *Required:* ACT, TOEFL for international students. **Application** *Deadline:* rolling (freshmen), rolling (transfer). *Notification:* continuous (freshmen). *Application fee:* $20.

Expenses (2004–05) *Tuition, state resident:* full-time $3076; part-time $187 per contact hour. *Tuition, nonresident:* full-time $9028; part-time $192 per contact hour. *International tuition:* $9028 full-time. *Room and board:* $4210; room only: $1600 per academic year. *Required fees:* full-time $710.

Financial Aid 82% of baccalaureate students in nursing programs received some form of financial aid in 2003–04. *Gift aid (need-based):* Federal Pell, FSEOG, state, private, college/university gift aid from institutional funds, Leveraging Educational Assistance Partnership Program (LEAPP). *Loans:* FFEL (Subsidized and Unsubsidized Stafford PLUS), Perkins, college/university, Federal Health Professions Student Loans. *Work-Study:* Federal Work-Study, part-time campus jobs. *Application deadline (priority):* 4/1.

Contact Ms. Linda F. Reid, Interim Director, School of Nursing, Nursing, University of Louisiana at Monroe, 700 University Avenue, Monroe, LA 71209-0460. *Telephone:* 318-342-1640. *Fax:* 318-342-1567. *E-mail:* reid@ulm.edu.

CONTINUING EDUCATION PROGRAM

Contact Mrs. Celia Laird, Coordinator of Continuing Education, Nursing, University of Louisiana at Monroe, 700 University Avenue, Monroe, LA 71209-0460. *Telephone:* 318-342-1679. *Fax:* 318-342-1567. *E-mail:* laird@ulm.edu.

University of Phoenix–Louisiana Campus

College of Health and Human Services
Metairie, Louisiana

Founded in 1976

DEGREES • BSN • MSN • MSN/MBA

Nursing Program Faculty 22 (27% with doctorates).

Baccalaureate Enrollment 16
Women 81% **Men** 19% **Minority** 14%

Graduate Enrollment 3
Women 100% **Minority** 33%

Nursing Student Activities Sigma Theta Tau.

Nursing Student Resources Academic advising; academic or career counseling; bookstore; computer lab; library services.

Library Facilities 27.1 million volumes; 11,648 periodical subscriptions (1,426 health-care related).

BACCALAUREATE PROGRAMS

Degree BSN

Available Programs ADN to Baccalaureate; Accelerated RN Baccalaureate.

Site Options Baton Rouge, LA; Lafayette, LA.

Study Options Full-time.

Program Entrance Requirements 1 letter of recommendation. Transfer students are accepted. **Standardized tests** *Required:* TOEFL for international students. **Application** *Deadline:* rolling (freshmen), rolling (transfer). *Application fee:* $100.

Advanced Placement Credit by examination available.

Expenses (2004–05) *Tuition:* full-time $9330; part-time $311 per credit hour. *International tuition:* $9330 full-time. *Required fees:* full-time $110.

Financial Aid 2% of baccalaureate students in nursing programs received some form of financial aid in 2003–04.

Contact Campus College Chair, Nursing, College of Health and Human Services, University of Phoenix–Louisiana Campus, One Galleria Boulevard, Suite 725, Metairie, LA 70001-2082. *Telephone:* 504-461-8852.

GRADUATE PROGRAMS

Expenses (2004–05) *Tuition:* full-time $8592; part-time $358 per credit hour. *International tuition:* $8592 full-time. *Required fees:* full-time $110.

Financial Aid 5% of graduate students in nursing programs received some form of financial aid in 2003–04.

Contact Campus College Chair, Nursing, College of Health and Human Services, University of Phoenix–Louisiana Campus, One Galleria Boulevard, Suite 725, Metairie, LA 70001-2082. *Telephone:* 504-461-8852.

MASTER'S DEGREE PROGRAM

Degrees MSN; MSN/MBA

Available Programs Master's.

Concentrations Available Health-care administration; nursing administration; nursing education. *Nurse practitioner programs in:* family health.

Site Options Baton Rouge, LA; Lafayette, LA.

Program Entrance Requirements Clinical experience, computer literacy, minimum overall college GPA of 2.5, transcript of college record. *Application deadline:* Applications are processed on a rolling basis. *Application fee:* $110.

Degree Requirements 39 total credit hours, thesis or project.

POST-MASTER'S PROGRAM

Areas of Study *Nurse practitioner programs in:* family health.

MAINE

Husson College

School of Nursing
Bangor, Maine

http://www.husson.edu

Founded in 1898

DEGREES • BSN • MSN

Nursing Program Faculty 26.

Baccalaureate Enrollment 182
Women 95% **Men** 5% **Minority** 3% **International** 6% **Part-time** 8%

Graduate Enrollment 36
Women 89% **Men** 11% **Minority** 8% **International** 8% **Part-time** 3%

Nursing Student Activities Sigma Theta Tau, Student Nurses' Association, nursing club.

Nursing Student Resources Bookstore; computer lab; computer-assisted instruction; interactive nursing skills videos; learning resource lab; library services; nursing audiovisuals.

Library Facilities 37,871 volumes (1,125 in health, 1,050 in nursing); 500 periodical subscriptions (70 health-care related).

BACCALAUREATE PROGRAMS

Degree BSN

Available Programs Generic Baccalaureate; RN Baccalaureate.

Study Options Full-time and part-time.

Program Entrance Requirements Minimum overall college GPA of 2.7, transcript of college record, written essay, health exam, high school biology, high school chemistry, 4 years high school math, 2 years high school science, high school transcript, immunizations, interview, 2 letters of recommendation, minimum high school GPA of 2.7, prerequisite course work. Transfer students are accepted. **Standardized tests** *Required:* SAT or ACT, TOEFL for international students. **Application** *Deadline:* 9/1 (freshmen), 9/1 (transfer). *Early decision:* 12/15. *Notification:* continuous (freshmen), 1/2 (early action). *Application fee:* $25.

Advanced Placement Credit by examination available. Credit given for nursing courses completed elsewhere dependent upon specific evaluations.

Expenses (2004–05) *Tuition:* full-time $10,800; part-time $360 per contact hour. *Room and board:* $2925 per academic year. *Required fees:* part-time $25 per credit.

Financial Aid 34% of baccalaureate students in nursing programs received some form of financial aid in 2003–04.

Contact Ms. Ann P. Ellis, Director, Undergraduate Nursing Program, School of Nursing, Husson College, One College Circle, Bangor, ME 04401-2999. *Telephone:* 207-941-7050. *Fax:* 207-941-7883. *E-mail:* ellisa@husson.edu.

GRADUATE PROGRAMS

Expenses (2004–05) *Tuition:* full-time $6480; part-time $360 per credit hour.

Financial Aid 46% of graduate students in nursing programs received some form of financial aid in 2003–04.

Contact Mr. George L. Case, Director, Family and Community Nurse Practitioner Program, School of Nursing, Husson College, One College Circle, Bangor, ME 04401-2999. *Telephone:* 207-941-7080. *Fax:* 207-941-7883. *E-mail:* caseg@husson.edu.

MASTER'S DEGREE PROGRAM

Degree MSN

Husson College (continued)

Available Programs Master's; Master's for Nurses with Non-Nursing Degrees; RN to Master's.

Concentrations Available *Clinical nurse specialist programs in:* psychiatric/mental health. *Nurse practitioner programs in:* acute care, family health, psychiatric/mental health.

Study Options Full-time and part-time.

Program Entrance Requirements Clinical experience, minimum overall college GPA of 3.0, transcript of college record, CPR certification, written essay, immunizations, interview, 3 letters of recommendation, prerequisite course work.

Advanced Placement Credit by examination available. Credit given for nursing courses completed elsewhere dependent upon specific evaluations.

Degree Requirements 43 total credit hours, thesis or project.

POST-MASTER'S PROGRAM

Areas of Study *Nurse practitioner programs in:* acute care.

Saint Joseph's College of Maine

Department of Nursing
Standish, Maine

Founded in 1912

DEGREES • BSN • MSN • MSN/MA

Nursing Program Faculty 40 (15% with doctorates).

Baccalaureate Enrollment 578
Women 95% **Men** 5% **Minority** 1% **Part-time** 58%

Graduate Enrollment 373
Women 96% **Men** 4% **Minority** 3% **International** 1% **Part-time** 100%

Nursing Student Activities Sigma Theta Tau, Student Nurses' Association.

Nursing Student Resources Academic advising; academic or career counseling; assistance for students with disabilities; bookstore; campus computer network; computer lab; computer-assisted instruction; e-mail services; interactive nursing skills videos; Internet; learning resource lab; library services; nursing audiovisuals; remedial services; resume preparation assistance; skills, simulation, or other laboratory; tutoring.

Library Facilities 98,626 volumes (1,473 in health, 1,295 in nursing); 11,461 periodical subscriptions (85 health-care related).

BACCALAUREATE PROGRAMS

Degree BSN

Available Programs RN Baccalaureate; RPN to Baccalaureate.

Study Options Full-time and part-time.

Program Entrance Requirements Minimum overall college GPA of 2.0, transcript of college record, written essay, health exam, health insurance, high school biology, high school chemistry, 3 years high school math, 2 years high school science, high school transcript, immunizations, 1 letter of recommendation, minimum high school GPA of 2.0. **Standardized tests** *Required:* SAT or ACT, TOEFL for international students. **Application** *Deadline:* rolling (freshmen), rolling (transfer). *Early decision:* 11/15. *Notification:* continuous (freshmen), 12/15 (early action). *Application fee:* $40.

Advanced Placement Credit given for nursing courses completed elsewhere dependent upon specific evaluations.

Expenses (2004–05) *Tuition:* full-time $16,150; part-time $250 per credit hour. *Room and board:* $6980 per academic year. *Required fees:* full-time $250.

Financial Aid 98% of baccalaureate students in nursing programs received some form of financial aid in 2003–04.

Contact Admissions Department, Department of Nursing, Saint Joseph's College of Maine, 278 Whites Bridge Road, Standish, ME 04084-5263. *Telephone:* 207-893-7830. *Fax:* 207-892-7423. *E-mail:* info@sjcme.edu.

GRADUATE PROGRAMS

Expenses (2004–05) *Tuition:* part-time $275 per credit hour.

Financial Aid 5% of graduate students in nursing programs received some form of financial aid in 2003–04. Institutionally sponsored loans available. Aid available to part-time students.

Contact Dr. Linda Conover, Director of Distance Nursing Education, Department of Nursing, Saint Joseph's College of Maine, 278 Whites Bridge Road, Standish, ME 04084-5263. *Telephone:* 207-893-7956. *Fax:* 207-893-7520. *E-mail:* lconover@sjcme.edu.

MASTER'S DEGREE PROGRAM

Degrees MSN; MSN/MA

Available Programs Master's; Master's for Nurses with Non-Nursing Degrees; RN to Master's.

Concentrations Available Nursing administration; nursing education.

Study Options Full-time and part-time.

Program Entrance Requirements Clinical experience, computer literacy, minimum overall college GPA of 3.0, transcript of college record, written essay, 3 letters of recommendation, prerequisite course work, resume, statistics course, MAT. *Application deadline:* Applications are processed on a rolling basis. *Application fee:* $50.

Advanced Placement Credit given for nursing courses completed elsewhere dependent upon specific evaluations.

Degree Requirements 40 total credit hours, thesis or project.

CONTINUING EDUCATION PROGRAM

Contact Dr. Linda Conover, Director of Distance Nursing Education, Department of Nursing, Saint Joseph's College of Maine, 278 Whites Bridge Road, Standish, ME 04084-5263. *Telephone:* 207-893-7956. *Fax:* 207-893-7520. *E-mail:* lconover@sjcme.edu.

University of Maine

School of Nursing
Orono, Maine

Founded in 1865

DEGREES • BSN • MSN

Nursing Program Faculty 19 (58% with doctorates).

Baccalaureate Enrollment 388
Women 93% **Men** 7% **Minority** 4% **International** 2% **Part-time** 9%

Graduate Enrollment 26
Women 85% **Men** 15% **Minority** 97% **Part-time** 50%

Nursing Student Activities Sigma Theta Tau, Student Nurses' Association.

Nursing Student Resources Academic advising; academic or career counseling; assistance for students with disabilities; bookstore; campus computer network; computer lab; daycare for children of students; e-mail services; employment services for current students; housing assistance; interactive nursing skills videos; Internet; learning resource lab; library services; nursing audiovisuals; skills, simulation, or other laboratory; tutoring.

Library Facilities 1 million volumes (826,648 in health); 13,041 periodical subscriptions (5,400 health-care related).

BACCALAUREATE PROGRAMS

Degree BSN

Available Programs Accelerated Baccalaureate; Generic Baccalaureate; RN Baccalaureate.

Site Options *Distance Learning:* Augusta, ME; Waterville, ME; Belfast, ME.

Study Options Full-time and part-time.

Program Entrance Requirements Minimum overall college GPA of 2.6, transcript of college record, CPR certification, health exam, high school biology, high school chemistry, high school foreign language, 3 years high school math, 3 years high school science, high school transcript, immunizations, minimum high school rank 30%. Transfer students are accepted. **Standardized tests** *Required:* SAT or ACT, TOEFL for international students. **Application** *Deadline:* rolling (freshmen), rolling (transfer). *Notification:* continuous until 12/15 (freshmen). *Application fee:* $40.

Advanced Placement Credit by examination available. Credit given for nursing courses completed elsewhere dependent upon specific evaluations.

Financial Aid 75% of baccalaureate students in nursing programs received some form of financial aid in 2002–03. *Gift aid (need-based):* Federal Pell, FSEOG, state, private, college/university gift aid from institutional funds. *Loans:* FFEL (Subsidized and Unsubsidized Stafford PLUS), Perkins, state, college/university. *Work-Study:* Federal Work-Study. *Application deadline (priority):* 3/1.

Contact Dr. Therese B. Shipps, Director, School of Nursing, University of Maine, 5724 Dunn Hall, Orono, ME 04469. *Telephone:* 207-581-2599. *Fax:* 207-581-2585. *E-mail:* tshipps@maine.edu.

GRADUATE PROGRAMS

Financial Aid 100% of graduate students in nursing programs received some form of financial aid in 2002–03. Career-related internships or fieldwork, Federal Work-Study, institutionally sponsored loans, and tuition waivers (full and partial) available. Aid available to part-time students. *Financial aid application deadline:* 3/1.

Contact Dr. Carol Wood, Coordinator, School of Nursing, University of Maine, 218 Dunn Hall, Orono, ME 04469. *Telephone:* 207-581-2605. *Fax:* 207-581-2585. *E-mail:* cwood@maine.edu.

MASTER'S DEGREE PROGRAM

Degree MSN

Available Programs Master's; RN to Master's.

Concentrations Available Health-care administration; nursing education. *Nurse practitioner programs in:* family health.

Study Options Full-time and part-time.

Program Entrance Requirements Clinical experience, minimum overall college GPA of 3.0, transcript of college record, CPR certification, written essay, immunizations, interview, 3 letters of recommendation, nursing research course, physical assessment course, statistics course, GRE General Test. *Application deadline:* Applications are processed on a rolling basis. *Application fee:* $50.

Advanced Placement Credit given for nursing courses completed elsewhere dependent upon specific evaluations.

Degree Requirements 47 total credit hours, thesis or project.

University of Maine at Fort Kent

Department of Nursing
Fort Kent, Maine

http://www.umfk.maine.edu/academics/programs/nursing/

Founded in 1878

DEGREE • BSN

Nursing Program Faculty 5 (20% with doctorates).

Baccalaureate Enrollment 296
Women 90% **Men** 10% **Minority** 2% **International** 2% **Part-time** 63%

Nursing Student Activities Nursing Honor Society, Student Nurses' Association, nursing club.

Nursing Student Resources Academic advising; academic or career counseling; assistance for students with disabilities; bookstore; campus computer network; career placement assistance; computer lab; computer-assisted instruction; e-mail services; housing assistance; interactive nursing skills videos; Internet; learning resource lab; library services; nursing audiovisuals; remedial services; resume preparation assistance; skills, simulation, or other laboratory; tutoring; unpaid internships.

Library Facilities 69,189 volumes (3,386 in health, 2,425 in nursing); 335 periodical subscriptions (73 health-care related).

BACCALAUREATE PROGRAMS

Degree BSN

Available Programs Accelerated Baccalaureate; Generic Baccalaureate; RN Baccalaureate.

Study Options Full-time and part-time.

Program Entrance Requirements Minimum overall college GPA of 2.5, CPR certification, health exam, health insurance, high school transcript, immunizations, prerequisite course work. Transfer students are accepted. **Standardized tests** *Required:* TOEFL for international students. *Recommended:* SAT and SAT Subject Tests or ACT. *Required for some:* SAT, SAT and SAT Subject Tests or ACT. **Application** *Deadline:* rolling (freshmen), rolling (transfer). *Notification:* continuous (freshmen). *Application fee:* $40.

Expenses (2004–05) *Tuition, state resident:* full-time $3960; part-time $132 per credit hour. *Tuition, nonresident:* full-time $9600; part-time $320 per credit hour. *International tuition:* $9600 full-time. *Room and board:* $5511; room only: $3026 per academic year. *Required fees:* full-time $554; part-time $19 per credit.

Financial Aid 80% of baccalaureate students in nursing programs received some form of financial aid in 2003–04.

Contact Ms. Jenny Radsma, Chair of Admission, Advisement, and Advancement Committee, Department of Nursing, University of Maine at Fort Kent, 23 University Drive, Fort Kent, ME 04743-1292. *Telephone:* 207-834-7586. *Fax:* 207-834-7577. *E-mail:* radsma@maine.edu.

University of New England

Department of Nursing
Biddeford, Maine

http://www.une.edu/chp/nursing/

Founded in 1831

DEGREE • BSN

Nursing Program Faculty 17 (41% with doctorates).

Baccalaureate Enrollment 24
Women 83% **Men** 17% **Minority** 8%

Nursing Student Activities Nursing Honor Society, Sigma Theta Tau, Student Nurses' Association, nursing club.

Nursing Student Resources Academic advising; academic or career counseling; assistance for students with disabilities; bookstore; campus computer network; career placement assistance; computer lab; computer-assisted instruction; e-mail services; employment services for current students; housing assistance; Internet; learning resource lab; library services; nursing audiovisuals; placement services for program completers; remedial services; resume preparation assistance; skills, simulation, or other laboratory; tutoring; unpaid internships.

Library Facilities 142,181 volumes (9,400 in health, 5,100 in nursing); 2,443 periodical subscriptions (1,200 health-care related).

BACCALAUREATE PROGRAMS

Degree BSN

Available Programs RN Baccalaureate.

Study Options Full-time and part-time.

Program Entrance Requirements Minimum overall college GPA of 2.5, transcript of college record, CPR certification, health exam, health insurance, high school biology, high school chemistry, 2 years high school math, 2 years high school science, high school transcript, immunizations, minimum high school GPA of 2.5, professional liability insurance/malpractice insurance. Transfer students are accepted. **Standardized tests** *Required:* SAT or ACT, TOEFL for international students. **Application** *Deadline:* rolling (freshmen), rolling (transfer). *Notification:* continuous (freshmen). *Application fee:* $40.

Advanced Placement Credit by examination available. Credit given for nursing courses completed elsewhere dependent upon specific evaluations.

Financial Aid 88% of baccalaureate students in nursing programs received some form of financial aid in 2003–04. *Gift aid (need-based):* Federal Pell, FSEOG, state, private, college/university gift aid from institutional funds. *Loans:* Federal Nursing Student Loans, FFEL (Subsidized and Unsubsidized Stafford PLUS), Perkins, state, college/university. *Work-Study:* Federal Work-Study. *Application deadline (priority):* 5/1.

Contact Karen T. Pardue, Interim Director, Department of Nursing, University of New England, Department of Nursing, 716 Stevens Avenue, Portland, ME 04103-7225. *Telephone:* 207-283-0171 Ext. 4476. *Fax:* 207-878-4895. *E-mail:* kpardue@une.edu.

University of New England (continued)

CONTINUING EDUCATION PROGRAM

Contact Nancy LaBrie, Office of Continuing Education, Department of Nursing, University of New England, 716 Stevens Avenue, Portland, ME 04103. *Telephone:* 207-797-7688 Ext. 4395. *Fax:* 207-878-4891. *E-mail:* nlabrie@une.edu.

University of Southern Maine

College of Nursing and Health Professions
Portland, Maine

http://www.usm.maine.edu/conhp

Founded in 1878

DEGREES • BS • MS • MS/MBA

Nursing Program Faculty 47 (32% with doctorates).

Baccalaureate Enrollment 612
Women 91% **Men** 9% **Minority** 5% **Part-time** 34%

Graduate Enrollment 94
Women 89% **Men** 11% **Minority** 2% **Part-time** 37%

Nursing Student Activities Sigma Theta Tau, Student Nurses' Association.

Nursing Student Resources Academic advising; academic or career counseling; assistance for students with disabilities; bookstore; campus computer network; computer lab; computer-assisted instruction; daycare for children of students; e-mail services; interactive nursing skills videos; Internet; learning resource lab; library services; nursing audiovisuals; remedial services; resume preparation assistance; skills, simulation, or other laboratory; tutoring.

Library Facilities 545,246 volumes (18,042 in health, 622 in nursing); 2,585 periodical subscriptions (230 health-care related).

BACCALAUREATE PROGRAMS

Degree BS

Available Programs ADN to Baccalaureate; Accelerated Baccalaureate for Second Degree; Generic Baccalaureate.

Site Options Lewiston, ME.

Study Options Full-time and part-time.

Program Entrance Requirements Minimum overall college GPA of 2.5, transcript of college record, written essay, high school biology, high school chemistry, 3 years high school math, 2 years high school science, high school transcript, immunizations. Transfer students are accepted. **Standardized tests** *Required:* SAT or ACT, TOEFL for international students. **Application** *Deadline:* 2/15 (freshmen), 2/15 (transfer). *Notification:* continuous (freshmen). *Application fee:* $40.

Advanced Placement Credit by examination available. Credit given for nursing courses completed elsewhere dependent upon specific evaluations.

Expenses (2004–05) *Tuition, state resident:* full-time $4620; part-time $154 per credit hour. *Tuition, nonresident:* full-time $12,780; part-time $426 per credit hour. *International tuition:* $12,780 full-time. *Room and board:* $6316; room only: $3386 per academic year. *Required fees:* full-time $1200; part-time $25 per credit; part-time $105 per term.

Financial Aid 96% of baccalaureate students in nursing programs received some form of financial aid in 2003–04. *Gift aid (need-based):* Federal Pell, FSEOG, state, college/university gift aid from institutional funds. *Loans:* Federal Nursing Student Loans, FFEL (Subsidized and Unsubsidized Stafford PLUS), Perkins, college/university. *Work-Study:* Federal Work-Study. *Application deadline (priority):* 2/15.

Contact Brenda Diane Webster, Coordinator of Nursing Student Services, College of Nursing and Health Professions, University of Southern Maine, PO Box 9300, Portland, ME 04104-9300. *Telephone:* 207-780-4802. *Fax:* 207-228-8177. *E-mail:* brenda@usm.maine.edu.

GRADUATE PROGRAMS

Expenses (2004–05) *Tuition, state resident:* full-time $4122; part-time $229 per credit hour. *Tuition, nonresident:* full-time $11,520; part-time $640 per credit hour. *International tuition:* $11,520 full-time. *Room and board:* $6290; room only: $3500 per academic year. *Required fees:* full-time $659; part-time $37 per credit; part-time $105 per term.

Financial Aid 75% of graduate students in nursing programs received some form of financial aid in 2003–04. 5 research assistantships with tuition reimbursements available (averaging $1,400 per year), 7 teaching assistantships with tuition reimbursements available (averaging $1,400 per year) were awarded; career-related internships or fieldwork, Federal Work-Study, scholarships, traineeships, tuition waivers (full and partial), and unspecified assistantships also available. Aid available to part-time students. *Financial aid application deadline:* 2/15.

Contact Dr. Marianne Rodgers, Chair of Nursing, College of Nursing and Health Professions, University of Southern Maine, PO Box 9300, Portland, ME 04104-9300. *Telephone:* 207-780-4808. *Fax:* 207-228-8177. *E-mail:* mrodgers@usm.maine.edu.

MASTER'S DEGREE PROGRAM

Degrees MS; MS/MBA

Available Programs Master's; Master's for Non-Nursing College Graduates; RN to Master's.

Concentrations Available *Clinical nurse specialist programs in:* medical-surgical, psychiatric/mental health. *Nurse practitioner programs in:* adult health, family health, psychiatric/mental health.

Study Options Full-time and part-time.

Program Entrance Requirements Minimum overall college GPA of 3.0, transcript of college record, written essay, immunizations, 2 letters of recommendation, physical assessment course, prerequisite course work, statistics course, GRE General Test or MAT. *Application deadline:* Applications are processed on a rolling basis. *Application fee:* $50.

Advanced Placement Credit given for nursing courses completed elsewhere dependent upon specific evaluations.

Degree Requirements 54 total credit hours.

POST-MASTER'S PROGRAM

Areas of Study *Clinical nurse specialist programs in:* medical-surgical, psychiatric/mental health. *Nurse practitioner programs in:* adult health, family health, psychiatric/mental health.

CONTINUING EDUCATION PROGRAM

Contact Ms. Molly Morrell, Senior Program Specialist, College of Nursing and Health Professions, University of Southern Maine, Center for Continuing Education, PO Box 9300, Portland, ME 04104-9300. *Telephone:* 207-780-5931. *Fax:* 207-780-5954. *E-mail:* mmorrell@usm.maine.edu.

MARYLAND

Bowie State University

Department of Nursing
Bowie, Maryland

http://www.bowiestate.edu/academics/nursing.htm

Founded in 1865

DEGREES • BSN • MSN

Nursing Program Faculty 13.

Nursing Student Activities Student Nurses' Association.

Nursing Student Resources Library services.

Library Facilities 331,640 volumes; 3,152 periodical subscriptions.

BACCALAUREATE PROGRAMS

Degree BSN

Available Programs RN Baccalaureate.

Study Options Full-time and part-time.

Program Entrance Requirements Minimum overall college GPA of 2.0, health exam, minimum high school GPA of 2.5, prerequisite course work, RN licensure. Transfer students are accepted. **Standardized tests** *Required:* SAT or ACT, TOEFL for international students. **Application** *Deadline:* 4/1 (freshmen), 4/1 (transfer). *Notification:* continuous (freshmen). *Application fee:* $40.

Advanced Placement Credit by examination available.

Contact Nursing Adviser, Department of Nursing, Bowie State University, 14000 Jericho Park Road, Robinson Hall Room 119, Bowie, MD 20715. *Telephone:* 301-860-3202. *Fax:* 301-860-3222.

GRADUATE PROGRAMS

Financial Aid Institutionally sponsored loans and traineeships available.

Contact Nursing Adviser, Department of Nursing, Bowie State University, 14000 Jericho Park Road, Bowie, MD 20715. *Telephone:* 301-860-4000. *Fax:* 301-860-3222.

MASTER'S DEGREE PROGRAM

Degree MSN

Available Programs Master's.

Concentrations Available Nursing administration; nursing education. *Nurse practitioner programs in:* family health.

Program Entrance Requirements Clinical experience, minimum overall college GPA of 2.5, CPR certification, written essay, 3 letters of recommendation, physical assessment course, professional liability insurance/malpractice insurance, resume, statistics course. *Application deadline:* For fall admission, 3/15. Applications are processed on a rolling basis. *Application fee:* $40.

Advanced Placement Credit by examination available. Credit given for nursing courses completed elsewhere dependent upon specific evaluations.

Degree Requirements 47 total credit hours, thesis or project, comprehensive exam.

College of Notre Dame of Maryland
Department of Nursing
Baltimore, Maryland

http://206.205.71.30/academics/departments/nd_aca_nursing.cfm

Founded in 1873

DEGREE • BS

Nursing Program Faculty 5 (60% with doctorates).

Nursing Student Resources Library services.

Library Facilities 400,000 volumes; 1,800 periodical subscriptions.

BACCALAUREATE PROGRAMS

Degree BS

Available Programs Accelerated RN Baccalaureate; RN Baccalaureate.

Site Options Frederick, MD; Aberdeen, MD.

Study Options Full-time and part-time.

Program Entrance Requirements Minimum overall college GPA of 2.5, transcript of college record, interview, minimum GPA in nursing prerequisites of 2.0, prerequisite course work, RN licensure. Transfer students are accepted. **Standardized tests** *Required:* SAT or ACT, TOEFL for international students. **Application** *Deadline:* 2/15 (freshmen), 2/15 (transfer). *Early decision:* 12/3. *Notification:* continuous until 6/30 (freshmen), 1/1 (early action). *Application fee:* $25.

Advanced Placement Credit by examination available. Credit given for nursing courses completed elsewhere dependent upon specific evaluations.

Contact Accelerated/Weekend College, Department of Nursing, College of Notre Dame of Maryland, 4701 North Charles Street, Baltimore, MD 21210-2476. *Telephone:* 410-532-5500. *E-mail:* accelerate@ndm.edu.

Columbia Union College
Nursing Department
Takoma Park, Maryland

Founded in 1904

DEGREE • BS

Nursing Program Faculty 7 (14% with doctorates).

Baccalaureate Enrollment 270
Women 90% **Men** 10% **Minority** 75% **International** 1% **Part-time** 10%

Nursing Student Activities Student Nurses' Association, nursing club.

Nursing Student Resources Academic advising; academic or career counseling; bookstore; campus computer network; computer lab; e-mail services; externships; interactive nursing skills videos; Internet; learning resource lab; library services; nursing audiovisuals; paid internships; remedial services; skills, simulation, or other laboratory; tutoring; unpaid internships.

Library Facilities 141,534 volumes; 9,000 periodical subscriptions.

BACCALAUREATE PROGRAMS

Degree BS

Available Programs Accelerated RN Baccalaureate; Generic Baccalaureate.

Study Options Full-time.

Program Entrance Requirements Minimum overall college GPA of 2.75, transcript of college record, CPR certification, written essay, health exam, immunizations, interview, 2 letters of recommendation, minimum GPA in nursing prerequisites of 2.75, prerequisite course work. Transfer students are accepted. **Standardized tests** *Required:* SAT or ACT. **Application** *Deadline:* 8/1 (freshmen), rolling (transfer). *Notification:* continuous (freshmen). *Application fee:* $25.

Advanced Placement Credit given for nursing courses completed elsewhere dependent upon specific evaluations.

Expenses (2004–05) *Tuition:* full-time $15,433; part-time $643 per credit hour. *Room and board:* $5560 per academic year. *Required fees:* full-time $1000.

Financial Aid 95% of baccalaureate students in nursing programs received some form of financial aid in 2003–04.

Contact Ms. Letetia H.P. Edmonds, Office Manager, Nursing Department, Columbia Union College, 7600 Flower Avenue, Takoma Park, MD 20912. *Telephone:* 301-891-4144. *Fax:* 301-891-4191. *E-mail:* ledmonds@cuc.edu.

CONTINUING EDUCATION PROGRAM

Contact Continuing Education Center, Nursing Department, Columbia Union College, 7600 Carroll Avenue, Takoma Park, MD 20912. *Telephone:* 301-891-5200.

Coppin State University
Helene Fuld School of Nursing
Baltimore, Maryland

http://www.coppin.edu/nursing

Founded in 1900

DEGREES • BSN • MSN

Nursing Program Faculty 15 (22% with doctorates).

Baccalaureate Enrollment 200
Women 96% **Men** 4% **Minority** 95% **International** 8% **Part-time** 6%

Graduate Enrollment 26
Women 93% **Men** 7% **Minority** 98% **International** 14% **Part-time** 35%

Nursing Student Activities Nursing Honor Society, Sigma Theta Tau, Student Nurses' Association.

Nursing Student Resources Academic advising; academic or career counseling; campus computer network; career placement assistance; computer lab; computer-assisted instruction; e-mail services; interactive nursing skills videos; Internet; learning resource lab; nursing audiovisuals; other; remedial services; skills, simulation, or other laboratory; tutoring.

Coppin State University (continued)
Library Facilities 134,983 volumes (1,339 in health, 1,298 in nursing); 665 periodical subscriptions (132 health-care related).

BACCALAUREATE PROGRAMS

Degree BSN

Available Programs ADN to Baccalaureate; Baccalaureate for Second Degree; Generic Baccalaureate; RN Baccalaureate.

Study Options Full-time.

Program Entrance Requirements Minimum overall college GPA of 2.5, transcript of college record, high school biology, high school chemistry, high school transcript, 3 letters of recommendation, minimum high school GPA of 2.5, minimum GPA in nursing prerequisites of 2.5. Transfer students are accepted. **Standardized tests** *Required:* SAT or ACT, TOEFL for international students. **Application** *Deadline:* 7/15 (freshmen), 7/15 (transfer). *Notification:* continuous (freshmen). *Application fee:* $35.

Expenses (2004–05) *Tuition, state resident:* full-time $4599; part-time $142 per credit hour. *Tuition, nonresident:* full-time $10,771; part-time $327 per credit hour. *International tuition:* $10,771 full-time. *Room and board:* $5600; room only: $3200 per academic year. *Required fees:* full-time $420; part-time $21 per credit; part-time $147 per term.

Financial Aid 90% of baccalaureate students in nursing programs received some form of financial aid in 2003–04. *Gift aid (need-based):* Federal Pell, FSEOG, state, private, college/university gift aid from institutional funds, Federal Nursing. *Loans:* Federal Direct (Subsidized and Unsubsidized Stafford), FFEL, Perkins. *Work-Study:* Federal Work-Study. *Application deadline (priority):* 3/4.

Contact Mr. Darryl A. Boyd, Nursing Admissions Coordinator/Recruiter, Helene Fuld School of Nursing, Coppin State University, 2500 W. North Avenue, Baltimore, MD 21216-3698. *Telephone:* 410-951-3988. *Fax:* 410-462-3032. *E-mail:* dboyd@coppin.edu.

GRADUATE PROGRAMS

Expenses (2004–05) *Tuition, state resident:* part-time $186 per credit hour. *Tuition, nonresident:* part-time $337 per credit hour. *International tuition:* $11,000 full-time. *Room and board:* $5600; room only: $3200 per academic year. *Required fees:* full-time $420; part-time $21 per credit; part-time $147 per term.

Financial Aid 70% of graduate students in nursing programs received some form of financial aid in 2003–04.

Contact Mr. Darryl A. Boyd, Nursing Admissions Coordinator/Recruiter, Helene Fuld School of Nursing, Coppin State University, 2500 West North Avenue, Baltimore, MD 21216-3698. *Telephone:* 410-951-3988. *Fax:* 410-462-3032. *E-mail:* dboyd@coppin.edu.

MASTER'S DEGREE PROGRAM

Degree MSN

Available Programs Master's.

Concentrations Available *Nurse practitioner programs in:* family health.

Study Options Full-time and part-time.

Program Entrance Requirements Clinical experience, computer literacy, minimum overall college GPA of 3.0, transcript of college record, CPR certification, written essay, immunizations, interview, 3 letters of recommendation, nursing research course, physical assessment course, statistics course.

Advanced Placement Credit given for nursing courses completed elsewhere dependent upon specific evaluations.

Degree Requirements 48 total credit hours, thesis or project, comprehensive exam.

POST-MASTER'S PROGRAM

Areas of Study *Nurse practitioner programs in:* family health.

The Johns Hopkins University

School of Nursing
Baltimore, Maryland

http://www.son.jhmi.edu
Founded in 1876
DEGREES • BS • MSN • MSN/MBA • MSN/MPH • MSN/PHD

Nursing Program Faculty 134 (62% with doctorates).

Baccalaureate Enrollment 306
Women 92% **Men** 8% **Minority** 20% **Part-time** 12%

Graduate Enrollment 263
Women 95% **Men** 5% **Minority** 23% **Part-time** 82%

Nursing Student Activities Nursing Honor Society, Sigma Theta Tau, Student Nurses' Association.

Nursing Student Resources Academic advising; academic or career counseling; assistance for students with disabilities; bookstore; campus computer network; computer lab; computer-assisted instruction; e-mail services; housing assistance; interactive nursing skills videos; Internet; learning resource lab; library services; nursing audiovisuals; resume preparation assistance; skills, simulation, or other laboratory.

Library Facilities 3.5 million volumes (350,000 in health, 2,500 in nursing); 30,023 periodical subscriptions (2,241 health-care related).

BACCALAUREATE PROGRAMS

Degree BS

Available Programs Accelerated Baccalaureate for Second Degree; Baccalaureate for Second Degree; Generic Baccalaureate; RN Baccalaureate.

Study Options Full-time and part-time.

Program Entrance Requirements Minimum overall college GPA of 3.0, transcript of college record, CPR certification, written essay, health exam, health insurance, immunizations, interview, 3 letters of recommendation, minimum GPA in nursing prerequisites of 3.0, prerequisite course work. Transfer students are accepted. **Standardized tests** *Required:* SAT or ACT, SAT II Writing Tests, TOEFL for international students. *Recommended:* SAT Subject Tests. **Application** *Deadline:* 1/1 (freshmen), 3/15 (transfer). *Early decision:* 11/15. *Notification:* 4/1 (freshmen), 12/15 (out-of-state freshmen), 12/15 (early decision). *Application fee:* $60.

Advanced Placement Credit by examination available. Credit given for nursing courses completed elsewhere dependent upon specific evaluations.

Expenses (2003–04) *Tuition:* full-time $20,776; part-time $866 per credit hour.

Financial Aid 85% of baccalaureate students in nursing programs received some form of financial aid in 2002–03.

Contact Ms. Mary O'Rourke, Director of Admissions and Student Services, School of Nursing, The Johns Hopkins University, 525 North Wolfe Street, Baltimore, MD 21205-2110. *Telephone:* 410-955-7548. *Fax:* 410-614-7086. *E-mail:* orourke@son.jhmi.edu.

GRADUATE PROGRAMS

Expenses (2003–04) *Tuition:* full-time $23,050; part-time $960 per credit hour.

Financial Aid 75% of graduate students in nursing programs received some form of financial aid in 2002–03. 3 research assistantships with full tuition reimbursements available (averaging $15,000 per year), 6 teaching assistantships with full tuition reimbursements available (averaging $7,500 per year) were awarded; fellowships, career-related internships or fieldwork, Federal Work-Study, institutionally sponsored loans, scholarships, and traineeships also available. Aid available to part-time students. *Financial aid application deadline:* 5/1.

Contact Ms. Mary O'Rourke, Director of Admissions and Student Services, School of Nursing, The Johns Hopkins University, 525 North Wolfe Street, Baltimore, MD 21205-2110. *Telephone:* 410-955-7548. *Fax:* 410-614-7086. *E-mail:* orourke@son.jhmi.edu.

MASTER'S DEGREE PROGRAM

Degrees MSN; MSN/MBA; MSN/MPH; MSN/PhD

Available Programs Master's.

Concentrations Available Nurse case management; nursing administration. *Clinical nurse specialist programs in:* acute care, adult health, cardiovascular, community health, critical care, family health, gerontology, home health care, maternity-newborn, medical-surgical, oncology, parent-child, pediatric, perinatal, public health, rehabilitation, school health, women's health. *Nurse practitioner programs in:* acute care, adult health, family health, pediatric.

Study Options Full-time and part-time.

Program Entrance Requirements Clinical experience, computer literacy, minimum overall college GPA of 3.0, transcript of college record, CPR certification, written essay, immunizations, interview, 3 letters of recommendation, nursing research course, physical assessment course, prerequisite course work, resume, statistics course, GRE. *Application deadline:* For fall admission, 3/1 (priority date); for winter and spring admission, 7/1 (priority date). Applications are processed on a rolling basis. *Application fee:* $50.

Advanced Placement Credit by examination available. Credit given for nursing courses completed elsewhere dependent upon specific evaluations.

Degree Requirements 36 total credit hours, thesis or project.

POST-MASTER'S PROGRAM

Areas of Study *Nurse practitioner programs in:* acute care, adult health, family health, pediatric.

DOCTORAL DEGREE PROGRAM

Degree PhD

Available Programs Doctorate.

Areas of Study Addiction/substance abuse, advanced practice nursing, aging, bio-behavioral research, biology of health and illness, clinical practice, community health, critical care, ethics, family health, gerontology, health policy, health promotion/disease prevention, health-care systems, human health and illness, illness and transition, individualized study, maternity-newborn, nurse case management, nursing administration, nursing policy, nursing research, nursing science, oncology, urban health, women's health.

Program Entrance Requirements Clinical experience, minimum overall college GPA of 3.0, interview by faculty committee, 3 letters of recommendation, MSN or equivalent, scholarly papers, statistics course, vita, writing sample, GRE. *Application deadline:* For fall admission, 3/1 (priority date); for winter and spring admission, 7/1 (priority date). Applications are processed on a rolling basis. *Application fee:* $50.

Degree Requirements 63 total credit hours, dissertation, oral exam, written exam.

POSTDOCTORAL PROGRAM

Areas of Study Health promotion/disease prevention, vulnerable population.

Postdoctoral Program Contact Dr. Jacquelyn Campbell, Associate Dean for Faculty Affairs, School of Nursing, The Johns Hopkins University, 525 North Wolfe Street, Baltimore, MD 21205-2110. *Telephone:* 410-955-2778. *Fax:* 410-614-8285. *E-mail:* jcampbel@son.jhmi.edu.

CONTINUING EDUCATION PROGRAM

Contact Kathleen Sabatier, Director, Institute for Johns Hopkins Nursing, School of Nursing, The Johns Hopkins University, 525 North Wolfe Street, Baltimore, MD 21205-2110. *Telephone:* 410-614-3160. *Fax:* 410-614-8972. *E-mail:* ksabatier@son.jhmi.edu.

See full description on page 504.

Salisbury University

Program in Nursing
Salisbury, Maryland

http://www.ssu.edu/Schools/Henson/NursingDept.html

Founded in 1925

DEGREES • BS • MS

Nursing Program Faculty 18 (67% with doctorates).

Baccalaureate Enrollment 402

Women 90% **Men** 10% **Minority** 15% **International** 3% **Part-time** 10%

Graduate Enrollment 27

Women 85% **Men** 15% **Minority** 10% **International** 5% **Part-time** 85%

Nursing Student Activities Nursing Honor Society, Sigma Theta Tau, Student Nurses' Association.

Nursing Student Resources Academic advising; academic or career counseling; assistance for students with disabilities; bookstore; campus computer network; career placement assistance; computer lab; computer-assisted instruction; e-mail services; employment services for current students; externships; housing assistance; interactive nursing skills videos; Internet; learning resource lab; library services; nursing audiovisuals; paid internships; resume preparation assistance; skills, simulation, or other laboratory; tutoring; unpaid internships.

Library Facilities 254,151 volumes (6,850 in health, 1,025 in nursing); 1,271 periodical subscriptions (145 health-care related).

BACCALAUREATE PROGRAMS

Degree BS

Available Programs ADN to Baccalaureate; Accelerated Baccalaureate for Second Degree; Accelerated RN Baccalaureate; Generic Baccalaureate.

Study Options Full-time and part-time.

Program Entrance Requirements Minimum overall college GPA, transcript of college record, CPR certification, health exam, high school biology, high school chemistry, 2 years high school math, high school transcript, immunizations, minimum GPA in nursing prerequisites, prerequisite course work. Transfer students are accepted. **Standardized tests** *Required:* SAT or ACT, TOEFL for international students. **Application** *Deadline:* 1/15 (freshmen), rolling (transfer). *Early decision:* 12/1. *Notification:* 3/15 (freshmen), 1/15 (early action). *Application fee:* $45.

Advanced Placement Credit given for nursing courses completed elsewhere dependent upon specific evaluations.

Expenses (2004–05) *Tuition, state resident:* full-time $4546; part-time $188 per credit hour. *Tuition, nonresident:* full-time $12,124; part-time $487 per credit hour. *International tuition:* $12,124 full-time. *Room and board:* $6600; room only: $3450 per academic year. *Required fees:* full-time $1430; part-time $8 per credit.

Financial Aid 90% of baccalaureate students in nursing programs received some form of financial aid in 2003–04. *Gift aid (need-based):* Federal Pell, FSEOG, state, college/university gift aid from institutional funds. *Loans:* Federal Direct (Subsidized and Unsubsidized Stafford PLUS), Perkins. *Work-Study:* Federal Work-Study, part-time campus jobs. *Application deadline (priority):* 2/1.

Contact Dr. Mary C. DiBartolo, RN, Associate Professor, Program in Nursing, Salisbury University, 1101 Camden Avenue, Salisbury, MD 21801. *Telephone:* 410-543-6403. *Fax:* 410-548-3313. *E-mail:* mcdibartolo@salisbury.edu.

GRADUATE PROGRAMS

Expenses (2004–05) *Tuition, state resident:* full-time $4248; part-time $236 per credit hour. *Tuition, nonresident:* full-time $9000; part-time $500 per credit hour. *International tuition:* $9000 full-time. *Required fees:* full-time $144; part-time $8 per credit.

Financial Aid 75% of graduate students in nursing programs received some form of financial aid in 2003–04. Career-related internships or fieldwork, scholarships, and unspecified assistantships available. Aid available to part-time students.

Contact Dr. Karin E. Johnson, RN, Director, Graduate Program, Program in Nursing, Salisbury University, 1101 Camden Avenue, Salisbury, MD 21801. *Telephone:* 410-543-6411. *Fax:* 410-548-3313. *E-mail:* kejohnson@salisbury.edu.

MASTER'S DEGREE PROGRAM

Degree MS

Available Programs Master's.

Concentrations Available Health-care administration; nursing administration. *Clinical nurse specialist programs in:* home health care. *Nurse practitioner programs in:* family health.

Study Options Full-time and part-time.

Program Entrance Requirements Minimum overall college GPA of 3.0, transcript of college record, CPR certification, written essay, interview, 2 letters of recommendation, resume. *Application deadline:* For fall admission, 2/15; for spring admission, 10/15. Applications are processed on a rolling basis. *Application fee:* $45.

Advanced Placement Credit given for nursing courses completed elsewhere dependent upon specific evaluations.

Degree Requirements 43 total credit hours, thesis or project.

Salisbury University (continued)

POST-MASTER'S PROGRAM

Areas of Study Health-care administration. *Nurse practitioner programs in:* family health.

Towson University

Department of Nursing
Towson, Maryland

http://www.towson.edu

Founded in 1866

DEGREES • BS • MS

Nursing Program Faculty 20 (75% with doctorates).

Baccalaureate Enrollment 190
Women 96% **Men** 4% **Minority** 24% **Part-time** 14%

Graduate Enrollment 24
Women 92% **Men** 8% **Minority** 21% **Part-time** 100%

Nursing Student Activities Sigma Theta Tau, Student Nurses' Association.

Nursing Student Resources Academic advising; academic or career counseling; assistance for students with disabilities; bookstore; campus computer network; career placement assistance; computer lab; computer-assisted instruction; daycare for children of students; e-mail services; employment services for current students; housing assistance; interactive nursing skills videos; Internet; learning resource lab; library services; nursing audiovisuals; remedial services; resume preparation assistance; skills, simulation, or other laboratory; tutoring.

Library Facilities 574,096 volumes (15,660 in health, 1,409 in nursing); 4,154 periodical subscriptions (550 health-care related).

BACCALAUREATE PROGRAMS

Degree BS

Available Programs Generic Baccalaureate; RN Baccalaureate.

Study Options Full-time and part-time.

Program Entrance Requirements Minimum overall college GPA of 2.5, transcript of college record, CPR certification, health exam, health insurance, immunizations, minimum GPA in nursing prerequisites, prerequisite course work. Transfer students are accepted. **Standardized tests** *Required:* SAT or ACT, TOEFL for international students. **Application** *Deadline:* 2/15 (freshmen). *Notification:* continuous (freshmen). *Application fee:* $45.

Advanced Placement Credit by examination available. Credit given for nursing courses completed elsewhere dependent upon specific evaluations.

Expenses (2004–05) *Tuition, state resident:* full-time $6672; part-time $281 per credit hour. *Tuition, nonresident:* full-time $15,352; part-time $577 per credit hour. *Room and board:* room only: $4000 per academic year.

Financial Aid 89% of baccalaureate students in nursing programs received some form of financial aid in 2003–04.

Contact Dr. Sharon B. Eifried, Undergraduate Program Director, Department of Nursing, Towson University, 8000 York Road, Towson, MD 21252-0001. *Telephone:* 410-704-4211. *Fax:* 410-704-4325. *E-mail:* seifried@towson.edu.

GRADUATE PROGRAMS

Expenses (2004–05) *Tuition, state resident:* part-time $327 per credit hour. *Tuition, nonresident:* part-time $608 per credit hour.

Contact Dr. Deborah L. Greener, Graduate Program Director, Department of Nursing, Towson University, 8000 York Road, Towson, MD 21252-0001. *Telephone:* 410-704-4203. *Fax:* 410-704-4325. *E-mail:* dlgreener@towson.edu.

MASTER'S DEGREE PROGRAM

Degree MS

Available Programs Master's.

Concentrations Available Health-care administration; nursing education.

Study Options Part-time.

Program Entrance Requirements Minimum overall college GPA of 3.0, transcript of college record, nursing research course, physical assessment course, resume, statistics course.

Degree Requirements 36 total credit hours.

University of Maryland

School of Nursing
Baltimore, Maryland

http://nursing.umaryland.edu

Founded in 1807

DEGREES • BSN • MS • MS/MBA • PHD

Nursing Program Faculty 137 (62% with doctorates).

Baccalaureate Enrollment 822
Women 88% **Men** 12% **Minority** 38% **International** 2% **Part-time** 9%

Graduate Enrollment 636
Women 91% **Men** 9% **Minority** 37% **International** 3% **Part-time** 61%

Nursing Student Activities Nursing Honor Society, Sigma Theta Tau, Student Nurses' Association.

Nursing Student Resources Academic advising; academic or career counseling; assistance for students with disabilities; bookstore; campus computer network; career placement assistance; computer lab; computer-assisted instruction; e-mail services; housing assistance; interactive nursing skills videos; Internet; learning resource lab; library services; nursing audiovisuals; remedial services; skills, simulation, or other laboratory; tutoring.

Library Facilities 340,000 volumes in health, 50 volumes in nursing; 2,300 periodical subscriptions health-care related.

BACCALAUREATE PROGRAMS

Degree BSN

Available Programs Accelerated Baccalaureate for Second Degree; Generic Baccalaureate; RN Baccalaureate.

Site Options Hagerstown, MD. *Distance Learning:* Cumberland, MD; Shady Grove, MD.

Study Options Full-time and part-time.

Program Entrance Requirements Minimum overall college GPA of 3.00, transcript of college record, CPR certification, written essay, health exam, immunizations, minimum GPA in nursing prerequisites of 3.00, prerequisite course work. Transfer students are accepted.

Advanced Placement Credit by examination available. Credit given for nursing courses completed elsewhere dependent upon specific evaluations.

Expenses (2004–05) *Tuition, state resident:* full-time $6506; part-time $285 per credit hour. *Tuition, nonresident:* full-time $16,745; part-time $427 per credit hour. *Required fees:* full-time $400; part-time $10 per credit; part-time $224 per term.

Financial Aid 90% of baccalaureate students in nursing programs received some form of financial aid in 2003–04.

Contact Candace Edwards, Assistant Director of Admissions, School of Nursing, University of Maryland, 655 West Lombard Street, Baltimore, MD 21201. *Telephone:* 410-706-0501. *Fax:* 410-706-7238. *E-mail:* Cedwards@son.umaryland.edu.

GRADUATE PROGRAMS

Expenses (2004–05) *Tuition, state resident:* full-time $7600; part-time $380 per credit hour. *Tuition, nonresident:* full-time $13,620; part-time $681 per credit hour. *Required fees:* full-time $450.

Financial Aid 45% of graduate students in nursing programs received some form of financial aid in 2003–04. Fellowships, research assistantships, teaching assistantships, career-related internships or fieldwork and traineeships available. Aid available to part-time students. *Financial aid application deadline:* 2/15.

Contact Mrs. Candace Edwards, Associate Director of Admissions and Student Affairs, School of Nursing, University of Maryland, 655 West Lombard Street, Room 102, Baltimore, MD 21201-1579. *Telephone:* 410-706-8346. *Fax:* 410-706-7238. *E-mail:* Cedwards@son.umaryland.edu.

MASTER'S DEGREE PROGRAM

Degrees MS; MS/MBA

Available Programs Master's; Master's for Nurses with Non-Nursing Degrees; RN to Master's.

Concentrations Available Health-care administration; nurse anesthesia; nurse-midwifery; nursing administration; nursing informatics. *Clinical nurse specialist programs in:* community health, psychiatric/mental health. *Nurse practitioner programs in:* acute care, adult health, family health, gerontology, neonatal health, oncology, pediatric, psychiatric/mental health, women's health.

Site Options *Distance Learning:* Cumberland, MD; Shady Grove, MD.

Study Options Full-time and part-time.

Program Entrance Requirements Minimum overall college GPA of 3.0, transcript of college record, CPR certification, written essay, immunizations, 2 letters of recommendation, nursing research course, physical assessment course, resume, GRE General Test. *Application fee:* $50.

Advanced Placement Credit by examination available. Credit given for nursing courses completed elsewhere dependent upon specific evaluations.

Degree Requirements 35 total credit hours, comprehensive exam.

POST-MASTER'S PROGRAM

Areas of Study Health-care administration; nursing administration; nursing education; nursing informatics. *Clinical nurse specialist programs in:* community health, psychiatric/mental health. *Nurse practitioner programs in:* acute care, adult health, family health, gerontology, neonatal health, oncology, pediatric, psychiatric/mental health, women's health.

DOCTORAL DEGREE PROGRAM

Degree PhD

Available Programs Doctorate; Post-Baccalaureate Doctorate.

Areas of Study Addiction/substance abuse, aging, bio-behavioral research, community health, critical care, family health, gerontology, health policy, health promotion/disease prevention, health-care systems, human health and illness, individualized study, information systems, maternity-newborn, nursing administration, nursing education, nursing policy, nursing research, nursing science, oncology, urban health, women's health.

Program Entrance Requirements Minimum overall college GPA of 3.0, interview by faculty committee, interview, 3 letters of recommendation, MSN or equivalent, statistics course, vita, writing sample, GRE General Test. *Application fee:* $50.

Degree Requirements 60 total credit hours, dissertation, oral exam, written exam, residency.

CONTINUING EDUCATION PROGRAM

Contact Dr. Kathryn Montgomery, Associate Dean for Organizational Partnership and Outreach, School of Nursing, University of Maryland, 655 West Lombard Street, Baltimore, MD 21201-1579. *Telephone:* 410-706-8198. *Fax:* 410-706-0018. *E-mail:* Montgomery@son.umaryland.edu.

See full description on page 560.

Villa Julie College

Nursing Division
Stevenson, Maryland

http://www4.vjc.edu/Nursing

Founded in 1952

DEGREE • BS

Nursing Program Faculty 40 (15% with doctorates).

Baccalaureate Enrollment 391

Women 93% **Men** 7% **Minority** 24% **Part-time** 47%

Nursing Student Activities Nursing Honor Society, Sigma Theta Tau, Student Nurses' Association.

Nursing Student Resources Academic advising; academic or career counseling; assistance for students with disabilities; bookstore; campus computer network; career placement assistance; computer lab; e-mail services; employment services for current students; Internet; learning resource lab; library services; nursing audiovisuals; placement services for program completers; remedial services; resume preparation assistance; skills, simulation, or other laboratory; tutoring.

Library Facilities 64,930 volumes (3,145 in health, 779 in nursing); 15,503 periodical subscriptions (604 health-care related).

■ The nursing curriculum builds on a foundation of liberal arts and science courses and provides graduates with the education to creatively meet the challenges and demands of nursing in the 21st century. A unique feature of this baccalaureate program is that nursing courses begin in the first semester. In addition to traditional day-division classes, there is an accelerated evening/weekend option for second bachelor's and adult students. The RN-BS option is also offered through an accelerated format.

BACCALAUREATE PROGRAMS

Degree BS

Available Programs ADN to Baccalaureate; Accelerated Baccalaureate for Second Degree; Accelerated RN Baccalaureate; Generic Baccalaureate; RN Baccalaureate.

Site Options Baltimore, MD. *Distance Learning:* Arnold, MD; Easton, MD.

Study Options Full-time and part-time.

Program Entrance Requirements Minimum overall college GPA of 3.0, transcript of college record, written essay, health exam, health insurance, high school biology, high school chemistry, 2 years high school math, high school transcript, immunizations, interview, minimum high school GPA of 3.0, minimum GPA in nursing prerequisites of 3.0. Transfer students are accepted. **Standardized tests** *Required:* SAT or ACT, TOEFL for international students. **Application** *Deadline:* 7/15 (freshmen), 7/15 (transfer). *Notification:* continuous (freshmen). *Application fee:* $25.

Advanced Placement Credit by examination available. Credit given for nursing courses completed elsewhere dependent upon specific evaluations.

Expenses (2004–05) *Tuition:* full-time $13,715; part-time $390 per credit hour. *International tuition:* $13,715 full-time. *Room and board:* room only: $6250 per academic year. *Required fees:* full-time $938; part-time $70 per term.

Financial Aid 80% of baccalaureate students in nursing programs received some form of financial aid in 2003–04. *Gift aid (need-based):* Federal Pell, FSEOG, state, private, college/university gift aid from institutional funds. *Loans:* FFEL (Subsidized and Unsubsidized Stafford PLUS), Perkins. *Work-Study:* Federal Work-Study. *Application deadline (priority):* 2/15.

Contact Dr. Judith A. Feustle, Nursing Department, Nursing Division, Villa Julie College, 1525 Greenspring Valley Road, Stevenson, MD 21153-0641. *Telephone:* 443-334-2312. *Fax:* 410-486-3552. *E-mail:* fac-feus@mail.vjc.edu.

MASSACHUSETTS

American International College

Division of Nursing
Springfield, Massachusetts

http://www.aic.edu/pages/315.html

Founded in 1885

DEGREES • BSN • MSN

American International College (continued)
Nursing Program Faculty 10.

Baccalaureate Enrollment 241
Women 95% **Men** 5% **Minority** 35% **International** 1% **Part-time** 5%

Nursing Student Activities Nursing Honor Society, Student Nurses' Association.

Nursing Student Resources Academic advising; academic or career counseling; assistance for students with disabilities; bookstore; campus computer network; career placement assistance; computer lab; e-mail services; employment services for current students; externships; housing assistance; interactive nursing skills videos; Internet; learning resource lab; library services; nursing audiovisuals; other; placement services for program completers; resume preparation assistance; skills, simulation, or other laboratory; tutoring.

Library Facilities 118,000 volumes (689 in health, 264 in nursing); 390 periodical subscriptions (50 health-care related).

■ The American International College (AIC) BSN program is accredited by the NLNAC. Nursing students are admitted directly into the program upon acceptance to the College. Clinical experiences start in the second semester of the sophomore year. Off-campus clinical sites include medical, surgical, maternity, pediatric, rehabilitation, and mental health units. One hundred percent of classes are faculty taught, with a student-faculty ratio of 12:1 in the classroom and 5:1 in clinical settings. Founded in 1885, AIC's campus is conveniently located in Springfield, Massachusetts, a metropolitan hub of a half-million people. It is 1½ hours from Boston and 2½ hours from New York City and is easily accessible by car, train, bus, or air service.

BACCALAUREATE PROGRAMS

Degree BSN

Available Programs Generic Baccalaureate; RN Baccalaureate.

Study Options Full-time and part-time.

Program Entrance Requirements Minimum overall college GPA of 2.0, transcript of college record, health exam, health insurance, high school biology, high school chemistry, 3 years high school math, 2 years high school science, high school transcript, immunizations, 1 letter of recommendation, minimum high school GPA of 2.0, professional liability insurance/malpractice insurance. Transfer students are accepted. **Standardized tests** *Required:* SAT or ACT, TOEFL for international students. **Application** *Deadline:* rolling (freshmen), rolling (transfer). *Notification:* continuous (freshmen). *Application fee:* $20.

Advanced Placement Credit by examination available. Credit given for nursing courses completed elsewhere dependent upon specific evaluations.

Expenses (2004–05) *Tuition:* full-time $18,000; part-time $405 per credit hour. *International tuition:* $18,000 full-time. *Room and board:* $8510 per academic year. *Required fees:* full-time $400.

Financial Aid 85% of baccalaureate students in nursing programs received some form of financial aid in 2003–04. *Gift aid (need-based):* Federal Pell, FSEOG, state, private, college/university gift aid from institutional funds. *Loans:* FFEL (Subsidized and Unsubsidized Stafford PLUS), Perkins, state, college/university, alternative loans. *Work-Study:* Federal Work-Study, part-time campus jobs. *Application deadline (priority):* 5/1.

Contact Mr. Peter J. Miller, Dean of Admissions, Division of Nursing, American International College, 1000 State Street, Springfield, MA 01109. *Telephone:* 413-205-3201. *Fax:* 413-205-3051. *E-mail:* pmiller@acad.aic.edu.

GRADUATE PROGRAMS

Expenses (2004–05) *Tuition:* full-time $9810; part-time $545 per credit hour. *Room and board:* $8510 per academic year.

Contact Dr. Anne Glanovsky, Director of Division of Nursing, Division of Nursing, American International College, 1000 State Street, Springfield, MA 01109. *Telephone:* 413-205-3519. *Fax:* 413-205-3957. *E-mail:* aglanovs@acad.aic.edu.

MASTER'S DEGREE PROGRAM

Degree MSN

Available Programs Master's.

Concentrations Available Nursing administration; nursing education.

Study Options Full-time and part-time.

Program Entrance Requirements Minimum overall college GPA of 3.0, transcript of college record, immunizations, interview, 2 letters of recommendation, nursing research course, professional liability insurance/malpractice insurance, prerequisite course work, resume, statistics course.

Advanced Placement Credit given for nursing courses completed elsewhere dependent upon specific evaluations.

Degree Requirements 36 total credit hours, thesis or project.

Anna Maria College
Department of Nursing
Paxton, Massachusetts

http://www.annamaria.edu
Founded in 1946

DEGREE • BSN

Nursing Program Faculty 7 (14% with doctorates).

Baccalaureate Enrollment 65
Women 99% **Men** 1% **Minority** 4% **Part-time** 99%

Nursing Student Activities Sigma Theta Tau.

Nursing Student Resources Academic advising; academic or career counseling; assistance for students with disabilities; bookstore; campus computer network; career placement assistance; computer lab; employment services for current students; Internet; library services; nursing audiovisuals; placement services for program completers; remedial services; resume preparation assistance; skills, simulation, or other laboratory; tutoring; unpaid internships.

Library Facilities 79,039 volumes (4,213 in health); 318 periodical subscriptions (44 health-care related).

BACCALAUREATE PROGRAMS

Degree BSN

Available Programs ADN to Baccalaureate; Baccalaureate for Second Degree.

Site Options Springfield, MA.

Study Options Full-time and part-time.

Program Entrance Requirements Minimum overall college GPA of 2.5, transcript of college record, interview, 2 letters of recommendation, minimum GPA in nursing prerequisites of 2.5. Transfer students are accepted. **Standardized tests** *Required:* SAT or ACT, TOEFL for international students. **Application** *Deadline:* rolling (freshmen). *Notification:* continuous (freshmen). *Application fee:* $40.

Advanced Placement Credit by examination available. Credit given for nursing courses completed elsewhere dependent upon specific evaluations.

Expenses (2003–04) *Tuition:* part-time $220 per credit hour.

Financial Aid 4% of baccalaureate students in nursing programs received some form of financial aid in 2002–03.

Contact Dr. Audrey Marie Silveri, Director, Department of Nursing, Anna Maria College, 50 Sunset Lane, Paxton, MA 01612-1198. *Telephone:* 508-829-3316 Ext. 316. *Fax:* 508-849-3343 Ext. 371. *E-mail:* asilveri@annamaria.edu.

CONTINUING EDUCATION PROGRAM

Contact Dr. Audrey Marie Silveri, Director of Nursing Program, Department of Nursing, Anna Maria College, 50 Sunset Lane, Paxton, MA 01612-1198. *Telephone:* 508-849-3316 Ext. 316. *Fax:* 508-849-3343 Ext. 371. *E-mail:* asilveri@annamaria.edu.

Atlantic Union College
Department of Nursing
South Lancaster, Massachusetts

http://www.atlanticuc.edu
Founded in 1882

DEGREE • BSN

Nursing Program Faculty 11.

Baccalaureate Enrollment 31
Women 90% **Men** 10% **Minority** 71% **Part-time** 71%

Nursing Student Activities Sigma Theta Tau.

Nursing Student Resources Academic advising; academic or career counseling; bookstore; campus computer network; career placement assistance; computer lab; computer-assisted instruction; e-mail services; employment services for current students; housing assistance; interactive nursing skills videos; Internet; learning resource lab; library services; nursing audiovisuals; placement services for program completers; remedial services; resume preparation assistance; skills, simulation, or other laboratory; tutoring.

Library Facilities 135,694 volumes (1,478 in health, 892 in nursing); 533 periodical subscriptions (76 health-care related).

BACCALAUREATE PROGRAMS

Degree BSN

Available Programs ADN to Baccalaureate; RN Baccalaureate.

Study Options Full-time and part-time.

Program Entrance Requirements Minimum overall college GPA of 2.5, transcript of college record, CPR certification, written essay, health exam, health insurance, high school biology, high school chemistry, high school foreign language, 3 years high school math, 2 years high school science, high school transcript, immunizations, interview, 2 letters of recommendation, minimum high school GPA of 2.5, minimum GPA in nursing prerequisites of 2.5, professional liability insurance/malpractice insurance, RN licensure. Transfer students are accepted. **Standardized tests** *Required:* TOEFL for international students. ***Placement:*** *Required:* SAT or ACT. *Recommended:* SAT. **Application** *Deadline:* 8/1 (freshmen), 8/1 (transfer). *Application fee:* $25.

Advanced Placement Credit by examination available. Credit given for nursing courses completed elsewhere dependent upon specific evaluations.

Expenses (2004–05) *Tuition:* full-time $12,000; part-time $250 per credit hour. *International tuition:* $12,000 full-time. *Room and board:* $3360; room only: $2100 per academic year.

Financial Aid 10% of baccalaureate students in nursing programs received some form of financial aid in 2003–04.

Contact Ms. Marguerite Rittenhouse, MSC, BS Coordinator, Department of Nursing, Atlantic Union College, 338 Main Street, PO Box 1000, South Lancaster, MA 01561. *Telephone:* 978-368-2402. *Fax:* 978-368-2518. *E-mail:* mrittenhouse@atlanticuc.edu.

CONTINUING EDUCATION PROGRAM

Contact Ms. Marguerite Rittenhouse, MSC, BS Coordinator, Department of Nursing, Atlantic Union College, 338 Main Street, PO Box 1000, South Lancaster, MA 01561. *Telephone:* 978-368-2402. *Fax:* 978-368-2518. *E-mail:* mrittenhouse@atlanticuc.edu.

Boston College

William F. Connell School of Nursing
Chestnut Hill, Massachusetts

http://www.bc.edu/nursing

Founded in 1863

DEGREES • BS • MS • MSN/MA • MSN/MBA • PHD

Nursing Program Faculty 73 (57% with doctorates).

Baccalaureate Enrollment 329
Women 95% **Men** 5% **Minority** 15%

Graduate Enrollment 231
Women 95% **Men** 5% **Minority** 4% **International** 3% **Part-time** 40%

Nursing Student Activities Nursing Honor Society, Sigma Theta Tau, Student Nurses' Association.

Nursing Student Resources Academic advising; academic or career counseling; assistance for students with disabilities; bookstore; campus computer network; career placement assistance; computer lab; computer-assisted instruction; e-mail services; employment services for current students; externships; housing assistance; interactive nursing skills videos; Internet; learning resource lab; library services; nursing audiovisuals; other; paid internships; placement services for program completers; remedial services; resume preparation assistance; skills, simulation, or other laboratory; tutoring; unpaid internships.

Library Facilities 2.2 million volumes (57,000 in health, 8,600 in nursing); 22,266 periodical subscriptions (700 health-care related).

BACCALAUREATE PROGRAMS

Degree BS

Available Programs Generic Baccalaureate.

Study Options Full-time.

Program Entrance Requirements Transcript of college record, written essay, health exam, high school biology, high school chemistry, high school foreign language, 4 years high school math, 3 years high school science, high school transcript, immunizations, 2 letters of recommendation. Transfer students are accepted. **Standardized tests** *Required:* SAT and SAT Subject Tests or ACT, SAT II Writing Tests, TOEFL for international students. **Application** *Deadline:* 1/2 (freshmen), 4/1 (transfer). *Early decision:* 11/1. *Notification:* 4/15 (freshmen), 12/24 (early action). *Application fee:* $60.

Advanced Placement Credit given for nursing courses completed elsewhere dependent upon specific evaluations.

Expenses (2004–05) *Tuition:* full-time $14,940. *International tuition:* $14,940 full-time. *Room and board:* $10,650; room only: $8000 per academic year. *Required fees:* full-time $400.

Financial Aid 83% of baccalaureate students in nursing programs received some form of financial aid in 2003–04.

Contact Ms. Maureen Eldredge, Administrative Coordinator, William F. Connell School of Nursing, Boston College, 140 Commonwealth Avenue, Chestnut Hill, MA 02467-3812. *Telephone:* 617-552-4925. *Fax:* 617-552-0745. *E-mail:* eldredgm@bc.edu.

GRADUATE PROGRAMS

Expenses (2004–05) *Tuition:* full-time $10,032; part-time $836 per credit hour. *International tuition:* $10,032 full-time. *Required fees:* full-time $110.

Financial Aid 80% of graduate students in nursing programs received some form of financial aid in 2003–04. 16 fellowships with full tuition reimbursements available (averaging $9,000 per year), 6 research assistantships, 4 teaching assistantships (averaging $10,500 per year) were awarded; Federal Work-Study, institutionally sponsored loans, scholarships, traineeships, and tuition waivers (partial) also available. Aid available to part-time students. *Financial aid application deadline:* 3/2.

Contact Ms. Kristin Parent, Graduate Programs Assistant, William F. Connell School of Nursing, Boston College, 140 Commonwealth Avenue, Chestnut Hill, MA 02467-3812. *Telephone:* 617-552-4059. *Fax:* 617-552-0745. *E-mail:* parentkr@bc.edu.

MASTER'S DEGREE PROGRAM

Degrees MS; MSN/MA; MSN/MBA

Available Programs Accelerated Master's for Non-Nursing College Graduates; Master's; RN to Master's.

Concentrations Available Nurse anesthesia. *Clinical nurse specialist programs in:* adult health, community health, gerontology, psychiatric/mental health. *Nurse practitioner programs in:* adult health, family health, gerontology, pediatric, women's health.

Study Options Full-time and part-time.

Program Entrance Requirements Minimum overall college GPA of 3.0, transcript of college record, written essay, immunizations, 3 letters of recommendation, statistics course, GRE General Test. *Application deadline:* For fall admission, 10/15; for spring admission, 3/15. *Application fee:* $40.

Advanced Placement Credit given for nursing courses completed elsewhere dependent upon specific evaluations.

Degree Requirements 45 total credit hours, comprehensive exam.

POST-MASTER'S PROGRAM

Areas of Study Nursing education. *Clinical nurse specialist programs in:* adult health, community health, gerontology, psychiatric/mental health. *Nurse practitioner programs in:* adult health, family health, gerontology, pediatric, women's health.

Boston College (continued)

DOCTORAL DEGREE PROGRAM

Degree PhD

Available Programs Doctorate.

Areas of Study Ethics, human health and illness, illness and transition, individualized study, nursing research, nursing science.

Program Entrance Requirements Minimum overall college GPA of 3.0, interview by faculty committee, interview, 3 letters of recommendation, MSN or equivalent, scholarly papers, statistics course, vita, writing sample, GRE General Test. *Application deadline:* For fall admission, 10/15; for spring admission, 3/15. *Application fee:* $40.

Degree Requirements 46 total credit hours, dissertation, oral exam, written exam.

CONTINUING EDUCATION PROGRAM

Contact Dr. Jean Weyman, Director of Continuing Education, William F. Connell School of Nursing, Boston College, 140 Commonwealth Avenue, Service Building 209, Chestnut Hill, MA 02467-3812. *Telephone:* 617-552-4256. *Fax:* 617-552-0745. *E-mail:* jean.weyman@bc.edu.

See full description on page 462.

Curry College

Division of Nursing
Milton, Massachusetts

http://www.curry.edu

Founded in 1879

DEGREE • BS

Nursing Program Faculty 37 (35% with doctorates).

Baccalaureate Enrollment 515
Women 95% **Men** 5% **Minority** 18% **Part-time** 55%

Nursing Student Activities Sigma Theta Tau, Student Nurses' Association.

Nursing Student Resources Academic advising; academic or career counseling; assistance for students with disabilities; bookstore; campus computer network; career placement assistance; computer lab; computer-assisted instruction; daycare for children of students; e-mail services; employment services for current students; housing assistance; interactive nursing skills videos; Internet; learning resource lab; library services; nursing audiovisuals; placement services for program completers; resume preparation assistance; skills, simulation, or other laboratory; tutoring.

Library Facilities 90,000 volumes (5,435 in health, 4,197 in nursing); 675 periodical subscriptions (142 health-care related).

■ Clinical experience begins in the sophomore year at Curry College. Boston and metropolitan hospitals and community agencies provide Curry students with a wide range of clinical experiences and the latest in professional nursing practice to enhance potential for employment. Boston clinical practice sites include Massachusetts General Hospital, Beth Israel/Deaconess Medical Center, Boston Medical Center, Brigham and Women's Hospital, and Children's Hospital Medical Center. The hallmark of a Curry education is personalized attention and respect for the individuality of every student. The College's commitment to the liberal arts and developmental learning, in combination with an intense professional clinical program, give Curry nursing students the advantage in synthesizing knowledge and applying current therapeutic techniques.

BACCALAUREATE PROGRAMS

Degree BS

Available Programs Accelerated Baccalaureate for Second Degree; Generic Baccalaureate; RN Baccalaureate.

Site Options Boston, MA; Plymouth, MA.

Study Options Full-time and part-time.

Program Entrance Requirements Minimum overall college GPA of 2.0, written essay, health exam, health insurance, high school biology, high school chemistry, 3 years high school math, 2 years high school science, high school transcript, immunizations, minimum high school GPA of 2.0. Transfer students are accepted. **Standardized tests** *Required:* TOEFL for international students. *Required for some:* SAT or ACT, Wechsler Adult Intelligence Scale-Revised for PAL candidates. **Application** *Deadline:* 4/1 (freshmen), 7/1 (transfer). *Early decision:* 12/1. *Notification:* continuous (freshmen), 12/15 (out-of-state freshmen), 12/15 (early decision). *Application fee:* $40.

Advanced Placement Credit by examination available. Credit given for nursing courses completed elsewhere dependent upon specific evaluations.

Expenses (2004–05) *Tuition:* full-time $20,860; part-time $288 per credit hour. *International tuition:* $20,860 full-time. *Room and board:* $9820; room only: $5880 per academic year. *Required fees:* full-time $935; part-time $265 per term.

Financial Aid 60% of baccalaureate students in nursing programs received some form of financial aid in 2003–04. *Gift aid (need-based):* Federal Pell, FSEOG, state, private, college/university gift aid from institutional funds. *Loans:* FFEL (Subsidized and Unsubsidized Stafford PLUS), Perkins, state. *Work-Study:* Federal Work-Study, part-time campus jobs. *Application deadline (priority):* 3/1.

Contact Miss Jane Fidler, Director of Admissions, Division of Nursing, Curry College, 1071 Blue Hill Avenue, Milton, MA 02186. *Telephone:* 800-669-0686. *Fax:* 617-333-2114. *E-mail:* jfidler0803@curry.edu.

CONTINUING EDUCATION PROGRAM

Contact Dr. Judith Stoessel, Dean for Graduate and Professional Studies, Division of Nursing, Curry College, 1071 Blue Hill Avenue, Milton, MA 02186. *Telephone:* 617-333-9674. *Fax:* 617-333-6860. *E-mail:* jstoesse0703@curry.edu.

Elms College

Division of Nursing
Chicopee, Massachusetts

Founded in 1928

DEGREE • BS

Nursing Program Faculty 13 (15% with doctorates).

Baccalaureate Enrollment 109
Women 93% **Men** 7% **Minority** 11% **Part-time** 24%

Nursing Student Activities Sigma Theta Tau, Student Nurses' Association.

Nursing Student Resources Academic advising; academic or career counseling; assistance for students with disabilities; bookstore; campus computer network; career placement assistance; computer lab; computer-assisted instruction; e-mail services; employment services for current students; externships; interactive nursing skills videos; Internet; learning resource lab; library services; nursing audiovisuals; paid internships; remedial services; resume preparation assistance; skills, simulation, or other laboratory; tutoring.

Library Facilities 111,379 volumes (3,832 in health, 3,000 in nursing); 529 periodical subscriptions (130 health-care related).

BACCALAUREATE PROGRAMS

Degree BS

Available Programs Generic Baccalaureate; RN Baccalaureate.

Study Options Full-time and part-time.

Program Entrance Requirements Minimum overall college GPA of 2.5, transcript of college record, CPR certification, written essay, health exam, health insurance, high school biology, high school chemistry, high school transcript, immunizations, interview, 2 letters of recommendation, minimum high school GPA of 3.3, minimum GPA in nursing prerequisites of 2.5, professional liability insurance/malpractice insurance. Transfer students are accepted. **Standardized tests** *Required:* SAT or ACT, TOEFL for international students. *Recommended:* SAT Subject Tests. **Application** *Deadline:* rolling (freshmen), rolling (transfer). *Notification:* continuous (freshmen). *Application fee:* $30.

Advanced Placement Credit given for nursing courses completed elsewhere dependent upon specific evaluations.

Expenses (2003–04) *Tuition:* full-time $8000. *Room and board:* $7100 per academic year.

Financial Aid 90% of baccalaureate students in nursing programs received some form of financial aid in 2002–03. *Gift aid (need-based):* Federal Pell, FSEOG, state, private, college/university gift aid from institutional funds. *Loans:* FFEL (Subsidized and Unsubsidized Stafford PLUS), Perkins, state, alternative loans, MEFA Loans, Key Alternative Loans, CitiAssist Loans, Signature Loans. *Work-Study:* Federal Work-Study. *Application deadline (priority):* 3/1.

Contact Dr. Kathleen B. Scoble, RN, Director of Nursing Department and Chair of Health Sciences Division, Division of Nursing, Elms College, The Elms College, 291 Springfield Street, Chicopee, MA 01013. *Telephone:* 413-265-2204. *Fax:* 413-594-2761. *E-mail:* scoblek@elms.edu.

CONTINUING EDUCATION PROGRAM

Contact Dr. Carla Oleska, Associate Academic Dean, Division of Nursing, Elms College, The Elms College, 291 Springfield Street, Chicopee, MA 01013. *Telephone:* 413-594-2761 Ext. 276. *Fax:* 413-592-4871. *E-mail:* oleskac@elms.edu.

Emmanuel College

Department of Nursing
Boston, Massachusetts

http://www.emmanuel.edu/gradprof

Founded in 1919

DEGREE • BSN

Nursing Program Faculty 11 (37% with doctorates).

Baccalaureate Enrollment 169
Women 96% **Men** 4% **Minority** 16% **Part-time** 98%

Nursing Student Activities Sigma Theta Tau.

Nursing Student Resources Academic advising; academic or career counseling; assistance for students with disabilities; bookstore; campus computer network; computer lab; computer-assisted instruction; e-mail services; interactive nursing skills videos; Internet; learning resource lab; library services; nursing audiovisuals; skills, simulation, or other laboratory.

Library Facilities 97,627 volumes (3,050 in health, 1,220 in nursing); 394 periodical subscriptions (92 health-care related).

■ The Emmanuel College NLNAC-accredited Nursing Program is designed specifically for the registered nurse. The faculty members believe that baccalaureate education builds on the prior educational and practice experiences of the registered nurse. The Nursing Program prepares a professional who thinks critically, communicates effectively, appreciates the diversity of human experience, and uses personal and professional values and standards in responsible ethical practice. Liberal transfer-credit policies, a strong advisement program, and outstanding individualized clinical placements ensure that the Nursing Program works for practicing nurses. Evening, weekend, and Saturday courses on 2 campus locations underpin the commitment to adult learners. Graduates report career and educational advancement.

BACCALAUREATE PROGRAMS

Degree BSN

Available Programs RN Baccalaureate.

Site Options Woburn, MA.

Study Options Full-time and part-time.

Program Entrance Requirements Transcript of college record, written essay, interview, 2 letters of recommendation, RN licensure. Transfer students are accepted. **Standardized tests** *Required:* SAT or ACT, TOEFL for international students. **Application** *Deadline:* rolling (freshmen), rolling (transfer). *Early decision:* 11/1. *Notification:* continuous (freshmen), 12/1 (out-of-state freshmen), 12/1 (early decision). *Application fee:* $40.

Advanced Placement Credit given for nursing courses completed elsewhere dependent upon specific evaluations.

Expenses (2004–05) *Tuition:* part-time $1192 per course.

Contact Dr. Joan M. Riley, Chair and Professor, Department of Nursing, Emmanuel College, 400 The Fenway, Boston, MA 02115. *Telephone:* 617-735-9935. *Fax:* 617-735-9797. *E-mail:* riley@emmanuel.edu.

Endicott College

Major in Nursing
Beverly, Massachusetts

http://www.endicott.edu

Founded in 1939

DEGREE • BS

Nursing Program Faculty 4.

Baccalaureate Enrollment 75
Women 95% **Men** 5% **Minority** 2%

Nursing Student Activities Student Nurses' Association.

Nursing Student Resources Academic advising; academic or career counseling; assistance for students with disabilities; bookstore; campus computer network; career placement assistance; computer lab; e-mail services; externships; interactive nursing skills videos; Internet; learning resource lab; library services; nursing audiovisuals; resume preparation assistance; skills, simulation, or other laboratory; tutoring; unpaid internships.

Library Facilities 121,000 volumes (2,828 in health, 624 in nursing); 3,500 periodical subscriptions (55 health-care related).

BACCALAUREATE PROGRAMS

Degree BS

Available Programs Generic Baccalaureate; RN Baccalaureate.

Site Options Beverly, MA.

Study Options Full-time.

Program Entrance Requirements Minimum overall college GPA of 2.5, transcript of college record, written essay, health exam, health insurance, high school biology, high school chemistry, 3 years high school math, 2 years high school science, high school transcript, immunizations, interview, 1 letter of recommendation, minimum high school GPA of 2.5, minimum high school rank 50%, minimum GPA in nursing prerequisites of 2.5. Transfer students are accepted. **Standardized tests** *Required:* SAT or ACT, TOEFL for international students. **Application** *Deadline:* 2/15 (freshmen), 2/15 (transfer). *Notification:* continuous (freshmen). *Application fee:* $40.

Advanced Placement Credit given for nursing courses completed elsewhere dependent upon specific evaluations.

Expenses (2003–04) *Tuition:* full-time $16,744. *Room and board:* $8858; room only: $6210 per academic year. *Required fees:* full-time $1014.

Financial Aid 88% of baccalaureate students in nursing programs received some form of financial aid in 2002–03. *Gift aid (need-based):* Federal Pell, FSEOG, state, private, college/university gift aid from institutional funds. *Loans:* FFEL (Subsidized and Unsubsidized Stafford PLUS), Perkins, state, college/university. *Work-Study:* Federal Work-Study. *Application deadline (priority):* 3/15.

Contact Mr. Thomas J. Redman, Vice President for Admissions and Financial Aid, Major in Nursing, Endicott College, 376 Hale Street, Beverly, MA 01915. *Telephone:* 978-921-1000. *Fax:* 978-232-2500. *E-mail:* admissio@endicott.edu.

CONTINUING EDUCATION PROGRAM

Contact Dr. Patricia A. Ottani, Dean School of Nursing and Health Sciences, Major in Nursing, Endicott College, 376 Hale Street, Beverly, MA 01915. *Telephone:* 978-232-2328. *Fax:* 978-232-3100. *E-mail:* pottani@endicott.edu.

Fitchburg State College

Department of Nursing
Fitchburg, Massachusetts

http://www.fsc.edu/nursing/

Founded in 1894

DEGREES • BSN • M SC

Nursing Program Faculty 25 (32% with doctorates).

Baccalaureate Enrollment 266
Women 93% **Men** 7% **Minority** 10% **Part-time** 2%

Graduate Enrollment 20
Women 100% **Part-time** 100%

Nursing Student Activities Sigma Theta Tau, Student Nurses' Association.

Nursing Student Resources Academic advising; academic or career counseling; assistance for students with disabilities; bookstore; campus computer network; computer lab; computer-assisted instruction; e-mail services; employment services for current students; housing assistance; interactive nursing skills videos; Internet; learning resource lab; library services; nursing audiovisuals; remedial services; skills, simulation, or other laboratory; tutoring.

Library Facilities 238,743 volumes (111 in health, 74 in nursing); 2,039 periodical subscriptions (1,218 health-care related).

BACCALAUREATE PROGRAMS

Degree BSN

Available Programs ADN to Baccalaureate; RN Baccalaureate.

Study Options Full-time.

Program Entrance Requirements Minimum overall college GPA of 2.5, transcript of college record, CPR certification, written essay, health exam, health insurance, high school chemistry, high school foreign language, high school transcript, immunizations, minimum high school GPA of 3.0, minimum GPA in nursing prerequisites of 2.5, prerequisite course work. Transfer students are accepted. **Standardized tests** *Required:* SAT or ACT, TOEFL for international students. **Application** *Notification:* continuous (freshmen). *Application fee:* $10.

Expenses (2004–05) *Tuition, area resident:* full-time $970; part-time $40 per credit hour. *Tuition, state resident:* full-time $1455; part-time $61 per credit hour. *Tuition, nonresident:* full-time $7050; part-time $294 per credit hour. *Room and board:* $3255; room only: $2165 per academic year. *Required fees:* full-time $3618; part-time $151 per credit; part-time $1809 per term.

Financial Aid 27% of baccalaureate students in nursing programs received some form of financial aid in 2003–04. *Gift aid (need-based):* Federal Pell, FSEOG, state, private, college/university gift aid from institutional funds. *Loans:* Federal Nursing Student Loans, Federal Direct (Subsidized and Unsubsidized Stafford PLUS), Perkins, state. *Work-Study:* Federal Work-Study. *Application deadline (priority):* 3/1.

Contact Office of Admissions, Department of Nursing, Fitchburg State College, 160 Pearl Street, Fitchburg, MA 01420-2697. *Telephone:* 978-665-3144. *Fax:* 978-665-4540. *E-mail:* admissions@fsc.edu.

GRADUATE PROGRAMS

Expenses (2004–05) *Tuition, state resident:* part-time $150 per credit hour. *Tuition, nonresident:* part-time $150 per credit hour. *Required fees:* part-time $65 per credit.

Contact Ms. Rachel Boersma, Chairperson, Department of Nursing, Fitchburg State College, 160 Pearl Street, Fitchburg, MA 01420-2697. *Telephone:* 978-665-3036. *Fax:* 978-665-3658. *E-mail:* rboersma@fsc.edu.

MASTER'S DEGREE PROGRAM

Degree M Sc

Available Programs Master's.

Concentrations Available *Clinical nurse specialist programs in:* forensic nursing.

Study Options Part-time.

Program Entrance Requirements Clinical experience, computer literacy, minimum overall college GPA of 2.8, transcript of college record, CPR certification, written essay, immunizations, 3 letters of recommendation, nursing research course, physical assessment course, prerequisite course work, resume, statistics course.

Degree Requirements 37 total credit hours, thesis or project.

Framingham State College

Department of Nursing
Framingham, Massachusetts

http://www.framingham.edu/nursing

Founded in 1839

DEGREE • BS

Nursing Program Faculty 4 (80% with doctorates).

Baccalaureate Enrollment 53
Women 94% **Men** 6% **Minority** 15% **International** 10% **Part-time** 90%

Graduate Enrollment 7
Women 100%

Nursing Student Activities Sigma Theta Tau.

Nursing Student Resources Academic advising; academic or career counseling; assistance for students with disabilities; bookstore; campus computer network; career placement assistance; computer lab; computer-assisted instruction; e-mail services; employment services for current students; housing assistance; Internet; learning resource lab; library services; nursing audiovisuals; placement services for program completers; remedial services; resume preparation assistance; skills, simulation, or other laboratory; tutoring.

Library Facilities 165,219 volumes; 409 periodical subscriptions.

BACCALAUREATE PROGRAMS

Degree BS

Available Programs ADN to Baccalaureate, Postbaccalaureate Certificate.

Study Options Full-time and part-time.

Program Entrance Requirements Transfer students are accepted. **Standardized tests** *Required:* SAT or ACT, TOEFL for international students. **Application** *Deadline:* 2/15 (freshmen), 2/15 (transfer). *Early decision:* 11/15. *Notification:* 3/31 (freshmen), 12/15 (early action). *Application fee:* $25.

Advanced Placement Credit by examination available. Credit given for nursing courses completed elsewhere dependent upon specific evaluations.

Expenses (2004–05) *Tuition, area resident:* full-time $485; part-time $162 per course. *Tuition, state resident:* full-time $485; part-time $1175 per course. *Tuition, nonresident:* full-time $3525; part-time $1175 per course. *International tuition:* $3525 full-time. *Room and board:* $2763; room only: $1783 per academic year. *Required fees:* full-time $1926; part-time $170 per credit; part-time $1842 per term.

Financial Aid 75% of baccalaureate students in nursing programs received some form of financial aid in 2003–04.

Contact Dr. Susan L. Conrad, RN, Chairperson and Professor, Department of Nursing, Framingham State College, 100 State Street H220, Framingham, MA 01701. *Telephone:* 508-626-4715. *Fax:* 508-626-4746. *E-mail:* sconrad@frc.mass.edu.

GRADUATE PROGRAMS

Expenses (2004–05) *Tuition, state resident:* part-time $710 per course. *Tuition, nonresident:* part-time $710 per course.

Contact Dr. Susan L. Conrad, RN, Chairperson and Professor, Department of Nursing, Framingham State College, 100 State Street H220, Framingham, MA 01701. *Telephone:* 508-626-4713. *Fax:* 508-626-4746. *E-mail:* sconrad@frc.mass.edu.

POST-MASTER'S PROGRAM

Areas of Study Nursing education.

MGH Institute of Health Professions

Program in Nursing
Boston, Massachusetts

http://www.mghihp.edu

Founded in 1977

DEGREE • MS

Nursing Program Faculty 36 (64% with doctorates).

Graduate Enrollment 221
Women 91% **Men** 9% **Minority** 12% **Part-time** 11%

Nursing Student Activities Student Nurses' Association.

Nursing Student Resources Academic advising; academic or career counseling; assistance for students with disabilities; bookstore; career placement assistance; computer lab; e-mail services; Internet; learning resource lab; library services; nursing audiovisuals; resume preparation assistance; skills, simulation, or other laboratory; tutoring.

GRADUATE PROGRAMS

Expenses (2004–05) *Tuition:* full-time $24,038; part-time $707 per credit hour. *International tuition:* $24,038 full-time. *Required fees:* full-time $800; part-time $200 per term.

Financial Aid 80% of graduate students in nursing programs received some form of financial aid in 2003–04. 1 research assistantship (averaging $1,200 per year), 2 teaching assistantships (averaging $1,200 per year) were awarded; career-related internships or fieldwork, scholarships, traineeships, tuition waivers (full and partial), and unspecified assistantships also available. Aid available to part-time students. *Financial aid application deadline:* 3/10.

Contact Office of Student Affairs, Program in Nursing, MGH Institute of Health Professions, PO Box 6357, Boston, MA 02114. *Telephone:* 617-726-3140. *Fax:* 617-726-8010. *E-mail:* admissions@mghihp.edu.

MASTER'S DEGREE PROGRAM

Degree MS

Available Programs Master's; Master's for Non-Nursing College Graduates; Master's for Nurses with Non-Nursing Degrees; RN to Master's.

Concentrations Available *Clinical nurse specialist programs in:* psychiatric/mental health. *Nurse practitioner programs in:* acute care, adult health, family health, gerontology, pediatric, primary care, psychiatric/mental health, women's health.

Site Options *Distance Learning:* Boston, MA.

Study Options Full-time and part-time.

Program Entrance Requirements Minimum overall college GPA of 3.0, transcript of college record, CPR certification, written essay, immunizations, 3 letters of recommendation, professional liability insurance/malpractice insurance, prerequisite course work, statistics course, GRE General Test. *Application deadline:* For fall admission, 8/2; for spring admission, 12/7. *Application fee:* $50.

Advanced Placement Credit by examination available. Credit given for nursing courses completed elsewhere dependent upon specific evaluations.

Degree Requirements Thesis or project.

POST-MASTER'S PROGRAM

Areas of Study *Clinical nurse specialist programs in:* psychiatric/mental health. *Nurse practitioner programs in:* acute care, adult health, gerontology, pediatric, primary care, psychiatric/mental health, women's health.

CONTINUING EDUCATION PROGRAM

Contact Nursing Program Office, Program in Nursing, MGH Institute of Health Professions, Charlestown Navy Yard, 36 1st Avenue, Boston, MA 02129. *Telephone:* 617-726-8053. *Fax:* 617-726-3152. *E-mail:* jblue@mghihp.edu.

See full description on page 520.

Northeastern University

School of Nursing
Boston, Massachusetts

http://www.bouve.neu.edu/Nursing

Founded in 1898

DEGREES • BSN • MS • MSN/MBA

Nursing Program Faculty 35 (65% with doctorates).

Baccalaureate Enrollment 586
Women 92% **Men** 8% **Minority** 31% **International** 1%

Graduate Enrollment 183
Women 90% **Men** 10% **Minority** 10% **Part-time** 38%

Nursing Student Activities Sigma Theta Tau, Student Nurses' Association.

Nursing Student Resources Academic advising; academic or career counseling; assistance for students with disabilities; bookstore; campus computer network; career placement assistance; computer lab; computer-assisted instruction; e-mail services; employment services for current students; externships; housing assistance; interactive nursing skills videos; Internet; learning resource lab; library services; nursing audiovisuals; other; paid internships; placement services for program completers; resume preparation assistance; skills, simulation, or other laboratory; tutoring.

Library Facilities 965,833 volumes (39,650 in health, 34,250 in nursing); 7,636 periodical subscriptions (1,200 health-care related).

BACCALAUREATE PROGRAMS

Degree BSN

Available Programs Generic Baccalaureate; RN Baccalaureate.

Study Options Full-time.

Program Entrance Requirements Transcript of college record, written essay, health exam, high school biology, high school chemistry, high school math, 2 years high school science, high school transcript, immunizations, 2 letters of recommendation, prerequisite course work. Transfer students are accepted. **Standardized tests** *Required:* SAT or ACT, TOEFL for international students. **Application** *Deadline:* 2/1 (freshmen), 5/1 (transfer). *Notification:* continuous until 4/1 (freshmen). *Application fee:* $50.

Advanced Placement Credit given for nursing courses completed elsewhere dependent upon specific evaluations.

Expenses (2004–05) *Tuition:* full-time $26,750. *Room and board:* $10,180; room only: $5440 per academic year. *Required fees:* full-time $330.

Financial Aid 50% of baccalaureate students in nursing programs received some form of financial aid in 2003–04. *Gift aid (need-based):* Federal Pell, FSEOG, state, private, college/university gift aid from institutional funds, Federal Nursing, Scholarships for Disadvantaged Students (SDS). *Loans:* Federal Nursing Student Loans, FFEL (Subsidized and Unsubsidized Stafford PLUS), Perkins, state, TERI Loans, Massachusetts No-Interest Loans (NIL), MEFA Loans, CitiAssist Loans. *Work-Study:* Federal Work-Study. *Application deadline (priority):* 2/15.

Contact Undergraduate Admissions, School of Nursing, Northeastern University, 150 Richards Hall, 360 Huntington Avenue, Boston, MA 02115. *Telephone:* 617-373-2200. *Fax:* 617-373-8780. *E-mail:* undergrad-admissions@neu.edu.

GRADUATE PROGRAMS

Expenses (2004–05) *Tuition:* part-time $825 per credit hour. *Room and board:* $4850 per academic year. *Required fees:* full-time $1688.

Financial Aid 65% of graduate students in nursing programs received some form of financial aid in 2003–04. 10 research assistantships with full tuition reimbursements available (averaging $13,866 per year), 7 teaching assistantships with full tuition reimbursements available (averaging $13,866 per year) were awarded; fellowships, career-related internships or fieldwork, institutionally sponsored loans, tuition waivers (full and partial), and unspecified assistantships also available. Aid available to part-time students. *Financial aid application deadline:* 7/1.

Contact Ms. Molly Schnabel, Director of Graduate Admissions and Student Services, School of Nursing, Northeastern University, 123 Behrakis Health Sciences Building, 360 Huntington Avenue, Boston, MA 02115. *Telephone:* 617-373-3501. *Fax:* 617-373-4701. *E-mail:* bouvegrad@neu.edu.

MASTER'S DEGREE PROGRAM

Degrees MS; MSN/MBA

Available Programs Accelerated RN to Master's; Master's; Master's for Non-Nursing College Graduates; RN to Master's.

Concentrations Available Nurse anesthesia; nursing administration. *Clinical nurse specialist programs in:* psychiatric/mental health. *Nurse practitioner programs in:* acute care, adult health, family health, gerontology, neonatal health, pediatric, primary care, psychiatric/mental health.

Study Options Full-time and part-time.

Northeastern University (continued)

Program Entrance Requirements Clinical experience, minimum overall college GPA of 3.0, transcript of college record, written essay, immunizations, 3 letters of recommendation, professional liability insurance/malpractice insurance, resume, statistics course, GRE General Test. *Application deadline:* Applications are processed on a rolling basis. *Application fee:* $50.

Advanced Placement Credit given for nursing courses completed elsewhere dependent upon specific evaluations.

Degree Requirements 43 total credit hours.

POST-MASTER'S PROGRAM

Areas of Study Nurse anesthesia; nursing administration. *Clinical nurse specialist programs in:* psychiatric/mental health. *Nurse practitioner programs in:* acute care, adult health, family health, gerontology, neonatal health, pediatric, primary care, psychiatric/mental health.

CONTINUING EDUCATION PROGRAM

Contact Ms. Lea Johnson, Director, Bouve Institute for Healthcare, School of Nursing, Northeastern University, 275 Ryder Hall, Boston, MA 02115. *Telephone:* 617-373-4237. *Fax:* 617-373-2325. *E-mail:* l.johnson@neu.edu.

See full description on page 530.

Regis College
Department of Nursing
Weston, Massachusetts

http://regisnet.regiscollege.edu/nursing/pro_ovrview.htm

Founded in 1927

DEGREES • BSN • MSN

Nursing Program Faculty 36 (75% with doctorates).

Baccalaureate Enrollment 69
Women 100%

Graduate Enrollment 292
Women 91% **Men** 9% **Minority** 14% **Part-time** 70%

Nursing Student Activities Sigma Theta Tau, Student Nurses' Association.

Nursing Student Resources Academic advising; academic or career counseling; assistance for students with disabilities; bookstore; campus computer network; computer lab; e-mail services; Internet; learning resource lab; library services; nursing audiovisuals; resume preparation assistance; skills, simulation, or other laboratory; tutoring.

Library Facilities 137,070 volumes (6,300 in health, 4,700 in nursing); 805 periodical subscriptions (228 health-care related).

BACCALAUREATE PROGRAMS

Degree BSN

Available Programs ADN to Baccalaureate; Accelerated Baccalaureate; Accelerated Baccalaureate for Second Degree; Accelerated RN Baccalaureate; Baccalaureate for Second Degree; Generic Baccalaureate; RN Baccalaureate.

Site Options Brighton, MA; Medford, MA; Boston, MA.

Study Options Full-time.

Program Entrance Requirements Written essay, health exam, health insurance, high school foreign language, 3 years high school math, 2 years high school science, high school transcript, immunizations, 2 letters of recommendation, minimum high school GPA of 3.0, minimum high school rank 40%, minimum GPA in nursing prerequisites. Transfer students are accepted. **Standardized tests** *Required:* SAT or ACT, TOEFL for international students. **Application** *Deadline:* rolling (freshmen), rolling (transfer). *Application fee:* $30.

Advanced Placement Credit by examination available. Credit given for nursing courses completed elsewhere dependent upon specific evaluations.

Expenses (2004–05) *Tuition:* full-time $22,500; part-time $395 per credit hour. *International tuition:* $22,500 full-time. *Room and board:* $9630 per academic year.

Financial Aid 85% of baccalaureate students in nursing programs received some form of financial aid in 2003–04. *Gift aid (need-based):* Federal Pell, FSEOG, state, private, college/university gift aid from institutional funds. *Loans:* FFEL (Subsidized and Unsubsidized Stafford PLUS), Perkins, state. *Work-Study:* Federal Work-Study, part-time campus jobs. *Application deadline (priority):* 2/15.

Contact Dr. Toni Hays, Center Director, Department of Nursing, Regis College, 235 Wellesley Street, Weston, MA 02493. *Telephone:* 781-768-7090. *Fax:* 781-768-7071. *E-mail:* antoinette.hays@regiscollege.edu.

GRADUATE PROGRAMS

Expenses (2004–05) *Tuition:* full-time $22,500; part-time $515 per credit hour. *International tuition:* $22,500 full-time.

Financial Aid 52% of graduate students in nursing programs received some form of financial aid in 2003–04. 7 research assistantships (averaging $4,762 per year) were awarded; Federal Work-Study, scholarships, traineeships, and unspecified assistantships also available. Aid available to part-time students.

Contact Ms. Claudia Christine Pouravelis, Graduate Admissions Counselor, Department of Nursing, Regis College, 235 Wellesley Street, Weston, MA 02493. *Telephone:* 781-768-7058. *Fax:* 781-768-7071. *E-mail:* claudia.pouravelis@regiscollege.edu.

MASTER'S DEGREE PROGRAM

Degree MSN

Available Programs Accelerated Master's for Non-Nursing College Graduates; Master's; Master's for Non-Nursing College Graduates; RN to Master's.

Concentrations Available Health-care administration; nursing administration. *Nurse practitioner programs in:* adult health, family health, pediatric, primary care, psychiatric/mental health.

Site Options Brighton, MA; Medford, MA; Boston, MA.

Study Options Full-time.

Program Entrance Requirements Computer literacy, minimum overall college GPA of 3.0, transcript of college record, CPR certification, written essay, immunizations, interview, 3 letters of recommendation, physical assessment course, professional liability insurance/malpractice insurance, prerequisite course work, resume, statistics course, GRE General Test or MAT. *Application deadline:* Applications are processed on a rolling basis. *Application fee:* $30.

Advanced Placement Credit by examination available. Credit given for nursing courses completed elsewhere dependent upon specific evaluations.

Degree Requirements 44 total credit hours, thesis or project.

POST-MASTER'S PROGRAM

Areas of Study Health-care administration; nursing administration; nursing education. *Nurse practitioner programs in:* adult health, family health, pediatric, primary care, psychiatric/mental health.

CONTINUING EDUCATION PROGRAM

Contact Dr. Antoinette Hays, Center of Health Sciences, Nursing, Department of Nursing, Regis College, 235 Wellesley Street, Weston, MA 02493. *Telephone:* 781-768-7090. *Fax:* 781-768-7089. *E-mail:* antoinette.hays@regiscollege.edu.

See full description on page 534.

Salem State College
Nursing Department
Salem, Massachusetts

http://www.salemstate.edu

Founded in 1854

DEGREES • BSN • MSN • MSN/MBA

Nursing Program Faculty 41 (25% with doctorates).

Nursing Student Activities Nursing Honor Society, Sigma Theta Tau, Student Nurses' Association.

Nursing Student Resources Academic advising; academic or career counseling; assistance for students with disabilities; bookstore; campus computer network; career placement assistance; computer lab; computer-assisted instruction; daycare for children of students; e-mail services; employment services for current students; externships; housing assistance; interactive nursing skills videos; Internet; learning resource lab; library services; nursing audiovisuals; paid internships; remedial services; resume preparation assistance; skills, simulation, or other laboratory; tutoring.

Library Facilities 217,842 volumes (2,000 in health, 1,600 in nursing); 1,914 periodical subscriptions (50 health-care related).

BACCALAUREATE PROGRAMS

Degree BSN

Available Programs ADN to Baccalaureate; Baccalaureate for Second Degree; Generic Baccalaureate; International Nurse to Baccalaureate; LPN to Baccalaureate; LPN to RN Baccalaureate.

Site Options Lawrence, MA.

Study Options Full-time and part-time.

Program Entrance Requirements Minimum overall college GPA of 2.75, transcript of college record, CPR certification, health exam, health insurance, high school biology, high school chemistry, 3 years high school math, high school science, high school transcript, immunizations, interview, minimum high school GPA of 2.7, professional liability insurance/malpractice insurance. Transfer students are accepted. **Standardized tests** *Required:* SAT or ACT, TOEFL for international students. **Application** *Deadline:* rolling (freshmen), rolling (transfer). *Notification:* continuous (freshmen). *Application fee:* $25.

Advanced Placement Credit given for nursing courses completed elsewhere dependent upon specific evaluations.

Expenses (2004–05) *Tuition, state resident:* full-time $910; part-time $105 per credit hour. *Tuition, nonresident:* full-time $7050; part-time $140 per credit hour. *Room and board:* $14,400; room only: $5200 per academic year. *Required fees:* full-time $4400.

Financial Aid 60% of baccalaureate students in nursing programs received some form of financial aid in 2003–04.

Contact Mr. Nate Bryant, Director of Admissions, Nursing Department, Salem State College, 352 Lafayette Street, Salem, MA 01970. *Telephone:* 978-542-6200. *E-mail:* admissions@salemstate.edu.

GRADUATE PROGRAMS

Expenses (2004–05) *Tuition, state resident:* full-time $3400; part-time $140 per credit hour. *Tuition, nonresident:* full-time $5520; part-time $230 per credit hour. *Required fees:* full-time $2040.

Financial Aid 25% of graduate students in nursing programs received some form of financial aid in 2003–04.

Contact Dr. Kathleen Skrabut, Coordinator, Graduate Program, Nursing Department, Salem State College, 352 Lafayette Street, Salem, MA 01970. *Telephone:* 978-542-7018. *Fax:* 978-542-2016. *E-mail:* kathleen.skrabut@salemstate.edu.

MASTER'S DEGREE PROGRAM

Degrees MSN; MSN/MBA

Available Programs Accelerated Master's for Non-Nursing College Graduates; Master's; Master's for Nurses with Non-Nursing Degrees; RN to Master's.

Concentrations Available Nursing administration; nursing education. *Clinical nurse specialist programs in:* adult health, community health, rehabilitation.

Study Options Full-time and part-time.

Program Entrance Requirements Clinical experience, computer literacy, minimum overall college GPA of 3.0, transcript of college record, CPR certification, written essay, immunizations, interview, 3 letters of recommendation, resume, statistics course, GRE General Test, MAT. *Application deadline:* Applications are processed on a rolling basis. *Application fee:* $25.

Advanced Placement Credit given for nursing courses completed elsewhere dependent upon specific evaluations.

Degree Requirements 39 total credit hours, thesis or project.

CONTINUING EDUCATION PROGRAM

Contact Ms. Linda A. Frontiero, Coordinator of Post-Licensure Evening Nursing Programs, Nursing Department, Salem State College, 352 Lafayette Street, Salem, MA 01970. *Telephone:* 978-542-6849. *Fax:* 978-542-2016. *E-mail:* linda.frontiero@salemstate.edu.

Simmons College
Department of Nursing
Boston, Massachusetts

http://www.simmons.edu/gshs/nursing/

Founded in 1899

DEGREES • BS • MS • MSN/MS

Nursing Program Faculty 50 (15% with doctorates).

Baccalaureate Enrollment 180
Women 100% **Minority** 20% **International** 21% **Part-time** 35%

Graduate Enrollment 105
Women 93% **Men** 7% **Minority** 7% **International** 1% **Part-time** 60%

Nursing Student Activities Sigma Theta Tau, Student Nurses' Association, nursing club.

Nursing Student Resources Academic advising; academic or career counseling; assistance for students with disabilities; bookstore; campus computer network; career placement assistance; computer lab; computer-assisted instruction; e-mail services; employment services for current students; housing assistance; interactive nursing skills videos; Internet; learning resource lab; library services; nursing audiovisuals; paid internships; placement services for program completers; remedial services; resume preparation assistance; skills, simulation, or other laboratory; tutoring.

Library Facilities 253,145 volumes (5,005 in health, 1,562 in nursing); 1,749 periodical subscriptions (196 health-care related).

BACCALAUREATE PROGRAMS

Degree BS

Available Programs ADN to Baccalaureate; Accelerated Baccalaureate; Accelerated Baccalaureate for Second Degree; Baccalaureate for Second Degree; Generic Baccalaureate; LPN to Baccalaureate; RN Baccalaureate.

Study Options Full-time and part-time.

Program Entrance Requirements Transcript of college record, written essay, health exam, health insurance, high school biology, high school chemistry, high school foreign language, 3 years high school math, 3 years high school science, high school transcript, immunizations, 2 letters of recommendation, minimum GPA in nursing prerequisites of 3.0, prerequisite course work. Transfer students are accepted. **Standardized tests** *Required:* SAT or ACT, TOEFL for international students. **Application** *Deadline:* 2/2 (freshmen), 4/1 (transfer). *Early decision:* 12/1. *Notification:* 4/15 (freshmen), 1/20 (early action). *Application fee:* $35.

Advanced Placement Credit given for nursing courses completed elsewhere dependent upon specific evaluations.

Expenses (2004–05) *Tuition:* full-time $23,760. *International tuition:* $23,760 full-time. *Room and board:* $9820 per academic year. *Required fees:* full-time $730.

Financial Aid 80% of baccalaureate students in nursing programs received some form of financial aid in 2003–04. *Gift aid (need-based):* Federal Pell, FSEOG, state, private, college/university gift aid from institutional funds. *Loans:* FFEL (Subsidized and Unsubsidized Stafford PLUS), Perkins, state, college/university. *Work-Study:* Federal Work-Study. *Application deadline (priority):* 2/1.

Contact Ms. Jennifer O'Loughlin Hieber, Director, Undergraduate Admission, Department of Nursing, Simmons College, 300 The Fenway, Boston, MA 02115. *Telephone:* 617-521-2051. *Fax:* 617-521-3190. *E-mail:* jennifer.oloughlin@simmons.edu.

GRADUATE PROGRAMS

Expenses (2004–05) *Tuition:* full-time $18,240; part-time $760 per credit hour. *International tuition:* $18,240 full-time. *Room and board:* $11,430; room only: $9820 per academic year.

Simmons College (continued)

Financial Aid 50% of graduate students in nursing programs received some form of financial aid in 2003–04.

Contact Dr. Judith Beal, Associate Dean,SHS, Chair, Nursing Dept., Department of Nursing, Simmons College, 300 The Fenway, Boston, MA 02115. *Telephone:* 617-521-2139. *Fax:* 617-521-3045. *E-mail:* judy.beal@simmons.edu.

MASTER'S DEGREE PROGRAM

Degrees MS; MSN/MS

Available Programs Accelerated AD/RN to Master's; Accelerated Master's; Accelerated Master's for Non-Nursing College Graduates; Accelerated Master's for Nurses with Non-Nursing Degrees; Accelerated RN to Master's; Master's; Master's for Non-Nursing College Graduates; Master's for Nurses with Non-Nursing Degrees; RN to Master's.

Concentrations Available Health-care administration; nursing education. *Nurse practitioner programs in:* adult health, family health, gerontology, occupational health, pediatric, primary care, school health, women's health.

Study Options Full-time and part-time.

Program Entrance Requirements Clinical experience, computer literacy, minimum overall college GPA of 3.0, transcript of college record, written essay, immunizations, 3 letters of recommendation, physical assessment course, professional liability insurance/malpractice insurance, prerequisite course work, resume, statistics course.

Advanced Placement Credit given for nursing courses completed elsewhere dependent upon specific evaluations.

Degree Requirements 64 total credit hours, thesis or project.

POST-MASTER'S PROGRAM

Areas of Study Health-care administration. *Nurse practitioner programs in:* adult health, family health, gerontology, pediatric, primary care, school health, women's health.

CONTINUING EDUCATION PROGRAM

Contact Ms. Kerry Vieira, Associate Director of Admission, Department of Nursing, Simmons College, Dix Scholar Program, 300 The Fenway, Boston, MA 02115. *Telephone:* 617-521-2051. *Fax:* 617-521-3190. *E-mail:* kerry.vieira@simmons.edu.

University of Massachusetts Amherst

School of Nursing
Amherst, Massachusetts

http://www.umass.edu/nursing

Founded in 1863

DEGREES • BS • MS • MS/MPH • PHD

Nursing Program Faculty 52 (42% with doctorates).

Baccalaureate Enrollment 623
Women 93% **Men** 7% **Minority** 19%

Graduate Enrollment 45
Women 89% **Men** 11% **Minority** 7%

Nursing Student Activities Nursing Honor Society, Sigma Theta Tau, Student Nurses' Association, nursing club.

Nursing Student Resources Academic advising; academic or career counseling; bookstore; campus computer network; career placement assistance; computer lab; computer-assisted instruction; e-mail services; interactive nursing skills videos; Internet; learning resource lab; library services; nursing audiovisuals; paid internships; resume preparation assistance; skills, simulation, or other laboratory; tutoring; unpaid internships.

Library Facilities 3.2 million volumes (260,319 in health, 27,875 in nursing); 37,716 periodical subscriptions (3,780 health-care related).

■ The University of Massachusetts Amherst School of Nursing is located in the picturesque Pioneer Valley. It is an exciting place to study. The School of Nursing is committed to educational excellence, career mobility, and lifelong learning. Traditional, prelicensure, second bachelor's, and RN-BS undergraduate programs are offered. On the graduate level, master's and doctoral programs are offered in family nurse practitioner studies, psychiatric/mental health nursing, gerontological nursing, and community/school health nursing. A joint MS/MPH dual-degree online program is also offered by the Schools of Nursing, Public Health, and Health Sciences, as is a collaborative PhD program with UMass Worcester. The University of Massachusetts is an Equal Opportunity Employer.

BACCALAUREATE PROGRAMS

Degree BS

Available Programs Accelerated Baccalaureate for Second Degree; Accelerated RN Baccalaureate; Generic Baccalaureate; RN Baccalaureate.

Study Options Full-time.

Program Entrance Requirements Minimum overall college GPA of 2.5, transcript of college record, CPR certification, written essay, health exam, health insurance, high school foreign language, 3 years high school math, 3 years high school science, high school transcript, immunizations, minimum high school GPA, minimum GPA in nursing prerequisites of 2.5, professional liability insurance/malpractice insurance, prerequisite course work. Transfer students are accepted. **Standardized tests** *Required:* SAT or ACT, TOEFL for international students. **Application** *Deadline:* 1/15 (freshmen), 4/15 (transfer). *Early decision:* 11/1. *Notification:* continuous (freshmen), 12/15 (early action). *Application fee:* $40.

Expenses (2004–05) *Tuition, state resident:* full-time $1714; part-time $175 per credit hour. *Tuition, nonresident:* full-time $9937; part-time $175 per credit hour. *International tuition:* $9937 full-time. *Room and board:* $6189; room only: $3428 per academic year. *Required fees:* full-time $4337; part-time $128 per credit; part-time $163 per term.

Financial Aid *Gift aid (need-based):* Federal Pell, FSEOG, state, private, college/university gift aid from institutional funds. *Loans:* Federal Direct (Subsidized and Unsubsidized Stafford PLUS), Perkins, state. *Work-Study:* Federal Work-Study. *Application deadline (priority):* 3/1.

Contact Miss Elizabeth Theroux, Academic Secretary, Office for the Advancement of Nursing Education, School of Nursing, University of Massachusetts Amherst, 219 Arnold House, 715 North Pleasant Street, Amherst, MA 01003-9304. *Telephone:* 413-545-5096. *Fax:* 413-577-2550. *E-mail:* etheroux@acad.umass.edu.

GRADUATE PROGRAMS

Expenses (2004–05) *Tuition, state resident:* full-time $1320; part-time $110 per credit hour. *Tuition, nonresident:* full-time $4968; part-time $414 per credit hour. *International tuition:* $4968 full-time. *Room and board:* $6305; room only: $3578 per academic year. *Required fees:* full-time $1873.

Financial Aid 29 fellowships (averaging $1,278 per year), 3 research assistantships (averaging $1,930 per year), 16 teaching assistantships (averaging $3,507 per year) were awarded; career-related internships or fieldwork, Federal Work-Study, scholarships, traineeships, tuition waivers (full), and unspecified assistantships also available.

Contact Ms. Karen Ayotte, Administrative Assistant for the Advancement of Nursing Education, School of Nursing, University of Massachusetts Amherst, 229 Arnold House, 715 North Pleasant Street, Amherst, MA 01003-9304. *Telephone:* 413-545-1302. *Fax:* 413-577-2550. *E-mail:* kayotte@nursing.umass.edu.

MASTER'S DEGREE PROGRAM

Degrees MS; MS/MPH

Available Programs Master's; Master's for Nurses with Non-Nursing Degrees.

Concentrations Available *Clinical nurse specialist programs in:* community health, gerontology, psychiatric/mental health, public health, school health. *Nurse practitioner programs in:* family health, psychiatric/mental health.

Study Options Full-time and part-time.

Program Entrance Requirements Minimum overall college GPA of 3.0, transcript of college record, written essay, immunizations, interview, 2 letters of recommendation, physical assessment course, statistics course, GRE General Test. *Application deadline:* For fall admission, 2/1 (priority date); for spring admission, 10/1. Applications are processed on a rolling basis. *Application fee:* $40 ($50 for international students).

Degree Requirements 45 total credit hours, thesis or project.

POST-MASTER'S PROGRAM

Areas of Study Nursing education. *Clinical nurse specialist programs in:* psychiatric/mental health, public health, school health. *Nurse practitioner programs in:* family health, psychiatric/mental health.

DOCTORAL DEGREE PROGRAM

Degree PhD

Available Programs Doctorate.

Areas of Study Advanced practice nursing, aging, community health, faculty preparation, family health, gerontology, health promotion/disease prevention, health-care systems, illness and transition, information systems, maternity-newborn, nursing education, nursing research, urban health.

Site Options *Distance Learning:* Worcester, MA.

Program Entrance Requirements Clinical experience, minimum overall college GPA of 3.0, interview, 2 letters of recommendation, MSN or equivalent, scholarly papers, statistics course, vita, writing sample. *Application deadline:* For fall admission, 2/1 (priority date); for spring admission, 10/1. Applications are processed on a rolling basis. *Application fee:* $40 ($50 for international students).

Degree Requirements 57 total credit hours, dissertation, oral exam, written exam, residency.

CONTINUING EDUCATION PROGRAM

Contact Ms. Karen Ayotte, Administrative Assistant for the Advancement of Nursing Education, School of Nursing, University of Massachusetts Amherst, 229 Arnold House, 715 North Pleasant Street, Amherst, MA 01003-9304. *Telephone:* 413-545-1302. *Fax:* 413-577-2550. *E-mail:* kayotte@nursing.umass.edu.

University of Massachusetts Boston

College of Nursing and Health Sciences
Boston, Massachusetts

http://www.cnhs.umb.edu/

Founded in 1964

DEGREES • BS • MS • PHD

Nursing Program Faculty 68 (37% with doctorates).

Baccalaureate Enrollment 536
Women 90% **Men** 10% **Minority** 30% **International** 2% **Part-time** 23%

Graduate Enrollment 112
Women 95% **Men** 5% **Minority** 14% **International** 3% **Part-time** 75%

Nursing Student Activities Nursing Honor Society, Sigma Theta Tau, Student Nurses' Association, nursing club.

Nursing Student Resources Academic advising; academic or career counseling; assistance for students with disabilities; bookstore; campus computer network; career placement assistance; computer lab; daycare for children of students; e-mail services; employment services for current students; housing assistance; interactive nursing skills videos; Internet; learning resource lab; library services; nursing audiovisuals; other; remedial services; resume preparation assistance; skills, simulation, or other laboratory; tutoring.

Library Facilities 584,015 volumes (3,400 in health, 1,260 in nursing); 25,575 periodical subscriptions.

BACCALAUREATE PROGRAMS

Degree BS

Available Programs Generic Baccalaureate; RN Baccalaureate.

Study Options Full-time and part-time.

Program Entrance Requirements Minimum overall college GPA of 2.75, transcript of college record, written essay, health insurance, high school biology, high school chemistry, high school foreign language, high school math, high school transcript, immunizations, 3 letters of recommendation, minimum high school GPA of 2.75, prerequisite course work. Transfer students are accepted. **Standardized tests** *Required:* SAT or ACT, TOEFL for international students. **Application** *Deadline:* rolling (freshmen), rolling (transfer). *Notification:* continuous (freshmen). *Application fee:* $40.

Expenses (2004–05) *Tuition, state resident:* full-time $4017; part-time $72 per credit hour. *Tuition, nonresident:* full-time $9383; part-time $407 per credit hour. *International tuition:* $9383 full-time. *Required fees:* full-time $3155; part-time $263 per credit; part-time $1578 per term.

Financial Aid 84% of baccalaureate students in nursing programs received some form of financial aid in 2003–04. *Gift aid (need-based):* Federal Pell, FSEOG, state, private, college/university gift aid from institutional funds. *Loans:* Federal Direct (Subsidized and Unsubsidized Stafford PLUS), Perkins, state. *Work-Study:* Federal Work-Study. *Application deadline (priority):* 3/1.

Contact Mr. Jon Hutton, Assistant Director of Enrollment Marketing and Information Service, College of Nursing and Health Sciences, University of Massachusetts Boston, 100 Morrissey Boulevard, Boston, MA 02125-3393. *Telephone:* 617-287-6000. *Fax:* 617-265-7173. *E-mail:* enrollment.information@umb.edu.

GRADUATE PROGRAMS

Expenses (2004–05) *Tuition, state resident:* full-time $4461; part-time $108 per credit hour. *Tuition, nonresident:* full-time $9389; part-time $407 per credit hour. *International tuition:* $9389 full-time. *Required fees:* full-time $3161; part-time $263 per credit; part-time $1578 per term.

Financial Aid 20% of graduate students in nursing programs received some form of financial aid in 2003–04. 3 research assistantships with full tuition reimbursements available (averaging $8,000 per year), 13 teaching assistantships with full tuition reimbursements available (averaging $5,000 per year) were awarded; career-related internships or fieldwork, Federal Work-Study, and unspecified assistantships also available. Aid available to part-time students. *Financial aid application deadline:* 3/1.

Contact Mr. Jon Hutton, Assistant Director of Enrollment Marketing and Information Service, College of Nursing and Health Sciences, University of Massachusetts Boston, 100 Morrissey Boulevard, Boston, MA 02125. *Telephone:* 617-287-6000. *Fax:* 617-265-7173. *E-mail:* enrollment.information@umb.edu.

MASTER'S DEGREE PROGRAM

Degree MS

Available Programs Master's.

Concentrations Available *Clinical nurse specialist programs in:* acute care, critical care. *Nurse practitioner programs in:* adult health, family health, gerontology.

Study Options Full-time and part-time.

Program Entrance Requirements Clinical experience, minimum overall college GPA of 2.75, transcript of college record, CPR certification, written essay, immunizations, 3 letters of recommendation, physical assessment course, prerequisite course work, statistics course. *Application deadline:* For fall admission, 3/1 (priority date); for spring admission, 11/1. *Application fee:* $25.

Degree Requirements 48 total credit hours, thesis or project.

POST-MASTER'S PROGRAM

Areas of Study *Nurse practitioner programs in:* adult health, family health, gerontology.

DOCTORAL DEGREE PROGRAM

Degree PhD

Available Programs Doctorate.

Areas of Study Health policy.

Program Entrance Requirements Clinical experience, minimum overall college GPA of 3.3, interview by faculty committee, interview, 3 letters of recommendation, MSN or equivalent, statistics course, vita, writing sample, GRE General Test. *Application deadline:* For fall admission, 3/1 (priority date); for spring admission, 11/1. *Application fee:* $25.

Degree Requirements 60 total credit hours, dissertation, oral exam, written exam, residency.

CONTINUING EDUCATION PROGRAM

Contact Ms. Wanda Willard, Director of Credit Programs, College of Nursing and Health Sciences, University of Massachusetts Boston, 100 Morrissey Boulevard, Boston, MA 02125-3393. *Telephone:* 617-287-7874. *Fax:* 617-287-7922. *E-mail:* wanda.willard@umb.edu.

University of Massachusetts Dartmouth

College of Nursing
North Dartmouth, Massachusetts

http://www.umassd.edu/nursing

Founded in 1895

DEGREES • BSN • MS

Nursing Program Faculty 43 (30% with doctorates).

Baccalaureate Enrollment 385
Women 90% **Men** 10% **Minority** 5% **Part-time** 22%

Graduate Enrollment 80
Women 95% **Men** 5% **Minority** 2%

Nursing Student Activities Sigma Theta Tau, nursing club.

Nursing Student Resources Academic advising; academic or career counseling; assistance for students with disabilities; bookstore; campus computer network; career placement assistance; computer lab; computer-assisted instruction; daycare for children of students; e-mail services; employment services for current students; externships; housing assistance; interactive nursing skills videos; Internet; learning resource lab; library services; nursing audiovisuals; placement services for program completers; resume preparation assistance; skills, simulation, or other laboratory; tutoring; unpaid internships.

Library Facilities 947,000 volumes (13,934 in nursing); 2,925 periodical subscriptions (221 health-care related).

■ The graduate of the University of Massachusetts Dartmouth College of Nursing understands the forces that have an impact on the health-care system as well as how these forces affect the delivery of nursing care to persons in the community. Critical judgment, the ability to apply research to practice, and therapeutic communications and leadership skills are fostered throughout the program of study. The commitment to humanism and the promotion of optimal levels of function for all members of society are important goals for the graduate of the College of Nursing.

BACCALAUREATE PROGRAMS

Degree BSN

Available Programs Generic Baccalaureate; RN Baccalaureate.

Site Options Fall River, MA.

Study Options Full-time and part-time.

Program Entrance Requirements Transcript of college record, CPR certification, written essay, health exam, health insurance, high school biology, high school chemistry, high school foreign language, 3 years high school math, 3 years high school science, high school transcript, immunizations, letters of recommendation, minimum high school GPA of 3.0, minimum high school rank 66%, professional liability insurance/malpractice insurance. Transfer students are accepted. **Standardized tests** *Required:* SAT or ACT, TOEFL for international students. **Application** *Deadline:* rolling (freshmen), rolling (transfer). *Early decision:* 11/15. *Notification:* continuous (freshmen), 12/15 (out-of-state freshmen), 12/15 (early decision). *Application fee:* $35, $55 for non-residents.

Advanced Placement Credit by examination available. Credit given for nursing courses completed elsewhere dependent upon specific evaluations.

Expenses (2003–04) *Tuition, state resident:* full-time $2834. *Tuition, nonresident:* full-time $16,198. *Room and board:* $7331; room only: $4565 per academic year.

Financial Aid 68% of baccalaureate students in nursing programs received some form of financial aid in 2002–03.

Contact Mr. Stephen T. Briggs, Director of Admissions, College of Nursing, University of Massachusetts Dartmouth, 285 Old Westport Road, North Dartmouth, MA 02747. *Telephone:* 508-999-8606. *Fax:* 508-999-8755. *E-mail:* sbriggs@umassd.edu.

GRADUATE PROGRAMS

Expenses (2003–04) *Tuition, state resident:* part-time $86 per credit hour. *Tuition, nonresident:* part-time $337 per credit hour.

Financial Aid 1% of graduate students in nursing programs received some form of financial aid in 2002–03. 4 research assistantships with full tuition reimbursements available (averaging $3,000 per year), 6 teaching assistantships with full tuition reimbursements available (averaging $3,600 per year) were awarded; Federal Work-Study, scholarships, and unspecified assistantships also available. Aid available to part-time students. *Financial aid application deadline:* 3/1.

Contact Prof. Jeanne Leffers, Director, Graduate Program, College of Nursing, University of Massachusetts Dartmouth, 285 Old Westport Road, North Dartmouth, MA 02747-2300. *Telephone:* 508-999-8581. *E-mail:* jleffers@umassd.edu.

MASTER'S DEGREE PROGRAM

Degree MS

Concentrations Available *Clinical nurse specialist programs in:* adult health, community health. *Nurse practitioner programs in:* adult health.

Study Options Full-time and part-time.

Program Entrance Requirements Clinical experience, computer literacy, minimum overall college GPA of 3.0, transcript of college record, CPR certification, written essay, immunizations, interview, 3 letters of recommendation, nursing research course, physical assessment course, professional liability insurance/malpractice insurance, statistics course, GRE General Test. *Application deadline:* For fall admission, 4/20; for spring admission, 11/15. *Application fee:* $35 ($55 for international students).

Advanced Placement Credit given for nursing courses completed elsewhere dependent upon specific evaluations.

Degree Requirements 39 total credit hours, thesis or project.

POST-MASTER'S PROGRAM

Areas of Study *Nurse practitioner programs in:* adult health.

CONTINUING EDUCATION PROGRAM

Contact Lorraine Fisher, Director, Division of Continuing Education, College of Nursing, University of Massachusetts Dartmouth, 285 Old Westport Road, North Dartmouth, MA 02747-2300. *Telephone:* 508-910-6929. *Fax:* 508-999-9127. *E-mail:* lfisher@umassd.edu.

University of Massachusetts Lowell

Department of Nursing
Lowell, Massachusetts

http://www.uml.edu/dept/nursing

Founded in 1894

DEGREES • BS • MS • PHD

Nursing Program Faculty 27 (95% with doctorates).

Baccalaureate Enrollment 299
Women 90% **Men** 10%

Graduate Enrollment 65
Women 90% **Men** 10%

Nursing Student Activities Sigma Theta Tau, Student Nurses' Association.

Nursing Student Resources Academic advising; academic or career counseling; assistance for students with disabilities; bookstore; campus computer network; career placement assistance; computer lab; computer-assisted instruction; e-mail services; employment services for current students; housing assistance; interactive nursing skills videos; Internet; learning resource lab; library services; nursing audiovisuals; placement services for program completers; resume preparation assistance; skills, simulation, or other laboratory; tutoring.

Library Facilities 549,243 volumes (29,100 in health, 4,465 in nursing); 350 periodical subscriptions health-care related.

BACCALAUREATE PROGRAMS

Degree BS

Available Programs Generic Baccalaureate; RN Baccalaureate.

Study Options Full-time and part-time.

Program Entrance Requirements Minimum overall college GPA of 2.5, transcript of college record, CPR certification, health exam, health insurance, high school chemistry, high school foreign language, 3 years high school math, 3 years high school science, high school transcript, immunizations, minimum high school GPA of 2.5, minimum GPA in nursing prerequisites of 2.5, professional liability insurance/malpractice insurance. Transfer students are accepted. **Standardized tests** *Required:* SAT or ACT, TOEFL for international students. **Application** *Deadline:* rolling (freshmen), rolling (transfer). *Notification:* continuous (freshmen). *Application fee:* $20.

Advanced Placement Credit by examination available.

Expenses (2004–05) *Tuition, state resident:* full-time $1454; part-time $61 per credit hour. *Tuition, nonresident:* full-time $8567; part-time $357 per credit hour. *Room and board:* $6001; room only: $3717 per academic year. *Required fees:* full-time $6437; part-time $280 per credit.

Financial Aid 68% of baccalaureate students in nursing programs received some form of financial aid in 2003–04.

Contact Office of Undergraduate Admissions, Department of Nursing, University of Massachusetts Lowell, 883 Broadway Street, Suite 110, Lowell, MA 01854-5104. *Telephone:* 800-410-4607. *E-mail:* admissions@uml.edu.

GRADUATE PROGRAMS

Expenses (2004–05) *Tuition, state resident:* full-time $273; part-time $91 per credit hour. *Tuition, nonresident:* full-time $1071; part-time $357 per credit hour. *International tuition:* $1211 full-time. *Required fees:* full-time $978; part-time $336 per credit.

Financial Aid 50% of graduate students in nursing programs received some form of financial aid in 2003–04. 37 fellowships with tuition reimbursements available, 10 teaching assistantships with full tuition reimbursements available were awarded; research assistantships with full tuition reimbursements available, career-related internships or fieldwork, Federal Work-Study, institutionally sponsored loans, scholarships, and traineeships also available. Aid available to part-time students. *Financial aid application deadline:* 4/1.

Contact Dr. May Futrell, Chair and Professor, Department of Nursing, University of Massachusetts Lowell, 3 Solomont Way, Suite 2, Lowell, MA 01854-5126. *Telephone:* 978-934-4467. *Fax:* 978-934-3006. *E-mail:* may_futrell@uml.edu.

MASTER'S DEGREE PROGRAM

Degree MS

Available Programs Master's.

Concentrations Available *Clinical nurse specialist programs in:* psychiatric/mental health. *Nurse practitioner programs in:* family health, gerontology, psychiatric/mental health.

Study Options Full-time and part-time.

Program Entrance Requirements Computer literacy, minimum overall college GPA of 3.0, transcript of college record, CPR certification, immunizations, interview, 3 letters of recommendation, professional liability insurance/malpractice insurance, statistics course, GRE General Test. *Application deadline:* For fall admission, 4/1 (priority date); for spring admission, 10/1. Applications are processed on a rolling basis. *Application fee:* $20 ($35 for international students).

Degree Requirements 42 total credit hours, thesis or project.

DOCTORAL DEGREE PROGRAM

Degree PhD

Available Programs Doctorate.

Areas of Study Health promotion/disease prevention.

Program Entrance Requirements Minimum overall college GPA of 3.4, interview by faculty committee, 3 letters of recommendation, MSN or equivalent, scholarly papers, statistics course, writing sample, GRE General Test. *Application deadline:* For fall admission, 4/1 (priority date); for spring admission, 10/1. Applications are processed on a rolling basis. *Application fee:* $20 ($35 for international students).

Degree Requirements 60 total credit hours, dissertation, oral exam, written exam.

University of Massachusetts Worcester

Graduate School of Nursing
Worcester, Massachusetts

http://www.umassmed.edu/gsn/

Founded in 1962

DEGREES • MS • PHD

Nursing Program Faculty 39 (67% with doctorates).

Graduate Enrollment 127

Women 93% **Men** 7% **Minority** 9% **International** 3% **Part-time** 44%

Nursing Student Activities Sigma Theta Tau, nursing club.

Nursing Student Resources Academic advising; academic or career counseling; assistance for students with disabilities; bookstore; computer lab; e-mail services; Internet; learning resource lab; library services; paid internships; remedial services; tutoring.

Library Facilities 258,800 volumes in health, 55,000 volumes in nursing; 20,000 periodical subscriptions health-care related.

GRADUATE PROGRAMS

Expenses (2004–05) *Tuition, state resident:* full-time $7920; part-time $110 per credit hour. *Tuition, nonresident:* full-time $29,568; part-time $410 per credit hour. *International tuition:* $29,568 full-time. *Required fees:* full-time $6361.

Financial Aid 40% of graduate students in nursing programs received some form of financial aid in 2003–04. Scholarships and traineeships available. Aid available to part-time students. *Financial aid application deadline:* 3/22.

Contact Ms. Lindsey Hall, Director of Recruitment and Retention, Graduate School of Nursing, University of Massachusetts Worcester, 55 Lake Avenue North, Worcester, MA 01655-0115. *Telephone:* 508-856-3488. *Fax:* 508-856-5851. *E-mail:* GSNAdmissions@umassmed.edu.

MASTER'S DEGREE PROGRAM

Degree MS

Available Programs Master's; Master's for Non-Nursing College Graduates.

Concentrations Available Nursing education. *Nurse practitioner programs in:* acute care, adult health, community health, gerontology.

Site Options *Distance Learning:* Worcester, MA.

Study Options Full-time and part-time.

Program Entrance Requirements Clinical experience, computer literacy, minimum overall college GPA of 3.0, transcript of college record, CPR certification, written essay, immunizations, interview, 3 letters of recommendation, physical assessment course, professional liability insurance/malpractice insurance, prerequisite course work, resume, statistics course, GRE General Test. *Application deadline:* For fall admission, 3/15. Applications are processed on a rolling basis. *Application fee:* $25 ($50 for international students).

Degree Requirements 42 total credit hours, thesis or project.

POST-MASTER'S PROGRAM

Areas of Study Nursing education. *Nurse practitioner programs in:* acute care, adult health, community health, family health, gerontology.

DOCTORAL DEGREE PROGRAM

Degree PhD

Available Programs Doctorate.

Areas of Study Nursing education, nursing research, nursing science.

Site Options *Distance Learning:* Worcester, MA.

Program Entrance Requirements Clinical experience, interview by faculty committee, interview, 2 letters of recommendation, MSN or equivalent, scholarly papers, statistics course, vita. *Application deadline:* For fall admission, 3/15. Applications are processed on a rolling basis. *Application fee:* $25 ($50 for international students).

Degree Requirements 54 total credit hours, dissertation, written exam, residency.

University of Massachusetts Worcester (continued)

CONTINUING EDUCATION PROGRAM

Contact Ms. Lindsey Hall, Director of Recruitment and Retention, Graduate School of Nursing, University of Massachusetts Worcester, 55 Lake Avenue North, Worcester, MA 01655-0115. *Telephone:* 508-856-5801. *E-mail:* GSNAdmissions@umassmed.edu.

See full description on page 562.

Worcester State College

Department of Nursing
Worcester, Massachusetts

http://www.worcester.edu

Founded in 1874

DEGREES • BS • MS

Nursing Program Faculty 17 (60% with doctorates).

Baccalaureate Enrollment 212
Women 95% **Men** 5% **Minority** 15% **International** 1%

Graduate Enrollment 10
Women 100% **Minority** 10% **International** 10% **Part-time** 100%

Nursing Student Activities Sigma Theta Tau, Student Nurses' Association, nursing club.

Nursing Student Resources Academic advising; academic or career counseling; assistance for students with disabilities; bookstore; career placement assistance; computer lab; computer-assisted instruction; e-mail services; employment services for current students; housing assistance; interactive nursing skills videos; Internet; learning resource lab; library services; nursing audiovisuals; paid internships; remedial services; resume preparation assistance; skills, simulation, or other laboratory; tutoring; unpaid internships.

Library Facilities 150,419 volumes (5,400 in health, 500 in nursing); 1,021 periodical subscriptions (85 health-care related).

BACCALAUREATE PROGRAMS

Degree BS

Available Programs Accelerated RN Baccalaureate; Generic Baccalaureate.

Study Options Full-time.

Program Entrance Requirements Minimum overall college GPA of 3.0, CPR certification, written essay, health exam, health insurance, high school chemistry, high school foreign language, 1 year of high school math, 2 years high school science, high school transcript, immunizations, interview, minimum high school GPA of 3.0, minimum GPA in nursing prerequisites of 3.0, professional liability insurance/malpractice insurance, prerequisite course work, RN licensure. Transfer students are accepted. **Standardized tests** *Required:* TOEFL for international students. *Required for some:* SAT or ACT. **Application** *Deadline:* 8/1 (freshmen), 6/1 (out-of-state freshmen), 6/1 (transfer). *Notification:* continuous (freshmen). *Application fee:* $20.

Advanced Placement Credit by examination available. Credit given for nursing courses completed elsewhere dependent upon specific evaluations.

Expenses (2004–05) *Tuition, state resident:* full-time $970; part-time $190 per credit hour. *Tuition, nonresident:* full-time $7050; part-time $444 per credit hour. *International tuition:* $7050 full-time. *Room and board:* $6282; room only: $3982 per academic year. *Required fees:* full-time $3609.

Financial Aid 45% of baccalaureate students in nursing programs received some form of financial aid in 2003–04. *Gift aid (need-based):* Federal Pell, FSEOG, state, private, college/university gift aid from institutional funds. *Loans:* FFEL (Subsidized and Unsubsidized Stafford PLUS), Perkins, Massachusetts No-Interest Loans (NIL). *Work-Study:* Federal Work-Study. *Application deadline (priority):* 3/1.

Contact Ms. Elizabeth Axelson, Associate Director, Admissions, Department of Nursing, Worcester State College, 486 Chandler Street, Worcester, MA 01602. *Telephone:* 508-929-8090. *Fax:* 508-929-8183. *E-mail:* baxelson@worcester.edu.

GRADUATE PROGRAMS

Expenses (2004–05) *Tuition, state resident:* full-time $2700; part-time $229 per credit hour. *Tuition, nonresident:* full-time $2700; part-time $229 per credit hour. *Required fees:* full-time $1422.

Financial Aid 40% of graduate students in nursing programs received some form of financial aid in 2003–04.

Contact Dr. Annmarie Samar, Coordinator, Department of Nursing, Worcester State College, 486 Chandler Street, Worcester, MA 01602. *Telephone:* 508-929-8685. *Fax:* 508-929-8168. *E-mail:* asamar@worcester.edu.

MASTER'S DEGREE PROGRAM

Degree MS

Available Programs Master's; Master's for Nurses with Non-Nursing Degrees.

Concentrations Available *Clinical nurse specialist programs in:* community health.

Study Options Part-time.

Program Entrance Requirements Clinical experience, transcript of college record, CPR certification, immunizations, interview, 1 letter of recommendation, nursing research course, professional liability insurance/malpractice insurance, prerequisite course work, resume, statistics course.

Advanced Placement Credit by examination available.

Degree Requirements 42 total credit hours, comprehensive exam.

MICHIGAN

Andrews University

Department of Nursing
Berrien Springs, Michigan

Founded in 1874

DEGREES • BS • MS

Nursing Program Faculty 11 (50% with doctorates).

Baccalaureate Enrollment 106

Graduate Enrollment 10

Nursing Student Activities Nursing Honor Society, Sigma Theta Tau, Student Nurses' Association.

Nursing Student Resources Academic advising; academic or career counseling; assistance for students with disabilities; bookstore; campus computer network; career placement assistance; computer lab; computer-assisted instruction; daycare for children of students; e-mail services; employment services for current students; externships; housing assistance; interactive nursing skills videos; Internet; learning resource lab; library services; nursing audiovisuals; paid internships; placement services for program completers; remedial services; resume preparation assistance; skills, simulation, or other laboratory; tutoring; unpaid internships.

Library Facilities 512,100 volumes (77,000 in health, 500 in nursing); 3,032 periodical subscriptions (700 health-care related).

BACCALAUREATE PROGRAMS

Degree BS

Available Programs ADN to Baccalaureate; Generic Baccalaureate.

Study Options Full-time.

Program Entrance Requirements Minimum overall college GPA of 2.5, transcript of college record, health exam, high school transcript, immunizations, minimum GPA in nursing prerequisites of 2.5. Transfer students are accepted. **Standardized tests** *Required:* SAT or ACT. *Recommended:* ACT. **Application** *Deadline:* rolling (freshmen), rolling (transfer). *Notification:* continuous (freshmen). *Application fee:* $30.

Expenses (2003–04) *Tuition:* full-time $18,950.

Contact Dr. Frances Johnson, Director of Undergraduate Programs, Department of Nursing, Andrews University, Berrien Springs, MI 49103. *Telephone:* 269-471-3192. *Fax:* 269-471-3454. *E-mail:* francesj@andrews.edu.

GRADUATE PROGRAMS

Expenses (2003–04) *Tuition:* part-time $585 per credit hour.

Financial Aid Institutionally sponsored loans available.

Contact Dr. Ruth Abbott, Director of Graduate Program, Department of Nursing, Andrews University, Berrien Springs, MI 49104. *Telephone:* 269-471-3337. *Fax:* 269-471-3454. *E-mail:* rabbott@andrews.edu.

MASTER'S DEGREE PROGRAM

Degree MS

Available Programs Master's.

Concentrations Available Nursing education.

Study Options Part-time.

Program Entrance Requirements Minimum overall college GPA of 3.0, transcript of college record, CPR certification, immunizations, 3 letters of recommendation. *Application deadline:* Applications are processed on a rolling basis. *Application fee:* $40.

Degree Requirements 38 total credit hours, thesis or project.

POST-MASTER'S PROGRAM

Areas of Study Nursing education.

Calvin College

Department of Nursing
Grand Rapids, Michigan

Founded in 1876

DEGREE • BSN

Nursing Program Faculty 20 (20% with doctorates).

Baccalaureate Enrollment 120
Women 95% **Men** 5% **Minority** 10% **International** 10%

Nursing Student Activities Sigma Theta Tau, Student Nurses' Association, nursing club.

Nursing Student Resources Academic advising; academic or career counseling; assistance for students with disabilities; bookstore; campus computer network; career placement assistance; computer lab; computer-assisted instruction; e-mail services; employment services for current students; externships; housing assistance; interactive nursing skills videos; Internet; learning resource lab; library services; nursing audiovisuals; paid internships; placement services for program completers; remedial services; resume preparation assistance; skills, simulation, or other laboratory; tutoring.

Library Facilities 824,806 volumes; 14,464 periodical subscriptions.

BACCALAUREATE PROGRAMS

Degree BSN

Available Programs Generic Baccalaureate.

Study Options Full-time.

Program Entrance Requirements CPR certification, health exam, health insurance, immunizations, 3 letters of recommendation, minimum GPA in nursing prerequisites of 2.0, professional liability insurance/malpractice insurance, prerequisite course work. Transfer students are accepted. **Standardized tests** *Required:* SAT or ACT, TOEFL for international students. **Application** *Deadline:* 8/15 (freshmen), rolling (transfer). *Notification:* continuous (freshmen). *Application fee:* $35.

Contact Dr. Mary Molewyk Doornbos, Chairperson and Professor of Nursing, Department of Nursing, Calvin College, 3201 Burton, SE, Grand Rapids, MI 49546. *Telephone:* 616-526-6268. *Fax:* 616-526-6501. *E-mail:* door@calvin.edu.

Eastern Michigan University

Department of Nursing
Ypsilanti, Michigan

http://www.emich.edu/nursing

Founded in 1849

DEGREES • BSN • MSN

Nursing Program Faculty 17 (53% with doctorates).

Baccalaureate Enrollment 334
Women 92% **Men** 8% **Minority** 28% **International** 4% **Part-time** 23%

Graduate Enrollment 52
Women 96% **Men** 4% **Minority** 27% **Part-time** 100%

Nursing Student Activities Nursing Honor Society, Sigma Theta Tau, Student Nurses' Association.

Nursing Student Resources Academic advising; academic or career counseling; assistance for students with disabilities; bookstore; campus computer network; career placement assistance; computer lab; computer-assisted instruction; daycare for children of students; e-mail services; employment services for current students; externships; housing assistance; interactive nursing skills videos; Internet; learning resource lab; library services; nursing audiovisuals; paid internships; placement services for program completers; remedial services; resume preparation assistance; skills, simulation, or other laboratory; tutoring.

Library Facilities 658,648 volumes; 4,457 periodical subscriptions.

BACCALAUREATE PROGRAMS

Degree BSN

Available Programs Baccalaureate for Second Degree; Generic Baccalaureate; RN Baccalaureate.

Site Options Jackson, MI; Detroit, MI; Livonia, MI.

Study Options Full-time and part-time.

Program Entrance Requirements CPR certification, health exam, health insurance, immunizations, minimum GPA in nursing prerequisites of 2.8, professional liability insurance/malpractice insurance, prerequisite course work. Transfer students are accepted. **Standardized tests** *Required:* SAT or ACT, TOEFL for international students. *Recommended:* ACT. **Application** *Deadline:* 6/30 (freshmen), rolling (transfer). *Notification:* continuous (freshmen). *Application fee:* $30.

Advanced Placement Credit given for nursing courses completed elsewhere dependent upon specific evaluations.

Expenses (2004–05) *Tuition, state resident:* full-time $2354; part-time $157 per credit hour. *Tuition, nonresident:* full-time $7357; part-time $490 per credit hour. *International tuition:* $7357 full-time. *Room and board:* $8068; room only: $4872 per academic year. *Required fees:* full-time $1128; part-time $40 per credit.

Financial Aid 48% of baccalaureate students in nursing programs received some form of financial aid in 2003–04. *Gift aid (need-based):* Federal Pell, FSEOG, state, private, college/university gift aid from institutional funds, Nursing Disadvantaged Student Grant. *Loans:* FFEL (Subsidized and Unsubsidized Stafford PLUS), Perkins, college/university. *Work-Study:* Federal Work-Study, part-time campus jobs. *Application deadline (priority):* 3/15.

Contact Miss Colleen Cotter, RN, BSN Coordinator, Department of Nursing, Eastern Michigan University, 309 Marshall Building, Ypsilanti, MI 48197. *Telephone:* 734-487-2334. *Fax:* 734-487-6946. *E-mail:* ccoter@emich.edu.

GRADUATE PROGRAMS

Expenses (2004–05) *Tuition, state resident:* full-time $4263; part-time $284 per credit hour. *Tuition, nonresident:* full-time $8630; part-time $575 per credit hour. *International tuition:* $8630 full-time. *Room and board:* $8068; room only: $4872 per academic year. *Required fees:* full-time $1128.

Financial Aid 27% of graduate students in nursing programs received some form of financial aid in 2003–04.

Contact Dr. Betty Beard, RN, Graduate Program Coordinator, Department of Nursing, Eastern Michigan University, 311 Marshall Building, Ypsilanti, MI 48197. *Telephone:* 734-487-2310. *Fax:* 734-487-2341.

MASTER'S DEGREE PROGRAM

Degree MSN

Available Programs Master's.

Eastern Michigan University (continued)

Concentrations Available *Clinical nurse specialist programs in:* adult health.

Site Options Livonia, MI.

Study Options Full-time and part-time.

Program Entrance Requirements Clinical experience, transcript of college record, CPR certification, written essay, immunizations, interview, 3 letters of recommendation, physical assessment course, professional liability insurance/malpractice insurance, statistics course.

Advanced Placement Credit by examination available. Credit given for nursing courses completed elsewhere dependent upon specific evaluations.

Degree Requirements 40 total credit hours, thesis or project.

Ferris State University

Department of Nursing and Dental Hygiene
Big Rapids, Michigan

Founded in 1884

DEGREE • BSN

Nursing Program Faculty 8.

Baccalaureate Enrollment 185

Nursing Student Activities Student Nurses' Association.

Nursing Student Resources Academic advising; academic or career counseling; assistance for students with disabilities; bookstore; campus computer network; career placement assistance; computer lab; computer-assisted instruction; daycare for children of students; e-mail services; employment services for current students; housing assistance; interactive nursing skills videos; Internet; library services; nursing audiovisuals; resume preparation assistance; tutoring.

Library Facilities 340,048 volumes (12,177 in health, 785 in nursing); 9,809 periodical subscriptions (515 health-care related).

BACCALAUREATE PROGRAMS

Degree BSN

Available Programs RN Baccalaureate.

Site Options Traverse City, MI; Grand Rapids , MI; Flint, MI.

Study Options Full-time and part-time.

Program Entrance Requirements Transcript of college record, minimum GPA in nursing prerequisites, prerequisite course work, RN licensure. Transfer students are accepted. **Standardized tests** *Required:* SAT or ACT, TOEFL for international students. **Application** *Deadline:* 8/1 (freshmen), 8/1 (transfer). *Notification:* continuous (freshmen). *Application fee:* $30.

Advanced Placement Credit by examination available. Credit given for nursing courses completed elsewhere dependent upon specific evaluations.

Expenses (2003–04) *Tuition, state resident:* full-time $6044; part-time $3022 per semester. *Tuition, nonresident:* full-time $12,088; part-time $6044 per semester. *Room and board:* $6326 per academic year.

Financial Aid 80% of baccalaureate students in nursing programs received some form of financial aid in 2002–03.

Contact Dr. Julie A. Coon, Department Head, Department of Nursing and Dental Hygiene, Ferris State University, 200 Ferris Drive, Room 400A, Big Rapids, MI 49307. *Telephone:* 231-591-2267. *Fax:* 231-591-2325. *E-mail:* coonj@ferris.edu.

Grand Valley State University

Russell B. Kirkhof School of Nursing
Allendale, Michigan

http://www4.gvsu.edu/kson/

Founded in 1960

DEGREES • BSN • MSN • MSN/MBA

Nursing Program Faculty 61 (34% with doctorates).

Nursing Student Activities Nursing Honor Society, Sigma Theta Tau, Student Nurses' Association.

Nursing Student Resources Skills, simulation, or other laboratory.

Library Facilities 634,000 volumes (15,000 in health, 3,000 in nursing); 5,000 periodical subscriptions (292 health-care related).

BACCALAUREATE PROGRAMS

Degree BSN

Available Programs Baccalaureate for Second Degree; Generic Baccalaureate; RN Baccalaureate.

Site Options *Distance Learning:* Muskegon, MI.

Study Options Full-time and part-time.

Program Entrance Requirements Minimum overall college GPA of 2.7, CPR certification, health exam, health insurance, immunizations, prerequisite course work. Transfer students are accepted. **Standardized tests** *Required:* SAT or ACT, TOEFL for international students. **Application** *Deadline:* 5/1 (freshmen), 7/25 (transfer). *Notification:* continuous until 5/1 (freshmen). *Application fee:* $30.

Advanced Placement Credit by examination available. Credit given for nursing courses completed elsewhere dependent upon specific evaluations.

Contact Dr. Kay Setter Kline, RN, Director of Undergraduate Program/Professor of Nursing, Russell B. Kirkhof School of Nursing, Grand Valley State University, Allendale, MI 49401-9403. *Telephone:* 616-331-3558. *Fax:* 616-331-2510.

GRADUATE PROGRAMS

Financial Aid 19 research assistantships were awarded; career-related internships or fieldwork, Federal Work-Study, institutionally sponsored loans, and traineeships also available.

Contact Dr. Jean Martin, Director of RN/BSN and MSN Programs/Assistant Professor of Nursing, Russell B. Kirkhof School of Nursing, Grand Valley State University, Allendale, MI 49401-9403. *Telephone:* 616-331-3558. *Fax:* 616-331-2510.

MASTER'S DEGREE PROGRAM

Degrees MSN; MSN/MBA

Available Programs Master's; Master's for Nurses with Non-Nursing Degrees; RN to Master's.

Concentrations Available Nurse case management; nursing administration; nursing education. *Clinical nurse specialist programs in:* acute care, adult health, family health, gerontology, pediatric, psychiatric/mental health, women's health. *Nurse practitioner programs in:* acute care, adult health, family health, gerontology, pediatric, primary care, psychiatric/mental health, women's health.

Site Options *Distance Learning:* Traverse City, MI.

Study Options Full-time and part-time.

Program Entrance Requirements Minimum overall college GPA of 3.0, transcript of college record, CPR certification, written essay, immunizations, interview, 3 letters of recommendation, physical assessment course, statistics course, GRE. *Application deadline:* For fall admission, 3/15 (priority date). Applications are processed on a rolling basis. *Application fee:* $30.

Advanced Placement Credit by examination available. Credit given for nursing courses completed elsewhere dependent upon specific evaluations.

Degree Requirements 43 total credit hours, thesis or project, comprehensive exam.

POST-MASTER'S PROGRAM

Areas of Study Nursing education. *Nurse practitioner programs in:* adult health, family health, gerontology, pediatric, women's health.

CONTINUING EDUCATION PROGRAM

Contact Kay Reick, RN, Coordinator for Continuing Nursing Education, Russell B. Kirkhof School of Nursing, Grand Valley State University, Allendale, MI 49401-9403. *Telephone:* 616-331-3558. *Fax:* 616-331-2510.

Hope College
Department of Nursing
Holland, Michigan

Founded in 1866

DEGREE • BSN

Library Facilities 358,329 volumes; 2,878 periodical subscriptions.

BACCALAUREATE PROGRAMS

Degree BSN

Available Programs Generic Baccalaureate.

Program Entrance Requirements Minimum overall college GPA of 2.5, transcript of college record, 3 letters of recommendation, minimum GPA in nursing prerequisites of 2.0. **Standardized tests** *Required:* SAT or ACT, TOEFL for international students. **Application** *Deadline:* rolling (freshmen), rolling (transfer). *Notification:* continuous (freshmen). *Application fee:* $35.

Contact Nursing Department, Department of Nursing, Hope College, 35 East 12th Street, Holland, MI 49422-9000. *Telephone:* 616-395-7420. *Fax:* 616-395-7163. *E-mail:* nursing@hope.edu.

Lake Superior State University
Department of Nursing
Sault Sainte Marie, Michigan

http://www.lssu.edu/academics/science/schools/nursing_health/nursdept/

Founded in 1946

DEGREE • BSN

Nursing Program Faculty 10 (1% with doctorates).

Nursing Student Activities Nursing Honor Society, Sigma Theta Tau, Student Nurses' Association.

Nursing Student Resources Academic advising; campus computer network; computer lab; computer-assisted instruction; e-mail services; employment services for current students; interactive nursing skills videos; learning resource lab; library services; nursing audiovisuals; skills, simulation, or other laboratory; tutoring.

Library Facilities 112,920 volumes (5,114 in health); 714 periodical subscriptions (72 health-care related).

BACCALAUREATE PROGRAMS

Degree BSN

Available Programs Generic Baccalaureate; RN Baccalaureate.

Site Options *Distance Learning:* Escanaba, MI; Alpena, MI; Petoskey, MI.

Study Options Full-time and part-time.

Program Entrance Requirements Minimum overall college GPA of 2.5, transcript of college record, CPR certification, health insurance, high school biology, high school chemistry, high school transcript, immunizations, minimum high school GPA of 2.0, minimum GPA in nursing prerequisites of 2.5, professional liability insurance/malpractice insurance, prerequisite course work. Transfer students are accepted. **Standardized tests** *Required:* ACT, TOEFL for international students. **Application** *Deadline:* 8/15 (freshmen), rolling (transfer). *Notification:* continuous (freshmen). *Application fee:* $20.

Advanced Placement Credit given for nursing courses completed elsewhere dependent upon specific evaluations.

Contact MaryAnne Shannon, Chair, Department of Nursing, Lake Superior State University, 650 West Easterday Avenue, Sault Sainte Marie, MI 49783. *Telephone:* 906-635-2147. *Fax:* 906-635-2266. *E-mail:* mshannon@lssu.edu.

Madonna University
College of Nursing and Health
Livonia, Michigan

http://www.madonna.edu

Founded in 1947

DEGREES • BSN • MSN • MSN/MSBA

Nursing Program Faculty 36 (17% with doctorates).

Baccalaureate Enrollment 348

Women 92% **Men** 8% **Minority** 15% **International** 1% **Part-time** 30%

Graduate Enrollment 42

Women 90% **Men** 10% **Minority** 5% **International** 5% **Part-time** 90%

Nursing Student Activities Sigma Theta Tau, Student Nurses' Association.

Nursing Student Resources Academic advising; academic or career counseling; assistance for students with disabilities; bookstore; campus computer network; career placement assistance; computer lab; computer-assisted instruction; e-mail services; interactive nursing skills videos; Internet; learning resource lab; library services; nursing audiovisuals; remedial services; resume preparation assistance; skills, simulation, or other laboratory; tutoring.

Library Facilities 199,144 volumes (106,387 in health, 6,290 in nursing); 1,679 periodical subscriptions (891 health-care related).

BACCALAUREATE PROGRAMS

Degree BSN

Available Programs ADN to Baccalaureate; Accelerated RN Baccalaureate; Baccalaureate for Second Degree; Generic Baccalaureate; LPN to RN Baccalaureate; RN Baccalaureate.

Site Options *Distance Learning:* Orchard Lake, MI; Gaylord, MI.

Study Options Full-time and part-time.

Program Entrance Requirements Minimum overall college GPA of 2.5, transcript of college record, CPR certification, health exam, high school biology, high school chemistry, 1 year of high school math, high school transcript, immunizations, minimum high school GPA of 2.75, minimum GPA in nursing prerequisites of 2.5, professional liability insurance/malpractice insurance. Transfer students are accepted. **Standardized tests** *Required:* SAT or ACT, TOEFL for international students. **Application** *Deadline:* rolling (freshmen), rolling (transfer). *Notification:* continuous (freshmen). *Application fee:* $25.

Advanced Placement Credit by examination available. Credit given for nursing courses completed elsewhere dependent upon specific evaluations.

Expenses (2004–05) *Tuition:* full-time $9600; part-time $362 per credit hour. *International tuition:* $12,000 full-time. *Room and board:* $5546; room only: $2550 per academic year. *Required fees:* full-time $220; part-time $110 per term.

Financial Aid 50% of baccalaureate students in nursing programs received some form of financial aid in 2003–04.

Contact Ms. Linda Smith, Nursing Admissions Counselor, College of Nursing and Health, Madonna University, 36600 Schoolcraft Road, Livonia, MI 48150-1173. *Telephone:* 734-432-5718. *Fax:* 734-432-5463. *E-mail:* lsmith@madonna.edu.

GRADUATE PROGRAMS

Expenses (2004–05) *Tuition:* full-time $6624; part-time $368 per credit hour. *International tuition:* $8280 full-time. *Room and board:* $5546; room only: $2505 per academic year. *Required fees:* full-time $260; part-time $130 per term.

Financial Aid 14% of graduate students in nursing programs received some form of financial aid in 2003–04.

Contact Dr. Nancy O'Connor, Chair of Graduate Nursing Program, College of Nursing and Health, Madonna University, 36600 Schoolcraft Road, Livonia, MI 48150-1173. *Telephone:* 734-432-5461. *Fax:* 734-432-5463. *E-mail:* noconnor@madonna.edu.

MASTER'S DEGREE PROGRAM

Degrees MSN; MSN/MSBA

Madonna University (continued)

Available Programs Accelerated AD/RN to Master's; Accelerated RN to Master's; Master's.

Concentrations Available Nursing administration. *Clinical nurse specialist programs in:* adult health. *Nurse practitioner programs in:* primary care.

Site Options *Distance Learning:* Orchard Lake, MI; Alpena, MI.

Study Options Full-time and part-time.

Program Entrance Requirements Computer literacy, minimum overall college GPA of 3.0, transcript of college record, CPR certification, immunizations, interview, 2 letters of recommendation, physical assessment course, professional liability insurance/malpractice insurance, resume, statistics course.

Degree Requirements 45 total credit hours.

POST-MASTER'S PROGRAM

Areas of Study Nursing education. *Clinical nurse specialist programs in:* adult health. *Nurse practitioner programs in:* primary care.

CONTINUING EDUCATION PROGRAM

Contact Ms. Susan Hasenau, Coordinator of Nursing Continuing Education, College of Nursing and Health, Madonna University, 36600 Schoolcraft Road, Livonia, MI 48150-1173. *Telephone:* 734-432-5863. *Fax:* 734-432-5463. *E-mail:* shasenau@madonna.edu.

Michigan State University

College of Nursing
East Lansing, Michigan

http://www.nursing.msu.edu/

Founded in 1855

DEGREES • BSN • MSN • PHD

Nursing Student Activities Sigma Theta Tau, Student Nurses' Association.

Nursing Student Resources Academic advising; academic or career counseling; computer lab; Internet; library services; nursing audiovisuals; remedial services; skills, simulation, or other laboratory; tutoring.

Library Facilities 4.4 million volumes; 29,470 periodical subscriptions.

■ Michigan State University (MSU) is a leader in community-based, technologically advanced nursing education. MSU offers highly competitive Bachelor of Science in Nursing (BSN) and Master of Science in Nursing (MSN) degree programs. Doctoral study (PhD), focused on health status and health outcomes, prepares clinical nurse researchers. Post-master's (PMSN) and postdoctoral programs are also available. Community-based clinical experiences are an essential component of nursing education at MSU, with many faculty members in active practice. International nursing education opportunities in Mexico, Ghana, and London further enhance the learning environment. Federally funded faculty research foci include chronic conditions and healthy families and communities.

BACCALAUREATE PROGRAMS

Degree BSN

Available Programs Accelerated Baccalaureate for Second Degree; Generic Baccalaureate; RN Baccalaureate.

Program Entrance Requirements Minimum overall college GPA of 2.5, letters of recommendation, minimum GPA in nursing prerequisites of 2.2, prerequisite course work. Transfer students are accepted. **Standardized tests** *Required:* SAT or ACT, TOEFL for international students. **Application** *Deadline:* rolling (freshmen). *Notification:* continuous until 9/1 (freshmen). *Application fee:* $35.

Contact Sharon Graver, Undergraduate Adviser, College of Nursing, Michigan State University, A-117 Life Sciences Building, East Lansing, MI 48824-1317. *Telephone:* 517-353-4827. *Fax:* 517-432-8251. *E-mail:* graver@msu.edu.

GRADUATE PROGRAMS

Financial Aid 33 fellowships (averaging $3,261 per year), 5 research assistantships (averaging $12,326 per year) were awarded; Federal Work-Study also available.

Contact Ms. Regina Traylor, Interim Director, Student Affairs, College of Nursing, Michigan State University, A-117 Life Sciences Building, East Lansing, MI 48824-1317. *Telephone:* 517-353-4827. *E-mail:* traylor1@msu.edu.

MASTER'S DEGREE PROGRAM

Degree MSN

Available Programs Master's.

Concentrations Available Nursing education. *Nurse practitioner programs in:* adult health, family health, gerontology.

Study Options Part-time.

Program Entrance Requirements Minimum overall college GPA of 3.0, written essay, 3 letters of recommendation, resume, statistics course, GRE General Test. *Application deadline:* For fall admission, 11/1. *Application fee:* $50.

Degree Requirements 47 total credit hours.

POST-MASTER'S PROGRAM

Areas of Study Nursing education. *Nurse practitioner programs in:* adult health, family health, gerontology.

DOCTORAL DEGREE PROGRAM

Degree PhD

Available Programs Doctorate; Post-Baccalaureate Doctorate.

Areas of Study Family health, health promotion/disease prevention, human health and illness, individualized study, nursing research.

Program Entrance Requirements Minimum overall college GPA of 3.5, interview by faculty committee, 3 letters of recommendation, statistics course, vita, GRE General Test. *Application deadline:* For fall admission, 11/1. *Application fee:* $50.

Degree Requirements 61 total credit hours, dissertation, oral exam, written exam, residency.

POSTDOCTORAL PROGRAM

Areas of Study Nursing research.

Postdoctoral Program Contact Dr. Audrey G. Gift, Professor and Associate Dean for Research and Doctoral Program, College of Nursing, Michigan State University, A-212 Life Sciences Building, East Lansing, MI 48824-1317. *Telephone:* 517-432-6220. *E-mail:* agift@msu.edu.

CONTINUING EDUCATION PROGRAM

Contact Katie Kessler, Coordinator of Professional Education, College of Nursing, Michigan State University, A-112 Life Sciences Building, East Lansing, MI 48824-1317. *Telephone:* 517-355-8539. *Fax:* 517-432-8131. *E-mail:* kessle24@msu.edu.

See full description on page 522.

Northern Michigan University

College of Nursing and Allied Health Science
Marquette, Michigan

http://www.nmu.edu/departments/nursing.html

Founded in 1899

DEGREES • BSN • MSN

Nursing Program Faculty 17 (50% with doctorates).

Baccalaureate Enrollment 185

Women 92% **Men** 8% **Minority** 6% **Part-time** 10%

Graduate Enrollment 23
Women 79% **Men** 21% **Minority** 9% **International** 4% **Part-time** 100%

Nursing Student Activities Sigma Theta Tau, Student Nurses' Association.

Nursing Student Resources Academic advising; academic or career counseling; assistance for students with disabilities; bookstore; campus computer network; career placement assistance; computer lab; computer-assisted instruction; e-mail services; employment services for current students; housing assistance; interactive nursing skills videos; Internet; learning resource lab; library services; nursing audiovisuals; other; paid internships; remedial services; resume preparation assistance; skills, simulation, or other laboratory; tutoring.

Library Facilities 592,689 volumes (34,466 in health, 3,608 in nursing); 2,588 periodical subscriptions (173 health-care related).

BACCALAUREATE PROGRAMS

Degree BSN

Available Programs ADN to Baccalaureate; Accelerated Baccalaureate; Accelerated LPN to Baccalaureate; Generic Baccalaureate; LPN to RN Baccalaureate.

Study Options Full-time and part-time.

Program Entrance Requirements Minimum overall college GPA of 2.75, transcript of college record, CPR certification, health exam, high school transcript, immunizations, minimum GPA in nursing prerequisites of 2.0, prerequisite course work. Transfer students are accepted. **Standardized tests** *Required:* SAT or ACT, TOEFL for international students. **Application** *Deadline:* rolling (freshmen), rolling (transfer). *Notification:* continuous (freshmen). *Application fee:* $30.

Advanced Placement Credit by examination available. Credit given for nursing courses completed elsewhere dependent upon specific evaluations.

Expenses (2004–05) *Tuition, state resident:* full-time $2388; part-time $199 per credit hour. *Tuition, nonresident:* full-time $4092; part-time $341 per credit hour. *International tuition:* $4092 full-time. *Room and board:* $6182 per academic year. *Required fees:* full-time $558.

Financial Aid 85% of baccalaureate students in nursing programs received some form of financial aid in 2003–04.

Contact Dr. Kerri Durnell Schuiling, Associate Director of BSN/MSN Programs, College of Nursing and Allied Health Science, Northern Michigan University, 1401 Presque Isle Avenue, 2302 New Science Facility, Marquette, MI 49855. *Telephone:* 906-227-2834. *Fax:* 906-227-1658. *E-mail:* kschuili@nmu.edu.

GRADUATE PROGRAMS

Expenses (2004–05) *Tuition, state resident:* full-time $2115; part-time $235 per credit hour. *Tuition, nonresident:* full-time $3267; part-time $363 per credit hour. *Room and board:* $6182 per academic year. *Required fees:* full-time $558.

Financial Aid 90% of graduate students in nursing programs received some form of financial aid in 2003–04. Career-related internships or fieldwork, Federal Work-Study, institutionally sponsored loans, and unspecified assistantships available. Aid available to part-time students. *Financial aid application deadline:* 3/1.

Contact Prof. Mary A. Wallace, Coordinator of MSN Program, College of Nursing and Allied Health Science, Northern Michigan University, 2310 New Science Facility, Marquette, MI 49855. *Telephone:* 906-227-2487. *Fax:* 906-227-1658. *E-mail:* mwallace@nmu.eduh.

MASTER'S DEGREE PROGRAM

Degree MSN

Available Programs Master's.

Concentrations Available *Nurse practitioner programs in:* family health.

Study Options Part-time.

Program Entrance Requirements Clinical experience, computer literacy, minimum overall college GPA of 3.0, transcript of college record, CPR certification, written essay, immunizations, 2 letters of recommendation, physical assessment course, professional liability insurance/malpractice insurance, GRE General Test. *Application deadline:* For spring admission, 11/1. Applications are processed on a rolling basis. *Application fee:* $25.

Degree Requirements 45 total credit hours, thesis or project, comprehensive exam.

POST-MASTER'S PROGRAM

Areas of Study *Nurse practitioner programs in:* family health.

CONTINUING EDUCATION PROGRAM

Contact Mr. Paul T. McKelvey, Director of Continuing Education and Sponsored Programs, College of Nursing and Allied Health Science, Northern Michigan University, 409 Cohodas Administration Center, Marquette, MI 49855. *Telephone:* 906-227-2302. *Fax:* 906-227-2308. *E-mail:* pmckelve@nmu.edu.

Oakland University

School of Nursing
Rochester, Michigan

http://www2.oakland.edu/nursing

Founded in 1957

DEGREES • BSN • MSN

Nursing Program Faculty 44 (50% with doctorates).

Baccalaureate Enrollment 462
Women 89% **Men** 11% **Minority** 12% **Part-time** 29%

Graduate Enrollment 123
Women 79% **Men** 21% **Minority** 11% **International** 1% **Part-time** 35%

Nursing Student Activities Nursing Honor Society, Sigma Theta Tau, Student Nurses' Association.

Nursing Student Resources Academic advising; academic or career counseling; assistance for students with disabilities; bookstore; campus computer network; career placement assistance; computer lab; computer-assisted instruction; e-mail services; employment services for current students; externships; housing assistance; interactive nursing skills videos; Internet; learning resource lab; library services; nursing audiovisuals; paid internships; placement services for program completers; remedial services; resume preparation assistance; skills, simulation, or other laboratory; tutoring; unpaid internships.

Library Facilities 12,652 volumes in health, 2,780 volumes in nursing; 375 periodical subscriptions health-care related.

BACCALAUREATE PROGRAMS

Degree BSN

Available Programs Generic Baccalaureate; RN Baccalaureate.

Site Options Royal Oak, MI.

Study Options Full-time and part-time.

Program Entrance Requirements Minimum overall college GPA of 3.0, transcript of college record, CPR certification, health exam, high school biology, high school chemistry, 2 years high school math, 1 year of high school science, high school transcript, immunizations, minimum high school GPA of 3.0, minimum GPA in nursing prerequisites of 3.0, professional liability insurance/malpractice insurance, prerequisite course work. Transfer students are accepted. **Standardized tests** *Required:* TOEFL for international students. ***Placement:*** *Required:* ACT. **Application** *Deadline:* rolling (freshmen), rolling (transfer). *Notification:* continuous (freshmen). *Application fee:* $40.

Advanced Placement Credit given for nursing courses completed elsewhere dependent upon specific evaluations.

Expenses (2003–04) *Tuition, state resident:* full-time $4511; part-time $174 per credit hour. *Tuition, nonresident:* full-time $7618; part-time $382 per credit hour. *Room and board:* $5540 per academic year. *Required fees:* full-time $400; part-time $80 per term.

Financial Aid 65% of baccalaureate students in nursing programs received some form of financial aid in 2002–03. *Gift aid (need-based):* Federal Pell, FSEOG, state, private, college/university gift aid from institutional funds. *Loans:* Federal Direct (Subsidized and Unsubsidized Stafford PLUS), Perkins, state, alternative loans. *Work-Study:* Federal Work-Study, part-time campus jobs. *Application deadline (priority):* 2/15.

Oakland University (continued)

Contact Joann K. Burrington, Special Projects Coordinator, School of Nursing, Oakland University, 428 O'Dowd Hall, Rochester, MI 48309-4401. *Telephone:* 248-370-4065. *Fax:* 248-370-4279. *E-mail:* burringt@oakland.edu.

GRADUATE PROGRAMS

Expenses (2003–04) *Tuition, state resident:* full-time $7600; part-time $293 per credit hour. *Tuition, nonresident:* full-time $13,870; part-time $533 per credit hour. *International tuition:* $13,870 full-time. *Required fees:* full-time $60; part-time $30 per term.

Financial Aid 60% of graduate students in nursing programs received some form of financial aid in 2002–03. Federal Work-Study, institutionally sponsored loans, and tuition waivers (full) available. *Financial aid application deadline:* 3/1.

Contact Sarah Mullin, Academic Adviser, School of Nursing, Oakland University, 444 O'Dowd Hall, Rochester, MI 48309-4401. *Telephone:* 248-370-4082. *Fax:* 248-370-2996. *E-mail:* mullin@oakland.edu.

MASTER'S DEGREE PROGRAM

Degree MSN

Available Programs Master's.

Concentrations Available Nurse anesthesia; nursing education. *Nurse practitioner programs in:* adult health, family health, gerontology.

Site Options Royal Oak, MI.

Study Options Full-time and part-time.

Program Entrance Requirements Clinical experience, minimum overall college GPA of 3.0, transcript of college record, CPR certification, written essay, immunizations, interview, 2 letters of recommendation, professional liability insurance/malpractice insurance, prerequisite course work, GRE General Test. *Application fee:* $30.

Advanced Placement Credit given for nursing courses completed elsewhere dependent upon specific evaluations.

Degree Requirements 45 total credit hours, thesis or project.

POST-MASTER'S PROGRAM

Areas of Study Nurse anesthesia; nursing education. *Nurse practitioner programs in:* adult health, family health, gerontology.

CONTINUING EDUCATION PROGRAM

Contact Dr. Pamela Marin, Director, Center for Professional Development, School of Nursing, Oakland University, 444 O'Dowd Hall, Rochester, MI 48309-4401. *Telephone:* 248-370-4013. *Fax:* 248-370-4279. *E-mail:* marin@oakland.edu.

Saginaw Valley State University

Crystal M. Lange College of Nursing and Health Sciences
University Center, Michigan

http://www.svsu.edu/acadprog/nhs/

Founded in 1963

DEGREES • BSN • MSN

Nursing Program Faculty 12 (50% with doctorates).

Nursing Student Activities Sigma Theta Tau, Student Nurses' Association.

Nursing Student Resources Academic advising; academic or career counseling; assistance for students with disabilities; bookstore; campus computer network; career placement assistance; computer lab; computer-assisted instruction; e-mail services; externships; interactive nursing skills videos; Internet; learning resource lab; library services; nursing audiovisuals; remedial services; resume preparation assistance; skills, simulation, or other laboratory; tutoring.

Library Facilities 226,952 volumes; 11,512 periodical subscriptions.

BACCALAUREATE PROGRAMS

Degree BSN

Available Programs Accelerated Baccalaureate for Second Degree; Baccalaureate for Second Degree; Generic Baccalaureate; RN Baccalaureate.

Site Options *Distance Learning:* Tawas, MI; Cass City, MI; Mt. Pleasant, MI.

Study Options Full-time and part-time.

Program Entrance Requirements Minimum overall college GPA of 2.5, transcript of college record, CPR certification, written essay, health exam, immunizations, interview, minimum GPA in nursing prerequisites of 2.5, professional liability insurance/malpractice insurance, prerequisite course work. Transfer students are accepted. **Standardized tests** *Required:* ACT, TOEFL for international students. **Application** *Deadline:* rolling (freshmen), rolling (transfer). *Application fee:* $25.

Advanced Placement Credit by examination available. Credit given for nursing courses completed elsewhere dependent upon specific evaluations.

Contact Ms. Ruth Gulliver, Administrative Secretary, Crystal M. Lange College of Nursing and Health Sciences, Saginaw Valley State University, Wickes 280, 7400 Bay Road, Saginaw Valley State University, University Center, MI 48710-0001. *Telephone:* 989-964-4145 Ext. 4145. *Fax:* 989-964-4024. *E-mail:* reg@svsu.edu.

GRADUATE PROGRAMS

Financial Aid Fellowships, research assistantships, Federal Work-Study available.

Contact Dr. Margaret Flatt, Assistant Dean, Crystal M. Lange College of Nursing and Health Sciences, Saginaw Valley State University, 7400 Bay Road, Saginaw Valley State University, University Center, MI 48710-0001. *Telephone:* 989-964-4145 Ext. 4145. *Fax:* 989-964-4024. *E-mail:* flatt@svsu.edu.

MASTER'S DEGREE PROGRAM

Degree MSN

Available Programs Master's; RN to Master's.

Concentrations Available Nursing administration; nursing education; nursing informatics. *Nurse practitioner programs in:* family health.

Study Options Full-time and part-time.

Program Entrance Requirements Clinical experience, minimum overall college GPA of 3.0, transcript of college record, written essay, interview, 3 letters of recommendation, professional liability insurance/malpractice insurance, resume, statistics course, GRE. *Application deadline:* Applications are processed on a rolling basis. *Application fee:* $25.

Advanced Placement Credit given for nursing courses completed elsewhere dependent upon specific evaluations.

Degree Requirements 39 total credit hours, thesis or project.

POST-MASTER'S PROGRAM

Areas of Study Nursing administration; nursing education; nursing informatics. *Nurse practitioner programs in:* family health.

CONTINUING EDUCATION PROGRAM

Contact CE Coordinator, Crystal M. Lange College of Nursing and Health Sciences, Saginaw Valley State University, 7400 Bay Road, Saginaw Valley State University, University Center, MI 48710. *Telephone:* 989-964-4145.

Spring Arbor University

Program in Nursing
Spring Arbor, Michigan

http://www.arbor.edu/bsn

Founded in 1873

DEGREE • BSN

Nursing Program Faculty 21 (10% with doctorates).

Baccalaureate Enrollment 38

Nursing Student Resources Academic advising; campus computer network; Internet; library services; nursing audiovisuals; other.

Library Facilities 100,094 volumes (1,000 in health, 350 in nursing); 667 periodical subscriptions (25 health-care related).

BACCALAUREATE PROGRAMS

Degree BSN

Available Programs ADN to Baccalaureate.

Site Options Battle Creek, MI; Jackson, MI; Toledo, OH.

Program Entrance Requirements Minimum overall college GPA of 2.5, transcript of college record, written essay, high school biology, high school chemistry, 1 year of high school math, 2 years high school science, high school transcript, minimum GPA in nursing prerequisites of 2.5, RN licensure. **Standardized tests** *Required:* SAT or ACT, TOEFL for international students. *Recommended:* ACT. **Application** *Deadline:* 8/1 (freshmen), rolling (transfer). *Notification:* continuous (freshmen). *Application fee:* $50.

Expenses (2003–04) *Tuition:* full-time $11,800.

Financial Aid 80% of baccalaureate students in nursing programs received some form of financial aid in 2002–03. *Gift aid (need-based):* Federal Pell, FSEOG, state, private, college/university gift aid from institutional funds. *Loans:* FFEL (Subsidized and Unsubsidized Stafford PLUS), Perkins, state, MI-Loan Program, alternative loans. *Work-Study:* Federal Work-Study, part-time campus jobs. *Application deadline (priority):* 3/1.

Contact Mrs. Cindy E. Meredith, RN, Director of Nursing, Program in Nursing, Spring Arbor University, Spring Arbor University—Suite #3, 106 East Main Street, Spring Arbor, MI 49283-9799. *Telephone:* 517-750-6344. *Fax:* 517-750-6602. *E-mail:* cemered@arbor.edu.

University of Detroit Mercy
McAuley School of Nursing
Detroit, Michigan

http://www.udmercy.edu/healthprof/nursing/

Founded in 1877

DEGREES • BSN • MSN

Nursing Program Faculty 28.

Baccalaureate Enrollment 630

Women 93% **Men** 7% **Minority** 17% **International** 3% **Part-time** 76%

Graduate Enrollment 37

Women 97% **Men** 3% **Minority** 28% **Part-time** 89%

Nursing Student Activities Sigma Theta Tau, Student Nurses' Association.

Nursing Student Resources Academic advising; academic or career counseling; bookstore; campus computer network; career placement assistance; computer lab; computer-assisted instruction; e-mail services; Internet; learning resource lab; library services; nursing audiovisuals; other; paid internships; placement services for program completers; remedial services; resume preparation assistance; skills, simulation, or other laboratory; tutoring.

Library Facilities 21,436 volumes in health, 3,100 volumes in nursing; 9,340 periodical subscriptions (585 health-care related).

BACCALAUREATE PROGRAMS

Degree BSN

Available Programs Generic Baccalaureate; RN Baccalaureate.

Site Options Dearborn, MI; Wayne, MI; Royal Oak, MI.

Study Options Full-time and part-time.

Program Entrance Requirements Minimum overall college GPA of 2.5, transcript of college record, CPR certification, health exam, health insurance, high school biology, high school chemistry, 2 years high school math, 2 years high school science, high school transcript, immunizations, minimum high school GPA of 2.5, minimum GPA in nursing prerequisites of 2.5, prerequisite course work. Transfer students are accepted. **Standardized tests** *Required:* SAT or ACT. **Application** *Deadline:* 7/1 (freshmen), 8/15 (transfer). *Notification:* continuous until 9/2 (freshmen). *Application fee:* $25.

Advanced Placement Credit given for nursing courses completed elsewhere dependent upon specific evaluations.

Financial Aid 38% of baccalaureate students in nursing programs received some form of financial aid in 2002–03. *Gift aid (need-based):* Federal Pell, FSEOG, state, private, college/university gift aid from institutional funds. *Loans:* Federal Nursing Student Loans, FFEL (Subsidized and Unsubsidized Stafford PLUS), Perkins, college/university. *Work-Study:* Federal Work-Study, part-time campus jobs. *Application deadline (priority):* 3/1.

Contact Denise Williams, Admissions Office, McAuley School of Nursing, University of Detroit Mercy, PO Box 19900, Detroit, MI 48219-0900. *Telephone:* 313-993-1245. *Fax:* 313-993-3325. *E-mail:* admissions@udmercy.edu.

GRADUATE PROGRAMS

Financial Aid 22% of graduate students in nursing programs received some form of financial aid in 2002–03.

Contact Janet Bairdi, McAuley School of Nursing, University of Detroit Mercy, PO Box 19900, Detroit, MI 48219-0900. *Telephone:* 313-993-6423. *Fax:* 313-993-6175. *E-mail:* baiardjm@udmercy.edu.

MASTER'S DEGREE PROGRAM

Degree MSN

Available Programs Accelerated AD/RN to Master's; Master's; Master's for Nurses with Non-Nursing Degrees.

Concentrations Available Nursing administration. *Nurse practitioner programs in:* family health.

Study Options Full-time and part-time.

Program Entrance Requirements Clinical experience, minimum overall college GPA of 3.0, transcript of college record, CPR certification, immunizations, interview, 3 letters of recommendation, resume.

Degree Requirements 50 total credit hours.

POST-MASTER'S PROGRAM

Areas of Study Nursing administration. *Nurse practitioner programs in:* family health.

University of Michigan
School of Nursing
Ann Arbor, Michigan

http://www.nursing.umich.edu

Founded in 1817

DEGREES • BSN • MS • MS/MBA • MS/MPH • PHD

Nursing Program Faculty 154 (56% with doctorates).

Baccalaureate Enrollment 631

Women 91% **Men** 9% **Minority** 13% **International** 1% **Part-time** 18%

Graduate Enrollment 234

Women 94% **Men** 6% **Minority** 13% **International** 7% **Part-time** 55%

Nursing Student Activities Nursing Honor Society, Sigma Theta Tau, Student Nurses' Association, nursing club.

Nursing Student Resources Academic advising; academic or career counseling; assistance for students with disabilities; bookstore; campus computer network; career placement assistance; computer lab; computer-assisted instruction; daycare for children of students; e-mail services; employment services for current students; externships; housing assistance; interactive nursing skills videos; Internet; learning resource lab; library services; nursing audiovisuals; placement services for program completers; resume preparation assistance; skills, simulation, or other laboratory; tutoring.

Library Facilities 8 million volumes (1.2 million in nursing); 67,554 periodical subscriptions.

BACCALAUREATE PROGRAMS

Degree BSN

Available Programs Accelerated Baccalaureate for Second Degree; Generic Baccalaureate; RN Baccalaureate.

Site Options *Distance Learning:* Kalamazoo, MI; Traverse City, MI.

Study Options Full-time and part-time.

University of Michigan (continued)

Program Entrance Requirements Minimum overall college GPA of 3.0, transcript of college record, written essay, high school chemistry, 2 years high school math, 2 years high school science, high school transcript, minimum high school GPA of 3.0, prerequisite course work. Transfer students are accepted. **Standardized tests** *Required:* SAT or ACT, TOEFL for international students. *Required for some:* SAT Subject Tests, SAT II Writing Tests. **Application** *Deadline:* 2/1 (freshmen), 3/1 (transfer). *Notification:* continuous until 4/1 (freshmen). *Application fee:* $40.

Advanced Placement Credit given for nursing courses completed elsewhere dependent upon specific evaluations.

Expenses (2004–05) *Tuition, state resident:* full-time $8968; part-time $670 per contact hour. *Tuition, nonresident:* full-time $27,584; part-time $1445 per contact hour. *International tuition:* $27,584 full-time. *Room and board:* $14,060 per academic year. *Required fees:* part-time $100 per term.

Financial Aid 60% of baccalaureate students in nursing programs received some form of financial aid in 2003–04. *Gift aid (need-based):* Federal Pell, FSEOG, state, private, college/university gift aid from institutional funds. *Loans:* Federal Nursing Student Loans, Federal Direct (Subsidized and Unsubsidized Stafford PLUS), Perkins, state, college/university, MI-Loan Program, Health Professions Student Loans (HPSL). *Work-Study:* Federal Work-Study, part-time campus jobs. *Application deadline:* 4/30 (priority: 2/15).

Contact Sheila Pantlind, Admissions Counselor, School of Nursing, University of Michigan, 1220 Student Activities Building, Ann Arbor, MI 48109. *Telephone:* 734-647-1443. *Fax:* 734-936-0740. *E-mail:* pantlin@umich.edu.

GRADUATE PROGRAMS

Expenses (2004–05) *Tuition, area resident:* full-time $13,820; part-time $1046 per contact hour. *Tuition, state resident:* full-time $13,820. *Tuition, nonresident:* full-time $27,984; part-time $1841 per contact hour. *International tuition:* $27,984 full-time. *Room and board:* $19,200; room only: $9600 per academic year. *Required fees:* full-time $200.

Financial Aid 80% of graduate students in nursing programs received some form of financial aid in 2003–04. 15 research assistantships with full and partial tuition reimbursements available, 28 teaching assistantships with full tuition reimbursements available were awarded; fellowships with full and partial tuition reimbursements available, Federal Work-Study, institutionally sponsored loans, scholarships, traineeships, and tuition waivers (partial) also available. Aid available to part-time students.

Contact Dr. Carol J. Loveland-Cherry, Professor and Executive Associate Dean, Academic Affairs, School of Nursing, University of Michigan, 400 North Ingalls Building, Room 1154, Ann Arbor, MI 48109-0482. *Telephone:* 734-764-7188. *Fax:* 734-647-1419. *E-mail:* loveland@umich.edu.

MASTER'S DEGREE PROGRAM

Degrees MS; MS/MBA; MS/MPH

Available Programs Accelerated RN to Master's; Master's; RN to Master's.

Concentrations Available Health-care administration; nurse-midwifery; nursing administration; nursing informatics. *Clinical nurse specialist programs in:* community health, gerontology, home health care, medical-surgical, occupational health, psychiatric/mental health. *Nurse practitioner programs in:* acute care, adult health, family health, gerontology, pediatric, primary care, psychiatric/mental health.

Study Options Full-time and part-time.

Program Entrance Requirements Computer literacy, minimum overall college GPA of 3.0, transcript of college record, written essay, interview, 3 letters of recommendation, resume, GRE General Test. *Application deadline:* For fall admission, 2/1 (priority date); for winter admission, 5/1 (priority date); for spring admission, 11/1 (priority date). Applications are processed on a rolling basis. *Application fee:* $55.

Advanced Placement Credit given for nursing courses completed elsewhere dependent upon specific evaluations.

Degree Requirements 36 total credit hours, thesis or project.

POST-MASTER'S PROGRAM

Areas of Study Health-care administration; nurse-midwifery; nursing administration; nursing informatics. *Clinical nurse specialist programs in:* community health, gerontology, home health care, medical-surgical, occupational health, psychiatric/mental health, women's health. *Nurse practitioner programs in:* acute care, adult health, family health, gerontology, pediatric, primary care, psychiatric/mental health, women's health.

DOCTORAL DEGREE PROGRAM

Degree PhD

Available Programs Doctorate; Post-Baccalaureate Doctorate.

Areas of Study Aging, bio-behavioral research, biology of health and illness, health policy, health promotion/disease prevention, health-care systems, individualized study, information systems, neuro-behavior, nursing administration, nursing policy, nursing research, nursing science, women's health.

Program Entrance Requirements Minimum overall college GPA of 3.0, interview, 3 letters of recommendation, scholarly papers, vita, writing sample, GRE General Test. *Application deadline:* For fall admission, 2/1 (priority date); for winter admission, 5/1 (priority date); for spring admission, 11/1 (priority date). Applications are processed on a rolling basis. *Application fee:* $55.

Degree Requirements 50 total credit hours, dissertation, oral exam, written exam, residency.

POSTDOCTORAL PROGRAM

Areas of Study Aging, gerontology, health promotion/disease prevention, individualized study, neuro-behavior, vulnerable population, women's health.

Postdoctoral Program Contact Dr. Richard Redman, Director, Doctoral and Postdoctoral Studies, School of Nursing, University of Michigan, 400 North Ingalls Building, Room 1305, Ann Arbor, MI 48109-0482. *Telephone:* 734-764-9454. *Fax:* 734-763-6668. *E-mail:* rwr@umich.edu.

See full description on page 564.

University of Michigan–Flint

Department of Nursing
Flint, Michigan

http://www.umflint.edu/nur

Founded in 1956

DEGREES • BSN • MSN

Nursing Program Faculty 47 (17% with doctorates).

Baccalaureate Enrollment 267
Women 90% **Men** 10% **Minority** 12% **Part-time** 36%

Graduate Enrollment 22
Women 95% **Men** 5% **Minority** 9% **Part-time** 100%

Nursing Student Activities Nursing Honor Society, Sigma Theta Tau, Student Nurses' Association.

Nursing Student Resources Academic advising; academic or career counseling; assistance for students with disabilities; bookstore; campus computer network; career placement assistance; computer lab; computer-assisted instruction; daycare for children of students; e-mail services; employment services for current students; externships; interactive nursing skills videos; Internet; library services; nursing audiovisuals; remedial services; resume preparation assistance; skills, simulation, or other laboratory; tutoring.

Library Facilities 253,182 volumes (8,264 in health, 5,330 in nursing); 900 periodical subscriptions (210 health-care related).

BACCALAUREATE PROGRAMS

Degree BSN

Available Programs Generic Baccalaureate; RN Baccalaureate.

Site Options *Distance Learning:* Flint, MI.

Study Options Full-time.

Program Entrance Requirements Minimum overall college GPA of 2.75, transcript of college record, CPR certification, written essay, health exam, health insurance, high school transcript, immunizations, 2 letters of recommendation, minimum GPA in nursing prerequisites of 2.75, prerequisite course work. Transfer students are accepted. **Standardized tests** *Required:* SAT or ACT, TOEFL for international students. **Application** *Deadline:* 11/1 (freshmen), 8/19 (transfer). *Notification:* continuous (freshmen). *Application fee:* $30.

Advanced Placement Credit given for nursing courses completed elsewhere dependent upon specific evaluations.

Expenses (2004–05) *Tuition, state resident:* full-time $5862; part-time $244 per credit hour. *Tuition, nonresident:* full-time $11,724; part-time $489 per contact hour. *International tuition:* $11,724 full-time. *Required fees:* full-time $296; part-time $231 per term.

Financial Aid 58% of baccalaureate students in nursing programs received some form of financial aid in 2003–04.

Contact Ms. Lynn M. Kruse, Department of Nursing, Department of Nursing, University of Michigan–Flint, 2180 William S. White Building, 303 East Kearsley, Flint, MI 48502-1950. *Telephone:* 810-762-3420. *Fax:* 810-766-6851. *E-mail:* nursing@list.flint.umich.edu.

GRADUATE PROGRAMS

Expenses (2004–05) *Tuition, state resident:* part-time $346 per credit hour. *Tuition, nonresident:* part-time $519 per credit hour. *Required fees:* part-time $116 per term.

Financial Aid 55% of graduate students in nursing programs received some form of financial aid in 2003–04.

Contact Margaret A. Hathaway, Administrative Assistant, Department of Nursing, University of Michigan–Flint, 2180 William S. White Building, 303 East Kearsley, Flint, MI 48502-1950. *Telephone:* 810-762-3420. *Fax:* 810-766-6851. *E-mail:* nursing@list.flint.umich.edu.

MASTER'S DEGREE PROGRAM

Degree MSN

Available Programs Master's; RN to Master's.

Concentrations Available *Nurse practitioner programs in:* adult health, family health, psychiatric/mental health.

Site Options *Distance Learning:* Flint, MI.

Study Options Part-time.

Program Entrance Requirements Minimum overall college GPA of 3.0, transcript of college record, CPR certification, written essay, immunizations, interview, 3 letters of recommendation, physical assessment course, professional liability insurance/malpractice insurance, prerequisite course work, resume, statistics course.

Advanced Placement Credit by examination available. Credit given for nursing courses completed elsewhere dependent upon specific evaluations.

Degree Requirements 39 total credit hours, thesis or project.

CONTINUING EDUCATION PROGRAM

Contact Ms. Lynn M. Kruse, Secretary, Nursing Development and Research, Department of Nursing, University of Michigan–Flint, 2180 William S. White Building, 303 East Kearsley, Flint, MI 48502-1950. *Telephone:* 810-762-3420. *Fax:* 810-766-6851. *E-mail:* nursing@list.flint.umich.edu.

University of Phoenix–Metro Detroit Campus

College of Health and Human Services
Southfield, Michigan

DEGREES • BSN • MSN • MSN/MBA

Nursing Program Faculty 36 (17% with doctorates).

Baccalaureate Enrollment 94
Women 96% **Men** 4% **Minority** 69%

Graduate Enrollment 48
Women 98% **Men** 2% **Minority** 57%

Nursing Student Activities Sigma Theta Tau.

Nursing Student Resources Academic advising; academic or career counseling; bookstore; computer lab; library services.

Library Facilities 27.1 million volumes; 11,648 periodical subscriptions (1,426 health-care related).

BACCALAUREATE PROGRAMS

Degree BSN

Available Programs ADN to Baccalaureate; Accelerated RN Baccalaureate.

Site Options Livonia, MI; Southfield, MI.

Study Options Full-time.

Program Entrance Requirements 1 letter of recommendation. Transfer students are accepted. **Standardized tests** *Required:* TOEFL for international students. **Application** *Deadline:* rolling (freshmen), rolling (transfer). *Application fee:* $100.

Advanced Placement Credit by examination available.

Expenses (2004–05) *Tuition:* full-time $11,550; part-time $385 per credit hour. *International tuition:* $11,550 full-time. *Required fees:* full-time $110.

Financial Aid 5% of baccalaureate students in nursing programs received some form of financial aid in 2003–04.

Contact Campus College Chair, Nursing, College of Health and Human Services, University of Phoenix–Metro Detroit Campus, 5480 Corporate Drive, Suite 240, Troy, MI 48098-2623. *Telephone:* 800-834-2438.

GRADUATE PROGRAMS

Expenses (2004–05) *Tuition:* full-time $11,256; part-time $439 per credit hour. *International tuition:* $11,256 full-time. *Required fees:* full-time $110.

Financial Aid 6% of graduate students in nursing programs received some form of financial aid in 2003–04.

Contact Campus College Chair, Nursing, College of Health and Human Services, University of Phoenix–Metro Detroit Campus, 5480 Corporate Drive, Suite 240, Troy, MI 48098-2623. *Telephone:* 800-834-2438.

MASTER'S DEGREE PROGRAM

Degrees MSN; MSN/MBA

Available Programs Master's.

Concentrations Available Health-care administration; nursing administration; nursing education. *Nurse practitioner programs in:* family health.

Site Options Livonia, MI; Southfield, MI.

Study Options Full-time.

Program Entrance Requirements Clinical experience, computer literacy, minimum overall college GPA of 2.5, transcript of college record. *Application deadline:* Applications are processed on a rolling basis. *Application fee:* $110.

Degree Requirements 39 total credit hours, thesis or project.

POST-MASTER'S PROGRAM

Areas of Study *Nurse practitioner programs in:* family health.

University of Phoenix–West Michigan Campus

College of Health and Human Services
Grand Rapids, Michigan

Founded in 2000

DEGREES • BSN • MSN • MSN/MBA

Nursing Program Faculty 22 (14% with doctorates).

Baccalaureate Enrollment 44
Women 100% **Minority** 5%

Graduate Enrollment 19
Women 100% **Minority** 6%

Nursing Student Activities Sigma Theta Tau.

Nursing Student Resources Academic advising; academic or career counseling; bookstore; computer lab; library services.

Library Facilities 27.1 million volumes; 11,648 periodical subscriptions (1,426 health-care related).

University of Phoenix–West Michigan Campus (continued)

BACCALAUREATE PROGRAMS

Degree BSN

Available Programs ADN to Baccalaureate; Accelerated Baccalaureate.

Site Options Portage, MI; Lansing, MI.

Study Options Full-time.

Program Entrance Requirements 1 letter of recommendation. Transfer students are accepted. **Standardized tests** *Required:* TOEFL for international students. **Application** *Deadline:* rolling (freshmen), rolling (transfer). *Application fee:* $85.

Advanced Placement Credit by examination available.

Expenses (2004–05) *Tuition:* full-time $11,520; part-time $384 per credit hour. *International tuition:* $11,520 full-time. *Required fees:* full-time $110.

Financial Aid 5% of baccalaureate students in nursing programs received some form of financial aid in 2003–04.

Contact Campus College Chair, Nursing, College of Health and Human Services, University of Phoenix–West Michigan Campus, 318 River Ridge Drive, NW, Grand Rapids, MI 49544-1683. *Telephone:* 888-345-9699.

GRADUATE PROGRAMS

Expenses (2004–05) *Tuition:* full-time $10,992; part-time $458 per credit hour. *International tuition:* $10,992 full-time. *Required fees:* full-time $110.

Financial Aid 19% of graduate students in nursing programs received some form of financial aid in 2003–04.

Contact Campus College Chair, Nursing, College of Health and Human Services, University of Phoenix–West Michigan Campus, 318 River Ridge Drive, NW, Grand Rapids, MI 49544-1683. *Telephone:* 888-345-9699.

MASTER'S DEGREE PROGRAM

Degrees MSN; MSN/MBA

Available Programs Master's.

Concentrations Available Health-care administration; nursing administration; nursing education. *Nurse practitioner programs in:* family health.

Site Options Portage, MI; Lansing, MI.

Study Options Full-time.

Program Entrance Requirements Clinical experience, computer literacy, minimum overall college GPA of 2.5, transcript of college record. *Application deadline:* Applications are processed on a rolling basis. *Application fee:* $110.

Degree Requirements 39 total credit hours, thesis or project.

POST-MASTER'S PROGRAM

Areas of Study *Nurse practitioner programs in:* family health.

Wayne State University

College of Nursing

Detroit, Michigan

http://www.nursing.wayne.edu

Founded in 1868

DEGREES • BSN • MSN • PHD

Nursing Program Faculty 83 (39% with doctorates).

Baccalaureate Enrollment 400

Women 85% **Men** 15% **Minority** 32% **International** 1% **Part-time** 61%

Graduate Enrollment 210

Women 93% **Men** 7% **Minority** 23% **International** 10% **Part-time** 65%

Nursing Student Activities Nursing Honor Society, Sigma Theta Tau, Student Nurses' Association.

Nursing Student Resources Academic advising; academic or career counseling; bookstore; campus computer network; computer lab; computer-assisted instruction; e-mail services; interactive nursing skills videos; Internet; learning resource lab; library services; nursing audiovisuals.

Library Facilities 1.9 million volumes (500,000 in health, 23,000 in nursing); 18,645 periodical subscriptions (5,000 health-care related).

BACCALAUREATE PROGRAMS

Degree BSN

Available Programs Accelerated Baccalaureate for Second Degree; Generic Baccalaureate; RN Baccalaureate.

Site Options Farmington Hills, MI; Clinton Township, MI.

Study Options Full-time.

Program Entrance Requirements Minimum overall college GPA of 2.0, transcript of college record, high school transcript, minimum high school GPA of 2.8, minimum GPA in nursing prerequisites of 2.5, prerequisite course work. Transfer students are accepted. **Standardized tests** *Required:* SAT or ACT, TOEFL for international students. **Application** *Deadline:* 8/1 (freshmen), 8/1 (transfer). *Notification:* continuous until 9/1 (freshmen). *Application fee:* $30.

Expenses (2004–05) *Room and board:* $1 per academic year.

Financial Aid 80% of baccalaureate students in nursing programs received some form of financial aid in 2003–04.

Contact Dr. Janet Harden, Director, Office of Student Affairs, College of Nursing, Wayne State University, 10 Cohn Building, 5557 Cass Avenue, Detroit, MI 48202. *Telephone:* 313-577-4082. *Fax:* 313-577-6949. *E-mail:* ac4961@wayne.edu.

GRADUATE PROGRAMS

Financial Aid 2 fellowships, 1 teaching assistantship were awarded; research assistantships, Federal Work-Study, institutionally sponsored loans, scholarships, and traineeships also available.

Contact Dr. Janet Harden, Interim Director for the Office of Student Affairs, College of Nursing, Wayne State University, 10 Cohn Building, 5557 Cass Avenue, Detroit, MI 48202. *Telephone:* 313-577-4082. *Fax:* 313-577-6949. *E-mail:* jharden@wayne.edu.

MASTER'S DEGREE PROGRAM

Degree MSN

Available Programs Accelerated AD/RN to Master's; Master's.

Concentrations Available *Clinical nurse specialist programs in:* community health, psychiatric/mental health. *Nurse practitioner programs in:* acute care, gerontology, neonatal health, pediatric, primary care, women's health.

Site Options *Distance Learning:* Detroit, MI.

Study Options Full-time and part-time.

Program Entrance Requirements Minimum overall college GPA of 2.8, transcript of college record, written essay, 3 letters of recommendation, GRE General Test. *Application deadline:* Applications are processed on a rolling basis. *Application fee:* $30 ($50 for international students).

Advanced Placement Credit given for nursing courses completed elsewhere dependent upon specific evaluations.

Degree Requirements 52 total credit hours, thesis or project.

POST-MASTER'S PROGRAM

Areas of Study *Clinical nurse specialist programs in:* psychiatric/mental health. *Nurse practitioner programs in:* acute care, gerontology, neonatal health, pediatric, primary care, women's health.

DOCTORAL DEGREE PROGRAM

Degree PhD

Available Programs Doctorate.

Areas of Study Nursing research.

Program Entrance Requirements Clinical experience, interview, 3 letters of recommendation, scholarly papers, vita, GRE General Test. *Application deadline:* Applications are processed on a rolling basis. *Application fee:* $30 ($50 for international students).

Degree Requirements 90 total credit hours, dissertation, oral exam, written exam, residency.

POSTDOCTORAL PROGRAM

Areas of Study Self-care, vulnerable population.

Postdoctoral Program Contact Professor and Director of Doctoral and Postdoctoral Programs, College of Nursing, Wayne State University, 319 Cohn Building, 5557 Cass Avenue, Detroit, MI 48202. *Telephone:* 313-577-4135. *Fax:* 313-577-5777. *E-mail:* ab5730@wayne.edu.

See full description on page 596.

Western Michigan University
College of Health and Human Services
Kalamazoo, Michigan

Founded in 1903

DEGREE • BS

Nursing Program Faculty 26 (31% with doctorates).

Baccalaureate Enrollment 397
Women 91% **Men** 9% **Minority** 10% **International** 2% **Part-time** 29%

Nursing Student Activities Student Nurses' Association.

Nursing Student Resources Academic advising; academic or career counseling; assistance for students with disabilities; bookstore; campus computer network; career placement assistance; computer lab; computer-assisted instruction; daycare for children of students; e-mail services; employment services for current students; externships; housing assistance; interactive nursing skills videos; Internet; learning resource lab; library services; nursing audiovisuals; placement services for program completers; remedial services; resume preparation assistance; skills, simulation, or other laboratory.

Library Facilities 2 million volumes (766 in nursing); 9,715 periodical subscriptions (362 health-care related).

BACCALAUREATE PROGRAMS

Degree BS

Available Programs ADN to Baccalaureate; Baccalaureate for Second Degree; Generic Baccalaureate; RN Baccalaureate.

Site Options St. Joseph, MI.

Study Options Full-time and part-time.

Program Entrance Requirements Minimum overall college GPA of 2.8, transcript of college record, CPR certification, written essay, high school biology, high school chemistry, 3 years high school math, 2 years high school science, high school transcript, immunizations, minimum high school GPA of 2.8, minimum GPA in nursing prerequisites of 2.8, prerequisite course work. Transfer students are accepted. **Standardized tests** *Required:* SAT or ACT, TOEFL for international students. **Application** *Deadline:* rolling (freshmen), 8/1 (transfer). *Notification:* continuous (freshmen). *Application fee:* $35.

Advanced Placement Credit given for nursing courses completed elsewhere dependent upon specific evaluations.

Expenses (2004–05) *Tuition, state resident:* full-time $4956; part-time $177 per credit hour. *Tuition, nonresident:* full-time $13,020; part-time $465 per credit hour. *International tuition:* $13,020 full-time. *Room and board:* $6496; room only: $3272 per academic year. *Required fees:* full-time $1150; part-time $472 per term.

Financial Aid 43% of baccalaureate students in nursing programs received some form of financial aid in 2003–04. *Gift aid (need-based):* Federal Pell, FSEOG, state, private, college/university gift aid from institutional funds. *Loans:* Federal Direct (Subsidized and Unsubsidized Stafford PLUS), Perkins, alternative loans. *Work-Study:* Federal Work-Study, part-time campus jobs. *Application deadline:* Continuous.

Contact Mrs. Marsha Ann Mahan, Student Advisor, College of Health and Human Services, Western Michigan University, 1903 West Michigan Avenue, Kalamazoo, MI 49008. *Telephone:* 269-387-8150. *Fax:* 269-387-8170. *E-mail:* marsha.mahan@wmich.edu.

MINNESOTA

Augsburg College
Program in Nursing
Minneapolis, Minnesota

http://www.augsburg.edu/nursing

Founded in 1869

DEGREES • BS • MA

Nursing Program Faculty 6 (50% with doctorates).

Baccalaureate Enrollment 169
Women 83% **Men** 17% **Part-time** 89%

Graduate Enrollment 42
Women 100% **Minority** 2% **Part-time** 90%

Nursing Student Resources Academic advising; academic or career counseling; assistance for students with disabilities; bookstore; campus computer network; computer lab; computer-assisted instruction; e-mail services; Internet; library services; tutoring.

Library Facilities 146,166 volumes (1,550 in health, 200 in nursing); 754 periodical subscriptions (70 health-care related).

BACCALAUREATE PROGRAMS

Degree BS

Site Options Rochester, MN.

Program Entrance Requirements Minimum overall college GPA of 2.5, transcript of college record, CPR certification, written essay, high school transcript, immunizations, professional liability insurance/malpractice insurance, prerequisite course work. Transfer students are accepted. **Standardized tests** *Required:* SAT or ACT, TOEFL for international students. **Application** *Deadline:* 8/15 (freshmen), 8/10 (transfer). *Notification:* continuous (freshmen). *Application fee:* $25.

Financial Aid *Gift aid (need-based):* Federal Pell, FSEOG, state, private, college/university gift aid from institutional funds, Federal Nursing. *Loans:* Federal Nursing Student Loans, FFEL (Subsidized and Unsubsidized Stafford PLUS), Perkins, state. *Work-Study:* Federal Work-Study, part-time campus jobs. *Application deadline:* 4/15.

Contact Luann Watson, Program Coordinator, Program in Nursing, Augsburg College, 2211 Riverside Avenue, South, Minneapolis, MN 55454. *Telephone:* 612-330-1204. *Fax:* 612-330-1649. *E-mail:* watson@augsburg.edu.

GRADUATE PROGRAMS

Contact Luann Watson, Program Coordinator, Program in Nursing, Augsburg College, 2211 Riverside Avenue, South, Minneapolis, MN 55454. *Telephone:* 612-330-1204. *Fax:* 612-330-1649. *E-mail:* watson@augsburg.edu.

MASTER'S DEGREE PROGRAM

Degree MA

Concentrations Available *Clinical nurse specialist programs in:* community health.

Site Options Rochester, MN.

Study Options Full-time and part-time.

Program Entrance Requirements Computer literacy, minimum overall college GPA of 3.0, transcript of college record, CPR certification, written essay, immunizations, 3 letters of recommendation, professional liability insurance/malpractice insurance, prerequisite course work, statistics course.

Advanced Placement Credit given for nursing courses completed elsewhere dependent upon specific evaluations.

Degree Requirements 48 total credit hours, thesis or project.

Bemidji State University
Department of Nursing
Bemidji, Minnesota

Founded in 1919

DEGREE • BS

Nursing Program Faculty 4 (25% with doctorates).

Baccalaureate Enrollment 63
Women 95% **Men** 5% **Minority** 6% **Part-time** 87%

Nursing Student Resources Academic advising; academic or career counseling; assistance for students with disabilities; bookstore; campus computer network; career placement assistance; computer lab; computer-assisted instruction; daycare for children of students; e-mail services; employment services for current students; housing assistance; Internet; library services; nursing audiovisuals; remedial services.

Library Facilities 554,087 volumes (9,000 in health, 1,000 in nursing); 991 periodical subscriptions (300 health-care related).

BACCALAUREATE PROGRAMS

Degree BS

Available Programs RN Baccalaureate.

Site Options *Distance Learning:* Hibbing, MN; Duluth, MN; Brainerd, MN.

Study Options Full-time and part-time.

Program Entrance Requirements Minimum overall college GPA, transcript of college record, immunizations, professional liability insurance/malpractice insurance. Transfer students are accepted. **Standardized tests** *Required:* ACT, TOEFL for international students. **Application** *Deadline:* rolling (freshmen), rolling (transfer). *Notification:* continuous (freshmen). *Application fee:* $20.

Advanced Placement Credit given for nursing courses completed elsewhere dependent upon specific evaluations.

Expenses (2003–04) *Tuition, state resident:* full-time $2169; part-time $158 per credit hour. *Tuition, nonresident:* full-time $4600; part-time $307 per credit hour. *Required fees:* part-time $7 per credit; part-time $245 per term.

Financial Aid 50% of baccalaureate students in nursing programs received some form of financial aid in 2002–03. *Gift aid (need-based):* Federal Pell, FSEOG, state, private, college/university gift aid from institutional funds. *Loans:* Federal Direct (Subsidized and Unsubsidized Stafford PLUS), Perkins, state, Alaska Loans, Canada Student Loans, Norwest Collegiate Loans, CitiAssist Loans and other alternative loans. *Work-Study:* Federal Work-Study, part-time campus jobs. *Application deadline (priority):* 5/15.

Contact Dr. Rochelle A. Scheela, Chair, Department of Nursing, Bemidji State University, Deputy Hall 105 Box 15, 1500 Birchmont Drive NE, Bemidji, MN 56601. *Telephone:* 218-755-3892. *Fax:* 218-755-4402. *E-mail:* rscheela@bemidjistate.edu.

CONTINUING EDUCATION PROGRAM

Contact Dr. Rochelle A. Scheela, Chair and Professor, Department of Nursing, Bemidji State University, Deputy Hall 105 Box 15, 1500 Birchmont Drive NE, Bemidji, MN 56601. *Telephone:* 218-755-3892. *Fax:* 218-755-4402. *E-mail:* rscheela@bemidjistate.edu.

Bethel University
Department of Nursing
St. Paul, Minnesota

http://www.bethel.edu/college/dept/nursing/index.html

Founded in 1871

DEGREES • BSN • MA

Nursing Program Faculty 27 (30% with doctorates).

Baccalaureate Enrollment 211
Women 93% **Men** 7% **Minority** 9%

Graduate Enrollment 49
Women 100% **Minority** 14% **International** 2% **Part-time** 29%

Nursing Student Resources Academic advising; academic or career counseling; assistance for students with disabilities; bookstore; campus computer network; career placement assistance; computer lab; computer-assisted instruction; daycare for children of students; e-mail services; employment services for current students; interactive nursing skills videos; Internet; learning resource lab; library services; nursing audiovisuals; paid internships; placement services for program completers; remedial services; resume preparation assistance; skills, simulation, or other laboratory; tutoring.

Library Facilities 194,000 volumes (5,366 in health, 4,700 in nursing); 18,000 periodical subscriptions (110 health-care related).

BACCALAUREATE PROGRAMS

Degree BSN

Available Programs Generic Baccalaureate; RN Baccalaureate.

Study Options Full-time and part-time.

Program Entrance Requirements Minimum overall college GPA of 2.5, transcript of college record, CPR certification, written essay, health exam, health insurance, high school transcript, immunizations, interview, 2 letters of recommendation, minimum GPA in nursing prerequisites of 2.5, professional liability insurance/malpractice insurance, prerequisite course work. Transfer students are accepted. **Standardized tests** *Required:* SAT or ACT, TOEFL for international students. **Application** *Deadline:* 3/1 (freshmen), 3/1 (transfer). *Early decision:* 12/1. *Notification:* 4/1 (freshmen), 1/15 (early action). *Application fee:* $25.

Advanced Placement Credit given for nursing courses completed elsewhere dependent upon specific evaluations.

Expenses (2003–04) *Tuition:* full-time $18,700; part-time $710 per credit hour. *Room and board:* $3790 per academic year. *Required fees:* full-time $205.

Financial Aid 80% of baccalaureate students in nursing programs received some form of financial aid in 2002–03.

Contact Ms. Elizabeth A. Peterson, Director, Pre-professional Program, Department of Nursing, Bethel University, 3900 Bethel Drive, St. Paul, MN 55112-6999. *Telephone:* 651-638-6455. *Fax:* 651-635-1965. *E-mail:* e-peterson@bethel.edu.

GRADUATE PROGRAMS

Expenses (2003–04) *Tuition:* part-time $340 per credit hour.

Financial Aid 30% of graduate students in nursing programs received some form of financial aid in 2002–03. Institutionally sponsored loans and scholarships available.

Contact Dr. Marjorie Schaffer, Professor, Department of Nursing, Bethel University, 3900 Bethel Drive, St. Paul, MN 55112. *Telephone:* 651-638-6298. *Fax:* 651-635-1965. *E-mail:* m-schaffer@bethel.edu.

MASTER'S DEGREE PROGRAM

Degree MA

Available Programs Master's.

Concentrations Available Nursing administration; nursing education.

Site Options *Distance Learning:* St. Paul, MN.

Study Options Full-time and part-time.

Program Entrance Requirements Clinical experience, computer literacy, minimum overall college GPA of 3.0, transcript of college record, written essay, immunizations, interview, 3 letters of recommendation, professional liability insurance/malpractice insurance, resume, statistics course, MAT. *Application deadline:* For fall admission, 3/20 (priority date). *Application fee:* $25.

Degree Requirements 42 total credit hours, thesis or project.

CONTINUING EDUCATION PROGRAM

Contact Ms. Kaye Cusick, Professional Development Coordinator, Department of Nursing, Bethel University, 3900 Bethel Drive, CGCS, St. Paul, MN 55112-6999. *Telephone:* 651-635-8013. *Fax:* 651-635-8004. *E-mail:* k-cusick@bethel.edu.

College of Saint Benedict
Department of Nursing
Saint Joseph, Minnesota

http://www.csbsju.edu/nursing/

Founded in 1887

DEGREE • BS

Nursing Program Faculty 15 (23% with doctorates).

Baccalaureate Enrollment 140

Women 95% **Men** 5% **Minority** 1% **Part-time** 4%

Nursing Student Activities Sigma Theta Tau, Student Nurses' Association, nursing club.

Nursing Student Resources Academic advising; academic or career counseling; assistance for students with disabilities; bookstore; campus computer network; career placement assistance; computer lab; computer-assisted instruction; e-mail services; interactive nursing skills videos; Internet; learning resource lab; nursing audiovisuals; placement services for program completers; skills, simulation, or other laboratory; tutoring.

Library Facilities 805,376 volumes (7,200 in health, 5,350 in nursing); 5,735 periodical subscriptions (335 health-care related).

BACCALAUREATE PROGRAMS

Degree BS

Available Programs Generic Baccalaureate.

Study Options Full-time.

Program Entrance Requirements Transcript of college record, CPR certification, written essay, health exam, health insurance, high school biology, high school chemistry, immunizations, 3 letters of recommendation, minimum GPA in nursing prerequisites of 2.5, professional liability insurance/malpractice insurance, prerequisite course work. **Standardized tests** *Required:* SAT or ACT, TOEFL for international students. **Application** *Deadline:* 12/1 (freshmen), rolling (transfer). *Notification:* continuous until 10/1 (freshmen).

Expenses (2004–05) *Tuition:* full-time $21,758; part-time $907 per credit hour. *International tuition:* $21,758 full-time. *Room and board:* $6208; room only: $3292 per academic year. *Required fees:* full-time $390; part-time $195 per term.

Financial Aid 90% of baccalaureate students in nursing programs received some form of financial aid in 2003–04. *Gift aid (need-based):* Federal Pell, FSEOG, state, private, college/university gift aid from institutional funds. *Loans:* FFEL (Subsidized and Unsubsidized Stafford PLUS), Perkins, state, alternative loans. *Work-Study:* Federal Work-Study, part-time campus jobs. *Application deadline (priority):* 3/15.

Contact Dr. Kathleen M. Twohy, Chairperson, Department of Nursing, College of Saint Benedict, 37 College Avenue South, St. Joseph, MN 56374. *Telephone:* 320-363-5404. *Fax:* 320-363-6099. *E-mail:* ktwohy@csbsju.edu.

College of St. Catherine
Department of Nursing
St. Paul, Minnesota

http://www.stkate.edu/offices/academic/nursing.nsf

Founded in 1905

DEGREES • BS • MA

Nursing Program Faculty 37 (38% with doctorates).

Baccalaureate Enrollment 216

Women 100% **Minority** 19% **International** 1% **Part-time** 1%

Graduate Enrollment 42

Women 98% **Men** 2% **Minority** 16% **Part-time** 14%

Nursing Student Activities Nursing Honor Society, Sigma Theta Tau, Student Nurses' Association.

Nursing Student Resources Academic advising; academic or career counseling; assistance for students with disabilities; bookstore; campus computer network; career placement assistance; computer lab; computer-assisted instruction; daycare for children of students; e-mail services; employment services for current students; housing assistance; Internet; learning resource lab; library services; nursing audiovisuals; placement services for program completers; remedial services; resume preparation assistance; skills, simulation, or other laboratory; tutoring; unpaid internships.

Library Facilities 263,495 volumes (71,100 in health, 17,775 in nursing); 1,141 periodical subscriptions (900 health-care related).

BACCALAUREATE PROGRAMS

Degree BS

Available Programs Baccalaureate for Second Degree; Generic Baccalaureate; RN Baccalaureate.

Site Options Minneapolis, MN.

Study Options Full-time.

Program Entrance Requirements Minimum overall college GPA of 2.75, transcript of college record, CPR certification, written essay, health insurance, immunizations, 2 letters of recommendation, minimum GPA in nursing prerequisites of 2.6, prerequisite course work. Transfer students are accepted. **Standardized tests** *Required:* SAT or ACT, TOEFL for international students. **Application** *Deadline:* 8/15 (freshmen), rolling (transfer). *Notification:* continuous (freshmen). *Application fee:* $20.

Expenses (2004–05) *Tuition:* full-time $14,640; part-time $610 per credit hour. *International tuition:* $14,640 full-time. *Room and board:* $5658; room only: $3258 per academic year. *Required fees:* part-time $475 per term.

Financial Aid 87% of baccalaureate students in nursing programs received some form of financial aid in 2003–04. *Gift aid (need-based):* Federal Pell, FSEOG, state, private, college/university gift aid from institutional funds, Federal Nursing. *Loans:* Federal Nursing Student Loans, FFEL (Subsidized and Unsubsidized Stafford PLUS), Perkins, state, college/university. *Work-Study:* Federal Work-Study, part-time campus jobs. *Application deadline (priority):* 4/15.

Contact Dr. Vicki Schug, Baccalaureate Program Director, Department of Nursing, College of St. Catherine, 2004 Randolph Avenue, St. Paul, MN 55105. *Telephone:* 651-690-6940. *Fax:* 651-690-6941. *E-mail:* vlschug@stkate.edu.

GRADUATE PROGRAMS

Expenses (2004–05) *Tuition:* part-time $550 per credit hour. *Room and board:* $5658; room only: $3258 per academic year. *Required fees:* part-time $30 per term.

Financial Aid 41% of graduate students in nursing programs received some form of financial aid in 2003–04.

Contact Dr. Ruth Brink, Graduate Program Director, Department of Nursing, College of St. Catherine, 2004 Randolph Avenue, F-22, St. Paul, MN 55105. *Telephone:* 651-690-6575. *Fax:* 651-690-6941. *E-mail:* rebrink@stkate.edu.

MASTER'S DEGREE PROGRAM

Degree MA

Available Programs Master's.

Concentrations Available Nursing education. *Nurse practitioner programs in:* adult health, gerontology, neonatal health, pediatric.

Study Options Full-time.

Program Entrance Requirements Clinical experience, minimum overall college GPA of 3.0, transcript of college record, CPR certification, written essay, immunizations, interview, 3 letters of recommendation, professional liability insurance/malpractice insurance, statistics course.

Degree Requirements 38 total credit hours, thesis or project.

POST-MASTER'S PROGRAM

Areas of Study Nursing education. *Nurse practitioner programs in:* adult health, gerontology, neonatal health, pediatric.

The College of St. Scholastica
Department of Nursing
Duluth, Minnesota

http://www.css.edu

Founded in 1912

DEGREES • BA • MA

Nursing Program Faculty 29 (21% with doctorates).

Baccalaureate Enrollment 213
Women 91% **Men** 9% **Minority** 9%

Graduate Enrollment 75
Women 95% **Men** 5% **Minority** 4% **International** 3% **Part-time** 75%

Nursing Student Activities Sigma Theta Tau, Student Nurses' Association.

Nursing Student Resources Academic advising; academic or career counseling; assistance for students with disabilities; bookstore; campus computer network; career placement assistance; computer lab; computer-assisted instruction; e-mail services; Internet; learning resource lab; library services; nursing audiovisuals; paid internships; placement services for program completers; resume preparation assistance; skills, simulation, or other laboratory; tutoring; unpaid internships.

Library Facilities 127,328 volumes (7,280 in health, 1,150 in nursing); 4,488 periodical subscriptions (291 health-care related).

BACCALAUREATE PROGRAMS

Degree BA

Available Programs Accelerated RN Baccalaureate; Generic Baccalaureate.

Site Options St. Cloud, MN; Brainerd, MN. *Distance Learning:* Duluth, MN.

Study Options Full-time and part-time.

Program Entrance Requirements Minimum overall college GPA of 3.0, transcript of college record, CPR certification, written essay, health exam, health insurance, high school transcript, immunizations, minimum GPA in nursing prerequisites of 2.0, prerequisite course work. Transfer students are accepted. **Standardized tests** *Required:* SAT or ACT, TOEFL for international students. **Application** *Deadline:* rolling (freshmen), rolling (transfer). *Notification:* continuous (freshmen). *Application fee:* $25.

Expenses (2004–05) *Tuition:* full-time $20,630; part-time $646 per credit hour. *International tuition:* $20,630 full-time. *Room and board:* $5916; room only: $2874 per academic year. *Required fees:* full-time $400; part-time $200 per term.

Financial Aid 98% of baccalaureate students in nursing programs received some form of financial aid in 2003–04.

Contact Ann Leja, RN, Director, Undergraduate Program in Nursing, Department of Nursing, The College of St. Scholastica, 1200 Kenwood Avenue, Duluth, MN 55811. *Telephone:* 218-723-6020. *Fax:* 218-723-6472. *E-mail:* aleja@css.edu.

GRADUATE PROGRAMS

Expenses (2004–05) *Tuition:* full-time $16,296; part-time $582 per credit hour. *International tuition:* $16,296 full-time. *Room and board:* $5916; room only: $2874 per academic year. *Required fees:* full-time $150; part-time $75 per term.

Financial Aid 90% of graduate students in nursing programs received some form of financial aid in 2003–04. Scholarships and traineeships available. Aid available to part-time students.

Contact Dr. Carleen Maynard, Graduate Program Director, Department of Nursing, The College of St. Scholastica, 1200 Kenwood Avenue, Duluth, MN 55811. *Telephone:* 218-723-6452. *Fax:* 218-723-6472. *E-mail:* cmaynard@css.edu.

MASTER'S DEGREE PROGRAM

Degree MA

Available Programs Master's.

Concentrations Available Nursing administration. *Clinical nurse specialist programs in:* adult health, gerontology. *Nurse practitioner programs in:* adult health, family health, psychiatric/mental health.

Site Options *Distance Learning:* Duluth, MN.

Study Options Full-time and part-time.

Program Entrance Requirements Clinical experience, computer literacy, minimum overall college GPA of 3.0, transcript of college record, CPR certification, written essay, immunizations, interview, 3 letters of recommendation, nursing research course, physical assessment course, professional liability insurance/malpractice insurance, resume, statistics course, GRE General Test or MAT. *Application deadline:* For fall admission, 5/1 (priority date). Applications are processed on a rolling basis. *Application fee:* $50.

Advanced Placement Credit given for nursing courses completed elsewhere dependent upon specific evaluations.

Degree Requirements 47 total credit hours, thesis or project.

POST-MASTER'S PROGRAM

Areas of Study Nursing administration. *Clinical nurse specialist programs in:* adult health, gerontology. *Nurse practitioner programs in:* adult health, family health, psychiatric/mental health.

Concordia College
Department of Nursing
Moorhead, Minnesota

http://www.cord.edu/dept/nursing/index.htm

Founded in 1891

DEGREES • BA • MS

Nursing Program Faculty 6 (33% with doctorates).

Baccalaureate Enrollment 82
Women 94% **Men** 6% **Minority** 7%

Graduate Enrollment 2
Women 100%

Nursing Student Activities Sigma Theta Tau, Student Nurses' Association.

Nursing Student Resources Academic advising; academic or career counseling; assistance for students with disabilities; bookstore; campus computer network; career placement assistance; computer lab; computer-assisted instruction; e-mail services; employment services for current students; externships; Internet; learning resource lab; library services; nursing audiovisuals; paid internships; placement services for program completers; remedial services; resume preparation assistance; skills, simulation, or other laboratory; tutoring; unpaid internships.

Library Facilities 306,644 volumes (2,135 in health, 837 in nursing); 3,460 periodical subscriptions (81 health-care related).

BACCALAUREATE PROGRAMS

Degree BA

Available Programs Accelerated Baccalaureate for Second Degree; Generic Baccalaureate.

Study Options Full-time.

Program Entrance Requirements Minimum overall college GPA of 2.5, transcript of college record, written essay, health exam, health insurance, immunizations, 2 letters of recommendation, minimum GPA in nursing prerequisites of 2.7, prerequisite course work. Transfer students are accepted. **Standardized tests** *Required:* SAT or ACT, TOEFL for international students. **Application** *Deadline:* rolling (freshmen), rolling (transfer). *Application fee:* $20.

Advanced Placement Credit by examination available. Credit given for nursing courses completed elsewhere dependent upon specific evaluations.

Expenses (2004–05) *Tuition:* full-time $17,620; part-time $2203 per unit. *International tuition:* $17,620 full-time. *Room and board:* $4065; room only: $2100 per academic year. *Required fees:* full-time $150; part-time $75 per term.

Financial Aid 89% of baccalaureate students in nursing programs received some form of financial aid in 2003–04. *Gift aid (need-based):* Federal Pell, FSEOG, state, private, college/university gift aid from institutional funds. *Loans:* FFEL (Subsidized and Unsubsidized Stafford PLUS), Perkins, state, college/university, alternative loans. *Work-Study:* Federal Work-Study, part-time campus jobs. *Application deadline:* Continuous.

Contact Ms. Connie L. Peterson, RN, Chair, Department of Nursing, Concordia College, 901 South 8th Street, Moorhead, MN 56562. *Telephone:* 218-299-4102. *Fax:* 218-299-4308. *E-mail:* cpeterso@cord.edu.

GRADUATE PROGRAMS

Expenses (2004–05) *Tuition:* full-time $7788; part-time $325 per credit hour. *International tuition:* $7788 full-time. *Room and board:* $4065; room only: $2100 per academic year. *Required fees:* full-time $648; part-time $27 per credit; part-time $324 per term.

Financial Aid 100% of graduate students in nursing programs received some form of financial aid in 2003–04.

Contact Ms. Connie L. Peterson, RN, Chair, Nursing Department, Department of Nursing, Concordia College, 901 South 8th Street, Moorhead, MN 56562. *Telephone:* 218-299-4102. *Fax:* 218-299-4308. *E-mail:* cpeterso@cord.edu.

MASTER'S DEGREE PROGRAM

Degree MS

Available Programs Master's; Master's for Nurses with Non-Nursing Degrees.

Concentrations Available Nursing education. *Clinical nurse specialist programs in:* adult health. *Nurse practitioner programs in:* family health.

Study Options Full-time and part-time.

Program Entrance Requirements Computer literacy, minimum overall college GPA of 3.0, transcript of college record, written essay, interview, 3 letters of recommendation.

Advanced Placement Credit given for nursing courses completed elsewhere dependent upon specific evaluations.

Degree Requirements 54 total credit hours, thesis or project, comprehensive exam.

Gustavus Adolphus College
Department of Nursing
St. Peter, Minnesota

Founded in 1862

DEGREE • BA

Nursing Program Faculty 9 (22% with doctorates).

Baccalaureate Enrollment 76
Women 96% **Men** 4% **Minority** 1% **International** 1%

Nursing Student Activities Sigma Theta Tau, Student Nurses' Association.

Nursing Student Resources Academic advising; academic or career counseling; assistance for students with disabilities; bookstore; campus computer network; e-mail services; Internet; library services; nursing audiovisuals; paid internships; remedial services; resume preparation assistance; skills, simulation, or other laboratory; tutoring; unpaid internships.

Library Facilities 288,685 volumes; 996 periodical subscriptions.

BACCALAUREATE PROGRAMS

Degree BA

Available Programs Generic Baccalaureate.

Study Options Full-time.

Program Entrance Requirements Minimum overall college GPA of 2.7, transcript of college record, written essay, high school transcript, immunizations, interview, prerequisite course work. Transfer students are accepted. **Standardized tests** *Required:* SAT or ACT, TOEFL for international students. ***Placement:*** *Required:* SAT or ACT. **Application** *Deadline:* 4/1 (freshmen), 4/1 (transfer). *Early decision:* 11/1. *Notification:* continuous until 5/1 (freshmen), 11/20 (early action).

Expenses (2004–05) *Tuition:* full-time $22,590. *Room and board:* $6810; room only: $3410 per academic year. *Required fees:* full-time $900.

Financial Aid 69% of baccalaureate students in nursing programs received some form of financial aid in 2003–04.

Contact Ms. Jane F. Coleman, Chair, Nursing Department, Department of Nursing, Gustavus Adolphus College, 800 West College Avenue, St. Peter, MN 56082-1498. *Telephone:* 507-933-6094. *Fax:* 507-933-6153. *E-mail:* jcw@gustavus.edu.

Metropolitan State University
School of Nursing
St. Paul, Minnesota

http://www.metrostate.edu

Founded in 1971

DEGREES • BSN • MSN

Nursing Program Faculty 22 (18% with doctorates).

Baccalaureate Enrollment 230
Women 91% **Men** 9% **Minority** 9% **Part-time** 96%

Graduate Enrollment 40
Women 95% **Men** 5% **Minority** 8% **Part-time** 23%

Nursing Student Activities Sigma Theta Tau, Student Nurses' Association.

Nursing Student Resources Academic advising; academic or career counseling; assistance for students with disabilities; bookstore; campus computer network; computer lab; e-mail services; externships; Internet; library services; skills, simulation, or other laboratory.

Library Facilities 29,385 volumes; 385 periodical subscriptions.

BACCALAUREATE PROGRAMS

Degree BSN

Site Options Minneapolis, MN.

Study Options Full-time and part-time.

Program Entrance Requirements Minimum overall college GPA of 2.5, transcript of college record, health insurance, immunizations, minimum GPA in nursing prerequisites of 3.0, professional liability insurance/malpractice insurance, prerequisite course work. Transfer students are accepted. **Standardized tests** *Required:* TOEFL for international students. *Required for some:* SAT or ACT. **Application** *Deadline:* 6/15 (freshmen), 6/15 (transfer). *Application fee:* $20.

Advanced Placement Credit given for nursing courses completed elsewhere dependent upon specific evaluations.

Expenses (2003–04) *Tuition, state resident:* full-time $2054; part-time $120 per credit hour. *Tuition, nonresident:* full-time $3046; part-time $266 per credit hour. *Required fees:* full-time $128; part-time $8 per credit.

Financial Aid 10% of baccalaureate students in nursing programs received some form of financial aid in 2002–03.

Contact Sandi Gerick, School of Nursing, Metropolitan State University, 700 East Seventh Street, St. Paul, MN 55106-5000. *Telephone:* 651-793-1379. *Fax:* 651-793-1382. *E-mail:* sandi.gerick@metrostate.edu.

GRADUATE PROGRAMS

Expenses (2003–04) *Tuition, state resident:* full-time $2820; part-time $235 per credit hour. *Tuition, nonresident:* full-time $4428; part-time $369 per credit hour. *Required fees:* full-time $128; part-time $8 per credit.

Financial Aid 10% of graduate students in nursing programs received some form of financial aid in 2002–03. Career-related internships or fieldwork, Federal Work-Study, and institutionally sponsored loans available.

Contact Ms. Lynda Zimmerman, Student/Faculty Services Coordinator, School of Nursing, Metropolitan State University, 700 East Seventh Street, St. Paul, MN 55106-5000. *Telephone:* 651-793-1378. *Fax:* 651-793-1382. *E-mail:* lynda.zimmerman@metrostate.edu.

MASTER'S DEGREE PROGRAM

Degree MSN

Available Programs Master's for Nurses with Non-Nursing Degrees; RN to Master's.

Concentrations Available Nursing administration. *Nurse practitioner programs in:* adult health, family health.

Metropolitan State University (continued)

Study Options Full-time and part-time.

Program Entrance Requirements Clinical experience, computer literacy, minimum overall college GPA of 3.0, transcript of college record, written essay, immunizations, interview, 3 letters of recommendation, professional liability insurance/malpractice insurance, resume, statistics course, GRE General Test or MAT. *Application deadline:* For fall admission, 1/15. *Application fee:* $20.

Advanced Placement Credit given for nursing courses completed elsewhere dependent upon specific evaluations.

Degree Requirements 42 total credit hours, thesis or project.

POST-MASTER'S PROGRAM

Areas of Study *Nurse practitioner programs in:* adult health, family health.

Minnesota Intercollegiate Nursing Consortium

Minnesota Intercollegiate Nursing Consortium
Northfield, Minnesota

DEGREE • BA

Nursing Program Faculty 10 (20% with doctorates).

Baccalaureate Enrollment 81

Women 94% **Men** 6% **Minority** 1%

Nursing Student Activities Sigma Theta Tau, Student Nurses' Association.

Nursing Student Resources Academic advising; academic or career counseling; assistance for students with disabilities; bookstore; campus computer network; career placement assistance; computer lab; computer-assisted instruction; e-mail services; employment services for current students; externships; interactive nursing skills videos; Internet; learning resource lab; library services; nursing audiovisuals; paid internships; resume preparation assistance; skills, simulation, or other laboratory; tutoring; unpaid internships.

BACCALAUREATE PROGRAMS

Degree BA

Available Programs Generic Baccalaureate.

Site Options Northfield, MN; St. Peter, MN.

Study Options Full-time.

Program Entrance Requirements Minimum overall college GPA of 2.7, transcript of college record, CPR certification, written essay, high school transcript, immunizations, interview, minimum GPA in nursing prerequisites of 2.7, prerequisite course work. Transfer students are accepted.

Contact Dr. Rita S. Glazebrook, Director, Minnesota Intercollegiate Nursing Consortium, 1520 St. Olaf Avenue, Northfield, MN 55057-1098. *Telephone:* 507-646-3265. *Fax:* 507-646-3733. *E-mail:* glazebro@stolaf.edu.

Minnesota State University Mankato

School of Nursing
Mankato, Minnesota

http://www.mnsu.edu/nursing/

Founded in 1868

DEGREES • BS • MSN

Nursing Program Faculty 46 (26% with doctorates).

Baccalaureate Enrollment 307

Women 93% **Men** 7% **Minority** 10% **Part-time** 13%

Graduate Enrollment 44

Women 95.5% **Men** 4.5% **Part-time** 56%

Nursing Student Activities Nursing Honor Society, Sigma Theta Tau, nursing club.

Nursing Student Resources Academic advising; academic or career counseling; assistance for students with disabilities; bookstore; campus computer network; career placement assistance; computer lab; computer-assisted instruction; daycare for children of students; e-mail services; employment services for current students; Internet; learning resource lab; library services; nursing audiovisuals; placement services for program completers; resume preparation assistance; skills, simulation, or other laboratory; tutoring.

Library Facilities 468,567 volumes (35,852 in health, 1,500 in nursing); 3,275 periodical subscriptions (156 health-care related).

BACCALAUREATE PROGRAMS

Degree BS

Available Programs Accelerated Baccalaureate for Second Degree; Generic Baccalaureate; RN Baccalaureate.

Study Options Full-time and part-time.

Program Entrance Requirements Minimum overall college GPA of 2.5, transcript of college record, minimum GPA in nursing prerequisites of 2.0, prerequisite course work. Transfer students are accepted. **Standardized tests** *Required:* ACT, TOEFL for international students. **Application** *Deadline:* rolling (freshmen), rolling (transfer). *Notification:* continuous (freshmen). *Application fee:* $20.

Advanced Placement Credit by examination available. Credit given for nursing courses completed elsewhere dependent upon specific evaluations.

Expenses (2004–05) *Tuition, state resident:* full-time $5088. *Tuition, nonresident:* full-time $9998. *International tuition:* $9998 full-time. *Required fees:* full-time $722.

Financial Aid 90% of baccalaureate students in nursing programs received some form of financial aid in 2003–04.

Contact Mrs. Julia Hebenstreit, Assistant Professor of Nursing, School of Nursing, Minnesota State University Mankato, 360 Wissink Hall, Mankato, MN 56001. *Telephone:* 507-389-6828. *Fax:* 507-389-6516. *E-mail:* julia.hebenstreit@mnsu.edu.

GRADUATE PROGRAMS

Expenses (2004–05) *Tuition, state resident:* full-time $6125. *Tuition, nonresident:* full-time $9626. *International tuition:* $9626 full-time. *Required fees:* full-time $754.

Contact Dr. Sonja J. Meiers, Graduate Program Director, School of Nursing, Minnesota State University Mankato, 360 Wissink Hall, Mankato, MN 56001. *Telephone:* 507-389-1317. *Fax:* 507-389-6516. *E-mail:* sonja.meiers@mnsu.edu.

MASTER'S DEGREE PROGRAM

Degree MSN

Available Programs Master's.

Concentrations Available *Clinical nurse specialist programs in:* family health. *Nurse practitioner programs in:* family health.

Study Options Full-time and part-time.

Program Entrance Requirements Clinical experience, computer literacy, minimum overall college GPA of 3.0, transcript of college record, written essay, 3 letters of recommendation, nursing research course, resume, statistics course.

Advanced Placement Credit given for nursing courses completed elsewhere dependent upon specific evaluations.

Degree Requirements 47 total credit hours, thesis or project.

POST-MASTER'S PROGRAM

Areas of Study *Nurse practitioner programs in:* family health.

CONTINUING EDUCATION PROGRAM

Contact Shirley Murray, Continuing Education Director, College of Allied Health and Nursing, School of Nursing, Minnesota State University Mankato, 360 Wissink Hall, Mankato, MN 56001. *Telephone:* 507-389-5194. *Fax:* 507-389-9516. *E-mail:* shirley.murray@mnsu.edu.

Minnesota State University Moorhead

Tri-College University Nursing Consortium
Moorhead, Minnesota

http://www.tri-college.org/nursing.htm

Founded in 1885

DEGREES • BSN • MS

Nursing Program Faculty 8 (62% with doctorates).

Baccalaureate Enrollment 88
Women 90% **Men** 10% **Part-time** 88%

Graduate Enrollment 33
Women 100% **Minority** 6% **Part-time** 30%

Nursing Student Activities Sigma Theta Tau.

Nursing Student Resources Academic advising; academic or career counseling; assistance for students with disabilities; bookstore; campus computer network; career placement assistance; computer lab; computer-assisted instruction; e-mail services; Internet; library services; nursing audiovisuals; remedial services; resume preparation assistance; tutoring; unpaid internships.

Library Facilities 367,334 volumes (4,903 in health, 682 in nursing); 1,539 periodical subscriptions (26 health-care related).

BACCALAUREATE PROGRAMS

Degree BSN

Available Programs RN Baccalaureate.

Site Options *Distance Learning:* St. Cloud, MN; Fergus Falls, MN; Alexandria, MN.

Study Options Full-time and part-time.

Program Entrance Requirements Minimum overall college GPA of 2.5, transcript of college record, CPR certification, written essay, health insurance, immunizations, 2 letters of recommendation, minimum GPA in nursing prerequisites of 2.25, professional liability insurance/malpractice insurance, prerequisite course work, RN licensure. Transfer students are accepted. **Standardized tests** *Required:* SAT or ACT, TOEFL for international students, PSAT. **Application** *Deadline:* 8/7 (freshmen), 8/7 (transfer). *Notification:* continuous (freshmen). *Application fee:* $20.

Expenses (2004–05) *Tuition, state resident:* full-time $3337; part-time $139 per credit hour. *Tuition, nonresident:* full-time $3337; part-time $139 per credit hour. *Room and board:* $2265; room only: $1457 per academic year. *Required fees:* full-time $1984; part-time $83 per credit; part-time $992 per term.

Financial Aid 85% of baccalaureate students in nursing programs received some form of financial aid in 2003–04. *Gift aid (need-based):* Federal Pell, FSEOG, state, private, college/university gift aid from institutional funds. *Loans:* Federal Direct (Subsidized and Unsubsidized Stafford PLUS), Perkins, state, alternative loans. *Work-Study:* Federal Work-Study, part-time campus jobs. *Application deadline (priority):* 3/1.

Contact Dr. Barbara Matthees, Director, Tri-College University Nursing Consortium, Minnesota State University Moorhead, 1104 7th Avenue, South, Moorhead, MN 56563. *Telephone:* 218-477-2695. *Fax:* 218-477-5990. *E-mail:* matthees@mnstate.edu.

GRADUATE PROGRAMS

Expenses (2004–05) *Tuition, state resident:* full-time $7788; part-time $325 per credit hour. *Tuition, nonresident:* full-time $7788; part-time $325 per credit hour. *International tuition:* $7788 full-time. *Room and board:* $2265; room only: $1457 per academic year. *Required fees:* full-time $648; part-time $27 per credit; part-time $324 per term.

Financial Aid 56% of graduate students in nursing programs received some form of financial aid in 2003–04.

Contact Dr. Jane Giedt, Chair, Graduate Nursing Program, Tri-College University Nursing Consortium, Minnesota State University Moorhead, 1104 7th Avenue, South, Moorhead, MN 56563. *Telephone:* 218-477-4699. *Fax:* 218-477-5990. *E-mail:* giedt@mnstate.edu.

MASTER'S DEGREE PROGRAM

Degree MS

Available Programs Master's; Master's for Nurses with Non-Nursing Degrees.

Concentrations Available Nursing education. *Clinical nurse specialist programs in:* adult health. *Nurse practitioner programs in:* family health.

Site Options *Distance Learning:* St. Cloud, MN; Fergus Falls, MN; Alexandria, MN.

Study Options Full-time and part-time.

Program Entrance Requirements Computer literacy, minimum overall college GPA of 3.0, transcript of college record, written essay, interview, 3 letters of recommendation.

Advanced Placement Credit given for nursing courses completed elsewhere dependent upon specific evaluations.

Degree Requirements 54 total credit hours, thesis or project, comprehensive exam.

St. Cloud State University

Department of Nursing Science
St. Cloud, Minnesota

Founded in 1869

DEGREE • BS

Nursing Program Faculty 12 (25% with doctorates).

Baccalaureate Enrollment 111

Nursing Student Activities Nursing club.

Nursing Student Resources Academic advising; academic or career counseling; assistance for students with disabilities; bookstore; campus computer network; career placement assistance; computer lab; computer-assisted instruction; daycare for children of students; e-mail services; interactive nursing skills videos; Internet; learning resource lab; library services; nursing audiovisuals; remedial services; resume preparation assistance; skills, simulation, or other laboratory; tutoring; unpaid internships.

Library Facilities 897,973 volumes (18,000 in health, 750 in nursing); 1,737 periodical subscriptions (100 health-care related).

BACCALAUREATE PROGRAMS

Degree BS

Available Programs Generic Baccalaureate.

Study Options Full-time.

Program Entrance Requirements Minimum overall college GPA of 2.75, transcript of college record, CPR certification, health exam, immunizations, 2 letters of recommendation, minimum GPA in nursing prerequisites of 2.75, prerequisite course work. **Standardized tests** *Required:* SAT or ACT, TOEFL for international students. **Application** *Deadline:* 6/1 (freshmen), 7/11 (transfer). *Notification:* continuous (freshmen). *Application fee:* $20.

Expenses (2004–05) *Tuition, state resident:* full-time $4882. *Tuition, nonresident:* full-time $10,597. *International tuition:* $10,597 full-time. *Room and board:* $4088; room only: $2800 per academic year. *Required fees:* full-time $625.

Financial Aid 86% of baccalaureate students in nursing programs received some form of financial aid in 2003–04. *Gift aid (need-based):* Federal Pell, FSEOG, state, college/university gift aid from institutional funds. *Loans:* FFEL (Subsidized and Unsubsidized Stafford PLUS), Perkins, state, college/university. *Work-Study:* Federal Work-Study, part-time campus jobs. *Application deadline (priority):* 5/1.

Contact Nursing Department, Department of Nursing Science, St. Cloud State University, 103 Mathematics and Science Center, St. Cloud, MN 56301. *Telephone:* 320-308-1749. *E-mail:* nursing@stcloudstate.edu.

St. Olaf College

Department of Nursing
Northfield, Minnesota

Founded in 1874

DEGREE • BA

St. Olaf College (continued)

Nursing Program Faculty 5 (40% with doctorates).

Baccalaureate Enrollment 40
Women 97% **Men** 3% **Minority** 3%

Nursing Student Activities Sigma Theta Tau, Student Nurses' Association.

Nursing Student Resources Academic advising; academic or career counseling; assistance for students with disabilities; bookstore; campus computer network; career placement assistance; computer lab; e-mail services; employment services for current students; Internet; learning resource lab; library services; nursing audiovisuals; paid internships; remedial services; resume preparation assistance; skills, simulation, or other laboratory; tutoring; unpaid internships.

Library Facilities 697,516 volumes; 2,149 periodical subscriptions.

BACCALAUREATE PROGRAMS

Degree BA

Available Programs Generic Baccalaureate.

Study Options Full-time.

Program Entrance Requirements Minimum overall college GPA of 2.7, transcript of college record, CPR certification, written essay, high school transcript, immunizations, interview, minimum GPA in nursing prerequisites of 2.7, prerequisite course work. Transfer students are accepted. **Standardized tests** *Required:* SAT or ACT, TOEFL for international students. **Application** *Deadline:* rolling (freshmen). *Early decision:* 11/15, 12/15. *Notification:* continuous (freshmen), 12/6 (out-of-state freshmen), 12/6 (early decision), 2/1 (early action). *Application fee:* $35.

Expenses (2004–05) *Tuition:* full-time $25,150; part-time $3140 per course. *International tuition:* $25,150 full-time. *Room and board:* $5800; room only: $2750 per academic year. *Required fees:* full-time $150.

Financial Aid 69% of baccalaureate students in nursing programs received some form of financial aid in 2003–04.

Contact Dr. Rita S. Glazebrook, Chair of the Department of Nursing, Department of Nursing, St. Olaf College, 1520 St. Olaf Avenue, Northfield, MN 55057-1098. *Telephone:* 507-646-3265. *Fax:* 507-646-3733. *E-mail:* glazebro@stolaf.edu.

University of Minnesota, Twin Cities Campus

School of Nursing
Minneapolis, Minnesota

http://www.nursing.umn.edu

Founded in 1851

DEGREES • BSN • MS • MS/MPH • PHD

Nursing Program Faculty 85 (90% with doctorates).

Baccalaureate Enrollment 365
Women 89% **Men** 11% **Minority** 10%

Graduate Enrollment 343
Women 98% **Men** 2% **Minority** 12% **International** 5% **Part-time** 44%

Nursing Student Activities Nursing Honor Society, Sigma Theta Tau, Student Nurses' Association.

Nursing Student Resources Academic advising; academic or career counseling; assistance for students with disabilities; bookstore; campus computer network; computer lab; computer-assisted instruction; daycare for children of students; e-mail services; employment services for current students; housing assistance; Internet; learning resource lab; library services; skills, simulation, or other laboratory.

Library Facilities 5.7 million volumes (4,000 in health, 1,500 in nursing); 45,000 periodical subscriptions (4,800 health-care related).

BACCALAUREATE PROGRAMS

Degree BSN

Available Programs Generic Baccalaureate.

Site Options Rochester, MN.

Study Options Full-time.

Program Entrance Requirements Minimum overall college GPA of 2.5, transcript of college record, CPR certification, written essay, health exam, health insurance, immunizations, minimum GPA in nursing prerequisites of 2.8, prerequisite course work. Transfer students are accepted. **Standardized tests** *Required:* SAT or ACT, TOEFL for international students. **Application** *Deadline:* rolling (freshmen), 3/1 (transfer). *Notification:* continuous (freshmen). *Application fee:* $45.

Expenses (2004–05) *Tuition, state resident:* full-time $3339; part-time $257 per credit hour. *Tuition, nonresident:* full-time $9154; part-time $704 per credit hour. *International tuition:* $9154 full-time. *Room and board:* $3500; room only: $2100 per academic year. *Required fees:* full-time $1572; part-time $51 per credit; part-time $110 per term.

Financial Aid 73% of baccalaureate students in nursing programs received some form of financial aid in 2003–04. *Gift aid (need-based):* Federal Pell, FSEOG, state, private, college/university gift aid from institutional funds, Federal Nursing. *Loans:* Federal Nursing Student Loans, Federal Direct (Subsidized and Unsubsidized Stafford PLUS), Perkins, state, college/university, Health Professions Loans, alternative loans. *Work-Study:* Federal Work-Study, part-time campus jobs. *Application deadline (priority):* 1/15.

Contact Office of Student Services, School of Nursing, University of Minnesota, Twin Cities Campus, 5-160 Weaver-Densford Hall, 308 Harvard Street, SE, Minneapolis, MN 55455-0213. *Telephone:* 612-624-4454. *Fax:* 612-624-3174. *E-mail:* nurseoss@umn.edu.

GRADUATE PROGRAMS

Expenses (2004–05) *Tuition, state resident:* full-time $4087; part-time $681 per credit hour. *Tuition, nonresident:* full-time $7637; part-time $1272 per credit hour. *International tuition:* $7637 full-time. *Room and board:* $3500; room only: $2100 per academic year. *Required fees:* full-time $1572; part-time $51 per credit; part-time $110 per term.

Financial Aid Fellowships, research assistantships, teaching assistantships, career-related internships or fieldwork and traineeships available.

Contact Office of Student Services, School of Nursing, University of Minnesota, Twin Cities Campus, 5-160 Weaver-Densford Hall, 308 Harvard Street, SE, Minneapolis, MN 55455-0213. *Telephone:* 612-624-4454. *Fax:* 612-624-3174. *E-mail:* nurseoss@umn.edu.

MASTER'S DEGREE PROGRAM

Degrees MS; MS/MPH

Available Programs Master's.

Concentrations Available Nurse anesthesia; nurse-midwifery; nursing administration; nursing education. *Clinical nurse specialist programs in:* adult health, gerontology, pediatric, psychiatric/mental health. *Nurse practitioner programs in:* family health, gerontology, pediatric, women's health.

Study Options Full-time and part-time.

Program Entrance Requirements Clinical experience, computer literacy, minimum overall college GPA of 3.0, transcript of college record, CPR certification, written essay, immunizations, interview, 2 letters of recommendation, statistics course. *Application deadline:* Applications are processed on a rolling basis. *Application fee:* $50 ($55 for international students).

Degree Requirements 33 total credit hours, thesis or project.

DOCTORAL DEGREE PROGRAM

Degree PhD

Available Programs Doctorate; Doctorate for Nurses with Non-Nursing Degrees; Post-Baccalaureate Doctorate.

Program Entrance Requirements Minimum overall college GPA of 3.0, interview by faculty committee, interview, 2 letters of recommendation, GRE General Test. *Application deadline:* Applications are processed on a rolling basis. *Application fee:* $50 ($55 for international students).

Degree Requirements 30 total credit hours, dissertation, oral exam, written exam, residency.

CONTINUING EDUCATION PROGRAM

Contact Office of Student Services, School of Nursing, University of Minnesota, Twin Cities Campus, 5-160 Weaver-Densford Hall, 308 Harvard Street, SE, Minneapolis, MN 55455-0213. *Telephone:* 612-624-4454. *Fax:* 612-624-3174. *E-mail:* nurseoss@umn.edu.

See full description on page 566.

Winona State University
College of Nursing
Winona, Minnesota

http://www.winona.edu/nursing/

Founded in 1858

DEGREES • BSN • MS

Nursing Program Faculty 39 (50% with doctorates).

Baccalaureate Enrollment 850
Women 88% **Men** 12% **Minority** 2% **International** 1% **Part-time** 5%

Graduate Enrollment 130
Women 96% **Men** 4% **Minority** 3% **International** 1%

Nursing Student Activities Sigma Theta Tau, Student Nurses' Association, nursing club.

Nursing Student Resources Academic advising; academic or career counseling; assistance for students with disabilities; bookstore; campus computer network; career placement assistance; computer lab; computer-assisted instruction; daycare for children of students; e-mail services; employment services for current students; externships; housing assistance; Internet; learning resource lab; library services; nursing audiovisuals; paid internships; placement services for program completers; remedial services; resume preparation assistance; skills, simulation, or other laboratory; tutoring.

Library Facilities 243,500 volumes (35,000 in nursing); 1,950 periodical subscriptions (200 health-care related).

BACCALAUREATE PROGRAMS

Degree BSN

Available Programs Generic Baccalaureate; RN Baccalaureate.

Site Options *Distance Learning:* Rochester, MN.

Study Options Full-time and part-time.

Program Entrance Requirements Minimum overall college GPA of 2.75, transcript of college record, CPR certification, health exam, health insurance, immunizations, professional liability insurance/malpractice insurance, prerequisite course work. Transfer students are accepted. **Standardized tests** *Required:* SAT or ACT, TOEFL for international students. **Application** *Deadline:* rolling (freshmen), 8/1 (transfer). *Notification:* continuous (freshmen). *Application fee:* $20.

Advanced Placement Credit given for nursing courses completed elsewhere dependent upon specific evaluations.

Expenses (2004–05) *Tuition, state resident:* full-time $2616; part-time $153 per credit hour. *Tuition, nonresident:* full-time $8562; part-time $285 per semester. *International tuition:* $8562 full-time. *Room and board:* $4880; room only: $3280 per academic year. *Required fees:* full-time $854; part-time $26 per credit.

Financial Aid 70% of baccalaureate students in nursing programs received some form of financial aid in 2003–04.

Contact Department of Nursing, College of Nursing, Winona State University, PO Box 5838, Winona, MN 55987-5838. *Telephone:* 507-457-5120. *Fax:* 507-457-5550. *E-mail:* nursing@winona.edu.

GRADUATE PROGRAMS

Expenses (2004–05) *Tuition, state resident:* part-time $234 per credit hour. *Tuition, nonresident:* part-time $353 per credit hour. *Required fees:* part-time $26 per credit.

Financial Aid 90% of graduate students in nursing programs received some form of financial aid in 2003–04. 3 research assistantships with partial tuition reimbursements available (averaging $6,000 per year) were awarded; Federal Work-Study, traineeships, and unspecified assistantships also available. Aid available to part-time students.

Contact Dr. William McBreen, Director, College of Nursing, Winona State University, 859 SE 30th Avenue, Rochester, MN 55904. *Telephone:* 507-285-7489. *Fax:* 507-292-5127. *E-mail:* wmcbreen@winona.msus.edu.

MASTER'S DEGREE PROGRAM

Degree MS

Available Programs Master's; RN to Master's.

Concentrations Available Nursing administration; nursing education. *Clinical nurse specialist programs in:* adult health. *Nurse practitioner programs in:* adult health, family health.

Site Options *Distance Learning:* Rochester, MN.

Study Options Full-time and part-time.

Program Entrance Requirements Clinical experience, computer literacy, minimum overall college GPA of 3.0, transcript of college record, written essay, immunizations, interview, 3 letters of recommendation, nursing research course, physical assessment course, professional liability insurance/malpractice insurance, statistics course. *Application deadline:* For fall admission, 2/1. *Application fee:* $20.

Advanced Placement Credit given for nursing courses completed elsewhere dependent upon specific evaluations.

Degree Requirements 43 total credit hours, thesis or project, comprehensive exam.

POST-MASTER'S PROGRAM

Areas of Study Nursing administration; nursing education. *Clinical nurse specialist programs in:* adult health. *Nurse practitioner programs in:* adult health, family health.

MISSISSIPPI

Alcorn State University
School of Nursing
Natchez, Mississippi

http://www.alcorn.edu/academic/academ/nurses.htm

Founded in 1871

DEGREES • BSN • MSN

Nursing Program Faculty 23 (33% with doctorates).

Baccalaureate Enrollment 63
Women 88.8% **Men** 11.2% **Minority** 42.8% **Part-time** 7.9%

Graduate Enrollment 56
Women 89.3% **Men** 10.7% **Minority** 35.7% **Part-time** 78.6%

Nursing Student Activities Nursing Honor Society, Sigma Theta Tau, Student Nurses' Association.

Nursing Student Resources Academic advising; computer lab; housing assistance; learning resource lab; library services; nursing audiovisuals; paid internships; skills, simulation, or other laboratory.

Library Facilities 210,036 volumes (2,082 in health, 1,385 in nursing); 1,046 periodical subscriptions (30 health-care related).

BACCALAUREATE PROGRAMS

Degree BSN

Available Programs Generic Baccalaureate; RN Baccalaureate.

Study Options Full-time and part-time.

Program Entrance Requirements Minimum overall college GPA of 2.5, transcript of college record, health exam, minimum high school GPA of 2.5, prerequisite course work. Transfer students are accepted. **Standardized tests** *Required:* SAT or ACT, TOEFL for international students. **Application** *Deadline:* rolling (freshmen), rolling (transfer). *Notification:* continuous (freshmen).

Advanced Placement Credit given for nursing courses completed elsewhere dependent upon specific evaluations.

Expenses (2004–05) *Tuition, state resident:* full-time $1866; part-time $155 per credit hour. *Tuition, nonresident:* full-time $4232; part-time $353 per credit hour. *Room and board:* $2309; room only: $2309 per academic year. *Required fees:* full-time $200.

Alcorn State University (continued)

Financial Aid 85% of baccalaureate students in nursing programs received some form of financial aid in 2003–04. *Gift aid (need-based):* Federal Pell, FSEOG, state, private, college/university gift aid from institutional funds. *Loans:* Federal Direct (Subsidized and Unsubsidized Stafford PLUS). *Work-Study:* Federal Work-Study. *Application deadline (priority):* 4/1.

Contact Mrs. Debra McDonough, Interim Chairperson, School of Nursing, Alcorn State University, 15 Campus Drive, P. O. Box 18399, Natchez, MS 39122. *Telephone:* 601-304-4305. *Fax:* 601-304-4398. *E-mail:* mcdonough@lorman.alcorn.edu.

GRADUATE PROGRAMS

Expenses (2004–05) *Tuition, state resident:* full-time $1732; part-time $193 per credit hour. *Tuition, nonresident:* full-time $4097; part-time $455 per credit hour. *Room and board:* $1008; room only: $1008 per academic year. *Required fees:* full-time $350.

Financial Aid 85% of graduate students in nursing programs received some form of financial aid in 2003–04.

Contact Dr. Diane Blanchar, Interim Chairperson, School of Nursing, Alcorn State University, 15 Campus Drive, P. O. Box 18399, Natchez, MS 39122. *Telephone:* 601-304-4303. *Fax:* 601-304-4398. *E-mail:* dianehb@lorman.alcorn.edu.

MASTER'S DEGREE PROGRAM

Degree MSN

Available Programs Master's.

Concentrations Available Nursing education. *Nurse practitioner programs in:* family health.

Study Options Full-time and part-time.

Program Entrance Requirements Computer literacy, minimum overall college GPA of 3.0, transcript of college record, written essay, 2 letters of recommendation, statistics course. *Application deadline:* For fall admission, 7/15 (priority date); for spring admission, 11/25. Applications are processed on a rolling basis. *Application fee:* $10 for international students).

Advanced Placement Credit given for nursing courses completed elsewhere dependent upon specific evaluations.

Degree Requirements 43 total credit hours, thesis or project.

POST-MASTER'S PROGRAM

Areas of Study Nursing education. *Nurse practitioner programs in:* family health, gerontology.

Delta State University

School of Nursing
Cleveland, Mississippi

http://www.deltastate.edu

Founded in 1924

DEGREES • BSN • MSN

Nursing Program Faculty 14 (29% with doctorates).

Baccalaureate Enrollment 38

Women 87% **Men** 13% **Minority** 34% **Part-time** 13%

Graduate Enrollment 23

Women 100% **Minority** 22% **Part-time** 35%

Nursing Student Activities Sigma Theta Tau, Student Nurses' Association.

Nursing Student Resources Academic advising; academic or career counseling; assistance for students with disabilities; bookstore; campus computer network; career placement assistance; computer lab; computer-assisted instruction; daycare for children of students; e-mail services; externships; housing assistance; interactive nursing skills videos; Internet; learning resource lab; library services; nursing audiovisuals; other; resume preparation assistance; skills, simulation, or other laboratory; tutoring.

Library Facilities 345,565 volumes (5,000 in health, 1,000 in nursing); 1,268 periodical subscriptions (120 health-care related).

BACCALAUREATE PROGRAMS

Degree BSN

Available Programs ADN to Baccalaureate; Generic Baccalaureate.

Site Options *Distance Learning:* Greenville, MS; Clarksdale, MS.

Study Options Full-time and part-time.

Program Entrance Requirements Transcript of college record, CPR certification, written essay, health exam, health insurance, immunizations, interview, 3 letters of recommendation, minimum GPA in nursing prerequisites of 2.5, professional liability insurance/malpractice insurance, prerequisite course work. Transfer students are accepted. **Standardized tests** *Required:* TOEFL for international students. **Application** *Deadline:* 8/1 (freshmen), 8/1 (transfer). *Notification:* continuous (freshmen).

Advanced Placement Credit given for nursing courses completed elsewhere dependent upon specific evaluations.

Expenses (2003–04) *Tuition, state resident:* full-time $3348; part-time $119 per credit hour. *Tuition, nonresident:* full-time $7965; part-time $311 per credit hour. *International tuition:* $7965 full-time. *Room and board:* $3594; room only: $3594 per academic year. *Required fees:* full-time $320; part-time $20 per credit; part-time $140 per term.

Financial Aid 95% of baccalaureate students in nursing programs received some form of financial aid in 2002–03. *Gift aid (need-based):* Federal Pell, FSEOG, state, private, college/university gift aid from institutional funds. *Loans:* FFEL (Subsidized and Unsubsidized Stafford PLUS), Perkins, college/university. *Work-Study:* Federal Work-Study. *Application deadline (priority):* 3/1.

Contact Mrs. Vicki L. Bingham, Coordinator of Academic Programs, School of Nursing, Delta State University, PO Box 3343, Cleveland, MS 38733. *Telephone:* 662-846-4255. *Fax:* 662-846-4267. *E-mail:* vbingham@deltastate.edu.

GRADUATE PROGRAMS

Expenses (2003–04) *Tuition, state resident:* full-time $3348; part-time $156 per credit hour. *Tuition, nonresident:* full-time $3348; part-time $156 per credit hour. *International tuition:* $3348 full-time. *Room and board:* $3594; room only: $3594 per academic year. *Required fees:* full-time $68; part-time $19 per credit; part-time $43 per term.

Financial Aid 25% of graduate students in nursing programs received some form of financial aid in 2002–03. Research assistantships, career-related internships or fieldwork, Federal Work-Study, and institutionally sponsored loans available. *Financial aid application deadline:* 6/1.

Contact Mrs. Vicki L. Bigham, Coordinator of Academic Programs, School of Nursing, Delta State University, PO Box 3343, Cleveland, MS 38733. *Telephone:* 662-846-4255. *Fax:* 662-846-4267. *E-mail:* vbingham@deltastate.edu.

MASTER'S DEGREE PROGRAM

Degree MSN

Available Programs Master's.

Concentrations Available Nursing administration; nursing education. *Nurse practitioner programs in:* family health.

Study Options Full-time and part-time.

Program Entrance Requirements Clinical experience, computer literacy, minimum overall college GPA of 3.0, transcript of college record, CPR certification, written essay, immunizations, 3 letters of recommendation, physical assessment course, professional liability insurance/malpractice insurance, prerequisite course work, statistics course, GRE General Test. *Application deadline:* For fall admission, 8/1 (priority date); for spring admission, 12/1 (priority date). Applications are processed on a rolling basis.

Advanced Placement Credit given for nursing courses completed elsewhere dependent upon specific evaluations.

Degree Requirements 43 total credit hours, thesis or project, comprehensive exam.

POST-MASTER'S PROGRAM

Areas of Study Nursing education. *Nurse practitioner programs in:* family health.

Mississippi College
School of Nursing
Clinton, Mississippi

http://www.mc.edu

Founded in 1826

DEGREE • BSN

Nursing Program Faculty 18 (28% with doctorates).

Baccalaureate Enrollment 123
Women 90% **Men** 10% **Minority** 25% **Part-time** 4%

Nursing Student Activities Sigma Theta Tau, Student Nurses' Association, nursing club.

Nursing Student Resources Academic advising; academic or career counseling; assistance for students with disabilities; bookstore; campus computer network; career placement assistance; computer lab; computer-assisted instruction; e-mail services; employment services for current students; externships; housing assistance; interactive nursing skills videos; Internet; learning resource lab; library services; nursing audiovisuals; other; paid internships; placement services for program completers; remedial services; resume preparation assistance; skills, simulation, or other laboratory; tutoring; unpaid internships.

Library Facilities 362,296 volumes (40,000 in health, 8,000 in nursing); 4,254 periodical subscriptions (290 health-care related).

BACCALAUREATE PROGRAMS

Degree BSN

Available Programs Generic Baccalaureate; RN Baccalaureate.

Study Options Full-time and part-time.

Program Entrance Requirements Minimum overall college GPA of 2.5, transcript of college record, high school biology, high school chemistry, high school transcript, immunizations, 2 letters of recommendation, minimum GPA in nursing prerequisites of 2.5, prerequisite course work. Transfer students are accepted. **Standardized tests** *Required:* SAT or ACT. **Application** *Deadline:* rolling (freshmen), rolling (transfer). *Early decision:* 12/15. *Notification:* continuous (freshmen), 12/31 (out-of-state freshmen), 12/31 (early decision). *Application fee:* $25.

Advanced Placement Credit given for nursing courses completed elsewhere dependent upon specific evaluations.

Expenses (2004–05) *Tuition:* full-time $11,200; part-time $355 per credit hour. *International tuition:* $11,200 full-time. *Room and board:* $5612; room only: $2944 per academic year. *Required fees:* full-time $600.

Financial Aid 80% of baccalaureate students in nursing programs received some form of financial aid in 2003–04.

Contact Dr. Mary Jean Padgett, RN, Dean, School of Nursing, Mississippi College, Box 4037, 200 South Capitol Street, Clinton, MS 39058. *Telephone:* 601-925-3278. *Fax:* 601-925-3379. *E-mail:* padgett@mc.edu.

Mississippi University for Women
Division of Nursing
Columbus, Mississippi

http://www.muw.edu/nursing

Founded in 1884

DEGREES • BSN • MSN

Nursing Program Faculty 37 (22% with doctorates).

Baccalaureate Enrollment 136
Women 90% **Men** 10% **Minority** 17%

Graduate Enrollment 40
Women 90% **Men** 10% **Minority** 20% **Part-time** 10%

Nursing Student Activities Sigma Theta Tau, Student Nurses' Association.

Nursing Student Resources Academic advising; academic or career counseling; assistance for students with disabilities; bookstore; campus computer network; career placement assistance; computer lab; computer-assisted instruction; e-mail services; externships; housing assistance; interactive nursing skills videos; Internet; learning resource lab; library services; nursing audiovisuals; paid internships; remedial services; resume preparation assistance; skills, simulation, or other laboratory; tutoring; unpaid internships.

Library Facilities 426,543 volumes (25,765 in nursing); 1,629 periodical subscriptions (210 health-care related).

BACCALAUREATE PROGRAMS

Degree BSN

Available Programs ADN to Baccalaureate; Generic Baccalaureate.

Site Options *Distance Learning:* Tupelo, MS.

Study Options Full-time.

Program Entrance Requirements Minimum overall college GPA of 2.0, transcript of college record, CPR certification, health exam, immunizations, minimum GPA in nursing prerequisites of 2.0, professional liability insurance/malpractice insurance, prerequisite course work. Transfer students are accepted. **Standardized tests** *Required:* TOEFL for international students. *Recommended:* SAT or ACT. *Required for some:* SAT or ACT. **Application** *Deadline:* rolling (freshmen), 9/6 (transfer). *Notification:* continuous (freshmen).

Advanced Placement Credit given for nursing courses completed elsewhere dependent upon specific evaluations.

Expenses (2004–05) *Tuition, state resident:* full-time $3495; part-time $146 per credit hour. *Tuition, nonresident:* full-time $8442; part-time $352 per credit hour. *Room and board:* $3778 per academic year. *Required fees:* full-time $400.

Financial Aid 80% of baccalaureate students in nursing programs received some form of financial aid in 2003–04. *Gift aid (need-based):* Federal Pell, FSEOG, state, private, college/university gift aid from institutional funds, United Negro College Fund. *Loans:* FFEL (Subsidized and Unsubsidized Stafford PLUS), Perkins. *Work-Study:* Federal Work-Study, part-time campus jobs. *Application deadline (priority):* 3/15.

Contact Dr. Linda Cox, Program Director, Division of Nursing, Mississippi University for Women, 1100 College Street, MUW-910, Columbus, MS 39701-5800. *Telephone:* 662-329-7302. *Fax:* 662-329-8555. *E-mail:* lcox@muw.edu.

GRADUATE PROGRAMS

Expenses (2004–05) *Tuition, state resident:* full-time $3495; part-time $194 per credit hour. *Tuition, nonresident:* full-time $8442; part-time $469 per credit hour. *Room and board:* $3778 per academic year. *Required fees:* full-time $500.

Financial Aid 95% of graduate students in nursing programs received some form of financial aid in 2003–04. Fellowships, Federal Work-Study, institutionally sponsored loans, and traineeships available. *Financial aid application deadline:* 4/1.

Contact Dr. Janice U. Davidson, Director of Graduate Nursing Program, Division of Nursing, Mississippi University for Women, 1100 College Street, MUW-910, Columbus, MS 39701-5800. *Telephone:* 662-329-7323 Ext. 7320. *Fax:* 662-329-7372. *E-mail:* jdavidson@muw.edu.

MASTER'S DEGREE PROGRAM

Degree MSN

Available Programs Master's.

Concentrations Available *Nurse practitioner programs in:* family health, pediatric.

Study Options Full-time and part-time.

Program Entrance Requirements Clinical experience, minimum overall college GPA of 3.0, transcript of college record, CPR certification, written essay, immunizations, interview, professional liability insurance/malpractice insurance, statistics course, GRE General Test. *Application deadline:* For fall admission, 4/1.

Advanced Placement Credit given for nursing courses completed elsewhere dependent upon specific evaluations.

Degree Requirements 39 total credit hours, thesis or project, comprehensive exam.

POST-MASTER'S PROGRAM

Areas of Study *Nurse practitioner programs in:* family health, pediatric.

University of Mississippi Medical Center

Program in Nursing
Jackson, Mississippi

http://son.umc.edu/

Founded in 1955

DEGREES • BSN • MSN • PHD

Nursing Program Faculty 51 (57% with doctorates).

Baccalaureate Enrollment 186
Women 85% **Men** 15% **Minority** 10% **Part-time** 5%

Graduate Enrollment 79
Women 86% **Men** 14% **Minority** 15% **Part-time** 35%

Nursing Student Activities Nursing Honor Society, Sigma Theta Tau, Student Nurses' Association, nursing club.

Nursing Student Resources Academic advising; academic or career counseling; assistance for students with disabilities; bookstore; campus computer network; computer lab; computer-assisted instruction; e-mail services; employment services for current students; externships; housing assistance; interactive nursing skills videos; Internet; learning resource lab; library services; nursing audiovisuals; remedial services; skills, simulation, or other laboratory; tutoring; unpaid internships.

Library Facilities 310,016 volumes (63,578 in health); 2,732 periodical subscriptions (150,333 health-care related).

BACCALAUREATE PROGRAMS

Degree BSN

Available Programs ADN to Baccalaureate; Generic Baccalaureate; RN Baccalaureate.

Site Options *Distance Learning:* Southaven, MS.

Study Options Full-time and part-time.

Program Entrance Requirements Minimum overall college GPA of 2.5, transcript of college record, CPR certification, written essay, health exam, health insurance, immunizations, interview, minimum GPA in nursing prerequisites of 2.5, professional liability insurance/malpractice insurance, prerequisite course work. Transfer students are accepted. **Application** *Deadline:* 2/15 (transfer). *Application fee:* $10.

Advanced Placement Credit given for nursing courses completed elsewhere dependent upon specific evaluations.

Expenses (2004–05) *Tuition, state resident:* full-time $1679; part-time $135 per credit hour. *Tuition, nonresident:* full-time $3357; part-time $288 per credit hour. *Required fees:* full-time $89.

Financial Aid 98% of baccalaureate students in nursing programs received some form of financial aid in 2003–04.

Contact Dr. Patricia Waltman, Assistant Dean for Undergraduate Programs, Program in Nursing, University of Mississippi Medical Center, 2500 North State Street, Jackson, MS 39216-4505. *Telephone:* 601-984-6255. *Fax:* 601-984-6206. *E-mail:* pwaltman@son.umsmed.edu.

GRADUATE PROGRAMS

Expenses (2004–05) *Tuition, state resident:* full-time $3091; part-time $171 per credit hour. *Tuition, nonresident:* full-time $6592; part-time $366 per credit hour.

Financial Aid 98% of graduate students in nursing programs received some form of financial aid in 2003–04. Institutionally sponsored loans and traineeships available. Aid available to part-time students. *Financial aid application deadline:* 4/1.

Contact Dr. Sharon Lobert, Assistant Dean for the Master's Program, Program in Nursing, University of Mississippi Medical Center, 2500 North State Street, Jackson, MS 39216-4505. *Telephone:* 601-984-6242. *Fax:* 601-984-6206. *E-mail:* slobert@son.umsmed.edu.

MASTER'S DEGREE PROGRAM

Degree MSN

Available Programs Accelerated Master's; Accelerated RN to Master's; Master's; RN to Master's.

Concentrations Available Health-care administration; nursing administration; nursing education. *Nurse practitioner programs in:* acute care, adult health, family health, neonatal health, psychiatric/mental health.

Study Options Full-time and part-time.

Program Entrance Requirements Clinical experience, computer literacy, minimum overall college GPA of 3.0, transcript of college record, CPR certification, immunizations, interview, 3 letters of recommendation, professional liability insurance/malpractice insurance, prerequisite course work, resume, statistics course, GRE. *Application deadline:* Applications are processed on a rolling basis. *Application fee:* $10.

Advanced Placement Credit given for nursing courses completed elsewhere dependent upon specific evaluations.

Degree Requirements 40 total credit hours, thesis or project.

POST-MASTER'S PROGRAM

Areas of Study *Nurse practitioner programs in:* acute care, adult health, family health, neonatal health, psychiatric/mental health.

DOCTORAL DEGREE PROGRAM

Degree PhD

Available Programs Doctorate.

Areas of Study Bio-behavioral research, nursing research, nursing science.

Program Entrance Requirements Clinical experience, minimum overall college GPA of 3.0, interview by faculty committee, interview, letters of recommendation, MSN or equivalent, statistics course, vita, writing sample, GRE. *Application deadline:* Applications are processed on a rolling basis. *Application fee:* $10.

Degree Requirements 34 total credit hours, dissertation, oral exam, written exam, residency.

CONTINUING EDUCATION PROGRAM

Contact Mrs. Renee Williams, Director of Continuing Education, Program in Nursing, University of Mississippi Medical Center, 2500 North State Street, Jackson, MS 39216-4505. *Telephone:* 601-984-6227. *Fax:* 601-984-6214. *E-mail:* rwilliams@son.umsmed.edu.

University of Southern Mississippi

School of Nursing
Hattiesburg, Mississippi

http://www.nursing.usm.edu

Founded in 1910

DEGREES • BSN • MSN • PHD

Nursing Program Faculty 48 (45% with doctorates).

Baccalaureate Enrollment 281
Women 77% **Men** 23% **Minority** 18.5% **Part-time** 3%

Graduate Enrollment 117
Women 85.5% **Men** 14.5% **Minority** 28% **International** .5% **Part-time** 26%

Nursing Student Activities Nursing Honor Society, Sigma Theta Tau, Student Nurses' Association.

Nursing Student Resources Academic advising; bookstore; career placement assistance; computer lab; computer-assisted instruction; e-mail services; externships; interactive nursing skills videos; Internet; learning resource lab; library services; nursing audiovisuals; skills, simulation, or other laboratory.

Library Facilities 1.4 million volumes; 21,259 periodical subscriptions (170 health-care related).

BACCALAUREATE PROGRAMS

Degree BSN

Available Programs ADN to Baccalaureate; Generic Baccalaureate; RN Baccalaureate.

Site Options Long Beach, MS; Meridian, MS.

Study Options Full-time.

Program Entrance Requirements Minimum overall college GPA of 2.5, transcript of college record, CPR certification, health exam, high school transcript, immunizations, minimum high school GPA of 2.0, minimum GPA in nursing prerequisites of 2.5, professional liability insurance/malpractice insurance, prerequisite course work. Transfer students are accepted. **Standardized tests** *Required:* SAT or ACT, TOEFL for international students. **Application** *Deadline:* rolling (freshmen), rolling (transfer). *Notification:* continuous (freshmen).

Expenses (2004–05) *Tuition, state resident:* full-time $2053; part-time $172 per credit hour. *Tuition, nonresident:* full-time $4368; part-time $172 per credit hour. *Room and board:* $4220; room only: $2880 per academic year. *Required fees:* full-time $115.

Financial Aid 85% of baccalaureate students in nursing programs received some form of financial aid in 2003–04. *Gift aid (need-based):* Federal Pell, FSEOG, state, private, college/university gift aid from institutional funds. *Loans:* Federal Nursing Student Loans, FFEL (Subsidized and Unsubsidized Stafford PLUS), Perkins, college/university. *Work-Study:* Federal Work-Study. *Application deadline (priority):* 3/15.

Contact Susan Kay Blackwell, Coordinator of Student Services, School of Nursing, University of Southern Mississippi, 118 College Drive, #5095, Hattiesburg, MS 39406-0001. *Telephone:* 601-266-5454. *Fax:* 601-266-5927. *E-mail:* susan.blackwell@usm.edu.

GRADUATE PROGRAMS

Financial Aid Research assistantships, Federal Work-Study and traineeships available.

Contact Ms. Shonna Breland, Program Contact, School of Nursing, University of Southern Mississippi, 118 College Dr. box 5095, Hattiesburg, MS 39406-5095. *Telephone:* 601-266-5456. *Fax:* 601-266-5927. *E-mail:* shonna.breland@usm.edu.

MASTER'S DEGREE PROGRAM

Degree MSN

Available Programs Master's; RN to Master's.

Concentrations Available Nursing administration. *Clinical nurse specialist programs in:* adult health, community health, psychiatric/mental health. *Nurse practitioner programs in:* family health, psychiatric/mental health.

Site Options Long Beach, MS; Meridian, MS.

Study Options Full-time and part-time.

Program Entrance Requirements Minimum overall college GPA of 3.0, transcript of college record, CPR certification, immunizations, 3 letters of recommendation, professional liability insurance/malpractice insurance, statistics course, GRE General Test. *Application deadline:* For fall admission, 3/15 (priority date); for spring admission, 11/1 (priority date). Applications are processed on a rolling basis. *Application fee:* $25.

Degree Requirements 45 total credit hours, thesis or project, comprehensive exam.

POST-MASTER'S PROGRAM

Areas of Study Nursing administration. *Clinical nurse specialist programs in:* adult health, community health, psychiatric/mental health. *Nurse practitioner programs in:* family health, psychiatric/mental health.

DOCTORAL DEGREE PROGRAM

Degree PhD

Available Programs Doctorate.

Areas of Study Ethics, health policy, nursing administration, nursing education.

Program Entrance Requirements Clinical experience, minimum overall college GPA of 3.50, interview by faculty committee, 3 letters of recommendation, MSN or equivalent, statistics course, vita, writing sample, GRE General Test. *Application deadline:* For fall admission, 3/15 (priority date); for spring admission, 11/1 (priority date). Applications are processed on a rolling basis. *Application fee:* $25.

Degree Requirements 72 total credit hours, dissertation, oral exam, written exam, residency.

William Carey College

School of Nursing
Hattiesburg, Mississippi

Founded in 1906

DEGREES • BSN • MSN

Nursing Program Faculty 23 (35% with doctorates).

Baccalaureate Enrollment 155
Women 94% **Men** 6% **Minority** 40% **International** 1% **Part-time** 5%

Graduate Enrollment 20

Nursing Student Activities Nursing Honor Society, Student Nurses' Association.

Nursing Student Resources Academic advising; academic or career counseling; assistance for students with disabilities; bookstore; campus computer network; computer lab; computer-assisted instruction; e-mail services; interactive nursing skills videos; Internet; learning resource lab; library services; nursing audiovisuals; resume preparation assistance; skills, simulation, or other laboratory; tutoring.

Library Facilities 98,139 volumes (450 in health, 450 in nursing); 472 periodical subscriptions (50 health-care related).

BACCALAUREATE PROGRAMS

Degree BSN

Available Programs ADN to Baccalaureate; Generic Baccalaureate.

Site Options New Orleans, LA; Gulfport, MS.

Study Options Full-time and part-time.

Program Entrance Requirements Minimum overall college GPA of 2.5, transcript of college record, CPR certification, health exam, high school transcript, immunizations, minimum GPA in nursing prerequisites, prerequisite course work. Transfer students are accepted. **Standardized tests** *Required:* SAT or ACT, TOEFL for international students. **Application** *Deadline:* rolling (freshmen), rolling (transfer). *Notification:* continuous until 8/15 (freshmen). *Application fee:* $20.

Advanced Placement Credit given for nursing courses completed elsewhere dependent upon specific evaluations.

Expenses (2004–05) *Tuition:* full-time $9360; part-time $260 per credit hour. *Room and board:* $3600; room only: $1750 per academic year. *Required fees:* full-time $300.

Financial Aid 85% of baccalaureate students in nursing programs received some form of financial aid in 2003–04. *Gift aid (need-based):* Federal Pell, FSEOG, state, private, college/university gift aid from institutional funds. *Loans:* FFEL (Subsidized and Unsubsidized Stafford PLUS), Perkins, college/university. *Work-Study:* Federal Work-Study, part-time campus jobs. *Application deadline (priority):* 3/1.

Contact Dr. Mary Stewart, Interim Dean, School of Nursing, School of Nursing, William Carey College, 498 Tuscan Avenue, Hattiesburg, MS 39401. *Telephone:* 601-318-6478. *E-mail:* mary.stewart@wmcarey.edu.

GRADUATE PROGRAMS

Expenses (2004–05) *Tuition:* full-time $7560; part-time $216 per credit hour. *Required fees:* full-time $100.

Financial Aid 50% of graduate students in nursing programs received some form of financial aid in 2003–04.

Contact Dr. Marilyn Cooksey, RN, Coordinator of MSN Program, School of Nursing, William Carey College, Gulfport Campus, 1856 Beach Drive, Gulfport, MS 39507. *Telephone:* 228-897-7200. *Fax:* 228-897-7202. *E-mail:* Marilyn.Cooksey@wmcarey.edu.

MASTER'S DEGREE PROGRAM

Degree MSN

Available Programs Master's.

Concentrations Available Nursing education.

Site Options Gulfport, MS.

Study Options Full-time and part-time.

Program Entrance Requirements Computer literacy, transcript of college record, CPR certification, immunizations, nursing research course, professional liability insurance/malpractice insurance, prerequisite course work, statistics course.

William Carey College (continued)
Advanced Placement Credit given for nursing courses completed elsewhere dependent upon specific evaluations.

Degree Requirements 35 total credit hours, thesis or project.

MISSOURI

Avila University
Department of Nursing
Kansas City, Missouri

http://www.avila.edu/catalog/degrees/nursing_.htm

Founded in 1916

DEGREE • BSN

Nursing Program Faculty 11 (36% with doctorates).

Baccalaureate Enrollment 56
Women 86% **Men** 14% **Minority** 29% **International** 1% **Part-time** 1%

Nursing Student Activities Nursing Honor Society, Sigma Theta Tau, Student Nurses' Association.

Nursing Student Resources Academic advising; academic or career counseling; assistance for students with disabilities; bookstore; campus computer network; computer lab; computer-assisted instruction; daycare for children of students; e-mail services; employment services for current students; interactive nursing skills videos; Internet; learning resource lab; library services; nursing audiovisuals; remedial services; resume preparation assistance; skills, simulation, or other laboratory; tutoring.

Library Facilities 80,865 volumes (2,325 in health, 1,525 in nursing); 7,179 periodical subscriptions (59 health-care related).

BACCALAUREATE PROGRAMS
Degree BSN

Available Programs Generic Baccalaureate.

Study Options Full-time.

Program Entrance Requirements Minimum overall college GPA of 2.5, transcript of college record, CPR certification, written essay, health exam, health insurance, immunizations, interview, minimum GPA in nursing prerequisites of 2.0, prerequisite course work. Transfer students are accepted. **Standardized tests** *Required:* SAT or ACT, TOEFL for international students. **Application** *Deadline:* rolling (freshmen), rolling (transfer). *Notification:* continuous (freshmen).

Advanced Placement Credit given for nursing courses completed elsewhere dependent upon specific evaluations.

Expenses (2004–05) *Tuition:* full-time $7800; part-time $365 per credit hour. *International tuition:* $7800 full-time. *Required fees:* full-time $370; part-time $12 per credit.

Financial Aid 95% of baccalaureate students in nursing programs received some form of financial aid in 2003–04. *Gift aid (need-based):* Federal Pell, FSEOG, state, private, college/university gift aid from institutional funds. *Loans:* FFEL (Subsidized and Unsubsidized Stafford PLUS), Perkins. *Work-Study:* Federal Work-Study, part-time campus jobs. *Application deadline:* Continuous.

Contact Office of Admissions, Department of Nursing, Avila University, 11901 Wornall Road, Kansas City, MO 64145-1698. *Telephone:* 816-501-2400. *Fax:* 816-501-2453. *E-mail:* admissions@mail.avila.edu.

Central Missouri State University
Department of Nursing
Warrensburg, Missouri

http://www.cmsu.edu/extcamp

Founded in 1871

DEGREES • BS • MS

Nursing Program Faculty 16 (7% with doctorates).

Baccalaureate Enrollment 87
Women 96% **Men** 4% **Minority** 5% **International** 4%

Graduate Enrollment 31
Women 96% **Men** 4% **Part-time** 95%

Nursing Student Activities Nursing club.

Nursing Student Resources Academic advising; academic or career counseling; assistance for students with disabilities; bookstore; campus computer network; career placement assistance; computer lab; computer-assisted instruction; daycare for children of students; e-mail services; employment services for current students; externships; housing assistance; interactive nursing skills videos; Internet; learning resource lab; library services; nursing audiovisuals; placement services for program completers; remedial services; resume preparation assistance; skills, simulation, or other laboratory; tutoring.

Library Facilities 1.3 million volumes (17,000 in health, 860 in nursing); 2,552 periodical subscriptions (250 health-care related).

BACCALAUREATE PROGRAMS
Degree BS

Available Programs Generic Baccalaureate; RN Baccalaureate.

Site Options *Distance Learning:* North Kansas City, MO; Lee's Summit, MO; Warrensburg, MO.

Study Options Full-time.

Program Entrance Requirements Minimum overall college GPA of 2.5, written essay, health exam, health insurance, immunizations, 2 letters of recommendation, minimum GPA in nursing prerequisites of 2.0, prerequisite course work. Transfer students are accepted. **Standardized tests** *Required:* ACT, TOEFL for international students. **Application** *Deadline:* rolling (freshmen), rolling (transfer). *Notification:* continuous (freshmen). *Application fee:* $30.

Advanced Placement Credit by examination available. Credit given for nursing courses completed elsewhere dependent upon specific evaluations.

Expenses (2004–05) *Tuition, state resident:* full-time $5340; part-time $178 per credit hour. *Tuition, nonresident:* full-time $10,260; part-time $342 per credit hour.

Contact Dr. Julie Ann Clawson, RN, Chair, Department of Nursing, Central Missouri State University, University Health Center, Room 106, Warrensburg, MO 64093. *Telephone:* 660-543-4775. *Fax:* 660-543-8304. *E-mail:* clawson@cmsu1.cmsu.edu.

GRADUATE PROGRAMS
Expenses (2004–05) *Tuition, state resident:* full-time $4230; part-time $235 per credit hour. *Tuition, nonresident:* full-time $4230; part-time $235 per credit hour.

Contact Dr. Novella Perrin, Dean, Department of Nursing, Central Missouri State University, Graduate Studies, WDE 1800, Warrensburg, MO 64093. *Telephone:* 660-543-4621. *E-mail:* perrin@cmsu1.cmsu.edu.

MASTER'S DEGREE PROGRAM
Degree MS

Available Programs Master's.

Concentrations Available Nursing education. *Nurse practitioner programs in:* family health.

Site Options *Distance Learning:* Lee's Summit, MO; Warrensburg, MO.

Study Options Full-time and part-time.

Program Entrance Requirements Clinical experience, minimum overall college GPA of 3.0, transcript of college record, CPR certification, written essay, immunizations, 2 letters of recommendation, professional liability insurance/malpractice insurance.

Advanced Placement Credit given for nursing courses completed elsewhere dependent upon specific evaluations.

Degree Requirements 32 total credit hours, thesis or project.

Culver-Stockton College

Blessing–Rieman College of Nursing
Canton, Missouri

http://www.culver.edu/

See description of programs under Blessing–Rieman College of Nursing (Quincy, Illinois).

Deaconess College of Nursing

Deaconess College of Nursing
St. Louis, Missouri

Founded in 1889

DEGREE • BSN

Nursing Program Faculty 14 (21% with doctorates).

Baccalaureate Enrollment 191
Women 96% **Men** 4% **Minority** 25%

Nursing Student Activities Student Nurses' Association.

Nursing Student Resources Academic advising; academic or career counseling; campus computer network; career placement assistance; computer lab; computer-assisted instruction; e-mail services; employment services for current students; housing assistance; Internet; learning resource lab; library services; nursing audiovisuals; placement services for program completers; skills, simulation, or other laboratory; tutoring.

Library Facilities 8,700 volumes (3,287 in health, 957 in nursing); 233 periodical subscriptions (182 health-care related).

BACCALAUREATE PROGRAMS

Degree BSN

Available Programs ADN to Baccalaureate; RN Baccalaureate; RPN to Baccalaureate.

Study Options Full-time and part-time.

Program Entrance Requirements Minimum overall college GPA of 2.5, transcript of college record, written essay, health exam, health insurance, high school biology, high school chemistry, 3 years high school math, 3 years high school science, high school transcript, immunizations, minimum high school GPA of 2.5, minimum high school rank 33%. Transfer students are accepted. **Standardized tests** *Required:* ACT, TOEFL for international students. **Application** *Deadline:* rolling (freshmen), rolling (transfer). *Notification:* continuous (freshmen). *Application fee:* $30.

Advanced Placement Credit by examination available. Credit given for nursing courses completed elsewhere dependent upon specific evaluations.

Expenses (2003–04) *Tuition:* part-time $415 per credit hour. *Room and board:* $2300 per academic year. *Required fees:* full-time $1300.

Financial Aid 77% of baccalaureate students in nursing programs received some form of financial aid in 2002–03.

Contact Mrs. Michelle McGrail, Dean of Enrollment and Student Services, Deaconess College of Nursing, 6150 Oakland Avenue, St. Louis, MO 63139. *Telephone:* 800-942-4310 Ext. 1. *Fax:* 314-768-3044 Ext. 1. *E-mail:* Michelle.McGrail@tenethealth.com.

Graceland University

School of Nursing
Independence, Missouri

http://www.graceland.edu/show.cfm?durki=26

Founded in 1895

DEGREES • BSN • MSN

Nursing Program Faculty 18 (16% with doctorates).

Baccalaureate Enrollment 435
Women 94% **Men** 6% **Minority** 7% **Part-time** 79%

Graduate Enrollment 116
Women 94% **Men** 6% **Minority** 6% **Part-time** 61%

Nursing Student Activities Nursing Honor Society, Sigma Theta Tau, Student Nurses' Association, nursing club.

Nursing Student Resources Academic advising; academic or career counseling; bookstore; campus computer network; computer lab; computer-assisted instruction; e-mail services; housing assistance; interactive nursing skills videos; Internet; learning resource lab; library services; nursing audiovisuals; resume preparation assistance; skills, simulation, or other laboratory; tutoring.

Library Facilities 193,109 volumes (2,336 in health, 1,968 in nursing); 503 periodical subscriptions (323 health-care related).

BACCALAUREATE PROGRAMS

Degree BSN

Available Programs ADN to Baccalaureate; Accelerated Baccalaureate; Accelerated Baccalaureate for Second Degree; Accelerated RN Baccalaureate; Generic Baccalaureate; RN Baccalaureate.

Site Options *Distance Learning:* Independence, MO.

Study Options Full-time and part-time.

Program Entrance Requirements Minimum overall college GPA of 2.5, transcript of college record, written essay, health exam, high school chemistry, high school transcript, immunizations, 2 letters of recommendation, minimum GPA in nursing prerequisites of 2.0, prerequisite course work. Transfer students are accepted. **Standardized tests** *Required:* SAT or ACT, TOEFL for international students. **Application** *Deadline:* rolling (freshmen), rolling (transfer). *Early decision:* 1/31. *Notification:* continuous (freshmen). *Application fee:* $50.

Advanced Placement Credit given for nursing courses completed elsewhere dependent upon specific evaluations.

Expenses (2003–04) *Tuition:* full-time $14,650; part-time $325 per credit hour. *Required fees:* full-time $235.

Financial Aid 96% of baccalaureate students in nursing programs received some form of financial aid in 2002–03.

Contact Mr. John D. Koehler, Admissions Counselor, School of Nursing, Graceland University, 1401 West Truman Road, Independence, MO 64050-3434. *Telephone:* 800-833-0524 Ext. 4804. *Fax:* 816-833-2990. *E-mail:* jkoehler@graceland.edu.

GRADUATE PROGRAMS

Expenses (2003–04) *Tuition:* part-time $425 per credit hour. *Required fees:* full-time $425.

Financial Aid 25% of graduate students in nursing programs received some form of financial aid in 2002–03.

Contact John D. Koehler, Admissions Counselor, School of Nursing, Graceland University, 1401 West Truman Road, Independence, MO 64050-3434. *Telephone:* 816-833-0524 Ext. 4804. *Fax:* 816-833-2990. *E-mail:* jkoehler@graceland.edu.

MASTER'S DEGREE PROGRAM

Degree MSN

Available Programs Master's; Master's for Nurses with Non-Nursing Degrees; RN to Master's.

Concentrations Available Health-care administration; nursing education. *Clinical nurse specialist programs in:* family health. *Nurse practitioner programs in:* family health.

Site Options *Distance Learning:* Independence, MO.

Study Options Full-time and part-time.

Graceland University (continued)

Program Entrance Requirements Clinical experience, minimum overall college GPA of 3.0, transcript of college record, written essay, 3 letters of recommendation, nursing research course, physical assessment course, prerequisite course work, statistics course.

Advanced Placement Credit given for nursing courses completed elsewhere dependent upon specific evaluations.

Degree Requirements 43 total credit hours, thesis or project, comprehensive exam.

POST-MASTER'S PROGRAM

Areas of Study Health-care administration. *Nurse practitioner programs in:* family health.

Jewish Hospital College of Nursing and Allied Health

Division of Nursing
St. Louis, Missouri

Founded in 1902

DEGREES • BSN • MSN

Nursing Program Faculty 29 (40% with doctorates).

Baccalaureate Enrollment 101
Women 90% **Men** 10% **Minority** 20% **Part-time** 80%

Graduate Enrollment 60
Women 95% **Men** 5% **Minority** 10% **Part-time** 60%

Nursing Student Activities Nursing Honor Society, Sigma Theta Tau, Student Nurses' Association.

Nursing Student Resources Academic advising; assistance for students with disabilities; bookstore; campus computer network; career placement assistance; computer lab; e-mail services; employment services for current students; externships; housing assistance; Internet; library services; placement services for program completers; remedial services; skills, simulation, or other laboratory; tutoring.

Library Facilities 3,765 volumes (11,000 in health, 8,100 in nursing); 232 periodical subscriptions (225 health-care related).

BACCALAUREATE PROGRAMS

Degree BSN

Available Programs RN Baccalaureate.

Study Options Full-time and part-time.

Program Entrance Requirements Minimum overall college GPA of 2.75, transcript of college record, CPR certification, health exam, high school biology, high school chemistry, high school math, high school transcript, immunizations, 2 letters of recommendation, minimum high school GPA of 2.75, prerequisite course work, RN licensure. Transfer students are accepted. **Standardized tests** *Required:* SAT or ACT. **Application** *Deadline:* rolling (freshmen), rolling (transfer). *Application fee:* $25.

Advanced Placement Credit by examination available. Credit given for nursing courses completed elsewhere dependent upon specific evaluations.

Expenses (2004–05) *Tuition:* full-time $11,010. *International tuition:* $11,010 full-time. *Room and board:* room only: $2550 per academic year. *Required fees:* full-time $200.

Financial Aid 95% of baccalaureate students in nursing programs received some form of financial aid in 2003–04. *Gift aid (need-based):* Federal Pell, FSEOG, state, private, college/university gift aid from institutional funds. *Loans:* FFEL (Subsidized and Unsubsidized Stafford PLUS), state, college/university. *Work-Study:* Federal Work-Study. *Application deadline (priority):* 4/1.

Contact Dr. Elizabeth A. Buck, Academic Dean, Nursing Division, Division of Nursing, Jewish Hospital College of Nursing and Allied Health, 306 South Kingshighway Boulevard, MS #90-30-625, St. Louis, MO 63110-1091. *Telephone:* 314-454-7064. *Fax:* 314-454-5239. *E-mail:* eab1458@bcj.org.

GRADUATE PROGRAMS

Expenses (2004–05) *Tuition:* full-time $4596. *International tuition:* $4596 full-time. *Room and board:* room only: $2550 per academic year.

Financial Aid 80% of graduate students in nursing programs received some form of financial aid in 2003–04. Institutionally sponsored loans and scholarships available. Aid available to part-time students. *Financial aid application deadline:* 4/15.

Contact Dr. Elizabeth A. Buck, Academic Dean, Nursing Division, Division of Nursing, Jewish Hospital College of Nursing and Allied Health, 306 South Kingshighway Boulevard, MS #90-30-625, St. Louis, MO 63110-1091. *Telephone:* 314-454-7064. *Fax:* 314-454-5239. *E-mail:* eab1458@bjc.org.

MASTER'S DEGREE PROGRAM

Degree MSN

Available Programs Master's; RN to Master's.

Concentrations Available Nurse anesthesia; nursing education. *Nurse practitioner programs in:* adult health, gerontology, neonatal health, oncology.

Study Options Full-time and part-time.

Program Entrance Requirements Computer literacy, minimum overall college GPA of 3.0, transcript of college record, CPR certification, immunizations, 3 letters of recommendation, nursing research course, physical assessment course, resume, statistics course. *Application deadline:* For fall admission, 6/1 (priority date); for spring admission, 11/1 (priority date). Applications are processed on a rolling basis. *Application fee:* $25.

Degree Requirements 34 total credit hours, thesis or project.

POST-MASTER'S PROGRAM

Areas of Study *Nurse practitioner programs in:* adult health, gerontology, neonatal health, oncology.

Lester L. Cox College of Nursing and Health Sciences

Department of Nursing
Springfield, Missouri

Founded in 1994

DEGREE • BSN

Nursing Program Faculty 20 (10% with doctorates).

Baccalaureate Enrollment 65

Nursing Student Activities Nursing Honor Society, Student Nurses' Association.

Nursing Student Resources Academic advising; academic or career counseling; assistance for students with disabilities; bookstore; campus computer network; computer lab; computer-assisted instruction; e-mail services; housing assistance; interactive nursing skills videos; Internet; learning resource lab; library services; nursing audiovisuals; remedial services; resume preparation assistance; skills, simulation, or other laboratory; tutoring.

Library Facilities 5,500 volumes in health, 1,900 volumes in nursing; 250 periodical subscriptions health-care related.

BACCALAUREATE PROGRAMS

Degree BSN

Available Programs ADN to Baccalaureate; Accelerated Baccalaureate for Second Degree; Generic Baccalaureate; RN Baccalaureate.

Study Options Full-time and part-time.

Program Entrance Requirements Minimum overall college GPA of 2.5, transcript of college record, CPR certification, health exam, high school biology, high school chemistry, 2 years high school math, high school transcript, minimum high school GPA of 3.0. Transfer students are accepted. **Standardized tests** *Required:* ACT. *Recommended:* ACT, SAT or ACT, SAT and SAT Subject Tests or ACT. **Application** *Deadline:* 2/1 (freshmen), 8/1 (transfer). *Early decision:* 11/1. *Notification:* 3/1 (freshmen), 12/1 (out-of-state freshmen), 12/1 (early decision). *Application fee:* $30.

Advanced Placement Credit given for nursing courses completed elsewhere dependent upon specific evaluations.

Expenses (2004–05) *Tuition:* full-time $8910; part-time $297 per credit hour. *International tuition:* $8910 full-time. *Room and board:* room only: $2000 per academic year. *Required fees:* full-time $1060; part-time $35 per credit.

Financial Aid 80% of baccalaureate students in nursing programs received some form of financial aid in 2003–04.

Contact Ms. Jennifer Plimmer, Admissions Coordinator, Department of Nursing, Lester L. Cox College of Nursing and Health Sciences, 1423 North Jefferson Avenue, Springfield, MO 65802. *Telephone:* 417-269-3038. *E-mail:* jplimme@coxcollege.edu.

Maryville University of Saint Louis
Nursing Program, School of Health Professions
St. Louis, Missouri

http://www.maryville.edu

Founded in 1872

DEGREES • BSN • MSN

Nursing Program Faculty 9 (50% with doctorates).

Baccalaureate Enrollment 275
Women 97% **Men** 3% **Minority** 8% **International** 2% **Part-time** 40%

Graduate Enrollment 25
Women 96% **Men** 4% **Minority** 2% **International** 2% **Part-time** 100%

Nursing Student Activities Sigma Theta Tau, Student Nurses' Association.

Nursing Student Resources Academic advising; academic or career counseling; assistance for students with disabilities; bookstore; campus computer network; computer lab; computer-assisted instruction; e-mail services; externships; interactive nursing skills videos; Internet; learning resource lab; library services; nursing audiovisuals; resume preparation assistance; skills, simulation, or other laboratory; tutoring.

Library Facilities 209,418 volumes (821 in health, 124 in nursing); 4,920 periodical subscriptions (110 health-care related).

BACCALAUREATE PROGRAMS

Degree BSN

Available Programs ADN to Baccalaureate; Generic Baccalaureate; LPN to Baccalaureate; RN Baccalaureate.

Study Options Full-time and part-time.

Program Entrance Requirements Minimum overall college GPA of 2.75, health exam, high school chemistry, high school transcript, immunizations, minimum high school GPA of 2.75, minimum GPA in nursing prerequisites of 2.75. Transfer students are accepted. **Standardized tests** *Required:* SAT or ACT, TOEFL for international students. **Application** *Deadline:* 8/15 (freshmen), rolling (transfer). *Notification:* continuous (freshmen). *Application fee:* $25.

Expenses (2003–04) *Tuition:* full-time $15,200; part-time $450 per credit hour. *International tuition:* $15,200 full-time. *Room and board:* $6650 per academic year. *Required fees:* full-time $240; part-time $45 per term.

Financial Aid 75% of baccalaureate students in nursing programs received some form of financial aid in 2002–03. *Gift aid (need-based):* Federal Pell, FSEOG, state, private, college/university gift aid from institutional funds. *Loans:* Federal Direct (Subsidized and Unsubsidized Stafford PLUS), Perkins, Sallie Mae Signature Loans, Keybank Loans, TERI Loans, Norwest Collegiate Loans, CitiAssist Loans, MOHELA ED Cash. *Work-Study:* Federal Work-Study, part-time campus jobs. *Application deadline (priority):* 4/1.

Contact Dr. Mary Curtis, Interim Director, Nursing Program, School of Health Professions, Maryville University of Saint Louis, 13550 Conway Road, St. Louis, MO 63141-7299. *Telephone:* 314-529-9478. *Fax:* 314-529-9139. *E-mail:* maryc@maryville.edu.

GRADUATE PROGRAMS

Expenses (2003–04) *Tuition:* full-time $15,200; part-time $465 per credit hour. *International tuition:* $15,200 full-time. *Room and board:* $6650 per academic year. *Required fees:* full-time $90; part-time $45 per term.

Financial Aid 75% of graduate students in nursing programs received some form of financial aid in 2002–03.

Contact Debbie Fritz, Coordinator of Graduate Program, Nursing Program, School of Health Professions, Maryville University of Saint Louis, 13550 Conway Road, St. Louis, MO 63141. *Telephone:* 314-529-9453. *Fax:* 314-529-9139. *E-mail:* fritz@maryville.edu.

MASTER'S DEGREE PROGRAM

Degree MSN

Available Programs Master's; RN to Master's.

Concentrations Available *Clinical nurse specialist programs in:* gerontology. *Nurse practitioner programs in:* adult health, gerontology, primary care.

Study Options Full-time and part-time.

Program Entrance Requirements Minimum overall college GPA of 3.0, transcript of college record, written essay, interview, 3 letters of recommendation, physical assessment course, resume, statistics course.

Advanced Placement Credit by examination available. Credit given for nursing courses completed elsewhere dependent upon specific evaluations.

Degree Requirements 60 total credit hours, thesis or project.

Missouri Southern State University
Department of Nursing
Joplin, Missouri

http://www.mssu.edu/nursing/

Founded in 1937

DEGREE • BSN

Nursing Program Faculty 9.

Baccalaureate Enrollment 99
Women 85% **Men** 15% **Minority** 3% **International** 1%

Nursing Student Activities Nursing Honor Society, Student Nurses' Association.

Nursing Student Resources Academic advising; academic or career counseling; assistance for students with disabilities; bookstore; campus computer network; career placement assistance; computer lab; computer-assisted instruction; daycare for children of students; e-mail services; employment services for current students; housing assistance; interactive nursing skills videos; Internet; learning resource lab; library services; nursing audiovisuals; remedial services; resume preparation assistance; skills, simulation, or other laboratory; tutoring.

Library Facilities 4,872 volumes in health, 4,470 volumes in nursing; 4,412 periodical subscriptions health-care related.

BACCALAUREATE PROGRAMS

Degree BSN

Available Programs ADN to Baccalaureate; Baccalaureate for Second Degree; Generic Baccalaureate; LPN to RN Baccalaureate; RN Baccalaureate.

Study Options Full-time.

Program Entrance Requirements Transcript of college record, CPR certification, health exam, health insurance, immunizations, minimum GPA in nursing prerequisites of 2.5, professional liability insurance/malpractice insurance, prerequisite course work. Transfer students are accepted. **Standardized tests** *Required:* SAT or ACT, TOEFL for international students. *Recommended:* ACT. *Required for some:* Michigan Test of English Language Proficiency. **Application** *Deadline:* 8/1 (freshmen), 8/1 (transfer). *Notification:* continuous (freshmen). *Application fee:* $15.

Advanced Placement Credit by examination available. Credit given for nursing courses completed elsewhere dependent upon specific evaluations.

Expenses (2004–05) *Tuition, state resident:* full-time $5267; part-time $1702 per semester. *Tuition, nonresident:* full-time $10,093; part-time $3226 per summer. *International tuition:* $10,093 full-time. *Room and board:* $4480 per academic year. *Required fees:* full-time $5267; part-time $1702 per credit.

Missouri Southern State University (continued)

Financial Aid 83% of baccalaureate students in nursing programs received some form of financial aid in 2003–04. *Gift aid (need-based):* Federal Pell, FSEOG, state, private, college/university gift aid from institutional funds. *Loans:* Federal Direct (Subsidized and Unsubsidized Stafford PLUS), Perkins, state. *Work-Study:* Federal Work-Study, part-time campus jobs. *Application deadline (priority):* 2/15.

Contact Dr. Barbara J. Box, Director, Department of Nursing, Missouri Southern State University, Kuhn Hall, Room 210B, 3950 East Newman Road, Joplin, MO 64801-1595. *Telephone:* 417-625-9322. *Fax:* 417-625-3186. *E-mail:* box-b@mssu.edu.

Missouri Western State College

Department of Nursing
St. Joseph, Missouri

http://www.mwsc.edu/nursing

Founded in 1915

DEGREE • BSN

Nursing Program Faculty 14 (28% with doctorates).

Baccalaureate Enrollment 213
Women 85% **Men** 15% **Minority** 3% **Part-time** 3%

Nursing Student Activities Sigma Theta Tau, Student Nurses' Association.

Nursing Student Resources Academic advising; academic or career counseling; assistance for students with disabilities; bookstore; campus computer network; career placement assistance; computer lab; computer-assisted instruction; daycare for children of students; e-mail services; employment services for current students; interactive nursing skills videos; Internet; library services; nursing audiovisuals; paid internships; remedial services; resume preparation assistance; skills, simulation, or other laboratory; tutoring; unpaid internships.

Library Facilities 147,509 volumes (8,607 in nursing); 1,068 periodical subscriptions (21 health-care related).

BACCALAUREATE PROGRAMS

Degree BSN

Available Programs Generic Baccalaureate; LPN to Baccalaureate; RN Baccalaureate.

Study Options Full-time and part-time.

Program Entrance Requirements Minimum overall college GPA of 2.5, transcript of college record, CPR certification, written essay, health exam, health insurance, high school transcript, immunizations, 3 letters of recommendation, minimum high school GPA of 2.5, minimum GPA in nursing prerequisites, prerequisite course work. Transfer students are accepted. **Standardized tests** *Required:* TOEFL for international students. ***Placement:*** *Required:* ACT. **Application** *Deadline:* 7/30 (freshmen), 7/30 (transfer). *Notification:* continuous until 8/10 (freshmen). *Application fee:* $15.

Advanced Placement Credit by examination available. Credit given for nursing courses completed elsewhere dependent upon specific evaluations.

Expenses (2004–05) *Tuition, state resident:* full-time $4780; part-time $188 per credit hour. *Tuition, nonresident:* full-time $8408; part-time $309 per credit hour.

Financial Aid *Gift aid (need-based):* Federal Pell, FSEOG, state, private, college/university gift aid from institutional funds. *Loans:* FFEL (Subsidized and Unsubsidized Stafford PLUS), Perkins. *Work-Study:* Federal Work-Study, part-time campus jobs. *Application deadline (priority):* 4/1.

Contact Department of Nursing, Missouri Western State College, 4525 Downs Drive, St. Joseph, MO 64507. *Telephone:* 816-271-4415. *Fax:* 816-271-5849. *E-mail:* nursing@mwsc.edu.

CONTINUING EDUCATION PROGRAM

Contact Dean, Western Institute, Department of Nursing, Missouri Western State College, 4525 Downs Drive, St. Joseph, MO 64507. *Telephone:* 816-271-4100.

Research College of Nursing

College of Nursing
Kansas City, Missouri

Founded in 1980

DEGREES • BSN • MSN

Nursing Program Faculty 45 (15% with doctorates).

Baccalaureate Enrollment 213
Women 98% **Men** 2% **Minority** 5% **International** 1% **Part-time** 4%

Graduate Enrollment 28
Women 95% **Men** 5% **Minority** 95% **International** 5% **Part-time** 96%

Nursing Student Activities Sigma Theta Tau, Student Nurses' Association.

Nursing Student Resources Academic advising; academic or career counseling; bookstore; campus computer network; career placement assistance; computer lab; computer-assisted instruction; daycare for children of students; e-mail services; housing assistance; Internet; learning resource lab; library services; resume preparation assistance; skills, simulation, or other laboratory; tutoring.

Library Facilities 150,000 volumes; 675 periodical subscriptions.

BACCALAUREATE PROGRAMS

Degree BSN

Available Programs Accelerated Baccalaureate; Accelerated Baccalaureate for Second Degree; Baccalaureate for Second Degree; Generic Baccalaureate.

Study Options Full-time.

Program Entrance Requirements Transcript of college record, high school chemistry, 3 years high school math, high school transcript, minimum GPA in nursing prerequisites of 2.7. Transfer students are accepted. **Standardized tests** *Required:* SAT or ACT, TOEFL for international students. **Application** *Deadline:* 6/30 (freshmen), 1/31 (transfer). *Notification:* continuous until 8/15 (freshmen). *Application fee:* $25.

Advanced Placement Credit given for nursing courses completed elsewhere dependent upon specific evaluations.

Expenses (2004–05) *Tuition:* full-time $17,500; part-time $600 per credit hour. *International tuition:* $17,500 full-time. *Room and board:* $6000; room only: $2500 per academic year. *Required fees:* full-time $550; part-time $55 per term.

Financial Aid 90% of baccalaureate students in nursing programs received some form of financial aid in 2003–04.

Contact Leslie Mendenhall, Director of Transfer and Graduate Admissions, College of Nursing, Research College of Nursing, 2300 East Meyer Boulevard, Kansas City, MO 64132-1199. *Telephone:* 816-276-4733. *Fax:* 816-276-3526. *E-mail:* leslie.mendenhall@hcamidwest.com.

GRADUATE PROGRAMS

Expenses (2004–05) *Tuition:* part-time $350 per credit hour. *Room and board:* room only: $2500 per academic year. *Required fees:* part-time $25 per credit; part-time $38 per term.

Financial Aid 15% of graduate students in nursing programs received some form of financial aid in 2003–04.

Contact Leslie Mendenhall, Director of Transfer and Graduate Admissions, College of Nursing, Research College of Nursing, 2300 East Meyer Boulevard, Kansas City, MO 64132-1199. *Telephone:* 816-276-4733. *Fax:* 816-276-3526. *E-mail:* leslie.mendenhall@hcamidwest.com.

MASTER'S DEGREE PROGRAM

Degree MSN

Available Programs Master's.

Concentrations Available Nursing administration; nursing education. *Nurse practitioner programs in:* family health.

Study Options Full-time and part-time.

Program Entrance Requirements Clinical experience, minimum overall college GPA of 3.0, transcript of college record, CPR certification, written essay, immunizations, interview, 3 letters of recommendation, physical assessment course, professional liability insurance/malpractice insurance, resume, statistics course.

Advanced Placement Credit given for nursing courses completed elsewhere dependent upon specific evaluations.

Degree Requirements 45 total credit hours, thesis or project.

Saint Louis University
School of Nursing
St. Louis, Missouri

http://www.slu.edu/colleges/NR

Founded in 1818

DEGREES • BSN • MSN • MSN/MPH • PHD

Nursing Program Faculty 54 (50% with doctorates).

Baccalaureate Enrollment 356
Women 93% **Men** 7% **Minority** 12% **Part-time** 5%

Graduate Enrollment 269
Women 94% **Men** 6% **Minority** 13% **International** 4% **Part-time** 89%

Nursing Student Activities Sigma Theta Tau, Student Nurses' Association.

Nursing Student Resources Academic advising; academic or career counseling; assistance for students with disabilities; bookstore; campus computer network; career placement assistance; computer lab; computer-assisted instruction; e-mail services; employment services for current students; housing assistance; interactive nursing skills videos; Internet; learning resource lab; library services; nursing audiovisuals; placement services for program completers; remedial services; resume preparation assistance; skills, simulation, or other laboratory; tutoring; unpaid internships.

Library Facilities 1.9 million volumes (112,581 in health, 41,034 in nursing); 13,999 periodical subscriptions (6,427 health-care related).

BACCALAUREATE PROGRAMS

Degree BSN

Available Programs Accelerated Baccalaureate; Accelerated Baccalaureate for Second Degree; Generic Baccalaureate; RN Baccalaureate.

Study Options Full-time and part-time.

Program Entrance Requirements Minimum overall college GPA of 2.5, transcript of college record, health exam, high school biology, high school chemistry, high school transcript, immunizations, minimum high school GPA of 2.5. Transfer students are accepted. **Standardized tests** *Required:* SAT or ACT. *Recommended:* TOEFL for international students. **Application** *Deadline:* rolling (freshmen). *Notification:* continuous until 8/1 (freshmen). *Application fee:* $25.

Advanced Placement Credit by examination available. Credit given for nursing courses completed elsewhere dependent upon specific evaluations.

Expenses (2004–05) *Tuition:* full-time $23,360; part-time $815 per credit hour. *International tuition:* $23,360 full-time. *Room and board:* $7960; room only: $4320 per academic year. *Required fees:* full-time $198; part-time $70 per term.

Financial Aid 75% of baccalaureate students in nursing programs received some form of financial aid in 2003–04. *Gift aid (need-based):* Federal Pell, FSEOG, state, private, college/university gift aid from institutional funds. *Loans:* Federal Nursing Student Loans, FFEL (Subsidized and Unsubsidized Stafford PLUS), Perkins, state, short term loans. *Work-Study:* Federal Work-Study, part-time campus jobs. *Application deadline (priority):* 3/1.

Contact Ms. Elaine Dempsey, Director of Marketing and Recruitment, School of Nursing, Saint Louis University, 3525 Caroline Mall, St. Louis, MO 63104. *Telephone:* 314-977-8921. *Fax:* 314-977-8949. *E-mail:* slunurse@slu.edu.

GRADUATE PROGRAMS

Expenses (2004–05) *Tuition:* part-time $745 per credit hour. *Required fees:* full-time $160; part-time $55 per term.

Financial Aid 50% of graduate students in nursing programs received some form of financial aid in 2003–04. 1 research assistantship with tuition reimbursement available, 2 teaching assistantships were awarded; traineeships and unspecified assistantships also available. *Financial aid application deadline:* 6/1.

Contact Dr. Margie Edel, Director, Master's Program in Nursing, School of Nursing, Saint Louis University, 3525 Caroline Mall, St. Louis, MO 63104. *Telephone:* 314-977-8931. *Fax:* 314-977-8949. *E-mail:* edele@slu.edu.

MASTER'S DEGREE PROGRAM

Degrees MSN; MSN/MPH

Available Programs Master's; Master's for Nurses with Non-Nursing Degrees; RN to Master's.

Concentrations Available Nursing education. *Clinical nurse specialist programs in:* adult health, gerontology, pediatric, perinatal, psychiatric/mental health. *Nurse practitioner programs in:* acute care, adult health, family health, gerontology, pediatric.

Site Options *Distance Learning:* St. Louis, MO.

Study Options Full-time and part-time.

Program Entrance Requirements Minimum overall college GPA of 3.0, transcript of college record, CPR certification, immunizations, 3 letters of recommendation, physical assessment course, resume, statistics course. *Application deadline:* For fall admission, 7/1; for spring admission, 11/1. Applications are processed on a rolling basis. *Application fee:* $40.

Advanced Placement Credit given for nursing courses completed elsewhere dependent upon specific evaluations.

Degree Requirements 36 total credit hours.

POST-MASTER'S PROGRAM

Areas of Study Nursing education. *Clinical nurse specialist programs in:* adult health, gerontology, pediatric, perinatal, psychiatric/mental health. *Nurse practitioner programs in:* acute care, adult health, family health, gerontology, pediatric, psychiatric/mental health.

DOCTORAL DEGREE PROGRAM

Degree PhD

Available Programs Doctorate.

Areas of Study Faculty preparation, gerontology, health promotion/disease prevention, human health and illness, maternity-newborn, nursing education, nursing research, nursing science, women's health.

Program Entrance Requirements Minimum overall college GPA of 3.25, 3 letters of recommendation, MSN or equivalent, statistics course, vita, writing sample, GRE General Test. *Application deadline:* For fall admission, 7/1; for spring admission, 11/1. Applications are processed on a rolling basis. *Application fee:* $40.

Degree Requirements 69 total credit hours, dissertation, oral exam, written exam, residency.

CONTINUING EDUCATION PROGRAM

Contact Ms. Kristine M. L'Ecuyer, Director, Continuing Education, School of Nursing, Saint Louis University, 3525 Caroline Mall, St. Louis, MO 63104. *Telephone:* 314-977-8975. *Fax:* 314-977-8949. *E-mail:* lecuyerk@slu.edu.

Saint Luke's College
Nursing College
Kansas City, Missouri

http://www.saintlukescollege.edu

Founded in 1903

DEGREE • BSN

Nursing Program Faculty 17 (18% with doctorates).

Baccalaureate Enrollment 115
Women 95% **Men** 5% **Minority** 10% **International** 1% **Part-time** 12%

Nursing Student Activities Student Nurses' Association.

Nursing Student Resources Academic advising; assistance for students with disabilities; bookstore; campus computer network; computer lab; computer-assisted instruction; e-mail services; employment services for current students; interactive nursing skills videos; Internet; learning resource lab; library services; nursing audiovisuals; skills, simulation, or other laboratory; tutoring.

Saint Luke's College (continued)

BACCALAUREATE PROGRAMS

Degree BSN

Available Programs Generic Baccalaureate.

Site Options Kansas City, MO.

Study Options Full-time and part-time.

Program Entrance Requirements Transcript of college record, CPR certification, written essay, health exam, health insurance, high school transcript, immunizations, interview, 3 letters of recommendation, minimum GPA in nursing prerequisites of 2.7, prerequisite course work. Transfer students are accepted. **Standardized tests** *Required:* TOEFL for international students. **Application** *Deadline:* 12/31 (transfer). *Application fee:* $20.

Advanced Placement Credit given for nursing courses completed elsewhere dependent upon specific evaluations.

Expenses (2004–05) *Tuition:* full-time $8850; part-time $295 per credit hour. *Required fees:* full-time $670; part-time $180 per term.

Financial Aid 95% of baccalaureate students in nursing programs received some form of financial aid in 2003–04. *Gift aid (need-based):* Federal Pell, FSEOG, state, private, college/university gift aid from institutional funds. *Loans:* Federal Nursing Student Loans, FFEL (Subsidized and Unsubsidized Stafford PLUS), Perkins, college/university. *Work-Study:* Federal Work-Study. *Application deadline:* Continuous.

Contact Lindsey Borgelt, Assistant Director of Admissions, Nursing College, Saint Luke's College, 8320 Ward Parkway, Suite 300, Kansas City, MO 64114. *Telephone:* 816-932-3372. *Fax:* 816-932-9064. *E-mail:* lborgelt@saint-lukes.org.

Southeast Missouri State University

Department of Nursing

Cape Girardeau, Missouri

http://www2.semo.edu/nursing

Founded in 1873

DEGREES • BSN • MSN

Nursing Program Faculty 24 (60% with doctorates).

Baccalaureate Enrollment 408

Women 95% **Men** 5% **Minority** 7% **Part-time** 20%

Graduate Enrollment 37

Women 80% **Men** 20% **Minority** 2% **Part-time** 65%

Nursing Student Activities Sigma Theta Tau, Student Nurses' Association.

Nursing Student Resources Academic advising; academic or career counseling; assistance for students with disabilities; bookstore; campus computer network; computer lab; computer-assisted instruction; daycare for children of students; e-mail services; employment services for current students; housing assistance; interactive nursing skills videos; Internet; learning resource lab; library services; nursing audiovisuals; remedial services; skills, simulation, or other laboratory; tutoring.

Library Facilities 411,992 volumes (450,750 in health, 16,145 in nursing); 2,781 periodical subscriptions (75 health-care related).

BACCALAUREATE PROGRAMS

Degree BSN

Available Programs Generic Baccalaureate; RN Baccalaureate.

Site Options *Distance Learning:* Poplar Bluff, MO; Kennett, MO.

Study Options Full-time.

Program Entrance Requirements Minimum overall college GPA of 2.5, transcript of college record, CPR certification, health exam, health insurance, high school transcript, immunizations, professional liability insurance/malpractice insurance, prerequisite course work. Transfer students are accepted. **Standardized tests** *Required:* ACT, TOEFL for international students. **Application** *Deadline:* 8/1 (freshmen). *Notification:* 10/1 (freshmen). *Application fee:* $20.

Expenses (2004–05) *Tuition, state resident:* full-time $4875; part-time $163 per credit hour. *Tuition, nonresident:* full-time $8460; part-time $282 per credit hour. *International tuition:* $8460 full-time. *Room and board:* $4554; room only: $3000 per academic year. *Required fees:* full-time $35; part-time $11 per credit; part-time $17 per term.

Financial Aid 65% of baccalaureate students in nursing programs received some form of financial aid in 2003–04. *Gift aid (need-based):* Federal Pell, FSEOG, state, private, college/university gift aid from institutional funds. *Loans:* FFEL (Subsidized and Unsubsidized Stafford PLUS), Perkins, state. *Work-Study:* Federal Work-Study, part-time campus jobs. *Application deadline (priority):* 3/1.

Contact Dr. Linda Bugle, Admissions Coordinator, Department of Nursing, Southeast Missouri State University, One University Plaza, Mail Stop 8300, Cape Girardeau, MO 63701-4799. *Telephone:* 573-651-2585. *Fax:* 573-651-2142. *E-mail:* lbugle@semo.edu.

GRADUATE PROGRAMS

Expenses (2004–05) *Tuition, state resident:* full-time $3382; part-time $188 per credit hour. *Tuition, nonresident:* full-time $5972; part-time $332 per credit hour. *International tuition:* $5972 full-time.

Financial Aid 50% of graduate students in nursing programs received some form of financial aid in 2003–04. 4 research assistantships with full tuition reimbursements available (averaging $6,100 per year), 2 teaching assistantships with full tuition reimbursements available (averaging $6,100 per year) were awarded.

Contact Dr. Elaine Jackson, Director, Graduate Studies, Department of Nursing, Southeast Missouri State University, One University Plaza, Mail Stop 8300, Cape Girardeau, MO 63701-4799. *Telephone:* 573-651-2871. *Fax:* 573-651-2142. *E-mail:* ejackson@semo.edu.

MASTER'S DEGREE PROGRAM

Degree MSN

Available Programs Master's.

Concentrations Available Nursing education. *Clinical nurse specialist programs in:* adult health. *Nurse practitioner programs in:* family health.

Site Options *Distance Learning:* Poplar Bluff, MO; Kennett, MO.

Study Options Full-time and part-time.

Program Entrance Requirements Clinical experience, minimum overall college GPA of 3.0, transcript of college record, CPR certification, written essay, immunizations, 2 letters of recommendation, physical assessment course, professional liability insurance/malpractice insurance, prerequisite course work, resume, statistics course. *Application deadline:* For fall admission, 4/1 (priority date); for spring admission, 11/1 (priority date). Applications are processed on a rolling basis. *Application fee:* $20 ($100 for international students).

Degree Requirements 45 total credit hours, thesis or project.

POST-MASTER'S PROGRAM

Areas of Study *Nurse practitioner programs in:* family health.

Southwest Baptist University

College of Nursing

Bolivar, Missouri

Founded in 1878

DEGREE • BSN

Nursing Program Faculty 3 (1% with doctorates).

Baccalaureate Enrollment 90

Women 90% **Men** 10% **Minority** 3% **International** 2% **Part-time** 50%

Nursing Student Activities Nursing Honor Society.

Nursing Student Resources Academic advising; bookstore; campus computer network; computer lab; computer-assisted instruction; e-mail services; interactive nursing skills videos; Internet; learning resource lab; library services; nursing audiovisuals; skills, simulation, or other laboratory.

Library Facilities 193,821 volumes; 10,939 periodical subscriptions.

BACCALAUREATE PROGRAMS

Degree BSN

Available Programs RN Baccalaureate.

Site Options Springfield, MO.

Study Options Full-time and part-time.

Program Entrance Requirements Minimum overall college GPA of 2.5, transcript of college record, CPR certification, health exam, high school transcript, immunizations, interview, minimum GPA in nursing prerequisites of 2.5, professional liability insurance/malpractice insurance, prerequisite course work. Transfer students are accepted. **Standardized tests** *Required:* SAT or ACT, TOEFL for international students. **Application** *Deadline:* rolling (freshmen), rolling (transfer). *Notification:* continuous (freshmen). *Application fee:* $25.

Advanced Placement Credit given for nursing courses completed elsewhere dependent upon specific evaluations.

Financial Aid 50% of baccalaureate students in nursing programs received some form of financial aid in 2002–03.

Contact Ms. Cartha C. Baker, Director, BSN program, College of Nursing, Southwest Baptist University, 4431 South Fremont, Springfield, MO 65804. *Telephone:* 417-820-5058. *Fax:* 417-887-4847. *E-mail:* mbaker@sbuniv.edu.

Southwest Missouri State University

Department of Nursing
Springfield, Missouri

http://www.smsu.edu/nursing

Founded in 1905

DEGREES • BSN • MSN

Nursing Program Faculty 11 (45% with doctorates).

Baccalaureate Enrollment 112
Women 90% **Men** 10% **Minority** 3% **International** 1% **Part-time** 40%

Graduate Enrollment 36
Women 94% **Men** 6% **Minority** 11% **Part-time** 62%

Nursing Student Activities Sigma Theta Tau, Student Nurses' Association.

Nursing Student Resources Academic advising; academic or career counseling; assistance for students with disabilities; bookstore; campus computer network; career placement assistance; computer lab; computer-assisted instruction; daycare for children of students; e-mail services; employment services for current students; externships; housing assistance; interactive nursing skills videos; Internet; learning resource lab; library services; nursing audiovisuals; paid internships; placement services for program completers; remedial services; resume preparation assistance; skills, simulation, or other laboratory; tutoring; unpaid internships.

Library Facilities 1.7 million volumes (10,500 in health, 3,516 in nursing); 4,238 periodical subscriptions (370 health-care related).

BACCALAUREATE PROGRAMS

Degree BSN

Available Programs ADN to Baccalaureate; Baccalaureate for Second Degree; Generic Baccalaureate; LPN to Baccalaureate.

Site Options *Distance Learning:* Branson, MO; West Plains, MO.

Study Options Full-time.

Program Entrance Requirements Minimum overall college GPA of 2.75, transcript of college record, CPR certification, health insurance, immunizations, prerequisite course work. Transfer students are accepted. **Standardized tests** *Required:* SAT or ACT, TOEFL for international students. **Application** *Deadline:* 7/20 (freshmen), 7/20 (transfer). *Notification:* continuous (freshmen). *Application fee:* $30.

Advanced Placement Credit given for nursing courses completed elsewhere dependent upon specific evaluations.

Expenses (2004–05) *Tuition, state resident:* full-time $4620; part-time $154 per credit hour. *Tuition, nonresident:* full-time $9240; part-time $308 per credit hour. *Room and board:* $2990; room only: $1649 per academic year. *Required fees:* full-time $508.

Financial Aid 30% of baccalaureate students in nursing programs received some form of financial aid in 2003–04. *Gift aid (need-based):* Federal Pell, FSEOG, state, private, college/university gift aid from institutional funds. *Loans:* FFEL (Subsidized and Unsubsidized Stafford PLUS), Perkins, state, college/university. *Work-Study:* Federal Work-Study, part-time campus jobs. *Application deadline (priority):* 3/30.

Contact Dr. Kathryn L. Hope, Head, Department of Nursing, Southwest Missouri State University, 901 South National, Springfield, MO 65804. *Telephone:* 417-836-5310. *Fax:* 417-836-5484. *E-mail:* kathrynhope@smsu.edu.

GRADUATE PROGRAMS

Expenses (2004–05) *Tuition, state resident:* full-time $2862; part-time $159 per credit hour. *Tuition, nonresident:* full-time $5724; part-time $318 per credit hour. *International tuition:* $5724 full-time. *Room and board:* $4800; room only: $3298 per academic year. *Required fees:* full-time $756.

Financial Aid 25% of graduate students in nursing programs received some form of financial aid in 2003–04. Research assistantships with full tuition reimbursements available (averaging $6,300 per year), 2 teaching assistantships with full tuition reimbursements available (averaging $6,300 per year) were awarded; Federal Work-Study and unspecified assistantships also available. *Financial aid application deadline:* 3/31.

Contact Dr. Kathryn L. Hope, Head, Department of Nursing, Southwest Missouri State University, 901 South National, Springfield, MO 65804. *Telephone:* 417-836-5310. *Fax:* 417-836-5484. *E-mail:* kathrynhope@smsu.edu.

MASTER'S DEGREE PROGRAM

Degree MSN

Available Programs Accelerated AD/RN to Master's; Master's; RN to Master's.

Concentrations Available Nursing education. *Nurse practitioner programs in:* family health.

Study Options Full-time and part-time.

Program Entrance Requirements Computer literacy, minimum overall college GPA of 3.0, transcript of college record, written essay, immunizations, interview, 2 letters of recommendation, nursing research course, physical assessment course, professional liability insurance/malpractice insurance, statistics course, GRE General Test. *Application deadline:* For fall admission, 8/5 (priority date); for spring admission, 12/20 (priority date). Applications are processed on a rolling basis. *Application fee:* $30.

Advanced Placement Credit given for nursing courses completed elsewhere dependent upon specific evaluations.

Degree Requirements 51 total credit hours, thesis or project, comprehensive exam.

POST-MASTER'S PROGRAM

Areas of Study Nursing education. *Nurse practitioner programs in:* family health.

CONTINUING EDUCATION PROGRAM

Contact Myra Miller, Program Coordinator for Health and Human Services, Department of Nursing, Southwest Missouri State University, Department of Continuing Education, 901 South National, Springfield, MO 65804. *Telephone:* 888-879-7678. *Fax:* 417-836-7674. *E-mail:* myramiller@smsu.edu.

Truman State University

Program in Nursing
Kirksville, Missouri

http://nursing.truman.edu

Founded in 1867

DEGREE • BSN

Nursing Program Faculty 12 (25% with doctorates).

Baccalaureate Enrollment 171
Women 93% **Men** 7% **Minority** 6% **International** 5%

Truman State University (continued)

Nursing Student Activities Nursing Honor Society, Sigma Theta Tau, Student Nurses' Association.

Nursing Student Resources Academic advising; academic or career counseling; assistance for students with disabilities; bookstore; campus computer network; career placement assistance; computer lab; computer-assisted instruction; daycare for children of students; e-mail services; employment services for current students; externships; interactive nursing skills videos; Internet; learning resource lab; library services; nursing audiovisuals; paid internships; placement services for program completers; remedial services; resume preparation assistance; skills, simulation, or other laboratory; tutoring; unpaid internships.

Library Facilities 492,916 volumes (6,848 in health, 1,877 in nursing); 3,468 periodical subscriptions (868 health-care related).

BACCALAUREATE PROGRAMS

Degree BSN

Available Programs Generic Baccalaureate; RN Baccalaureate.

Site Options St. Louis, MO.

Study Options Full-time.

Program Entrance Requirements Minimum overall college GPA of 2.75, transcript of college record, written essay, high school biology, high school chemistry, high school foreign language, 3 years high school math, 3 years high school science, high school transcript, minimum GPA in nursing prerequisites of 2.75. Transfer students are accepted. **Standardized tests** *Required:* SAT or ACT, TOEFL for international students. *Recommended:* ACT. **Application** *Deadline:* 3/1 (freshmen), rolling (transfer). *Early decision:* 11/15. *Notification:* continuous (freshmen), 12/15 (early action).

Advanced Placement Credit by examination available.

Expenses (2004–05) *Tuition, state resident:* full-time $5410. *Tuition, nonresident:* full-time $9510. *International tuition:* $9510 full-time. *Room and board:* $5250; room only: $4850 per academic year. *Required fees:* full-time $50.

Financial Aid 46% of baccalaureate students in nursing programs received some form of financial aid in 2003–04.

Contact Dr. Stephanie A. Powelson, Director, Program in Nursing, Truman State University, Barnett Hall 223, 100 East Normal Street, Kirksville, MO 63501. *Telephone:* 660-785-4557. *Fax:* 660-785-7424. *E-mail:* spowelso@truman.edu.

University of Missouri–Columbia
Sinclair School of Nursing
Columbia, Missouri

http://www.muhealth.org/

Founded in 1839

DEGREES • BSN • MS • PHD

Nursing Program Faculty 50 (23% with doctorates).

Baccalaureate Enrollment 219
Women 95% **Men** 5% **Minority** 9%

Graduate Enrollment 145
Women 96% **Men** 4% **Minority** 5% **International** 5% **Part-time** 53%

Nursing Student Activities Sigma Theta Tau, Student Nurses' Association, nursing club.

Nursing Student Resources Academic advising; academic or career counseling; campus computer network; computer lab; computer-assisted instruction; e-mail services; externships; interactive nursing skills videos; Internet; learning resource lab; library services; nursing audiovisuals; paid internships; resume preparation assistance; skills, simulation, or other laboratory; tutoring; unpaid internships.

Library Facilities 3.2 million volumes (253,271 in health); 15,808 periodical subscriptions.

BACCALAUREATE PROGRAMS

Degree BSN

Available Programs Accelerated Baccalaureate for Second Degree; Generic Baccalaureate; RN Baccalaureate.

Study Options Full-time and part-time.

Program Entrance Requirements Minimum overall college GPA of 2.5, transcript of college record, CPR certification, high school biology, high school chemistry, 4 years high school math, high school science, high school transcript, immunizations, minimum GPA in nursing prerequisites of 2.5, prerequisite course work. Transfer students are accepted. **Standardized tests** *Required:* SAT or ACT, TOEFL for international students. **Application** *Deadline:* rolling (freshmen), rolling (transfer). *Notification:* continuous (freshmen). *Application fee:* $35.

Advanced Placement Credit by examination available. Credit given for nursing courses completed elsewhere dependent upon specific evaluations.

Expenses (2004–05) *Room and board:* $6131 per academic year. *Required fees:* full-time $6276; part-time $209 per credit.

Financial Aid 85% of baccalaureate students in nursing programs received some form of financial aid in 2003–04. *Gift aid (need-based):* Federal Pell, FSEOG, state, private, college/university gift aid from institutional funds, Federal Nursing. *Loans:* Federal Nursing Student Loans, Federal Direct (Subsidized and Unsubsidized Stafford PLUS), Perkins, state, college/university, Health Professions Loans, Primary Care Loans, alternative loans. *Work-Study:* Federal Work-Study. *Application deadline (priority):* 3/1.

Contact Ms. Jackie Vendt, Undergraduate Academic Advisor, Sinclair School of Nursing, University of Missouri–Columbia, S235, Columbia, MO 65211. *Telephone:* 573-882-0277. *Fax:* 573-884-4544. *E-mail:* vendtJ@missouri.edu.

GRADUATE PROGRAMS

Expenses (2004–05) *Room and board:* $7390 per academic year. *Required fees:* full-time $5772; part-time $254 per credit.

Financial Aid 65% of graduate students in nursing programs received some form of financial aid in 2003–04. Fellowships, research assistantships, teaching assistantships, career-related internships or fieldwork, institutionally sponsored loans, traineeships, and tuition waivers (full) available.

Contact Ms. Nancy Lee Johnson, Coordinator of Student Affairs, Sinclair School of Nursing, University of Missouri–Columbia, S235, Columbia, MO 65211. *Telephone:* 573-882-0277. *Fax:* 573-884-4544. *E-mail:* johnsonn@missouri.edu.

MASTER'S DEGREE PROGRAM

Degree MS

Available Programs Master's.

Concentrations Available Nursing administration; nursing education. *Clinical nurse specialist programs in:* adult health, cardiovascular, critical care, gerontology, home health care, medical-surgical, oncology, pediatric, public health, rehabilitation, school health, women's health. *Nurse practitioner programs in:* family health, gerontology, pediatric, psychiatric/mental health.

Program Entrance Requirements Minimum overall college GPA of 3.0, transcript of college record, CPR certification, immunizations, interview, 2 letters of recommendation, statistics course, GRE General Test. *Application deadline:* For fall admission, 2/1 (priority date). Applications are processed on a rolling basis. *Application fee:* $45 ($60 for international students).

Degree Requirements 42 total credit hours, comprehensive exam.

POST-MASTER'S PROGRAM

Areas of Study Nursing administration; nursing education. *Clinical nurse specialist programs in:* adult health, cardiovascular, critical care, gerontology, home health care, medical-surgical, oncology, pediatric, public health, rehabilitation, school health, women's health. *Nurse practitioner programs in:* family health, gerontology, pediatric, psychiatric/mental health.

DOCTORAL DEGREE PROGRAM

Degree PhD

Available Programs Doctorate.

Areas of Study Health promotion/disease prevention, health-care systems, nursing administration, nursing policy, nursing research, nursing science.

Program Entrance Requirements Minimum overall college GPA of 3.5, interview by faculty committee, interview, 3 letters of recommendation, vita, writing sample. *Application deadline:* For fall admission, 2/1 (priority date). Applications are processed on a rolling basis. *Application fee:* $45 ($60 for international students).

Degree Requirements 72 total credit hours, dissertation, oral exam, written exam, residency.

CONTINUING EDUCATION PROGRAM

Contact Dr. Shirley Farrah, Assistant Dean, Nursing Outreach and Distance Education, Sinclair School of Nursing, University of Missouri–Columbia, S266B, Columbia, MO 65211. *Telephone:* 573-882-0215. *Fax:* 573-884-4544. *E-mail:* farrahs@missouri.edu.

University of Missouri–Kansas City

School of Nursing
Kansas City, Missouri

Founded in 1929

DEGREES • BSN • MSN • PHD

Nursing Program Faculty 46 (50% with doctorates).

Baccalaureate Enrollment 227
Women 93% **Men** 7% **Minority** 24% **Part-time** 11%

Graduate Enrollment 225
Women 96% **Men** 4% **Minority** 12% **Part-time** 94%

Nursing Student Activities Sigma Theta Tau, Student Nurses' Association.

Nursing Student Resources Academic advising; academic or career counseling; assistance for students with disabilities; bookstore; campus computer network; career placement assistance; computer lab; computer-assisted instruction; e-mail services; housing assistance; interactive nursing skills videos; Internet; learning resource lab; library services; nursing audiovisuals; other; placement services for program completers; remedial services; resume preparation assistance; skills, simulation, or other laboratory; tutoring.

Library Facilities 1.3 million volumes (81,000 in health, 10,530 in nursing); 7,222 periodical subscriptions (796 health-care related).

BACCALAUREATE PROGRAMS

Degree BSN

Available Programs Generic Baccalaureate; RN Baccalaureate.

Study Options Full-time.

Program Entrance Requirements Minimum overall college GPA of 2.75, transcript of college record, CPR certification, written essay, health insurance, high school foreign language, 4 years high school math, 4 years high school science, high school transcript, immunizations, minimum GPA in nursing prerequisites of 2.75, prerequisite course work. Transfer students are accepted. **Standardized tests** *Required:* SAT or ACT, TOEFL for international students. **Application** *Deadline:* rolling (freshmen), rolling (transfer). *Notification:* continuous (freshmen). *Application fee:* $35.

Expenses (2004–05) *Tuition, state resident:* full-time $6276; part-time $209 per credit hour. *Tuition, nonresident:* full-time $15,723; part-time $524 per credit hour. *International tuition:* $15,723 full-time. *Room and board:* $8275 per academic year. *Required fees:* full-time $3004; part-time $50 per credit; part-time $662 per term.

Financial Aid 45% of baccalaureate students in nursing programs received some form of financial aid in 2003–04. *Gift aid (need-based):* Federal Pell, FSEOG, state, private, college/university gift aid from institutional funds, United Negro College Fund, Federal Nursing. *Loans:* FFEL (Subsidized and Unsubsidized Stafford PLUS), Perkins, state, college/university. *Work-Study:* Federal Work-Study. *Application deadline (priority):* 3/1.

Contact Ms. Judy A. Jellison, Manager, Nursing Student Services, School of Nursing, University of Missouri–Kansas City, 2220 Holmes Street, Kansas City, MO 64108. *Telephone:* 816-235-1740. *Fax:* 816-235-1701. *E-mail:* jellisonj@umkc.edu.

GRADUATE PROGRAMS

Expenses (2004–05) *Tuition, state resident:* full-time $6203; part-time $254 per credit hour. *Tuition, nonresident:* full-time $15,861; part-time $657 per credit hour. *International tuition:* $15,861 full-time. *Room and board:* $8000 per academic year. *Required fees:* full-time $1286; part-time $52 per credit.

Financial Aid 35% of graduate students in nursing programs received some form of financial aid in 2003–04. Fellowships, teaching assistantships, career-related internships or fieldwork, Federal Work-Study, institutionally sponsored loans, and tuition waivers (full and partial) available. Aid available to part-time students. *Financial aid application deadline:* 6/30.

Contact Ms. Judy A. Jellison, Manager, Nursing Student Services, School of Nursing, University of Missouri–Kansas City, 2220 Holmes Street, Kansas City, MO 64108. *Telephone:* 816-235-1740. *Fax:* 816-235-1701. *E-mail:* jellisonj@umkc.edu.

MASTER'S DEGREE PROGRAM

Degree MSN

Available Programs Master's.

Concentrations Available Nursing administration; nursing education. *Clinical nurse specialist programs in:* pediatric. *Nurse practitioner programs in:* adult health, family health, neonatal health, pediatric, women's health.

Site Options *Distance Learning:* Joplin, MO; St. Joseph, MO.

Study Options Full-time and part-time.

Program Entrance Requirements Clinical experience, computer literacy, minimum overall college GPA of 3.2, transcript of college record, CPR certification, immunizations, physical assessment course, resume, statistics course, California Critical Thinking Skills Test. *Application deadline:* For fall admission, 2/1 (priority date); for spring admission, 9/15 (priority date). *Application fee:* $25.

Degree Requirements 42 total credit hours, thesis or project.

POST-MASTER'S PROGRAM

Areas of Study Nursing administration; nursing education. *Clinical nurse specialist programs in:* pediatric. *Nurse practitioner programs in:* adult health, family health, neonatal health, pediatric, women's health.

DOCTORAL DEGREE PROGRAM

Degree PhD

Available Programs Doctorate; Post-Baccalaureate Doctorate.

Areas of Study Health promotion/disease prevention, health-care systems.

Program Entrance Requirements Minimum overall college GPA of 3.5, interview by faculty committee, interview, 3 letters of recommendation, MSN or equivalent, vita, writing sample, GRE. *Application deadline:* For fall admission, 2/1 (priority date); for spring admission, 9/15 (priority date). *Application fee:* $25.

Degree Requirements 82 total credit hours, dissertation, oral exam, written exam, residency.

University of Missouri–St. Louis

College of Nursing
St. Louis, Missouri

Founded in 1963

DEGREES • BSN • MSN • PHD

Nursing Program Faculty 35 (54% with doctorates).

Baccalaureate Enrollment 507
Women 93% **Men** 7% **Minority** 19% **International** 1% **Part-time** 32%

Graduate Enrollment 177
Women 96% **Men** 4% **Minority** 21% **International** 2% **Part-time** 92%

Nursing Student Activities Sigma Theta Tau, Student Nurses' Association.

Nursing Student Resources Academic advising; academic or career counseling; assistance for students with disabilities; bookstore; campus computer network; career placement assistance; computer lab; computer-assisted instruction; daycare for children of students; e-mail services; employment services for current students; externships; interactive nursing skills videos; Internet; learning resource lab; library services; nursing audiovisuals; resume preparation assistance; skills, simulation, or other laboratory; tutoring; unpaid internships.

University of Missouri–St. Louis (continued)

Library Facilities 782,431 volumes (15,530 in health, 8,450 in nursing); 3,570 periodical subscriptions (485 health-care related).

BACCALAUREATE PROGRAMS

Degree BSN

Available Programs Accelerated Baccalaureate; Generic Baccalaureate; RN Baccalaureate.

Site Options *Distance Learning:* St. Charles, MO; Florissant.

Study Options Full-time and part-time.

Program Entrance Requirements Minimum overall college GPA of 2.5, transcript of college record, CPR certification, health exam, 4 years high school math, 3 years high school science, high school transcript, immunizations, minimum high school GPA of 2.5, minimum high school rank 67%. Transfer students are accepted. **Standardized tests** *Required:* SAT or ACT, TOEFL for international students. **Application** *Deadline:* rolling (freshmen), 8/1 (transfer). *Notification:* continuous (freshmen). *Application fee:* $35.

Advanced Placement Credit given for nursing courses completed elsewhere dependent upon specific evaluations.

Expenses (2004–05) *Tuition, state resident:* full-time $11,311; part-time $359 per credit hour. *Tuition, nonresident:* full-time $16,034; part-time $577 per semester. *Room and board:* $1715 per academic year.

Financial Aid 70% of baccalaureate students in nursing programs received some form of financial aid in 2003–04. *Gift aid (need-based):* Federal Pell, FSEOG, state, private, college/university gift aid from institutional funds, Federal Nursing. *Loans:* Federal Nursing Student Loans, FFEL (Subsidized and Unsubsidized Stafford PLUS), Perkins, state, college/university. *Work-Study:* Federal Work-Study. *Application deadline (priority):* 4/1.

Contact Ms. Kathern Furgason, Director of Student Services, College of Nursing, University of Missouri–St. Louis, One University Boulevard, St. Louis, MO 63121-4499. *Telephone:* 314-516-7087. *Fax:* 314-516-7519. *E-mail:* furgason@umsl.edu.

GRADUATE PROGRAMS

Expenses (2004–05) *Tuition, state resident:* full-time $5521; part-time $307 per credit hour. *Tuition, nonresident:* full-time $12,406; part-time $709 per credit hour. *Room and board:* $1715; room only: $1715 per academic year. *Required fees:* part-time $2680 per term.

Financial Aid 45% of graduate students in nursing programs received some form of financial aid in 2003–04. Research assistantships with full and partial tuition reimbursements available, teaching assistantships with full and partial tuition reimbursements available available.

Contact Ms. Kathern Furgason, Director of Student Services, College of Nursing, University of Missouri–St. Louis, One University Boulevard, St. Louis, MO 63121-4499. *Telephone:* 314-516-7087. *Fax:* 314-516-7519. *E-mail:* furgason@umsl.edu.

MASTER'S DEGREE PROGRAM

Degree MSN

Available Programs RN to Master's.

Concentrations Available Nursing administration; nursing education. *Clinical nurse specialist programs in:* adult health, pediatric, women's health. *Nurse practitioner programs in:* adult health, family health, pediatric, women's health.

Site Options *Distance Learning:* Park Hill, MO; St. Charles, MO.

Study Options Full-time and part-time.

Program Entrance Requirements Clinical experience, minimum overall college GPA of 3.0, transcript of college record, CPR certification, immunizations, 2 letters of recommendation, physical assessment course, statistics course. *Application deadline:* For fall admission, 7/1 (priority date); for spring admission, 10/1. Applications are processed on a rolling basis. *Application fee:* $35 ($40 for international students).

Advanced Placement Credit given for nursing courses completed elsewhere dependent upon specific evaluations.

Degree Requirements 36 total credit hours.

DOCTORAL DEGREE PROGRAM

Degree PhD

Available Programs Doctorate.

Areas of Study Nursing administration, nursing education, nursing policy, nursing research.

Program Entrance Requirements Minimum overall college GPA of 3.2, interview, 3 letters of recommendation, vita, writing sample, GRE General Test. *Application deadline:* For fall admission, 7/1 (priority date); for spring admission, 10/1. Applications are processed on a rolling basis. *Application fee:* $35 ($40 for international students).

Degree Requirements 72 total credit hours, dissertation, oral exam, written exam, residency.

Webster University

Department of Nursing
St. Louis, Missouri

http://www.webster.edu/depts/artsci/nursing/nursing.html

Founded in 1915

DEGREES • BSN • MSN

Nursing Program Faculty 11 (72% with doctorates).

Baccalaureate Enrollment 135
Women 93% **Men** 7% **Minority** 14% **International** 1% **Part-time** 90%

Graduate Enrollment 34
Women 90% **Men** 10% **Minority** 20% **International** 10% **Part-time** 100%

Nursing Student Activities Nursing Honor Society, Sigma Theta Tau.

Nursing Student Resources Academic advising; academic or career counseling; assistance for students with disabilities; bookstore; campus computer network; career placement assistance; computer lab; e-mail services; employment services for current students; Internet; library services; nursing audiovisuals; placement services for program completers; remedial services; resume preparation assistance; skills, simulation, or other laboratory; tutoring.

Library Facilities 271,047 volumes (7,030 in health, 3,114 in nursing); 1,598 periodical subscriptions (108 health-care related).

BACCALAUREATE PROGRAMS

Degree BSN

Available Programs ADN to Baccalaureate; RN Baccalaureate.

Site Options Kansas City, MO.

Program Entrance Requirements Minimum overall college GPA of 2.5, transcript of college record, immunizations, interview, prerequisite course work, RN licensure. Transfer students are accepted. **Standardized tests** *Required:* SAT or ACT, TOEFL for international students. **Application** *Deadline:* 6/1 (freshmen), 8/1 (transfer). *Notification:* continuous (freshmen). *Application fee:* $25.

Financial Aid 53% of baccalaureate students in nursing programs received some form of financial aid in 2003–04. *Gift aid (need-based):* Federal Pell, FSEOG, state, private, college/university gift aid from institutional funds. *Loans:* FFEL (Subsidized and Unsubsidized Stafford PLUS), Perkins. *Work-Study:* Federal Work-Study, part-time campus jobs. *Application deadline (priority):* 4/1.

Contact Dr. Anne E. Schappe, Chair, Department of Nursing, Webster University, 470 East Lockwood Avenue, St. Louis, MO 63119-3194. *Telephone:* 314-968-7483. *Fax:* 314-963-6101. *E-mail:* schappan@webster.edu.

GRADUATE PROGRAMS

Financial Aid 40% of graduate students in nursing programs received some form of financial aid in 2003–04. Federal Work-Study available. Aid available to part-time students. *Financial aid application deadline:* 4/1.

Contact Dr. Jennifer Broeder, Coordinator, MSN Program, Department of Nursing, Webster University, 470 East Lockwood Avenue, St. Louis, MO 63119-3194. *Telephone:* 314-968-7483. *Fax:* 314-963-6101. *E-mail:* jbroeder@webster.edu.

MASTER'S DEGREE PROGRAM

Degree MSN

Available Programs Master's.

Concentrations Available Nursing education. *Clinical nurse specialist programs in:* family health.

Site Options Kansas City, MO.

Study Options Part-time.

Program Entrance Requirements Clinical experience, minimum overall college GPA of 3.0, transcript of college record, written essay, immunizations, interview, 3 letters of recommendation, nursing research course, physical assessment course, resume, statistics course. *Application deadline:* Applications are processed on a rolling basis. *Application fee:* $25 ($50 for international students).

Advanced Placement Credit given for nursing courses completed elsewhere dependent upon specific evaluations.

Degree Requirements 36 total credit hours, thesis or project.

William Jewell College

Department of Nursing
Liberty, Missouri

http://www.jewell.edu

Founded in 1849

DEGREE • BS

Nursing Program Faculty 20 (25% with doctorates).

Baccalaureate Enrollment 191
Women 90% **Men** 10% **Minority** 2% **International** 2%

Nursing Student Activities Sigma Theta Tau, Student Nurses' Association.

Nursing Student Resources Academic advising; academic or career counseling; bookstore; campus computer network; career placement assistance; computer lab; computer-assisted instruction; e-mail services; employment services for current students; externships; housing assistance; interactive nursing skills videos; Internet; learning resource lab; library services; nursing audiovisuals; placement services for program completers; resume preparation assistance; skills, simulation, or other laboratory; tutoring; unpaid internships.

Library Facilities 260,119 volumes (4,000 in health, 1,000 in nursing); 868 periodical subscriptions (250 health-care related).

BACCALAUREATE PROGRAMS

Degree BS

Available Programs Accelerated Baccalaureate; Generic Baccalaureate.

Study Options Full-time and part-time.

Program Entrance Requirements Minimum overall college GPA of 2.5, transcript of college record, CPR certification, written essay, health exam, health insurance, high school transcript, immunizations, minimum high school GPA, minimum GPA in nursing prerequisites of 2.5, professional liability insurance/malpractice insurance, prerequisite course work. Transfer students are accepted. **Standardized tests** *Required:* SAT or ACT, TOEFL for international students. *Required for some:* SAT Subject Tests. **Application** *Deadline:* rolling (freshmen), rolling (transfer). *Early decision:* 11/15. *Notification:* continuous (freshmen), 12/1 (early action). *Application fee:* $25.

Financial Aid 98% of baccalaureate students in nursing programs received some form of financial aid in 2003–04. *Gift aid (need-based):* Federal Pell, FSEOG, state, private, college/university gift aid from institutional funds. *Loans:* Federal Nursing Student Loans, FFEL (Subsidized and Unsubsidized Stafford PLUS), Perkins. *Work-Study:* Federal Work-Study, part-time campus jobs. *Application deadline (priority):* 3/1.

Contact Dr. Nelda S. Godfrey, Associate Professor and Chair, Department of Nursing, William Jewell College, 500 College Hill, Box 2002, Liberty, MO 64068. *Telephone:* 816-415-7605. *Fax:* 816-415-5024. *E-mail:* godfreyn@william.jewell.edu.

MONTANA

Carroll College

Department of Nursing
Helena, Montana

http://www.carroll.edu

Founded in 1909

DEGREE • BA

Nursing Program Faculty 13 (15% with doctorates).

Baccalaureate Enrollment 118
Women 94% **Men** 6% **Minority** 5% **International** 1% **Part-time** 2%

Nursing Student Activities Sigma Theta Tau, Student Nurses' Association.

Nursing Student Resources Academic advising; academic or career counseling; assistance for students with disabilities; bookstore; campus computer network; career placement assistance; computer lab; computer-assisted instruction; e-mail services; employment services for current students; externships; housing assistance; interactive nursing skills videos; Internet; learning resource lab; library services; nursing audiovisuals; paid internships; placement services for program completers; remedial services; resume preparation assistance; skills, simulation, or other laboratory; tutoring; unpaid internships.

Library Facilities 89,003 volumes (38,000 in health); 2,721 periodical subscriptions (152 health-care related).

BACCALAUREATE PROGRAMS

Degree BA

Available Programs Generic Baccalaureate.

Study Options Full-time and part-time.

Program Entrance Requirements Transcript of college record, high school transcript, immunizations, minimum GPA in nursing prerequisites of 2.75, prerequisite course work. Transfer students are accepted. **Standardized tests** *Required:* SAT or ACT, TOEFL for international students. *Required for some:* SAT Subject Tests, SAT II Writing Tests. **Application** *Deadline:* 6/1 (freshmen), 6/1 (transfer). *Notification:* continuous (freshmen). *Application fee:* $35.

Advanced Placement Credit given for nursing courses completed elsewhere dependent upon specific evaluations.

Expenses (2004–05) *Tuition:* full-time $15,550; part-time $518 per credit hour. *Room and board:* $6000 per academic year. *Required fees:* full-time $250.

Financial Aid 96% of baccalaureate students in nursing programs received some form of financial aid in 2003–04.

Contact Mike Brown, Associate Director, Admissions, Department of Nursing, Carroll College, 1601 North Benton Avenue, Helena, MT 59625. *Telephone:* 406-447-5482. *Fax:* 406-447-4533. *E-mail:* mbrown@carroll.edu.

CONTINUING EDUCATION PROGRAM

Contact Dr. Cynthia Z. Gustafson, Director of Parish Nursing Program, Department of Nursing, Carroll College, 1601 North Benton Avenue, Helena, MT 59625. *Telephone:* 406-447-5494. *Fax:* 406-447-5476. *E-mail:* cgustafs@carroll.edu.

Montana State University–Bozeman

College of Nursing
Bozeman, Montana

http://www.montana.edu/wwwnu/index.html

Founded in 1893

DEGREES • BSN • MN

Montana State University–Bozeman (continued)

Nursing Program Faculty 85 (23% with doctorates).

Baccalaureate Enrollment 781
Women 90% **Men** 10% **Minority** 7% **Part-time** 20%

Graduate Enrollment 25
Men 8% **Minority** 4% **Part-time** 24%

Nursing Student Activities Nursing Honor Society, Sigma Theta Tau, Student Nurses' Association.

Nursing Student Resources Academic advising; academic or career counseling; assistance for students with disabilities; bookstore; campus computer network; career placement assistance; computer lab; computer-assisted instruction; e-mail services; employment services for current students; Internet; library services; placement services for program completers; resume preparation assistance; skills, simulation, or other laboratory; tutoring.

Library Facilities 574,634 volumes (78,178 in health, 11,383 in nursing); 6,643 periodical subscriptions (1,117 health-care related).

BACCALAUREATE PROGRAMS

Degree BSN

Available Programs LPN to Baccalaureate; RN Baccalaureate.

Site Options *Distance Learning:* Billings, MT; Great Falls, MT; Missoula, MT.

Study Options Full-time and part-time.

Program Entrance Requirements Minimum overall college GPA of 2.5, transcript of college record, CPR certification, health exam, high school transcript, immunizations, minimum high school GPA of 2.5, minimum high school rank 50%, professional liability insurance/malpractice insurance, prerequisite course work. Transfer students are accepted. **Standardized tests** *Required:* SAT or ACT, TOEFL for international students. **Application** *Deadline:* rolling (freshmen), rolling (transfer). *Notification:* continuous (freshmen). *Application fee:* $30.

Advanced Placement Credit by examination available. Credit given for nursing courses completed elsewhere dependent upon specific evaluations.

Expenses (2004–05) *Tuition, state resident:* full-time $4386; part-time $183 per credit hour. *Tuition, nonresident:* full-time $13,898; part-time $579 per credit hour. *Room and board:* $11,000; room only: $6200 per academic year. *Required fees:* full-time $2176; part-time $147 per credit.

Financial Aid *Gift aid (need-based):* Federal Pell, FSEOG, state, private, college/university gift aid from institutional funds, Federal Nursing. *Loans:* Federal Nursing Student Loans, Federal Direct (Subsidized and Unsubsidized Stafford PLUS), Perkins, college/university, Freeborn Loans. *Work-Study:* Federal Work-Study, part-time campus jobs. *Application deadline (priority):* 3/1.

Contact Dr. A. Gretchen McNeely, Associate Dean, College of Nursing, Montana State University–Bozeman, Sherrick Hall, PO Box 173560, Bozeman, MT 59717-3560. *Telephone:* 406-994-3784. *Fax:* 406-994-6020. *E-mail:* gmcneely@montana.edu.

GRADUATE PROGRAMS

Expenses (2004–05) *Tuition, state resident:* full-time $2193; part-time $183 per credit hour. *Tuition, nonresident:* full-time $6950; part-time $579 per credit hour. *Required fees:* full-time $2177; part-time $148 per credit.

Financial Aid 72% of graduate students in nursing programs received some form of financial aid in 2003–04. 2 research assistantships (averaging $6,656 per year), 6 teaching assistantships with partial tuition reimbursements available (averaging $5,120 per year) were awarded; institutionally sponsored loans, scholarships, traineeships, and unspecified assistantships also available. Aid available to part-time students. *Financial aid application deadline:* 3/1.

Contact Dr. A. Gretchen McNeely, Associate Dean, College of Nursing, Montana State University–Bozeman, Sherrick Hall, PO Box 173560, Bozeman, MT 59717-3560. *Telephone:* 406-994-3784. *Fax:* 406-994-6020. *E-mail:* gmcneely@montana.edu.

MASTER'S DEGREE PROGRAM

Degree MN

Available Programs Master's.

Concentrations Available *Clinical nurse specialist programs in:* community health, medical-surgical. *Nurse practitioner programs in:* family health.

Site Options *Distance Learning:* Billings, MT; Great Falls, MT; Missoula, MT.

Study Options Full-time and part-time.

Program Entrance Requirements Computer literacy, minimum overall college GPA of 3.0, transcript of college record, interview, 3 letters of recommendation, nursing research course, physical assessment course, statistics course, GRE General Test. *Application deadline:* For fall admission, 7/15 (priority date); for spring admission, 12/1 (priority date). Applications are processed on a rolling basis. *Application fee:* $50.

Degree Requirements 59 total credit hours, thesis or project, comprehensive exam.

POST-MASTER'S PROGRAM

Areas of Study *Nurse practitioner programs in:* family health.

Montana State University–Northern

College of Nursing
Havre, Montana

http://www.msun.edu/academics/nursing

Founded in 1929

DEGREE • BSN

Nursing Program Faculty 9.

Baccalaureate Enrollment 43
Women 92% **Men** 8% **Minority** 15%

Nursing Student Activities Nursing club.

Nursing Student Resources Academic advising; academic or career counseling; assistance for students with disabilities; bookstore; campus computer network; career placement assistance; computer lab; computer-assisted instruction; daycare for children of students; e-mail services; employment services for current students; housing assistance; interactive nursing skills videos; Internet; learning resource lab; library services; nursing audiovisuals; remedial services; resume preparation assistance; skills, simulation, or other laboratory; tutoring.

Library Facilities 128,000 volumes (2,600 in health, 2,600 in nursing); 1,729 periodical subscriptions (50 health-care related).

BACCALAUREATE PROGRAMS

Degree BSN

Available Programs ADN to Baccalaureate; RN Baccalaureate.

Site Options *Distance Learning:* Great Falls, MT; Lewistown, MT.

Study Options Full-time and part-time.

Program Entrance Requirements Minimum overall college GPA of 2.25, transcript of college record, CPR certification, health exam, health insurance, immunizations, professional liability insurance/malpractice insurance, prerequisite course work. Transfer students are accepted. **Standardized tests** *Required:* TOEFL for international students. ***Placement:*** *Required:* ACT. **Application** *Deadline:* rolling (freshmen), rolling (transfer). *Notification:* continuous (freshmen). *Application fee:* $30.

Advanced Placement Credit given for nursing courses completed elsewhere dependent upon specific evaluations.

Expenses (2004–05) *Tuition, state resident:* full-time $11,240; part-time $624 per course. *Tuition, nonresident:* full-time $26,025; part-time $1446 per course. *Required fees:* full-time $200.

Financial Aid 75% of baccalaureate students in nursing programs received some form of financial aid in 2003–04.

Contact Ms. Renae Munson, Administrative Support, College of Nursing, Montana State University–Northern, 2100 16th Avenue South, PO Box 6010, Great Falls, MT 59406. *Telephone:* 800-446-2698 Ext. 4437. *Fax:* 406-771-4426. *E-mail:* munsonr@msun.edu.

CONTINUING EDUCATION PROGRAM

Contact Ms. Sharon Keeley, Administrative Associate, College of Nursing, Montana State University–Northern, PO Box 7751, Havre, MT 59501. *Telephone:* 800-662-6132 Ext. 4196. *Fax:* 406-265-3772. *E-mail:* skeeley@msun.edu.

NEBRASKA

Clarkson College
Department of Nursing
Omaha, Nebraska

http://www.clarksoncollege.edu
Founded in 1888

DEGREES • BSN • MSN

Nursing Program Faculty 17 (24% with doctorates).

Baccalaureate Enrollment 281
Women 95% **Men** 5% **Minority** 8% **Part-time** 20%

Graduate Enrollment 83
Women 99% **Men** 1% **Minority** 5% **Part-time** 100%

Nursing Student Activities Sigma Theta Tau, Student Nurses' Association.

Nursing Student Resources Academic advising; academic or career counseling; assistance for students with disabilities; bookstore; campus computer network; career placement assistance; computer lab; computer-assisted instruction; e-mail services; employment services for current students; interactive nursing skills videos; Internet; learning resource lab; library services; nursing audiovisuals; placement services for program completers; resume preparation assistance; skills, simulation, or other laboratory; tutoring.

Library Facilities 8,807 volumes (7,500 in health, 2,193 in nursing); 262 periodical subscriptions (583 health-care related).

BACCALAUREATE PROGRAMS

Degree BSN

Available Programs ADN to Baccalaureate; Accelerated Baccalaureate; Baccalaureate for Second Degree; Generic Baccalaureate; LPN to Baccalaureate.

Study Options Full-time and part-time.

Program Entrance Requirements Minimum overall college GPA of 2.5, transcript of college record, CPR certification, written essay, health exam, health insurance, 2 years high school math, 2 years high school science, high school transcript, immunizations, minimum high school GPA of 2.5, minimum high school rank 50%. Transfer students are accepted. **Standardized tests** *Required for some:* SAT or ACT. **Application** *Deadline:* rolling (freshmen), rolling (transfer). *Notification:* continuous (freshmen). *Application fee:* $15.

Advanced Placement Credit given for nursing courses completed elsewhere dependent upon specific evaluations.

Expenses (2004–05) *Tuition:* part-time $325 per credit hour. *Required fees:* full-time $5000.

Financial Aid 78% of baccalaureate students in nursing programs received some form of financial aid in 2003–04.

Contact Ms. Anne Folkers, Admissions Coordinator, Department of Nursing, Clarkson College, 101 South 42nd Street, Omaha, NE 68131-2739. *Telephone:* 402-552-3100. *Fax:* 402-552-6057. *E-mail:* folkers@clarksoncollege.edu.

GRADUATE PROGRAMS

Expenses (2004–05) *Tuition:* part-time $370 per credit hour.

Financial Aid 40% of graduate students in nursing programs received some form of financial aid in 2003–04. Federal Work-Study, institutionally sponsored loans, and scholarships available. Aid available to part-time students. *Financial aid application deadline:* 4/1.

Contact Ms. Anne Folkers, Admissions Coordinator, Department of Nursing, Clarkson College, 101 South 42nd Street, Omaha, NE 68131-2739. *Telephone:* 800-647-5500. *Fax:* 402-552-6057. *E-mail:* admiss@clarksoncollege.edu.

MASTER'S DEGREE PROGRAM

Degree MSN

Available Programs Master's.

Concentrations Available Nursing administration; nursing education. *Nurse practitioner programs in:* family health.

Study Options Full-time and part-time.

Program Entrance Requirements Clinical experience, minimum overall college GPA of 3.0, transcript of college record, CPR certification, written essay, immunizations, 2 letters of recommendation, resume. *Application deadline:* For fall admission, 7/13; for spring admission, 1/5. Applications are processed on a rolling basis. *Application fee:* $15.

Advanced Placement Credit given for nursing courses completed elsewhere dependent upon specific evaluations.

Degree Requirements 38 total credit hours, thesis or project, comprehensive exam.

POST-MASTER'S PROGRAM

Areas of Study Nursing administration; nursing education. *Nurse practitioner programs in:* family health.

CONTINUING EDUCATION PROGRAM

Contact Ms. Judi Dunn, Director, Professional Development, Department of Nursing, Clarkson College, 101 South 42nd Street, Omaha, NE 68131-2739. *Telephone:* 402-552-3100 Ext. 26123. *Fax:* 402-552-6058. *E-mail:* dunn@clarksoncollege.edu.

College of Saint Mary
Division of Health Care Professions
Omaha, Nebraska

Founded in 1923

DEGREE • BSN

Nursing Program Faculty 18 (6% with doctorates).

Baccalaureate Enrollment 26
Women 100% **Minority** 10% **Part-time** 65%

Nursing Student Activities Nursing Honor Society, Sigma Theta Tau, Student Nurses' Association, nursing club.

Nursing Student Resources Academic advising; academic or career counseling; bookstore; campus computer network; career placement assistance; computer lab; computer-assisted instruction; e-mail services; Internet; learning resource lab; library services; nursing audiovisuals; other; placement services for program completers; resume preparation assistance; skills, simulation, or other laboratory; tutoring.

Library Facilities 81,268 volumes; 12,800 periodical subscriptions (100 health-care related).

BACCALAUREATE PROGRAMS

Degree BSN

Available Programs ADN to Baccalaureate; Generic Baccalaureate.

Study Options Full-time and part-time.

Program Entrance Requirements Minimum overall college GPA of 2.5, transcript of college record, 2 letters of recommendation, minimum GPA in nursing prerequisites of 2.5, prerequisite course work. Transfer students are accepted. **Standardized tests** *Required:* SAT or ACT, TOEFL for international students. **Application** *Deadline:* rolling (freshmen), rolling (transfer). *Notification:* continuous until 8/24 (freshmen). *Application fee:* $30.

Advanced Placement Credit given for nursing courses completed elsewhere dependent upon specific evaluations.

Expenses (2003–04) *Tuition:* full-time $15,770; part-time $325 per credit hour. *Room and board:* $2600 per academic year.

Financial Aid 81% of baccalaureate students in nursing programs received some form of financial aid in 2002–03.

Contact Dr. Peggy L. Hawkins, RN, Nursing Programs Director, Division of Health Care Professions, College of Saint Mary, 1901 South 72nd Street, Omaha, NE 68124. *Telephone:* 402-399-2636. *Fax:* 402-399-2654. *E-mail:* phawkins@csm.edu.

Creighton University

School of Nursing
Omaha, Nebraska

http://nursing.creighton.edu/

Founded in 1878

DEGREES • BSN • MS

Nursing Program Faculty 51 (27% with doctorates).

Baccalaureate Enrollment 461
Women 90% **Men** 10% **Minority** 11% **Part-time** 7%

Graduate Enrollment 73
Women 88% **Men** 12% **Minority** 7% **Part-time** 55%

Nursing Student Activities Nursing Honor Society, Sigma Theta Tau, Student Nurses' Association.

Nursing Student Resources Academic advising; academic or career counseling; assistance for students with disabilities; bookstore; campus computer network; career placement assistance; computer lab; computer-assisted instruction; daycare for children of students; e-mail services; employment services for current students; Internet; learning resource lab; library services; nursing audiovisuals; remedial services; resume preparation assistance; skills, simulation, or other laboratory; tutoring; unpaid internships.

Library Facilities 481,848 volumes (243,924 in health, 3,617 in nursing); 1,666 periodical subscriptions (2,813 health-care related).

BACCALAUREATE PROGRAMS

Degree BSN

Available Programs Accelerated Baccalaureate for Second Degree; Generic Baccalaureate; RN Baccalaureate.

Site Options *Distance Learning:* Hastings, NE.

Study Options Full-time and part-time.

Program Entrance Requirements Minimum overall college GPA of 2.0, transcript of college record, health insurance, high school chemistry, 3 years high school math, 2 years high school science, high school transcript, immunizations, 1 letter of recommendation, minimum high school GPA of 2.75, minimum high school rank 50%, minimum GPA in nursing prerequisites of 2.0. Transfer students are accepted. **Standardized tests** *Required:* SAT or ACT, TOEFL for international students. **Application** *Deadline:* 8/1 (freshmen), rolling (transfer). *Notification:* continuous (freshmen). *Application fee:* $40.

Advanced Placement Credit given for nursing courses completed elsewhere dependent upon specific evaluations.

Expenses (2004–05) *Tuition:* full-time $20,354; part-time $636 per credit hour. *International tuition:* $20,354 full-time. *Room and board:* $6826; room only: $4080 per academic year. *Required fees:* full-time $764; part-time $64 per term.

Financial Aid 85% of baccalaureate students in nursing programs received some form of financial aid in 2003–04.

Contact Dr. Linda L. Lazure, RN, Associate Dean for Student Affairs, School of Nursing, Creighton University, 2500 California Plaza, Omaha, NE 68178. *Telephone:* 402-280-2001. *Fax:* 402-280-2045. *E-mail:* llazure@creighton.edu.

GRADUATE PROGRAMS

Expenses (2004–05) *Tuition:* full-time $13,608; part-time $567 per credit hour. *International tuition:* $13,608 full-time. *Room and board:* $6826; room only: $4080 per academic year. *Required fees:* full-time $764; part-time $64 per term.

Financial Aid 85% of graduate students in nursing programs received some form of financial aid in 2003–04. Career-related internships or fieldwork, Federal Work-Study, institutionally sponsored loans, and traineeships available.

Contact Dr. Brenda Bergman-Evans, RN, Chair of Advanced Practice, School of Nursing, Creighton University, 2500 California Plaza, Omaha, NE 68178. *Telephone:* 402-280-2041. *Fax:* 402-280-2045. *E-mail:* bbevans@creighton.edu.

MASTER'S DEGREE PROGRAM

Degree MS

Available Programs Master's.

Concentrations Available Nursing education. *Clinical nurse specialist programs in:* cardiovascular, community health, gerontology, psychiatric/mental health. *Nurse practitioner programs in:* adult health, family health, gerontology, neonatal health.

Site Options *Distance Learning:* Hastings, NE.

Study Options Full-time and part-time.

Program Entrance Requirements Clinical experience, minimum overall college GPA of 3.0, transcript of college record, CPR certification, written essay, immunizations, 3 letters of recommendation, physical assessment course, prerequisite course work, statistics course. *Application deadline:* For fall admission, 3/15 (priority date); for spring admission, 10/15 (priority date). Applications are processed on a rolling basis. *Application fee:* $30.

Advanced Placement Credit given for nursing courses completed elsewhere dependent upon specific evaluations.

Degree Requirements 43 total credit hours, thesis or project.

POST-MASTER'S PROGRAM

Areas of Study *Clinical nurse specialist programs in:* cardiovascular, community health, gerontology, psychiatric/mental health. *Nurse practitioner programs in:* adult health, family health, neonatal health.

Midland Lutheran College

Department of Nursing
Fremont, Nebraska

http://www.mlc.edu

Founded in 1883

DEGREE • BSN

Nursing Program Faculty 11 (27% with doctorates).

Baccalaureate Enrollment 70
Women 93% **Men** 7%

Nursing Student Activities Sigma Theta Tau, Student Nurses' Association.

Nursing Student Resources Academic advising; academic or career counseling; assistance for students with disabilities; bookstore; campus computer network; career placement assistance; computer lab; e-mail services; employment services for current students; interactive nursing skills videos; Internet; learning resource lab; library services; nursing audiovisuals; paid internships; placement services for program completers; remedial services; resume preparation assistance; skills, simulation, or other laboratory; tutoring; unpaid internships.

Library Facilities 110,000 volumes (3,600 in health, 1,900 in nursing); 900 periodical subscriptions (250 health-care related).

BACCALAUREATE PROGRAMS

Degree BSN

Available Programs Generic Baccalaureate; LPN to RN Baccalaureate; RN Baccalaureate.

Study Options Full-time and part-time.

Program Entrance Requirements Minimum overall college GPA of 2.5, transcript of college record, CPR certification, written essay, health exam, health insurance, high school foreign language, high school transcript, immunizations, interview, 2 letters of recommendation, minimum GPA in nursing prerequisites of 2.5, professional liability insurance/malpractice insurance, prerequisite course work. Transfer students are accepted. **Standardized tests** *Required:* SAT or ACT, TOEFL for international students. **Application** *Deadline:* rolling (freshmen), rolling (transfer). *Notification:* continuous until 9/1 (freshmen). *Application fee:* $30.

Advanced Placement Credit given for nursing courses completed elsewhere dependent upon specific evaluations.

Expenses (2004–05) *Tuition:* full-time $17,210; part-time $430 per credit hour. *Room and board:* $4560 per academic year. *Required fees:* full-time $250.

Financial Aid 98% of baccalaureate students in nursing programs received some form of financial aid in 2003–04. *Gift aid (need-based):* Federal Pell, FSEOG, state, private, college/university gift aid from institutional funds. *Loans:* FFEL (Subsidized and Unsubsidized Stafford PLUS), Perkins, college/university. *Work-Study:* Federal Work-Study, part-time campus jobs. *Application deadline:* Continuous.

Contact Dean Obenauer, Director of Financial Aid, Department of Nursing, Midland Lutheran College, 900 North Clarkson, Fremont, NE 68025. *Telephone:* 402-721-5480 Ext. 6519. *Fax:* 402-721-0250. *E-mail:* obenauer@mlc.edu.

CONTINUING EDUCATION PROGRAM

Contact Dr. Nancy A. Harms, RN, Chair, Department of Nursing, Midland Lutheran College, 900 North Clarkson, Fremont, NE 68025. *Telephone:* 402-721-5480 Ext. 6280. *Fax:* 402-941-6279. *E-mail:* harms@mlc.edu.

Nebraska Methodist College
Department of Nursing
Omaha, Nebraska

http://www.methodistcollege.edu

Founded in 1891

DEGREES • BSN • MSN

Nursing Program Faculty 33 (25% with doctorates).

Baccalaureate Enrollment 327
Women 88% **Men** 12% **Minority** 5% **Part-time** 25%

Graduate Enrollment 26
Women 100%

Nursing Student Activities Nursing Honor Society, Student Nurses' Association.

Nursing Student Resources Academic advising; academic or career counseling; assistance for students with disabilities; bookstore; campus computer network; career placement assistance; computer lab; computer-assisted instruction; e-mail services; employment services for current students; interactive nursing skills videos; learning resource lab; library services; nursing audiovisuals; remedial services; resume preparation assistance; skills, simulation, or other laboratory; tutoring.

Library Facilities 8,656 volumes (10,000 in health); 475 periodical subscriptions (640 health-care related).

BACCALAUREATE PROGRAMS

Degree BSN

Available Programs ADN to Baccalaureate; Accelerated Baccalaureate for Second Degree; Generic Baccalaureate; LPN to Baccalaureate.

Site Options *Distance Learning:* Omaha, NE.

Study Options Full-time and part-time.

Program Entrance Requirements Minimum overall college GPA of 2.0, transcript of college record, written essay, high school biology, high school chemistry, 2 years high school math, 2 years high school science, high school transcript, interview, 1 letter of recommendation, minimum high school GPA of 2.0, minimum GPA in nursing prerequisites of 2.0. Transfer students are accepted. **Standardized tests** *Required:* SAT or ACT, TOEFL for international students. **Application** *Deadline:* 4/1 (freshmen), 4/1 (transfer). *Notification:* 4/15 (freshmen). *Application fee:* $25.

Advanced Placement Credit given for nursing courses completed elsewhere dependent upon specific evaluations.

Expenses (2004–05) *Tuition:* full-time $9960; part-time $332 per credit hour. *International tuition:* $9960 full-time. *Room and board:* room only: $1665 per academic year. *Required fees:* full-time $600; part-time $20 per credit.

Financial Aid 90% of baccalaureate students in nursing programs received some form of financial aid in 2003–04. *Gift aid (need-based):* Federal Pell, FSEOG, state, private, college/university gift aid from institutional funds. *Loans:* Federal Nursing Student Loans, FFEL (Subsidized and Unsubsidized Stafford PLUS), Perkins, college/university, alternative loans. *Work-Study:* part-time campus jobs. *Application deadline (priority):* 5/1.

Contact Dr. Marilyn Valerio, Chairperson, Department of Nursing, Nebraska Methodist College, 8501 West Dodge Road, Omaha, NE 68114-3426. *Telephone:* 402-354-2270. *Fax:* 402-354-8875. *E-mail:* Marilyn.Valerio@methodistcollege.edu.

GRADUATE PROGRAMS

Expenses (2004–05) *Tuition:* full-time $7200; part-time $401 per credit hour. *International tuition:* $7200 full-time. *Room and board:* room only: $2740 per academic year. *Required fees:* full-time $450; part-time $25 per credit.

Financial Aid 40% of graduate students in nursing programs received some form of financial aid in 2003–04.

Contact Dr. Linda Foley, Associate Chairperson, Department of Nursing, Nebraska Methodist College, 8501 West Dodge Road, Omaha, NE 68114-3426. *Telephone:* 402-354-4930. *Fax:* 402-354-8875. *E-mail:* Linda.Foley@methodistcollege.edu.

MASTER'S DEGREE PROGRAM

Degree MSN

Available Programs Master's.

Concentrations Available Nursing education.

Site Options *Distance Learning:* Omaha, NE.

Study Options Full-time and part-time.

Program Entrance Requirements Clinical experience, computer literacy, minimum overall college GPA of 3.0, transcript of college record, CPR certification, written essay, interview, 3 letters of recommendation, nursing research course, physical assessment course, prerequisite course work, statistics course.

Advanced Placement Credit given for nursing courses completed elsewhere dependent upon specific evaluations.

Degree Requirements 38 total credit hours, thesis or project.

POST-MASTER'S PROGRAM

Areas of Study Nursing education.

CONTINUING EDUCATION PROGRAM

Contact Ms. Susan Jeffrey, Coordinator, Nursing Programs, Department of Nursing, Nebraska Methodist College, 515 South 26th Street, Omaha, NE 68105. *Telephone:* 402-354-6538. *Fax:* 402-354-6550. *E-mail:* Susan.Jeffrey@methodistcollege.edu.

Nebraska Wesleyan University
Department of Nursing
Lincoln, Nebraska

http://www.nebrwesleyan.edu

Founded in 1887

DEGREES • BSN • MSN

Nursing Program Faculty 9 (50% with doctorates).

Baccalaureate Enrollment 86
Women 97% **Men** 3% **Minority** 2% **Part-time** 100%

Graduate Enrollment 52
Women 94% **Men** 6% **Minority** 2% **Part-time** 100%

Nursing Student Activities Sigma Theta Tau.

Nursing Student Resources Academic advising; academic or career counseling; assistance for students with disabilities; bookstore; campus computer network; career placement assistance; computer lab; e-mail services; employment services for current students; interactive nursing skills videos; Internet; library services; nursing audiovisuals; placement services for program completers; remedial services; resume preparation assistance; tutoring; unpaid internships.

Library Facilities 178,531 volumes (3,700 in health, 3,700 in nursing); 743 periodical subscriptions (38 health-care related).

BACCALAUREATE PROGRAMS

Degree BSN

Available Programs ADN to Baccalaureate; International Nurse to Baccalaureate; RN Baccalaureate.

Site Options Omaha, NE.

Study Options Full-time and part-time.

Program Entrance Requirements Minimum overall college GPA of 2.5, transcript of college record, CPR certification, immunizations, 3 letters of recommendation, minimum GPA in nursing prerequisites of 2.5, professional liability insurance/malpractice insurance, prerequisite course work, RN licensure. Transfer students are accepted. **Standardized tests** *Required:* SAT or ACT, TOEFL for international students. **Application**

Nebraska Wesleyan University (continued)
Deadline: 8/15 (freshmen), 8/15 (transfer). *Early decision:* 11/15. *Notification:* continuous (freshmen), 12/15 (out-of-state freshmen), 12/15 (early decision). *Application fee:* $20.

Advanced Placement Credit by examination available. Credit given for nursing courses completed elsewhere dependent upon specific evaluations.

Expenses (2003–04) *Tuition:* part-time $185 per credit hour. *Room and board:* $4720; room only: $4000 per academic year.

Financial Aid 85% of baccalaureate students in nursing programs received some form of financial aid in 2002–03. *Gift aid (need-based):* Federal Pell, FSEOG, state, private, college/university gift aid from institutional funds. *Loans:* FFEL (Subsidized and Unsubsidized Stafford PLUS), Perkins. *Work-Study:* Federal Work-Study, part-time campus jobs. *Application deadline:* Continuous.

Contact Dr. Jeri L. Brandt, Program Director, Department of Nursing, Nebraska Wesleyan University, 5000 St. Paul Avenue, Lincoln, NE 68504. *Telephone:* 402-465-2333. *Fax:* 402-465-2179. *E-mail:* jlb@nebrwesleyan.edu.

GRADUATE PROGRAMS

Expenses (2003–04) *Tuition:* part-time $250 per credit hour. *Room and board:* $4750; room only: $4000 per academic year.

Financial Aid 65% of graduate students in nursing programs received some form of financial aid in 2002–03.

Contact Dr. Jeri L. Brandt, RN, Program Director, Department of Nursing, Nebraska Wesleyan University, 5000 St. Paul Avenue, Lincoln, NE 68504. *Telephone:* 402-465-2336. *Fax:* 402-465-2179. *E-mail:* jlb@nebrwesleyan.edu.

MASTER'S DEGREE PROGRAM

Degree MSN

Available Programs Master's.

Concentrations Available Nursing administration; nursing education.

Site Options Omaha, NE.

Study Options Part-time.

Program Entrance Requirements Minimum overall college GPA of 3.0, transcript of college record, written essay, 2 letters of recommendation, nursing research course, resume, statistics course.

Advanced Placement Credit given for nursing courses completed elsewhere dependent upon specific evaluations.

Degree Requirements 36 total credit hours, thesis or project.

Union College
Division of Health Sciences
Lincoln, Nebraska

http://www.ucollege.edu
Founded in 1891

DEGREE • BSN

Nursing Program Faculty 10.

Baccalaureate Enrollment 79
Women 85% **Men** 15% **Minority** 8% **International** 13%

Nursing Student Activities Sigma Theta Tau, Student Nurses' Association, nursing club.

Nursing Student Resources Academic advising; academic or career counseling; bookstore; campus computer network; career placement assistance; computer lab; computer-assisted instruction; daycare for children of students; e-mail services; externships; housing assistance; interactive nursing skills videos; Internet; learning resource lab; library services; nursing audiovisuals; skills, simulation, or other laboratory; tutoring; unpaid internships.

Library Facilities 147,813 volumes (450 in health, 350 in nursing); 1,357 periodical subscriptions (50 health-care related).

BACCALAUREATE PROGRAMS

Degree BSN

Available Programs ADN to Baccalaureate; Generic Baccalaureate; LPN to Baccalaureate.

Study Options Full-time and part-time.

Program Entrance Requirements Minimum overall college GPA of 2.75, transcript of college record, CPR certification, written essay, health exam, health insurance, high school transcript, immunizations, 3 letters of recommendation, minimum GPA in nursing prerequisites of 2.5, professional liability insurance/malpractice insurance, prerequisite course work. Transfer students are accepted. **Standardized tests** *Required:* ACT. **Application** *Deadline:* rolling (freshmen), rolling (transfer). *Notification:* continuous (freshmen).

Advanced Placement Credit by examination available. Credit given for nursing courses completed elsewhere dependent upon specific evaluations.

Expenses (2004–05) *Tuition:* full-time $13,380; part-time $558 per credit hour. *International tuition:* $13,380 full-time. *Room and board:* $4366; room only: $2576 per academic year. *Required fees:* full-time $730; part-time $365 per term.

Financial Aid 85% of baccalaureate students in nursing programs received some form of financial aid in 2003–04. *Gift aid (need-based):* Federal Pell, FSEOG, state, private, college/university gift aid from institutional funds. *Loans:* Federal Nursing Student Loans, FFEL (Subsidized and Unsubsidized Stafford PLUS), Perkins, college/university. *Work-Study:* Federal Work-Study. *Application deadline (priority):* 5/1.

Contact Mrs. Karen W. Minear, Office Manager, Division of Health Sciences, Union College, 3800 South 48th Street, Lincoln, NE 68506. *Telephone:* 402-486-2524. *Fax:* 402-486-2559. *E-mail:* kaminear@ucollege.edu.

University of Nebraska Medical Center
College of Nursing
Omaha, Nebraska

http://www.unmc.edu/nursing/
Founded in 1869

DEGREES • BSN • MSN • PHD

Nursing Program Faculty 112 (60% with doctorates).

Baccalaureate Enrollment 600

Graduate Enrollment 300

Nursing Student Activities Nursing Honor Society, Sigma Theta Tau, Student Nurses' Association, nursing club.

Nursing Student Resources Academic advising; academic or career counseling; assistance for students with disabilities; bookstore; campus computer network; career placement assistance; computer lab; computer-assisted instruction; daycare for children of students; e-mail services; employment services for current students; externships; housing assistance; interactive nursing skills videos; Internet; learning resource lab; library services; nursing audiovisuals; other; paid internships; placement services for program completers; remedial services; resume preparation assistance; skills, simulation, or other laboratory; tutoring.

Library Facilities 241,551 volumes (240,000 in health, 3,500 in nursing); 4,280 periodical subscriptions (2,200 health-care related).

BACCALAUREATE PROGRAMS

Degree BSN

Available Programs ADN to Baccalaureate; Accelerated Baccalaureate; Accelerated Baccalaureate for Second Degree; Accelerated RN Baccalaureate; Baccalaureate for Second Degree; Generic Baccalaureate; International Nurse to Baccalaureate; LPN to Baccalaureate; RN Baccalaureate; RPN to Baccalaureate.

Site Options *Distance Learning:* Scottsbluff, NE; Kearney, NE; Lincoln, NE.

Study Options Full-time.

Program Entrance Requirements Minimum overall college GPA of 2.5, transcript of college record, CPR certification, health insurance, high school transcript, immunizations, 2 letters of recommendation, prerequisite course work. Transfer students are accepted. **Standardized tests** *Required:* TOEFL for international students. **Application** *Deadline:* rolling (transfer). *Application fee:* $45.

Advanced Placement Credit by examination available. Credit given for nursing courses completed elsewhere dependent upon specific evaluations.

Expenses (2004–05) *Tuition, state resident:* full-time $4914. *Tuition, nonresident:* full-time $14,391. *Required fees:* full-time $1522.

Financial Aid 88% of baccalaureate students in nursing programs received some form of financial aid in 2003–04. *Gift aid (need-based):* Federal Pell, FSEOG, state, private, college/university gift aid from institutional funds. *Loans:* Federal Nursing Student Loans, FFEL (Subsidized and Unsubsidized Stafford PLUS), Perkins, state, college/university. *Work-Study:* Federal Work-Study. *Application deadline (priority):* 2/1.

Contact Larry D. Hewitt, Director of Student Services, College of Nursing, University of Nebraska Medical Center, 985330 Nebraska Medical Center, Omaha, NE 68198-5330. *Telephone:* 402-559-5102. *E-mail:* lhewitt@unmc.edu.

GRADUATE PROGRAMS

Expenses (2004–05) *Tuition, state resident:* part-time $206 per credit hour. *Tuition, nonresident:* part-time $576 per credit hour. *Required fees:* part-time $396 per term.

Contact Dani Eveloff, RN, Recruitment Coordinator, College of Nursing, University of Nebraska Medical Center, 985330 Nebraska Medical Center, Omaha, NE 68198-5330. *Telephone:* 402-559-5184. *E-mail:* develoff@unmc.edu.

MASTER'S DEGREE PROGRAM

Degree MSN

Available Programs Master's; Master's for Non-Nursing College Graduates; RN to Master's.

Concentrations Available Health-care administration; nurse case management; nursing administration; nursing education; nursing informatics. *Clinical nurse specialist programs in:* acute care, adult health, cardiovascular, community health, critical care, family health, gerontology, maternity-newborn, medical-surgical, oncology, parent-child, pediatric, perinatal, psychiatric/mental health, public health, women's health. *Nurse practitioner programs in:* acute care, adult health, community health, family health, gerontology, neonatal health, oncology, pediatric, primary care, psychiatric/mental health, women's health.

Site Options *Distance Learning:* Scottsbluff, NE; Kearney, NE; Lincoln, NE.

Study Options Full-time and part-time.

Program Entrance Requirements Computer literacy, minimum overall college GPA of 3.0, transcript of college record, CPR certification, immunizations, interview, 3 letters of recommendation, nursing research course, statistics course.

Advanced Placement Credit given for nursing courses completed elsewhere dependent upon specific evaluations.

Degree Requirements 45 total credit hours.

POST-MASTER'S PROGRAM

Areas of Study Health-care administration; nurse case management; nursing administration; nursing education; nursing informatics. *Clinical nurse specialist programs in:* acute care, adult health, cardiovascular, community health, critical care, family health, gerontology, maternity-newborn, medical-surgical, oncology, parent-child, pediatric, perinatal, psychiatric/mental health, public health, women's health. *Nurse practitioner programs in:* acute care, adult health, community health, family health, gerontology, neonatal health, oncology, pediatric, primary care, psychiatric/mental health, women's health.

DOCTORAL DEGREE PROGRAM

Degree PhD

Available Programs Doctorate; Doctorate for Nurses with Non-Nursing Degrees; Post-Baccalaureate Doctorate.

Areas of Study Health promotion/disease prevention, health-care systems, human health and illness, nursing research.

Site Options *Distance Learning:* Scottsbluff, NE; Kearney, NE; Lincoln, NE.

Program Entrance Requirements Minimum overall college GPA of 3.2, interview by faculty committee, interview, 3 letters of recommendation, scholarly papers, statistics course, vita, writing sample.

Degree Requirements Dissertation, oral exam, written exam.

POSTDOCTORAL PROGRAM

Areas of Study Health promotion/disease prevention, individualized study, nursing interventions, nursing research.

Postdoctoral Program Contact Dr. Margaret Wilson, Associate Dean for Graduate Programs, College of Nursing, University of Nebraska Medical Center, 985330 Nebraska Medical Center, Omaha, NE 68198-5330. *Telephone:* 402-559-7457. *Fax:* 410-706-0945. *E-mail:* mwilson@unmc.edu.

CONTINUING EDUCATION PROGRAM

Contact Catherine A. Bevil, Director of Continuing Education-Evaluation and Professor, College of Nursing, University of Nebraska Medical Center, 985330 Nebraska Medical Center, Omaha, NE 68198-5330. *Telephone:* 402-559-6412. *E-mail:* cbevil@unmc.edu.

NEVADA

University of Nevada, Las Vegas
Department of Nursing
Las Vegas, Nevada

Founded in 1957

DEGREES • BSN • MSN • PHD

Nursing Program Faculty 25 (52% with doctorates).

Baccalaureate Enrollment 170
Women 92% **Men** 8% **Minority** 40% **International** 2% **Part-time** 7%

Graduate Enrollment 43
Women 93% **Men** 7% **Minority** 23% **International** 1% **Part-time** 35%

Nursing Student Activities Sigma Theta Tau, Student Nurses' Association.

Nursing Student Resources Academic advising; academic or career counseling; assistance for students with disabilities; bookstore; career placement assistance; computer lab; daycare for children of students; e-mail services; learning resource lab; nursing audiovisuals; remedial services; skills, simulation, or other laboratory; tutoring.

Library Facilities 1 million volumes (25,737 in health, 12,000 in nursing); 9,536 periodical subscriptions (305 health-care related).

BACCALAUREATE PROGRAMS

Degree BSN

Available Programs ADN to Baccalaureate; Accelerated RN Baccalaureate; Generic Baccalaureate.

Study Options Full-time and part-time.

Program Entrance Requirements Minimum overall college GPA of 3.0, transcript of college record, CPR certification, health exam, health insurance, high school biology, high school chemistry, 1 year of high school math, high school transcript, immunizations, minimum GPA in nursing prerequisites of 3.0, prerequisite course work. Transfer students are accepted. **Standardized tests** *Required:* TOEFL for international students. *Recommended:* SAT or ACT. *Required for some:* SAT or ACT. **Application** *Deadline:* 4/2 (freshmen), 4/1 (transfer). *Notification:* continuous (freshmen). *Application fee:* $60.

Advanced Placement Credit by examination available. Credit given for nursing courses completed elsewhere dependent upon specific evaluations.

Expenses (2004–05) *Tuition, state resident:* full-time $2912; part-time $91 per credit hour. *Tuition, nonresident:* full-time $11,586; part-time $100 per credit hour. *International tuition:* $11,586 full-time. *Room and board:* $8400; room only: $5200 per academic year. *Required fees:* full-time $150; part-time $75 per credit.

Financial Aid 60% of baccalaureate students in nursing programs received some form of financial aid in 2003–04. *Gift aid (need-based):* Federal Pell, FSEOG, state, private, college/university gift aid from institutional funds. *Loans:* Federal Direct (Subsidized and Unsubsidized Stafford PLUS), Perkins, state, college/university. *Work-Study:* Federal Work-Study, part-time campus jobs. *Application deadline (priority):* 2/1.

University of Nevada, Las Vegas (continued)

Contact Mrs. Deborah Warner, RN, Pre-Nursing Advisor, Department of Nursing, University of Nevada, Las Vegas, 4505 Maryland Parkway, Las Vegas, NV 89154-3018. *Telephone:* 702-895-3360. *Fax:* 702-895-4807. *E-mail:* dwarner@ccmail.nevada.edu.

GRADUATE PROGRAMS

Expenses (2004–05) *Tuition, state resident:* full-time $2470; part-time $124 per credit hour. *Tuition, nonresident:* full-time $11,144; part-time $259 per credit hour. *International tuition:* $11,144 full-time. *Room and board:* $8400; room only: $5200 per academic year. *Required fees:* full-time $70; part-time $35 per credit.

Financial Aid 60% of graduate students in nursing programs received some form of financial aid in 2003–04. 1 research assistantship with partial tuition reimbursement available (averaging $10,000 per year), 3 teaching assistantships with partial tuition reimbursements available (averaging $10,000 per year) were awarded. *Financial aid application deadline:* 3/1.

Contact Dr. Cheryl Bowles, Coordinator, Graduate Programs, Department of Nursing, University of Nevada, Las Vegas, 4505 Maryland Parkway, Las Vegas, NV 89154-3018. *Telephone:* 702-895-3360. *Fax:* 702-895-4807. *E-mail:* cbowles@ccmail.nevada.edu.

MASTER'S DEGREE PROGRAM

Degree MSN

Available Programs Master's; RN to Master's.

Concentrations Available Nursing education. *Nurse practitioner programs in:* family health.

Study Options Full-time and part-time.

Program Entrance Requirements Clinical experience, computer literacy, minimum overall college GPA of 3.0, transcript of college record, CPR certification, written essay, immunizations, 2 letters of recommendation, nursing research course, physical assessment course, professional liability insurance/malpractice insurance, prerequisite course work, resume, statistics course, GRE General Test. *Application deadline:* For fall admission, 4/15. *Application fee:* $60 ($75 for international students).

Advanced Placement Credit given for nursing courses completed elsewhere dependent upon specific evaluations.

Degree Requirements 40 total credit hours, thesis or project, comprehensive exam.

POST-MASTER'S PROGRAM

Areas of Study Nursing education. *Nurse practitioner programs in:* family health.

DOCTORAL DEGREE PROGRAM

Degree PhD

Available Programs Doctorate.

Areas of Study Nursing education.

Program Entrance Requirements Clinical experience, minimum overall college GPA of 3.0, interview by faculty committee, 2 letters of recommendation, MSN or equivalent, statistics course, vita, writing sample. *Application deadline:* For fall admission, 4/15. *Application fee:* $60 ($75 for international students).

Degree Requirements 60 total credit hours, dissertation, oral exam.

CONTINUING EDUCATION PROGRAM

Contact Dr. Rosemary Witt, Senior Academic Coordinator, Department of Nursing, University of Nevada, Las Vegas, School of Nursing, 4505 Maryland Parkway, Las Vegas, NV 89154-3018. *Telephone:* 702-895-3360. *Fax:* 702-895-4807. *E-mail:* rwitt@ccmail.nevada.edu.

University of Nevada, Reno

Orvis School of Nursing
Reno, Nevada

http://www.unr.edu/bcs/osn

Founded in 1874

DEGREES • BSN • MS • MSN/MPH

Nursing Program Faculty 27 (40% with doctorates).

Baccalaureate Enrollment 149

Women 60% **Men** 40% **Minority** 16% **International** 5% **Part-time** 20%

Graduate Enrollment 35

Women 90% **Men** 10% **Minority** 1% **Part-time** 85%

Nursing Student Activities Nursing Honor Society, Sigma Theta Tau, Student Nurses' Association.

Nursing Student Resources Academic advising; academic or career counseling; assistance for students with disabilities; bookstore; campus computer network; computer lab; computer-assisted instruction; e-mail services; Internet; learning resource lab; library services; nursing audiovisuals; remedial services; skills, simulation, or other laboratory.

Library Facilities 1.1 million volumes (5,000 in health, 3,000 in nursing); 15,000 periodical subscriptions (172 health-care related).

BACCALAUREATE PROGRAMS

Degree BSN

Available Programs ADN to Baccalaureate; Accelerated Baccalaureate; Generic Baccalaureate; RN Baccalaureate.

Site Options Reno , NV.

Study Options Full-time.

Program Entrance Requirements Transcript of college record, CPR certification, health exam, health insurance, immunizations, minimum GPA in nursing prerequisites of 3.0, professional liability insurance/malpractice insurance, prerequisite course work. Transfer students are accepted. **Standardized tests** *Required:* TOEFL for international students. **Application** *Deadline:* rolling (freshmen), rolling (transfer). *Early decision:* 11/15. *Notification:* continuous (freshmen). *Application fee:* $60.

Advanced Placement Credit given for nursing courses completed elsewhere dependent upon specific evaluations.

Expenses (2003–04) *Tuition, state resident:* full-time $2700; part-time $678 per term. *Tuition, nonresident:* full-time $5228; part-time $1307 per term. *International tuition:* $5228 full-time. *Room and board:* $7940; room only: $4750 per academic year. *Required fees:* full-time $300.

Financial Aid 50% of baccalaureate students in nursing programs received some form of financial aid in 2002–03. *Gift aid (need-based):* Federal Pell, FSEOG, private, college/university gift aid from institutional funds. *Loans:* FFEL (Subsidized and Unsubsidized Stafford PLUS), Perkins, college/university. *Work-Study:* Federal Work-Study, part-time campus jobs. *Application deadline (priority):* 2/1.

Contact Pam Schueler, Coordinator, Undergraduate Program, Orvis School of Nursing, University of Nevada, Reno, Mail Stop 134, Reno, NV 89557. *Telephone:* 775-784-6841. *Fax:* 775-784-4262. *E-mail:* pschuele@unr.edu.

GRADUATE PROGRAMS

Expenses (2003–04) *Tuition, state resident:* full-time $1998; part-time $667 per semester. *Tuition, nonresident:* full-time $5228; part-time $1307 per semester. *International tuition:* $5228 full-time. *Room and board:* $7940; room only: $4750 per academic year. *Required fees:* full-time $100.

Financial Aid 90% of graduate students in nursing programs received some form of financial aid in 2002–03. 3 research assistantships were awarded; teaching assistantships. *Financial aid application deadline:* 3/1.

Contact Pat Holden-Huchton, Coordinator, Graduate Program, Orvis School of Nursing, University of Nevada, Reno, Mail Stop 134, Reno, NV 89557. *Telephone:* 775-784-6841 Ext. 242. *Fax:* 775-784-4262. *E-mail:* pathh@unr.edu.

MASTER'S DEGREE PROGRAM

Degrees MS; MSN/MPH

Available Programs Master's.

Concentrations Available Nursing education. *Clinical nurse specialist programs in:* acute care, adult health, community health, gerontology, medical-surgical, oncology, parent-child, psychiatric/mental health, school health. *Nurse practitioner programs in:* family health.

Study Options Full-time and part-time.

Program Entrance Requirements Computer literacy, minimum overall college GPA of 3.0, transcript of college record, CPR certification, written essay, immunizations, interview, 3 letters of recommendation, physical assessment course, professional liability insurance/malpractice insurance, statistics course, GRE General Test or MAT. *Application deadline:* For fall admission, 3/1 (priority date). Applications are processed on a rolling basis. *Application fee:* $60 ($95 for international students).

Degree Requirements 58 total credit hours, thesis or project, comprehensive exam.

POST-MASTER'S PROGRAM

Areas of Study Nursing education. *Nurse practitioner programs in:* family health.

NEW HAMPSHIRE

Colby-Sawyer College

Department of Nursing
New London, New Hampshire

http://www.colby-sawyer.edu/academic/nursing

Founded in 1837

DEGREE • BS

Nursing Program Faculty 7 (14% with doctorates).

Baccalaureate Enrollment 122

Women 93% **Men** 7% **Minority** 2% **Part-time** 2%

Nursing Student Activities Nursing Honor Society, Student Nurses' Association.

Nursing Student Resources Academic advising; academic or career counseling; assistance for students with disabilities; bookstore; campus computer network; career placement assistance; computer lab; computer-assisted instruction; e-mail services; employment services for current students; housing assistance; interactive nursing skills videos; Internet; learning resource lab; library services; nursing audiovisuals; remedial services; resume preparation assistance; skills, simulation, or other laboratory; tutoring.

Library Facilities 90,305 volumes (9,130 in health, 743 in nursing); 467 periodical subscriptions (95 health-care related).

BACCALAUREATE PROGRAMS

Degree BS

Available Programs Generic Baccalaureate.

Study Options Full-time and part-time.

Program Entrance Requirements Minimum overall college GPA of 2.5, transcript of college record, CPR certification, written essay, health exam, health insurance, high school foreign language, 3 years high school math, 2 years high school science, high school transcript, immunizations, 2 letters of recommendation, minimum GPA in nursing prerequisites of 2.0, prerequisite course work. Transfer students are accepted. **Standardized tests** *Required:* SAT or ACT, TOEFL for international students. **Application** *Deadline:* rolling (freshmen). *Early decision:* 12/15. *Notification:* continuous (freshmen), 1/15 (early action). *Application fee:* $40.

Advanced Placement Credit by examination available. Credit given for nursing courses completed elsewhere dependent upon specific evaluations.

Expenses (2004–05) *Tuition:* full-time $23,310; part-time $780 per credit hour. *International tuition:* $23,310 full-time. *Room and board:* $8950; room only: $4980 per academic year.

Financial Aid 88% of baccalaureate students in nursing programs received some form of financial aid in 2003–04.

Contact Joan Huber, Assistant Acting Interim Chair, Nursing Department, Department of Nursing, Colby-Sawyer College, 541 Main Street, New London, NH 03257-4648. *Telephone:* 603-526-3649. *Fax:* 603-526-3452. *E-mail:* jhuber@colby-sawyer.edu.

See full description on page 466.

Rivier College

Department of Nursing and Health Sciences
Nashua, New Hampshire

Founded in 1933

DEGREES • BS • MS • MS/MBA

Nursing Program Faculty 24 (25% with doctorates).

Baccalaureate Enrollment 250

Women 97% **Men** 3% **Minority** 3% **Part-time** 75%

Graduate Enrollment 43

Women 95% **Men** 5% **Minority** 3% **Part-time** 84%

Nursing Student Activities Nursing Honor Society, Student Nurses' Association.

Nursing Student Resources Academic advising; academic or career counseling; assistance for students with disabilities; bookstore; campus computer network; career placement assistance; computer lab; computer-assisted instruction; e-mail services; employment services for current students; externships; housing assistance; interactive nursing skills videos; Internet; learning resource lab; library services; nursing audiovisuals; other; placement services for program completers; remedial services; resume preparation assistance; skills, simulation, or other laboratory; tutoring.

Library Facilities 92,000 volumes (4,400 in health, 3,800 in nursing); 500 periodical subscriptions (275 health-care related).

BACCALAUREATE PROGRAMS

Degree BS

Available Programs ADN to Baccalaureate; RN Baccalaureate.

Site Options Lowell, MA; Manchester, NH.

Study Options Full-time and part-time.

Program Entrance Requirements Transcript of college record, written essay, health exam, health insurance, high school chemistry, high school foreign language, 2 years high school math, high school transcript, immunizations, 2 letters of recommendation, minimum high school GPA of 2.5, minimum high school rank 80%, prerequisite course work. Transfer students are accepted. **Standardized tests** *Required:* SAT or ACT, TOEFL for international students. *Required for some:* nursing exam. **Application** *Deadline:* rolling (freshmen), rolling (transfer). *Early decision:* 11/15. *Notification:* continuous (freshmen), 12/1 (early action). *Application fee:* $25.

Advanced Placement Credit by examination available. Credit given for nursing courses completed elsewhere dependent upon specific evaluations.

Expenses (2004–05) *Tuition:* full-time $19,200. *Room and board:* $7273 per academic year. *Required fees:* full-time $300.

Financial Aid 67% of baccalaureate students in nursing programs received some form of financial aid in 2003–04. *Gift aid (need-based):* Federal Pell, FSEOG, state, private, college/university gift aid from institutional funds. *Loans:* FFEL (Subsidized and Unsubsidized Stafford PLUS), Perkins. *Work-Study:* Federal Work-Study, part-time campus jobs. *Application deadline (priority):* 3/1.

Contact Dr. Susan A. Murphy, Program Director, Department of Nursing and Health Sciences, Rivier College, 420 Main Street, Nashua, NH 03060-5086. *Telephone:* 603-897-8627. *Fax:* 603-897-8884. *E-mail:* smurphy@rivier.edu.

GRADUATE PROGRAMS

Expenses (2004–05) *Tuition:* part-time $640 per credit hour.

Financial Aid 29% of graduate students in nursing programs received some form of financial aid in 2003–04. Available to part-time students. *Application deadline:* 2/1.

Contact Dr. Susan A. Murphy, Program Director, Department of Nursing and Health Sciences, Rivier College, 420 Main Street, Nashua, NH 03060-5086. *Telephone:* 603-897-8627. *Fax:* 603-897-8884. *E-mail:* smurphy@rivier.edu.

MASTER'S DEGREE PROGRAM

Degrees MS; MS/MBA

Available Programs Master's; Master's for Nurses with Non-Nursing Degrees.

Rivier College (continued)
Concentrations Available Health-care administration; nursing education. *Clinical nurse specialist programs in:* psychiatric/mental health. *Nurse practitioner programs in:* family health, psychiatric/mental health.

Study Options Full-time and part-time.

Program Entrance Requirements Clinical experience, transcript of college record, written essay, immunizations, interview, 2 letters of recommendation, resume, statistics course, GRE, MAT. *Application deadline:* Applications are processed on a rolling basis. *Application fee:* $25.

Advanced Placement Credit given for nursing courses completed elsewhere dependent upon specific evaluations.

Degree Requirements 43 total credit hours, thesis or project.

POST-MASTER'S PROGRAM

Areas of Study Nursing education. *Clinical nurse specialist programs in:* psychiatric/mental health. *Nurse practitioner programs in:* family health, psychiatric/mental health.

Saint Anselm College
Department of Nursing
Manchester, New Hampshire

Founded in 1889

DEGREE • BS

Nursing Program Faculty 17 (35% with doctorates).

Baccalaureate Enrollment 194
Women 95% **Men** 5% **Minority** 2% **International** 1% **Part-time** 1%

Nursing Student Activities Student Nurses' Association.

Nursing Student Resources Academic advising; academic or career counseling; assistance for students with disabilities; bookstore; campus computer network; career placement assistance; computer lab; computer-assisted instruction; e-mail services; employment services for current students; externships; housing assistance; interactive nursing skills videos; Internet; learning resource lab; library services; nursing audiovisuals; resume preparation assistance; skills, simulation, or other laboratory; tutoring.

Library Facilities 222,000 volumes (7,127 in health); 1,900 periodical subscriptions (292 health-care related).

BACCALAUREATE PROGRAMS

Degree BS

Available Programs RN Baccalaureate.

Study Options Full-time and part-time.

Program Entrance Requirements Minimum overall college GPA of 3.0, transcript of college record, written essay, health exam, health insurance, high school biology, high school chemistry, high school foreign language, 4 years high school math, 4 years high school science, high school transcript, immunizations, 2 letters of recommendation, minimum high school GPA of 3.0, minimum high school rank 40%, professional liability insurance/malpractice insurance. Transfer students are accepted. **Standardized tests** *Required:* SAT or ACT, TOEFL for international students. **Application** *Deadline:* rolling (freshmen), rolling (transfer). *Early decision:* 12/1. *Notification:* continuous (freshmen), 12/15 (out-of-state freshmen), 12/15 (early decision). *Application fee:* $50.

Advanced Placement Credit by examination available. Credit given for nursing courses completed elsewhere dependent upon specific evaluations.

Expenses (2003–04) *Tuition:* full-time $21,410. *International tuition:* $21,410 full-time. *Room and board:* $8090 per academic year. *Required fees:* full-time $750.

Financial Aid 83% of baccalaureate students in nursing programs received some form of financial aid in 2002–03.

Contact Nancy Davis Griffin, Director of Admission, Department of Nursing, Saint Anselm College, 100 Saint Anselm Drive, Manchester, NH 03102-1310. *Telephone:* 603-641-7500. *Fax:* 603-641-7550. *E-mail:* ngriffin@anselm.edu.

CONTINUING EDUCATION PROGRAM

Contact Jill Howard, Conference Coordinator, Continuing Nursing Education, Department of Nursing, Saint Anselm College, 100 Saint Anselm Drive, #1745, Manchester, NH 03102-1310. *Telephone:* 603-641-7085. *Fax:* 603-641-7089. *E-mail:* jhoward@anselm.edu.

University of New Hampshire
Department of Nursing
Durham, New Hampshire

http://www.unh.edu/ur-nurs.html

Founded in 1866

DEGREES • BS • MS

Nursing Program Faculty 13 (75% with doctorates).

Baccalaureate Enrollment 268
Women 91% **Men** 9% **Minority** 1%

Graduate Enrollment 54
Women 95% **Men** 5% **Minority** 1%

Nursing Student Activities Nursing Honor Society, Sigma Theta Tau, Student Nurses' Association.

Nursing Student Resources Academic advising; academic or career counseling; assistance for students with disabilities; bookstore; campus computer network; computer lab; computer-assisted instruction; daycare for children of students; e-mail services; housing assistance; interactive nursing skills videos; Internet; learning resource lab; nursing audiovisuals; paid internships; resume preparation assistance; skills, simulation, or other laboratory; tutoring.

Library Facilities 1.8 million volumes; 25,962 periodical subscriptions.

BACCALAUREATE PROGRAMS

Degree BS

Available Programs Generic Baccalaureate; RN Baccalaureate.

Study Options Full-time and part-time.

Program Entrance Requirements High school transcript, prerequisite course work. Transfer students are accepted. **Standardized tests** *Required:* SAT, TOEFL for international students. **Application** *Deadline:* 2/1 (freshmen), 3/1 (transfer). *Early decision:* 12/1. *Notification:* 4/15 (freshmen), 1/15 (early action). *Application fee:* $45.

Expenses (2003–04) *Tuition, state resident:* full-time $8664. *Tuition, nonresident:* full-time $19,024. *Room and board:* $6234 per academic year.

Contact Dr. Raelene Shippee-Rice, Chairperson and Undergraduate Program, Director, Department of Nursing, University of New Hampshire, University of New Hampshire, Hewitt Hall/ 4 Library Way, Durham, NH 03824-3563. *Telephone:* 603-862-4715. *Fax:* 603-862-4771. *E-mail:* rvs@cisunix.unh.edu.

GRADUATE PROGRAMS

Financial Aid 7 fellowships, 2 teaching assistantships were awarded; Federal Work-Study, scholarships, and tuition waivers (full and partial) also available.

Contact Gene Harkless, Graduate Director, Department of Nursing, University of New Hampshire, University of New Hampshire, Hewitt Hall/4 Library Way, Durham, NH 03824-3563. *Telephone:* 603-862-2285. *Fax:* 603-862-4771. *E-mail:* geh@cisunix.unh.edu.

MASTER'S DEGREE PROGRAM

Degree MS

Available Programs Master's; Master's for Nurses with Non-Nursing Degrees.

Concentrations Available *Clinical nurse specialist programs in:* adult health. *Nurse practitioner programs in:* adult health, family health.

Program Entrance Requirements GRE General Test or MAT. *Application deadline:* For fall admission, 4/1 (priority date); for winter admission, 12/1. Applications are processed on a rolling basis. *Application fee:* $50.

Degree Requirements 45 total credit hours, thesis or project, comprehensive exam.

POST-MASTER'S PROGRAM

Areas of Study *Clinical nurse specialist programs in:* adult health. *Nurse practitioner programs in:* adult health, family health.

NEW JERSEY

Bloomfield College
Division of Nursing
Bloomfield, New Jersey

http://www.bloomfield.edu
Founded in 1868

DEGREE • BSN

Nursing Program Faculty 18 (22% with doctorates).

Baccalaureate Enrollment 128

Women 88% **Men** 12% **Minority** 55% **International** 2% **Part-time** 38%

Nursing Student Activities Student Nurses' Association.

Nursing Student Resources Academic advising; academic or career counseling; assistance for students with disabilities; bookstore; campus computer network; career placement assistance; computer lab; computer-assisted instruction; e-mail services; employment services for current students; externships; interactive nursing skills videos; Internet; learning resource lab; library services; nursing audiovisuals; placement services for program completers; remedial services; resume preparation assistance; skills, simulation, or other laboratory; tutoring.

Library Facilities 60,000 volumes (5,000 in health, 627 in nursing); 375 periodical subscriptions (53 health-care related).

BACCALAUREATE PROGRAMS

Degree BSN

Available Programs Generic Baccalaureate; RN Baccalaureate.

Site Options *Distance Learning:* Toms River, NJ.

Study Options Full-time and part-time.

Program Entrance Requirements Minimum overall college GPA of 2.5, transcript of college record, CPR certification, health exam, health insurance, high school biology, high school chemistry, high school transcript, immunizations, 2 letters of recommendation, minimum high school GPA of 2.5, minimum GPA in nursing prerequisites of 2.5, professional liability insurance/malpractice insurance, prerequisite course work. Transfer students are accepted. **Standardized tests** *Required:* SAT or ACT, TOEFL for international students. **Application** *Deadline:* 8/1 (freshmen), 8/1 (transfer). *Early decision:* 1/7. *Notification:* continuous (freshmen), 1/21 (early action). *Application fee:* $35.

Advanced Placement Credit given for nursing courses completed elsewhere dependent upon specific evaluations.

Expenses (2004–05) *Tuition:* full-time $13,700; part-time $1380 per course. *International tuition:* $13,700 full-time. *Room and board:* $6750; room only: $3375 per academic year. *Required fees:* full-time $200; part-time $25 per term.

Financial Aid 59% of baccalaureate students in nursing programs received some form of financial aid in 2003–04. *Gift aid (need-based):* Federal Pell, FSEOG, state, private, college/university gift aid from institutional funds. *Loans:* FFEL (Subsidized and Unsubsidized Stafford PLUS), state. *Work-Study:* Federal Work-Study, part-time campus jobs. *Application deadline (priority):* 6/1.

Contact Ms. Lourdes Delgado, Vice President of Enrollment Management/Dean of Admission, Division of Nursing, Bloomfield College, 1 Park Place, Bloomfield, NJ 07003. *Telephone:* 973-748-9000 Ext. 392. *Fax:* 973-748-0916. *E-mail:* lourdes_delgado@bloomfield.edu.

The College of New Jersey
School of Nursing
Ewing, New Jersey

http://www.tcnj.edu/~nursing
Founded in 1855

DEGREES • BSN • MSN

Nursing Program Faculty 15 (60% with doctorates).

Baccalaureate Enrollment 258

Women 93% **Men** 7% **Minority** 34% **Part-time** 2%

Graduate Enrollment 47

Women 98% **Men** 2% **Minority** 23% **Part-time** 2%

Nursing Student Activities Sigma Theta Tau, Student Nurses' Association.

Nursing Student Resources Academic advising; academic or career counseling; assistance for students with disabilities; computer lab; computer-assisted instruction; e-mail services; interactive nursing skills videos; Internet; learning resource lab; library services; nursing audiovisuals; skills, simulation, or other laboratory.

Library Facilities 550,000 volumes (30,000 in health, 18,800 in nursing); 7,900 periodical subscriptions (228 health-care related).

BACCALAUREATE PROGRAMS

Degree BSN

Available Programs Generic Baccalaureate.

Study Options Full-time and part-time.

Program Entrance Requirements Written essay, health exam, high school transcript, immunizations. Transfer students are accepted. **Standardized tests** *Required:* SAT or ACT, TOEFL for international students. **Application** *Deadline:* 2/15 (freshmen), 2/15 (transfer). *Early decision:* 11/15. *Notification:* continuous until 4/1 (freshmen), 12/15 (out-of-state freshmen), 12/15 (early decision). *Application fee:* $50.

Advanced Placement Credit by examination available. Credit given for nursing courses completed elsewhere dependent upon specific evaluations.

Expenses (2004–05) *Tuition, state resident:* full-time $6621; part-time $217 per credit hour. *Tuition, nonresident:* full-time $11,562; part-time $379 per credit hour. *International tuition:* $11,562 full-time. *Room and board:* $5724 per academic year. *Required fees:* full-time $2367; part-time $72 per credit.

Financial Aid 42% of baccalaureate students in nursing programs received some form of financial aid in 2003–04. *Gift aid (need-based):* Federal Pell, FSEOG, state, private, college/university gift aid from institutional funds, Federal Nursing. *Loans:* Federal Nursing Student Loans, FFEL (Subsidized and Unsubsidized Stafford PLUS), Perkins, state. *Work-Study:* Federal Work-Study, part-time campus jobs. *Application deadline (priority):* 3/1.

Contact Mr. Patrick Roger-Gordon, Assistant Dean for Student Services, School of Nursing, The College of New Jersey, PO Box 7718, 2000 Pennington Road, Ewing, NJ 08628-0718. *Telephone:* 609-771-2669. *Fax:* 609-637-5159. *E-mail:* roger@tcnj.edu.

GRADUATE PROGRAMS

Expenses (2004–05) *Tuition, state resident:* full-time $8219; part-time $423 per credit hour. *Tuition, nonresident:* full-time $11,502; part-time $592 per credit hour. *International tuition:* $11,502 full-time. *Room and board:* $5724 per academic year. *Required fees:* full-time $1323; part-time $67 per credit; part-time $662 per term.

Financial Aid 8% of graduate students in nursing programs received some form of financial aid in 2003–04. Unspecified assistantships available. *Financial aid application deadline:* 5/1.

Contact Dr. Claire Lindberg, Chair, Division of Advanced Nursing Education and Practice, School of Nursing, The College of New Jersey, PO Box 7718, 2000 Pennington Road, Ewing, NJ 08628-0718. *Telephone:* 609-771-2591. *Fax:* 609-637-5159. *E-mail:* lindberg@tcnj.edu.

MASTER'S DEGREE PROGRAM

Degree MSN

The College of New Jersey (continued)

Available Programs Master's; Master's for Nurses with Non-Nursing Degrees; RN to Master's.

Concentrations Available *Clinical nurse specialist programs in:* adult health. *Nurse practitioner programs in:* family health, neonatal health.

Study Options Full-time and part-time.

Program Entrance Requirements Computer literacy, minimum overall college GPA of 3.0, transcript of college record, written essay, immunizations, interview, 3 letters of recommendation, nursing research course, physical assessment course, statistics course, GRE General Test. *Application deadline:* For fall admission, 3/15. *Application fee:* $50.

Advanced Placement Credit given for nursing courses completed elsewhere dependent upon specific evaluations.

Degree Requirements 42 total credit hours, comprehensive exam.

POST-MASTER'S PROGRAM

Areas of Study *Clinical nurse specialist programs in:* adult health. *Nurse practitioner programs in:* family health.

College of Saint Elizabeth

Department of Nursing
Morristown, New Jersey

http://www.cse.edu/sgcs_continuingstudies.htm

Founded in 1899

DEGREE • BSN

Nursing Program Faculty 8 (50% with doctorates).

Baccalaureate Enrollment 166

Women 95% **Men** 5% **Minority** 45% **Part-time** 99%

Nursing Student Activities Nursing Honor Society, Sigma Theta Tau, nursing club.

Nursing Student Resources Academic advising; academic or career counseling; assistance for students with disabilities; bookstore; campus computer network; career placement assistance; computer lab; computer-assisted instruction; e-mail services; employment services for current students; interactive nursing skills videos; Internet; learning resource lab; library services; nursing audiovisuals; other; remedial services; resume preparation assistance; skills, simulation, or other laboratory; tutoring.

Library Facilities 110,230 volumes (4,246 in health, 702 in nursing); 852 periodical subscriptions (194 health-care related).

BACCALAUREATE PROGRAMS

Degree BSN

Available Programs ADN to Baccalaureate; Accelerated RN Baccalaureate; International Nurse to Baccalaureate; RN Baccalaureate.

Site Options Hoboken, NJ; Randolph, NJ; Elizabeth , NJ.

Study Options Part-time.

Program Entrance Requirements Minimum overall college GPA of 2.0, transcript of college record, CPR certification, health exam, immunizations, prerequisite course work, RN licensure. Transfer students are accepted. **Standardized tests** *Required:* SAT or ACT, TOEFL for international students. **Application** *Deadline:* 8/15 (freshmen), rolling (transfer). *Notification:* 11/15 (freshmen). *Application fee:* $35.

Advanced Placement Credit by examination available. Credit given for nursing courses completed elsewhere dependent upon specific evaluations.

Expenses (2004–05) *Tuition:* full-time $17,437; part-time $549 per credit hour. *International tuition:* $17,437 full-time. *Room and board:* $8618 per academic year. *Required fees:* full-time $900; part-time $30 per credit; part-time $480 per term.

Financial Aid 20% of baccalaureate students in nursing programs received some form of financial aid in 2003–04.

Contact Dr. Ellen Ehrlich, Chairperson, Department of Nursing, College of Saint Elizabeth, 2 Convent Road, Morristown, NJ 07960-6989. *Telephone:* 973-290-4056. *Fax:* 973-290-4177. *E-mail:* eehrlich@cse.edu.

CONTINUING EDUCATION PROGRAM

Contact Dr. Eileen Specchio, Assistant Professor, Department of Nursing, College of Saint Elizabeth, 2 Convent Road, Morristown, NJ 07960-6989. *Telephone:* 973-290-4073. *Fax:* 973-290-4177. *E-mail:* especchio@cse.edu.

Fairleigh Dickinson University, Metropolitan Campus

Henry P. Becton School of Nursing and Allied Health
Teaneck, New Jersey

http://fduinfo.com/depts/ucnah.php

Founded in 1942

DEGREES • BSN • MSN

Nursing Program Faculty 25 (28% with doctorates).

Baccalaureate Enrollment 191

Women 90% **Men** 10% **Minority** 56% **International** 2% **Part-time** 31%

Graduate Enrollment 30

Women 97% **Men** 3% **Minority** 53% **Part-time** 97%

Nursing Student Activities Nursing Honor Society, Sigma Theta Tau, Student Nurses' Association.

Nursing Student Resources Academic advising; academic or career counseling; assistance for students with disabilities; bookstore; campus computer network; career placement assistance; computer lab; computer-assisted instruction; e-mail services; employment services for current students; externships; housing assistance; interactive nursing skills videos; Internet; learning resource lab; library services; nursing audiovisuals; other; paid internships; remedial services; resume preparation assistance; skills, simulation, or other laboratory; tutoring; unpaid internships.

Library Facilities 2,166 volumes in nursing; 104 periodical subscriptions health-care related.

BACCALAUREATE PROGRAMS

Degree BSN

Available Programs Accelerated Baccalaureate; Accelerated Baccalaureate for Second Degree; Baccalaureate for Second Degree; Generic Baccalaureate; RN Baccalaureate.

Site Options *Distance Learning:* Madison, NJ; Teaneck, NJ.

Study Options Full-time and part-time.

Program Entrance Requirements Minimum overall college GPA of 2.7, health exam, high school biology, high school chemistry, 2 years high school math, 2 years high school science, high school transcript, immunizations, 2 letters of recommendation. Transfer students are accepted. **Standardized tests** *Required:* SAT and SAT Subject Tests or ACT, TOEFL for international students. *Recommended:* SAT II Writing Tests. **Application** *Notification:* continuous (freshmen). *Application fee:* $40.

Advanced Placement Credit given for nursing courses completed elsewhere dependent upon specific evaluations.

Expenses (2004–05) *Tuition:* full-time $21,224; part-time $681 per credit hour. *International tuition:* $21,224 full-time. *Room and board:* $7630 per academic year. *Required fees:* full-time $510; part-time $122 per term.

Financial Aid 75% of baccalaureate students in nursing programs received some form of financial aid in 2003–04. *Gift aid (need-based):* Federal Pell, FSEOG, state, private, college/university gift aid from institutional funds, United Negro College Fund, Federal Nursing. *Loans:* Federal Nursing Student Loans, FFEL (Subsidized and Unsubsidized Stafford PLUS), Perkins, state. *Work-Study:* Federal Work-Study. *Application deadline:* Continuous.

Contact Prof. Carol Jasko, Associate Director, Undergraduate Nursing, Henry P. Becton School of Nursing and Allied Health, Fairleigh Dickinson University, Metropolitan Campus, Henry P. Becton School of Nursing & Allied Health, 1000 River Road H-DH4-02, Teaneck, NJ 07666-1914. *Telephone:* 201-692-2880. *Fax:* 201-692-2388. *E-mail:* clj@fdu.edu.

GRADUATE PROGRAMS

Expenses (2004–05) *Tuition:* part-time $740 per credit hour.

Contact Dr. Susan Warren, Associate Director of Graduate Programs, Henry P. Becton School of Nursing and Allied Health, Fairleigh Dickinson University, Metropolitan Campus, Henry P. Becton School of Nursing & Allied Health, 1000 River Road H-DH4-02, H444A, Teaneck, NJ 07666-1914. *Telephone:* 201-692-2881. *Fax:* 201-692-2388. *E-mail:* warren@fdu.edu.

MASTER'S DEGREE PROGRAM

Degree MSN

Available Programs Master's; Master's for Nurses with Non-Nursing Degrees; RN to Master's.

Concentrations Available Nursing administration; nursing education; nursing informatics. *Nurse practitioner programs in:* adult health, psychiatric/mental health.

Site Options *Distance Learning:* Teaneck, NJ.

Study Options Full-time and part-time.

Program Entrance Requirements Computer literacy, minimum overall college GPA of 3.0, transcript of college record, written essay, 2 letters of recommendation, nursing research course, physical assessment course, professional liability insurance/malpractice insurance, statistics course.

Advanced Placement Credit given for nursing courses completed elsewhere dependent upon specific evaluations.

Degree Requirements 45 total credit hours, thesis or project.

POST-MASTER'S PROGRAM

Areas of Study Nursing administration; nursing education; nursing informatics. *Nurse practitioner programs in:* adult health.

See full description on page 488.

Felician College

Department of Professional Nursing–BSN
Lodi, New Jersey

http://www.felician.edu/academics/nabp/nursing.asp

Founded in 1942

DEGREES • BSN • MSN

Nursing Program Faculty 15 (33% with doctorates).

Nursing Student Activities Nursing Honor Society, Sigma Theta Tau, Student Nurses' Association.

Nursing Student Resources Academic advising; academic or career counseling; assistance for students with disabilities; bookstore; campus computer network; computer lab; computer-assisted instruction; daycare for children of students; e-mail services; externships; interactive nursing skills videos; Internet; learning resource lab; library services; nursing audiovisuals; paid internships; remedial services; resume preparation assistance; skills, simulation, or other laboratory; tutoring.

Library Facilities 101,040 volumes; 563 periodical subscriptions.

BACCALAUREATE PROGRAMS

Degree BSN

Available Programs Accelerated RN Baccalaureate; Generic Baccalaureate; RN Baccalaureate.

Site Options Pompton Plains, NJ.

Study Options Full-time and part-time.

Program Entrance Requirements Transcript of college record, CPR certification, health exam, health insurance, high school biology, high school chemistry, 2 years high school math, 2 years high school science, high school transcript, immunizations, 2 letters of recommendation, minimum high school GPA of 2.75, minimum GPA in nursing prerequisites of 2.75, professional liability insurance/malpractice insurance. Transfer students are accepted. **Standardized tests** *Required:* SAT, SAT or ACT, TOEFL for international students. *Required for some:* ACT, SAT Subject Tests. **Application** *Application fee:* $30.

Advanced Placement Credit given for nursing courses completed elsewhere dependent upon specific evaluations.

Expenses (2004–05) *Tuition:* full-time $16,000; part-time $570 per credit hour. *Room and board:* $8000 per academic year. *Required fees:* full-time $1600.

Contact Office of Undergraduate Admissions, Department of Professional Nursing–BSN, Felician College, 262 South Main Street, Lodi, NJ 07644-2117. *Telephone:* 201-559-6131. *Fax:* 201-559-6138.

GRADUATE PROGRAMS

Expenses (2004–05) *Tuition:* part-time $570 per credit hour.

Contact Director of Adult Education and Graduate Admission, Department of Professional Nursing–BSN, Felician College, 262 South Main Street, Lodi, NJ 07644-2117. *Telephone:* 201-559-6055.

MASTER'S DEGREE PROGRAM

Degree MSN

Available Programs Master's; RN to Master's.

Concentrations Available *Nurse practitioner programs in:* adult health, family health.

Program Entrance Requirements Computer literacy, transcript of college record, written essay, letters of recommendation, nursing research course, physical assessment course, prerequisite course work, statistics course.

Advanced Placement Credit given for nursing courses completed elsewhere dependent upon specific evaluations.

Degree Requirements 43 total credit hours, thesis or project.

POST-MASTER'S PROGRAM

Areas of Study *Nurse practitioner programs in:* adult health, family health.

Kean University

Department of Nursing
Union, New Jersey

http://www.kean.edu/~nursing/

Founded in 1855

DEGREES • BSN • MSN • MSN/MPA

Nursing Program Faculty 18 (88% with doctorates).

Baccalaureate Enrollment 174
Women 93% **Men** 7% **Minority** 60% **Part-time** 90%

Graduate Enrollment 103
Women 93% **Men** 7% **Minority** 62% **Part-time** 87%

Nursing Student Activities Nursing Honor Society, Sigma Theta Tau, nursing club.

Nursing Student Resources Academic advising; academic or career counseling; assistance for students with disabilities; bookstore; campus computer network; career placement assistance; computer lab; computer-assisted instruction; daycare for children of students; e-mail services; employment services for current students; housing assistance; Internet; learning resource lab; library services; nursing audiovisuals; placement services for program completers; remedial services; resume preparation assistance; skills, simulation, or other laboratory; tutoring; unpaid internships.

Library Facilities 280,000 volumes; 16,053 periodical subscriptions.

BACCALAUREATE PROGRAMS

Degree BSN

Available Programs ADN to Baccalaureate; RN Baccalaureate.

Site Options Raritan, NJ; Plainfield, NJ; Perth Amboy, NJ.

Study Options Full-time and part-time.

Program Entrance Requirements Minimum overall college GPA of 2.0, written essay, 2 letters of recommendation, prerequisite course work, RN licensure. Transfer students are accepted. **Standardized tests** *Required:* SAT or ACT. **Application** *Deadline:* 5/31 (freshmen), 8/1 (transfer). *Notification:* continuous until 9/1 (freshmen). *Application fee:* $50.

Kean University (continued)

Advanced Placement Credit by examination available. Credit given for nursing courses completed elsewhere dependent upon specific evaluations.

Expenses (2004–05) *Tuition, state resident:* full-time $4665; part-time $156 per credit hour. *Tuition, nonresident:* full-time $7170; part-time $239 per credit hour. *International tuition:* $7170 full-time. *Required fees:* full-time $2486; part-time $84 per credit.

Financial Aid 80% of baccalaureate students in nursing programs received some form of financial aid in 2003–04.

Contact Dr. Susan W. Salmond, Chairperson, Department of Nursing, Kean University, 1000 Morris Avenue, Townsend 112, Union, NJ 07083-0411. *Telephone:* 908-737-3385. *Fax:* 908-737-3393. *E-mail:* ssalmond@kean.edu.

GRADUATE PROGRAMS

Expenses (2004–05) *Tuition, state resident:* full-time $3936; part-time $328 per credit hour. *Tuition, nonresident:* full-time $5004; part-time $417 per credit hour.

Financial Aid 80% of graduate students in nursing programs received some form of financial aid in 2003–04. Research assistantships with full tuition reimbursements available available.

Contact Dr. Dula Pacquiao, Graduate Coordinator, Department of Nursing, Kean University, 1000 Morris Avenue, Townsend 112, Union, NJ 07083-0411. *Telephone:* 908-737-3386. *Fax:* 908-737-3393. *E-mail:* dulafp@aol.com.

MASTER'S DEGREE PROGRAM

Degrees MSN; MSN/MPA

Available Programs Accelerated Master's for Nurses with Non-Nursing Degrees; Master's; Master's for Nurses with Non-Nursing Degrees.

Concentrations Available Health-care administration; nursing administration. *Clinical nurse specialist programs in:* community health, school health.

Study Options Full-time and part-time.

Program Entrance Requirements Clinical experience, computer literacy, minimum overall college GPA of 3.0, transcript of college record, written essay, immunizations, interview, 2 letters of recommendation, nursing research course, professional liability insurance/malpractice insurance, statistics course, GRE General Test or MAT. *Application deadline:* For fall admission, 6/15; for spring admission, 11/15. *Application fee:* $60.

Advanced Placement Credit given for nursing courses completed elsewhere dependent upon specific evaluations.

Degree Requirements 36 total credit hours, thesis or project.

CONTINUING EDUCATION PROGRAM

Contact Dr. Susan W. Salmond, Chairperson, Department of Nursing, Kean University, 1000 Morris Avenue, Townsend 112, Union, NJ 07083-0411. *Telephone:* 908-737-3385. *Fax:* 908-737-3393. *E-mail:* ssalmond@kean.edu.

Monmouth University

Marjorie K. Unterberg School of Nursing
West Long Branch, New Jersey

http://www.monmouth.edu

Founded in 1933

DEGREES • BSN • MSN

Nursing Program Faculty 16 (45% with doctorates).

Baccalaureate Enrollment 60
Women 95% **Men** 5% **Minority** 12% **Part-time** 97%

Graduate Enrollment 224
Women 97% **Men** 3% **Minority** 12% **Part-time** 96%

Nursing Student Activities Sigma Theta Tau, Student Nurses' Association.

Nursing Student Resources Academic advising; academic or career counseling; assistance for students with disabilities; bookstore; campus computer network; career placement assistance; computer lab; computer-assisted instruction; e-mail services; employment services for current students; housing assistance; interactive nursing skills videos; Internet; learning resource lab; library services; nursing audiovisuals; paid internships; resume preparation assistance; skills, simulation, or other laboratory; tutoring.

Library Facilities 260,400 volumes (250,000 in health); 16,000 periodical subscriptions (98 health-care related).

BACCALAUREATE PROGRAMS

Degree BSN

Available Programs ADN to Baccalaureate; RN Baccalaureate.

Study Options Full-time and part-time.

Program Entrance Requirements Transcript of college record, health exam, immunizations, 2 letters of recommendation, minimum GPA in nursing prerequisites of 2.0, professional liability insurance/malpractice insurance, prerequisite course work, RN licensure. Transfer students are accepted. **Standardized tests** *Required:* SAT or ACT, TOEFL for international students. **Application** *Deadline:* 3/1 (freshmen), 1/1 (transfer). *Early decision:* 12/1, 12/15. *Notification:* 4/1 (freshmen), 1/1 (out-of-state freshmen), 1/1 (early decision), 1/15 (early action). *Application fee:* $35.

Advanced Placement Credit by examination available. Credit given for nursing courses completed elsewhere dependent upon specific evaluations.

Expenses (2004–05) *Tuition:* full-time $19,108; part-time $533 per credit hour. *Room and board:* $7000; room only: $4000 per academic year. *Required fees:* full-time $533; part-time $284 per term.

Financial Aid 80% of baccalaureate students in nursing programs received some form of financial aid in 2003–04.

Contact Dr. Cira Fraser, Associate Professor, Marjorie K. Unterberg School of Nursing, Monmouth University, West Long Branch, NJ 07764. *Telephone:* 732-571-3443. *Fax:* 732-263-5131. *E-mail:* cfraser@monmouth.edu.

GRADUATE PROGRAMS

Expenses (2004–05) *Tuition:* part-time $605 per credit hour. *Room and board:* $7000; room only: $4000 per academic year. *Required fees:* full-time $568; part-time $284 per term.

Financial Aid 80% of graduate students in nursing programs received some form of financial aid in 2003–04.

Contact Dr. Janet Mahoney, Director of MSN Program, Associate Dean, Marjorie K. Unterberg School of Nursing, Monmouth University, West Long Branch, NJ 07764. *Telephone:* 732-571-3443. *Fax:* 732-263-5131. *E-mail:* jmahoney@monmouth.edu.

MASTER'S DEGREE PROGRAM

Degree MSN

Available Programs Master's; Master's for Nurses with Non-Nursing Degrees.

Concentrations Available Forensic nursing; nursing administration; nursing education. *Nurse practitioner programs in:* adult health, family health, school health.

Study Options Full-time and part-time.

Program Entrance Requirements Clinical experience, minimum overall college GPA of 2.75, transcript of college record, immunizations, 2 letters of recommendation, physical assessment course, professional liability insurance/malpractice insurance.

Advanced Placement Credit given for nursing courses completed elsewhere dependent upon specific evaluations.

Degree Requirements 40 total credit hours.

POST-MASTER'S PROGRAM

Areas of Study Forensic nursing; nursing administration; nursing education. *Nurse practitioner programs in:* adult health, family health.

CONTINUING EDUCATION PROGRAM

Contact Ms. Barbara Paskewich, RN, Special Projects Coordinator, Marjorie K. Unterberg School of Nursing, Monmouth University, West Long Branch, NJ 07764. *Telephone:* 732-571-3694. *Fax:* 732-263-5131. *E-mail:* bpaskewi@monmouth.edu.

New Jersey City University

Department of Nursing
Jersey City, New Jersey

http://www.njcu.edu/dept/ProfStudies/nursing2/rnbsn.htm

Founded in 1927

DEGREES • BSN • MS

Nursing Program Faculty 4 (75% with doctorates).

Baccalaureate Enrollment 110
Women 90% **Men** 10% **Minority** 75% **Part-time** 90%

Graduate Enrollment 36
Women 95% **Men** 5% **Minority** 15% **Part-time** 100%

Nursing Student Activities Nursing Honor Society, Sigma Theta Tau, Student Nurses' Association.

Nursing Student Resources Academic advising; academic or career counseling; bookstore; campus computer network; computer lab; computer-assisted instruction; daycare for children of students; e-mail services; interactive nursing skills videos; Internet; learning resource lab; library services; nursing audiovisuals.

Library Facilities 212,786 volumes; 1,260 periodical subscriptions.

BACCALAUREATE PROGRAMS

Degree BSN

Available Programs RN Baccalaureate.

Site Options Montclair, NJ; East Orange, NJ; Newark, NJ.

Program Entrance Requirements Transfer students are accepted. **Standardized tests** *Required:* SAT or ACT, TOEFL for international students. *Recommended:* SAT. **Application** *Deadline:* 4/1 (freshmen), rolling (transfer). *Notification:* continuous (freshmen). *Application fee:* $35.

Expenses (2003–04) *Tuition, state resident:* part-time $152 per credit hour. *Tuition, nonresident:* part-time $296 per credit hour.

Contact Dr. Pat Joffe, Assistant Professor, Department of Nursing, New Jersey City University, 2039 Kennedy Boulevard, P449, Jersey City, NJ 07305. *Telephone:* 201-200-3157. *Fax:* 201-200-3222. *E-mail:* pjoffe@njcu.edu.

GRADUATE PROGRAMS

Expenses (2003–04) *Tuition, state resident:* part-time $341 per credit hour. *Tuition, nonresident:* part-time $561 per credit hour.

Contact Dr. Gloria Boseman, Interim Chair, Department of Nursing, New Jersey City University, 2039 Kennedy Boulevard, P449, Jersey City, NJ 07305. *Telephone:* 201-200-3157. *Fax:* 201-200-3222. *E-mail:* gboseman@njcu.edu.

MASTER'S DEGREE PROGRAM

Degree MS

Study Options Part-time.

Program Entrance Requirements Minimum overall college GPA of 3.3, transcript of college record, interview, 2 letters of recommendation.

Degree Requirements 36 total credit hours, thesis or project.

The Richard Stockton College of New Jersey

Program in Nursing
Pomona, New Jersey

http://talon.stockton.edu/eyos/page.cfm?siteID=14&pageID=48

Founded in 1969

DEGREES • BSN • MSN

Nursing Program Faculty 6 (66% with doctorates).

Baccalaureate Enrollment 69
Women 98% **Men** 2% **Minority** 10% **Part-time** 80%

Graduate Enrollment 20
Women 90% **Men** 10% **Minority** 15% **Part-time** 95%

Nursing Student Activities Sigma Theta Tau.

Nursing Student Resources Academic advising; academic or career counseling; assistance for students with disabilities; bookstore; campus computer network; computer lab; computer-assisted instruction; daycare for children of students; e-mail services; housing assistance; Internet; learning resource lab; library services; nursing audiovisuals; resume preparation assistance; skills, simulation, or other laboratory; tutoring.

Library Facilities 258,822 volumes (9,761 in health, 1,258 in nursing); 16,826 periodical subscriptions (83 health-care related).

BACCALAUREATE PROGRAMS

Degree BSN

Available Programs RN Baccalaureate.

Site Options *Distance Learning:* Vineland, NJ.

Study Options Full-time and part-time.

Program Entrance Requirements Transfer students are accepted. **Standardized tests** *Required:* SAT or ACT, TOEFL for international students. **Application** *Deadline:* 5/1 (freshmen), 6/1 (transfer). *Early decision:* 2/1. *Notification:* continuous until 5/15 (freshmen). *Application fee:* $50.

Advanced Placement Credit given for nursing courses completed elsewhere dependent upon specific evaluations.

Expenses (2003–04) *Tuition, state resident:* full-time $6224; part-time $195 per credit hour. *Tuition, nonresident:* full-time $9168; part-time $287 per credit hour. *Room and board:* $6804; room only: $4425 per academic year.

Financial Aid 50% of baccalaureate students in nursing programs received some form of financial aid in 2002–03.

Contact Office of Enrollment Management, Program in Nursing, The Richard Stockton College of New Jersey, PO Box 195, Pomona, NJ 08240. *Telephone:* 609-652-4837. *E-mail:* admissions@stockton.edu.

GRADUATE PROGRAMS

Expenses (2003–04) *Tuition, state resident:* part-time $372 per credit hour. *Tuition, nonresident:* part-time $500 per credit hour.

Financial Aid 10% of graduate students in nursing programs received some form of financial aid in 2002–03. Career-related internships or fieldwork and Federal Work-Study available. Aid available to part-time students. *Financial aid application deadline:* 3/1.

Contact Nursing Program Coordinator, Program in Nursing, The Richard Stockton College of New Jersey, Pomona, NJ 08240. *Telephone:* 609-652-4501.

MASTER'S DEGREE PROGRAM

Degree MSN

Concentrations Available *Nurse practitioner programs in:* adult health.

Study Options Full-time and part-time.

Program Entrance Requirements Clinical experience, computer literacy, minimum overall college GPA of 3.0, transcript of college record, CPR certification, written essay, immunizations, 2 letters of recommendation, nursing research course, physical assessment course, professional liability insurance/malpractice insurance, statistics course, GRE General Test. *Application deadline:* For fall admission, 6/1. Applications are processed on a rolling basis. *Application fee:* $35.

Advanced Placement Credit given for nursing courses completed elsewhere dependent upon specific evaluations.

Degree Requirements 42 total credit hours, thesis or project.

Rutgers, The State University of New Jersey, Camden College of Arts and Sciences

Department of Nursing
Camden, New Jersey

Founded in 1927

DEGREES • BS • MS

Rutgers, The State University of New Jersey, Camden College of Arts and Sciences (continued)

Nursing Program Faculty 10 (50% with doctorates).

Baccalaureate Enrollment 95
Women 90% **Men** 10% **Minority** 25%

Nursing Student Activities Sigma Theta Tau, Student Nurses' Association.

Nursing Student Resources Academic advising; academic or career counseling; bookstore; campus computer network; career placement assistance; computer lab; computer-assisted instruction; e-mail services; employment services for current students; externships; housing assistance; interactive nursing skills videos; Internet; learning resource lab; library services; nursing audiovisuals; placement services for program completers; remedial services; resume preparation assistance; skills, simulation, or other laboratory; tutoring.

Library Facilities 6.4 million volumes; 28,934 periodical subscriptions.

BACCALAUREATE PROGRAMS

Degree BS

Available Programs Accelerated RN Baccalaureate; Baccalaureate for Second Degree; Generic Baccalaureate.

Program Entrance Requirements CPR certification, health exam, immunizations, professional liability insurance/malpractice insurance, prerequisite course work. Transfer students are accepted. **Standardized tests** *Required:* SAT or ACT, TOEFL for international students. *Required for some:* SAT Subject Tests. **Application** *Deadline:* 12/15 (freshmen), 3/1 (transfer). *Notification:* continuous until 2/27 (freshmen). *Application fee:* $50.

Financial Aid 75% of baccalaureate students in nursing programs received some form of financial aid in 2003–04.

Contact Dr. Mary E. Greipp, RN, Professor and Chairperson, Department of Nursing, Rutgers, The State University of New Jersey, Camden College of Arts and Sciences, 311 North Fifth Street, Camden, NJ 08102. *Telephone:* 856-225-6226. *Fax:* 856-225-6250. *E-mail:* greipp@camden.rutgers.edu.

GRADUATE PROGRAMS

Contact Dr. Wendy Nehring, RN, Graduate Program, Department of Nursing, Rutgers, The State University of New Jersey, Camden College of Arts and Sciences, 102 Ackerson Hall, 180 University Avenue, Newark, NJ 07102. *Telephone:* 973-353-5293 Ext. 606. *Fax:* 973-353-1277. *E-mail:* nehring@nightingale.rutgers.edu.

MASTER'S DEGREE PROGRAM

Degree MS

Available Programs Master's.

Rutgers, The State University of New Jersey, College of Nursing

Rutgers, The State University of New Jersey, College of Nursing
Newark, New Jersey

http://www.rutgers.edu/

Founded in 1956

DEGREES • BS • MS • MS/MPH • PHD

Nursing Program Faculty 35 (80% with doctorates).

Baccalaureate Enrollment 502
Women 90% **Men** 10% **Minority** 52% **International** 1% **Part-time** 10%

Graduate Enrollment 225
Women 98% **Men** 2% **Minority** 20% **Part-time** 90%

Nursing Student Activities Nursing Honor Society, Sigma Theta Tau, Student Nurses' Association, nursing club.

Nursing Student Resources Academic advising; academic or career counseling; assistance for students with disabilities; bookstore; campus computer network; career placement assistance; computer lab; computer-assisted instruction; e-mail services; externships; interactive nursing skills videos; Internet; learning resource lab; library services; nursing audiovisuals; paid internships; resume preparation assistance; skills, simulation, or other laboratory; tutoring; unpaid internships.

Library Facilities 6.4 million volumes; 28,934 periodical subscriptions.

BACCALAUREATE PROGRAMS

Degree BS

Available Programs Baccalaureate for Second Degree; Generic Baccalaureate; RN Baccalaureate.

Site Options Camden, NJ; Freehold, NJ; New Brunswick, NJ.

Study Options Full-time and part-time.

Program Entrance Requirements Minimum overall college GPA of 3.0, transcript of college record, health exam, high school biology, high school chemistry, 3 years high school math, 2 years high school science, high school transcript, immunizations, minimum high school GPA of 3.0, minimum high school rank 20%. Transfer students are accepted. **Standardized tests** *Required:* SAT or ACT, TOEFL for international students. *Required for some:* SAT Subject Tests. **Application** *Deadline:* 12/15 (freshmen), 3/1 (transfer). *Notification:* continuous until 2/27 (freshmen). *Application fee:* $50.

Advanced Placement Credit by examination available. Credit given for nursing courses completed elsewhere dependent upon specific evaluations.

Expenses (2003–04) *Tuition, state resident:* full-time $6290; part-time $202 per credit hour. *Tuition, nonresident:* full-time $12,804; part-time $415 per credit hour.

Financial Aid 53% of baccalaureate students in nursing programs received some form of financial aid in 2002–03.

Contact Ms. Hanna Roth, Coordinator of Recruitment, Rutgers, The State University of New Jersey, College of Nursing, 180 University Avenue, Newark, NJ 07102-1803. *Telephone:* 973-353-5293 Ext. 630. *E-mail:* hanna@nightingale.rutgers.edu.

GRADUATE PROGRAMS

Financial Aid 15% of graduate students in nursing programs received some form of financial aid in 2002–03.

Contact Dr. Elaine Dolinsky, Associate Dean for Student Affairs, Rutgers, The State University of New Jersey, College of Nursing, 180 University Avenue, Newark, NJ 07102-1803. *Telephone:* 973-353-5293 Ext. 611. *Fax:* 973-353-1277. *E-mail:* dolinsky@nightingale.rutgers.edu.

MASTER'S DEGREE PROGRAM

Degrees MS; MS/MPH

Available Programs Master's.

Concentrations Available *Clinical nurse specialist programs in:* community health, psychiatric/mental health. *Nurse practitioner programs in:* acute care, adult health, family health, pediatric, women's health.

Site Options Camden, NJ; Freehold, NJ.

Study Options Full-time and part-time.

Program Entrance Requirements Minimum overall college GPA of 3.0, transcript of college record, written essay, immunizations, 3 letters of recommendation, physical assessment course, professional liability insurance/malpractice insurance, resume, statistics course.

Advanced Placement Credit given for nursing courses completed elsewhere dependent upon specific evaluations.

Degree Requirements 42 total credit hours.

POST-MASTER'S PROGRAM

Areas of Study Nursing administration; nursing education; nursing informatics. *Clinical nurse specialist programs in:* community health, psychiatric/mental health. *Nurse practitioner programs in:* acute care, family health, pediatric, women's health.

DOCTORAL DEGREE PROGRAM

Degree PhD

Available Programs Doctorate.

Areas of Study Nursing research.

Program Entrance Requirements Minimum overall college GPA of 3.2, interview by faculty committee, interview, 3 letters of recommendation, MSN or equivalent, scholarly papers, statistics course, vita, writing sample.

Degree Requirements 59 total credit hours, dissertation, oral exam, written exam, residency.

CONTINUING EDUCATION PROGRAM

Contact Dr. Gayle Pearson, Assistant Dean, Center for Professional Development, Rutgers, The State University of New Jersey, College of Nursing, 175 University Avenue, Newark, NJ 07102. *Telephone:* 973-353-5895. *Fax:* 973-353-1700. *E-mail:* pearson@nightingale.rutgers.edu.

Saint Peter's College

Nursing Program
Jersey City, New Jersey

Founded in 1872

DEGREES • BSN • MSN

Nursing Program Faculty 15 (73% with doctorates).

Baccalaureate Enrollment 70
Women 99% **Men** 1% **Minority** 40%

Graduate Enrollment 54
Women 99% **Men** 1% **Minority** 45%

Nursing Student Activities Nursing Honor Society, Sigma Theta Tau, Student Nurses' Association.

Nursing Student Resources Academic advising; academic or career counseling; bookstore; campus computer network; computer lab; computer-assisted instruction; e-mail services; interactive nursing skills videos; Internet; library services; nursing audiovisuals; paid internships; remedial services; resume preparation assistance; skills, simulation, or other laboratory; tutoring.

Library Facilities 178,587 volumes (7,200 in health); 1,741 periodical subscriptions (1,586 health-care related).

BACCALAUREATE PROGRAMS

Degree BSN

Available Programs ADN to Baccalaureate; RN Baccalaureate.

Site Options Englewood Cliffs, NJ.

Program Entrance Requirements Minimum overall college GPA of 2.0, transcript of college record, written essay, health exam, immunizations, minimum GPA in nursing prerequisites of 2.0, professional liability insurance/malpractice insurance, RN licensure. Transfer students are accepted. **Standardized tests** *Required:* SAT or ACT, TOEFL for international students. **Application** *Deadline:* rolling (freshmen), 8/1 (transfer). *Notification:* continuous (freshmen). *Application fee:* $40.

Expenses (2004–05) *Tuition:* part-time $470 per credit hour.

Financial Aid 30% of baccalaureate students in nursing programs received some form of financial aid in 2003–04.

Contact Mrs. Shelly Most, Assistant Dean of Englewood Cliffs Campus, Nursing Program, Saint Peter's College, Hudson Terrace, Englewood Cliffs, NJ 07632. *Telephone:* 201-568-7730 Ext. 209. *E-mail:* rmost@spc.edu.

GRADUATE PROGRAMS

Financial Aid 25% of graduate students in nursing programs received some form of financial aid in 2003–04. 2 research assistantships with partial tuition reimbursements available were awarded.

Contact Dr. Marylou Yam, Associate Dean of Nursing, Nursing Program, Saint Peter's College, Hudson Terrace, Englewood Cliffs, NJ 07632. *Telephone:* 201-568-5208. *Fax:* 201-569-1254. *E-mail:* myam@spc.edu.

MASTER'S DEGREE PROGRAM

Degree MSN

Available Programs Master's; Master's for Nurses with Non-Nursing Degrees.

Concentrations Available Nurse case management. *Nurse practitioner programs in:* adult health.

Site Options Englewood Cliffs, NJ.

Study Options Part-time.

Program Entrance Requirements Clinical experience, minimum overall college GPA of 3.0, transcript of college record, written essay, immunizations, 3 letters of recommendation, nursing research course, physical assessment course, professional liability insurance/malpractice insurance, statistics course, GRE or MAT. *Application deadline:* For fall admission, 8/1 (priority date). Applications are processed on a rolling basis. *Application fee:* $20.

Degree Requirements 39 total credit hours, thesis or project.

POST-MASTER'S PROGRAM

Areas of Study *Nurse practitioner programs in:* adult health.

Seton Hall University

College of Nursing
South Orange, New Jersey

http://nursing.shu.edu/

Founded in 1856

DEGREES • BSN • MSN • MSN/MA • MSN/MBA

Nursing Program Faculty 50 (65% with doctorates).

Baccalaureate Enrollment 425
Women 92% **Men** 8%

Graduate Enrollment 225
Women 86% **Men** 14%

Nursing Student Activities Sigma Theta Tau, Student Nurses' Association.

Nursing Student Resources Academic advising; assistance for students with disabilities; bookstore; campus computer network; computer lab; computer-assisted instruction; e-mail services; housing assistance; interactive nursing skills videos; Internet; learning resource lab; library services; nursing audiovisuals; paid internships; remedial services; resume preparation assistance; skills, simulation, or other laboratory; tutoring.

Library Facilities 506,042 volumes (26,000 in health, 4,100 in nursing); 1,475 periodical subscriptions (300 health-care related).

BACCALAUREATE PROGRAMS

Degree BSN

Available Programs Accelerated Baccalaureate for Second Degree; Baccalaureate for Second Degree; Generic Baccalaureate; RN Baccalaureate.

Site Options *Distance Learning:* Lakewood, NJ; Brick, NJ; Toms River, NJ.

Study Options Full-time and part-time.

Program Entrance Requirements Minimum overall college GPA of 2.5, transcript of college record, written essay, high school biology, high school chemistry, high school foreign language, 3 years high school math, 2 years high school science, high school transcript, minimum high school GPA of 2.5, minimum high school rank 50%. Transfer students are accepted. **Standardized tests** *Required:* SAT or ACT, TOEFL for international students. **Application** *Deadline:* 3/1 (freshmen), 6/1 (transfer). *Notification:* continuous until 12/1 (freshmen). *Application fee:* $45.

Expenses (2004–05) *Tuition:* full-time $20,700; part-time $689 per credit hour. *Room and board:* $9700; room only: $7700 per academic year. *Required fees:* full-time $650; part-time $185 per term.

Financial Aid 68% of baccalaureate students in nursing programs received some form of financial aid in 2003–04. *Gift aid (need-based):* Federal Pell, FSEOG, state, private, college/university gift aid from institutional funds. *Loans:* FFEL (Subsidized and Unsubsidized Stafford PLUS), Perkins, state. *Work-Study:* Federal Work-Study, part-time campus jobs. *Application deadline:* Continuous.

Contact Mary Jo Bugel, RN, Director of Recruitment, College of Nursing, Seton Hall University, 400 South Orange Avenue, Schwartz Hall, South Orange, NJ 07079-2693. *Telephone:* 973-761-9285. *Fax:* 973-761-9607. *E-mail:* bugelmar@shu.edu.

GRADUATE PROGRAMS

Expenses (2004–05) *Tuition:* part-time $701 per credit hour. *Room and board:* $9700; room only: $7700 per academic year. *Required fees:* full-time $725.

Seton Hall University (continued)

Financial Aid 68% of graduate students in nursing programs received some form of financial aid in 2003–04. Institutionally sponsored loans, traineeships, tuition waivers (partial), and unspecified assistantships available. Aid available to part-time students. *Financial aid application deadline:* 7/15.

Contact Mary Jo Bugel, RN, Director of Recruitment, College of Nursing, Seton Hall University, 400 South Orange Avenue, Schwartz Hall, South Orange, NJ 07079-2693. *Telephone:* 973-761-9285. *Fax:* 973-761-9607. *E-mail:* bugelmar@shu.edu.

MASTER'S DEGREE PROGRAM

Degrees MSN; MSN/MA; MSN/MBA

Available Programs Master's; RN to Master's.

Concentrations Available Health-care administration; nurse case management; nursing administration; nursing education. *Nurse practitioner programs in:* acute care, adult health, gerontology, pediatric, primary care, school health, women's health.

Site Options *Distance Learning:* Toms River, NJ.

Study Options Full-time and part-time.

Program Entrance Requirements Minimum overall college GPA of 3.0, transcript of college record, CPR certification, written essay, 2 letters of recommendation, nursing research course, physical assessment course, professional liability insurance/malpractice insurance, resume, statistics course, GRE or MAT. *Application deadline:* For fall admission, 5/15 (priority date); for spring admission, 11/15. Applications are processed on a rolling basis. *Application fee:* $50.

Degree Requirements 43 total credit hours, thesis or project.

POST-MASTER'S PROGRAM

Areas of Study Health-care administration; nurse case management; nursing administration; nursing education. *Nurse practitioner programs in:* acute care, adult health, gerontology, pediatric, primary care, school health, women's health.

CONTINUING EDUCATION PROGRAM

Contact Mary Jo Bugel, Director of Recruitment, College of Nursing, Seton Hall University, 400 South Orange Avenue, South Orange, NJ 07079. *Telephone:* 973-7619285. *E-mail:* Bugelmar@shu.edu.

Thomas Edison State College
Program in Nursing
Trenton, New Jersey

http://www.tesc.edu

Nursing program started in 1983

DEGREE • BSN for RNs

Nursing Student Resources Students have the opportunity to earn degrees through traditional and nontraditional methods which take into consideration the personal needs and interests of each student. Online courses are designed and delivered as mentored, independent study courses via the Internet using MyEdison, the College's online course management system that utilizes the Blackboard platform. Students in these courses communicate with mentors and fellow students using e-mail and submit assignments to mentors through the Internet. Students may earn credit toward a degree by demonstrating college-level knowledge through testing and assessment of prior learning; by transfer credit for courses taken through other regionally accredited institutions; through the College's e-Pack® courses; and, for licenses, certificates, and courses taken at work or through military training, if approved and recommended for academic credit.

Nursing Program Faculty The nursing program utilizes off-site nurse educators from a variety of nursing education and service settings to develop, implement, and evaluate the program. All nursing educators have a minimum of a master's degree in nursing, with approximately 80 percent prepared at the doctoral level and many tenured at their home institution. As a distance learning program, the BSN degree program has the opportunity to draw nurse educators from throughout the United States, resulting in a very diverse and experienced group of online nurse educators. The program is accredited by the New Jersey Board of Nursing and the National League for Nursing Accrediting Commission.

BACCALAUREATE PROGRAM

Degree BSN for RNs

Study Options Self-paced; all nursing courses offered quarterly online; multiple options for credit earning; no time limit for degree completion; no residency requirement with maximum flexibility in transfer credit.

Program Entrance Requirements The Bachelor of Science in Nursing program, an online distance learning program for registered nurses who are currently licensed in the United States, and who want an alternative to campus-based instruction, has open and rolling admissions. In addition to the submission of a notarized copy of their current RN license, applicants must submit a completed College application and $75 fee along with the BSN Credential Review form and fee of $300. The program requires a minimum of 120 semester hours of credit: 60 in general education, 48 in nursing and 12 in free electives. RNs who have completed an associate degree nursing program or an RN diploma program will have 20 credits applied from previous nursing course work toward the 48-credit nursing component. A total of 80 credits may be accepted from a community college, and up to 60 credits awarded to diploma graduates based on current licensure. There is no age restriction on credits transferred in to meet general education requirements or lower-division nursing requirements. All upper-division nursing credits must be from an accredited baccalaureate or higher degree nursing program, and newer than 10 years if completed prior to application to Thomas Edison State College. All credits used in the nursing component must have a grade equivalent of "C" or better.

Expenses (2004–05) $260 per credit for New Jersey residents; $374 per credit for out-of-state residents for all Thomas Edison State College methods of credit earning.

Financial Aid Two percent of the RNs in the baccalaureate nursing program received some form of financial aid in 2003–04.

Contact Thomas Edison State College, 101 West State Street, Trenton, NJ 08608-1176. *Telephone:* (888) 442-8372, *E-mail:* info@tesc.edu.

See full description on page 542.

University of Medicine and Dentistry of New Jersey
School of Nursing
Newark, New Jersey

http://sn.umdnj.edu/

Founded in 1954

DEGREES • BSN • MSN

Nursing Program Faculty 46 (25% with doctorates).

Baccalaureate Enrollment 333
Women 82% **Men** 18% **Minority** 50% **Part-time** 4%

Graduate Enrollment 243
Women 87% **Men** 13% **Minority** 49% **Part-time** 90%

Nursing Student Activities Sigma Theta Tau, Student Nurses' Association.

Nursing Student Resources Academic advising; academic or career counseling; assistance for students with disabilities; bookstore; campus computer network; computer lab; computer-assisted instruction; daycare for children of students; e-mail services; interactive nursing skills videos; Internet; learning resource lab; library services; nursing audiovisuals; skills, simulation, or other laboratory; tutoring.

BACCALAUREATE PROGRAMS

Degree BSN

Available Programs Accelerated Baccalaureate for Second Degree; Generic Baccalaureate; RN Baccalaureate.

Site Options Glassboro, NJ; Mahwah, NJ.

Study Options Full-time and part-time.

Program Entrance Requirements Minimum overall college GPA of 2.5, transcript of college record, CPR certification, written essay, health exam, health insurance, high school transcript, immunizations, 3 letters of recommendation, minimum high school rank 40%, RN licensure. Transfer students are accepted.

Advanced Placement Credit given for nursing courses completed elsewhere dependent upon specific evaluations.

Contact Mr. Victor Marques, Marketing Representative/Recruiter, School of Nursing, University of Medicine and Dentistry of New Jersey, 65 Bergen Street, Room 1130, Newark, NJ 07101. *Telephone:* 973-972-7445. *Fax:* 973-972-7453. *E-mail:* marquevm@umdnj.edu.

GRADUATE PROGRAMS

Expenses (2004–05) *Tuition, state resident:* part-time $355 per credit hour. *Tuition, nonresident:* part-time $504 per credit hour.

Financial Aid Teaching assistantships, institutionally sponsored loans and scholarships available.

Contact Ms. Debra Savage, Nurse Student Recruiter, School of Nursing, University of Medicine and Dentistry of New Jersey, 65 Bergen Street, Room 1126, Newark, NJ 07101. *Telephone:* 973-972-9245. *Fax:* 973-972-7453. *E-mail:* savageda@umdnj.edu.

MASTER'S DEGREE PROGRAM

Degree MSN

Available Programs Master's.

Concentrations Available Nurse anesthesia; nursing education; nursing informatics. *Clinical nurse specialist programs in:* acute care, critical care, oncology, psychiatric/mental health. *Nurse practitioner programs in:* acute care, adult health, family health, gerontology, oncology, psychiatric/mental health, women's health.

Site Options Stratford, NJ.

Study Options Full-time and part-time.

Program Entrance Requirements Clinical experience, minimum overall college GPA of 3.0, transcript of college record, CPR certification, 3 letters of recommendation, physical assessment course, prerequisite course work, statistics course, GRE. *Application deadline:* For fall admission, 4/15; for spring admission, 10/15. Applications are processed on a rolling basis. *Application fee:* $30.

Advanced Placement Credit given for nursing courses completed elsewhere dependent upon specific evaluations.

Degree Requirements 40 total credit hours.

POST-MASTER'S PROGRAM

Areas of Study Nurse anesthesia; nursing education; nursing informatics. *Clinical nurse specialist programs in:* acute care, critical care, oncology, psychiatric/mental health. *Nurse practitioner programs in:* acute care, adult health, family health, gerontology, oncology, psychiatric/mental health, women's health.

CONTINUING EDUCATION PROGRAM

Contact Mr. Lesley A. Perry, Associate Professor and Associate Dean for Academic Affairs, School of Nursing, University of Medicine and Dentistry of New Jersey, 65 Bergen Street, Room 1143, Newark, NJ 07107. *Telephone:* 973-972-4288. *Fax:* 973-972-3225. *E-mail:* perryle@umdnj.edu.

William Paterson University of New Jersey

Department of Nursing
Wayne, New Jersey

http://www.wpunj.edu/cos/nursing/

Founded in 1855

DEGREES • BSN • MSN

Nursing Program Faculty 29 (73% with doctorates).

Baccalaureate Enrollment 450

Women 90% **Men** 10% **Minority** 51% **International** 5% **Part-time** 25%

Graduate Enrollment 60

Women 98% **Men** 2% **Minority** 18% **Part-time** 90%

Nursing Student Activities Sigma Theta Tau, Student Nurses' Association.

Nursing Student Resources Academic advising; academic or career counseling; assistance for students with disabilities; bookstore; campus computer network; career placement assistance; computer lab; computer-assisted instruction; daycare for children of students; e-mail services; employment services for current students; housing assistance; interactive nursing skills videos; Internet; learning resource lab; library services; nursing audiovisuals; placement services for program completers; remedial services; resume preparation assistance; skills, simulation, or other laboratory; tutoring.

Library Facilities 305,155 volumes (15,000 in health, 12,700 in nursing); 4,112 periodical subscriptions (120 health-care related).

BACCALAUREATE PROGRAMS

Degree BSN

Available Programs ADN to Baccalaureate; Accelerated Baccalaureate for Second Degree; Generic Baccalaureate; RN Baccalaureate.

Study Options Full-time and part-time.

Program Entrance Requirements Minimum overall college GPA of 2.5, transcript of college record, CPR certification, health exam, health insurance, high school biology, high school chemistry, 1 year of high school math, 2 years high school science, high school transcript, immunizations, minimum GPA in nursing prerequisites of 2.5. Transfer students are accepted. **Standardized tests** *Required:* SAT or ACT, TOEFL for international students. **Application** *Deadline:* 5/1 (freshmen), 5/1 (transfer). *Early decision:* 3/10. *Notification:* continuous (freshmen). *Application fee:* $50.

Expenses (2004–05) *Tuition, state resident:* full-time $7952; part-time $255 per credit hour. *Tuition, nonresident:* full-time $12,690; part-time $410 per credit hour. *Room and board:* $4000; room only: $2750 per academic year. *Required fees:* part-time $7 per credit; part-time $21 per term.

Financial Aid *Gift aid (need-based):* Federal Pell, FSEOG, state, college/university gift aid from institutional funds. *Loans:* Federal Direct (Subsidized and Unsubsidized Stafford PLUS), Perkins, NJ Class Loans. *Work-Study:* Federal Work-Study, part-time campus jobs. *Application deadline (priority):* 4/1.

Contact Dr. Julie Beshore Bliss, Chairperson, Department of Nursing, William Paterson University of New Jersey, 300 Pompton Road-W106, Wayne, NJ 07470. *Telephone:* 973-720-2673. *Fax:* 973-720-2668. *E-mail:* blissj@wpunj.edu.

GRADUATE PROGRAMS

Expenses (2004–05) *Tuition, state resident:* part-time $436 per credit hour. *Tuition, nonresident:* part-time $659 per credit hour. *Room and board:* $8000; room only: $5400 per academic year.

Financial Aid Research assistantships, unspecified assistantships available.

Contact Dr. Kem Louie, RN, Director, Graduate Program, Department of Nursing, William Paterson University of New Jersey, 300 Pompton Road-W240, Wayne, NJ 07470. *Telephone:* 973-720-3511. *Fax:* 973-720-3517. *E-mail:* louiek@wpunj.edu.

MASTER'S DEGREE PROGRAM

Degree MSN

Available Programs Master's; Master's for Nurses with Non-Nursing Degrees.

Concentrations Available Nursing administration; nursing education. *Clinical nurse specialist programs in:* community health. *Nurse practitioner programs in:* adult health.

Study Options Full-time and part-time.

Program Entrance Requirements Clinical experience, minimum overall college GPA of 3.0, transcript of college record, written essay, 3 letters of recommendation, nursing research course, physical assessment course, professional liability insurance/malpractice insurance, statistics course, GRE General Test. *Application deadline:* Applications are processed on a rolling basis. *Application fee:* $35.

Advanced Placement Credit given for nursing courses completed elsewhere dependent upon specific evaluations.

Degree Requirements 40 total credit hours, thesis or project.

William Paterson University of New Jersey (continued)

POST-MASTER'S PROGRAM

Areas of Study *Clinical nurse specialist programs in:* school health. *Nurse practitioner programs in:* adult health.

NEW MEXICO

Eastern New Mexico University

Department of Allied Health—Nursing
Portales, New Mexico

http://www.enmu.edu/academics/undergrad/colleges/las/disorders-nursing

Founded in 1934

DEGREE • BSN

Nursing Program Faculty 4 (25% with doctorates).

Nursing Student Resources Academic advising; academic or career counseling; assistance for students with disabilities; bookstore; campus computer network; computer lab; computer-assisted instruction; daycare for children of students; e-mail services; housing assistance; interactive nursing skills videos; Internet; learning resource lab; library services; nursing audiovisuals; other; resume preparation assistance; skills, simulation, or other laboratory; tutoring.

Library Facilities 305,108 volumes (100 in health, 50 in nursing); 7,621 periodical subscriptions (15 health-care related).

BACCALAUREATE PROGRAMS

Degree BSN

Available Programs RN Baccalaureate.

Site Options *Distance Learning:* Hobbs, NM; Clovis.

Study Options Full-time and part-time.

Program Entrance Requirements Minimum overall college GPA of 2.0, transcript of college record, CPR certification, written essay, high school biology, high school chemistry, 2 years high school math, 2 years high school science, high school transcript, interview, 3 letters of recommendation, minimum high school GPA of 2.5, minimum GPA in nursing prerequisites of 2.0, professional liability insurance/malpractice insurance, prerequisite course work, RN licensure. Transfer students are accepted. **Standardized tests** *Required:* SAT or ACT, TOEFL for international students. **Application** *Deadline:* rolling (freshmen), rolling (transfer).

Advanced Placement Credit given for nursing courses completed elsewhere dependent upon specific evaluations.

Contact Dr. Ellen E. Bral, RN, Director, Department of Allied Health—Nursing, Eastern New Mexico University, Station #12, Portales, NM 88130. *Telephone:* 505-562-2403. *Fax:* 505-562-2293. *E-mail:* ellen.bral@enmu.edu.

New Mexico State University

Department of Nursing
Las Cruces, New Mexico

http://www.nmsu.edu/~nursing

Founded in 1888

DEGREES • BSN • MSN

Nursing Program Faculty 35 (40% with doctorates).

Baccalaureate Enrollment 273
Women 87% **Men** 13% **Minority** 46% **International** 1% **Part-time** 16%

Graduate Enrollment 53
Women 91% **Men** 9% **Minority** 36% **International** 2% **Part-time** 55%

Nursing Student Activities Sigma Theta Tau, Student Nurses' Association.

Nursing Student Resources Academic advising; academic or career counseling; assistance for students with disabilities; bookstore; campus computer network; computer lab; computer-assisted instruction; daycare for children of students; e-mail services; housing assistance; interactive nursing skills videos; Internet; learning resource lab; library services; nursing audiovisuals; paid internships; remedial services; skills, simulation, or other laboratory; tutoring.

Library Facilities 1.6 million volumes (31,000 in health, 16,500 in nursing); 5,975 periodical subscriptions (620 health-care related).

BACCALAUREATE PROGRAMS

Degree BSN

Available Programs Accelerated Baccalaureate for Second Degree; Accelerated RN Baccalaureate; Generic Baccalaureate.

Site Options *Distance Learning:* Carlsbad, NM; Deming, NM; Alamagordo, NM.

Study Options Full-time and part-time.

Program Entrance Requirements Transcript of college record, CPR certification, health exam, health insurance, immunizations, minimum GPA in nursing prerequisites of 2.5, prerequisite course work. Transfer students are accepted. **Standardized tests** *Required:* SAT or ACT, TOEFL for international students. **Application** *Deadline:* 8/19 (freshmen), 8/14 (transfer). *Notification:* continuous (freshmen). *Application fee:* $15.

Advanced Placement Credit given for nursing courses completed elsewhere dependent upon specific evaluations.

Expenses (2004–05) *Tuition, state resident:* full-time $3666; part-time $153 per credit hour. *Tuition, nonresident:* full-time $12,210; part-time $509 per credit hour. *International tuition:* $12,210 full-time. *Room and board:* $2600; room only: $1500 per academic year. *Required fees:* full-time $200; part-time $100 per term.

Financial Aid 80% of baccalaureate students in nursing programs received some form of financial aid in 2003–04.

Contact Lissa Kirby, Advising Coordinator, Department of Nursing, New Mexico State University, PO Box 30001, MSC 3446, Las Cruces, NM 88003-8001. *Telephone:* 505-646-3534. *Fax:* 505-646-6166.

GRADUATE PROGRAMS

Expenses (2004–05) *Tuition, state resident:* full-time $3936; part-time $164 per credit hour. *Tuition, nonresident:* full-time $12,534; part-time $522 per credit hour. *International tuition:* $12,534 full-time. *Room and board:* $2600; room only: $1500 per academic year. *Required fees:* full-time $250; part-time $150 per term.

Financial Aid 70% of graduate students in nursing programs received some form of financial aid in 2003–04. 2 teaching assistantships were awarded; fellowships, research assistantships, career-related internships or fieldwork, Federal Work-Study, scholarships, and traineeships also available. *Financial aid application deadline:* 3/1.

Contact Dr. Mary M. Hoke, Academic Department Head, Department of Nursing, New Mexico State University, PO Box 30001, Department 3185, Las Cruces, NM 88003-8001. *Telephone:* 505-646-8170. *Fax:* 505-646-2167. *E-mail:* aksky@nmsu.edu.

MASTER'S DEGREE PROGRAM

Degree MSN

Available Programs Master's.

Concentrations Available Nursing administration. *Clinical nurse specialist programs in:* community health, medical-surgical, psychiatric/mental health. *Nurse practitioner programs in:* psychiatric/mental health.

Study Options Full-time and part-time.

Program Entrance Requirements Minimum overall college GPA of 3.0, transcript of college record, CPR certification, written essay, immunizations, 3 letters of recommendation, statistics course. *Application deadline:* For fall admission, 7/1 (priority date); for spring admission, 11/1 (priority date). Applications are processed on a rolling basis. *Application fee:* $30 ($50 for international students).

Advanced Placement Credit given for nursing courses completed elsewhere dependent upon specific evaluations.

Degree Requirements 50 total credit hours, thesis or project, comprehensive exam.

POST-MASTER'S PROGRAM

Areas of Study Nursing administration. *Clinical nurse specialist programs in:* community health, medical-surgical, psychiatric/mental health. *Nurse practitioner programs in:* psychiatric/mental health.

CONTINUING EDUCATION PROGRAM

Contact Dr. Mary Hoyte Sizemore, Local Monitoring Program Chair, Department of Nursing, New Mexico State University, PO Box 30001, Department 3185, Las Cruces, NM 88003-8001. *Telephone:* 505-646-3812. *Fax:* 505-646-2167. *E-mail:* masizemo@nmsu.edu.

University of New Mexico
College of Nursing
Albuquerque, New Mexico

http://hsc.unm.edu/consg/

Founded in 1889

DEGREES • BSN • MSN • MSN/MALAS • MSN/MPA • MSN/MPH • PHD

Nursing Program Faculty 50 (46% with doctorates).

Baccalaureate Enrollment 342
Women 89% **Men** 11% **Minority** 45% **Part-time** 35%

Graduate Enrollment 127
Women 94% **Men** 6% **Minority** 24% **Part-time** 65%

Nursing Student Activities Sigma Theta Tau, Student Nurses' Association.

Nursing Student Resources Academic advising; assistance for students with disabilities; bookstore; campus computer network; career placement assistance; computer lab; computer-assisted instruction; daycare for children of students; e-mail services; housing assistance; interactive nursing skills videos; Internet; learning resource lab; library services; nursing audiovisuals; remedial services; skills, simulation, or other laboratory.

Library Facilities 2.7 million volumes (176,055 in health, 5,081 in nursing); 592,243 periodical subscriptions (1,567 health-care related).

BACCALAUREATE PROGRAMS

Degree BSN

Available Programs Accelerated Baccalaureate for Second Degree; Generic Baccalaureate; RN Baccalaureate.

Study Options Full-time.

Program Entrance Requirements Minimum overall college GPA of 2.5, transcript of college record, minimum GPA in nursing prerequisites of 2.5, prerequisite course work. Transfer students are accepted. **Standardized tests** *Required:* SAT or ACT, TOEFL for international students. *Required for some:* SAT and SAT Subject Tests or ACT, SAT Subject Tests, SAT II Writing Tests. **Application** *Deadline:* 6/15 (freshmen), 6/15 (transfer). *Notification:* continuous (freshmen). *Application fee:* $20.

Advanced Placement Credit given for nursing courses completed elsewhere dependent upon specific evaluations.

Expenses (2004–05) *Tuition, state resident:* full-time $3738; part-time $156 per credit hour. *Tuition, nonresident:* full-time $12,500; part-time $520 per credit hour. *International tuition:* $12,500 full-time. *Room and board:* $7100; room only: $4500 per academic year. *Required fees:* full-time $600; part-time $40 per credit; part-time $300 per term.

Financial Aid 70% of baccalaureate students in nursing programs received some form of financial aid in 2003–04.

Contact Ms. Ann Marie Oechsler, Director of Student Services, College of Nursing, University of New Mexico, MSCS09 5350, 1 University of New Mexico, Albuquerque, NM 87131-5688. *Telephone:* 505-272-4223. *Fax:* 505-272-3970. *E-mail:* aoechsler@salud.unm.edu.

GRADUATE PROGRAMS

Expenses (2004–05) *Tuition, state resident:* full-time $4070; part-time $171 per credit hour. *Tuition, nonresident:* full-time $12,810; part-time $521 per credit hour. *International tuition:* $12,810 full-time. *Room and board:* $7100; room only: $4500 per academic year. *Required fees:* full-time $500; part-time $40 per credit; part-time $250 per term.

Financial Aid 40% of graduate students in nursing programs received some form of financial aid in 2003–04. 1 research assistantship (averaging $2,620 per year), 12 teaching assistantships (averaging $3,545 per year) were awarded; scholarships, traineeships, and tuition waivers (full) also available. *Financial aid application deadline:* 3/1.

Contact Ms. Elizabeth Rowe, Senior Academic Advisor, College of Nursing, University of New Mexico, MSC09 5350, NRPH Building, Room 152, 1 University of New Mexico, Albuquerque, NM 87131-0001. *Telephone:* 505-272-4223. *Fax:* 505-272-3970. *E-mail:* erowe@salud.unm.edu.

MASTER'S DEGREE PROGRAM

Degrees MSN; MSN/MALAS; MSN/MPA; MSN/MPH

Available Programs Master's; Master's for Nurses with Non-Nursing Degrees.

Concentrations Available Nurse-midwifery; nursing administration; nursing education. *Clinical nurse specialist programs in:* adult health, gerontology, pediatric, psychiatric/mental health, women's health. *Nurse practitioner programs in:* acute care, family health, primary care.

Study Options Full-time and part-time.

Program Entrance Requirements Clinical experience, minimum overall college GPA of 3.0, transcript of college record, 3 letters of recommendation, resume, GRE General Test. *Application deadline:* For fall admission, 6/15; for spring admission, 10/15. *Application fee:* $40.

Advanced Placement Credit by examination available. Credit given for nursing courses completed elsewhere dependent upon specific evaluations.

Degree Requirements 30 total credit hours, thesis or project, comprehensive exam.

POST-MASTER'S PROGRAM

Areas of Study Nurse-midwifery; nursing administration; nursing education. *Clinical nurse specialist programs in:* adult health, gerontology, pediatric, psychiatric/mental health, women's health. *Nurse practitioner programs in:* acute care, family health, primary care.

DOCTORAL DEGREE PROGRAM

Degree PhD

Available Programs Doctorate.

Areas of Study Nursing education, nursing research.

Program Entrance Requirements Clinical experience, minimum overall college GPA of 3.0, interview by faculty committee, 3 letters of recommendation, MSN or equivalent, scholarly papers, vita. *Application deadline:* For fall admission, 6/15; for spring admission, 10/15. *Application fee:* $40.

Degree Requirements 66 total credit hours, dissertation.

University of Phoenix–New Mexico Campus
College of Health and Human Services
Albuquerque, New Mexico

DEGREES • BSN • MSN • MSN/MBA

Nursing Program Faculty 35 (17% with doctorates).

Baccalaureate Enrollment 61
Women 88.5% **Men** 11.5% **Minority** 37%

Graduate Enrollment 55
Women 91% **Men** 9% **Minority** 51%

Nursing Student Activities Sigma Theta Tau.

Nursing Student Resources Academic advising; academic or career counseling; bookstore; computer lab; library services.

Library Facilities 27.1 million volumes; 11,648 periodical subscriptions (1,426 health-care related).

BACCALAUREATE PROGRAMS

Degree BSN

Available Programs ADN to Baccalaureate; Accelerated Baccalaureate.

University of Phoenix–New Mexico Campus (continued)

Site Options Santa Fe, NM; Santa Teresa, NM.

Study Options Full-time.

Program Entrance Requirements 1 letter of recommendation. Transfer students are accepted. **Standardized tests** *Required:* TOEFL for international students. **Application** *Deadline:* rolling (freshmen), rolling (transfer). *Application fee:* $85.

Advanced Placement Credit by examination available.

Expenses (2004–05) *Tuition:* full-time $8940; part-time $298 per credit hour. *International tuition:* $8940 full-time. *Required fees:* full-time $110.

Financial Aid 3% of baccalaureate students in nursing programs received some form of financial aid in 2003–04.

Contact Campus College Chair, Nursing, College of Health and Human Services, University of Phoenix–New Mexico Campus, 7471 Pan American Freeway, NE, Albuquerque, NM 87109-4645. *Telephone:* 505-821-4800.

GRADUATE PROGRAMS

Expenses (2004–05) *Tuition:* full-time $8280; part-time $345 per credit hour. *International tuition:* $8280 full-time. *Required fees:* full-time $110.

Financial Aid 7% of graduate students in nursing programs received some form of financial aid in 2003–04.

Contact Campus College Chair, Nursing, College of Health and Human Services, University of Phoenix–New Mexico Campus, 7471 Pan American Freeway, NE, Albuquerque, NM 87109-4645. *Telephone:* 505-821-4800.

MASTER'S DEGREE PROGRAM

Degrees MSN; MSN/MBA

Available Programs Master's.

Concentrations Available Health-care administration; nursing administration; nursing education. *Nurse practitioner programs in:* family health.

Site Options Santa Fe, NM; Santa Teresa, NM.

Study Options Full-time.

Program Entrance Requirements Clinical experience, computer literacy, minimum overall college GPA of 2.5, transcript of college record. *Application deadline:* Applications are processed on a rolling basis. *Application fee:* $110.

Degree Requirements 39 total credit hours, thesis or project.

POST-MASTER'S PROGRAM

Areas of Study *Nurse practitioner programs in:* family health.

NEW YORK

Adelphi University

School of Nursing
Garden City, New York

Founded in 1896

DEGREES • BS • MS • MS/MBA

Nursing Program Faculty 73 (25% with doctorates).

Baccalaureate Enrollment 510

Women 90% **Men** 10% **Minority** 40% **International** 1% **Part-time** 30%

Graduate Enrollment 140

Women 96% **Men** 4% **Minority** 36% **Part-time** 99%

Nursing Student Activities Nursing Honor Society, Sigma Theta Tau, Student Nurses' Association, nursing club.

Nursing Student Resources Academic advising; academic or career counseling; assistance for students with disabilities; bookstore; campus computer network; career placement assistance; computer lab; computer-assisted instruction; e-mail services; employment services for current students; externships; housing assistance; interactive nursing skills videos; Internet; learning resource lab; library services; nursing audiovisuals; paid internships; remedial services; resume preparation assistance; skills, simulation, or other laboratory; tutoring; unpaid internships.

Library Facilities 631,023 volumes (27,862 in health, 2,686 in nursing); 1,642 periodical subscriptions (371 health-care related).

BACCALAUREATE PROGRAMS

Degree BS

Available Programs Accelerated Baccalaureate; Accelerated Baccalaureate for Second Degree; Baccalaureate for Second Degree; Generic Baccalaureate; RN Baccalaureate.

Site Options Forest Hills , NY; Glen Cove, NY.

Study Options Full-time and part-time.

Program Entrance Requirements Minimum overall college GPA of 2.8, transcript of college record, written essay, health exam, high school foreign language, 3 years high school math, 3 years high school science, high school transcript, immunizations, interview, 2 letters of recommendation, minimum high school GPA of 2.8. Transfer students are accepted. **Standardized tests** *Required:* SAT or ACT, TOEFL for international students. **Application** *Deadline:* rolling (freshmen), rolling (transfer). *Early decision:* 12/1. *Notification:* continuous (freshmen), 12/31 (early action). *Application fee:* $35.

Advanced Placement Credit by examination available.

Expenses (2004–05) *Tuition:* full-time $19,650; part-time $580 per credit hour. *International tuition:* $19,650 full-time. *Room and board:* $8500; room only: $5700 per academic year. *Required fees:* full-time $1040; part-time $520 per term.

Financial Aid 92% of baccalaureate students in nursing programs received some form of financial aid in 2003–04.

Contact Mr. Joseph Posillico, Director of Admissions, School of Nursing, Adelphi University, One South Avenue, Levermore Hall, Garden City, NY 11530. *Telephone:* 516-877-3052. *Fax:* 516-877-3039. *E-mail:* posillic@adelphi.edu.

GRADUATE PROGRAMS

Expenses (2004–05) *Tuition:* full-time $14,760; part-time $615 per credit hour. *International tuition:* $14,760 full-time. *Room and board:* $8500; room only: $5700 per academic year. *Required fees:* full-time $500; part-time $250 per term.

Financial Aid 23% of graduate students in nursing programs received some form of financial aid in 2003–04. Research assistantships, teaching assistantships, career-related internships or fieldwork and graduate achievement awards available. Aid available to part-time students. *Financial aid application deadline:* 2/15.

Contact Mr. Joseph Posillico, Director of Admissions, School of Nursing, Adelphi University, One South Avenue, Levermore Hall, Garden City, NY 11530. *Telephone:* 516-877-3052. *Fax:* 516-877-3039. *E-mail:* posillic@adelphi.edu.

MASTER'S DEGREE PROGRAM

Degrees MS; MS/MBA

Available Programs Master's; Master's for Nurses with Non-Nursing Degrees.

Concentrations Available Nursing administration. *Nurse practitioner programs in:* adult health.

Site Options West Islip, NY; Glen Cove, NY.

Study Options Full-time and part-time.

Program Entrance Requirements Clinical experience, minimum overall college GPA of 3.0, transcript of college record, CPR certification, written essay, immunizations, interview, 2 letters of recommendation, physical assessment course, professional liability insurance/malpractice insurance, resume, statistics course. *Application deadline:* For fall admission, 8/15 (priority date); for spring admission, 1/15 (priority date). Applications are processed on a rolling basis. *Application fee:* $50.

Advanced Placement Credit by examination available. Credit given for nursing courses completed elsewhere dependent upon specific evaluations.

Degree Requirements 48 total credit hours, thesis or project.

POST-MASTER'S PROGRAM

Areas of Study Nursing administration. *Nurse practitioner programs in:* adult health.

CONTINUING EDUCATION PROGRAM

Contact Karen Pappas, Director, Professional Development and Lifelong Learning, School of Nursing, Adelphi University, One South Avenue, Garden City, NY 11530. *Telephone:* 516-877-4554. *Fax:* 516-877-4558. *E-mail:* pappas@adelphi.edu.

College of Mount Saint Vincent

Division of Nursing
Riverdale, New York

http://www.mountsaintvincent.edu/academics/majors_and_programs/nursing2/nursing.htm

Founded in 1911

DEGREES • BS • MSN

Nursing Program Faculty 30 (40% with doctorates).

Nursing Student Resources Library services.

Library Facilities 160,696 volumes (5,304 in nursing); 362 periodical subscriptions.

BACCALAUREATE PROGRAMS

Degree BS

Available Programs ADN to Baccalaureate; Baccalaureate for Second Degree; Generic Baccalaureate.

Site Options Manhattan, NY; Queens, NY.

Study Options Full-time and part-time.

Program Entrance Requirements Minimum overall college GPA of 2.3, transcript of college record, CPR certification, written essay, health exam, health insurance, high school biology, high school chemistry, 3 years high school math, 3 years high school science, high school transcript, immunizations, 1 letter of recommendation, minimum high school GPA of 2.5, minimum GPA in nursing prerequisites of 2.75, prerequisite course work. Transfer students are accepted. **Standardized tests** *Required:* SAT or ACT, TOEFL for international students. **Application** *Deadline:* rolling (freshmen), rolling (transfer). *Early decision:* 11/15. *Notification:* continuous (freshmen), 12/1 (early action). *Application fee:* $35.

Advanced Placement Credit given for nursing courses completed elsewhere dependent upon specific evaluations.

Contact Harriet Rothman, RN, Nurse Recruiter, Division of Nursing, College of Mount Saint Vincent, 6301 Riverdale Avenue, Riverdale, NY 10471. *Telephone:* 718-405-3365. *Fax:* 718-405-3286. *E-mail:* harriet.rothman@mountsaintvincent.edu.

GRADUATE PROGRAMS

Financial Aid Career-related internships or fieldwork available.

Contact Dr. Susan Apold, Chairperson, Graduate Program of Nursing, Division of Nursing, College of Mount Saint Vincent, 6301 Riverdale Avenue, Riverdale, NY 10471-1093. *Telephone:* 718-405-3354. *Fax:* 718-405-3286. *E-mail:* susan.apold@mountsaintvincent.edu.

MASTER'S DEGREE PROGRAM

Degree MSN

Available Programs Master's; Master's for Nurses with Non-Nursing Degrees.

Concentrations Available Nursing administration. *Clinical nurse specialist programs in:* adult health, gerontology. *Nurse practitioner programs in:* adult health, family health.

Study Options Part-time.

Program Entrance Requirements Clinical experience, computer literacy, minimum overall college GPA of 3.0, transcript of college record, written essay, immunizations, interview, 2 letters of recommendation, nursing research course, physical assessment course, professional liability insurance/malpractice insurance, prerequisite course work, statistics course. *Application deadline:* For fall admission, 6/1; for spring admission, 11/1. Applications are processed on a rolling basis. *Application fee:* $50.

Degree Requirements 42 total credit hours.

POST-MASTER'S PROGRAM

Areas of Study *Nurse practitioner programs in:* adult health, family health.

The College of New Rochelle

School of Nursing
New Rochelle, New York

Founded in 1904

DEGREES • BSN • MS

Nursing Program Faculty 47 (82% with doctorates).

Baccalaureate Enrollment 520
Women 95% **Men** 5% **Minority** 67% **International** 1% **Part-time** 60%

Graduate Enrollment 75
Women 95% **Men** 5% **Minority** 18% **International** 1%

Nursing Student Activities Nursing Honor Society, Sigma Theta Tau, Student Nurses' Association, nursing club.

Nursing Student Resources Academic advising; academic or career counseling; assistance for students with disabilities; bookstore; campus computer network; career placement assistance; computer lab; computer-assisted instruction; e-mail services; housing assistance; interactive nursing skills videos; Internet; learning resource lab; library services; nursing audiovisuals; other; remedial services; resume preparation assistance; skills, simulation, or other laboratory; tutoring.

Library Facilities 220,000 volumes (8,700 in health, 8,700 in nursing); 1,450 periodical subscriptions (165 health-care related).

BACCALAUREATE PROGRAMS

Degree BSN

Available Programs Accelerated Baccalaureate for Second Degree; Baccalaureate for Second Degree; Generic Baccalaureate; RN Baccalaureate.

Study Options Full-time and part-time.

Program Entrance Requirements Transcript of college record, CPR certification, written essay, health exam, health insurance, high school biology, high school chemistry, high school transcript, immunizations, professional liability insurance/malpractice insurance. Transfer students are accepted. **Standardized tests** *Required:* SAT or ACT, TOEFL for international students. **Application** *Deadline:* rolling (freshmen), rolling (transfer). *Early decision:* 11/1. *Notification:* continuous (freshmen), 12/15 (out-of-state freshmen), 12/15 (early decision). *Application fee:* $20.

Advanced Placement Credit by examination available. Credit given for nursing courses completed elsewhere dependent upon specific evaluations.

Expenses (2004–05) *Tuition:* full-time $19,100; part-time $643 per credit hour. *Room and board:* $7400 per academic year.

Financial Aid 80% of baccalaureate students in nursing programs received some form of financial aid in 2003–04. *Gift aid (need-based):* Federal Pell, FSEOG, state, private, college/university gift aid from institutional funds. *Loans:* Federal Nursing Student Loans, Federal Direct (Subsidized and Unsubsidized Stafford), FFEL, Perkins. *Work-Study:* Federal Work-Study, part-time campus jobs. *Application deadline:* Continuous.

Contact Ms. Nancy Cole, Director of Academic Programs, School of Nursing, The College of New Rochelle, 29 Castle Place, New Rochelle, NY 10805-2308. *Telephone:* 914-654-5802. *Fax:* 914-654-5994. *E-mail:* ncole@cnr.edu.

GRADUATE PROGRAMS

Expenses (2004–05) *Tuition:* part-time $530 per credit hour.

Financial Aid 75% of graduate students in nursing programs received some form of financial aid in 2003–04.

Contact Dr. Mary Alice Donius, Coordinator of Graduate Programs, School of Nursing, The College of New Rochelle, 29 Castle Place, New Rochelle, NY 10805-2308. *Telephone:* 914-654-5803. *Fax:* 914-654-5994. *E-mail:* mdonius@cnr.edu.

MASTER'S DEGREE PROGRAM

Degree MS

Available Programs Master's.

The College of New Rochelle (continued)

Concentrations Available Nursing administration. *Nurse practitioner programs in:* acute care, family health.

Site Options Bronx, NY.

Study Options Part-time.

Program Entrance Requirements Clinical experience, minimum overall college GPA of 3.0, transcript of college record, written essay, immunizations, interview, 2 letters of recommendation, professional liability insurance/malpractice insurance, resume, statistics course.

Advanced Placement Credit given for nursing courses completed elsewhere dependent upon specific evaluations.

Degree Requirements 40 total credit hours, thesis or project.

POST-MASTER'S PROGRAM

Areas of Study Health-care administration; nursing education. *Nurse practitioner programs in:* acute care, family health.

See full description on page 468.

College of Staten Island of the City University of New York

Department of Nursing
Staten Island, New York

http://www.csi.cuny.edu/nursing

Founded in 1955

DEGREES • BS • MS

Nursing Program Faculty 40 (30% with doctorates).

Baccalaureate Enrollment 150

Women 83% **Men** 17% **Minority** 32% **International** 5% **Part-time** 90%

Graduate Enrollment 40

Women 98% **Men** 2% **Minority** 35% **International** 5% **Part-time** 99%

Nursing Student Activities Nursing Honor Society, Sigma Theta Tau, Student Nurses' Association, nursing club.

Nursing Student Resources Academic advising; academic or career counseling; assistance for students with disabilities; bookstore; campus computer network; career placement assistance; computer lab; computer-assisted instruction; daycare for children of students; e-mail services; employment services for current students; externships; interactive nursing skills videos; Internet; learning resource lab; library services; nursing audiovisuals; placement services for program completers; remedial services; resume preparation assistance; skills, simulation, or other laboratory; tutoring.

Library Facilities 220,025 volumes; 18,796 periodical subscriptions.

BACCALAUREATE PROGRAMS

Degree BS

Available Programs ADN to Baccalaureate; RN Baccalaureate.

Study Options Full-time and part-time.

Program Entrance Requirements Minimum overall college GPA of 2.0, transcript of college record, CPR certification, health exam, health insurance, high school transcript, immunizations, minimum GPA in nursing prerequisites, professional liability insurance/malpractice insurance, prerequisite course work, RN licensure. Transfer students are accepted. **Standardized tests** *Required:* TOEFL for international students. *Required for some:* SAT or ACT, SAT Subject Tests. **Application** *Deadline:* rolling (freshmen), rolling (transfer). *Notification:* 12/15 (freshmen). *Application fee:* $60.

Advanced Placement Credit by examination available. Credit given for nursing courses completed elsewhere dependent upon specific evaluations.

Expenses (2003–04) *Tuition, area resident:* full-time $4000; part-time $170 per credit hour. *Tuition, state resident:* full-time $5000; part-time $360 per credit hour. *Tuition, nonresident:* full-time $5000; part-time $360 per credit hour. *International tuition:* $5000 full-time. *Required fees:* full-time $350; part-time $175 per credit.

Financial Aid 40% of baccalaureate students in nursing programs received some form of financial aid in 2002–03. *Gift aid (need-based):* Federal Pell, FSEOG, state, private, college/university gift aid from institutional funds, Federal Nursing. *Loans:* Federal Direct PLUS), Perkins. *Work-Study:* Federal Work-Study, part-time campus jobs. *Application deadline:* Continuous.

Contact Prof. Linda E. Reese, RN, Chairperson, Department of Nursing, College of Staten Island of the City University of New York, 2800 Victory Boulevard, Marcus Hall, 5S-213, Staten Island, NY 10314. *Telephone:* 718-982-3810. *Fax:* 718-982-3813. *E-mail:* reese@mail.csi.cuny.edu.

GRADUATE PROGRAMS

Expenses (2003–04) *Tuition, area resident:* full-time $5440; part-time $230 per credit hour. *Tuition, state resident:* full-time $5440; part-time $425 per credit hour. *Tuition, nonresident:* full-time $5440; part-time $425 per credit hour. *International tuition:* $5440 full-time. *Required fees:* full-time $310; part-time $200 per term.

Financial Aid 20% of graduate students in nursing programs received some form of financial aid in 2002–03.

Contact Dr. Margaret Lunney, Director, Graduate Program, Department of Nursing, College of Staten Island of the City University of New York, 2800 Victory Boulevard, Staten island, NY 10314. *Telephone:* 718-982-3845. *Fax:* 718-982-3813. *E-mail:* lunney@postbox.csi.cuny.edu.

MASTER'S DEGREE PROGRAM

Degree MS

Available Programs Master's.

Concentrations Available *Clinical nurse specialist programs in:* adult health. *Nurse practitioner programs in:* adult health, gerontology.

Study Options Full-time and part-time.

Program Entrance Requirements Clinical experience, minimum overall college GPA of 3.0, transcript of college record, written essay, immunizations, interview, 2 letters of recommendation, nursing research course, physical assessment course, professional liability insurance/malpractice insurance, prerequisite course work, statistics course.

Advanced Placement Credit given for nursing courses completed elsewhere dependent upon specific evaluations.

Degree Requirements 48 total credit hours, thesis or project.

POST-MASTER'S PROGRAM

Areas of Study *Nurse practitioner programs in:* adult health, gerontology.

Columbia University

School of Nursing
New York, New York

http://www.nursing.hs.columbia.edu

Founded in 1754

DEGREES • BS • DN SC • MS • MS/MBA • MS/MPH

Nursing Program Faculty 56 (25% with doctorates).

Baccalaureate Enrollment 161

Women 90% **Men** 10% **Minority** 39% **International** 1% **Part-time** 2%

Graduate Enrollment 337

Women 91% **Men** 9% **Minority** 38% **International** 7% **Part-time** 75%

Nursing Student Activities Sigma Theta Tau.

Nursing Student Resources Academic advising; academic or career counseling; assistance for students with disabilities; bookstore; campus computer network; career placement assistance; computer lab; computer-assisted instruction; daycare for children of students; e-mail services; employment services for current students; housing assistance; interactive nursing skills videos; Internet; learning resource lab; library services; resume preparation assistance; skills, simulation, or other laboratory.

Library Facilities 469,000 volumes in health; 4,352 periodical subscriptions health-care related.

BACCALAUREATE PROGRAMS

Degree BS

Available Programs Accelerated Baccalaureate for Second Degree.

Study Options Full-time.

Program Entrance Requirements Minimum overall college GPA of 3.0, transcript of college record, CPR certification, written essay, health exam, immunizations, 3 letters of recommendation, minimum GPA in nursing prerequisites, prerequisite course work.

Expenses (2004–05) *Tuition:* full-time $57,128; part-time $907 per credit hour.

Financial Aid 90% of baccalaureate students in nursing programs received some form of financial aid in 2003–04.

Contact Amy Duschenchuk, Manager, Student Services, School of Nursing, Columbia University, 630 West 168th Street, Box 6, New York, NY 10032. *Telephone:* 212-305-5756. *Fax:* 212-305-3680. *E-mail:* nursing@columbia.edu.

GRADUATE PROGRAMS

Expenses (2004–05) *Tuition:* full-time $32,281; part-time $907 per credit hour.

Financial Aid 50% of graduate students in nursing programs received some form of financial aid in 2003–04. Research assistantships, teaching assistantships, Federal Work-Study and institutionally sponsored loans available. Aid available to part-time students.

Contact Amy Duschenchuk, Manager, Student Services, School of Nursing, Columbia University, 630 West 168th Street, Box 6, New York, NY 10032. *Telephone:* 212-305-5756. *Fax:* 212-305-3680. *E-mail:* nursing@columbia.edu.

MASTER'S DEGREE PROGRAM

Degrees MS; MS/MBA; MS/MPH

Available Programs Accelerated AD/RN to Master's; Accelerated Master's for Non-Nursing College Graduates; Accelerated Master's for Nurses with Non-Nursing Degrees; Master's; Master's for Non-Nursing College Graduates.

Concentrations Available Nurse anesthesia; nurse-midwifery. *Nurse practitioner programs in:* acute care, adult health, family health, gerontology, neonatal health, oncology, pediatric, psychiatric/mental health, women's health.

Site Options New York, NY.

Study Options Full-time and part-time.

Program Entrance Requirements Clinical experience, computer literacy, minimum overall college GPA of 3.0, transcript of college record, CPR certification, written essay, immunizations, 3 letters of recommendation, physical assessment course, professional liability insurance/malpractice insurance, prerequisite course work, statistics course, GRE General Test. *Application deadline:* Applications are processed on a rolling basis. *Application fee:* $75.

Advanced Placement Credit by examination available. Credit given for nursing courses completed elsewhere dependent upon specific evaluations.

Degree Requirements 45 total credit hours, thesis or project, comprehensive exam.

POST-MASTER'S PROGRAM

Areas of Study Nurse anesthesia. *Nurse practitioner programs in:* acute care, adult health, family health, gerontology, neonatal health, oncology, pediatric, psychiatric/mental health, women's health.

DOCTORAL DEGREE PROGRAM

Degree DN Sc

Available Programs Doctorate; Doctorate for Nurses with Non-Nursing Degrees; Post-Baccalaureate Doctorate.

Areas of Study Addiction/substance abuse, advanced practice nursing, aging, bio-behavioral research, biology of health and illness, clinical practice, community health, critical care, ethics, faculty preparation, family health, gerontology, health policy, health promotion/disease prevention, health-care systems, human health and illness, illness and transition, individualized study, information systems, maternity-newborn, neurobehavior, nurse case management, nursing administration, nursing education, nursing policy, nursing research, nursing science, oncology, urban health, women's health.

Program Entrance Requirements Clinical experience, minimum overall college GPA of 3.5, interview by faculty committee, interview, 3 letters of recommendation, MSN or equivalent, scholarly papers, statistics course, vita, writing sample, GRE General Test. *Application deadline:* Applications are processed on a rolling basis. *Application fee:* $75.

Degree Requirements 45 total credit hours, dissertation, oral exam, written exam.

CONTINUING EDUCATION PROGRAM

Contact Sarah Cook, Vice Dean, School of Nursing, Columbia University, 630 West 168th Street, Box 6, New York, NY 10032. *Telephone:* 212-305-3582. *Fax:* 212-305-1116. *E-mail:* ssc3@columbia.edu.

See full description on page 472.

Daemen College
Department of Nursing
Amherst, New York

http://www.daemen.edu

Founded in 1947

DEGREES • BS • MSN

Nursing Program Faculty 15 (60% with doctorates).

Baccalaureate Enrollment 200
Women 96% **Men** 4% **Minority** 3% **International** 2% **Part-time** 90%

Graduate Enrollment 50
Women 98% **Men** 2% **International** 6% **Part-time** 50%

Nursing Student Activities Sigma Theta Tau, nursing club.

Nursing Student Resources Academic advising; academic or career counseling; assistance for students with disabilities; bookstore; campus computer network; career placement assistance; computer lab; computer-assisted instruction; e-mail services; Internet; learning resource lab; library services; nursing audiovisuals; placement services for program completers; remedial services; resume preparation assistance; skills, simulation, or other laboratory; tutoring.

Library Facilities 127,232 volumes (10,000 in health, 4,000 in nursing); 889 periodical subscriptions (250 health-care related).

BACCALAUREATE PROGRAMS

Degree BS

Available Programs ADN to Baccalaureate; Accelerated RN Baccalaureate; RN Baccalaureate.

Site Options *Distance Learning:* Olean, NY; North Hornell, NY; Jamestown, NY.

Study Options Full-time and part-time.

Program Entrance Requirements Minimum overall college GPA of 2.0, transcript of college record, high school transcript, immunizations. Transfer students are accepted. **Standardized tests** *Required:* SAT or ACT, TOEFL for international students. **Application** *Deadline:* rolling (freshmen), rolling (transfer). *Early decision:* 8/30. *Notification:* continuous (freshmen), 9/1 (early action). *Application fee:* $25.

Expenses (2004–05) *Tuition:* full-time $7785; part-time $260 per credit hour. *International tuition:* $7785 full-time. *Room and board:* $6870 per academic year. *Required fees:* full-time $250; part-time $75 per term.

Financial Aid 100% of baccalaureate students in nursing programs received some form of financial aid in 2003–04. *Gift aid (need-based):* Federal Pell, FSEOG, state, private, college/university gift aid from institutional funds. *Loans:* FFEL (Subsidized and Unsubsidized Stafford PLUS), Perkins, college/university, alternative loans. *Work-Study:* Federal Work-Study, part-time campus jobs. *Application deadline (priority):* 2/15.

Contact Dr. Mary Lou Rusin, Professor and Chair, Department of Nursing, Daemen College, 4380 Main Street, Amherst, NY 14226. *Telephone:* 716-839-8387. *Fax:* 716-839-8403. *E-mail:* mrusin@daemen.edu.

GRADUATE PROGRAMS

Expenses (2004–05) *Tuition:* full-time $5310; part-time $590 per credit hour. *International tuition:* $5310 full-time. *Room and board:* $6870 per academic year. *Required fees:* part-time $15 per credit.

Daemen College (continued)

Financial Aid 75% of graduate students in nursing programs received some form of financial aid in 2003–04. Scholarships and tuition waivers (partial) available. Aid available to part-time students. *Financial aid application deadline:* 2/15.

Contact Dr. Mary Lou Rusin, Professor and Chair, Department of Nursing, Daemen College, 4380 Main Street, Amherst, NY 14226. *Telephone:* 716-839-8387. *Fax:* 716-839-8403. *E-mail:* mrusin@daemen.edu.

MASTER'S DEGREE PROGRAM

Degree MSN

Available Programs Accelerated AD/RN to Master's; Accelerated RN to Master's; Master's; RN to Master's.

Concentrations Available Health-care administration; palliative care. *Nurse practitioner programs in:* adult health.

Study Options Full-time and part-time.

Program Entrance Requirements Clinical experience, minimum overall college GPA of 3.25, transcript of college record, written essay, immunizations, interview, 3 letters of recommendation, statistics course. *Application deadline:* For fall admission, 3/1 (priority date); for spring admission, 10/1 (priority date). Applications are processed on a rolling basis. *Application fee:* $25.

Advanced Placement Credit given for nursing courses completed elsewhere dependent upon specific evaluations.

Degree Requirements 30 total credit hours, thesis or project.

POST-MASTER'S PROGRAM

Areas of Study Health-care administration; palliative care. *Nurse practitioner programs in:* adult health.

Dominican College

Division of Nursing
Orangeburg, New York

Founded in 1952

DEGREES • BSN • MS

Nursing Program Faculty 14.

Nursing Student Activities Nursing Honor Society, Sigma Theta Tau.

Library Facilities 103,350 volumes (5,650 in health); 650 periodical subscriptions (235 health-care related).

BACCALAUREATE PROGRAMS

Degree BSN

Available Programs Accelerated Baccalaureate for Second Degree; Accelerated LPN to Baccalaureate; Accelerated RN Baccalaureate; Generic Baccalaureate; LPN to Baccalaureate; RN Baccalaureate.

Study Options Full-time and part-time.

Program Entrance Requirements Minimum overall college GPA of 2.7, transcript of college record, CPR certification, health exam, health insurance, high school transcript, immunizations, minimum GPA in nursing prerequisites of 2.0, professional liability insurance/malpractice insurance, prerequisite course work. Transfer students are accepted. **Standardized tests** *Required:* SAT or ACT, TOEFL for international students. **Application** *Deadline:* rolling (freshmen), rolling (transfer). *Notification:* continuous (freshmen). *Application fee:* $35.

Advanced Placement Credit by examination available. Credit given for nursing courses completed elsewhere dependent upon specific evaluations.

Contact Division of Nursing, Division of Nursing, Dominican College, 470 Western Highway, Orangeburg, NY 10962. *Telephone:* 845-398-4998. *Fax:* 845-398-4999.

GRADUATE PROGRAMS

Contact Coordinator of Family Nurse Practitioner Program, Division of Nursing, Dominican College, Casey Hall, 470 Western Highway, Orangeburg, NY 10962. *Telephone:* 845-359-7800 Ext. 342. *Fax:* 845-398-4999.

MASTER'S DEGREE PROGRAM

Degree MS

Available Programs Master's.

Concentrations Available *Nurse practitioner programs in:* family health.

Study Options Full-time and part-time.

Program Entrance Requirements Clinical experience, minimum overall college GPA of 3.0, transcript of college record, written essay, immunizations, 3 letters of recommendation, nursing research course, physical assessment course, professional liability insurance/malpractice insurance, prerequisite course work, statistics course, GRE General Test or MAT. *Application deadline:* Applications are processed on a rolling basis. *Application fee:* $50.

Degree Requirements 42 total credit hours, thesis or project.

D'Youville College

Department of Nursing
Buffalo, New York

Founded in 1908

DEGREES • BSN • MS

Nursing Program Faculty 16 (38% with doctorates).

Baccalaureate Enrollment 150

Women 95% **Men** 5% **Minority** 20% **International** 1% **Part-time** 30%

Graduate Enrollment 145

Women 97% **Men** 3% **Minority** 28% **International** 2% **Part-time** 30%

Nursing Student Activities Sigma Theta Tau, Student Nurses' Association.

Nursing Student Resources Academic advising; academic or career counseling; assistance for students with disabilities; bookstore; campus computer network; career placement assistance; computer lab; computer-assisted instruction; e-mail services; interactive nursing skills videos; Internet; learning resource lab; library services; nursing audiovisuals; paid internships; placement services for program completers; remedial services; resume preparation assistance; skills, simulation, or other laboratory; tutoring.

Library Facilities 122,057 volumes (14,000 in health); 665 periodical subscriptions (720 health-care related).

■ A current worldwide shortage in nursing leaves the door wide open for qualified nurses. D'Youville College has been educating nurses since 1942, and its nursing program is one of the largest 4-year, private-college nursing programs in the country. The faculty members are hardworking and dedicated. Classes are small, which permits much individualized attention. Baccalaureate graduates who wish to continue their education can choose from 3 master's programs at D'Youville College. Registered nurses enrolled in the BSN program have the option of completing some of their major courses via distance learning. D'Youville also offers a combined bachelor's/master's program for RNs and traditional students.

BACCALAUREATE PROGRAMS

Degree BSN

Available Programs ADN to Baccalaureate; Baccalaureate for Second Degree; Generic Baccalaureate; RN Baccalaureate.

Site Options *Distance Learning:* Buffalo, NY.

Study Options Full-time and part-time.

Program Entrance Requirements Minimum overall college GPA of 2.5, transcript of college record, health exam, health insurance, high school biology, high school chemistry, 1 year of high school math, 1 year of high school science, high school transcript, immunizations, minimum high school GPA of 2.0, minimum high school rank 50%, minimum GPA in nursing prerequisites of 2.0, professional liability insurance/malpractice insurance, prerequisite course work. Transfer students are accepted. **Standardized tests** *Required:* SAT or ACT, TOEFL for international students. **Application** *Deadline:* rolling (freshmen), rolling (transfer). *Notification:* continuous (freshmen). *Application fee:* $25.

Advanced Placement Credit given for nursing courses completed elsewhere dependent upon specific evaluations.

Expenses (2004–05) *Tuition:* full-time $14,690; part-time $405 per credit hour. *Room and board:* $7340 per academic year. *Required fees:* full-time $200; part-time $32 per term.

Financial Aid 95% of baccalaureate students in nursing programs received some form of financial aid in 2003–04. *Gift aid (need-based):* Federal Pell, FSEOG, state, private, college/university gift aid from institutional funds. *Loans:* Federal Nursing Student Loans, FFEL (Subsidized and Unsubsidized Stafford PLUS), Perkins, college/university. *Work-Study:* Federal Work-Study, part-time campus jobs. *Application deadline (priority):* 3/1.

Contact Mr. Ron Dannecker, Director of Admissions, Department of Nursing, D'Youville College, 320 Porter Avenue, Buffalo, NY 14201. *Telephone:* 716-881-7600. *Fax:* 716-515-0679. *E-mail:* admiss@dyc.edu.

GRADUATE PROGRAMS

Expenses (2004–05) *Tuition:* part-time $520 per credit hour. *Required fees:* full-time $200; part-time $32 per term.

Financial Aid 85% of graduate students in nursing programs received some form of financial aid in 2003–04. 1 research assistantship with partial tuition reimbursement available (averaging $3,000 per year) was awarded; Federal Work-Study and scholarships also available. Aid available to part-time students. *Financial aid application deadline:* 3/1.

Contact Miss Linda Fisher, Director of Graduate Admissions, Department of Nursing, D'Youville College, 320 Porter Avenue, Buffalo, NY 14201. *Telephone:* 716-881-7744. *Fax:* 716-515-0679. *E-mail:* fisherl@dyc.edu.

MASTER'S DEGREE PROGRAM

Degree MS

Available Programs Accelerated AD/RN to Master's; Master's; RN to Master's.

Concentrations Available Nursing education. *Clinical nurse specialist programs in:* community health. *Nurse practitioner programs in:* family health.

Study Options Full-time and part-time.

Program Entrance Requirements Clinical experience, computer literacy, transcript of college record, CPR certification, written essay, immunizations, interview, 2 letters of recommendation, nursing research course, physical assessment course, professional liability insurance/malpractice insurance, prerequisite course work, resume, statistics course. *Application deadline:* Applications are processed on a rolling basis. *Application fee:* $25.

Advanced Placement Credit given for nursing courses completed elsewhere dependent upon specific evaluations.

Degree Requirements 39 total credit hours, thesis or project.

POST-MASTER'S PROGRAM

Areas of Study *Nurse practitioner programs in:* family health.

See full description on page 482.

Elmira College

Program in Nursing Education
Elmira, New York

Founded in 1855

DEGREE • BS

Nursing Program Faculty 11.

Baccalaureate Enrollment 64
Women 96% **Men** 4% **Minority** 3% **Part-time** 24%

Nursing Student Activities Sigma Theta Tau, nursing club.

Nursing Student Resources Academic advising; academic or career counseling; assistance for students with disabilities; bookstore; campus computer network; career placement assistance; computer lab; e-mail services; housing assistance; Internet; learning resource lab; library services; nursing audiovisuals; placement services for program completers; resume preparation assistance; skills, simulation, or other laboratory; tutoring; unpaid internships.

Library Facilities 391,038 volumes (7,461 in health, 5,200 in nursing); 859 periodical subscriptions (72 health-care related).

■ Many features distinguish the Elmira College nursing program from other nursing programs. Students in the Elmira College nursing program begin clinical experiences of 6 to 17 hours per week in the sophomore year. Students are admitted directly to the nursing program and do not have to qualify again. Clinical nursing experiences take place in a variety of community-based health-care agencies as well as in acute-care hospitals. Curriculum emphasis is on health maintenance within the community. Extracurricular activities and intercollegiate athletic participation are encouraged by the nursing faculty. A strong liberal arts component and a required community service experience ensure a well-rounded graduate.

BACCALAUREATE PROGRAMS

Degree BS

Available Programs ADN to Baccalaureate; Generic Baccalaureate; RN Baccalaureate.

Study Options Full-time and part-time.

Program Entrance Requirements Minimum overall college GPA of 2.0, transcript of college record, written essay, health exam, health insurance, high school biology, high school chemistry, 3 years high school math, 3 years high school science, high school transcript, immunizations, 2 letters of recommendation, minimum high school GPA of 2.5. Transfer students are accepted. **Standardized tests** *Required:* SAT or ACT, TOEFL for international students. **Application** *Deadline:* 4/15 (freshmen). *Early decision:* 11/15 (for plan 1), 1/15 (for plan 2). *Notification:* continuous until 4/30 (freshmen), 12/15 (out-of-state freshmen), 12/15 (early decision plan 1), 2/1 (early decision plan 2). *Application fee:* $50.

Advanced Placement Credit by examination available. Credit given for nursing courses completed elsewhere dependent upon specific evaluations.

Expenses (2004–05) *Tuition:* full-time $26,130. *International tuition:* $26,130 full-time. *Room and board:* $8330 per academic year. *Required fees:* full-time $900.

Financial Aid 94% of baccalaureate students in nursing programs received some form of financial aid in 2003–04.

Contact Mr. Gary Fallis, Dean of Admissions, Program in Nursing Education, Elmira College, One Park Place, Elmira, NY 14901. *Telephone:* 607-735-1724. *Fax:* 607-735-1718. *E-mail:* gfallis@elmira.edu.

CONTINUING EDUCATION PROGRAM

Contact Dr. Lois Schoener, Professor of Nursing/Director of Nurse Education, Program in Nursing Education, Elmira College, One Park Place, Elmira, NY 14901. *Telephone:* 607-735-1890. *Fax:* 607-735-1758. *E-mail:* lschoener@elmira.edu.

Excelsior College

School of Nursing
Albany, New York

http://www.excelsior.edu

Founded in 1970

DEGREES • BSN • MS

Nursing Program Faculty 280 (32% with doctorates).

Excelsior College (continued)

Baccalaureate Enrollment 1,881 **Women** 84% **Men** 16% **Minority** 25% **Part-time** 100%

Graduate Enrollment 251
Women 87% **Men** 13% **Minority** 20% **Part-time** 100%

Nursing Student Activities Sigma Theta Tau.

Nursing Student Resources Academic advising; academic or career counseling; assistance for students with disabilities; bookstore; computer-assisted instruction; e-mail services; Internet; learning resource lab; library services; nursing audiovisuals; skills, simulation, or other laboratory.

BACCALAUREATE PROGRAMS

Degree BSN

Available Programs RN Baccalaureate.

Site Options *Distance Learning:* Albany, NY.

Study Options Part-time.

Program Entrance Requirements Transcript of college record, high school transcript, RN licensure. Transfer students are accepted. **Application** *Deadline:* rolling (freshmen), rolling (transfer). *Notification:* continuous (freshmen). *Application fee:* $50.

Advanced Placement Credit by examination available. Credit given for nursing courses completed elsewhere dependent upon specific evaluations.

Expenses (2004–05) *Required fees:* full-time $995.

Financial Aid 4% of baccalaureate students in nursing programs received some form of financial aid in 2003–04. *Gift aid (need-based):* state, private, college/university gift aid from institutional funds. *Loans:* alternative loans, PLATO Loans, Excel. *Application deadline (priority):* 7/1.

Contact Admissions Office, School of Nursing, Excelsior College, 7 Columbia Circle, Albany, NY 12203. *Telephone:* 518-464-8500. *Fax:* 518-464-8777. *E-mail:* admissions@excelsior.edu.

GRADUATE PROGRAMS

Expenses (2004–05) *Required fees:* part-time $350 per credit.

Financial Aid 15% of graduate students in nursing programs received some form of financial aid in 2003–04. Scholarships and traineeships available. Aid available to part-time students. *Financial aid application deadline:* 9/15.

Contact Dr. Patricia Edwards, RN, Director, Master of Science in Nursing, School of Nursing, Excelsior College, 7 Columbia Circle, Albany, NY 12203. *Telephone:* 518-464-8500. *Fax:* 518-464-8777. *E-mail:* msn@excelsior.edu.

MASTER'S DEGREE PROGRAM

Degree MS

Available Programs Master's; RN to Master's.

Concentrations Available Health-care administration; nursing informatics.

Site Options *Distance Learning:* Albany, NY.

Study Options Full-time and part-time.

Program Entrance Requirements Computer literacy, minimum overall college GPA of 3.0, transcript of college record, written essay, resume. *Application deadline:* Applications are processed on a rolling basis. *Application fee:* $50.

Advanced Placement Credit given for nursing courses completed elsewhere dependent upon specific evaluations.

Degree Requirements 44 total credit hours, thesis or project.

See full description on page 486.

Hartwick College
Department of Nursing
Oneonta, New York

http://www.hartwick.edu

Founded in 1797

DEGREE • BS

Nursing Program Faculty 9 (11% with doctorates).

Baccalaureate Enrollment 80
Women 88% **Men** 12% **Minority** 8% **Part-time** 7%

Nursing Student Activities Sigma Theta Tau, Student Nurses' Association.

Nursing Student Resources Academic advising; academic or career counseling; assistance for students with disabilities; bookstore; campus computer network; career placement assistance; computer lab; computer-assisted instruction; e-mail services; employment services for current students; externships; housing assistance; interactive nursing skills videos; Internet; learning resource lab; library services; nursing audiovisuals; placement services for program completers; remedial services; resume preparation assistance; skills, simulation, or other laboratory; tutoring; unpaid internships.

Library Facilities 353,776 volumes (5,691 in health, 1,152 in nursing); 571 periodical subscriptions (184 health-care related).

BACCALAUREATE PROGRAMS

Degree BS

Available Programs Accelerated Baccalaureate; Accelerated Baccalaureate for Second Degree; Generic Baccalaureate; RN Baccalaureate.

Site Options Albany, NY; Cooperstown, NY.

Study Options Full-time and part-time.

Program Entrance Requirements Minimum overall college GPA of 2.0, written essay, health exam, high school biology, high school chemistry, high school foreign language, 3 years high school math, 2 years high school science, high school transcript, immunizations, 2 letters of recommendation, minimum GPA in nursing prerequisites of 2.0. Transfer students are accepted. **Standardized tests** *Required:* TOEFL for international students. *Recommended:* SAT or ACT. **Application** *Deadline:* 2/15 (freshmen), 8/1 (transfer). *Early decision:* 1/15, 1/1. *Notification:* 3/5 (freshmen), 2/22 (early action). *Application fee:* $35.

Advanced Placement Credit given for nursing courses completed elsewhere dependent upon specific evaluations.

Expenses (2003–04) *Tuition:* full-time $27,400; part-time $840 per credit hour. *Room and board:* $7250; room only: $3750 per academic year. *Required fees:* full-time $1400.

Financial Aid 78% of baccalaureate students in nursing programs received some form of financial aid in 2002–03.

Contact Sharon D. Dettenrieder, RN, Professor and Chair, Department of Nursing, Hartwick College, One Hartwick College Drive, Miller Science Center, Oneonta, NY 13820. *Telephone:* 607-431-4780. *Fax:* 607-431-4850. *E-mail:* dettenriedes@hartwick.edu.

Hunter College of the City University of New York
Hunter-Bellevue School of Nursing
New York, New York

http://www.hunter.cuny.edu/schoolhp/nursing

Founded in 1870

DEGREES • BS • MS • MS/MPH

Nursing Program Faculty 22 (56% with doctorates).

Nursing Student Activities Sigma Theta Tau.

Nursing Student Resources Academic advising; academic or career counseling; assistance for students with disabilities; bookstore; campus computer network; computer lab; computer-assisted instruction; e-mail services; interactive nursing skills videos; Internet; learning resource lab; library services; nursing audiovisuals.

Library Facilities 789,718 volumes (39,245 in health, 4,295 in nursing); 4,282 periodical subscriptions (375 health-care related).

BACCALAUREATE PROGRAMS

Degree BS

Available Programs Generic Baccalaureate; RN Baccalaureate.

Study Options Full-time.

Program Entrance Requirements Minimum overall college GPA of 2.5, CPR certification, health exam, immunizations, professional liability insurance/malpractice insurance, prerequisite course work. Transfer students are accepted. **Standardized tests** *Required:* SAT or ACT, TOEFL for international students. **Application** *Deadline:* 10/1 (freshmen), 3/1 (transfer). *Notification:* continuous until 1/3 (freshmen). *Application fee:* $50.

Contact Dr. Susan Neville, RN, Assistant Professor and Director of Undergraduate Programs, Generic and RN Pathways, Hunter-Bellevue School of Nursing, Hunter College of the City University of New York, 425 East 25th Street, New York, NY 10010. *Telephone:* 212-481-7598. *Fax:* 212-481-4427. *E-mail:* sneville@hunter.cuny.edu.

GRADUATE PROGRAMS

Financial Aid Federal Work-Study, scholarships, traineeships, and tuition waivers (partial) available.

Contact Dr. Violet M. Malinski, RN, Director of Graduate Program, Hunter-Bellevue School of Nursing, Hunter College of the City University of New York, 425 East 25th Street, New York, NY 10010. *Telephone:* 212-481-4465. *Fax:* 212-481-4427. *E-mail:* vmalinsk@hunter.cuny.edu.

MASTER'S DEGREE PROGRAM

Degrees MS; MS/MPH

Available Programs Master's.

Concentrations Available *Clinical nurse specialist programs in:* community health, medical-surgical, parent-child, psychiatric/mental health. *Nurse practitioner programs in:* adult health, gerontology, pediatric.

Study Options Full-time and part-time.

Program Entrance Requirements Clinical experience, minimum overall college GPA of 3.0, transcript of college record, written essay, immunizations, 2 letters of recommendation, resume, statistics course. *Application deadline:* For fall admission, 4/1; for spring admission, 11/1. Applications are processed on a rolling basis. *Application fee:* $50.

Degree Requirements 42 total credit hours, thesis or project.

POST-MASTER'S PROGRAM

Areas of Study *Nurse practitioner programs in:* pediatric.

CONTINUING EDUCATION PROGRAM

Contact Continuing Education, Hunter-Bellevue School of Nursing, Hunter College of the City University of New York, 695 East Park Avenue, East Building, 10th Floor, New York, NY 10021. *Telephone:* 212-650-3850. *Fax:* 212-772-3402. *E-mail:* ce@hunter.cuny.edu.

Keuka College

Division of Nursing
Keuka Park, New York

http://www.keuka.edu/asap/nursing.htm

Founded in 1890

DEGREE • BS

Nursing Program Faculty 6 (34% with doctorates).

Baccalaureate Enrollment 100

Nursing Student Activities Student Nurses' Association.

Nursing Student Resources Academic advising; academic or career counseling; assistance for students with disabilities; bookstore; campus computer network; computer lab; computer-assisted instruction; e-mail services; employment services for current students; housing assistance; interactive nursing skills videos; Internet; learning resource lab; library services; nursing audiovisuals; resume preparation assistance; skills, simulation, or other laboratory; tutoring.

Library Facilities 117,192 volumes (986 in health, 532 in nursing); 48 periodical subscriptions health-care related.

BACCALAUREATE PROGRAMS

Degree BS

Available Programs RN Baccalaureate.

Site Options *Distance Learning:* Canandaigua, NY; Geneva, NY.

Study Options Full-time and part-time.

Program Entrance Requirements Minimum overall college GPA of 2.5, transcript of college record, CPR certification, health exam, high school transcript, immunizations, minimum GPA in nursing prerequisites of 2.5, prerequisite course work, RN licensure. Transfer students are accepted. **Standardized tests** *Required:* SAT or ACT, TOEFL for international students. **Application** *Deadline:* rolling (freshmen), rolling (transfer). *Application fee:* $30.

Advanced Placement Credit by examination available. Credit given for nursing courses completed elsewhere dependent upon specific evaluations.

Expenses (2003–04) *Tuition:* part-time $360 per credit hour.

Contact Dr. Linda R. Rossi, RN, Chair, Division of Nursing, Keuka College, PO Box 98, Keuka Park, NY 14478-0098. *Telephone:* 315-536-5273. *Fax:* 315-531-5660. *E-mail:* lrrossi@mail.keuka.edu.

Lehman College of the City University of New York

Department of Nursing
Bronx, New York

http://www.lehman.cuny.edu/departments/

Founded in 1931

DEGREES • BS • MS

Nursing Program Faculty 17 (65% with doctorates).

Baccalaureate Enrollment 300
Women 75% **Men** 25% **Minority** 85% **International** 30%

Graduate Enrollment 100
Women 90% **Men** 10% **Minority** 75% **Part-time** 75%

Nursing Student Activities Sigma Theta Tau, Student Nurses' Association, nursing club.

Nursing Student Resources Academic advising; academic or career counseling; assistance for students with disabilities; bookstore; campus computer network; career placement assistance; computer lab; computer-assisted instruction; daycare for children of students; e-mail services; externships; interactive nursing skills videos; Internet; learning resource lab; library services; nursing audiovisuals; paid internships; resume preparation assistance; skills, simulation, or other laboratory; tutoring; unpaid internships.

Library Facilities 541,944 volumes; 1,350 periodical subscriptions.

BACCALAUREATE PROGRAMS

Degree BS

Available Programs Generic Baccalaureate; RN Baccalaureate.

Site Options Queens, NY.

Study Options Full-time.

Program Entrance Requirements Minimum overall college GPA of 2.0, transcript of college record, written essay, high school transcript, immunizations, minimum GPA in nursing prerequisites of 2.75, prerequisite course work. Transfer students are accepted. **Standardized tests** *Required:* SAT or ACT, TOEFL for international students. **Application** *Deadline:* rolling (freshmen), rolling (transfer). *Notification:* continuous (freshmen). *Application fee:* $50.

Advanced Placement Credit given for nursing courses completed elsewhere dependent upon specific evaluations.

Expenses (2004–05) *Tuition, state resident:* full-time $3200; part-time $135 per credit hour. *Tuition, nonresident:* full-time $6800; part-time $285 per credit hour. *International tuition:* $6800 full-time. *Required fees:* part-time $35 per credit.

Financial Aid 50% of baccalaureate students in nursing programs received some form of financial aid in 2003–04.

Contact Director of Undergraduate Programs, Department of Nursing, Lehman College of the City University of New York, 250 Bedford Park Boulevard, West, Bronx, NY 10468. *Telephone:* 718-960-8373. *Fax:* 718-960-8488.

Lehman College of the City University of New York (continued)

GRADUATE PROGRAMS

Expenses (2004–05) *Tuition, state resident:* full-time $4350; part-time $185 per credit hour. *Tuition, nonresident:* full-time $7600; part-time $320 per credit hour. *International tuition:* $7600 full-time. *Required fees:* full-time $60; part-time $40 per credit.

Financial Aid 25% of graduate students in nursing programs received some form of financial aid in 2003–04. Career-related internships or fieldwork, Federal Work-Study, and tuition waivers (partial) available. Aid available to part-time students. *Financial aid application deadline:* 5/15.

Contact Graduate Program, Department of Nursing, Lehman College of the City University of New York, 250 Bedford Park Boulevard, West, Bronx, NY 10468. *Telephone:* 718-960-8373. *Fax:* 718-960-8488.

MASTER'S DEGREE PROGRAM

Degree MS

Available Programs Master's.

Concentrations Available Nursing administration; nursing education. *Clinical nurse specialist programs in:* adult health, gerontology, parent-child. *Nurse practitioner programs in:* pediatric.

Site Options New York, NY.

Study Options Full-time and part-time.

Program Entrance Requirements Clinical experience, transcript of college record, written essay, immunizations, interview, 2 letters of recommendation, prerequisite course work. *Application deadline:* For fall admission, 4/1; for spring admission, 11/1. Applications are processed on a rolling basis. *Application fee:* $40.

Degree Requirements 43 total credit hours.

Long Island University, Brooklyn Campus

School of Nursing
Brooklyn, New York

http://www.liunet.edu

Founded in 1926

DEGREES • BS • MS

Nursing Program Faculty 54 (25% with doctorates).

Baccalaureate Enrollment 600
Women 94% **Men** 6% **Minority** 85% **Part-time** 20%

Graduate Enrollment 130
Women 90% **Men** 10% **Minority** 85% **Part-time** 83%

Nursing Student Activities Nursing Honor Society, Student Nurses' Association.

Nursing Student Resources Academic advising; academic or career counseling; assistance for students with disabilities; bookstore; campus computer network; computer lab; daycare for children of students; e-mail services; employment services for current students; interactive nursing skills videos; Internet; learning resource lab; library services; nursing audiovisuals; paid internships; remedial services; skills, simulation, or other laboratory; tutoring.

Library Facilities 11,000 volumes in health, 850 volumes in nursing; 230 periodical subscriptions health-care related.

BACCALAUREATE PROGRAMS

Degree BS

Available Programs Generic Baccalaureate; International Nurse to Baccalaureate; RN Baccalaureate.

Study Options Full-time and part-time.

Program Entrance Requirements Minimum overall college GPA of 2.5, transcript of college record, CPR certification, health exam, high school transcript, interview, minimum high school GPA of 3.0, minimum GPA in nursing prerequisites of 2.5. Transfer students are accepted. **Standardized tests** *Required:* TOEFL for international students. *Required for some:* SAT or ACT. **Application** *Deadline:* rolling (freshmen), rolling (transfer). *Application fee:* $30.

Expenses (2004–05) *Tuition:* full-time $20,000; part-time $651 per credit hour. *International tuition:* $20,000 full-time. *Room and board:* $2000 per academic year. *Required fees:* full-time $1000; part-time $500 per term.

Financial Aid 94% of baccalaureate students in nursing programs received some form of financial aid in 2003–04. *Gift aid (need-based):* Federal Pell, FSEOG, state, private, college/university gift aid from institutional funds, Scholarships for Disadvantaged Students (Nursing and Pharmacy). *Loans:* Federal Direct (Subsidized and Unsubsidized Stafford PLUS), Perkins, Federal Health Professions Student Loans, alternative loans. *Work-Study:* Federal Work-Study, part-time campus jobs. *Application deadline:* Continuous.

Contact Prof. Dawn F. Kilts, Dean, School of Nursing, Long Island University, Brooklyn Campus, 1 University Plaza, Brooklyn, NY 11201. *Telephone:* 718-488-1509. *Fax:* 718-780-4019. *E-mail:* Dawn.Kilts@liu.edu.

GRADUATE PROGRAMS

Expenses (2004–05) *Tuition:* full-time $13,000; part-time $705 per credit hour. *International tuition:* $13,000 full-time. *Room and board:* $2000 per academic year. *Required fees:* full-time $1000; part-time $500 per term.

Financial Aid 75% of graduate students in nursing programs received some form of financial aid in 2003–04. Scholarships and unspecified assistantships available. Aid available to part-time students.

Contact Prof. Susanne Flower, Director, School of Nursing, Long Island University, Brooklyn Campus, 1 University Plaza, Brooklyn, NY 11201. *Telephone:* 718-488-1059. *Fax:* 718-780-4019. *E-mail:* Susanne.Flower@liu.edu.

MASTER'S DEGREE PROGRAM

Degree MS

Available Programs Master's; RN to Master's.

Concentrations Available Nursing administration. *Nurse practitioner programs in:* adult health, family health, gerontology.

Study Options Full-time and part-time.

Program Entrance Requirements Clinical experience, minimum overall college GPA of 3.0, transcript of college record, immunizations, interview, 3 letters of recommendation, nursing research course, physical assessment course, professional liability insurance/malpractice insurance, resume, statistics course. *Application deadline:* Applications are processed on a rolling basis. *Application fee:* $30.

Degree Requirements 43 total credit hours, thesis or project.

POST-MASTER'S PROGRAM

Areas of Study *Nurse practitioner programs in:* adult health, family health, gerontology.

See full description on page 512.

Long Island University, C.W. Post Campus

Program in Nursing
Brookville, New York

http://www.cwpost.liu.edu/cwis/cwp/health/nursing

Founded in 1954

DEGREES • BS • MS

Nursing Program Faculty 12 (66% with doctorates).

Baccalaureate Enrollment 70
Women 95% **Men** 5% **Minority** 40% **International** 5% **Part-time** 100%

Graduate Enrollment 51
Women 96% **Men** 4% **Minority** 35% **International** 11% **Part-time** 100%

Nursing Student Activities Student Nurses' Association.

Nursing Student Resources Academic advising; academic or career counseling; assistance for students with disabilities; bookstore; campus computer network; career placement assistance; computer lab; computer-assisted instruction; e-mail services; employment services for current students; housing assistance; interactive nursing skills videos; Internet; library services; nursing audiovisuals; placement services for program completers; remedial services; resume preparation assistance; skills, simulation, or other laboratory; tutoring.

Library Facilities 20,000 volumes in health, 15,000 volumes in nursing; 3,100 periodical subscriptions health-care related.

BACCALAUREATE PROGRAMS

Degree BS

Available Programs RN Baccalaureate.

Site Options Brentwood, NY; Southampton, NY; Manhasset, NY.

Study Options Full-time and part-time.

Program Entrance Requirements Minimum overall college GPA of 2.5, transcript of college record, health exam, health insurance, immunizations, minimum GPA in nursing prerequisites of 2.5, professional liability insurance/malpractice insurance, prerequisite course work, RN licensure. Transfer students are accepted. **Standardized tests** *Required:* SAT or ACT, TOEFL for international students. **Application** *Deadline:* rolling (freshmen). *Notification:* continuous (freshmen). *Application fee:* $30.

Advanced Placement Credit by examination available. Credit given for nursing courses completed elsewhere dependent upon specific evaluations.

Expenses (2004–05) *Tuition:* part-time $651 per credit hour. *Room and board:* $6590; room only: $5150 per academic year. *Required fees:* part-time $195 per term.

Financial Aid 10% of baccalaureate students in nursing programs received some form of financial aid in 2003–04.

Contact Dr. Minna Kapp, Chair, Program in Nursing, Long Island University, C.W. Post Campus, Life Science/Room 270, 720 Northern Boulevard, Brookville, NY 11548-1300. *Telephone:* 516-299-3065. *Fax:* 516-299-2352. *E-mail:* minna.kapp@liu.edu.

GRADUATE PROGRAMS

Expenses (2004–05) *Tuition:* part-time $705 per credit hour. *Room and board:* $6590; room only: $5150 per academic year. *Required fees:* part-time $195 per term.

Financial Aid 10% of graduate students in nursing programs received some form of financial aid in 2003–04. Federal Work-Study and unspecified assistantships available. Aid available to part-time students. *Financial aid application deadline:* 5/15.

Contact Dr. Minna Kapp, Chair, Program in Nursing, Long Island University, C.W. Post Campus, Life Science/Room 270, 720 Northern Boulevard, Brookville, NY 11548-1300. *Telephone:* 516-299-3065. *Fax:* 516-299-2352. *E-mail:* minna.kapp@liu.edu.

MASTER'S DEGREE PROGRAM

Degree MS

Available Programs Accelerated Master's; Master's.

Concentrations Available *Clinical nurse specialist programs in:* adult health, medical-surgical, parent-child. *Nurse practitioner programs in:* family health.

Study Options Part-time.

Program Entrance Requirements Clinical experience, minimum overall college GPA of 3.0, transcript of college record, written essay, immunizations, interview, 2 letters of recommendation, nursing research course, physical assessment course, professional liability insurance/malpractice insurance, prerequisite course work. *Application deadline:* Applications are processed on a rolling basis. *Application fee:* $30.

Degree Requirements 46 total credit hours, thesis or project.

POST-MASTER'S PROGRAM

Areas of Study *Nurse practitioner programs in:* family health.

Medgar Evers College of the City University of New York

Department of Nursing
Brooklyn, New York

http://www.mec.cuny.edu/academic_affairs/science_tech_school/nursing/nurse_home.htm

Founded in 1969

DEGREE • BSN

Nursing Program Faculty 18.

Library Facilities 111,000 volumes; 24,410 periodical subscriptions.

BACCALAUREATE PROGRAMS

Degree BSN

Available Programs ADN to Baccalaureate; Accelerated RN Baccalaureate.

Study Options Full-time and part-time.

Program Entrance Requirements Minimum overall college GPA of 2.5, transcript of college record, CPR certification, health exam, health insurance, immunizations, professional liability insurance/malpractice insurance, prerequisite course work, RN licensure. Transfer students are accepted. **Standardized tests** *Required:* TOEFL for international students. *Required for some:* SAT and SAT Subject Tests or ACT. **Application** *Deadline:* rolling (freshmen), rolling (transfer). *Notification:* continuous (freshmen). *Application fee:* $60.

Advanced Placement Credit given for nursing courses completed elsewhere dependent upon specific evaluations.

Contact Dr. Eileen McCarroll, Coordinator, BSN Program, Department of Nursing, Medgar Evers College of the City University of New York, C-200, Brooklyn, NY 11225. *Telephone:* 718-270-6230. *Fax:* 718-270-6235. *E-mail:* emccarroll@mec.cuny.edu.

Mercy College

Program in Nursing
Dobbs Ferry, New York

Founded in 1951

DEGREES • BSCN • MS

Nursing Program Faculty 12 (50% with doctorates).

Baccalaureate Enrollment 176
Women 96% **Men** 4% **Minority** 75% **International** 1% **Part-time** 88%

Graduate Enrollment 86
Women 99% **Men** 1% **Minority** 50% **Part-time** 75%

Nursing Student Activities Sigma Theta Tau.

Nursing Student Resources Academic advising; academic or career counseling; assistance for students with disabilities; career placement assistance; computer lab; computer-assisted instruction; e-mail services; Internet; learning resource lab; library services; nursing audiovisuals; resume preparation assistance; skills, simulation, or other laboratory; tutoring.

Library Facilities 322,610 volumes (10,000 in health, 550 in nursing); 1,765 periodical subscriptions (180 health-care related).

BACCALAUREATE PROGRAMS

Degree BScN

Available Programs RN Baccalaureate.

Site Options Manhattan, NY; Dobbs Ferry, NY.

Study Options Full-time and part-time.

Mercy College (continued)

Program Entrance Requirements Transfer students are accepted. **Standardized tests** *Recommended:* SAT, TOEFL for international students. **Application** *Deadline:* rolling (freshmen), rolling (transfer). *Notification:* continuous (freshmen). *Application fee:* $35.

Expenses (2003–04) *Tuition:* full-time $10,700; part-time $450 per credit hour.

Contact Dr. Mary McGuinness, Director, Undergraduate Program, Program in Nursing, Mercy College, 555 Broadway, Dobbs Ferry, NY 10522. *Telephone:* 914-674-9331 Ext. 550. *Fax:* 914-674-9280. *E-mail:* mmcguiness@mercy.edu.

GRADUATE PROGRAMS

Expenses (2003–04) *Tuition:* full-time $9180; part-time $510 per credit hour.

Financial Aid Career-related internships or fieldwork, Federal Work-Study, and institutionally sponsored loans available.

Contact Dr. Joan Paternoster, RN, Director, Graduate Nursing, Program in Nursing, Mercy College, Mercy College, 555 Broadway, Dobbs Ferry, NY 10522. *Telephone:* 914-674-9331 Ext. 694. *Fax:* 914-674-9280. *E-mail:* jpaternoster@mercy.edu.

MASTER'S DEGREE PROGRAM

Degree MS

Available Programs Master's; Master's for Nurses with Non-Nursing Degrees.

Concentrations Available Health-care administration; nursing education. *Clinical nurse specialist programs in:* family health. *Nurse practitioner programs in:* adult health.

Site Options Dobbs Ferry, NY.

Study Options Full-time and part-time.

Program Entrance Requirements Clinical experience, minimum overall college GPA of 3.0, transcript of college record, written essay, immunizations, interview, 2 letters of recommendation, professional liability insurance/malpractice insurance, GRE General Test or MAT. *Application deadline:* For fall admission, 8/15 (priority date); for spring admission, 2/15. Applications are processed on a rolling basis. *Application fee:* $35.

Advanced Placement Credit given for nursing courses completed elsewhere dependent upon specific evaluations.

Degree Requirements 37 total credit hours, thesis or project, comprehensive exam.

POST-MASTER'S PROGRAM

Areas of Study *Nurse practitioner programs in:* adult health.

CONTINUING EDUCATION PROGRAM

Contact Rena Murtha, Director, Continuing Education, Program in Nursing, Mercy College, 555 Broadway, Dobbs Ferry, NY 10522. *Telephone:* 914-693-4500 Ext. 7758. *E-mail:* rmurtha@mercy.edu.

Molloy College

Department of Nursing
Rockville Centre, New York

Founded in 1955

DEGREES • BS • MS

Nursing Program Faculty 74.

Baccalaureate Enrollment 774
Women 90% **Men** 10% **Minority** 48% **International** 1% **Part-time** 44%

Graduate Enrollment 222
Women 96% **Men** 4% **Minority** 36% **Part-time** 96%

Nursing Student Activities Sigma Theta Tau, Student Nurses' Association.

Nursing Student Resources Academic advising; academic or career counseling; assistance for students with disabilities; bookstore; campus computer network; computer lab; computer-assisted instruction; e-mail services; interactive nursing skills videos; Internet; learning resource lab; library services; nursing audiovisuals; resume preparation assistance; tutoring.

Library Facilities 135,000 volumes (9,600 in health, 7,100 in nursing); 295 periodical subscriptions health-care related.

■ **Undergraduate programs in nursing are designed to prepare the nurse generalist for practice in a variety of health-care settings. Eligible students may pursue one of the following options: baccalaureate degree in nursing, registered nurse baccalaureate completion program, and dual-degree programs for both second-degree students and registered nurse students. The Master of Science degree program combines academic, clinical, and research activities that educate graduate nurses for advanced clinical practice and role functions. Preparation as adult, pediatric, psychiatric, and family nurse practitioner is offered in both the master's and post-master's certificate programs. In addition, the post-master's program is available for role functions in education or administration.**

BACCALAUREATE PROGRAMS

Degree BS

Available Programs Accelerated RN Baccalaureate; Generic Baccalaureate; LPN to Baccalaureate; RN Baccalaureate.

Site Options Plainview, NY.

Study Options Full-time and part-time.

Program Entrance Requirements Minimum overall college GPA of 3.0, transcript of college record, written essay, high school biology, high school chemistry, 3 years high school math, high school transcript, immunizations, minimum high school GPA of 3.0, minimum high school rank 40%. Transfer students are accepted. **Standardized tests** *Required:* SAT or ACT, TOEFL for international students. **Application** *Deadline:* rolling (freshmen), rolling (transfer). *Early decision:* 11/1. *Notification:* continuous (freshmen), 12/1 (out-of-state freshmen), 12/1 (early decision). *Application fee:* $30.

Advanced Placement Credit given for nursing courses completed elsewhere dependent upon specific evaluations.

Expenses (2003–04) *Tuition:* full-time $14,430; part-time $480 per credit hour.

Financial Aid 85% of baccalaureate students in nursing programs received some form of financial aid in 2002–03. *Gift aid (need-based):* Federal Pell, FSEOG, state, private, college/university gift aid from institutional funds. *Loans:* FFEL (Subsidized and Unsubsidized Stafford PLUS), Perkins. *Work-Study:* Federal Work-Study. *Application deadline (priority):* 5/1.

Contact Marguerite Lane, Director of Admissions, Department of Nursing, Molloy College, 1000 Hempstead Avenue, PO Box 5002, Rockville Centre, NY 11571-5002. *Telephone:* 516-678-5000 Ext. 6233. *E-mail:* mlane@molloy.edu.

GRADUATE PROGRAMS

Expenses (2003–04) *Tuition:* part-time $555 per credit hour.

Financial Aid 1 research assistantship was awarded; teaching assistantships, institutionally sponsored loans, scholarships, and unspecified assistantships also available.

Contact Dr. Freida Pemberton, Director, Graduate Program, Department of Nursing, Molloy College, 1000 Hempstead Avenue, PO Box 5002, Rockville Centre, NY 11571-5002. *Telephone:* 516-256-2218. *Fax:* 516-678-9718. *E-mail:* fpemberton@molloy.edu.

MASTER'S DEGREE PROGRAM

Degree MS

Concentrations Available Nursing administration; nursing education. *Clinical nurse specialist programs in:* adult health. *Nurse practitioner programs in:* adult health, family health, pediatric, psychiatric/mental health.

Site Options New Hyde Park, NY.

Study Options Full-time and part-time.

Program Entrance Requirements Clinical experience, minimum overall college GPA of 3.0, transcript of college record, written essay, interview, 3 letters of recommendation, nursing research course, prerequisite course work, statistics course. *Application deadline:* For fall admission, 9/2 (priority date); for spring admission, 1/20 (priority date). Applications are processed on a rolling basis. *Application fee:* $60.

Degree Requirements 49 total credit hours, thesis or project.

POST-MASTER'S PROGRAM

Areas of Study *Clinical nurse specialist programs in:* adult health. *Nurse practitioner programs in:* adult health, family health, pediatric, psychiatric/mental health.

CONTINUING EDUCATION PROGRAM

Contact Virginia Hackett, RN, Associate Director, Continuing Education, Department of Nursing, Molloy College, 1000 Hempstead Avenue, Rockville Centre, NY 11570. *Telephone:* 516-678-5000 Ext. 6106. *Fax:* 516-678-7295. *E-mail:* vhackett@molloy.edu.

Mount Saint Mary College

Division of Nursing
Newburgh, New York

Founded in 1960

DEGREES • BSN • MS

Nursing Program Faculty 10 (20% with doctorates).

Nursing Student Activities Sigma Theta Tau, Student Nurses' Association, nursing club.

Nursing Student Resources Academic advising; academic or career counseling; assistance for students with disabilities; bookstore; campus computer network; career placement assistance; computer lab; computer-assisted instruction; e-mail services; employment services for current students; externships; housing assistance; interactive nursing skills videos; Internet; learning resource lab; library services; nursing audiovisuals; paid internships; remedial services; resume preparation assistance; skills, simulation, or other laboratory; tutoring.

Library Facilities 113,676 volumes (7,035 in health, 4,385 in nursing); 870 periodical subscriptions (150 health-care related).

BACCALAUREATE PROGRAMS

Degree BSN

Available Programs Accelerated Baccalaureate; Accelerated RN Baccalaureate; Generic Baccalaureate; RN Baccalaureate.

Study Options Full-time and part-time.

Program Entrance Requirements Minimum overall college GPA of 2.75, transcript of college record, CPR certification, health exam, high school biology, high school chemistry, 3 years high school math, high school transcript, immunizations, interview. Transfer students are accepted. **Standardized tests** *Required:* SAT or ACT, TOEFL for international students. **Application** *Deadline:* rolling (freshmen), rolling (transfer). *Notification:* continuous (freshmen). *Application fee:* $35.

Advanced Placement Credit by examination available. Credit given for nursing courses completed elsewhere dependent upon specific evaluations.

Contact Director, Admissions, Division of Nursing, Mount Saint Mary College, 330 Powell Avenue, Newburgh, NY 12550. *Telephone:* 845-569-3248. *Fax:* 845-562-6762. *E-mail:* admissions@msmc.edu.

GRADUATE PROGRAMS

Financial Aid Scholarships, traineeships, and nursing lab assistant available.

Contact Sr. Leona DeBoer, Graduate Nursing Program Coordinator and Professor, Division of Nursing, Mount Saint Mary College, 330 Powell Avenue, Newburgh, NY 12550. *Telephone:* 845-569-3138. *Fax:* 845-562-6762. *E-mail:* deboer@msmc.edu.

MASTER'S DEGREE PROGRAM

Degree MS

Available Programs Master's.

Concentrations Available *Clinical nurse specialist programs in:* adult health. *Nurse practitioner programs in:* adult health.

Program Entrance Requirements Clinical experience, computer literacy, minimum overall college GPA of 3.0, transcript of college record, written essay, immunizations, interview, 3 letters of recommendation, nursing research course, physical assessment course, professional liability insurance/malpractice insurance, resume, statistics course. *Application deadline:* For fall admission, 6/3 (priority date); for spring admission, 10/31 (priority date). Applications are processed on a rolling basis. *Application fee:* $35.

Degree Requirements 48 total credit hours.

POST-MASTER'S PROGRAM

Areas of Study Nursing administration; nursing education.

See full description on page 526.

Nazareth College of Rochester

Department of Nursing
Rochester, New York

http://www.naz.edu

Founded in 1924

DEGREES • BS • MS

Nursing Program Faculty 14 (50% with doctorates).

Baccalaureate Enrollment 119
Women 91% **Men** 9% **Minority** 12% **Part-time** 45%

Graduate Enrollment 12
Women 98% **Men** 2% **Minority** 1% **Part-time** 98%

Nursing Student Activities Nursing Honor Society, Sigma Theta Tau, nursing club.

Nursing Student Resources Academic advising; academic or career counseling; assistance for students with disabilities; bookstore; campus computer network; career placement assistance; computer lab; computer-assisted instruction; daycare for children of students; e-mail services; employment services for current students; housing assistance; interactive nursing skills videos; Internet; learning resource lab; library services; nursing audiovisuals; resume preparation assistance; skills, simulation, or other laboratory.

Library Facilities 162,593 volumes (12,522 in health, 8,506 in nursing); 1,888 periodical subscriptions (155 health-care related).

■ Nazareth College in Rochester, New York, offers a 4-year BS in nursing, an RN-BS, and a master's degree in gerontological nurse practitioner program. The mission of the Department of Nursing is to educate students in the profession within a transcultural context and to advance students' abilities to integrate the liberal arts and sciences within the discipline. The faculty members, who are all doctorally prepared, are committed to preparing students for culturally competent nursing practice, leadership in service to the community, and commitment to a life informed by intellectual, ethical, and aesthetic values.

BACCALAUREATE PROGRAMS

Degree BS

Available Programs Generic Baccalaureate; LPN to Baccalaureate; RN Baccalaureate.

Site Options Geneva, NY; Rochester , NY.

Study Options Full-time and part-time.

Program Entrance Requirements Minimum overall college GPA of 2.5, transcript of college record, written essay, health exam, high school chemistry, high school transcript, immunizations, 1 letter of recommendation, minimum high school GPA of 2.5, minimum GPA in nursing prerequisites of 2.5, prerequisite course work. Transfer students are accepted. **Standardized tests** *Required:* SAT or ACT, TOEFL for international students. **Application** *Deadline:* 2/15 (freshmen), 3/15 (transfer).

Nazareth College of Rochester (continued)
Early decision: 11/15, 12/15. *Notification:* continuous (freshmen), 12/15 (out-of-state freshmen), 12/15 (early decision), 1/15 (early action). *Application fee:* $40.

Advanced Placement Credit given for nursing courses completed elsewhere dependent upon specific evaluations.

Expenses (2004–05) *Tuition:* full-time $18,040; part-time $439 per credit hour. *International tuition:* $18,040 full-time. *Room and board:* $4474; room only: $3000 per academic year. *Required fees:* full-time $137.

Financial Aid 91% of baccalaureate students in nursing programs received some form of financial aid in 2003–04. *Gift aid (need-based):* Federal Pell, FSEOG, state, private, college/university gift aid from institutional funds. *Loans:* FFEL (Subsidized and Unsubsidized Stafford PLUS), Perkins. *Work-Study:* Federal Work-Study. *Application deadline (priority):* 2/15.

Contact Dr. Georgia Millor, RN, Associate Professor and Coordinator of Recruitment, Department of Nursing, Nazareth College of Rochester, 4245 East Avenue, Rochester, NY 14618-3790. *Telephone:* 585-389-2718. *Fax:* 585-389-2714. *E-mail:* gmillor3@naz.edu.

GRADUATE PROGRAMS

Expenses (2004–05) *Tuition:* part-time $522 per credit hour. *Room and board:* room only: $3000 per academic year.

Financial Aid 50% of graduate students in nursing programs received some form of financial aid in 2003–04. Research assistantships with partial tuition reimbursements available, career-related internships or fieldwork available. Aid available to part-time students.

Contact Dr. Georgia Millor, RN, Associate Professor and Coordinator of Recruitment, Department of Nursing, Nazareth College of Rochester, 4245 East Avenue, Rochester, NY 14618-3790. *Telephone:* 585-389-2718. *Fax:* 585-389-2714. *E-mail:* gmillor3@naz.edu.

MASTER'S DEGREE PROGRAM

Degree MS

Available Programs Master's.

Concentrations Available *Nurse practitioner programs in:* gerontology.

Study Options Full-time and part-time.

Program Entrance Requirements Minimum overall college GPA of 3.0, transcript of college record, written essay, immunizations, interview, 2 letters of recommendation, physical assessment course, statistics course. *Application deadline:* For fall admission, 4/1 (priority date); for spring admission, 10/1. Applications are processed on a rolling basis. *Application fee:* $40.

Degree Requirements 42 total credit hours, thesis or project.

CONTINUING EDUCATION PROGRAM

Contact Mrs. Helene Lovett, Secretary, Department of Nursing, Nazareth College of Rochester, 4245 East Avenue, Rochester, NY 14618-3790. *Telephone:* 585-389-2709. *Fax:* 585-389-2714. *E-mail:* hlovett8@naz.edu.

New York University

Division of Nursing
New York, New York

http://www.nyu.edu/education/nursing

Founded in 1831

DEGREES • BS • MA • MS/MA • PHD

Nursing Program Faculty 32 (72% with doctorates).

Baccalaureate Enrollment 443
Women 94% **Men** 6% **Minority** 38% **International** 2% **Part-time** 20%

Graduate Enrollment 379
Women 95% **Men** 5% **Minority** 35% **International** 3% **Part-time** 95%

Nursing Student Activities Sigma Theta Tau, Student Nurses' Association, nursing club.

Nursing Student Resources Academic advising; academic or career counseling; assistance for students with disabilities; bookstore; campus computer network; computer lab; computer-assisted instruction; e-mail services; employment services for current students; housing assistance; interactive nursing skills videos; Internet; learning resource lab; library services; nursing audiovisuals; resume preparation assistance; skills, simulation, or other laboratory; tutoring.

Library Facilities 5.2 million volumes (102,448 in health, 62,781 in nursing); 48,958 periodical subscriptions (4,658 health-care related).

BACCALAUREATE PROGRAMS

Degree BS

Available Programs Accelerated Baccalaureate; Accelerated Baccalaureate for Second Degree; Baccalaureate for Second Degree; Generic Baccalaureate; RN Baccalaureate.

Study Options Full-time and part-time.

Program Entrance Requirements Transcript of college record, written essay, health exam, high school biology, high school chemistry, 3 years high school math, 3 years high school science, high school transcript, immunizations, 2 letters of recommendation, minimum high school GPA of 2.8. Transfer students are accepted. **Standardized tests** *Required:* SAT or ACT, TOEFL for international students. *Recommended:* SAT Subject Tests, SAT II Writing Tests. *Required for some:* SAT Subject Tests. **Application** *Deadline:* 1/15 (freshmen), 4/1 (transfer). *Early decision:* 11/1. *Notification:* 4/1 (freshmen), 12/15 (out-of-state freshmen), 12/15 (early decision). *Application fee:* $65.

Advanced Placement Credit by examination available. Credit given for nursing courses completed elsewhere dependent upon specific evaluations.

Expenses (2004–05) *Tuition:* full-time $28,328; part-time $835 per unit. *Room and board:* $11,390 per academic year. *Required fees:* full-time $1420; part-time $52 per credit; part-time $537 per term.

Financial Aid 79% of baccalaureate students in nursing programs received some form of financial aid in 2003–04. *Gift aid (need-based):* Federal Pell, FSEOG, state, private, college/university gift aid from institutional funds. *Loans:* Federal Nursing Student Loans, FFEL (Subsidized and Unsubsidized Stafford PLUS), Perkins. *Work-Study:* Federal Work-Study. *Application deadline (priority):* 2/15.

Contact Ms. Temi S. Pedro, Undergraduate Recruitment Coordinator, Division of Nursing, New York University, 246 Greene Street, New York, NY 10003. *Telephone:* 212-998-5336. *Fax:* 212-995-4302. *E-mail:* tp18@is2.nyu.edu.

GRADUATE PROGRAMS

Expenses (2004–05) *Tuition:* full-time $22,824; part-time $951 per unit. *Room and board:* $15,614 per academic year. *Required fees:* part-time $52 per credit.

Financial Aid 30% of graduate students in nursing programs received some form of financial aid in 2003–04. 2 research assistantships with full and partial tuition reimbursements available were awarded; fellowships with full and partial tuition reimbursements available, career-related internships or fieldwork, Federal Work-Study, institutionally sponsored loans, scholarships, and tuition waivers (partial) also available. Aid available to part-time students. *Financial aid application deadline:* 2/1.

Contact Mrs. Vida Samuel-Wheeler, Graduate and Doctoral Recruitment Coordinator, Division of Nursing, New York University, 246 Greene Street, New York, NY 10003. *Telephone:* 212-992-9418. *Fax:* 212-995-4302. *E-mail:* nursing.programs@nyu.edu.

MASTER'S DEGREE PROGRAM

Degrees MA; MS/MA

Available Programs Master's; RN to Master's.

Concentrations Available Nurse-midwifery; nursing administration; nursing education; nursing informatics. *Clinical nurse specialist programs in:* acute care, adult health, critical care, gerontology, home health care, pediatric, psychiatric/mental health. *Nurse practitioner programs in:* acute care, adult health, gerontology, pediatric, primary care, psychiatric/mental health.

Study Options Full-time and part-time.

Program Entrance Requirements Minimum overall college GPA of 3.0, transcript of college record, written essay, 2 letters of recommendation, resume, statistics course. *Application deadline:* For fall admission, 2/1 (priority date); for spring admission, 12/1. Applications are processed on a rolling basis. *Application fee:* $40 ($60 for international students).

Advanced Placement Credit given for nursing courses completed elsewhere dependent upon specific evaluations.

Degree Requirements 48 total credit hours, comprehensive exam.

POST-MASTER'S PROGRAM

Areas of Study Nurse-midwifery; nursing administration; nursing education; nursing informatics. *Clinical nurse specialist programs in:* acute care, adult health, critical care, gerontology, home health care, pediatric, psychiatric/mental health. *Nurse practitioner programs in:* acute care, adult health, gerontology, pediatric, primary care, psychiatric/mental health.

DOCTORAL DEGREE PROGRAM

Degree PhD

Available Programs Doctorate.

Areas of Study Nursing research.

Program Entrance Requirements Minimum overall college GPA of 3.0, interview, 3 letters of recommendation, MSN or equivalent, vita, writing sample, GRE General Test. *Application deadline:* For fall admission, 2/1 (priority date); for spring admission, 12/1. Applications are processed on a rolling basis. *Application fee:* $40 ($60 for international students).

Degree Requirements 54 total credit hours, dissertation, oral exam.

CONTINUING EDUCATION PROGRAM

Contact Dr. Hila Richardson, Continuing Education Director, Division of Nursing, New York University, 246 Greene Street, New York, NY 10003. *Telephone:* 212-998-5329. *E-mail:* nursing.programs@nyu.edu.

See full description on page 528.

Pace University
Lienhard School of Nursing
New York, New York

http://appserv.pace.edu/execute/page.cfm?doc_id=558

Founded in 1906

DEGREES • BS • MS

Nursing Program Faculty 105 (40% with doctorates).

Baccalaureate Enrollment 425

Women 87% **Men** 13% **Minority** 46% **International** 2% **Part-time** 25%

Graduate Enrollment 142

Women 94% **Men** 6% **Minority** 41% **International** 4% **Part-time** 88%

Nursing Student Activities Nursing Honor Society, Sigma Theta Tau, Student Nurses' Association.

Nursing Student Resources Academic advising; academic or career counseling; assistance for students with disabilities; bookstore; campus computer network; career placement assistance; computer lab; computer-assisted instruction; e-mail services; employment services for current students; housing assistance; interactive nursing skills videos; Internet; learning resource lab; library services; nursing audiovisuals; placement services for program completers; resume preparation assistance; skills, simulation, or other laboratory.

Library Facilities 813,997 volumes (4,330 in health, 2,996 in nursing); 1,729 periodical subscriptions (190 health-care related).

BACCALAUREATE PROGRAMS

Degree BS

Available Programs Accelerated Baccalaureate for Second Degree; Accelerated RN Baccalaureate; Generic Baccalaureate.

Site Options *Distance Learning:* Pleasantville, NY.

Study Options Full-time and part-time.

Program Entrance Requirements Transcript of college record, CPR certification, written essay, health exam, health insurance, high school biology, high school chemistry, high school foreign language, 4 years high school math, 2 years high school science, high school transcript, immunizations, 2 letters of recommendation, minimum GPA in nursing prerequisites of 2.75. Transfer students are accepted. **Standardized tests** *Required:* SAT or ACT. *Recommended:* TOEFL for international students.

Application *Deadline:* rolling (freshmen), rolling (transfer). *Early decision:* 11/1. *Notification:* continuous (freshmen), 12/15 (early action). *Application fee:* $45.

Advanced Placement Credit by examination available. Credit given for nursing courses completed elsewhere dependent upon specific evaluations.

Expenses (2004–05) *Tuition:* full-time $22,100; part-time $634 per credit hour. *International tuition:* $22,100 full-time. *Room and board:* $8400 per academic year. *Required fees:* full-time $612.

Financial Aid 79% of baccalaureate students in nursing programs received some form of financial aid in 2003–04. *Gift aid (need-based):* Federal Pell, FSEOG, state, private, college/university gift aid from institutional funds, United Negro College Fund, Federal Nursing. *Loans:* Federal Nursing Student Loans, Federal Direct (Subsidized and Unsubsidized Stafford PLUS), Perkins. *Work-Study:* Federal Work-Study. *Application deadline (priority):* 2/15.

Contact Dr. Donna Hallas, Chairperson, Lienhard School of Nursing, Pace University, 861 Bedford Road, Pleasantville, NY 10570. *Telephone:* 914-773-3323. *Fax:* 914-773-3345. *E-mail:* dhallas@pace.edu.

GRADUATE PROGRAMS

Expenses (2004–05) *Tuition:* part-time $660 per credit hour. *Room and board:* room only: $6000 per academic year. *Required fees:* full-time $460.

Financial Aid 29% of graduate students in nursing programs received some form of financial aid in 2003–04. Research assistantships, career-related internships or fieldwork, Federal Work-Study, and tuition waivers (partial) available. Aid available to part-time students.

Contact Dr. Marie Truglio-Londrigan, Chairperson, Lienhard School of Nursing, Pace University, 861 Bedford Road, Pleasantville, NY 10570. *Telephone:* 914-773-3709. *Fax:* 914-773-3345. *E-mail:* mlondrigan@pace.edu.

MASTER'S DEGREE PROGRAM

Degree MS

Available Programs Accelerated AD/RN to Master's; Accelerated RN to Master's; Master's; Master's for Nurses with Non-Nursing Degrees; RN to Master's.

Concentrations Available Nursing administration; nursing education; nursing informatics. *Nurse practitioner programs in:* family health, women's health.

Site Options *Distance Learning:* Pleasantville, NY.

Study Options Full-time and part-time.

Program Entrance Requirements Computer literacy, minimum overall college GPA of 3.0, transcript of college record, CPR certification, immunizations, 2 letters of recommendation, nursing research course, professional liability insurance/malpractice insurance, resume, statistics course, GRE General Test or MAT. *Application deadline:* For fall admission, 7/31 (priority date); for spring admission, 11/30. Applications are processed on a rolling basis. *Application fee:* $65.

Advanced Placement Credit by examination available. Credit given for nursing courses completed elsewhere dependent upon specific evaluations.

Degree Requirements 42 total credit hours, comprehensive exam.

POST-MASTER'S PROGRAM

Areas of Study Nursing administration; nursing education; nursing informatics. *Nurse practitioner programs in:* family health.

CONTINUING EDUCATION PROGRAM

Contact Ms. Judy Valarelli, Director, Lienhard School of Nursing, Pace University, 861 Bedford Road, Pleasantville, NY 10570. *Telephone:* 914-773-3726. *Fax:* 914-773-3376. *E-mail:* cenurse@pace.edu.

Roberts Wesleyan College
Division of Nursing
Rochester, New York

http://www.roberts.edu/Nursing/

Founded in 1866

DEGREE • BS

Roberts Wesleyan College (continued)

Nursing Program Faculty 12 (25% with doctorates).

Baccalaureate Enrollment 192
Women 90% **Men** 10% **Minority** 5%

Nursing Student Activities Nursing Honor Society, nursing club.

Nursing Student Resources Academic advising; academic or career counseling; assistance for students with disabilities; bookstore; campus computer network; career placement assistance; computer lab; computer-assisted instruction; e-mail services; employment services for current students; externships; housing assistance; interactive nursing skills videos; Internet; learning resource lab; library services; nursing audiovisuals; paid internships; placement services for program completers; remedial services; resume preparation assistance; skills, simulation, or other laboratory; tutoring; unpaid internships.

Library Facilities 123,434 volumes (6,749 in health, 1,850 in nursing); 1,057 periodical subscriptions (1,750 health-care related).

BACCALAUREATE PROGRAMS

Degree BS

Available Programs Accelerated RN Baccalaureate; Generic Baccalaureate; RN Baccalaureate.

Site Options Dansville, NY; Weedsport, NY; Buffalo, NY.

Study Options Full-time and part-time.

Program Entrance Requirements Minimum overall college GPA of 2.25, transcript of college record, written essay, high school biology, high school chemistry, high school transcript, 2 letters of recommendation, minimum GPA in nursing prerequisites of 2.25, prerequisite course work. Transfer students are accepted. **Standardized tests** *Required:* SAT or ACT, TOEFL for international students. **Application** *Deadline:* 2/1 (freshmen), rolling (transfer). *Application fee:* $35.

Advanced Placement Credit by examination available. Credit given for nursing courses completed elsewhere dependent upon specific evaluations.

Expenses (2004–05) *Tuition:* full-time $17,182; part-time $356 per credit hour. *International tuition:* $17,182 full-time. *Room and board:* $6604; room only: $4708 per academic year. *Required fees:* full-time $658.

Financial Aid 91% of baccalaureate students in nursing programs received some form of financial aid in 2003–04.

Contact Mr. Kirk Kettinger, Director of Admissions, Division of Nursing, Roberts Wesleyan College, Office of Admissions, 2301 Westside Drive, Rochester, NY 14624. *Telephone:* 585-594-6400. *Fax:* 585-549-6371. *E-mail:* admissions@roberts.edu.

CONTINUING EDUCATION PROGRAM

Contact Dr. Susanne M Mohnkern, RN, Chairperson and Professor, Division of Nursing, Division of Nursing, Roberts Wesleyan College, 2301 Westside Drive, Rochester, NY 14624-1997. *Telephone:* 585-594-6330. *Fax:* 585-594-6593. *E-mail:* mohnkerns@roberts.edu.

The Sage Colleges
Division of Nursing
Troy, New York

http://www.sage.edu/departments/nur

DEGREES • BS • MS • MS/MBA

Nursing Student Resources Library services.

Library Facilities 4,003 volumes in health, 2,516 volumes in nursing; 400 periodical subscriptions health-care related.

BACCALAUREATE PROGRAMS

Degree BS

Available Programs Generic Baccalaureate; RN Baccalaureate.

Study Options Full-time and part-time.

Program Entrance Requirements Minimum overall college GPA of 2.5, transcript of college record, written essay, health exam, high school biology, high school chemistry, high school foreign language, 3 years high school math, 3 years high school science, high school transcript, immunizations, interview, 2 letters of recommendation, minimum high school GPA of 3.0, professional liability insurance/malpractice insurance. Transfer students are accepted.

Advanced Placement Credit by examination available. Credit given for nursing courses completed elsewhere dependent upon specific evaluations.

Contact Kathleen Kennedy, Program Contact, Division of Nursing, The Sage Colleges, Troy, NY 12180-4115. *Telephone:* 518-244-2231. *Fax:* 518-244-2009. *E-mail:* nursing@sage.edu.

GRADUATE PROGRAMS

Financial Aid Career-related internships or fieldwork, Federal Work-Study, scholarships, and unspecified assistantships available.

Contact Linda C. Peterson, EdD, MS Program, Division of Nursing, The Sage Colleges, Troy, NY 12180-4115. *Telephone:* 518-244-2384. *Fax:* 518-244-2009. *E-mail:* nursing@sage.edu.

MASTER'S DEGREE PROGRAM

Degrees MS; MS/MBA

Concentrations Available *Clinical nurse specialist programs in:* psychiatric/mental health. *Nurse practitioner programs in:* acute care, adult health, community health, family health, gerontology, psychiatric/mental health.

Study Options Full-time and part-time.

Program Entrance Requirements Minimum overall college GPA of 2.75, transcript of college record, CPR certification, written essay, 2 letters of recommendation, physical assessment course, professional liability insurance/malpractice insurance, resume. *Application fee:* $40.

Degree Requirements Thesis or project.

POST-MASTER'S PROGRAM

Areas of Study *Nurse practitioner programs in:* acute care, adult health, community health, family health, gerontology.

St. John Fisher College
Nursing Program
Rochester, New York

http://www.sjfc.edu

Founded in 1948

DEGREES • BS • MS

Nursing Program Faculty 12 (25% with doctorates).

Baccalaureate Enrollment 181
Women 91% **Men** 9% **Minority** 12% **Part-time** 10%

Graduate Enrollment 45
Women 93% **Men** 7% **Minority** 7% **Part-time** 9%

Nursing Student Activities Sigma Theta Tau, Student Nurses' Association.

Nursing Student Resources Academic advising; academic or career counseling; assistance for students with disabilities; bookstore; campus computer network; career placement assistance; computer lab; computer-assisted instruction; daycare for children of students; e-mail services; employment services for current students; interactive nursing skills videos; Internet; learning resource lab; library services; nursing audiovisuals; resume preparation assistance; skills, simulation, or other laboratory; tutoring.

Library Facilities 190,903 volumes (28,837 in health, 4,600 in nursing); 8,964 periodical subscriptions (75 health-care related).

BACCALAUREATE PROGRAMS

Degree BS

Available Programs Baccalaureate for Second Degree; Generic Baccalaureate; RN Baccalaureate.

Study Options Full-time and part-time.

Program Entrance Requirements Minimum overall college GPA of 2.75, transcript of college record, CPR certification, written essay, health exam, health insurance, high school chemistry, 1 year of high school math, high school transcript, immunizations, 2 letters of recommendation, minimum high school GPA of 2.0, minimum GPA in nursing prerequisites of 2.75, prerequisite course work. Transfer students are accepted. **Standardized tests** *Required:* SAT or ACT, TOEFL for international students. **Application** *Deadline:* rolling (freshmen), rolling (transfer). *Early decision:* 12/1. *Notification:* continuous until 9/1 (freshmen), 12/15 (out-of-state freshmen), 12/15 (early decision). *Application fee:* $25.

Advanced Placement Credit by examination available. Credit given for nursing courses completed elsewhere dependent upon specific evaluations.

Expenses (2004–05) *Tuition:* full-time $18,200; part-time $500 per credit hour. *International tuition:* $18,200 full-time. *Room and board:* $7900 per academic year. *Required fees:* full-time $160; part-time $50 per term.

Financial Aid 95% of baccalaureate students in nursing programs received some form of financial aid in 2003–04.

Contact Dr. Dianne Cooney Miner, Chairperson, Nursing Program, St. John Fisher College, 3690 East Avenue, Rochester, NY 14618. *Telephone:* 585-385-8241. *Fax:* 585-385-8466. *E-mail:* dcooney-miner@sjfc.edu.

GRADUATE PROGRAMS

Expenses (2004–05) *Tuition:* part-time $550 per credit hour.

Financial Aid 20% of graduate students in nursing programs received some form of financial aid in 2003–04. Federal Work-Study and scholarships available. *Financial aid application deadline:* 2/15.

Contact Dr. Dianne Cooney Miner, Graduate Program Director, Nursing Program, St. John Fisher College, 3690 East Avenue, Rochester, NY 14618. *Telephone:* 585-385-8472. *Fax:* 585-385-8466. *E-mail:* dcooney-miner@sjfc.edu.

MASTER'S DEGREE PROGRAM

Degree MS

Available Programs Master's; RN to Master's.

Concentrations Available *Nurse practitioner programs in:* family health.

Study Options Full-time and part-time.

Program Entrance Requirements Minimum overall college GPA of 3.0, transcript of college record, CPR certification, written essay, immunizations, 2 letters of recommendation, nursing research course, physical assessment course, resume, statistics course. *Application deadline:* For fall admission, 8/1; for spring admission, 11/15. *Application fee:* $30.

Advanced Placement Credit given for nursing courses completed elsewhere dependent upon specific evaluations.

Degree Requirements 39 total credit hours.

POST-MASTER'S PROGRAM

Areas of Study *Nurse practitioner programs in:* family health.

St. Joseph's College, New York

Department of Nursing
Brooklyn, New York

http://www.sjcny.edu

Founded in 1916

DEGREE • BSN

Nursing Program Faculty 9 (55% with doctorates).

Baccalaureate Enrollment 257

Women 93% **Men** 7% **Minority** 53% **Part-time** 92%

Nursing Student Activities Nursing Honor Society, nursing club.

Nursing Student Resources Academic advising; academic or career counseling; assistance for students with disabilities; bookstore; campus computer network; computer lab; computer-assisted instruction; e-mail services; Internet; learning resource lab; library services; nursing audiovisuals; resume preparation assistance; skills, simulation, or other laboratory; tutoring.

Library Facilities 100,000 volumes (9,022 in health, 4,219 in nursing); 432 periodical subscriptions (700 health-care related).

BACCALAUREATE PROGRAMS

Degree BSN

Available Programs RN Baccalaureate.

Site Options Patchogue, NY.

Program Entrance Requirements Minimum overall college GPA of 2.5, transcript of college record, CPR certification, written essay, health exam, health insurance, immunizations, 2 letters of recommendation, minimum GPA in nursing prerequisites of 2.5, professional liability insurance/malpractice insurance, prerequisite course work, RN licensure. Transfer students are accepted. **Standardized tests** *Required:* SAT or ACT, TOEFL for international students. **Application** *Deadline:* 8/15 (freshmen), 8/15 (transfer). *Notification:* continuous until 8/30 (freshmen). *Application fee:* $25.

Expenses (2004–05) *Tuition:* full-time $11,078; part-time $357 per credit hour. *International tuition:* $11,078 full-time. *Required fees:* full-time $472; part-time $11 per credit; part-time $236 per term.

Financial Aid 15% of baccalaureate students in nursing programs received some form of financial aid in 2003–04.

Contact Dr. Barbara L. Sands, Director, Department of Nursing, St. Joseph's College, New York, 245 Clinton Avenue, Brooklyn, NY 11205-3688. *Telephone:* 718-399-0185. *Fax:* 718-638-8839. *E-mail:* bsands@sjcny.edu.

State University of New York at Binghamton

Decker School of Nursing
Binghamton, New York

http://dson.binghamton.edu

Founded in 1946

DEGREES • BS • MS • PHD

Nursing Program Faculty 43 (40% with doctorates).

Baccalaureate Enrollment 300

Graduate Enrollment 150

Nursing Student Activities Sigma Theta Tau, Student Nurses' Association.

Nursing Student Resources Campus computer network; computer lab; skills, simulation, or other laboratory.

Library Facilities 1.9 million volumes (7,000 in health); 8,915 periodical subscriptions (9,300 health-care related).

BACCALAUREATE PROGRAMS

Degree BS

Available Programs Accelerated RN Baccalaureate; Generic Baccalaureate.

Study Options Full-time and part-time.

Program Entrance Requirements Minimum overall college GPA of 2.7, transcript of college record, CPR certification, written essay, health exam, high school biology, high school chemistry, high school foreign language, 3 years high school math, 2 years high school science, high school transcript, minimum high school GPA of 3.0, prerequisite course work. Transfer students are accepted. **Standardized tests** *Required:* SAT or ACT. **Application** *Deadline:* rolling (freshmen), rolling (transfer). *Early decision:* 11/15. *Notification:* continuous (freshmen), 12/22 (early action). *Application fee:* $40.

Advanced Placement Credit by examination available. Credit given for nursing courses completed elsewhere dependent upon specific evaluations.

Expenses (2003–04) *Tuition, state resident:* full-time $4350; part-time $181 per credit hour. *Tuition, nonresident:* full-time $10,300; part-time $429 per credit hour. *Room and board:* $7100 per academic year. *Required fees:* full-time $1340; part-time $105 per credit.

Contact Ms. Fran Srnka-Debnar, MS, RN, Clinical Instructor and Coordinator, Student Services, Decker School of Nursing, State University of New York at Binghamton, PO Box 6000, Binghamton, NY 13902. *Telephone:* 607-777-4954. *Fax:* 607-777-4440. *E-mail:* fsrnka@binghamton.edu.

State University of New York at Binghamton (continued)

GRADUATE PROGRAMS

Expenses (2003–04) *Tuition, state resident:* full-time $6900; part-time $288 per credit hour. *Tuition, nonresident:* full-time $10,500; part-time $438 per credit hour.

Financial Aid 7 fellowships (averaging $7,743 per year), 3 research assistantships (averaging $7,233 per year), 12 teaching assistantships (averaging $6,325 per year) were awarded; career-related internships or fieldwork, Federal Work-Study, institutionally sponsored loans, traineeships, tuition waivers (full and partial), and unspecified assistantships also available.

Contact Dr. Joyce Ferrario, Associate Dean and Coordinator, Graduate Program, Decker School of Nursing, State University of New York at Binghamton, PO Box 6000, Binghamton, NY 13902-6000. *Telephone:* 607-777-4964. *Fax:* 607-777-4440. *E-mail:* jferrari@binghamton.edu.

MASTER'S DEGREE PROGRAM

Degree MS

Available Programs Master's.

Concentrations Available Nursing administration; nursing education. *Clinical nurse specialist programs in:* community health, family health, gerontology. *Nurse practitioner programs in:* community health, family health, gerontology, primary care.

Study Options Full-time and part-time.

Program Entrance Requirements Minimum overall college GPA of 3.0, transcript of college record, written essay, 2 letters of recommendation, statistics course, GRE General Test. *Application deadline:* For fall admission, 4/15 (priority date); for spring admission, 11/1. Applications are processed on a rolling basis.

Advanced Placement Credit given for nursing courses completed elsewhere dependent upon specific evaluations.

Degree Requirements 48 total credit hours, thesis or project, comprehensive exam.

POST-MASTER'S PROGRAM

Areas of Study *Nurse practitioner programs in:* community health, family health, gerontology.

DOCTORAL DEGREE PROGRAM

Degree PhD

Available Programs Doctorate.

Program Entrance Requirements Clinical experience, interview by faculty committee, interview, 3 letters of recommendation, MSN or equivalent, scholarly papers, statistics course, vita, writing sample. *Application deadline:* For fall admission, 4/15 (priority date); for spring admission, 11/1. Applications are processed on a rolling basis.

Degree Requirements 66 total credit hours, dissertation, written exam.

CONTINUING EDUCATION PROGRAM

Contact Dean's Office, Decker School of Nursing, State University of New York at Binghamton, PO Box 6000, Binghamton, NY 13902-6000. *Telephone:* 607-777-4954. *Fax:* 607-777-4440.

State University of New York at New Paltz

Department of Nursing
New Paltz, New York

http://www.newpaltz.edu/nursing

Founded in 1828

DEGREES • BSN • MSN

Nursing Program Faculty 10 (90% with doctorates).

Nursing Student Activities Nursing Honor Society, Sigma Theta Tau, Student Nurses' Association.

Nursing Student Resources Academic advising; academic or career counseling; assistance for students with disabilities; bookstore; campus computer network; computer lab; computer-assisted instruction; daycare for children of students; e-mail services; interactive nursing skills videos; Internet; learning resource lab; library services; nursing audiovisuals; remedial services; resume preparation assistance; skills, simulation, or other laboratory; tutoring.

Library Facilities 525,296 volumes; 1,253 periodical subscriptions.

BACCALAUREATE PROGRAMS

Degree BSN

Available Programs ADN to Baccalaureate; Generic Baccalaureate; RN Baccalaureate.

Site Options Middletown, NY; Suffern, NY.

Study Options Full-time and part-time.

Program Entrance Requirements Transcript of college record, written essay, health exam, immunizations, 3 letters of recommendation, professional liability insurance/malpractice insurance, prerequisite course work. Transfer students are accepted. **Standardized tests** *Required:* SAT or ACT, TOEFL for international students. **Application** *Deadline:* 3/31 (freshmen), 5/1 (transfer). *Early decision:* 11/15. *Notification:* continuous until 12/15 (freshmen), 1/1 (early action). *Application fee:* $40.

Expenses (2003–04) *Tuition, state resident:* full-time $4350; part-time $181 per credit hour. *Tuition, nonresident:* full-time $10,300; part-time $429 per credit hour. *Room and board:* $6480; room only: $3880 per academic year. *Required fees:* full-time $795; part-time $25 per credit.

Contact Dr. Ellen Abate, Director, Department of Nursing, State University of New York at New Paltz, WSB 03D, New Paltz, NY 12561. *Telephone:* 845-257-2963. *Fax:* 845-257-2926. *E-mail:* abatee@newpaltz.edu.

GRADUATE PROGRAMS

Expenses (2003–04) *Tuition, state resident:* full-time $6900; part-time $288 per credit hour. *Tuition, nonresident:* full-time $10,500; part-time $438 per credit hour.

Contact Dr. Sharon Holmberg, Graduate Coordinator, Department of Nursing, State University of New York at New Paltz, WSB 01B, New Paltz, NY 12561. *Telephone:* 845-257-2949. *Fax:* 845-257-2926. *E-mail:* holmbers@newpaltz.edu.

MASTER'S DEGREE PROGRAM

Degree MSN

Concentrations Available *Clinical nurse specialist programs in:* family health, gerontology.

Program Entrance Requirements Clinical experience, minimum overall college GPA of 3.0, transcript of college record, 2 letters of recommendation, nursing research course, physical assessment course, resume, GRE General Test. *Application deadline:* For fall admission, 5/15 (priority date); for spring admission, 11/15. *Application fee:* $50.

Degree Requirements 42 total credit hours, thesis or project.

State University of New York at Plattsburgh

Department of Nursing
Plattsburgh, New York

http://www.plattsburgh.edu/nursing

Founded in 1889

DEGREE • BS

Nursing Program Faculty 9 (50% with doctorates).

Baccalaureate Enrollment 215
Women 95% **Men** 5%

Nursing Student Activities Nursing Honor Society, Sigma Theta Tau, Student Nurses' Association.

Nursing Student Resources Academic advising; academic or career counseling; assistance for students with disabilities; bookstore; campus computer network; career placement assistance; computer lab; computer-assisted instruction; e-mail services; employment services for current students; Internet; learning resource lab; library services; nursing audiovisuals; remedial services; resume preparation assistance; skills, simulation, or other laboratory; tutoring.

Library Facilities 378,020 volumes (19,450 in health, 200 in nursing); 1,412 periodical subscriptions (174 health-care related).

BACCALAUREATE PROGRAMS

Degree BS

Available Programs ADN to Baccalaureate; Generic Baccalaureate; RN Baccalaureate.

Site Options *Distance Learning:* Glens Falls, NY; Johnstown, NY; Potsdam, NY.

Study Options Full-time and part-time.

Program Entrance Requirements Minimum overall college GPA of 2.5, transcript of college record, CPR certification, health exam, high school biology, high school chemistry, high school math, high school transcript, immunizations, minimum GPA in nursing prerequisites of 2.5. Transfer students are accepted. **Standardized tests** *Required:* SAT or ACT, TOEFL for international students. **Application** *Deadline:* 8/1 (freshmen), rolling (transfer). *Early decision:* 11/15. *Notification:* continuous (freshmen), 12/15 (out-of-state freshmen), 12/15 (early decision). *Application fee:* $40.

Advanced Placement Credit given for nursing courses completed elsewhere dependent upon specific evaluations.

Financial Aid *Gift aid (need-based):* Federal Pell, FSEOG, state, private, college/university gift aid from institutional funds, Scholarships for Disadvantaged Students (SDS), Empire State Minority Honors Scholarships. *Loans:* Federal Nursing Student Loans, Federal Direct (Subsidized and Unsubsidized Stafford PLUS), Perkins, college/university, alternative loans, short-term emergency loans from Student Association. *Work-Study:* Federal Work-Study. *Application deadline (priority):* 3/1.

Contact Mr. David G. Curry, RN, Chairperson for Nursing, Department of Nursing, State University of New York at Plattsburgh, 101 Broad Street, Hawkins Hall 209B, Plattsburgh, NY 12901. *Telephone:* 518-564-4245. *Fax:* 518-564-3100. *E-mail:* david.curry@plattsburgh.edu.

CONTINUING EDUCATION PROGRAM

Contact Mr. David G. Curry, RN, Chairperson for Nursing, Department of Nursing, State University of New York at Plattsburgh, 101 Broad Street, Hawkins Hall 209B, Plattsburgh, NY 12901. *Telephone:* 518-564-4245. *Fax:* 518-564-3100. *E-mail:* david.curry@plattsburgh.edu.

State University of New York College at Brockport

Department of Nursing
Brockport, New York

http://www.brockport.edu

Founded in 1867

DEGREE • BSN

Nursing Program Faculty 21 (20% with doctorates).

Baccalaureate Enrollment 121
Women 94% **Men** 6% **Minority** 17% **Part-time** 9%

Nursing Student Activities Nursing Honor Society, Sigma Theta Tau, Student Nurses' Association.

Nursing Student Resources Academic advising; academic or career counseling; assistance for students with disabilities; bookstore; campus computer network; career placement assistance; computer lab; computer-assisted instruction; e-mail services; interactive nursing skills videos; Internet; learning resource lab; library services; nursing audiovisuals; remedial services; resume preparation assistance.

Library Facilities 584,687 volumes (18,952 in health, 1,065 in nursing); 1,800 periodical subscriptions (257 health-care related).

BACCALAUREATE PROGRAMS

Degree BSN

Available Programs ADN to Baccalaureate; Baccalaureate for Second Degree; Generic Baccalaureate; LPN to Baccalaureate; RN Baccalaureate.

Study Options Full-time and part-time.

Program Entrance Requirements Minimum overall college GPA of 2.5, transcript of college record, CPR certification, written essay, health exam, high school foreign language, high school transcript, immunizations, 3 letters of recommendation, minimum GPA in nursing prerequisites of 2.5, professional liability insurance/malpractice insurance, prerequisite course work. Transfer students are accepted. **Standardized tests** *Required:* SAT or ACT, TOEFL for international students. **Application** *Deadline:* rolling (freshmen), 8/1 (transfer). *Notification:* continuous (freshmen). *Application fee:* $40.

Advanced Placement Credit by examination available. Credit given for nursing courses completed elsewhere dependent upon specific evaluations.

Expenses (2003–04) *Tuition, state resident:* full-time $4350; part-time $181 per credit hour. *Tuition, nonresident:* full-time $10,300; part-time $429 per credit hour. *Room and board:* $4240; room only: $2200 per academic year. *Required fees:* full-time $870; part-time $36 per credit; part-time $435 per term.

Financial Aid 66% of baccalaureate students in nursing programs received some form of financial aid in 2002–03. *Gift aid (need-based):* Federal Pell, FSEOG, state, private, college/university gift aid from institutional funds. *Loans:* Federal Nursing Student Loans, Federal Direct (Subsidized and Unsubsidized Stafford PLUS), Perkins, alternative loans. *Work-Study:* Federal Work-Study, part-time campus jobs. *Application deadline (priority):* 3/15.

Contact Ms. Sheila Myer, RN, Interim Chairperson, Department of Nursing, State University of New York College at Brockport, 350 New Campus Drive, Brockport, NY 14420-2988. *Telephone:* 585-395-2355. *Fax:* 585-395-5312. *E-mail:* smyer@brockport.edu.

State University of New York Downstate Medical Center

College of Nursing
Brooklyn, New York

http://sls.downstate.edu/admissions/nursing/index.html

Founded in 1858

DEGREES • BS • MS • MS/MPH

Nursing Program Faculty 13 (62% with doctorates).

Baccalaureate Enrollment 133
Women 93% **Men** 7% **Minority** 80% **Part-time** 77%

Graduate Enrollment 192
Women 83% **Men** 17% **Minority** 79% **Part-time** 74%

Nursing Student Activities Student Nurses' Association.

Nursing Student Resources Academic advising; academic or career counseling; assistance for students with disabilities; bookstore; campus computer network; computer lab; computer-assisted instruction; e-mail services; housing assistance; interactive nursing skills videos; Internet; learning resource lab; library services; nursing audiovisuals; skills, simulation, or other laboratory.

Library Facilities 357,209 volumes (357,209 in health, 2,679 in nursing); 2,104 periodical subscriptions (619 health-care related).

BACCALAUREATE PROGRAMS

Degree BS

Available Programs Accelerated Baccalaureate for Second Degree; RN Baccalaureate.

Study Options Full-time.

Program Entrance Requirements Minimum overall college GPA of 3.0, transcript of college record, written essay, health exam, interview, 2 letters of recommendation, professional liability insurance/malpractice insurance, prerequisite course work. Transfer students are accepted. **Application** *Deadline:* 5/1 (transfer). *Application fee:* $30.

State University of New York Downstate Medical Center (continued)

Expenses (2003–04) *Tuition, state resident:* full-time $4685. *Tuition, nonresident:* full-time $10,635. *Room and board:* $1264 per academic year.

Contact Dr. Nellie Bailey, Associate Dean, College of Nursing, State University of New York Downstate Medical Center, 450 Clarkson Avenue, Box 22, Brooklyn, NY 11203. *Telephone:* 718-270-7617. *Fax:* 718-270-7636. *E-mail:* nellie.bailey@downstate.edu.

GRADUATE PROGRAMS

Financial Aid Traineeships and health workforce retraining available.

Contact Dr. Laila N. Sedhom, Associate Dean, College of Nursing, State University of New York Downstate Medical Center, 450 Clarkson Avenue, Box 22, Brooklyn, NY 11203-2098. *Telephone:* 718-270-7605. *Fax:* 718-270-7636. *E-mail:* laila.sedhom@downstate.edu.

MASTER'S DEGREE PROGRAM

Degrees MS; MS/MPH

Concentrations Available Nurse anesthesia; nurse-midwifery. *Clinical nurse specialist programs in:* adult health, maternity-newborn. *Nurse practitioner programs in:* family health, women's health.

Study Options Full-time and part-time.

Program Entrance Requirements Clinical experience, minimum overall college GPA of 3.0, transcript of college record, CPR certification, written essay, interview, 2 letters of recommendation, nursing research course, physical assessment course, professional liability insurance/malpractice insurance, prerequisite course work, resume, statistics course, GRE. *Application deadline:* For fall admission, 4/1 (priority date). Applications are processed on a rolling basis. *Application fee:* $35.

Advanced Placement Credit by examination available. Credit given for nursing courses completed elsewhere dependent upon specific evaluations.

Degree Requirements Thesis or project.

POST-MASTER'S PROGRAM

Areas of Study *Nurse practitioner programs in:* family health, women's health.

CONTINUING EDUCATION PROGRAM

Contact Edna Lewis, Director of Continuing Education, College of Nursing, State University of New York Downstate Medical Center, 450 Clarkson Avenue, Box 22, Brooklyn, NY 11203. *Telephone:* 718-270-7616. *Fax:* 718-270-7636. *E-mail:* edna.lewis@downstate.edu.

State University of New York Institute of Technology

School of Nursing and Health Systems
Utica, New York

http://www.sunyit.edu

Founded in 1966

DEGREES • BS • MS

Nursing Program Faculty 10 (70% with doctorates).

Baccalaureate Enrollment 230
Women 96% **Men** 4% **Minority** 5% **Part-time** 82%

Graduate Enrollment 28
Women 96.5% **Men** 3.5% **Minority** 11% **Part-time** 61%

Nursing Student Activities Nursing Honor Society, Sigma Theta Tau, Student Nurses' Association.

Nursing Student Resources Academic advising; academic or career counseling; assistance for students with disabilities; bookstore; campus computer network; career placement assistance; computer lab; computer-assisted instruction; e-mail services; employment services for current students; externships; housing assistance; interactive nursing skills videos; Internet; learning resource lab; library services; nursing audiovisuals; other; placement services for program completers; remedial services; resume preparation assistance; skills, simulation, or other laboratory; tutoring; unpaid internships.

Library Facilities 193,682 volumes (14,000 in health, 8,500 in nursing); 1,090 periodical subscriptions (335 health-care related).

BACCALAUREATE PROGRAMS

Degree BS

Available Programs ADN to Baccalaureate; Accelerated RN Baccalaureate; RN Baccalaureate.

Site Options Albany, NY.

Study Options Full-time and part-time.

Program Entrance Requirements Minimum overall college GPA of 2.0, transcript of college record, CPR certification, minimum GPA in nursing prerequisites of 2.0, prerequisite course work. Transfer students are accepted. **Standardized tests** *Required:* TOEFL for international students.
Application *Deadline:* rolling (freshmen), rolling (transfer). *Notification:* continuous (freshmen). *Application fee:* $30.

Advanced Placement Credit given for nursing courses completed elsewhere dependent upon specific evaluations.

Expenses (2003–04) *Tuition, state resident:* full-time $4350; part-time $181 per credit hour. *Tuition, nonresident:* full-time $10,300; part-time $429 per credit hour. *International tuition:* $10,300 full-time. *Room and board:* $3500 per academic year. *Required fees:* full-time $804; part-time $31 per credit.

Financial Aid 33% of baccalaureate students in nursing programs received some form of financial aid in 2002–03. *Gift aid (need-based):* Federal Pell, FSEOG, state. *Loans:* Federal Nursing Student Loans, Federal Direct (Subsidized and Unsubsidized Stafford PLUS), Perkins, college/university. *Work-Study:* Federal Work-Study, part-time campus jobs. *Application deadline:* Continuous.

Contact Marybeth Lyons, Director of Admissions, School of Nursing and Health Systems, State University of New York Institute of Technology, PO Box 3050, Utica, NY 13504-3050. *Telephone:* 315-792-7500. *Fax:* 315-792-7837. *E-mail:* admissions@sunyit.edu.

GRADUATE PROGRAMS

Expenses (2003–04) *Tuition, state resident:* full-time $6900; part-time $288 per credit hour. *Tuition, nonresident:* full-time $10,500; part-time $438 per credit hour. *Room and board:* $3500 per academic year. *Required fees:* full-time $764; part-time $31 per credit.

Financial Aid 60% of graduate students in nursing programs received some form of financial aid in 2002–03. Federal Work-Study, scholarships, and unspecified assistantships available.

Contact Ms. Nancy Rickard, Staff Assistant, School of Nursing and Health Systems, State University of New York Institute of Technology, PO Box 3050, Utica, NY 13504-3050. *Telephone:* 315-792-7295. *Fax:* 315-792-7555. *E-mail:* snlr@sunyit.edu.

MASTER'S DEGREE PROGRAM

Degree MS

Available Programs Accelerated AD/RN to Master's; Accelerated RN to Master's; Master's.

Concentrations Available Nursing administration. *Nurse practitioner programs in:* adult health, family health.

Site Options Albany, NY.

Study Options Full-time and part-time.

Program Entrance Requirements Clinical experience, computer literacy, minimum overall college GPA of 3.0, transcript of college record, written essay, interview, 2 letters of recommendation, nursing research course, physical assessment course, prerequisite course work, statistics course, GRE General Test. *Application deadline:* For fall admission, 6/15 (priority date). Applications are processed on a rolling basis. *Application fee:* $50.

Advanced Placement Credit given for nursing courses completed elsewhere dependent upon specific evaluations.

Degree Requirements 45 total credit hours, comprehensive exam.

POST-MASTER'S PROGRAM

Areas of Study Nursing administration. *Nurse practitioner programs in:* adult health, family health.

CONTINUING EDUCATION PROGRAM

Contact Dr. Esther G. Bankert, Interim Dean and Professor, School of Nursing and Health Systems, State University of New York Institute of Technology, School of Nursing and Health Systems, PO Box 3050, Utica, NY 13504-3050. *Telephone:* 315-792-7295. *Fax:* 315-792-7555. *E-mail:* fegb@suny.edu.

State University of New York Upstate Medical University
College of Nursing
Syracuse, New York

http://www.upstate.edu/con

Founded in 1950

DEGREES • BS • MS

Nursing Program Faculty 12 (30% with doctorates).

Baccalaureate Enrollment 109
Women 93% **Men** 7% **Minority** 4% **Part-time** 80%

Graduate Enrollment 99
Women 98% **Men** 2% **Minority** 2% **Part-time** 70%

Nursing Student Activities Sigma Theta Tau, Student Nurses' Association.

Nursing Student Resources Academic advising; academic or career counseling; assistance for students with disabilities; bookstore; campus computer network; computer lab; computer-assisted instruction; daycare for children of students; e-mail services; Internet; learning resource lab; library services; skills, simulation, or other laboratory; tutoring.

Library Facilities 132,500 volumes (219,261 in health); 1,800 periodical subscriptions (3,856 health-care related).

BACCALAUREATE PROGRAMS

Degree BS

Available Programs ADN to Baccalaureate.

Program Entrance Requirements Transcript of college record, CPR certification, written essay, health exam, health insurance, immunizations, 2 letters of recommendation, prerequisite course work, RN licensure. **Application** *Deadline:* rolling (transfer). *Application fee:* $30.

Expenses (2004–05) *Tuition, state resident:* full-time $4350; part-time $181 per credit hour. *Tuition, nonresident:* full-time $10,610; part-time $442 per credit hour. *International tuition:* $10,610 full-time. *Room and board:* room only: $4500 per academic year. *Required fees:* full-time $25; part-time $1 per credit.

Financial Aid 33% of baccalaureate students in nursing programs received some form of financial aid in 2003–04. *Gift aid (need-based):* Federal Pell, FSEOG, state, college/university gift aid from institutional funds. *Loans:* FFEL (Subsidized and Unsubsidized Stafford PLUS), Perkins. *Work-Study:* Federal Work-Study. *Application deadline:* 4/1 (priority: 3/1).

Contact Mrs. Debora E. Kirsch, Director, Undergraduate Program, College of Nursing, State University of New York Upstate Medical University, 750 East Adams Street, Syracuse, NY 13210. *Telephone:* 315-464-4276. *Fax:* 315-464-5168. *E-mail:* kirschde@upstate.edu.

GRADUATE PROGRAMS

Expenses (2004–05) *Tuition, state resident:* full-time $6900; part-time $288 per credit hour. *Tuition, nonresident:* full-time $10,920; part-time $455 per credit hour. *International tuition:* $10,920 full-time. *Room and board:* room only: $4500 per academic year. *Required fees:* full-time $25; part-time $1 per credit.

Financial Aid 33% of graduate students in nursing programs received some form of financial aid in 2003–04. Federal Work-Study, institutionally sponsored loans, and scholarships available. Aid available to part-time students. *Financial aid application deadline:* 3/1.

Contact Dr. Carol Gavan, Associate Professor/Associate Dean and Director, Graduate Program, College of Nursing, State University of New York Upstate Medical University, 750 East Adams Street, Syracuse, NY 13210. *Telephone:* 315-464-4276. *Fax:* 315-464-5168. *E-mail:* gavanc@upstate.edu.

MASTER'S DEGREE PROGRAM

Degree MS

Available Programs Master's.

Concentrations Available *Clinical nurse specialist programs in:* adult health. *Nurse practitioner programs in:* adult health, family health, pediatric.

Program Entrance Requirements Clinical experience, minimum overall college GPA of 3.0, transcript of college record, CPR certification, written essay, immunizations, 3 letters of recommendation, nursing research course, physical assessment course, statistics course, GRE General Test, GRE Subject Test. *Application deadline:* For fall admission, 3/1 (priority date). Applications are processed on a rolling basis. *Application fee:* $40.

Degree Requirements 47 total credit hours, comprehensive exam.

POST-MASTER'S PROGRAM

Areas of Study *Nurse practitioner programs in:* adult health, family health, pediatric.

CONTINUING EDUCATION PROGRAM

Contact Ms. Barbara Black, Director, Continuing Nursing Education, College of Nursing, State University of New York Upstate Medical University, 750 East Adams Street, Syracuse, NY 13210. *Telephone:* 315-464-4276. *Fax:* 315-464-5168. *E-mail:* blackb@upstate.edu.

Stony Brook University, State University of New York
School of Nursing
Stony Brook, New York

Founded in 1957

DEGREES • BS • MS

Nursing Program Faculty 79 (50% with doctorates).

Baccalaureate Enrollment 223
Women 82% **Men** 18% **Minority** 44% **International** 17% **Part-time** 57%

Graduate Enrollment 601
Women 91% **Men** 9% **Minority** 25% **International** 9%

Library Facilities 2.2 million volumes; 29,091 periodical subscriptions.

BACCALAUREATE PROGRAMS

Degree BS

Study Options Full-time and part-time.

Program Entrance Requirements Minimum overall college GPA of 2.5, transcript of college record, CPR certification, written essay, health insurance, immunizations, 3 letters of recommendation, minimum GPA in nursing prerequisites of 2.5, professional liability insurance/malpractice insurance. Transfer students are accepted. **Standardized tests** *Required:* SAT or ACT, TOEFL for international students. *Recommended:* SAT Subject Tests. **Application** *Deadline:* 3/1 (freshmen), 4/15 (transfer). *Early decision:* 11/15. *Notification:* continuous (freshmen), 1/1 (early action). *Application fee:* $40.

Advanced Placement Credit by examination available. Credit given for nursing courses completed elsewhere dependent upon specific evaluations.

Financial Aid *Gift aid (need-based):* Federal Pell, FSEOG, state, private, college/university gift aid from institutional funds. *Loans:* FFEL (Subsidized and Unsubsidized Stafford PLUS), Perkins. *Work-Study:* Federal Work-Study, part-time campus jobs. *Application deadline (priority):* 3/1.

Contact The Office of Student Affairs, School of Nursing, Stony Brook University, State University of New York, Health Sciences Center, Stony Brook, NY 11974-8240. *Telephone:* 631-444-3200. *Fax:* 631-444-6628.

GRADUATE PROGRAMS

Financial Aid Fellowships, research assistantships, teaching assistantships, career-related internships or fieldwork, Federal Work-Study, institutionally sponsored loans, and traineeships available.

Contact The Office of Student Affairs, School of Nursing, Stony Brook University, State University of New York, Health Sciences Center, Stony Brook, NY 11794-8240. *Telephone:* 631-444-3200. *Fax:* 631-444-6628.

MASTER'S DEGREE PROGRAM

Degree MS

Stony Brook University, State University of New York (continued)

Concentrations Available Nurse-midwifery. *Clinical nurse specialist programs in:* adult health, community health, critical care, family health, parent-child, pediatric, perinatal, psychiatric/mental health, women's health. *Nurse practitioner programs in:* adult health, family health, neonatal health, pediatric, psychiatric/mental health, women's health.

Study Options Full-time and part-time.

Program Entrance Requirements Clinical experience, computer literacy, minimum overall college GPA of 3.0, transcript of college record, CPR certification, written essay, immunizations, interview, 3 letters of recommendation, physical assessment course, professional liability insurance/malpractice insurance, prerequisite course work, resume, statistics course. *Application deadline:* For fall admission, 1/15. *Application fee:* $50.

Advanced Placement Credit given for nursing courses completed elsewhere dependent upon specific evaluations.

Degree Requirements 45 total credit hours.

POST-MASTER'S PROGRAM

Areas of Study Nurse-midwifery. *Clinical nurse specialist programs in:* adult health, community health, critical care, family health, parent-child, pediatric, perinatal, psychiatric/mental health, women's health. *Nurse practitioner programs in:* adult health, family health, neonatal health, pediatric, psychiatric/mental health, women's health.

CONTINUING EDUCATION PROGRAM

Contact Mrs. Valerie R. DiGiovannai, Assistant to the Dean for Student Affairs/Continuing Education, School of Nursing, Stony Brook University, State University of New York, Health Sciences Center Level 2, Room 218, Stony Brook, NY 11794-8240. *Telephone:* 631-444-3481. *Fax:* 631-444-6628. *E-mail:* valerie.digiovanni@sunysb.edu.

Teachers College Columbia University

Department of Health and Behavioral Studies
New York, New York

http://www.tc.edu/academic/hbs/nurseed

Founded in 1887

DEGREE • EDD

Nursing Program Faculty 8 (100% with doctorates).

Graduate Enrollment 18

Women 100% **Minority** 28% **Part-time** 100%

Nursing Student Activities Sigma Theta Tau.

Nursing Student Resources Academic advising; assistance for students with disabilities; bookstore; campus computer network; computer lab; e-mail services; employment services for current students; housing assistance; Internet; library services.

GRADUATE PROGRAMS

Expenses (2004–05) *Tuition:* full-time $21,000; part-time $875 per credit hour. *International tuition:* $21,000 full-time. *Room and board:* $4800 per academic year. *Required fees:* full-time $1069; part-time $689 per term.

Financial Aid 70% of graduate students in nursing programs received some form of financial aid in 2003–04. Fellowships, research assistantships, teaching assistantships, career-related internships or fieldwork, Federal Work-Study, institutionally sponsored loans, and tuition waivers (full and partial) available. Aid available to part-time students. *Financial aid application deadline:* 2/1.

Contact Dr. Kathleen A. O'Connell, Program Contact, Department of Health and Behavioral Studies, Teachers College Columbia University, 525 West 120th Street, Box 35, New York, NY 10027. *Telephone:* 212-678-3120. *Fax:* 212-678-4048. *E-mail:* oconnell@tc.columbia.edu.

MASTER'S DEGREE PROGRAM

Program Entrance Requirements *Application deadline:* For fall admission, 5/15. *Application fee:* $50.

DOCTORAL DEGREE PROGRAM

Degree EdD

Available Programs Doctorate.

Areas of Study Bio-behavioral research, faculty preparation, health promotion/disease prevention, nursing research.

Program Entrance Requirements Minimum overall college GPA of 3.4, interview, 2 letters of recommendation, MSN or equivalent, vita, writing sample. *Application deadline:* For fall admission, 5/15. *Application fee:* $50.

Degree Requirements 90 total credit hours, dissertation, written exam.

University at Buffalo, The State University of New York

School of Nursing
Buffalo, New York

http://nursing.buffalo.edu

Founded in 1846

DEGREES • BS • MS • PHD

Nursing Program Faculty 47 (70% with doctorates).

Baccalaureate Enrollment 346

Women 91% **Men** 9% **Minority** 24% **International** 2% **Part-time** 12%

Graduate Enrollment 176

Women 83% **Men** 17% **Minority** 11% **International** 8% **Part-time** 41%

Nursing Student Activities Nursing Honor Society, Sigma Theta Tau, Student Nurses' Association, nursing club.

Nursing Student Resources Academic advising; academic or career counseling; assistance for students with disabilities; bookstore; campus computer network; career placement assistance; computer lab; computer-assisted instruction; daycare for children of students; e-mail services; employment services for current students; housing assistance; interactive nursing skills videos; Internet; learning resource lab; library services; nursing audiovisuals; paid internships; placement services for program completers; remedial services; resume preparation assistance; skills, simulation, or other laboratory; tutoring.

Library Facilities 3.4 million volumes (250,000 in health, 25,000 in nursing); 34,126 periodical subscriptions (2,500 health-care related).

BACCALAUREATE PROGRAMS

Degree BS

Available Programs ADN to Baccalaureate; Accelerated Baccalaureate for Second Degree; Generic Baccalaureate; International Nurse to Baccalaureate.

Study Options Full-time.

Program Entrance Requirements Minimum overall college GPA of 2.5, transcript of college record, CPR certification, health exam, health insurance, high school chemistry, high school transcript, immunizations, minimum GPA in nursing prerequisites of 2.5, prerequisite course work. Transfer students are accepted. **Standardized tests** *Required:* SAT or ACT, TOEFL for international students. **Application** *Deadline:* rolling (freshmen), rolling (transfer). *Early decision:* 11/1. *Notification:* 12/15 (out-of-state freshmen), 12/15 (early decision). *Application fee:* $40.

Advanced Placement Credit by examination available. Credit given for nursing courses completed elsewhere dependent upon specific evaluations.

Expenses (2004–05) *Tuition, state resident:* full-time $4350; part-time $181 per credit hour. *Tuition, nonresident:* full-time $10,300; part-time $429 per credit hour. *International tuition:* $10,300 full-time. *Room and board:* $6816; room only: $4036 per academic year. *Required fees:* full-time $808; part-time $66 per credit.

Financial Aid 72% of baccalaureate students in nursing programs received some form of financial aid in 2003–04.

Contact Dr. Elaine R. Cusker, Assistant Dean, School of Nursing, University at Buffalo, The State University of New York, 1040 Kimball Tower, 3435 Main Street, Building #37, Buffalo, NY 14214-3079. *Telephone:* 716-829-3314. *Fax:* 716-829-2021. *E-mail:* nurse-studentaffairs@buffalo.edu.

GRADUATE PROGRAMS

Expenses (2004–05) *Tuition, state resident:* full-time $7500; part-time $288 per credit hour. *Tuition, nonresident:* full-time $10,500; part-time $439 per credit hour. *International tuition:* $10,500 full-time. *Room and board:* $6816; room only: $4036 per academic year. *Required fees:* full-time $595; part-time $51 per credit.

Financial Aid 78% of graduate students in nursing programs received some form of financial aid in 2003–04. 2 fellowships with full tuition reimbursements available (averaging $10,000 per year), 16 teaching assistantships with full tuition reimbursements available (averaging $8,625 per year) were awarded; Federal Work-Study, scholarships, traineeships, tuition waivers (partial), and unspecified assistantships also available. *Financial aid application deadline:* 3/15.

Contact Dr. Elaine R. Cusker, Assistant Dean, School of Nursing, University at Buffalo, The State University of New York, 1040 Kimball Tower, 3435 Main Street, Building #37, Buffalo, NY 14214-3079. *Telephone:* 716-829-3314. *Fax:* 716-829-2021. *E-mail:* nurse-studentaffairs@buffalo.edu.

MASTER'S DEGREE PROGRAM

Degree MS

Available Programs Accelerated AD/RN to Master's; Master's.

Concentrations Available Nurse anesthesia; nursing education; nursing informatics. *Clinical nurse specialist programs in:* acute care, critical care, gerontology, medical-surgical. *Nurse practitioner programs in:* acute care, adult health, family health, gerontology, neonatal health, pediatric, psychiatric/mental health, women's health.

Site Options *Distance Learning:* Syracuse, NY.

Study Options Full-time and part-time.

Program Entrance Requirements Computer literacy, minimum overall college GPA of 3.0, transcript of college record, CPR certification, written essay, immunizations, interview, 3 letters of recommendation, physical assessment course, statistics course, GRE General Test if overall GPA is below 3.0. *Application deadline:* For fall admission, 8/1 (priority date); for spring admission, 12/15. Applications are processed on a rolling basis. *Application fee:* $35.

Advanced Placement Credit given for nursing courses completed elsewhere dependent upon specific evaluations.

Degree Requirements 42 total credit hours, thesis or project, comprehensive exam.

POST-MASTER'S PROGRAM

Areas of Study *Nurse practitioner programs in:* acute care, adult health, family health, gerontology, neonatal health, pediatric, psychiatric/mental health, women's health.

DOCTORAL DEGREE PROGRAM

Degree PhD

Available Programs Doctorate; Post-Baccalaureate Doctorate.

Areas of Study Advanced practice nursing, aging, clinical practice, critical care, ethics, faculty preparation, family health, gerontology, health policy, health promotion/disease prevention, health-care systems, individualized study, information systems, maternity-newborn, nurse case management, nursing administration, nursing education, nursing policy, nursing research, nursing science, oncology, women's health.

Program Entrance Requirements Minimum overall college GPA of 3.25, interview by faculty committee, interview, 3 letters of recommendation, scholarly papers, statistics course, vita, writing sample, GRE General Test. *Application deadline:* For fall admission, 8/1 (priority date); for spring admission, 12/15. Applications are processed on a rolling basis. *Application fee:* $35.

Degree Requirements 60 total credit hours, dissertation, written exam, residency.

University of Rochester

School of Nursing
Rochester, New York

http://www.urmc.rochester.edu/son

Founded in 1850

DEGREES • BS • MS • MSN/PHD

Nursing Program Faculty 67 (43% with doctorates).

Baccalaureate Enrollment 135

Women 83% **Men** 17% **Minority** 10% **Part-time** 55%

Graduate Enrollment 170

Women 85% **Men** 15% **Minority** 9% **International** 2% **Part-time** 76%

Nursing Student Activities Sigma Theta Tau, Student Nurses' Association.

Nursing Student Resources Academic advising; academic or career counseling; assistance for students with disabilities; bookstore; campus computer network; career placement assistance; computer lab; computer-assisted instruction; e-mail services; housing assistance; interactive nursing skills videos; Internet; learning resource lab; library services; nursing audiovisuals; resume preparation assistance; skills, simulation, or other laboratory.

Library Facilities 3 million volumes (220,000 in health); 11,254 periodical subscriptions (1,600 health-care related).

BACCALAUREATE PROGRAMS

Degree BS

Available Programs ADN to Baccalaureate; Accelerated Baccalaureate for Second Degree; Accelerated RN Baccalaureate; Baccalaureate for Second Degree; RN Baccalaureate.

Study Options Full-time and part-time.

Program Entrance Requirements Minimum overall college GPA of 3.0, transcript of college record, written essay, health exam, health insurance, immunizations, 2 letters of recommendation, prerequisite course work. **Standardized tests** *Required:* SAT or ACT. *Recommended:* SAT Subject Tests. **Application** *Deadline:* 1/20 (freshmen), rolling (transfer). *Early decision:* 11/1 (for plan 1), 1/20 (for plan 2). *Notification:* 4/1 (freshmen), 12/15 (out-of-state freshmen), 12/15 (early decision plan 1), 4/1 (early decision plan 2). *Application fee:* $50.

Expenses (2004–05) *Tuition:* full-time $27,440; part-time $880 per credit hour. *International tuition:* $27,440 full-time. *Room and board:* $9000; room only: $5000 per academic year. *Required fees:* full-time $350; part-time $100 per term.

Financial Aid 95% of baccalaureate students in nursing programs received some form of financial aid in 2003–04. *Gift aid (need-based):* Federal Pell, FSEOG, state, private, college/university gift aid from institutional funds. *Loans:* Federal Nursing Student Loans, Federal Direct (Subsidized and Unsubsidized Stafford PLUS), Perkins, college/university, alternative loans. *Work-Study:* Federal Work-Study. *Application deadline (priority):* 2/1.

Contact Ms. Elaine M. Andolina, Director of Admissions, School of Nursing, School of Nursing, University of Rochester, Box SON, 601 Elmwood Avenue, Rochester, NY 14642. *Telephone:* 585-275-2375. *Fax:* 585-756-8299. *E-mail:* son_admissions@urmc.rochester.edu.

GRADUATE PROGRAMS

Expenses (2004–05) *Tuition:* full-time $18,500; part-time $880 per credit hour. *International tuition:* $18,500 full-time. *Room and board:* $9000; room only: $5000 per academic year. *Required fees:* full-time $250.

Financial Aid 95% of graduate students in nursing programs received some form of financial aid in 2003–04. 14 fellowships with full and partial tuition reimbursements available (averaging $12,250 per year), 11 research assistantships with full and partial tuition reimbursements available (averaging $9,360 per year), 3 teaching assistantships with full and partial tuition reimbursements available (averaging $2,800 per year) were awarded; scholarships, traineeships, and unspecified assistantships also available. Aid available to part-time students. *Financial aid application deadline:* 6/30.

Contact Ms. Elaine M. Andolina, RN, Director of Admissions, School of Nursing, School of Nursing, University of Rochester, Box SON, 601 Elmwood Avenue, Rochester, NY 14642. *Telephone:* 585-275-2375. *Fax:* 585-756-8299. *E-mail:* son_admissions@urmc.rochester.edu.

MASTER'S DEGREE PROGRAM

Degrees MS; MSN/PhD

Available Programs Accelerated AD/RN to Master's; Accelerated Master's for Non-Nursing College Graduates; Accelerated RN to Master's; Master's; Master's for Non-Nursing College Graduates; Master's for Nurses with Non-Nursing Degrees.

University of Rochester (continued)

Concentrations Available Health-care administration. *Nurse practitioner programs in:* acute care, adult health, family health, gerontology, neonatal health, pediatric, psychiatric/mental health.

Study Options Full-time and part-time.

Program Entrance Requirements Minimum overall college GPA of 3.0, transcript of college record, CPR certification, written essay, immunizations, interview, 2 letters of recommendation, statistics course. *Application deadline:* For fall admission, 11/1 (priority date). *Application fee:* $25.

Advanced Placement Credit given for nursing courses completed elsewhere dependent upon specific evaluations.

Degree Requirements 41 total credit hours, comprehensive exam.

POST-MASTER'S PROGRAM

Areas of Study *Nurse practitioner programs in:* acute care, adult health, family health, gerontology, neonatal health, pediatric, psychiatric/mental health.

DOCTORAL DEGREE PROGRAM

Degree PhD

Available Programs Doctorate; Post-Baccalaureate Doctorate.

Areas of Study Advanced practice nursing, aging, family health, gerontology, individualized study, nursing research.

Program Entrance Requirements Minimum overall college GPA of 3.5, interview by faculty committee, interview, 3 letters of recommendation, MSN or equivalent, statistics course, vita, writing sample, GRE General Test. *Application deadline:* For fall admission, 11/1 (priority date). *Application fee:* $25.

Degree Requirements 60 total credit hours, dissertation, oral exam, residency.

POSTDOCTORAL PROGRAM

Areas of Study Adolescent health, aging, family health, gerontology, individualized study, nursing interventions, nursing research, outcomes, vulnerable population.

Postdoctoral Program Contact Dr. Harriet Kitzman, Associate Dean for Research, School of Nursing, University of Rochester, Box SON, 601 Elmwood Avenue, Rochester, NY 14642. *Telephone:* 585-275-8874. *Fax:* 585-273-1258. *E-mail:* harriet_kitzman@urmc.rochester.edu.

CONTINUING EDUCATION PROGRAM

Contact Ms. Pamela Smith, RN, Administrator, Center for Lifelong Learning, School of Nursing, University of Rochester, Box SON, 601 Elmwood Avenue, Rochester, NY 14642. *Telephone:* 585-273-5456. *Fax:* 585-461-4488. *E-mail:* pamela_smith@urmc.rochester.edu.

Utica College

Department of Nursing
Utica, New York

http://www.utica.edu

Founded in 1946

DEGREE • BS

Nursing Program Faculty 10 (20% with doctorates).

Baccalaureate Enrollment 130
Women 91% **Men** 9% **Minority** 30% **Part-time** 9%

Nursing Student Activities Student Nurses' Association.

Nursing Student Resources Academic advising; academic or career counseling; assistance for students with disabilities; bookstore; campus computer network; career placement assistance; computer lab; computer-assisted instruction; e-mail services; employment services for current students; externships; housing assistance; interactive nursing skills videos; Internet; learning resource lab; library services; nursing audiovisuals; paid internships; placement services for program completers; remedial services; resume preparation assistance; skills, simulation, or other laboratory; tutoring; unpaid internships.

Library Facilities 183,559 volumes (2,598 in health, 1,120 in nursing); 1,279 periodical subscriptions (140 health-care related).

BACCALAUREATE PROGRAMS

Degree BS

Available Programs Generic Baccalaureate; RN Baccalaureate.

Site Options Syracuse, NY.

Study Options Full-time and part-time.

Program Entrance Requirements Minimum overall college GPA of 2.3, transcript of college record, written essay, health exam, health insurance, high school biology, high school chemistry, 3 years high school math, 3 years high school science, high school transcript, immunizations, 3 letters of recommendation, minimum high school GPA of 2.5, minimum high school rank 25%, minimum GPA in nursing prerequisites of 2.0. Transfer students are accepted. **Standardized tests** *Required:* TOEFL for international students. *Recommended:* SAT or ACT. *Required for some:* SAT or ACT. **Application** *Deadline:* rolling (freshmen), rolling (transfer). *Notification:* 9/1 (freshmen). *Application fee:* $40.

Advanced Placement Credit by examination available. Credit given for nursing courses completed elsewhere dependent upon specific evaluations.

Expenses (2004–05) *Tuition:* full-time $20,980; part-time $234 per credit hour. *International tuition:* $20,980 full-time. *Room and board:* $8700; room only: $4500 per academic year. *Required fees:* full-time $290.

Financial Aid 97% of baccalaureate students in nursing programs received some form of financial aid in 2003–04. *Gift aid (need-based):* Federal Pell, FSEOG, state, private, college/university gift aid from institutional funds, Federal Nursing. *Loans:* Federal Direct (Subsidized and Unsubsidized Stafford PLUS), Perkins, GATE Loans. *Work-Study:* Federal Work-Study, part-time campus jobs. *Application deadline (priority):* 2/15.

Contact Mr. Patrick A. Quinn, Vice President for Enrollment Management, Department of Nursing, Utica College, 1600 Burrstone Road, Utica, NY 13502-4892. *Telephone:* 315-792-3006. *Fax:* 315-792-3003. *E-mail:* pquinn@utica.edu.

CONTINUING EDUCATION PROGRAM

Contact Ms. Evelyn Fazekas, Director of Credit Programs, Continuing Education, Department of Nursing, Utica College, 1600 Burrstone Road, Utica, NY 13502-4892. *Telephone:* 315-792-3001. *Fax:* 315-792-3292. *E-mail:* efazekas@utica.edu.

Wagner College

Department of Nursing
Staten Island, New York

http://www.wagner.edu/programs/nursing.html

Founded in 1883

DEGREES • BS • MSN

Nursing Program Faculty 17 (90% with doctorates).

Baccalaureate Enrollment 60
Women 82% **Men** 18% **Minority** 20% **International** 10% **Part-time** 5%

Graduate Enrollment 63
Women 90% **Men** 10% **Minority** 10% **Part-time** 95%

Nursing Student Activities Nursing Honor Society, Sigma Theta Tau, Student Nurses' Association.

Nursing Student Resources Academic advising; academic or career counseling; assistance for students with disabilities; bookstore; campus computer network; career placement assistance; computer lab; computer-assisted instruction; e-mail services; externships; housing assistance; interactive nursing skills videos; Internet; learning resource lab; library services; nursing audiovisuals; remedial services; skills, simulation, or other laboratory; tutoring; unpaid internships.

Library Facilities 310,000 volumes (4,505 in health, 859 in nursing); 1,000 periodical subscriptions (87 health-care related).

BACCALAUREATE PROGRAMS

Degree BS

Available Programs Baccalaureate for Second Degree; Generic Baccalaureate.

Study Options Full-time.

Program Entrance Requirements Minimum overall college GPA of 3.0, written essay, health exam, health insurance, high school chemistry, high school transcript, immunizations, letters of recommendation, minimum high school GPA of 2.7, minimum GPA in nursing prerequisites of 3.0, prerequisite course work. Transfer students are accepted. **Standardized tests** *Required:* TOEFL for international students. *Recommended:* SAT II Writing Tests. **Application** *Deadline:* 2/15 (freshmen), 5/1 (transfer). *Early decision:* 1/1. *Notification:* 3/1 (freshmen), 1/10 (out-of-state freshmen), 1/10 (early decision). *Application fee:* $50.

Advanced Placement Credit by examination available. Credit given for nursing courses completed elsewhere dependent upon specific evaluations.

Expenses (2003–04) *Tuition:* full-time $22,600; part-time $760 per credit hour. *Room and board:* $7300 per academic year.

Financial Aid 55% of baccalaureate students in nursing programs received some form of financial aid in 2002–03. *Gift aid (need-based):* Federal Pell, FSEOG, state, private, college/university gift aid from institutional funds. *Loans:* Federal Nursing Student Loans, FFEL (Subsidized and Unsubsidized Stafford PLUS), Perkins, alternative loans. *Work-Study:* Federal Work-Study, part-time campus jobs. *Application deadline (priority):* 2/15.

Contact Dr. Paula Tropello, Professor and Department Chair, Department of Nursing, Wagner College, 1 Campus Road, Campus Hall, 3rd Floor, Staten Island, NY 10301. *Telephone:* 718-390-3452. *Fax:* 718-420-4009. *E-mail:* ptropell@wagner.edu.

GRADUATE PROGRAMS

Expenses (2003–04) *Tuition:* part-time $780 per credit hour.

Financial Aid 20% of graduate students in nursing programs received some form of financial aid in 2002–03. 8 teaching assistantships with partial tuition reimbursements available (averaging $1,200 per year) were awarded; fellowships, Federal Work-Study, traineeships, tuition waivers (partial), and alumni fellowships also available.

Contact Dr. Kathleen Ahern, Director, Graduate Studies, Department of Nursing, Wagner College, 1 Campus Road, Campus Hall, 3rd Floor, Staten Island, NY 10301. *Telephone:* 718-390-3444. *Fax:* 718-420-4009. *E-mail:* kahern@wagner.edu.

MASTER'S DEGREE PROGRAM

Degree MSN

Concentrations Available Nursing education. *Nurse practitioner programs in:* family health.

Study Options Full-time and part-time.

Program Entrance Requirements Clinical experience, minimum overall college GPA of 2.7, transcript of college record, CPR certification, immunizations, interview, 2 letters of recommendation, nursing research course, professional liability insurance/malpractice insurance, resume. *Application deadline:* For fall admission, 8/1 (priority date); for spring admission, 12/10. Applications are processed on a rolling basis. *Application fee:* $50 ($85 for international students).

Degree Requirements 44 total credit hours.

POST-MASTER'S PROGRAM

Areas of Study *Nurse practitioner programs in:* family health.

York College of the City University of New York

Program in Nursing
Jamaica, New York

http://www.york.cuny.edu/~healthsci/nuprogram.html

Founded in 1967

DEGREE • BS

Nursing Program Faculty 5 (60% with doctorates).

Library Facilities 179,022 volumes (8,714 in health, 567 in nursing); 1,962 periodical subscriptions.

BACCALAUREATE PROGRAMS

Degree BS

Available Programs ADN to Baccalaureate; RN Baccalaureate.

Program Entrance Requirements Minimum overall college GPA of 2.5, transcript of college record, CPR certification, health exam, immunizations, minimum GPA in nursing prerequisites, professional liability insurance/malpractice insurance, prerequisite course work, RN licensure. Transfer students are accepted. **Standardized tests** *Required:* SAT or ACT, TOEFL for international students. **Application** *Deadline:* rolling (freshmen), rolling (transfer). *Notification:* continuous (freshmen). *Application fee:* $60.

Advanced Placement Credit by examination available. Credit given for nursing courses completed elsewhere dependent upon specific evaluations.

Contact Admissions Office, Program in Nursing, York College of the City University of New York, 94-20 Guy R. Brewer Boulevard, Jamaica, NY 11451. *Telephone:* 718-262-2165. *E-mail:* admissions@york.cuny.edu.

NORTH CAROLINA

Barton College

School of Nursing
Wilson, North Carolina

http://www.barton.edu/nursing

Founded in 1902

DEGREE • BSN

Nursing Program Faculty 8.

Baccalaureate Enrollment 120

Nursing Student Activities Nursing Honor Society, Sigma Theta Tau, Student Nurses' Association.

Nursing Student Resources Academic advising; academic or career counseling; assistance for students with disabilities; bookstore; campus computer network; career placement assistance; computer lab; computer-assisted instruction; e-mail services; externships; interactive nursing skills videos; Internet; learning resource lab; library services; nursing audiovisuals; paid internships; placement services for program completers; remedial services; resume preparation assistance; skills, simulation, or other laboratory; tutoring; unpaid internships.

Library Facilities 169,836 volumes (2,500 in health, 2,125 in nursing); 13,437 periodical subscriptions (80 health-care related).

BACCALAUREATE PROGRAMS

Degree BSN

Available Programs Generic Baccalaureate.

Site Options Smithfield, NC; Goldsboro, NC; Raleigh, NC.

Study Options Full-time and part-time.

Program Entrance Requirements Minimum overall college GPA of 2.5, transcript of college record, CPR certification, health exam, health insurance, high school chemistry, immunizations, minimum GPA in nursing prerequisites of 2.5, professional liability insurance/malpractice insurance, prerequisite course work. Transfer students are accepted. **Standardized tests** *Required:* SAT or ACT, TOEFL for international students. **Application** *Deadline:* rolling (freshmen), rolling (transfer). *Application fee:* $25.

Advanced Placement Credit given for nursing courses completed elsewhere dependent upon specific evaluations.

Expenses (2003–04) *Tuition:* full-time $13,000. *Room and board:* $4000 per academic year.

Barton College (continued)

Contact Prof. Kim L. Larson, RN, Dean, School of Nursing, Barton College, PO Box 5000, Wilson, NC 27893-7000. *Telephone:* 252-399-6400. *Fax:* 252-399-6416. *E-mail:* klarson@barton.edu.

Cabarrus College of Health Sciences

Louise Harkey School of Nursing
Concord, North Carolina

http://www.cabarruscollege.edu

Founded in 1942

DEGREE • BSN

Nursing Program Faculty 3 (50% with doctorates).

Baccalaureate Enrollment 22
Women 100% **Minority** 2% **Part-time** 98%

Nursing Student Activities Nursing Honor Society, Student Nurses' Association, nursing club.

Nursing Student Resources Academic advising; academic or career counseling; assistance for students with disabilities; bookstore; campus computer network; career placement assistance; computer lab; computer-assisted instruction; e-mail services; externships; interactive nursing skills videos; Internet; library services; skills, simulation, or other laboratory; unpaid internships.

Library Facilities 7,676 volumes (500 in health, 300 in nursing); 2,127 periodical subscriptions (300 health-care related).

BACCALAUREATE PROGRAMS

Degree BSN

Available Programs RN Baccalaureate.

Program Entrance Requirements Transcript of college record, CPR certification, health exam, immunizations, 2 letters of recommendation, RN licensure. Transfer students are accepted. **Standardized tests** *Required:* SAT or ACT. *Required for some:* ACT ASSET. **Application** *Deadline:* 3/1 (freshmen), 3/1 (transfer). *Notification:* 4/15 (freshmen). *Application fee:* $35.

Expenses (2003–04) *Tuition:* part-time $170 per credit hour. *Required fees:* full-time $225.

Financial Aid 62% of baccalaureate students in nursing programs received some form of financial aid in 2002–03. *Gift aid (need-based):* Federal Pell, FSEOG, state, private, college/university gift aid from institutional funds. *Loans:* FFEL (Subsidized and Unsubsidized Stafford PLUS), state. *Work-Study:* Federal Work-Study. *Application deadline (priority):* 4/15.

Contact Dr. Ernestine Small, EdD, Chair, Baccalaureate Programs, Louise Harkey School of Nursing, Cabarrus College of Health Sciences, 401 Medical Park Drive, Concord, NC 28025-2405. *Telephone:* 704-783-1756. *Fax:* 704-783-2077. *E-mail:* esmall@cabarruscollege.edu.

Duke University

School of Nursing
Durham, North Carolina

http://www.nursing.duke.edu

Founded in 1838

DEGREES • BSN • MSN • MSN/MBA • MSN/MCM

Nursing Program Faculty 46 (57% with doctorates).

Baccalaureate Enrollment 105
Women 86% **Men** 14% **Minority** 14% **International** 1%

Graduate Enrollment 339
Women 90% **Men** 10% **Minority** 11% **International** 2% **Part-time** 54%

Nursing Student Activities Sigma Theta Tau, Student Nurses' Association.

Nursing Student Resources Academic advising; academic or career counseling; assistance for students with disabilities; bookstore; campus computer network; career placement assistance; computer lab; computer-assisted instruction; e-mail services; Internet; library services; nursing audiovisuals; skills, simulation, or other laboratory.

Library Facilities 5.5 million volumes (272,767 in health, 40,915 in nursing); 36,995 periodical subscriptions (2,781 health-care related).

BACCALAUREATE PROGRAMS

Degree BSN

Available Programs Accelerated Baccalaureate for Second Degree.

Site Options Durham, NC.

Study Options Full-time.

Program Entrance Requirements Minimum overall college GPA of 3.0, transcript of college record, written essay, health exam, health insurance, immunizations, interview, 3 letters of recommendation, prerequisite course work. **Standardized tests** *Required:* SAT and SAT Subject Tests or ACT, TOEFL for international students. *Required for some:* SAT II Writing Tests. **Application** *Deadline:* 1/2 (freshmen), 3/15 (transfer). *Early decision:* 11/1. *Notification:* 4/1 (freshmen), 12/15 (out-of-state freshmen), 12/15 (early decision). *Application fee:* $70.

Advanced Placement Credit by examination available.

Expenses (2004–05) *Tuition:* full-time $35,000. *Room and board:* $10,500; room only: $5820 per academic year. *Required fees:* full-time $1252.

Financial Aid 94% of baccalaureate students in nursing programs received some form of financial aid in 2003–04. *Gift aid (need-based):* Federal Pell, FSEOG, state, private, college/university gift aid from institutional funds. *Loans:* FFEL (Subsidized and Unsubsidized Stafford PLUS), Perkins, college/university, alternative loans. *Work-Study:* Federal Work-Study, part-time campus jobs. *Application deadline:* 2/1.

Contact Ms. Shaunda P. Fennell, Admissions Officer, School of Nursing, Duke University, 811 Ninth Street, Suite 200, Durham, NC 27705. *Telephone:* 919-286-5617 Ext. 223. *Fax:* 919-681-8899. *E-mail:* fenne007@mc.duke.edu.

GRADUATE PROGRAMS

Expenses (2004–05) *Tuition:* full-time $18,873; part-time $4194 per semester. *International tuition:* $18,873 full-time. *Room and board:* $10,500; room only: $5820 per academic year. *Required fees:* full-time $2088.

Financial Aid 62% of graduate students in nursing programs received some form of financial aid in 2003–04. Career-related internships or fieldwork, institutionally sponsored loans, scholarships, and traineeships available. Aid available to part-time students. *Financial aid application deadline:* 6/30.

Contact Jennifer Avery, Admissions Officer, School of Nursing, Duke University, Box 3322, Durham, NC 27710. *Telephone:* 877-415-3853. *Fax:* 919-681-8899. *E-mail:* admissions@son3.mc.duke.edu.

MASTER'S DEGREE PROGRAM

Degrees MSN; MSN/MBA; MSN/MCM

Available Programs Master's; RN to Master's.

Concentrations Available Health-care administration; nurse anesthesia; nurse case management; nursing administration; nursing education; nursing informatics. *Clinical nurse specialist programs in:* cardiovascular, critical care, gerontology, maternity-newborn, oncology, pediatric. *Nurse practitioner programs in:* acute care, adult health, family health, gerontology, neonatal health, oncology, pediatric, primary care.

Site Options *Distance Learning:* Durham, NC.

Study Options Full-time and part-time.

Program Entrance Requirements Clinical experience, computer literacy, minimum overall college GPA of 3.0, transcript of college record, written essay, immunizations, interview, 3 letters of recommendation, prerequisite course work, resume, statistics course, GRE General Test or MAT. *Application deadline:* For fall admission, 3/1 (priority date); for spring admission, 10/1 (priority date). Applications are processed on a rolling basis. *Application fee:* $50.

Advanced Placement Credit given for nursing courses completed elsewhere dependent upon specific evaluations.

Degree Requirements 39 total credit hours, thesis or project.

POST-MASTER'S PROGRAM

Areas of Study Health-care administration; nurse anesthesia; nurse case management; nursing administration; nursing education; nursing informatics. *Clinical nurse specialist programs in:* cardiovascular, critical care, gerontology, maternity-newborn, oncology, pediatric. *Nurse practitioner programs in:* acute care, adult health, family health, gerontology, neonatal health, oncology, pediatric, primary care.

See full description on page 478.

East Carolina University

School of Nursing
Greenville, North Carolina

Founded in 1907

DEGREES • BSN • MSN • PHD

Nursing Program Faculty 72 (37% with doctorates).

Baccalaureate Enrollment 483
Women 91% **Men** 9% **Minority** 18% **International** 1% **Part-time** 19%

Graduate Enrollment 248
Women 90% **Men** 10% **Minority** 15% **Part-time** 47%

Nursing Student Activities Sigma Theta Tau, Student Nurses' Association.

Nursing Student Resources Academic advising; academic or career counseling; assistance for students with disabilities; bookstore; campus computer network; career placement assistance; computer lab; computer-assisted instruction; e-mail services; employment services for current students; externships; housing assistance; interactive nursing skills videos; Internet; learning resource lab; library services; nursing audiovisuals; paid internships; remedial services; resume preparation assistance; skills, simulation, or other laboratory.

Library Facilities 1.3 million volumes (67,627 in health, 6,692 in nursing); 4,453 periodical subscriptions (848 health-care related).

BACCALAUREATE PROGRAMS

Degree BSN

Available Programs ADN to Baccalaureate; Accelerated RN Baccalaureate; Baccalaureate for Second Degree; Generic Baccalaureate; RN Baccalaureate.

Site Options *Distance Learning:* New Bern, NC.

Study Options Full-time and part-time.

Program Entrance Requirements Minimum overall college GPA of 2.2, transcript of college record, CPR certification, health exam, health insurance, immunizations, minimum GPA in nursing prerequisites, professional liability insurance/malpractice insurance, prerequisite course work. Transfer students are accepted. **Standardized tests** *Required:* SAT or ACT, TOEFL for international students. **Application** *Deadline:* 3/15 (freshmen). *Notification:* continuous (freshmen). *Application fee:* $50.

Advanced Placement Credit given for nursing courses completed elsewhere dependent upon specific evaluations.

Expenses (2004–05) *Tuition, state resident:* full-time $2135. *Tuition, nonresident:* full-time $12,349. *International tuition:* $12,349 full-time. *Room and board:* $3320; room only: $1475 per academic year. *Required fees:* full-time $3280; part-time $200 per term.

Financial Aid 60% of baccalaureate students in nursing programs received some form of financial aid in 2003–04. *Gift aid (need-based):* Federal Pell, FSEOG, state, private, college/university gift aid from institutional funds. *Loans:* Federal Nursing Student Loans, FFEL (Subsidized and Unsubsidized Stafford PLUS), Perkins. *Work-Study:* Federal Work-Study, part-time campus jobs. *Application deadline (priority):* 4/15.

Contact Karen Krupa, RN, Director of Student Services, School of Nursing, East Carolina University, Rivers Building, Room 108A, Greenville, NC 27858-4353. *Telephone:* 252-328-6075. *Fax:* 252-328-6075. *E-mail:* krupak@mail.ecu.edu.

GRADUATE PROGRAMS

Expenses (2004–05) *Tuition, state resident:* full-time $2216; part-time $831 per semester. *Tuition, nonresident:* full-time $12,532; part-time $4699 per semester. *International tuition:* $12,532 full-time. *Room and board:* room only: $3690 per academic year. *Required fees:* full-time $1319; part-time $659 per term.

Financial Aid 49% of graduate students in nursing programs received some form of financial aid in 2003–04. Research assistantships with partial tuition reimbursements available, teaching assistantships with partial tuition reimbursements available, Federal Work-Study available. Aid available to part-time students. *Financial aid application deadline:* 6/1.

Contact Dr. Sylvia Brown, Associate Dean, School of Nursing, East Carolina University, Rivers Building, Room 130, Greenville, NC 27858-4353. *Telephone:* 252-328-4302. *Fax:* 252-328-4300. *E-mail:* brownsy@mail.ecu.edu.

MASTER'S DEGREE PROGRAM

Degree MSN

Available Programs Master's; Master's for Nurses with Non-Nursing Degrees; RN to Master's.

Concentrations Available Nurse anesthesia; nurse-midwifery; nursing administration; nursing education. *Clinical nurse specialist programs in:* adult health, community health, oncology. *Nurse practitioner programs in:* family health, neonatal health.

Study Options Full-time and part-time.

Program Entrance Requirements Clinical experience, computer literacy, minimum overall college GPA of 3.0, transcript of college record, CPR certification, written essay, immunizations, interview, 3 letters of recommendation, nursing research course, physical assessment course, professional liability insurance/malpractice insurance, statistics course, GRE General Test or MAT. *Application deadline:* For fall admission, 6/1 (priority date). Applications are processed on a rolling basis. *Application fee:* $50.

Advanced Placement Credit by examination available. Credit given for nursing courses completed elsewhere dependent upon specific evaluations.

Degree Requirements 49 total credit hours, comprehensive exam.

POST-MASTER'S PROGRAM

Areas of Study Nurse anesthesia; nurse-midwifery; nursing education. *Nurse practitioner programs in:* family health, neonatal health.

DOCTORAL DEGREE PROGRAM

Degree PhD

Available Programs Doctorate.

Areas of Study Nursing science.

Program Entrance Requirements Minimum overall college GPA of 3.2, interview by faculty committee, 3 letters of recommendation, MSN or equivalent, scholarly papers, statistics course, vita, writing sample. *Application deadline:* For fall admission, 6/1 (priority date). Applications are processed on a rolling basis. *Application fee:* $50.

Degree Requirements 54 total credit hours, dissertation, oral exam, written exam.

Fayetteville State University

Southeastern North Carolina Nursing Consortium
Fayetteville, North Carolina

http://www.uncfsu.edu/conted

See description of programs under Southeastern North Carolina Nursing Consortium (Pembroke, North Carolina).

Gardner-Webb University
School of Nursing
Boiling Springs, North Carolina

http://www.nursing.gardner-webb.edu/index.html
Founded in 1905

DEGREES • BSN • MSN • MSN/MBA

Nursing Student Activities Nursing Honor Society, Student Nurses' Association.

Library Facilities 230,000 volumes; 12,500 periodical subscriptions.

BACCALAUREATE PROGRAMS

Degree BSN

Available Programs RN Baccalaureate.

Site Options Statesville, NC; Charlotte, NC; Cabarrus, NC.

Study Options Full-time and part-time.

Program Entrance Requirements Minimum overall college GPA of 2.5, transcript of college record, minimum GPA in nursing prerequisites of 2.5, prerequisite course work, RN licensure. Transfer students are accepted. **Standardized tests** *Required:* SAT or ACT, TOEFL for international students. **Application** *Deadline:* rolling (freshmen), rolling (transfer). *Application fee:* $25.

Contact Dr. Shirley P. Toney, RN, Dean, School of Nursing, Gardner-Webb University, PO Box 7268, Boiling Springs, NC 28017. *Telephone:* 704-406-4360. *Fax:* 704-406-3919. *E-mail:* stoney@gardner-webb.edu.

GRADUATE PROGRAMS

Contact Dr. Rebecca Beck-Little, RN, Director of MSN Program, School of Nursing, Gardner-Webb University, PO Box 7268, Boiling Springs, NC 28017. *Telephone:* 704-406-4358. *Fax:* 704-406-3919. *E-mail:* rbeck-little@gardner-webb.edu.

MASTER'S DEGREE PROGRAM

Degrees MSN; MSN/MBA

Available Programs Master's; RN to Master's.

Concentrations Available Nursing administration; nursing education.

Program Entrance Requirements Minimum overall college GPA of 2.7, transcript of college record, immunizations, 3 letters of recommendation, statistics course.

Degree Requirements 30 total credit hours.

Lees-McRae College
Nursing Program
Banner Elk, North Carolina

http://www.lmc.edu/lmcAcademics/Outreach/OffCampusPrograms/Mayland_Nursing.htm
Founded in 1900

DEGREE • BSN

Nursing Program Faculty 3.

Baccalaureate Enrollment 32
Women 97% **Men** 3% **Minority** 3% **Part-time** 3%

Nursing Student Resources Academic advising; academic or career counseling; bookstore; computer lab; computer-assisted instruction; e-mail services; Internet; learning resource lab; library services; nursing audiovisuals; skills, simulation, or other laboratory.

Library Facilities 88,756 volumes; 429 periodical subscriptions.

BACCALAUREATE PROGRAMS

Degree BSN

Available Programs ADN to Baccalaureate.

Site Options Spruce Pine, NC.

Program Entrance Requirements Transcript of college record, immunizations, 2 letters of recommendation, prerequisite course work, RN licensure. Transfer students are accepted. **Standardized tests** *Required:* SAT or ACT. **Application** *Deadline:* 8/15 (freshmen), 8/15 (transfer). *Notification:* continuous until 8/30 (freshmen). *Application fee:* $25.

Contact Martha Hartley, RN, Director of RN to BSN Completion Program, Nursing Program, Lees-McRae College, 375 College Drive, PO Box 128, Banner Elk, NC 28604. *Telephone:* 828-765-2667. *Fax:* 828-898-8814. *E-mail:* Hartley@lmc.edu.

Lenoir-Rhyne College
Program in Nursing
Hickory, North Carolina

http://www.lrc.edu
Founded in 1891

DEGREE • BS

Nursing Program Faculty 24 (13% with doctorates).

Baccalaureate Enrollment 212
Women 91% **Men** 9% **Minority** 15% **Part-time** 92%

Nursing Student Activities Sigma Theta Tau, Student Nurses' Association.

Nursing Student Resources Academic advising; academic or career counseling; assistance for students with disabilities; bookstore; campus computer network; career placement assistance; computer lab; computer-assisted instruction; e-mail services; employment services for current students; externships; housing assistance; interactive nursing skills videos; Internet; learning resource lab; library services; nursing audiovisuals; placement services for program completers; remedial services; resume preparation assistance; skills, simulation, or other laboratory; tutoring; unpaid internships.

Library Facilities 275,961 volumes (5,000 in health, 4,200 in nursing); 445 periodical subscriptions (219 health-care related).

BACCALAUREATE PROGRAMS

Degree BS

Available Programs ADN to Baccalaureate; Generic Baccalaureate.

Study Options Full-time and part-time.

Program Entrance Requirements Minimum overall college GPA of 2.5, transcript of college record, health exam, high school chemistry, 3 years high school math, high school transcript, immunizations, minimum high school GPA of 2.5, minimum GPA in nursing prerequisites of 2.5. Transfer students are accepted. **Standardized tests** *Required:* SAT or ACT, TOEFL for international students. **Application** *Deadline:* rolling (freshmen), 9/1 (transfer). *Notification:* continuous (freshmen), 9/1 (early action). *Application fee:* $25.

Advanced Placement Credit by examination available. Credit given for nursing courses completed elsewhere dependent upon specific evaluations.

Expenses (2004–05) *Tuition:* full-time $17,120; part-time $430 per credit hour. *International tuition:* $17,120 full-time. *Room and board:* $5815 per academic year. *Required fees:* full-time $800; part-time $400 per term.

Financial Aid 100% of baccalaureate students in nursing programs received some form of financial aid in 2003–04.

Contact Dr. Linda W. Reece, Head, Program in Nursing, Lenoir-Rhyne College, PO Box 7292, Hickory, NC 28603. *Telephone:* 828-328-7282. *Fax:* 828-328-7284. *E-mail:* reecel@lrc.edu.

North Carolina Agricultural and Technical State University
School of Nursing
Greensboro, North Carolina

http://www.ncat.edu/~nursing/index.html
Founded in 1891

DEGREE • BSN

Nursing Program Faculty 24 (46% with doctorates).

Baccalaureate Enrollment 519

Women 97% **Men** 3% **Minority** 97% **International** 1% **Part-time** 10%

Nursing Student Activities Nursing Honor Society, Sigma Theta Tau, Student Nurses' Association, nursing club.

Nursing Student Resources Academic advising; academic or career counseling; assistance for students with disabilities; bookstore; campus computer network; career placement assistance; computer lab; e-mail services; interactive nursing skills videos; Internet; learning resource lab; nursing audiovisuals; other; paid internships; remedial services; resume preparation assistance; skills, simulation, or other laboratory; tutoring; unpaid internships.

Library Facilities 541,403 volumes (14,000 in health, 2,769 in nursing); 31,674 periodical subscriptions (85 health-care related).

BACCALAUREATE PROGRAMS

Degree BSN

Available Programs Generic Baccalaureate; LPN to Baccalaureate; RN Baccalaureate.

Study Options Full-time and part-time.

Program Entrance Requirements Minimum overall college GPA of 2.6, transcript of college record, CPR certification, written essay, health exam, health insurance, 3 years high school math, 3 years high school science, high school transcript, immunizations, 3 letters of recommendation, minimum high school GPA of 3.0, minimum GPA in nursing prerequisites of 2.6, professional liability insurance/malpractice insurance, prerequisite course work. Transfer students are accepted. **Standardized tests** *Required:* TOEFL for international students. *Recommended:* SAT or ACT. **Application** *Deadline:* 6/1 (freshmen), 6/1 (transfer). *Notification:* continuous (freshmen). *Application fee:* $35.

Advanced Placement Credit by examination available. Credit given for nursing courses completed elsewhere dependent upon specific evaluations.

Expenses (2004–05) *Tuition, state resident:* full-time $2788; part-time $551 per semester. *Tuition, nonresident:* full-time $12,788; part-time $3897 per semester. *International tuition:* $12,788 full-time. *Room and board:* $4968 per academic year. *Required fees:* full-time $1315; part-time $1131 per term.

Financial Aid 94% of baccalaureate students in nursing programs received some form of financial aid in 2003–04. *Gift aid (need-based):* Federal Pell, FSEOG, state, private, college/university gift aid from institutional funds, United Negro College Fund, Federal Nursing. *Loans:* Federal Direct (Subsidized and Unsubsidized Stafford PLUS), Perkins, alternative loans. *Work-Study:* Federal Work-Study, part-time campus jobs. *Application deadline (priority):* 3/15.

Contact Ms. Dawn F. Murphy, Student Services Director, School of Nursing, North Carolina Agricultural and Technical State University, Noble Hall, 1601 East Market Street, Greensboro, NC 27411. *Telephone:* 336-334-7752. *Fax:* 336-334-7637. *E-mail:* dmurphy@ncat.edu.

North Carolina Central University

Department of Nursing
Durham, North Carolina

http://www.nccu.edu/artsci/nursing/

Founded in 1910

DEGREE • BSN

Nursing Program Faculty 30 (4% with doctorates).

Nursing Student Activities Sigma Theta Tau.

Nursing Student Resources Academic advising; academic or career counseling; assistance for students with disabilities; bookstore; campus computer network; career placement assistance; computer lab; computer-assisted instruction; e-mail services; employment services for current students; externships; housing assistance; interactive nursing skills videos; Internet; learning resource lab; library services; nursing audiovisuals; paid internships; placement services for program completers; resume preparation assistance; skills, simulation, or other laboratory; tutoring.

Library Facilities 500,712 volumes; 1,934 periodical subscriptions.

BACCALAUREATE PROGRAMS

Degree BSN

Available Programs Generic Baccalaureate.

Site Options *Distance Learning:* Henderson, NC.

Study Options Full-time.

Program Entrance Requirements Minimum overall college GPA of 2.0, transcript of college record, health exam, immunizations, minimum GPA in nursing prerequisites of 2.5, professional liability insurance/malpractice insurance, prerequisite course work. Transfer students are accepted. **Standardized tests** *Required:* SAT or ACT, TOEFL for international students. **Application** *Deadline:* 8/1 (freshmen), 8/1 (transfer). *Notification:* continuous until 10/15 (freshmen). *Application fee:* $30.

Advanced Placement Credit given for nursing courses completed elsewhere dependent upon specific evaluations.

Contact Dr. Betty P. Dennis, RN, Chairperson, Department of Nursing, North Carolina Central University, 234 Miller Morgan Building, Durham, NC 27707. *Telephone:* 919-530-5336. *Fax:* 919-530-5343. *E-mail:* bpdennis@wpo.nccu.edu.

Queens University of Charlotte

Division of Nursing
Charlotte, North Carolina

http://www.queens.edu

Founded in 1857

DEGREES • BSN • MSN • MSN/MBA

Nursing Program Faculty 13 (33% with doctorates).

Baccalaureate Enrollment 100

Women 96% **Men** 4% **Minority** 12% **International** 2% **Part-time** 30%

Graduate Enrollment 35

Women 97% **Men** 3% **Minority** 12% **Part-time** 90%

Nursing Student Activities Sigma Theta Tau, Student Nurses' Association.

Nursing Student Resources Academic advising; academic or career counseling; assistance for students with disabilities; bookstore; campus computer network; career placement assistance; computer lab; computer-assisted instruction; e-mail services; employment services for current students; externships; housing assistance; interactive nursing skills videos; Internet; learning resource lab; library services; nursing audiovisuals; placement services for program completers; resume preparation assistance; skills, simulation, or other laboratory; tutoring; unpaid internships.

Library Facilities 126,242 volumes (6,000 in health, 1,000 in nursing); 592 periodical subscriptions (500 health-care related).

BACCALAUREATE PROGRAMS

Degree BSN

Available Programs ADN to Baccalaureate; Baccalaureate for Second Degree; Generic Baccalaureate; LPN to Baccalaureate.

Study Options Full-time and part-time.

Program Entrance Requirements Minimum overall college GPA of 2.5, transcript of college record, CPR certification, health exam, health insurance, high school transcript, immunizations, minimum GPA in nursing prerequisites of 2.5, prerequisite course work. Transfer students are accepted. **Standardized tests** *Required:* SAT or ACT, TOEFL for international students. **Application** *Deadline:* rolling (freshmen), rolling (transfer). *Notification:* continuous (freshmen). *Application fee:* $40.

Advanced Placement Credit given for nursing courses completed elsewhere dependent upon specific evaluations.

Expenses (2004–05) *Tuition:* full-time $17,008; part-time $270 per credit hour. *International tuition:* $17,008 full-time. *Room and board:* $6190 per academic year.

Financial Aid 85% of baccalaureate students in nursing programs received some form of financial aid in 2003–04.

Queens University of Charlotte (continued)

Contact Dr. Joan S. McGill, RN, Chair and Professor, Division of Nursing, Queens University of Charlotte, 1900 Selwyn Avenue, Charlotte, NC 28274. *Telephone:* 704-337-2276. *Fax:* 704-337-2477. *E-mail:* mcgillj@queens.edu.

GRADUATE PROGRAMS

Expenses (2004–05) *Tuition:* part-time $280 per credit hour.

Financial Aid 70% of graduate students in nursing programs received some form of financial aid in 2003–04.

Contact Dr. Joan S. McGill, RN, Chair and Professor, Division of Nursing, Queens University of Charlotte, 1900 Selwyn Avenue, Charlotte, NC 28274. *Telephone:* 704-337-2295. *Fax:* 704-337-2477. *E-mail:* mcgillj@queens.edu.

MASTER'S DEGREE PROGRAM

Degrees MSN; MSN/MBA

Available Programs Accelerated RN to Master's; Master's; RN to Master's.

Concentrations Available Nursing administration.

Study Options Full-time and part-time.

Program Entrance Requirements Minimum overall college GPA of 3.0, transcript of college record, 2 letters of recommendation, resume. *Application deadline:* Applications are processed on a rolling basis. *Application fee:* $40.

Advanced Placement Credit given for nursing courses completed elsewhere dependent upon specific evaluations.

Degree Requirements 39 total credit hours, thesis or project.

POST-MASTER'S PROGRAM

Areas of Study Nursing administration.

Southeastern North Carolina Nursing Consortium

Southeastern North Carolina Nursing Consortium
Pembroke, North Carolina

DEGREE • BSN

Nursing Program Faculty 7 (56% with doctorates).

Baccalaureate Enrollment 107
Women 98% **Men** 2% **Minority** 10% **Part-time** 80%

Nursing Student Resources Academic advising; academic or career counseling; assistance for students with disabilities; bookstore; campus computer network; career placement assistance; computer lab; computer-assisted instruction; e-mail services; Internet; learning resource lab; library services; nursing audiovisuals; resume preparation assistance; tutoring.

Library Facilities 433,164 volumes in health.

BACCALAUREATE PROGRAMS

Degree BSN

Available Programs RN Baccalaureate.

Site Options Pinehurst, NC; Fayetteville, NC.

Study Options Full-time and part-time.

Program Entrance Requirements Minimum overall college GPA of 2.0, CPR certification, immunizations, professional liability insurance/malpractice insurance, RN licensure. Transfer students are accepted.

Advanced Placement Credit by examination available. Credit given for nursing courses completed elsewhere dependent upon specific evaluations.

Contact Ms. Tonya E. Locklear, Administrative Secretary, Southeastern North Carolina Nursing Consortium, PO Box 1510, Pembroke, NC 28372. *Telephone:* 910-521-6522. *Fax:* 910-521-6178. *E-mail:* tonya.locklear@uncp.edu.

The University of North Carolina at Chapel Hill

School of Nursing
Chapel Hill, North Carolina

http://nursing.unc.edu/

Founded in 1789

DEGREES • BSN • MSN • MSN/MS • PHD

Nursing Program Faculty 112 (70% with doctorates).

Baccalaureate Enrollment 307
Women 92% **Men** 8% **Minority** 11%

Graduate Enrollment 174
Women 90% **Men** 10% **Minority** 20%

Nursing Student Activities Nursing Honor Society, Sigma Theta Tau, Student Nurses' Association, nursing club.

Nursing Student Resources Academic advising; academic or career counseling; assistance for students with disabilities; bookstore; campus computer network; career placement assistance; computer lab; computer-assisted instruction; e-mail services; employment services for current students; housing assistance; interactive nursing skills videos; Internet; learning resource lab; library services; nursing audiovisuals; other; remedial services; resume preparation assistance; skills, simulation, or other laboratory; tutoring.

Library Facilities 5.5 million volumes (315,000 in health); 40,597 periodical subscriptions (4,000 health-care related).

BACCALAUREATE PROGRAMS

Degree BSN

Available Programs ADN to Baccalaureate; Accelerated Baccalaureate for Second Degree; Generic Baccalaureate; RN Baccalaureate.

Site Options *Distance Learning:* Smithfield, NC; High Point, NC.

Study Options Full-time.

Program Entrance Requirements Minimum overall college GPA of 2.0, transcript of college record, CPR certification, written essay, health exam, health insurance, high school transcript, immunizations, 2 letters of recommendation, minimum GPA in nursing prerequisites of 2.0, prerequisite course work. Transfer students are accepted. **Standardized tests** *Required:* SAT or ACT, TOEFL for international students. **Application** *Deadline:* 1/15 (freshmen), 3/1 (transfer). *Early decision:* 11/1. *Notification:* 3/31 (freshmen), 1/31 (early action). *Application fee:* $60.

Advanced Placement Credit by examination available. Credit given for nursing courses completed elsewhere dependent upon specific evaluations.

Financial Aid 40% of baccalaureate students in nursing programs received some form of financial aid in 2002–03.

Contact Ms. Anna Terry, Undergraduate Admissions Assistant, School of Nursing, The University of North Carolina at Chapel Hill, CB #7460, Chapel Hill, NC 27599-7460. *Telephone:* 919-966-4260. *Fax:* 919-966-3540. *E-mail:* terry@email.unc.edu.

GRADUATE PROGRAMS

Financial Aid 8 fellowships, 6 research assistantships (averaging $8,000 per year), 10 teaching assistantships (averaging $8,000 per year) were awarded; scholarships, traineeships, and unspecified assistantships also available.

Contact Ms. Katherine Moore, RN, Director, Office of Admissions and Student Services, School of Nursing, The University of North Carolina at Chapel Hill, CB #7460, Chapel Hill, NC 27599-7460. *Telephone:* 919-966-4260. *Fax:* 919-966-3540. *E-mail:* kathy_moore@unc.edu.

MASTER'S DEGREE PROGRAM

Degrees MSN; MSN/MS

Available Programs Master's for Nurses with Non-Nursing Degrees; RN to Master's.

Concentrations Available Nurse case management; nursing administration; nursing education; nursing informatics. *Clinical nurse specialist programs in:* maternity-newborn, pediatric, psychiatric/mental health, women's health. *Nurse practitioner programs in:* adult health, family health, neonatal health, pediatric, primary care, psychiatric/mental health, women's health.

Study Options Full-time and part-time.

Program Entrance Requirements Clinical experience, minimum overall college GPA of 3.0, transcript of college record, CPR certification, written essay, immunizations, 3 letters of recommendation, physical assessment course, professional liability insurance/malpractice insurance, resume, statistics course, GRE General Test. *Application deadline:* For fall admission, 3/31; for spring admission, 10/15. *Application fee:* $55.

Advanced Placement Credit given for nursing courses completed elsewhere dependent upon specific evaluations.

Degree Requirements 40 total credit hours, thesis or project, comprehensive exam.

POST-MASTER'S PROGRAM

Areas of Study Nurse case management; nursing administration; nursing education; nursing informatics. *Clinical nurse specialist programs in:* maternity-newborn, pediatric, psychiatric/mental health, women's health. *Nurse practitioner programs in:* adult health, family health, neonatal health, pediatric, primary care, psychiatric/mental health, women's health.

DOCTORAL DEGREE PROGRAM

Degree PhD

Available Programs Doctorate.

Areas of Study Nursing research.

Program Entrance Requirements Minimum overall college GPA of 3.0, interview by faculty committee, 3 letters of recommendation, scholarly papers, statistics course, vita, writing sample, GRE General Test. *Application deadline:* For fall admission, 3/31; for spring admission, 10/15. *Application fee:* $55.

Degree Requirements 48 total credit hours, dissertation, oral exam, written exam, residency.

POSTDOCTORAL PROGRAM

Areas of Study Adolescent health, aging, cancer care, chronic illness, community health, family health, gerontology, health promotion/disease prevention, individualized study, information systems, neuro-behavior, nursing informatics, nursing interventions, nursing research, nursing science, outcomes, self-care, vulnerable population, women's health.

Postdoctoral Program Contact Dr. Merle Mishel, Professor, School of Nursing, The University of North Carolina at Chapel Hill, 433 Carrington Hall, CB #7460, Chapel Hill, NC 27599-7460. *Telephone:* 919-966-5294. *Fax:* 919-966-3540. *E-mail:* mishel@email.unc.edu.

CONTINUING EDUCATION PROGRAM

Contact Dr. Barbara Jo Foley, Director of Continuing Education, School of Nursing, The University of North Carolina at Chapel Hill, 433 Carrington Hall, CB #7460, Chapel Hill, NC 27599-7460. *Telephone:* 919-966-3638. *Fax:* 919-966-7298. *E-mail:* bfoley@email.unc.edu.

The University of North Carolina at Charlotte

School of Nursing
Charlotte, North Carolina

http://www.health.uncc.edu

Founded in 1946

DEGREES • BSN • MSN • MSN/MHA

Nursing Program Faculty 45 (53% with doctorates).

Baccalaureate Enrollment 260
Women 90% **Men** 10% **Minority** 15%

Graduate Enrollment 177
Women 80% **Men** 20% **Minority** 10% **Part-time** 75%

Nursing Student Activities Sigma Theta Tau, Student Nurses' Association.

Nursing Student Resources Academic advising; academic or career counseling; assistance for students with disabilities; bookstore; campus computer network; career placement assistance; computer lab; computer-assisted instruction; e-mail services; externships; interactive nursing skills videos; Internet; learning resource lab; library services; nursing audiovisuals; skills, simulation, or other laboratory.

Library Facilities 916,218 volumes (39,000 in health, 2,400 in nursing); 10,599 periodical subscriptions (160 health-care related).

BACCALAUREATE PROGRAMS

Degree BSN

Available Programs ADN to Baccalaureate; Generic Baccalaureate; RN Baccalaureate.

Study Options Full-time.

Program Entrance Requirements Minimum overall college GPA of 2.5, transcript of college record, CPR certification, health exam, health insurance, high school biology, high school chemistry, high school foreign language, 3 years high school math, 3 years high school science, high school transcript, immunizations, minimum GPA in nursing prerequisites of 2.5, prerequisite course work. Transfer students are accepted. **Standardized tests** *Required:* SAT or ACT, TOEFL for international students. **Application** *Deadline:* 7/1 (freshmen), 7/1 (transfer). *Early decision:* 10/15. *Notification:* continuous (freshmen). *Application fee:* $50.

Expenses (2003–04) *Tuition, state resident:* full-time $3122; part-time $406 per course. *Tuition, nonresident:* full-time $13,158; part-time $1661 per course.

Financial Aid 50% of baccalaureate students in nursing programs received some form of financial aid in 2002–03.

Contact Ms. Martha Sloss, Academic Adviser, School of Nursing, The University of North Carolina at Charlotte, 9201 University City Boulevard, Charlotte, NC 28223-0001. *Telephone:* 704-687-4682. *Fax:* 704-687-3180. *E-mail:* mksloss@email.uncc.edu.

GRADUATE PROGRAMS

Expenses (2003–04) *Tuition, state resident:* full-time $3197; part-time $415 per course. *Tuition, nonresident:* full-time $13,329; part-time $1682 per course.

Financial Aid 75% of graduate students in nursing programs received some form of financial aid in 2002–03.

Contact Ms. Martha Sloss, Academic Adviser, School of Nursing, The University of North Carolina at Charlotte, 9201 University City Boulevard, Charlotte, NC 28223-0001. *Telephone:* 704-687-4682. *Fax:* 704-687-3180. *E-mail:* mksloss@email.uncc.edu.

MASTER'S DEGREE PROGRAM

Degrees MSN; MSN/MHA

Available Programs Master's; RN to Master's.

Concentrations Available Health-care administration; nurse anesthesia. *Clinical nurse specialist programs in:* adult health, community health, psychiatric/mental health. *Nurse practitioner programs in:* adult health, family health.

Site Options *Distance Learning:* Gastonia, NC; Salisbury, NC.

Program Entrance Requirements Clinical experience, computer literacy, minimum overall college GPA of 3.0, transcript of college record, CPR certification, written essay, immunizations, interview, 3 letters of recommendation, nursing research course, professional liability insurance/malpractice insurance, resume, statistics course.

POST-MASTER'S PROGRAM

Areas of Study Nurse anesthesia; nursing administration. *Nurse practitioner programs in:* family health.

CONTINUING EDUCATION PROGRAM

Contact Dr. Lienne Edwards, Director of Continuing Education, School of Nursing, The University of North Carolina at Charlotte, 9201 University City Boulevard, Charlotte, NC 28223-0001. *Telephone:* 704-687-4675. *Fax:* 704-687-3180. *E-mail:* ledward@email.uncc.edu.

The University of North Carolina at Greensboro

School of Nursing
Greensboro, North Carolina

http://www.uncg.edu/nur/

Founded in 1891

DEGREES • BSN • MSN • MSN/MBA • PHD

The University of North Carolina at Greensboro (continued)

Nursing Program Faculty 54 (60% with doctorates).

Baccalaureate Enrollment 1,094 **Women** 93% **Men** 7% **Minority** 29% **International** 4% **Part-time** 33%

Graduate Enrollment 275
Women 80% **Men** 20% **Minority** 18% **International** 4% **Part-time** 30%

Nursing Student Activities Nursing Honor Society, Sigma Theta Tau, Student Nurses' Association.

Nursing Student Resources Academic advising; academic or career counseling; assistance for students with disabilities; bookstore; campus computer network; career placement assistance; computer lab; computer-assisted instruction; e-mail services; externships; Internet; learning resource lab; library services; nursing audiovisuals; paid internships; placement services for program completers; remedial services; resume preparation assistance; skills, simulation, or other laboratory; tutoring; unpaid internships.

Library Facilities 844,448 volumes; 8,714 periodical subscriptions.

BACCALAUREATE PROGRAMS

Degree BSN

Available Programs ADN to Baccalaureate; Baccalaureate for Second Degree; Generic Baccalaureate; LPN to Baccalaureate; LPN to RN Baccalaureate; RN Baccalaureate.

Site Options Hickory, NC; Greensboro, NC.

Study Options Full-time.

Program Entrance Requirements Minimum overall college GPA of 2.7, transcript of college record, CPR certification, health exam, immunizations, minimum GPA in nursing prerequisites of 2.7, professional liability insurance/malpractice insurance, prerequisite course work. Transfer students are accepted. **Standardized tests** *Required:* SAT or ACT, TOEFL for international students. **Application** *Deadline:* 8/1 (freshmen), 8/1 (transfer). *Notification:* continuous (freshmen). *Application fee:* $35.

Expenses (2004–05) *Tuition, state resident:* full-time $1014; part-time $254 per course. *Tuition, nonresident:* full-time $12,996; part-time $1625 per course. *International tuition:* $12,996 full-time. *Room and board:* $4800; room only: $2600 per academic year. *Required fees:* full-time $1407; part-time $50 per credit.

Financial Aid *Gift aid (need-based):* Federal Pell, FSEOG, state, private, college/university gift aid from institutional funds. *Loans:* FFEL (Subsidized and Unsubsidized Stafford PLUS), Perkins, college/university. *Work-Study:* Federal Work-Study. *Application deadline (priority):* 3/1.

Contact Dr. Virginia B. Karb, Associate Dean, School of Nursing, The University of North Carolina at Greensboro, PO Box 26170, Greensboro, NC 27402-6170. *Telephone:* 336-334-5280. *Fax:* 336-334-3628. *E-mail:* virginia_karb@uncg.edu.

GRADUATE PROGRAMS

Expenses (2004–05) *Tuition, state resident:* full-time $2112; part-time $528 per course. *Tuition, nonresident:* full-time $13,162; part-time $3290 per course. *International tuition:* $13,162 full-time. *Room and board:* $4200; room only: $2340 per academic year. *Required fees:* full-time $1105; part-time $50 per credit.

Financial Aid 90% of graduate students in nursing programs received some form of financial aid in 2003–04. 16 research assistantships with full tuition reimbursements available (averaging $4,883 per year) were awarded; career-related internships or fieldwork, Federal Work-Study, scholarships, and traineeships also available. Aid available to part-time students.

Contact Eileen Kohlenberg, Associate Dean and Director of Graduate Studies, School of Nursing, The University of North Carolina at Greensboro, PO Box 26170, Greensboro, NC 27402-6170. *Telephone:* 336-334-5561. *Fax:* 336-334-3628. *E-mail:* eileen_kohlenberg@uncg.edu.

MASTER'S DEGREE PROGRAM

Degrees MSN; MSN/MBA

Available Programs Master's.

Concentrations Available Nurse anesthesia; nursing administration; nursing education. *Clinical nurse specialist programs in:* adult health. *Nurse practitioner programs in:* adult health, gerontology.

Site Options Hickory, NC.

Study Options Full-time and part-time.

Program Entrance Requirements Clinical experience, minimum overall college GPA of 3.0, transcript of college record, CPR certification, immunizations, 3 letters of recommendation, physical assessment course, professional liability insurance/malpractice insurance, prerequisite course work, statistics course, GRE General Test or MAT. *Application fee:* $35.

Advanced Placement Credit given for nursing courses completed elsewhere dependent upon specific evaluations.

Degree Requirements Thesis or project, comprehensive exam.

POST-MASTER'S PROGRAM

Areas of Study Nurse anesthesia. *Nurse practitioner programs in:* adult health, gerontology.

DOCTORAL DEGREE PROGRAM

Degree PhD

Available Programs Doctorate.

Areas of Study Aging, faculty preparation, gerontology, health policy, health promotion/disease prevention, nursing administration, nursing education, nursing research, nursing science, women's health.

Program Entrance Requirements Minimum overall college GPA of 3.0, interview by faculty committee, 3 letters of recommendation, MSN or equivalent, writing sample. *Application fee:* $35.

Degree Requirements 57 total credit hours, dissertation, oral exam, written exam, residency.

The University of North Carolina at Pembroke

Southeastern North Carolina Nursing Consortium
Pembroke, North Carolina

See description of programs under Southeastern North Carolina Nursing Consortium (Pembroke, North Carolina).

The University of North Carolina at Wilmington

School of Nursing
Wilmington, North Carolina

http://www.uncwil.edu/inside

Founded in 1947

DEGREES • BS • MSN

Nursing Program Faculty 23 (52% with doctorates).

Baccalaureate Enrollment 151
Women 90% **Men** 10% **Minority** 7% **Part-time** 13%

Graduate Enrollment 22
Women 95% **Men** 5% **Minority** 27% **Part-time** 55%

Nursing Student Activities Sigma Theta Tau, Student Nurses' Association.

Nursing Student Resources Academic advising; academic or career counseling; assistance for students with disabilities; bookstore; campus computer network; career placement assistance; computer lab; computer-assisted instruction; e-mail services; employment services for current students; externships; housing assistance; interactive nursing skills videos; Internet; learning resource lab; library services; nursing audiovisuals; placement services for program completers; remedial services; resume preparation assistance; skills, simulation, or other laboratory; unpaid internships.

Library Facilities 530,368 volumes (13,000 in health, 7,000 in nursing); 3,668 periodical subscriptions (370 health-care related).

BACCALAUREATE PROGRAMS

Degree BS

Available Programs Generic Baccalaureate; RN Baccalaureate.

Study Options Full-time.

Program Entrance Requirements Minimum overall college GPA of 2.5, transcript of college record, CPR certification, written essay, health exam, health insurance, immunizations, minimum GPA in nursing prerequisites of 2.0, professional liability insurance/malpractice insurance, prerequisite course work. Transfer students are accepted. **Standardized tests** *Required:* SAT or ACT, TOEFL for international students. **Application** *Deadline:* 2/1 (freshmen), 3/15 (transfer). *Early decision:* 11/1. *Notification:* 4/1 (freshmen), 1/19 (early action). *Application fee:* $45.

Advanced Placement Credit given for nursing courses completed elsewhere dependent upon specific evaluations.

Expenses (2004–05) *Tuition, state resident:* full-time $1928. *Tuition, nonresident:* full-time $11,638. *Room and board:* $6524 per academic year. *Required fees:* full-time $1698.

Financial Aid 65% of baccalaureate students in nursing programs received some form of financial aid in 2003–04.

Contact Ms. Nancy L. McLemore, Student Services Director, School of Nursing, The University of North Carolina at Wilmington, 601 South College Road, Wilmington, NC 28403-5995. *Telephone:* 910-962-3208. *Fax:* 910-962-3723. *E-mail:* nursing@uncwil.edu.

GRADUATE PROGRAMS

Expenses (2004–05) *Tuition, state resident:* full-time $3438. *Tuition, nonresident:* full-time $13,140. *Room and board:* $6524 per academic year. *Required fees:* full-time $1659.

Financial Aid 88% of graduate students in nursing programs received some form of financial aid in 2003–04. 2 teaching assistantships were awarded. *Financial aid application deadline:* 3/15.

Contact Ms. Nancy L. McLemore, Student Services Director, School of Nursing, The University of North Carolina at Wilmington, 601 South College Road, Wilmington, NC 28403-5995. *Telephone:* 910-962-3208. *Fax:* 910-962-3723. *E-mail:* nursing@uncwil.edu.

MASTER'S DEGREE PROGRAM

Degree MSN

Available Programs Master's; RN to Master's.

Concentrations Available Nursing education. *Nurse practitioner programs in:* family health.

Study Options Full-time and part-time.

Program Entrance Requirements Clinical experience, computer literacy, minimum overall college GPA of 3.0, transcript of college record, CPR certification, written essay, immunizations, 3 letters of recommendation, nursing research course, physical assessment course, professional liability insurance/malpractice insurance, prerequisite course work, resume, statistics course, GRE General Test. *Application deadline:* For fall admission, 3/1. Applications are processed on a rolling basis. *Application fee:* $45.

Advanced Placement Credit given for nursing courses completed elsewhere dependent upon specific evaluations.

Degree Requirements 47 total credit hours, thesis or project, comprehensive exam.

Western Carolina University

Department of Nursing
Cullowhee, North Carolina

Founded in 1889

DEGREES • BSN • MSN

Nursing Program Faculty 18 (45% with doctorates).

Baccalaureate Enrollment 114
Women 97% **Men** 3% **Minority** 2%

Graduate Enrollment 30
Women 100%

Nursing Student Activities Sigma Theta Tau, Student Nurses' Association.

Nursing Student Resources Academic advising; academic or career counseling; assistance for students with disabilities; bookstore; campus computer network; career placement assistance; computer lab; computer-assisted instruction; daycare for children of students; e-mail services; externships; housing assistance; interactive nursing skills videos; Internet; learning resource lab; library services; nursing audiovisuals; resume preparation assistance; skills, simulation, or other laboratory; tutoring.

Library Facilities 694,530 volumes (10,000 in health, 900 in nursing); 3,330 periodical subscriptions (70 health-care related).

BACCALAUREATE PROGRAMS

Degree BSN

Available Programs Generic Baccalaureate; RN Baccalaureate.

Site Options *Distance Learning:* Enka, NC.

Study Options Full-time.

Program Entrance Requirements Transcript of college record, CPR certification, written essay, health exam, immunizations, minimum GPA in nursing prerequisites of 2.0, professional liability insurance/malpractice insurance, prerequisite course work. Transfer students are accepted. **Standardized tests** *Required:* SAT or ACT, TOEFL for international students. **Application** *Deadline:* 8/1 (freshmen), 8/1 (transfer). *Notification:* continuous (freshmen). *Application fee:* $40.

Advanced Placement Credit given for nursing courses completed elsewhere dependent upon specific evaluations.

Expenses (2003–04) *Tuition, state resident:* full-time $3060; part-time $225 per credit hour. *Tuition, nonresident:* full-time $11,000; part-time $1139 per credit hour. *Room and board:* $3826; room only: $2026 per academic year. *Required fees:* full-time $1500.

Financial Aid 50% of baccalaureate students in nursing programs received some form of financial aid in 2002–03.

Contact Dr. Vincent P. Hall, Department Head, Department of Nursing, Western Carolina University, 209 Moore Building, Cullowhee, NC 28723. *Telephone:* 828-227-7467. *Fax:* 828-227-7052.

GRADUATE PROGRAMS

Expenses (2003–04) *Tuition, state resident:* full-time $713; part-time $219 per credit hour. *Tuition, nonresident:* full-time $5254; part-time $1355 per degree program. *Room and board:* $3826; room only: $2026 per academic year. *Required fees:* full-time $3405.

Financial Aid 30% of graduate students in nursing programs received some form of financial aid in 2002–03.

Contact Dr. Valerie Matthiesen, RN, Director of MSN Program, Department of Nursing, Western Carolina University, AB Tech Campus—Suite 33, 1459 Sand Hill Road, Enka, NC 28715. *Telephone:* 828-670-8810 Ext. 222. *Fax:* 828-670-8807. *E-mail:* matthiesen@email.wcu.edu.

MASTER'S DEGREE PROGRAM

Degree MSN

Available Programs Master's.

Concentrations Available Nursing education. *Nurse practitioner programs in:* family health.

Site Options *Distance Learning:* Enka, NC.

Study Options Full-time and part-time.

Program Entrance Requirements Minimum overall college GPA of 3.0, transcript of college record, CPR certification, immunizations, 2 letters of recommendation, physical assessment course, professional liability insurance/malpractice insurance, statistics course.

Advanced Placement Credit given for nursing courses completed elsewhere dependent upon specific evaluations.

Degree Requirements Thesis or project, comprehensive exam.

POST-MASTER'S PROGRAM

Areas of Study Nursing education. *Nurse practitioner programs in:* family health.

POSTDOCTORAL PROGRAM

Postdoctoral Program Contact Dr. Sandra Grenieiicki, Head, Department of Nursing, Western Carolina University, Cullowhee, NC 28723. *Telephone:* 828-227-7467. *Fax:* 828-227-7071. *E-mail:* grenwicki@wcu.edu.

Winston-Salem State University

Department of Nursing
Winston-Salem, North Carolina

http://www.wssu.edu

Founded in 1892

DEGREES • BSN • MSN

Nursing Program Faculty 25 (24% with doctorates).

Baccalaureate Enrollment 229

Women 77% **Men** 23% **Minority** 75% **Part-time** 17%

Graduate Enrollment 15

Nursing Student Activities Nursing Honor Society, Sigma Theta Tau, Student Nurses' Association.

Nursing Student Resources Academic advising; campus computer network; computer lab; interactive nursing skills videos; learning resource lab; nursing audiovisuals; skills, simulation, or other laboratory.

Library Facilities 197,765 volumes (10,664 in nursing); 1,010 periodical subscriptions (182 health-care related).

BACCALAUREATE PROGRAMS

Degree BSN

Available Programs ADN to Baccalaureate; Baccalaureate for Second Degree; Generic Baccalaureate; RN Baccalaureate.

Site Options *Distance Learning:* Wilkesboro, NC; Salisbury, NC; Boone, NC.

Study Options Full-time.

Program Entrance Requirements Minimum overall college GPA of 2.6, transcript of college record, CPR certification, health exam, immunizations, professional liability insurance/malpractice insurance, prerequisite course work. Transfer students are accepted. **Standardized tests** *Required:* SAT or ACT, TOEFL for international students. **Application** *Deadline:* rolling (freshmen), rolling (transfer). *Application fee:* $30.

Advanced Placement Credit by examination available. Credit given for nursing courses completed elsewhere dependent upon specific evaluations.

Expenses (2003–04) *Tuition, state resident:* full-time $1226; part-time $153 per credit hour. *Tuition, nonresident:* full-time $9491; part-time $1186 per credit hour. *Room and board:* $2446; room only: $1443 per academic year. *Required fees:* full-time $1168; part-time $154 per credit.

Financial Aid 80% of baccalaureate students in nursing programs received some form of financial aid in 2002–03. *Gift aid (need-based):* Federal Pell, FSEOG, state, private, college/university gift aid from institutional funds, United Negro College Fund. *Loans:* FFEL (Subsidized and Unsubsidized Stafford PLUS), Perkins, state, college/university. *Work-Study:* Federal Work-Study, part-time campus jobs. *Application deadline:* 4/1 (priority: 3/1).

Contact Ms. Nancy McInnis, Assistant to the Dean, Department of Nursing, Winston-Salem State University, 601 Martin Luther King Jr. Drive, Winston-Salem, NC 27110. *Telephone:* 336-750-2560. *Fax:* 336-750-2599. *E-mail:* mcinnisn@wssn.edu.

GRADUATE PROGRAMS

Expenses (2003–04) *Tuition, state resident:* full-time $1285; part-time $161 per credit hour. *Tuition, nonresident:* full-time $9703; part-time $1213 per credit hour. *Required fees:* full-time $1168; part-time $154 per credit.

Contact Bonnie Pope, RN, Interim Chair MSN Program, Department of Nursing, Winston-Salem State University, 601 Martin Luther King Jr. Drive, Winston-Salem, NC 27110. *Telephone:* 336-750-2298. *Fax:* 336-750-2599. *E-mail:* popeb@wssu.edu.

MASTER'S DEGREE PROGRAM

Degree MSN

Available Programs Master's.

Concentrations Available *Nurse practitioner programs in:* family health, psychiatric/mental health.

Study Options Full-time and part-time.

Program Entrance Requirements Clinical experience, transcript of college record, CPR certification, immunizations, interview, 3 letters of recommendation, physical assessment course, professional liability insurance/malpractice insurance, resume.

Advanced Placement Credit given for nursing courses completed elsewhere dependent upon specific evaluations.

Degree Requirements 50 total credit hours, thesis or project.

CONTINUING EDUCATION PROGRAM

Contact Ms. Nancy McInnis, Assistant to the Dean, Department of Nursing, Winston-Salem State University, 601 Martin Luther King Jr. Drive, Winston-Salem, NC 27110. *Telephone:* 336-750-2560. *Fax:* 336-750-2599. *E-mail:* McInnisN@wssu.edu.

NORTH DAKOTA

Dickinson State University

Department of Nursing
Dickinson, North Dakota

http://www.dsu.nodak.edu/Catalog/nursing.htm

Founded in 1918

DEGREE • BSN

Nursing Program Faculty 4.

Baccalaureate Enrollment 35

Women 96% **Men** 4% **Part-time** 10%

Nursing Student Activities Student Nurses' Association.

Nursing Student Resources Academic advising; academic or career counseling; assistance for students with disabilities; bookstore; campus computer network; career placement assistance; computer lab; computer-assisted instruction; e-mail services; employment services for current students; housing assistance; Internet; learning resource lab; library services; nursing audiovisuals; placement services for program completers; remedial services; resume preparation assistance; skills, simulation, or other laboratory; tutoring.

Library Facilities 105,713 volumes (3,158 in health, 595 in nursing); 823 periodical subscriptions (1,538 health-care related).

BACCALAUREATE PROGRAMS

Degree BSN

Available Programs ADN to Baccalaureate; LPN to Baccalaureate; RN Baccalaureate.

Study Options Full-time and part-time.

Program Entrance Requirements Minimum overall college GPA of 2.5, transcript of college record, health exam, immunizations, minimum GPA in nursing prerequisites of 2.5, prerequisite course work, RN licensure. Transfer students are accepted. **Standardized tests** *Required:* SAT or ACT, TOEFL for international students. **Application** *Deadline:* rolling (freshmen), rolling (transfer). *Notification:* continuous (freshmen). *Application fee:* $35.

Advanced Placement Credit given for nursing courses completed elsewhere dependent upon specific evaluations.

Expenses (2004–05) *Tuition, state resident:* full-time $3799; part-time $158 per credit hour. *Tuition, nonresident:* full-time $8876; part-time $180 per credit hour. *International tuition:* $8876 full-time. *Room and board:* $2258; room only: $1260 per academic year.

Financial Aid 90% of baccalaureate students in nursing programs received some form of financial aid in 2003–04. *Gift aid (need-based):* Federal Pell, FSEOG, state, college/university gift aid from institutional funds, National Guard tuition waivers, staff waivers. *Loans:* Federal Nursing Student Loans, FFEL (Subsidized and Unsubsidized Stafford PLUS), Perkins, state, college/university, Alaska Loans, alternative loans. *Work-Study:* Federal Work-Study, part-time campus jobs. *Application deadline (priority):* 3/15.

Contact Ms. Mary Anne Marsh, Chair, Department of Nursing, Dickinson State University, 291 Campus Drive, Dickinson, ND 58601-4896. *Telephone:* 701-483-2133. *Fax:* 701-483-2524.

Jamestown College
Department of Nursing
Jamestown, North Dakota

Founded in 1883

DEGREE • BSN

Nursing Program Faculty 11 (9% with doctorates).

Baccalaureate Enrollment 80

Nursing Student Activities Sigma Theta Tau, Student Nurses' Association.

Nursing Student Resources Academic advising; academic or career counseling; bookstore; campus computer network; computer lab; computer-assisted instruction; e-mail services; externships; interactive nursing skills videos; Internet; learning resource lab; library services; nursing audiovisuals; resume preparation assistance; skills, simulation, or other laboratory; tutoring.

Library Facilities 121,382 volumes (990 in health, 983 in nursing); 630 periodical subscriptions (163 health-care related).

BACCALAUREATE PROGRAMS

Degree BSN

Study Options Full-time and part-time.

Program Entrance Requirements Minimum overall college GPA of 3.0, transcript of college record, written essay, high school transcript, immunizations, prerequisite course work. Transfer students are accepted. **Standardized tests** *Required:* SAT and SAT Subject Tests or ACT, TOEFL for international students. *Recommended:* SAT or ACT. **Application** *Deadline:* rolling (freshmen), rolling (transfer). *Application fee:* $20.

Advanced Placement Credit given for nursing courses completed elsewhere dependent upon specific evaluations.

Financial Aid 90% of baccalaureate students in nursing programs received some form of financial aid in 2002–03.

Contact Admissions Department, Department of Nursing, Jamestown College, 6081 College Lane, Jamestown, ND 58405. *Telephone:* 701-252-3467 Ext. 2562. *Fax:* 701-253-4318.

Medcenter One College of Nursing
Medcenter One College of Nursing
Bismarck, North Dakota

http://www.college.medcenterone.com

Founded in 1988

DEGREE • BSN

Nursing Program Faculty 14.

Baccalaureate Enrollment 88

Women 92% **Men** 8% **Minority** 8% **Part-time** 2%

Nursing Student Activities Sigma Theta Tau, Student Nurses' Association.

Nursing Student Resources Academic advising; assistance for students with disabilities; bookstore; computer lab; computer-assisted instruction; e-mail services; Internet; library services; nursing audiovisuals; placement services for program completers; resume preparation assistance; skills, simulation, or other laboratory; tutoring.

Library Facilities 28,470 volumes (30,118 in health); 331 periodical subscriptions (327 health-care related).

BACCALAUREATE PROGRAMS

Degree BSN

Available Programs ADN to Baccalaureate; LPN to RN Baccalaureate; RN Baccalaureate.

Study Options Full-time and part-time.

Program Entrance Requirements Minimum overall college GPA of 2.5, transcript of college record, CPR certification, written essay, health exam, high school transcript, immunizations, interview, minimum GPA in nursing prerequisites of 2.5, prerequisite course work. Transfer students are accepted. **Application** *Deadline:* 11/7 (transfer). *Application fee:* $40.

Advanced Placement Credit given for nursing courses completed elsewhere dependent upon specific evaluations.

Expenses (2004–05) *Tuition:* full-time $8000; part-time $334 per credit hour. *Room and board:* room only: $1800 per academic year. *Required fees:* full-time $620.

Financial Aid 98% of baccalaureate students in nursing programs received some form of financial aid in 2003–04. *Gift aid (need-based):* Federal Pell, FSEOG, state, private, college/university gift aid from institutional funds. *Loans:* Federal Nursing Student Loans, FFEL (Subsidized and Unsubsidized Stafford PLUS), Perkins, college/university. *Work-Study:* Federal Work-Study. *Application deadline (priority):* 5/1.

Contact Ms. Mary Smith, RN, Director of Student Services, Medcenter One College of Nursing, 512 North 7th Street, Bismarck, ND 58501. *Telephone:* 701-323-6271. *Fax:* 701-323-6967. *E-mail:* msmith@mohs.org.

Minot State University
Department of Nursing
Minot, North Dakota

http://www.minotstateu.edu/nursing/index.html

Founded in 1913

DEGREE • BSN

Nursing Program Faculty 15 (13% with doctorates).

Baccalaureate Enrollment 130

Women 94% **Men** 6% **Minority** 10% **International** 78% **Part-time** 22%

Nursing Student Activities Sigma Theta Tau, Student Nurses' Association.

Nursing Student Resources Academic advising; academic or career counseling; assistance for students with disabilities; bookstore; campus computer network; career placement assistance; computer lab; computer-assisted instruction; e-mail services; housing assistance; interactive nursing skills videos; Internet; learning resource lab; library services; nursing audiovisuals; paid internships; resume preparation assistance; skills, simulation, or other laboratory; tutoring.

Library Facilities 420,971 volumes (6,926 in health, 1,385 in nursing); 752 periodical subscriptions (56 health-care related).

BACCALAUREATE PROGRAMS

Degree BSN

Available Programs Generic Baccalaureate; LPN to Baccalaureate; RN Baccalaureate.

Study Options Full-time.

Program Entrance Requirements Minimum overall college GPA of 2.5, transcript of college record, minimum GPA in nursing prerequisites of 2.0, prerequisite course work. Transfer students are accepted. **Standardized tests** *Required:* SAT or ACT, TOEFL for international students. **Application** *Deadline:* rolling (freshmen), rolling (transfer). *Notification:* continuous (freshmen). *Application fee:* $35.

Advanced Placement Credit given for nursing courses completed elsewhere dependent upon specific evaluations.

Expenses (2004–05) *Tuition, state resident:* full-time $3160. *Tuition, nonresident:* full-time $8437. *Required fees:* full-time $552.

Financial Aid *Gift aid (need-based):* Federal Pell, FSEOG, state, college/university gift aid from institutional funds, Federal Nursing. *Loans:* Federal Nursing Student Loans, FFEL (Subsidized and Unsubsidized Stafford PLUS), Perkins, college/university. *Work-Study:* Federal Work-Study. *Application deadline (priority):* 3/15.

Contact Dr. Elizabeth Pross, RN, Department Chair, Department of Nursing, Minot State University, 500 University Avenue West, Minot, ND 58707-0002. *Telephone:* 701-858-3101. *Fax:* 701-858-4309. *E-mail:* Elizabeth.Pross@minotstateu.edu.

North Dakota State University
Tri-College University Nursing Consortium
Fargo, North Dakota

http://www.ndsu.nodak.edu/instruct/nysveen/nursing

Founded in 1890

DEGREES • BSN • MS

Nursing Program Faculty 12 (49% with doctorates).

Baccalaureate Enrollment 107
Women 88% **Men** 12% **Minority** 7% **Part-time** 9%

Graduate Enrollment 19
Women 100% **Part-time** 80%

Nursing Student Activities Sigma Theta Tau, Student Nurses' Association.

Nursing Student Resources Academic advising; academic or career counseling; assistance for students with disabilities; bookstore; campus computer network; career placement assistance; computer lab; computer-assisted instruction; daycare for children of students; e-mail services; employment services for current students; externships; interactive nursing skills videos; Internet; learning resource lab; library services; nursing audiovisuals; paid internships; placement services for program completers; remedial services; resume preparation assistance; skills, simulation, or other laboratory; tutoring; unpaid internships.

Library Facilities 303,274 volumes (8,524 in health, 1,779 in nursing); 4,497 periodical subscriptions (100 health-care related).

BACCALAUREATE PROGRAMS

Degree BSN

Available Programs Generic Baccalaureate; LPN to Baccalaureate.

Study Options Full-time.

Program Entrance Requirements Minimum overall college GPA of 2.8, transcript of college record, 2 letters of recommendation, minimum GPA in nursing prerequisites of 2.8, prerequisite course work. Transfer students are accepted. **Standardized tests** *Required:* SAT or ACT, TOEFL for international students. **Application** *Deadline:* 8/15 (freshmen), 8/15 (transfer). *Notification:* continuous (freshmen). *Application fee:* $35.

Advanced Placement Credit by examination available. Credit given for nursing courses completed elsewhere dependent upon specific evaluations.

Expenses (2004–05) *Tuition, state resident:* full-time $3981; part-time $166 per credit hour. *Tuition, nonresident:* full-time $10,629. *International tuition:* $16,808 full-time. *Room and board:* $4727 per academic year. *Required fees:* full-time $1436; part-time $200 per credit.

Financial Aid 90% of baccalaureate students in nursing programs received some form of financial aid in 2003–04.

Contact Ms. Gloria J. Nysveen, Administrative Secretary, Tri-College University Nursing Consortium, North Dakota State University, 136 Sudro Hall, PO Box 5055, Fargo, ND 58105-5055. *Telephone:* 701-231-7395. *Fax:* 701-231-7606. *E-mail:* Gloria.Nysveen@ndsu.nodak.edu.

GRADUATE PROGRAMS

Expenses (2004–05) *Tuition, state resident:* part-time $350 per credit hour. *Tuition, nonresident:* part-time $350 per credit hour. *Required fees:* part-time $30 per credit.

Financial Aid 35% of graduate students in nursing programs received some form of financial aid in 2003–04.

Contact Dr. Jane Giedt, RN, Director, Graduate Program, Tri-College University Nursing Consortium, North Dakota State University, 214 Murray Commons, 1104 7th Avenue South, Moorhead, MN 56563. *Telephone:* 218-477-4699. *Fax:* 218-477-5990. *E-mail:* giedt@mnstate.edu.

MASTER'S DEGREE PROGRAM

Degree MS

Available Programs Master's.

Concentrations Available Nursing education. *Clinical nurse specialist programs in:* adult health. *Nurse practitioner programs in:* family health.

Site Options Moorhead, MN.

Study Options Full-time and part-time.

Program Entrance Requirements Computer literacy, minimum overall college GPA of 3.0, transcript of college record, CPR certification, immunizations, interview, 3 letters of recommendation, nursing research course, physical assessment course, professional liability insurance/malpractice insurance, resume, statistics course.

Advanced Placement Credit given for nursing courses completed elsewhere dependent upon specific evaluations.

Degree Requirements 54 total credit hours, thesis or project, comprehensive exam.

POST-MASTER'S PROGRAM

Areas of Study *Nurse practitioner programs in:* family health.

CONTINUING EDUCATION PROGRAM

Contact Dr. Mary Margaret Mooney, PBVM, Professor and Chair.

University of Mary
Division of Nursing
Bismarck, North Dakota

http://www.umary.edu/AcadInfo/NurDiv

Founded in 1959

DEGREES • BSN • MSN

Nursing Program Faculty 21 (10% with doctorates).

Library Facilities 65,842 volumes (10,425 in health, 3,000 in nursing); 584 periodical subscriptions (125 health-care related).

BACCALAUREATE PROGRAMS

Degree BSN

Available Programs Generic Baccalaureate; LPN to Baccalaureate; RN Baccalaureate.

Study Options Full-time and part-time.

Program Entrance Requirements Minimum overall college GPA of 2.5, transcript of college record, CPR certification, written essay, health exam, high school transcript, immunizations, 2 letters of recommendation, minimum GPA in nursing prerequisites of 2.0, professional liability insurance/malpractice insurance, prerequisite course work. Transfer students are accepted. **Standardized tests** *Required:* SAT or ACT, TOEFL for international students. **Application** *Deadline:* rolling (freshmen), rolling (transfer). *Application fee:* $25.

Advanced Placement Credit by examination available. Credit given for nursing courses completed elsewhere dependent upon specific evaluations.

Expenses (2003–04) *Tuition:* full-time $9600; part-time $60 per credit hour.

Contact Admissions Office, Division of Nursing, University of Mary, 7500 University Drive, Bismarck, ND 58504. *Telephone:* 701-255-7500. *Fax:* 701-255-7687.

GRADUATE PROGRAMS

Expenses (2003–04) *Tuition:* part-time $365 per credit hour.

Financial Aid 14 fellowships, 3 teaching assistantships were awarded; institutionally sponsored loans also available.

Contact Chairperson, Division of Nursing, University of Mary, 7500 University Drive, Bismarck, ND 58504. *Telephone:* 701-255-7500. *Fax:* 701-255-7687.

MASTER'S DEGREE PROGRAM

Degree MSN

Available Programs Master's.

Concentrations Available Nursing education. *Nurse practitioner programs in:* family health.

Study Options Full-time and part-time.

Program Entrance Requirements Clinical experience, minimum overall college GPA of 3.0, transcript of college record, CPR certification, written essay, immunizations, interview, 3 letters of recommendation, physical assessment course. *Application deadline:* For fall admission, 4/15 (priority date). Applications are processed on a rolling basis. *Application fee:* $40.

Degree Requirements 39 total credit hours, thesis or project, comprehensive exam.

University of North Dakota

College of Nursing
Grand Forks, North Dakota

http://www.und.nodak.edu/dept/nursing

Founded in 1883

DEGREES • BSN • MS • PHD

Nursing Program Faculty 54 (33% with doctorates).

Baccalaureate Enrollment 303
Women 91% **Men** 9% **Minority** 11% **International** 1% **Part-time** 22%

Graduate Enrollment 75
Women 90% **Men** 10% **Minority** 7% **International** 3% **Part-time** 60%

Nursing Student Activities Sigma Theta Tau, Student Nurses' Association.

Nursing Student Resources Academic advising; academic or career counseling; assistance for students with disabilities; bookstore; campus computer network; career placement assistance; computer lab; computer-assisted instruction; daycare for children of students; e-mail services; employment services for current students; externships; housing assistance; interactive nursing skills videos; Internet; learning resource lab; library services; nursing audiovisuals; paid internships; remedial services; resume preparation assistance; skills, simulation, or other laboratory; tutoring.

Library Facilities 925,367 volumes (83,000 in health, 2,368 in nursing); 18,955 periodical subscriptions (1,074 health-care related).

BACCALAUREATE PROGRAMS

Degree BSN

Available Programs ADN to Baccalaureate; Generic Baccalaureate; LPN to Baccalaureate; LPN to RN Baccalaureate; RN Baccalaureate.

Site Options *Distance Learning:* Grand Forks, ND.

Study Options Full-time and part-time.

Program Entrance Requirements Minimum overall college GPA of 2.5, transcript of college record, CPR certification, written essay, health insurance, immunizations, minimum GPA in nursing prerequisites of 2.5, prerequisite course work. Transfer students are accepted. **Standardized tests** *Required:* SAT or ACT, TOEFL for international students. *Recommended:* ACT. **Application** *Deadline:* 7/1 (freshmen), rolling (transfer). *Notification:* continuous (freshmen). *Application fee:* $35.

Advanced Placement Credit by examination available. Credit given for nursing courses completed elsewhere dependent upon specific evaluations.

Expenses (2004–05) *Tuition, state resident:* full-time $4009; part-time $222 per credit hour. *Tuition, nonresident:* full-time $6832; part-time $306 per credit hour. *International tuition:* $11,522 full-time. *Room and board:* $4398 per academic year. *Required fees:* full-time $1119.

Financial Aid 89% of baccalaureate students in nursing programs received some form of financial aid in 2003–04. *Gift aid (need-based):* Federal Pell, FSEOG, state, private, college/university gift aid from institutional funds. *Loans:* Federal Nursing Student Loans, FFEL (Subsidized and Unsubsidized Stafford PLUS), Perkins. *Work-Study:* Federal Work-Study. *Application deadline (priority):* 3/15.

Contact Mr. Marlys Escobar, Director of Student and Alumni Affairs, College of Nursing, University of North Dakota, UND College of Nursing, PO Box 9025, Grand Forks, ND 58202-9025. *Telephone:* 701-777-4548. *Fax:* 701-777-4096. *E-mail:* marlysescobar@mail.und.nodak.edu.

GRADUATE PROGRAMS

Expenses (2004–05) *Tuition, state resident:* full-time $6468; part-time $180 per credit hour. *Tuition, nonresident:* full-time $17,277; part-time $480 per credit hour. *International tuition:* $17,973 full-time. *Room and board:* $4454; room only: $1824 per academic year. *Required fees:* full-time $2729; part-time $97 per credit; part-time $909 per term.

Financial Aid 65% of graduate students in nursing programs received some form of financial aid in 2003–04. 6 research assistantships (averaging $9,747 per year), 9 teaching assistantships with full tuition reimbursements available (averaging $10,655 per year) were awarded; fellowships, Federal Work-Study, institutionally sponsored loans, scholarships, traineeships, and tuition waivers (full and partial) also available. Aid available to part-time students. *Financial aid application deadline:* 3/15.

Contact Dr. Ginny W. Guido, Director of Graduate Studies, College of Nursing, University of North Dakota, PO Box 9025, Grand Forks, ND 58202-9025. *Telephone:* 701-777-4552. *Fax:* 701-777-4096. *E-mail:* ginnyguido@mail.und.nodak.edu.

MASTER'S DEGREE PROGRAM

Degree MS

Available Programs Master's.

Concentrations Available Nurse anesthesia; nursing administration; nursing education. *Clinical nurse specialist programs in:* acute care, adult health, community health, family health, gerontology, home health care, psychiatric/mental health. *Nurse practitioner programs in:* family health, psychiatric/mental health.

Site Options *Distance Learning:* Grand Forks, ND.

Study Options Full-time and part-time.

Program Entrance Requirements Clinical experience, minimum overall college GPA of 3.0, transcript of college record, CPR certification, written essay, immunizations, interview, 3 letters of recommendation, prerequisite course work, resume, statistics course. *Application deadline:* For fall admission, 12/15. *Application fee:* $35.

Advanced Placement Credit given for nursing courses completed elsewhere dependent upon specific evaluations.

Degree Requirements 36 total credit hours, thesis or project.

POST-MASTER'S PROGRAM

Areas of Study Nurse anesthesia; nursing education. *Clinical nurse specialist programs in:* psychiatric/mental health. *Nurse practitioner programs in:* family health, psychiatric/mental health.

DOCTORAL DEGREE PROGRAM

Degree PhD

Available Programs Doctorate.

Areas of Study Faculty preparation, health promotion/disease prevention, nursing research.

Site Options *Distance Learning:* Grand Forks, ND.

Program Entrance Requirements Minimum overall college GPA of 3.5, interview by faculty committee, interview, 3 letters of recommendation, MSN or equivalent, statistics course, vita, GRE or MAT. *Application deadline:* For fall admission, 12/15. *Application fee:* $35.

Degree Requirements 90 total credit hours, dissertation, oral exam, written exam, residency.

OHIO

Ashland University

Department of Nursing
Ashland, Ohio

http://www.ashland.edu

Founded in 1878

DEGREE • BSN

Nursing Program Faculty 5 (50% with doctorates).

Baccalaureate Enrollment 50
Women 96% **Men** 4% **Minority** 12% **Part-time** 96%

Nursing Student Activities Sigma Theta Tau.

Ashland University (continued)

Nursing Student Resources Academic advising; academic or career counseling; assistance for students with disabilities; bookstore; campus computer network; career placement assistance; computer lab; computer-assisted instruction; e-mail services; Internet; library services; nursing audiovisuals; placement services for program completers; remedial services; resume preparation assistance; skills, simulation, or other laboratory; tutoring.

Library Facilities 205,200 volumes; 1,625 periodical subscriptions.

BACCALAUREATE PROGRAMS

Degree BSN

Available Programs RN Baccalaureate.

Site Options Middleburg Heights, OH; Mansfield, OH; Canton, OH.

Study Options Full-time and part-time.

Program Entrance Requirements Minimum overall college GPA of 2.0, transcript of college record, minimum GPA in nursing prerequisites of 2.0, prerequisite course work. Transfer students are accepted. **Standardized tests** *Required:* SAT or ACT, TOEFL for international students. **Application** *Deadline:* rolling (freshmen), rolling (transfer). *Notification:* continuous (freshmen). *Application fee:* $25.

Advanced Placement Credit by examination available. Credit given for nursing courses completed elsewhere dependent upon specific evaluations.

Expenses (2004–05) *Tuition:* part-time $363 per credit hour. *Required fees:* part-time $45 per term.

Financial Aid 45% of baccalaureate students in nursing programs received some form of financial aid in 2003–04. *Gift aid (need-based):* Federal Pell, FSEOG, state, private, college/university gift aid from institutional funds. *Loans:* Federal Direct (Subsidized and Unsubsidized Stafford PLUS), Perkins, college/university. *Work-Study:* Federal Work-Study, part-time campus jobs. *Application deadline:* 3/15.

Contact Dr. Dorothy A. Stitzlein, Chair, Department of Nursing, Ashland University, 401 College Avenue, Ashland, OH 44805. *Telephone:* 419-289-5242. *Fax:* 419-289-5989. *E-mail:* dstitzle@ashland.edu.

Capital University
School of Nursing
Columbus, Ohio

http://www.capital.edu/nursing/nurshome.shtml

Founded in 1830

DEGREES • BSN • MSN

Nursing Program Faculty 35 (40% with doctorates).

Baccalaureate Enrollment 250
Women 95% **Men** 5% **Minority** 6% **International** 2% **Part-time** 25%

Graduate Enrollment 80
Women 95% **Men** 5% **Minority** 4% **Part-time** 75%

Nursing Student Activities Sigma Theta Tau, Student Nurses' Association.

Nursing Student Resources Academic advising; academic or career counseling; assistance for students with disabilities; bookstore; campus computer network; computer lab; computer-assisted instruction; e-mail services; interactive nursing skills videos; Internet; learning resource lab; library services; nursing audiovisuals; resume preparation assistance; skills, simulation, or other laboratory; tutoring.

Library Facilities 187,281 volumes (6,209 in health); 3,741 periodical subscriptions (82 health-care related).

BACCALAUREATE PROGRAMS

Degree BSN

Available Programs Accelerated Baccalaureate for Second Degree; Generic Baccalaureate; RN Baccalaureate.

Site Options Dayton, OH.

Study Options Full-time.

Program Entrance Requirements Minimum overall college GPA of 2.5, transcript of college record, CPR certification, health exam, high school biology, high school chemistry, high school foreign language, 3 years high school math, 3 years high school science, high school transcript, immunizations, minimum high school GPA of 3.0, professional liability insurance/malpractice insurance. Transfer students are accepted. **Standardized tests** *Required:* SAT or ACT, TOEFL for international students. **Application** *Deadline:* 4/15 (freshmen), rolling (transfer). *Early decision:* 9/22. *Notification:* 9/15 (freshmen), 10/2 (early action). *Application fee:* $25.

Advanced Placement Credit by examination available. Credit given for nursing courses completed elsewhere dependent upon specific evaluations.

Financial Aid 95% of baccalaureate students in nursing programs received some form of financial aid in 2003–04. *Gift aid (need-based):* Federal Pell, FSEOG, state, private, college/university gift aid from institutional funds. *Loans:* Federal Nursing Student Loans, FFEL (Subsidized and Unsubsidized Stafford PLUS), Perkins, state, college/university. *Work-Study:* Federal Work-Study, part-time campus jobs. *Application deadline (priority):* 2/28.

Contact Dr. Elaine F. Haynes, Dean and Professor, School of Nursing, Capital University, 2199 East Main Street, Columbus, OH 43209-2394. *Telephone:* 614-236-6703. *Fax:* 614-236-6157. *E-mail:* ehaynes@capital.edu.

GRADUATE PROGRAMS

Financial Aid Career-related internships or fieldwork available.

Contact Dr. Elaine F. Haynes, Dean and Professor, School of Nursing, Capital University, 2199 East Main Street, Columbus, OH 43209-2394. *Telephone:* 614-236-6703. *Fax:* 614-236-6157. *E-mail:* ehaynes@capital.edu.

MASTER'S DEGREE PROGRAM

Degree MSN

Available Programs Master's; RN to Master's.

Concentrations Available Nursing administration; nursing education. *Clinical nurse specialist programs in:* community health, family health, occupational health, school health.

Study Options Full-time and part-time.

Program Entrance Requirements Computer literacy, minimum overall college GPA of 3.0, transcript of college record, CPR certification, written essay, immunizations, 3 letters of recommendation, nursing research course, physical assessment course, professional liability insurance/malpractice insurance, prerequisite course work, resume, statistics course. *Application deadline:* For fall admission, 8/1 (priority date); for spring admission, 12/1. Applications are processed on a rolling basis. *Application fee:* $25.

Advanced Placement Credit given for nursing courses completed elsewhere dependent upon specific evaluations.

Degree Requirements 36 total credit hours, thesis or project.

Case Western Reserve University
Frances Payne Bolton School of Nursing
Cleveland, Ohio

http://fpb.case.edu

Founded in 1826

DEGREES • BSN • MSN • MSN/MA • MSN/MBA • MSN/MPH • MSN/PHD

Nursing Program Faculty 81 (55% with doctorates).

Baccalaureate Enrollment 222
Women 89% **Men** 11% **Minority** 18%

Graduate Enrollment 493
Women 87% **Men** 13% **Minority** 25% **International** 9% **Part-time** 56%

Nursing Student Activities Nursing Honor Society, Sigma Theta Tau, Student Nurses' Association.

Nursing Student Resources Academic advising; academic or career counseling; assistance for students with disabilities; bookstore; campus computer network; career placement assistance; computer lab; computer-assisted instruction; e-mail services; employment services for current students; housing assistance; interactive nursing skills videos; Internet; learning resource lab; library services; nursing audiovisuals; placement services for program completers; remedial services; resume preparation assistance; skills, simulation, or other laboratory; tutoring.

Library Facilities 2.5 million volumes (475,000 in health); 20,678 periodical subscriptions (2,500 health-care related).

BACCALAUREATE PROGRAMS

Degree BSN

Available Programs ADN to Baccalaureate; Generic Baccalaureate; RN Baccalaureate.

Study Options Full-time.

Program Entrance Requirements Transcript of college record, CPR certification, written essay, high school biology, high school chemistry, 2 years high school science, high school transcript, immunizations, 2 letters of recommendation, minimum high school GPA of 3.0, professional liability insurance/malpractice insurance. Transfer students are accepted. **Standardized tests** *Required:* SAT or ACT, TOEFL for international students. *Recommended:* SAT Subject Tests. **Application** *Deadline:* 1/15 (freshmen), 5/15 (transfer). *Early decision:* 11/15. *Notification:* 3/1 (freshmen), 1/15 (early action). *Application fee:* $35.

Advanced Placement Credit given for nursing courses completed elsewhere dependent upon specific evaluations.

Expenses (2004–05) *Tuition:* full-time $26,500; part-time $1104 per credit hour. *International tuition:* $26,500 full-time. *Room and board:* $7802; room only: $4710 per academic year. *Required fees:* full-time $2206; part-time $50 per term.

Financial Aid 100% of baccalaureate students in nursing programs received some form of financial aid in 2003–04. *Gift aid (need-based):* Federal Pell, FSEOG, state, private, college/university gift aid from institutional funds. *Loans:* Federal Nursing Student Loans, Federal Direct (Subsidized and Unsubsidized Stafford), FFEL, Perkins, state, college/university. *Work-Study:* Federal Work-Study. *Application deadline (priority):* 2/15.

Contact Office of Student Services, Frances Payne Bolton School of Nursing, Case Western Reserve University, 10900 Euclid Avenue, Cleveland, OH 44106-4904. *Telephone:* 216-368-2529. *Fax:* 216-368-0124. *E-mail:* admissions@fpb.case.edu.

GRADUATE PROGRAMS

Expenses (2004–05) *Tuition:* part-time $1104 per credit hour. *Room and board:* $7802; room only: $4710 per academic year. *Required fees:* part-time $115 per term.

Financial Aid 90% of graduate students in nursing programs received some form of financial aid in 2003–04. 3 research assistantships, 6 teaching assistantships were awarded; fellowships, Federal Work-Study, institutionally sponsored loans, scholarships, and tuition waivers (partial) also available. Aid available to part-time students. *Financial aid application deadline:* 6/30.

Contact Office of Student Services, Frances Payne Bolton School of Nursing, Case Western Reserve University, 10900 Euclid Avenue, Cleveland, OH 44106-4904. *Telephone:* 216-368-2529. *Fax:* 216-368-3542. *E-mail:* admissions@fbp.case.edu.

MASTER'S DEGREE PROGRAM

Degrees MSN; MSN/MA; MSN/MBA; MSN/MPH; MSN/PhD

Available Programs Accelerated AD/RN to Master's; Accelerated Master's for Non-Nursing College Graduates; Accelerated Master's for Nurses with Non-Nursing Degrees; Master's; Master's for Non-Nursing College Graduates; Master's for Nurses with Non-Nursing Degrees.

Concentrations Available Nurse anesthesia; nurse-midwifery; nursing administration; nursing informatics. *Clinical nurse specialist programs in:* acute care, adult health, cardiovascular, community health, critical care, family health, gerontology, maternity-newborn, medical-surgical, oncology, pediatric, psychiatric/mental health, women's health. *Nurse practitioner programs in:* acute care, adult health, family health, gerontology, neonatal health, pediatric, psychiatric/mental health, women's health.

Study Options Full-time and part-time.

Program Entrance Requirements Minimum overall college GPA of 3.0, transcript of college record, CPR certification, written essay, 3 letters of recommendation, nursing research course, professional liability insurance/malpractice insurance, resume, statistics course, MAT or GRE General Test. *Application deadline:* For spring admission, 10/1. Applications are processed on a rolling basis. *Application fee:* $75.

Advanced Placement Credit given for nursing courses completed elsewhere dependent upon specific evaluations.

Degree Requirements 40 total credit hours.

POST-MASTER'S PROGRAM

Areas of Study Nurse anesthesia; nurse-midwifery; nursing education; nursing informatics. *Clinical nurse specialist programs in:* acute care, adult health, cardiovascular, community health, critical care, family health, maternity-newborn, medical-surgical, oncology, pediatric, psychiatric/mental health, women's health. *Nurse practitioner programs in:* acute care, adult health, family health, gerontology, neonatal health, pediatric, psychiatric/mental health, women's health.

DOCTORAL DEGREE PROGRAM

Degree PhD

Available Programs Doctorate; Doctorate for Nurses with Non-Nursing Degrees; Post-Baccalaureate Doctorate.

Areas of Study Aging, bio-behavioral research, community health, critical care, ethics, faculty preparation, family health, gerontology, health policy, health promotion/disease prevention, human health and illness, illness and transition, individualized study, maternity-newborn, nursing education, nursing research, nursing science, oncology, women's health.

Site Options Los Angeles, CA.

Program Entrance Requirements Minimum overall college GPA of 3.0, interview by faculty committee, interview, 3 letters of recommendation, statistics course, writing sample, GRE General Test, MAT (ND). *Application deadline:* For spring admission, 10/1. Applications are processed on a rolling basis. *Application fee:* $75.

Degree Requirements 36 total credit hours, dissertation, oral exam, residency.

POSTDOCTORAL PROGRAM

Areas of Study Aging, cancer care, chronic illness, community health, family health, gerontology, health promotion/disease prevention, individualized study, information systems, nursing interventions, nursing research, nursing science, outcomes, self-care, vulnerable population, women's health.

Postdoctoral Program Contact Dr. Shirley M. Moore, Professor and Associate Dean for Research, Frances Payne Bolton School of Nursing, Case Western Reserve University, 10900 Euclid Avenue, Cleveland, OH 44106-4904. *Telephone:* 216-368-5978. *Fax:* 216-368-3542. *E-mail:* shirley.moore@case.edu.

CONTINUING EDUCATION PROGRAM

Contact JoAnn Glick, RN, Lecturer of Nursing, Frances Payne Bolton School of Nursing, Case Western Reserve University, 10900 Euclid Avenue, Cleveland, OH 44106-4904. *Telephone:* 216-368-0480. *Fax:* 216-368-5303. *E-mail:* JoAnn.Glick@case.edu.

Cedarville University

Department of Nursing
Cedarville, Ohio

Founded in 1887

DEGREE • BSN

Nursing Program Faculty 25 (40% with doctorates).

Baccalaureate Enrollment 331
Women 91% **Men** 9% **Minority** 6%

Nursing Student Activities Nursing Honor Society, Sigma Theta Tau, Student Nurses' Association.

Nursing Student Resources Academic advising; academic or career counseling; assistance for students with disabilities; bookstore; campus computer network; career placement assistance; computer lab; computer-assisted instruction; e-mail services; housing assistance; interactive nursing skills videos; Internet; library services; nursing audiovisuals; paid internships; resume preparation assistance; skills, simulation, or other laboratory.

Library Facilities 162,195 volumes (4,754 in health, 979 in nursing); 5,250 periodical subscriptions (114 health-care related).

Cedarville University (continued)

BACCALAUREATE PROGRAMS

Degree BSN

Available Programs RN Baccalaureate.

Study Options Full-time.

Program Entrance Requirements Minimum overall college GPA of 2.5, transcript of college record, CPR certification, written essay, health exam, health insurance, high school biology, high school chemistry, high school foreign language, 4 years high school math, 4 years high school science, high school transcript, immunizations, 1 letter of recommendation, minimum high school GPA of 3.0, minimum high school rank 50%, minimum GPA in nursing prerequisites of 2.5, professional liability insurance/malpractice insurance, prerequisite course work. Transfer students are accepted. **Standardized tests** *Required:* SAT or ACT, SAT and SAT Subject Tests or ACT, TOEFL for international students. **Application** *Deadline:* rolling (freshmen). *Notification:* continuous (freshmen). *Application fee:* $30.

Advanced Placement Credit given for nursing courses completed elsewhere dependent upon specific evaluations.

Expenses (2004–05) *Tuition:* full-time $16,032. *Room and board:* $5010; room only: $2684 per academic year.

Financial Aid 89% of baccalaureate students in nursing programs received some form of financial aid in 2003–04. *Gift aid (need-based):* Federal Pell, FSEOG, state, private, college/university gift aid from institutional funds. *Loans:* Federal Nursing Student Loans, FFEL (Subsidized and Unsubsidized Stafford PLUS), Perkins, college/university. *Work-Study:* Federal Work-Study, part-time campus jobs. *Application deadline (priority):* 3/1.

Contact Mr. Roscoe Smith, Admissions, Department of Nursing, Cedarville University, 251 North Main Street, Cedarville, OH 45314-0601. *Telephone:* 800-233-2784. *Fax:* 937-766-7575. *E-mail:* admissions@cedarville.edu.

Cleveland State University

Department of Nursing
Cleveland, Ohio

http://www.csuohio.edu

Founded in 1964

DEGREES • BSN • MSN • MSN/MBA

Nursing Program Faculty 17 (60% with doctorates).

Baccalaureate Enrollment 195

Women 91% **Men** 9% **Minority** 26% **International** 1% **Part-time** 1%

Graduate Enrollment 17

Women 88% **Men** 12% **Minority** 24% **Part-time** 60%

Nursing Student Activities Sigma Theta Tau, Student Nurses' Association.

Nursing Student Resources Academic advising; bookstore; campus computer network; computer lab; e-mail services; interactive nursing skills videos; Internet; learning resource lab; nursing audiovisuals; skills, simulation, or other laboratory.

Library Facilities 484,914 volumes (6,000 in health, 70 in nursing); 6,186 periodical subscriptions (70 health-care related).

BACCALAUREATE PROGRAMS

Degree BSN

Available Programs ADN to Baccalaureate; Accelerated Baccalaureate; Accelerated Baccalaureate for Second Degree; Generic Baccalaureate; RN Baccalaureate.

Site Options Kirkland, OH.

Study Options Full-time and part-time.

Program Entrance Requirements Minimum overall college GPA of 2.5, transcript of college record, CPR certification, written essay, health exam, health insurance, high school transcript, immunizations, minimum GPA in nursing prerequisites of 2.5, professional liability insurance/malpractice insurance, prerequisite course work. Transfer students are accepted. **Standardized tests** *Required:* SAT or ACT, TOEFL for international students. **Application** *Deadline:* rolling (freshmen), 7/15 (transfer). *Notification:* continuous (freshmen). *Application fee:* $30.

Advanced Placement Credit given for nursing courses completed elsewhere dependent upon specific evaluations.

Expenses (2003–04) *Tuition, state resident:* full-time $6072; part-time $253 per credit hour. *Tuition, nonresident:* full-time $11,940; part-time $457 per credit hour. *International tuition:* $11,940 full-time. *Required fees:* part-time $75 per term.

Financial Aid 80% of baccalaureate students in nursing programs received some form of financial aid in 2002–03. *Gift aid (need-based):* Federal Pell, FSEOG, state, private, college/university gift aid from institutional funds. *Loans:* FFEL (Subsidized and Unsubsidized Stafford PLUS), Perkins, state, alternative loans. *Work-Study:* Federal Work-Study, part-time campus jobs. *Application deadline (priority):* 2/15.

Contact Mr. Ronald Mickler, Jr., Recruiter and Advisor, Department of Nursing, Cleveland State University, 2121 Euclid Avenue (RT 915), Cleveland, OH 44115. *Telephone:* 216-687-3810. *Fax:* 216-687-3556. *E-mail:* nurse.adviser@csuohio.edu.

GRADUATE PROGRAMS

Expenses (2003–04) *Tuition, state resident:* full-time $7680; part-time $320 per credit hour. *Tuition, nonresident:* full-time $15,156; part-time $631 per credit hour. *International tuition:* $15,156 full-time.

Contact Dr. Sharon Radzyminski, Graduate Program Director, Department of Nursing, Cleveland State University, 2121 Euclid Avenue (RT 915), Cleveland, OH 44115. *Telephone:* 216-687-3558. *Fax:* 216-687-3556. *E-mail:* s.radzyminski@csuohio.edu.

MASTER'S DEGREE PROGRAM

Degrees MSN; MSN/MBA

Available Programs Master's.

Concentrations Available Health-care administration.

Study Options Full-time and part-time.

Program Entrance Requirements Clinical experience, computer literacy, minimum overall college GPA of 3.0, transcript of college record, CPR certification, written essay, immunizations, 2 letters of recommendation, physical assessment course, professional liability insurance/malpractice insurance, resume, statistics course.

Advanced Placement Credit given for nursing courses completed elsewhere dependent upon specific evaluations.

Degree Requirements 38 total credit hours, thesis or project.

CONTINUING EDUCATION PROGRAM

Contact Dr. Vida Svarcas, Director, Nursing and Health Science Continuing Education, Department of Nursing, Cleveland State University, Euclid Building 103, 1824 East 24th Street, Cleveland, OH 44115. *Telephone:* 216-687-4843. *Fax:* 216-687-9399. *E-mail:* v.svarcas@csuohio.edu.

College of Mount St. Joseph

Department of Nursing
Cincinnati, Ohio

Founded in 1920

DEGREES • BSN • MN

Nursing Program Faculty 20 (40% with doctorates).

Baccalaureate Enrollment 177

Women 90% **Men** 10% **Minority** 20% **International** 2% **Part-time** 30%

Nursing Student Activities Nursing Honor Society, Sigma Theta Tau, Student Nurses' Association.

Nursing Student Resources Academic advising; academic or career counseling; assistance for students with disabilities; bookstore; campus computer network; career placement assistance; computer lab; computer-assisted instruction; daycare for children of students; e-mail services; employment services for current students; externships; housing assistance; interactive nursing skills videos; Internet; learning resource lab; library services; nursing audiovisuals; paid internships; placement services for program completers; remedial services; resume preparation assistance; skills, simulation, or other laboratory; tutoring.

Library Facilities 98,849 volumes (2,700 in health, 2,100 in nursing); 429 periodical subscriptions (1,800 health-care related).

BACCALAUREATE PROGRAMS

Degree BSN

Available Programs Accelerated RN Baccalaureate; Generic Baccalaureate.

Site Options Cincinnati, OH.

Study Options Full-time and part-time.

Program Entrance Requirements Minimum overall college GPA of 2.5, transcript of college record, CPR certification, health exam, health insurance, high school chemistry, 2 years high school math, 2 years high school science, high school transcript, immunizations, interview, minimum high school GPA of 2.25, minimum high school rank 60%, minimum GPA in nursing prerequisites of 2.5, professional liability insurance/malpractice insurance, prerequisite course work. Transfer students are accepted. **Standardized tests** *Required:* SAT or ACT, TOEFL for international students. **Application** *Deadline:* 8/15 (freshmen), 8/15 (transfer). *Notification:* continuous (freshmen). *Application fee:* $25.

Advanced Placement Credit by examination available. Credit given for nursing courses completed elsewhere dependent upon specific evaluations.

Expenses (2003–04) *Tuition:* full-time $16,000; part-time $400 per credit hour. *Room and board:* $5750; room only: $2875 per academic year. *Required fees:* full-time $840.

Financial Aid 85% of baccalaureate students in nursing programs received some form of financial aid in 2002–03.

Contact Dr. Darla Vale, Chairperson, Department of Nursing, College of Mount St. Joseph, 5701 Delhi Road, Cincinnati, OH 45233-1670. *Telephone:* 513-244-4511. *Fax:* 513-451-2547. *E-mail:* darla_vale@mail.msj.edu.

GRADUATE PROGRAMS

Expenses (2003–04) *Tuition:* full-time $24,000; part-time $32,000 per degree program. *Room and board:* $5750; room only: $2875 per academic year.

Contact Dr. Darla Vale, Chairperson, Department of Nursing, College of Mount St. Joseph, 5701 Delhi Road, Cincinnati, OH 45233. *Telephone:* 513-244-4322. *Fax:* 513-451-2547. *E-mail:* darla_vale@mail.msj.edu.

MASTER'S DEGREE PROGRAM

Degree MN

Available Programs Accelerated Master's; Accelerated Master's for Nurses with Non-Nursing Degrees.

Study Options Full-time.

Program Entrance Requirements Minimum overall college GPA of 3.0, transcript of college record, CPR certification, written essay, immunizations, interview, prerequisite course work, statistics course.

Advanced Placement Credit by examination available. Credit given for nursing courses completed elsewhere dependent upon specific evaluations.

Degree Requirements 64 total credit hours, thesis or project.

Franciscan University of Steubenville

Department of Nursing
Steubenville, Ohio

Founded in 1946

DEGREES • BSN • MSN

Nursing Program Faculty 15 (20% with doctorates).

Baccalaureate Enrollment 177
Women 91% **Men** 9% **Minority** 5% **International** 1% **Part-time** 5%

Graduate Enrollment 23
Women 78% **Men** 22% **Minority** 4% **Part-time** 83%

Nursing Student Activities Student Nurses' Association.

Nursing Student Resources Academic advising; academic or career counseling; assistance for students with disabilities; bookstore; campus computer network; computer lab; e-mail services; Internet; learning resource lab; library services; resume preparation assistance; tutoring.

Library Facilities 231,176 volumes (29,761 in health, 8,946 in nursing); 578 periodical subscriptions (178 health-care related).

BACCALAUREATE PROGRAMS

Degree BSN

Available Programs Generic Baccalaureate; RN Baccalaureate; RPN to Baccalaureate.

Study Options Full-time and part-time.

Program Entrance Requirements Minimum overall college GPA of 2.5, transcript of college record, health exam, health insurance, high school biology, high school chemistry, 2 years high school science, high school transcript, immunizations, 2 letters of recommendation, minimum high school GPA of 2.4, minimum GPA in nursing prerequisites of 2.5, professional liability insurance/malpractice insurance, prerequisite course work. Transfer students are accepted. **Standardized tests** *Required:* SAT or ACT, TOEFL for international students. **Application** *Deadline:* 5/1 (freshmen), rolling (transfer). *Notification:* 9/1 (freshmen). *Application fee:* $20.

Advanced Placement Credit by examination available. Credit given for nursing courses completed elsewhere dependent upon specific evaluations.

Expenses (2004–05) *Tuition:* full-time $21,050; part-time $505 per credit hour. *International tuition:* $21,050 full-time. *Room and board:* $2675 per academic year. *Required fees:* full-time $380; part-time $10 per credit.

Financial Aid 78% of baccalaureate students in nursing programs received some form of financial aid in 2003–04. *Gift aid (need-based):* Federal Pell, FSEOG, state, private, college/university gift aid from institutional funds. *Loans:* FFEL (Subsidized and Unsubsidized Stafford PLUS), Perkins, alternative loans. *Work-Study:* Federal Work-Study, part-time campus jobs. *Application deadline (priority):* 4/15.

Contact Dr. Carolyn Miller, Chairman, Department of Nursing, Franciscan University of Steubenville, Steubenville, OH 43952. *Telephone:* 740-283-6324. *Fax:* 740-283-6449. *E-mail:* cmiller@franciscan.edu.

GRADUATE PROGRAMS

Expenses (2004–05) *Tuition:* full-time $6480; part-time $360 per credit hour. *International tuition:* $6480 full-time. *Required fees:* full-time $180; part-time $10 per credit.

Financial Aid 50% of graduate students in nursing programs received some form of financial aid in 2003–04.

Contact Dr. Carolyn Miller, Director, Graduate Nursing, Department of Nursing, Franciscan University of Steubenville, 1235 University Boulevard, Steubenville, OH 43952-1763. *Telephone:* 740-284-7245. *Fax:* 740-283-6449. *E-mail:* cmiller@franciscan.edu.

MASTER'S DEGREE PROGRAM

Degree MSN

Available Programs Master's; RN to Master's.

Concentrations Available Nursing education. *Nurse practitioner programs in:* family health.

Study Options Full-time and part-time.

Program Entrance Requirements Clinical experience, minimum overall college GPA of 3.0, transcript of college record, interview, 2 letters of recommendation, nursing research course, physical assessment course, professional liability insurance/malpractice insurance, prerequisite course work, statistics course.

Advanced Placement Credit given for nursing courses completed elsewhere dependent upon specific evaluations.

Degree Requirements 48 total credit hours, thesis or project.

Kent State University

College of Nursing
Kent, Ohio

http://www.kent.edu/nursing

Founded in 1910

DEGREES • BSN • MSN • MSN/MBA • MSN/MPA • PHD

Kent State University (continued)
Nursing Program Faculty 65 (48% with doctorates).

Baccalaureate Enrollment 642
Women 89% **Men** 11% **Minority** 8% **International** 1% **Part-time** 12%

Nursing Student Activities Sigma Theta Tau, Student Nurses' Association.

Nursing Student Resources Academic advising; academic or career counseling; assistance for students with disabilities; bookstore; campus computer network; career placement assistance; computer lab; computer-assisted instruction; e-mail services; employment services for current students; externships; housing assistance; interactive nursing skills videos; Internet; learning resource lab; library services; nursing audiovisuals; other; placement services for program completers; remedial services; resume preparation assistance; skills, simulation, or other laboratory; tutoring.

Library Facilities 2.3 million volumes; 11,139 periodical subscriptions.

BACCALAUREATE PROGRAMS

Degree BSN

Available Programs ADN to Baccalaureate; Accelerated Baccalaureate; Accelerated Baccalaureate for Second Degree; Accelerated RN Baccalaureate; Baccalaureate for Second Degree; Generic Baccalaureate; LPN to Baccalaureate; RN Baccalaureate.

Site Options *Distance Learning:* Salem, OH; Warren, OH; Canton, OH.

Study Options Full-time and part-time.

Program Entrance Requirements Transcript of college record, written essay, immunizations, interview, letters of recommendation, minimum high school GPA, minimum GPA in nursing prerequisites of 2.5. Transfer students are accepted. **Standardized tests** *Required:* SAT or ACT, TOEFL for international students. **Application** *Deadline:* 5/1 (freshmen). *Application fee:* $30.

Advanced Placement Credit given for nursing courses completed elsewhere dependent upon specific evaluations.

Financial Aid 85% of baccalaureate students in nursing programs received some form of financial aid in 2003–04. *Gift aid (need-based):* Federal Pell, FSEOG, state, private, college/university gift aid from institutional funds. *Loans:* Federal Nursing Student Loans, Federal Direct (Subsidized and Unsubsidized Stafford PLUS), Perkins, state, college/university, alternative loans. *Work-Study:* Federal Work-Study. *Application deadline (priority):* 3/1.

Contact Connie Stopper, Assistant Dean, College of Nursing, Kent State University, PO Box 5190, Kent, OH 44242-0001. *Telephone:* 330-672-7930. *Fax:* 330-672-2433. *E-mail:* cstopper@kent.edu.

GRADUATE PROGRAMS

Financial Aid 10 research assistantships, 10 teaching assistantships were awarded; Federal Work-Study, institutionally sponsored loans, traineeships, tuition waivers (full), and unspecified assistantships also available.

Contact Dr. DIana Diordi, Assistant Dean, College of Nursing, Kent State University, PO Box 5190, Kent, OH 44242-0001. *Telephone:* 330-672-2234. *Fax:* 330-672-2433. *E-mail:* dbiordi@kent.edu.

MASTER'S DEGREE PROGRAM

Degrees MSN; MSN/MBA; MSN/MPA

Available Programs Accelerated RN to Master's; Master's.

Concentrations Available Health-care administration; nurse case management; nursing administration. *Clinical nurse specialist programs in:* adult health, gerontology, maternity-newborn, parent-child, pediatric, psychiatric/mental health, women's health. *Nurse practitioner programs in:* adult health, gerontology, pediatric, primary care, women's health.

Study Options Full-time and part-time.

Program Entrance Requirements Minimum overall college GPA of 3.0, transcript of college record, written essay, immunizations, interview, nursing research course, professional liability insurance/malpractice insurance, GRE if undergraduate GPA is less than 3.0. *Application deadline:* For fall admission, 7/12; for spring admission, 11/29. Applications are processed on a rolling basis. *Application fee:* $30.

Advanced Placement Credit given for nursing courses completed elsewhere dependent upon specific evaluations.

POST-MASTER'S PROGRAM

Areas of Study Nursing education. *Nurse practitioner programs in:* adult health, family health, gerontology, pediatric, primary care, psychiatric/mental health, women's health.

DOCTORAL DEGREE PROGRAM

Degree PhD

Available Programs Doctorate.

Areas of Study Health policy, health-care systems, individualized study, nursing policy, nursing research, nursing science.

Program Entrance Requirements Minimum overall college GPA of 3.0, interview, 3 letters of recommendation, MSN or equivalent, scholarly papers, statistics course, writing sample, GRE. *Application deadline:* For fall admission, 7/12; for spring admission, 11/29. Applications are processed on a rolling basis. *Application fee:* $30.

Degree Requirements 72 total credit hours, dissertation, written exam.

CONTINUING EDUCATION PROGRAM

Contact Betty Freund, Coordinator of Continuing Nursing Education, College of Nursing, Kent State University, PO Box 5190, Kent, OH 44242-0001. *Telephone:* 330-672-8810. *Fax:* 330-672-2433. *E-mail:* bfreund@kent.edu.

See full description on page 508.

Kettering College of Medical Arts
Division of Nursing
Kettering, Ohio

http://www.kcma.edu
Founded in 1967

DEGREE • BSN

Nursing Program Faculty 5 (40% with doctorates).

Baccalaureate Enrollment 15
Women 100% **Part-time** 100%

Nursing Student Resources Academic advising; academic or career counseling; assistance for students with disabilities; bookstore; campus computer network; computer lab; computer-assisted instruction; e-mail services; Internet; learning resource lab; library services; nursing audiovisuals; remedial services; resume preparation assistance; skills, simulation, or other laboratory; tutoring.

Library Facilities 29,390 volumes (4,060 in health, 1,073 in nursing); 266 periodical subscriptions (173 health-care related).

BACCALAUREATE PROGRAMS

Degree BSN

Available Programs RN Baccalaureate.

Study Options Full-time and part-time.

Program Entrance Requirements Transcript of college record, health exam, immunizations, 3 letters of recommendation, RN licensure. Transfer students are accepted. **Standardized tests** *Required:* ACT, TOEFL for international students. *Recommended:* SAT. **Application** *Deadline:* rolling (freshmen), rolling (transfer). *Notification:* continuous (freshmen). *Application fee:* $25.

Advanced Placement Credit given for nursing courses completed elsewhere dependent upon specific evaluations.

Expenses (2003–04) *Tuition:* part-time $230 per credit hour. *Required fees:* full-time $340; part-time $170 per term.

Financial Aid 42% of baccalaureate students in nursing programs received some form of financial aid in 2002–03. *Gift aid (need-based):* Federal Pell, state, private, college/university gift aid from institutional funds. *Loans:* Federal Nursing Student Loans, Federal Direct (Subsidized and Unsubsidized Stafford PLUS), Perkins, college/university. *Work-Study:* Federal Work-Study, part-time campus jobs. *Application deadline (priority):* 3/31.

Contact Ms. Sharon Millard, Chair, BSN Completion Program, Division of Nursing, Kettering College of Medical Arts, 3737 Southern Boulevard, Kettering, OH 45429. *Telephone:* 937-395-8642. *Fax:* 937-395-8810. *E-mail:* sharon.millard@kcma.edu.

Lourdes College
Nursing Department
Sylvania, Ohio

http://www.lourdes.edu

Founded in 1958

DEGREE • BSN

Nursing Program Faculty 15 (20% with doctorates).

Baccalaureate Enrollment 298
Women 95% **Men** 5% **Minority** 17% **Part-time** 24%

Nursing Student Activities Sigma Theta Tau, Student Nurses' Association.

Nursing Student Resources Academic advising; academic or career counseling; assistance for students with disabilities; bookstore; campus computer network; computer lab; computer-assisted instruction; e-mail services; employment services for current students; interactive nursing skills videos; Internet; learning resource lab; library services; nursing audiovisuals; remedial services; resume preparation assistance; skills, simulation, or other laboratory; tutoring.

Library Facilities 58,633 volumes (1,200 in health, 700 in nursing); 448 periodical subscriptions (101 health-care related).

BACCALAUREATE PROGRAMS

Degree BSN

Available Programs Generic Baccalaureate; LPN to Baccalaureate; RN Baccalaureate.

Site Options Sandusky, OH.

Study Options Full-time and part-time.

Program Entrance Requirements Minimum overall college GPA of 2.0, transcript of college record, CPR certification, health exam, health insurance, high school biology, high school chemistry, high school transcript, immunizations, 3 letters of recommendation, minimum GPA in nursing prerequisites of 2.5, professional liability insurance/malpractice insurance, prerequisite course work. Transfer students are accepted. **Standardized tests** *Required:* TOEFL for international students. *Required for some:* SAT or ACT. **Application** *Deadline:* rolling (freshmen), rolling (transfer). *Notification:* continuous (freshmen). *Application fee:* $25.

Advanced Placement Credit by examination available. Credit given for nursing courses completed elsewhere dependent upon specific evaluations.

Expenses (2004–05) *Tuition:* full-time $8544; part-time $356 per credit hour. *International tuition:* $8544 full-time. *Required fees:* full-time $960; part-time $40 per credit.

Financial Aid 98% of baccalaureate students in nursing programs received some form of financial aid in 2003–04. *Gift aid (need-based):* Federal Pell, FSEOG, state, private, college/university gift aid from institutional funds. *Loans:* FFEL (Subsidized and Unsubsidized Stafford PLUS), Perkins, state, college/university, alternative loans. *Work-Study:* Federal Work-Study. *Application deadline (priority):* 3/1.

Contact Ms. Kerry Loe, RN, Nursing Advisor/Recruiter, Nursing Department, Lourdes College, 6832 Convent Boulevard, Sylvania, OH 43560. *Telephone:* 419-824-3793. *Fax:* 419-824-3985. *E-mail:* kloe@lourdes.edu.

Malone College
School of Nursing
Canton, Ohio

http://www.malone.edu

Founded in 1892

DEGREES • BSN • MSN

Nursing Program Faculty 23 (22% with doctorates).

Baccalaureate Enrollment 252
Women 86% **Men** 14% **Minority** 8% **Part-time** 24%

Graduate Enrollment 30
Women 100% **Minority** 7%

Nursing Student Activities Nursing Honor Society, Sigma Theta Tau, Student Nurses' Association.

Nursing Student Resources Academic advising; academic or career counseling; assistance for students with disabilities; bookstore; campus computer network; career placement assistance; computer lab; computer-assisted instruction; e-mail services; employment services for current students; interactive nursing skills videos; Internet; learning resource lab; library services; nursing audiovisuals; placement services for program completers; remedial services; resume preparation assistance; skills, simulation, or other laboratory; tutoring.

Library Facilities 238,830 volumes (4,408 in health, 1,172 in nursing); 1,385 periodical subscriptions (290 health-care related).

BACCALAUREATE PROGRAMS

Degree BSN

Available Programs Generic Baccalaureate; LPN to RN Baccalaureate; RN Baccalaureate.

Study Options Full-time and part-time.

Program Entrance Requirements Minimum overall college GPA of 2.0, transcript of college record, CPR certification, written essay, health exam, health insurance, high school biology, high school chemistry, 3 years high school math, 3 years high school science, high school transcript, immunizations, minimum high school GPA of 2.5, professional liability insurance/malpractice insurance, prerequisite course work. Transfer students are accepted. **Standardized tests** *Required:* SAT or ACT, TOEFL for international students. **Application** *Deadline:* 7/1 (freshmen), 7/1 (transfer). *Notification:* continuous (freshmen). *Application fee:* $20.

Advanced Placement Credit by examination available. Credit given for nursing courses completed elsewhere dependent upon specific evaluations.

Expenses (2004–05) *Tuition:* full-time $15,630; part-time $320 per credit hour. *International tuition:* $15,630 full-time. *Room and board:* $6000; room only: $3250 per academic year. *Required fees:* full-time $680; part-time $155 per term.

Financial Aid 96% of baccalaureate students in nursing programs received some form of financial aid in 2003–04.

Contact Mr. John Chopka, Dean of Admissions, School of Nursing, Malone College, 515 25th Street, NW, Canton, OH 44709. *Telephone:* 330-471-8145. *Fax:* 330-454-6977. *E-mail:* admissions@malone.edu.

GRADUATE PROGRAMS

Expenses (2004–05) *Tuition:* full-time $11,683; part-time $425 per credit hour. *International tuition:* $11,683 full-time.

Financial Aid 60% of graduate students in nursing programs received some form of financial aid in 2003–04.

Contact Dr. Loretta M. Reinhart, RN, Dean and Professor, School of Nursing, Malone College, 515 25th Street, NW, Canton, OH 44709. *Telephone:* 330-471-8366. *Fax:* 330-471-8478. *E-mail:* lreinhart2@malone.edu.

MASTER'S DEGREE PROGRAM

Degree MSN

Available Programs Master's.

Concentrations Available *Clinical nurse specialist programs in:* medical-surgical. *Nurse practitioner programs in:* family health.

Study Options Full-time.

Program Entrance Requirements Clinical experience, computer literacy, minimum overall college GPA of 3.0, transcript of college record, CPR certification, written essay, immunizations, interview, 2 letters of recommendation, nursing research course, physical assessment course, professional liability insurance/malpractice insurance, resume.

Degree Requirements 48 total credit hours, thesis or project.

CONTINUING EDUCATION PROGRAM

Contact Dr. Loretta M. Reinhart, RN, Dean and Professor, School of Nursing, Malone College, 515 25th Street, NW, Canton, OH 44709. *Telephone:* 330-471-8366. *Fax:* 330-471-8478. *E-mail:* lreinhart2@malone.edu.

Medical College of Ohio
School of Nursing
Toledo, Ohio

http://www.mco.edu/snur/index.html
Founded in 1964

DEGREES • BSN • MSN

Nursing Program Faculty 60 (40% with doctorates).

Baccalaureate Enrollment 347
Women 90% **Men** 10% **Minority** 9% **International** 5% **Part-time** 16%

Graduate Enrollment 115
Women 97% **Men** 3% **Minority** 4% **Part-time** 85%

Nursing Student Activities Sigma Theta Tau, Student Nurses' Association.

Nursing Student Resources Academic advising; academic or career counseling; assistance for students with disabilities; bookstore; campus computer network; computer lab; computer-assisted instruction; daycare for children of students; e-mail services; interactive nursing skills videos; Internet; learning resource lab; library services; nursing audiovisuals; resume preparation assistance; skills, simulation, or other laboratory; tutoring.

Library Facilities 2,400 volumes in health, 91 volumes in nursing; 1,435 periodical subscriptions health-care related.

BACCALAUREATE PROGRAMS

Degree BSN

Available Programs ADN to Baccalaureate; Generic Baccalaureate.

Site Options *Distance Learning:* Lima, OH; Archbold, OH; Huron, OH.

Study Options Full-time and part-time.

Program Entrance Requirements Minimum overall college GPA of 2.5, transcript of college record, CPR certification, health exam, high school biology, high school chemistry, high school foreign language, 3 years high school math, 3 years high school science, high school transcript, immunizations, minimum high school GPA of 2.5, minimum GPA in nursing prerequisites of 2.0, professional liability insurance/malpractice insurance, prerequisite course work. Transfer students are accepted.

Advanced Placement Credit given for nursing courses completed elsewhere dependent upon specific evaluations.

Expenses (2003–04) *Tuition, state resident:* full-time $7408; part-time $308 per credit hour. *Tuition, nonresident:* full-time $14,368; part-time $598 per credit hour. *Room and board:* $5892; room only: $3642 per academic year. *Required fees:* full-time $205.

Financial Aid 60% of baccalaureate students in nursing programs received some form of financial aid in 2002–03.

Contact Paula Ballmer, RN, Admissions Representative, School of Nursing, Medical College of Ohio, Howard L. Collier Building, 3015 Arlington Avenue, Toledo, OH 43614. *Telephone:* 419-383-5839. *Fax:* 419-383-5894. *E-mail:* pballmer@mco.edu.

GRADUATE PROGRAMS

Expenses (2003–04) *Tuition, state resident:* full-time $6560; part-time $275 per credit hour. *Tuition, nonresident:* full-time $14,950; part-time $625 per credit hour. *Required fees:* full-time $760; part-time $250 per term.

Financial Aid 36% of graduate students in nursing programs received some form of financial aid in 2002–03. Federal Work-Study, institutionally sponsored loans, and scholarships available.

Contact Dr. Janet H. Robinson, Associate Dean, Graduate Program, School of Nursing, Medical College of Ohio, 3015 Arlington Avenue, Toledo, OH 43614-5803. *Telephone:* 419-383-5892. *Fax:* 419-383-5894. *E-mail:* jrobinson@mco.edu.

MASTER'S DEGREE PROGRAM

Degree MSN

Available Programs Master's; Master's for Non-Nursing College Graduates.

Concentrations Available Nursing education. *Clinical nurse specialist programs in:* adult health, pediatric, psychiatric/mental health. *Nurse practitioner programs in:* adult health, family health, pediatric.

Study Options Full-time and part-time.

Program Entrance Requirements Computer literacy, minimum overall college GPA of 3.0, transcript of college record, CPR certification, written essay, 2 letters of recommendation, professional liability insurance/malpractice insurance, resume, statistics course, GRE General Test. *Application deadline:* For fall admission, 5/1; for spring admission, 9/1. *Application fee:* $30.

Advanced Placement Credit given for nursing courses completed elsewhere dependent upon specific evaluations.

Degree Requirements 47 total credit hours, thesis or project.

POST-MASTER'S PROGRAM

Areas of Study *Nurse practitioner programs in:* adult health, family health, pediatric.

CONTINUING EDUCATION PROGRAM

Contact Dr. Dianne Smolen, Director, Continuing Nursing Education, School of Nursing, Medical College of Ohio, Collier Building, 3015 Arlington Avenue, Toledo, OH 43614-5803. *Telephone:* 419-383-5812. *Fax:* 419-383-5894. *E-mail:* smolen@mco.edu.

Mercy College of Northwest Ohio
Division of Nursing
Toledo, Ohio

Founded in 1993

DEGREE • BSN

Library Facilities 5,900 volumes; 171 periodical subscriptions.

BACCALAUREATE PROGRAMS

Degree BSN

Available Programs Generic Baccalaureate; RN Baccalaureate.

Program Entrance Requirements Minimum overall college GPA of 2.5, immunizations, minimum high school GPA of 2.5, RN licensure. **Standardized tests** *Recommended:* SAT or ACT. *Required for some:* SAT or ACT. **Application** *Deadline:* rolling (freshmen), rolling (transfer). *Notification:* continuous (freshmen). *Application fee:* $25.

Contact Nursing Department, Division of Nursing, Mercy College of Northwest Ohio, 2221 Madison Avenue, Toledo, OH 43624. *Telephone:* 888-806-3729. *Fax:* 419-251-1313.

Miami University
Department of Nursing
Hamilton, Ohio

http://www.ham.muohio.edu/nursing/
Founded in 1809

DEGREE • BSN

Nursing Program Faculty 6 (75% with doctorates).

Baccalaureate Enrollment 69
Women 98% **Men** 2% **Minority** 7% **Part-time** 56%

Nursing Student Activities Sigma Theta Tau.

Nursing Student Resources Academic advising; academic or career counseling; assistance for students with disabilities; bookstore; campus computer network; computer lab; daycare for children of students; e-mail services; interactive nursing skills videos; Internet; learning resource lab; library services; nursing audiovisuals; resume preparation assistance; tutoring.

Library Facilities 2.7 million volumes (29,000 in nursing); 14,089 periodical subscriptions (852 health-care related).

BACCALAUREATE PROGRAMS

Degree BSN

Available Programs Accelerated RN Baccalaureate; RN Baccalaureate.

Site Options Hamilton, OH; Middletown, OH.

Study Options Full-time and part-time.

Program Entrance Requirements Minimum overall college GPA of 2.5, transcript of college record, health exam, health insurance, immunizations, professional liability insurance/malpractice insurance, prerequisite course work, RN licensure. Transfer students are accepted. **Standardized tests** *Required:* SAT or ACT, TOEFL for international students. **Application** *Deadline:* 1/31 (freshmen), 5/1 (transfer). *Early decision:* 11/1. *Notification:* 3/15 (freshmen), 12/15 (out-of-state freshmen), 12/15 (early decision). *Application fee:* $45.

Advanced Placement Credit given for nursing courses completed elsewhere dependent upon specific evaluations.

Expenses (2004–05) *Tuition, state resident:* full-time $2934; part-time $243 per credit hour. *Tuition, nonresident:* full-time $8224; part-time $684 per credit hour. *Required fees:* full-time $36; part-time $18 per term.

Financial Aid 40% of baccalaureate students in nursing programs received some form of financial aid in 2003–04. *Gift aid (need-based):* Federal Pell, FSEOG, state, private, college/university gift aid from institutional funds. *Loans:* Federal Nursing Student Loans, Federal Direct (Subsidized and Unsubsidized Stafford PLUS), Perkins, college/university, alternative loans. *Work-Study:* Federal Work-Study. *Application deadline (priority):* 2/15.

Contact Dr. Paulette I. Worcester, Interim Chair/Associate Professor, Department of Nursing, Miami University, 1601 University Boulevard, Hamilton, OH 45011. *Telephone:* 513-785-7751. *Fax:* 513-785-7767. *E-mail:* worcesp@muohio.edu.

Mount Carmel College of Nursing

Baccalaureate Nursing Program
Columbus, Ohio

http://www.mccn.edu/index.html

DEGREES • BSN • MS

Nursing Program Faculty 51 (10% with doctorates).

Baccalaureate Enrollment 539
Women 92% **Men** 8% **Minority** 14% **Part-time** 22%

Graduate Enrollment 23
Women 96% **Men** 4% **Minority** 22%

Nursing Student Activities Nursing Honor Society, Sigma Theta Tau, Student Nurses' Association, nursing club.

Nursing Student Resources Academic advising; academic or career counseling; assistance for students with disabilities; campus computer network; career placement assistance; computer lab; computer-assisted instruction; employment services for current students; interactive nursing skills videos; Internet; learning resource lab; library services; nursing audiovisuals; placement services for program completers; remedial services; resume preparation assistance; skills, simulation, or other laboratory; tutoring.

Library Facilities 15,000 volumes in health, 1,500 volumes in nursing; 20,000 periodical subscriptions health-care related.

BACCALAUREATE PROGRAMS

Degree BSN

Available Programs Generic Baccalaureate; RN Baccalaureate.

Study Options Full-time and part-time.

Program Entrance Requirements Minimum overall college GPA of 2.5, transcript of college record, written essay, health exam, high school biology, high school chemistry, high school foreign language, 3 years high school math, 2 years high school science, high school transcript, immunizations, minimum high school GPA of 2.5. Transfer students are accepted. **Application** *Deadline:* rolling (freshmen). *Application fee:* $30.

Advanced Placement Credit given for nursing courses completed elsewhere dependent upon specific evaluations.

Expenses (2004–05) *Tuition:* full-time $14,520; part-time $372 per credit hour. *Room and board:* room only: $1870 per academic year. *Required fees:* full-time $292; part-time $146 per term.

Financial Aid 88% of baccalaureate students in nursing programs received some form of financial aid in 2003–04. *Gift aid (need-based):* Federal Pell, FSEOG, state, private, college/university gift aid from institutional funds. *Loans:* Federal Nursing Student Loans, FFEL (Subsidized and Unsubsidized Stafford PLUS), Perkins, state, college/university. *Work-Study:* part-time campus jobs. *Application deadline:* Continuous.

Contact Merchel Menefield, Director of Admissions, Baccalaureate Nursing Program, Mount Carmel College of Nursing, 127 South Davis Avenue, Columbus, OH 43222-1504. *Telephone:* 614-234-5144. *Fax:* 614-234-2875. *E-mail:* mmenefield@mchs.com.

GRADUATE PROGRAMS

Expenses (2004–05) *Tuition:* full-time $4860; part-time $324 per credit hour. *Room and board:* room only: $1870 per academic year.

Financial Aid 19% of graduate students in nursing programs received some form of financial aid in 2003–04.

Contact Kip Sexton, MSN Program Coordinator, Baccalaureate Nursing Program, Mount Carmel College of Nursing, 127 South Davis Avenue, Columbus, OH 43222. *Telephone:* 614-234-5800. *Fax:* 614-234-2875. *E-mail:* esexton@mchs.com.

MASTER'S DEGREE PROGRAM

Degree MS

Available Programs Master's.

Concentrations Available *Clinical nurse specialist programs in:* adult health.

Study Options Full-time and part-time.

Program Entrance Requirements Minimum overall college GPA of 3.0, transcript of college record, CPR certification, written essay, immunizations, 3 letters of recommendation, professional liability insurance/malpractice insurance, resume.

Degree Requirements 30 total credit hours.

POST-MASTER'S PROGRAM

Areas of Study Nursing education.

See full description on page 524.

The Ohio State University

College of Nursing
Columbus, Ohio

http://www.nursing.osu.edu

Founded in 1870

DEGREES • BSN • MS • PHD

Nursing Program Faculty 69 (43% with doctorates).

Baccalaureate Enrollment 474
Women 91% **Men** 9% **Minority** 13% **Part-time** 15%

Graduate Enrollment 243
Women 93% **Men** 7% **Minority** 8% **International** 1% **Part-time** 38%

Nursing Student Activities Nursing Honor Society, Sigma Theta Tau, Student Nurses' Association, nursing club.

Nursing Student Resources Academic advising; academic or career counseling; assistance for students with disabilities; bookstore; campus computer network; career placement assistance; computer lab; computer-assisted instruction; daycare for children of students; e-mail services; employment services for current students; externships; housing assistance; interactive nursing skills videos; Internet; learning resource lab; library services; nursing audiovisuals; other; paid internships; placement services for program completers; remedial services; resume preparation assistance; skills, simulation, or other laboratory; tutoring; unpaid internships.

Library Facilities 5.6 million volumes (188,602 in health, 4,198 in nursing); 43,086 periodical subscriptions (5,060 health-care related).

BACCALAUREATE PROGRAMS

Degree BSN

The Ohio State University (continued)

Available Programs Accelerated RN Baccalaureate; Generic Baccalaureate.

Study Options Full-time and part-time.

Program Entrance Requirements Minimum overall college GPA of 2.75, transcript of college record, CPR certification, written essay, health insurance, high school biology, high school chemistry, high school foreign language, 3 years high school math, 2 years high school science, high school transcript, immunizations, professional liability insurance/malpractice insurance, prerequisite course work. Transfer students are accepted. **Standardized tests** *Required:* SAT or ACT, TOEFL for international students. **Application** *Deadline:* 2/1 (freshmen), 6/25 (transfer). *Notification:* continuous (freshmen). *Application fee:* $40.

Advanced Placement Credit by examination available. Credit given for nursing courses completed elsewhere dependent upon specific evaluations.

Expenses (2004–05) *Tuition, state resident:* full-time $7542. *Tuition, nonresident:* full-time $18,129. *International tuition:* $18,129 full-time. *Room and board:* $8016; room only: $5961 per academic year.

Financial Aid 70% of baccalaureate students in nursing programs received some form of financial aid in 2003–04.

Contact Ms. Susan Mills Potter, Coordinator, Nursing Student Affairs, College of Nursing, The Ohio State University, 236 Newton Hall, 1585 Neil Avenue, Columbus, OH 43210-1289. *Telephone:* 614-292-4041. *Fax:* 614-292-9399. *E-mail:* potter.99@osu.edu.

GRADUATE PROGRAMS

Expenses (2004–05) *Tuition, state resident:* full-time $8250. *Tuition, nonresident:* full-time $20,133. *International tuition:* $20,133 full-time.

Financial Aid Fellowships, research assistantships, teaching assistantships, Federal Work-Study, institutionally sponsored loans, and unspecified assistantships available.

Contact Ms. Jackie Min, Graduate Outreach Coordinator, College of Nursing, The Ohio State University, 1585 Neil Avenue, Columbus, OH 43210-1289. *Telephone:* 614-688-8145. *Fax:* 614-292-9399. *E-mail:* Min.37@osu.edu.

MASTER'S DEGREE PROGRAM

Degree MS

Available Programs Accelerated Master's; Accelerated Master's for Non-Nursing College Graduates; Master's; Master's for Non-Nursing College Graduates.

Concentrations Available Nurse-midwifery; nursing administration. *Clinical nurse specialist programs in:* adult health, cardiovascular, community health, oncology, parent-child, perinatal, psychiatric/mental health, public health, women's health. *Nurse practitioner programs in:* adult health, family health, neonatal health, pediatric, primary care, psychiatric/mental health, school health, women's health.

Study Options Full-time and part-time.

Program Entrance Requirements Minimum overall college GPA of 3.0, transcript of college record, CPR certification, written essay, 3 letters of recommendation, resume, GRE General Test. *Application deadline:* For fall admission, 5/1 (priority date); for spring admission, 2/1. Applications are processed on a rolling basis. *Application fee:* $40 ($50 for international students).

Advanced Placement Credit given for nursing courses completed elsewhere dependent upon specific evaluations.

Degree Requirements 50 total credit hours, thesis or project, comprehensive exam.

POST-MASTER'S PROGRAM

Areas of Study Nurse-midwifery; nursing administration. *Clinical nurse specialist programs in:* adult health, cardiovascular, community health, oncology, parent-child, psychiatric/mental health, public health, women's health. *Nurse practitioner programs in:* adult health, family health, neonatal health, pediatric, primary care, psychiatric/mental health, school health, women's health.

DOCTORAL DEGREE PROGRAM

Degree PhD

Available Programs Doctorate.

Areas of Study Addiction/substance abuse, aging, bio-behavioral research, biology of health and illness, clinical practice, community health, critical care, ethics, family health, gerontology, health policy, health promotion/disease prevention, health-care systems, illness and transition, individualized study, maternity-newborn, neuro-behavior, nursing policy, nursing research, nursing science, oncology, women's health.

Program Entrance Requirements Minimum overall college GPA of 3.3, 3 letters of recommendation, MSN or equivalent, statistics course, vita, writing sample, GRE General Test. *Application deadline:* For fall admission, 5/1 (priority date); for spring admission, 2/1. Applications are processed on a rolling basis. *Application fee:* $40 ($50 for international students).

Degree Requirements 90 total credit hours, dissertation, oral exam, written exam, residency.

Ohio University
School of Nursing
Athens, Ohio

http://www.ohio.edu/nursing/

Founded in 1804

DEGREES • BSN • MSN

Nursing Program Faculty 9 (89% with doctorates).

Nursing Student Activities Nursing Honor Society, Sigma Theta Tau.

Nursing Student Resources Academic or career counseling; career placement assistance; computer lab; e-mail services; Internet; library services.

Library Facilities 2.6 million volumes; 25,557 periodical subscriptions.

BACCALAUREATE PROGRAMS

Degree BSN

Available Programs RN Baccalaureate.

Study Options Full-time and part-time.

Program Entrance Requirements Minimum overall college GPA of 2.0, transcript of college record, CPR certification, high school transcript, immunizations, professional liability insurance/malpractice insurance, prerequisite course work. Transfer students are accepted. **Standardized tests** *Required:* SAT or ACT. **Application** *Deadline:* 2/1 (freshmen), 5/15 (transfer). *Notification:* continuous (freshmen). *Application fee:* $45.

Advanced Placement Credit by examination available. Credit given for nursing courses completed elsewhere dependent upon specific evaluations.

Expenses (2003–04) *Tuition, state resident:* full-time $7128. *Tuition, nonresident:* full-time $15,351. *Room and board:* $7320; room only: $3600 per academic year.

Contact Emily Harman, RN, Interim Director, School of Nursing, Ohio University, Grover Center E365, Athens, OH 45701. *Telephone:* 740-593-4494. *Fax:* 740-593-0286. *E-mail:* nursing@ohio.edu.

GRADUATE PROGRAMS

Expenses (2003–04) *Tuition, state resident:* part-time $328 per credit hour. *Tuition, nonresident:* part-time $632 per credit hour.

Contact Graduate Coordinator, School of Nursing, Ohio University, School of Nursing/Ohio University, Grover Center E365, Athens, OH 45701-2979. *Telephone:* 740-593-4494. *Fax:* 740-593-0144. *E-mail:* nursing@ohio.edu.

MASTER'S DEGREE PROGRAM

Degree MSN

Concentrations Available Nursing administration; nursing education. *Nurse practitioner programs in:* family health.

Study Options Full-time and part-time.

Program Entrance Requirements Minimum overall college GPA of 3.0, transcript of college record, written essay, 3 letters of recommendation, resume, statistics course.

Advanced Placement Credit given for nursing courses completed elsewhere dependent upon specific evaluations.

Degree Requirements 55 total credit hours.

Otterbein College

Program in Nursing
Westerville, Ohio

http://www.otterbein.edu/dept/NURS

Founded in 1847

DEGREES • BSN • MSN

Nursing Student Activities Nursing Honor Society, Sigma Theta Tau.

Library Facilities 182,629 volumes; 1,012 periodical subscriptions.

BACCALAUREATE PROGRAMS

Degree BSN

Available Programs Accelerated RN Baccalaureate; Generic Baccalaureate; LPN to Baccalaureate; RN Baccalaureate.

Site Options *Distance Learning:* Newark, OH; Nelsonville, OH.

Program Entrance Requirements Transfer students are accepted. **Standardized tests** *Required:* SAT or ACT, TOEFL for international students. **Application** *Deadline:* 3/1 (freshmen), rolling (transfer). *Notification:* continuous (freshmen). *Application fee:* $25.

Advanced Placement Credit by examination available. Credit given for nursing courses completed elsewhere dependent upon specific evaluations.

Contact Program Contact, Program in Nursing, Otterbein College, Westerville, OH 43081. *Telephone:* 614-823-1614. *Fax:* 614-823-3131. *E-mail:* lbrantch@otterbein.edu.

GRADUATE PROGRAMS

Financial Aid Traineeships available.

Contact Program Contact, Program in Nursing, Otterbein College, Westerville, OH 43081. *Telephone:* 614-823-1614. *E-mail:* sbuxton@otterbein.edu.

MASTER'S DEGREE PROGRAM

Degree MSN

Available Programs Master's.

Concentrations Available Nursing administration; nursing education. *Clinical nurse specialist programs in:* adult health. *Nurse practitioner programs in:* adult health, family health.

Site Options *Distance Learning:* Newark, OH; Nelsonville, OH; Hillsboro, OH.

Study Options Part-time.

Program Entrance Requirements *Application deadline:* Applications are processed on a rolling basis.

POST-MASTER'S PROGRAM

Areas of Study Nursing education. *Nurse practitioner programs in:* adult health, family health.

CONTINUING EDUCATION PROGRAM

Contact Linda Brantch, Program Contact, Program in Nursing, Otterbein College, Westerville, OH 43081. *Telephone:* 614-823-1614. *E-mail:* lbrantch@otterbein.edu.

Shawnee State University

Department of Nursing
Portsmouth, Ohio

http://www.shawnee.edu/acadamics/bsc/nurs/index.html

Founded in 1986

DEGREE • BSN

Nursing Program Faculty 9.

Nursing Student Activities Student Nurses' Association.

Nursing Student Resources Academic advising; academic or career counseling; assistance for students with disabilities; bookstore; campus computer network; career placement assistance; computer lab; computer-assisted instruction; daycare for children of students; e-mail services; employment services for current students; housing assistance; interactive nursing skills videos; Internet; learning resource lab; library services; nursing audiovisuals; other; placement services for program completers; remedial services; resume preparation assistance; skills, simulation, or other laboratory; tutoring.

Library Facilities 150,661 volumes (8,273 in health, 870 in nursing); 13,820 periodical subscriptions (1,798 health-care related).

BACCALAUREATE PROGRAMS

Degree BSN

Available Programs ADN to Baccalaureate; RN Baccalaureate.

Study Options Full-time and part-time.

Program Entrance Requirements Minimum overall college GPA of 2.5, transcript of college record, CPR certification, health exam, health insurance, high school transcript, immunizations, professional liability insurance/malpractice insurance, prerequisite course work, RN licensure. Transfer students are accepted. **Standardized tests** *Required:* TOEFL for international students. ***Placement:*** *Recommended:* ACT. **Application** *Deadline:* rolling (freshmen), rolling (transfer). *Notification:* continuous (freshmen).

Advanced Placement Credit given for nursing courses completed elsewhere dependent upon specific evaluations.

Contact Chaiperson, Department of Nursing, Department of Nursing, Shawnee State University, 940 Second Street, Portsmouth, OH 45662. *Telephone:* 740-351-3378. *Fax:* 740-351-3354.

CONTINUING EDUCATION PROGRAM

Contact Mrs. Ginnie Moore, Director, University Outreach Services, Department of Nursing, Shawnee State University, 940 Second Street, Portsmouth, OH 45662. *Telephone:* 740-351-3281. *E-mail:* gmoore@shawnee.edu.

The University of Akron

College of Nursing
Akron, Ohio

http://www.uakron.edu/nursing

Founded in 1870

DEGREES • BSN • MSN • PHD

Nursing Program Faculty 42 (60% with doctorates).

Baccalaureate Enrollment 400
Women 90% **Men** 10% **Minority** 13% **Part-time** 19%

Graduate Enrollment 200
Women 80% **Men** 20% **Minority** 9% **International** 5% **Part-time** 71%

Nursing Student Activities Sigma Theta Tau, Student Nurses' Association, nursing club.

Nursing Student Resources Academic advising; academic or career counseling; assistance for students with disabilities; bookstore; campus computer network; career placement assistance; computer lab; computer-assisted instruction; daycare for children of students; e-mail services; employment services for current students; interactive nursing skills videos; Internet; learning resource lab; library services; nursing audiovisuals; remedial services; resume preparation assistance; skills, simulation, or other laboratory; tutoring.

Library Facilities 1.2 million volumes (32,000 in health, 7,286 in nursing); 12,849 periodical subscriptions (1,662 health-care related).

■ A joint PhD in nursing is offered in conjunction with Kent State University for those students interested in becoming nurse scholars. The RN to Master of Science in Nursing program meets the needs of registered nurses whose goal

The University of Akron (continued)

is graduate study for advanced practice. The accelerated BSN program provides the opportunity for postbaccalaureate students from other majors to earn a nursing degree in 15 months. Postbaccalaureate certificate programs in nursing education and in nursing management and business are also available.

BACCALAUREATE PROGRAMS

Degree BSN

Available Programs ADN to Baccalaureate; Accelerated Baccalaureate for Second Degree; Generic Baccalaureate; LPN to Baccalaureate; RN Baccalaureate.

Site Options *Distance Learning:* Orville, OH; Lorain, OH.

Study Options Full-time and part-time.

Program Entrance Requirements Transcript of college record, CPR certification, health exam, immunizations, minimum GPA in nursing prerequisites of 2.75, prerequisite course work. Transfer students are accepted. **Standardized tests** *Required:* SAT or ACT, TOEFL for international students. **Application** *Deadline:* 8/15 (freshmen), 8/15 (transfer). *Early decision:* 2/1. *Notification:* continuous (freshmen), 3/15 (early action). *Application fee:* $30.

Advanced Placement Credit given for nursing courses completed elsewhere dependent upon specific evaluations.

Expenses (2004–05) *Tuition, state resident:* full-time $7510; part-time $313 per credit hour. *Tuition, nonresident:* full-time $15,740; part-time $587 per credit hour. *Required fees:* full-time $1000.

Financial Aid 80% of baccalaureate students in nursing programs received some form of financial aid in 2003–04. *Gift aid (need-based):* Federal Pell, FSEOG, state. *Loans:* Federal Nursing Student Loans, FFEL (Subsidized and Unsubsidized Stafford PLUS), Perkins, college/university. *Work-Study:* Federal Work-Study, part-time campus jobs. *Application deadline:* 3/1 (priority: 2/1).

Contact Dr. Rita Klein, Director, Office of Student Affairs, College of Nursing, The University of Akron, Akron, OH 44325-3701. *Telephone:* 330-972-5103. *Fax:* 330-972-5493. *E-mail:* rklein@uakron.edu.

GRADUATE PROGRAMS

Expenses (2004–05) *Tuition, state resident:* part-time $328 per credit hour. *Tuition, nonresident:* part-time $545 per credit hour.

Financial Aid 80% of graduate students in nursing programs received some form of financial aid in 2003–04. 15 fellowships with full tuition reimbursements available, 13 research assistantships with full tuition reimbursements available, 5 teaching assistantships with full tuition reimbursements available were awarded; career-related internships or fieldwork, Federal Work-Study, and tuition waivers (full) also available. *Financial aid application deadline:* 5/15.

Contact Dr. Irene Glanville, Coordinator, Master's Program, College of Nursing, The University of Akron, Akron, OH 44325-3701. *Telephone:* 330-972-7733. *Fax:* 330-972-5737. *E-mail:* glanvil@uakron.edu.

MASTER'S DEGREE PROGRAM

Degree MSN

Available Programs Master's; RN to Master's.

Concentrations Available Nurse anesthesia; nursing administration. *Clinical nurse specialist programs in:* adult health, gerontology, pediatric, psychiatric/mental health. *Nurse practitioner programs in:* adult health, gerontology, pediatric, psychiatric/mental health.

Site Options *Distance Learning:* Orville, OH; Lorain, OH.

Study Options Full-time and part-time.

Program Entrance Requirements Clinical experience, computer literacy, minimum overall college GPA of 3.0, transcript of college record, CPR certification, written essay, immunizations, interview, 3 letters of recommendation, physical assessment course, professional liability insurance/malpractice insurance, resume, statistics course, GRE or MAT. *Application deadline:* For fall admission, 8/15. Applications are processed on a rolling basis. *Application fee:* $40 ($60 for international students).

Advanced Placement Credit given for nursing courses completed elsewhere dependent upon specific evaluations.

Degree Requirements 37 total credit hours.

POST-MASTER'S PROGRAM

Areas of Study Nurse anesthesia. *Clinical nurse specialist programs in:* adult health, gerontology, pediatric, psychiatric/mental health. *Nurse practitioner programs in:* adult health, gerontology, pediatric, psychiatric/mental health.

DOCTORAL DEGREE PROGRAM

Degree PhD

Available Programs Doctorate.

Areas of Study Aging, ethics, gerontology, health policy, health promotion/disease prevention, health-care systems, human health and illness, illness and transition, individualized study, nursing administration, nursing policy, nursing research, nursing science, women's health.

Program Entrance Requirements Minimum overall college GPA of 3.0, interview, 3 letters of recommendation, MSN or equivalent, vita, writing sample, GRE. *Application deadline:* For fall admission, 8/15. Applications are processed on a rolling basis. *Application fee:* $40 ($60 for international students).

Degree Requirements 72 total credit hours, dissertation, oral exam, written exam, residency.

CONTINUING EDUCATION PROGRAM

Contact Dr. Marlene Huff, Coordinator, Educational Progression Program, College of Nursing, The University of Akron, Akron, OH 44325-3701. *Telephone:* 330-972-5930. *Fax:* 330-972-5737. *E-mail:* mhuff@uakron.edu.

See full description on page 546.

University of Cincinnati
College of Nursing
Cincinnati, Ohio

http://www.nursing.uc.edu

Founded in 1819

DEGREES • BSN • MSN • MSN/MBA • PHD

Nursing Program Faculty 72 (49% with doctorates).

Baccalaureate Enrollment 651
Women 91% **Men** 9% **Minority** 20% **Part-time** 13%

Graduate Enrollment 219
Women 86% **Men** 14% **Minority** 26% **International** .08% **Part-time** 15%

Nursing Student Activities Sigma Theta Tau, Student Nurses' Association.

Nursing Student Resources Academic advising; academic or career counseling; assistance for students with disabilities; bookstore; campus computer network; computer lab; computer-assisted instruction; e-mail services; employment services for current students; externships; housing assistance; interactive nursing skills videos; Internet; learning resource lab; library services; nursing audiovisuals; paid internships; remedial services; resume preparation assistance; skills, simulation, or other laboratory; tutoring; unpaid internships.

Library Facilities 221,630 volumes in health, 21,306 volumes in nursing; 16,560 periodical subscriptions (2,384 health-care related).

BACCALAUREATE PROGRAMS

Degree BSN

Available Programs Generic Baccalaureate; RN Baccalaureate.

Site Options Cincinnati, OH.

Study Options Full-time and part-time.

Program Entrance Requirements Minimum overall college GPA of 2.5, transcript of college record, CPR certification, health insurance, high school biology, high school chemistry, 3 years high school math, high school transcript, immunizations, minimum GPA in nursing prerequisites of 2.5, prerequisite course work. Transfer students are accepted. **Standardized tests** *Required:* SAT or ACT, SAT Subject Tests, TOEFL for international students. **Application** *Deadline:* rolling (freshmen), rolling (transfer). *Notification:* continuous until 11/1 (freshmen). *Application fee:* $35.

Advanced Placement Credit by examination available. Credit given for nursing courses completed elsewhere dependent upon specific evaluations.

Expenses (2004–05) *Tuition, state resident:* full-time $8379; part-time $233 per credit hour. *Tuition, nonresident:* full-time $21,351; part-time $594 per credit hour. *Room and board:* $7425; room only: $4455 per academic year.

Financial Aid 65% of baccalaureate students in nursing programs received some form of financial aid in 2003–04. *Gift aid (need-based):* Federal Pell, FSEOG, state, private, college/university gift aid from institutional funds, Federal Nursing. *Loans:* Federal Nursing Student Loans, FFEL (Subsidized and Unsubsidized Stafford PLUS), Perkins, state, college/university. *Work-Study:* Federal Work-Study. *Application deadline:* Continuous.

Contact Ms. Brandy Rayburn, Baccalaureate Academic Advisor, College of Nursing, University of Cincinnati, PO Box 210038, Cincinnati, OH 45221-0038. *Telephone:* 513-558-5070. *Fax:* 513-558-7523. *E-mail:* brandy.rayburn@uc.edu.

GRADUATE PROGRAMS

Expenses (2004–05) *Tuition, state resident:* full-time $2867; part-time $333 per credit hour. *Tuition, nonresident:* full-time $5677; part-time $614 per credit hour. *Room and board:* $8163; room only: $5193 per academic year.

Financial Aid 70% of graduate students in nursing programs received some form of financial aid in 2003–04. 11 research assistantships with full tuition reimbursements available (averaging $12,000 per year), 4 teaching assistantships with full tuition reimbursements available (averaging $12,000 per year) were awarded; Federal Work-Study, scholarships, traineeships, and tuition waivers (partial) also available. Aid available to part-time students. *Financial aid application deadline:* 2/1.

Contact Mr. Loren Carter, Graduate Academic Advisor, College of Nursing, University of Cincinnati, PO Box 210038, Cincinnati, OH 45221-0038. *Telephone:* 513-558-5072. *Fax:* 513-558-7523. *E-mail:* loren.carter@uc.edu.

MASTER'S DEGREE PROGRAM

Degrees MSN; MSN/MBA

Available Programs Accelerated Master's for Non-Nursing College Graduates; Accelerated RN to Master's; Master's.

Concentrations Available Nurse anesthesia; nurse-midwifery; nursing administration. *Clinical nurse specialist programs in:* acute care, adult health, community health, occupational health. *Nurse practitioner programs in:* acute care, adult health, family health, gerontology, neonatal health, pediatric, psychiatric/mental health, women's health.

Study Options Full-time and part-time.

Program Entrance Requirements Clinical experience, computer literacy, minimum overall college GPA of 3.0, transcript of college record, CPR certification, written essay, immunizations, interview, 3 letters of recommendation, physical assessment course, professional liability insurance/malpractice insurance, resume, statistics course, GRE General Test. *Application deadline:* For fall admission, 2/1 (priority date). Applications are processed on a rolling basis. *Application fee:* $30.

Advanced Placement Credit given for nursing courses completed elsewhere dependent upon specific evaluations.

Degree Requirements 60 total credit hours, thesis or project.

POST-MASTER'S PROGRAM

Areas of Study *Nurse practitioner programs in:* acute care, adult health, family health, gerontology, neonatal health, pediatric, psychiatric/mental health, women's health.

DOCTORAL DEGREE PROGRAM

Degree PhD

Available Programs Doctorate; Post-Baccalaureate Doctorate.

Areas of Study Addiction/substance abuse, community health, critical care, ethics, faculty preparation, family health, health promotion/disease prevention, health-care systems, human health and illness, illness and transition, individualized study, maternity-newborn, nursing administration, nursing research, nursing science, oncology, women's health.

Program Entrance Requirements Minimum overall college GPA of 3.0, interview, 3 letters of recommendation, statistics course, vita, writing sample, GRE General Test. *Application deadline:* For fall admission, 2/1 (priority date). Applications are processed on a rolling basis. *Application fee:* $30.

Degree Requirements 135 total credit hours, dissertation, written exam, residency.

CONTINUING EDUCATION PROGRAM

Contact Ms. Elizabeth Karle, Program Coordinator, Continuing Education, College of Nursing, University of Cincinnati, PO Box 210038, Cincinnati, OH 45221-0038. *Telephone:* 513-558-5311. *Fax:* 513-558-5054. *E-mail:* elizabeth.karle@uc.edu.

See full description on page 552.

University of Phoenix–Cleveland Campus

College of Health and Human Services
Independence, Ohio

Founded in 2000

DEGREES • BSN • MSN

Library Facilities 27.1 million volumes; 11,648 periodical subscriptions.

BACCALAUREATE PROGRAMS

Degree BSN

Available Programs RN Baccalaureate.

Program Entrance Requirements Transcript of college record, high school transcript, prerequisite course work, RN licensure. Transfer students are accepted. **Standardized tests** *Required:* TOEFL for international students. **Application** *Deadline:* rolling (freshmen), rolling (transfer). *Application fee:* $100.

Advanced Placement Credit given for nursing courses completed elsewhere dependent upon specific evaluations.

Contact Campus College Chair, Nursing, College of Health and Human Services, University of Phoenix–Cleveland Campus, 5005 Rockside Road, Suite 130, Independence, OH 44131. *Telephone:* 216-447-8807.

GRADUATE PROGRAMS

Contact Campus College Chair, Nursing, College of Health and Human Services, University of Phoenix–Cleveland Campus, 5005 Rockside Road, Suite 130, Independence, OH 44131. *Telephone:* 216-447-8807.

MASTER'S DEGREE PROGRAM

Degree MSN

Available Programs Master's; Master's for Non-Nursing College Graduates.

Program Entrance Requirements Minimum overall college GPA of 2.5, transcript of college record, prerequisite course work. *Application deadline:* Applications are processed on a rolling basis. *Application fee:* $110.

Degree Requirements 39 total credit hours.

Ursuline College

The Breen School of Nursing
Pepper Pike, Ohio

http://www.ursuline.edu

Founded in 1871

DEGREES • BSN • MSN

Nursing Program Faculty 25 (28% with doctorates).

Baccalaureate Enrollment 325

Graduate Enrollment 70

Nursing Student Activities Sigma Theta Tau, Student Nurses' Association.

Ursuline College (continued)

Nursing Student Resources Academic advising; academic or career counseling; assistance for students with disabilities; bookstore; campus computer network; career placement assistance; computer lab; computer-assisted instruction; e-mail services; employment services for current students; externships; housing assistance; interactive nursing skills videos; Internet; learning resource lab; library services; nursing audiovisuals; placement services for program completers; remedial services; resume preparation assistance; skills, simulation, or other laboratory; tutoring.

Library Facilities 108,699 volumes; 12,989 periodical subscriptions.

BACCALAUREATE PROGRAMS

Degree BSN

Available Programs Accelerated Baccalaureate for Second Degree; Accelerated LPN to Baccalaureate; Accelerated RN Baccalaureate; Generic Baccalaureate.

Site Options Cleveland, OH; Garfield Heights, OH.

Study Options Full-time and part-time.

Program Entrance Requirements Minimum overall college GPA of 2.5, transcript of college record, written essay, health exam, health insurance, high school biology, high school chemistry, 1 year of high school math, 2 years high school science, high school transcript, immunizations, 1 letter of recommendation, minimum high school GPA of 2.5, minimum GPA in nursing prerequisites of 2.5. Transfer students are accepted. **Standardized tests** *Required:* SAT or ACT, TOEFL for international students. **Application** *Deadline:* rolling (freshmen), rolling (transfer). *Early decision:* 11/15. *Notification:* continuous (freshmen), 2/15 (early action). *Application fee:* $25.

Advanced Placement Credit by examination available. Credit given for nursing courses completed elsewhere dependent upon specific evaluations.

Expenses (2004–05) *Tuition:* part-time $599 per credit hour.

Contact Sarah Carr, Director of Admission, The Breen School of Nursing, Ursuline College, 2550 Lander Road, Pepper Pike, OH 44124-4398. *Telephone:* 440-646-4203. *Fax:* 440-684-6138.

GRADUATE PROGRAMS

Expenses (2004–05) *Tuition:* part-time $639 per credit hour.

Contact Dr. Carol H. Waggoner, RN, Director, Graduate Program, The Breen School of Nursing, Ursuline College, 2550 Lander Road, Pepper Pike, OH 44124-4398. *Telephone:* 440-449-3425. *Fax:* 440-449-4267. *E-mail:* cwaggoner@ursuline.edu.

MASTER'S DEGREE PROGRAM

Degree MSN

Available Programs Accelerated Master's; Master's.

Concentrations Available Nurse case management. *Clinical nurse specialist programs in:* adult health, family health. *Nurse practitioner programs in:* adult health, family health.

Study Options Full-time and part-time.

Program Entrance Requirements Clinical experience, minimum overall college GPA of 3.0, transcript of college record, CPR certification, immunizations, 3 letters of recommendation, nursing research course, physical assessment course, statistics course.

Advanced Placement Credit given for nursing courses completed elsewhere dependent upon specific evaluations.

Degree Requirements 39 total credit hours, thesis or project.

POST-MASTER'S PROGRAM

Areas of Study Nurse case management. *Clinical nurse specialist programs in:* adult health, family health. *Nurse practitioner programs in:* adult health, family health.

See full description on page 586.

Walsh University

Department of Nursing
North Canton, Ohio

http://www.walsh.edu/

Founded in 1958

DEGREE • BSN

Nursing Program Faculty 7 (12% with doctorates).

Baccalaureate Enrollment 160

Women 90% **Men** 10% **Minority** 6% **Part-time** 10%

Nursing Student Activities Nursing Honor Society, Student Nurses' Association.

Nursing Student Resources Academic advising; academic or career counseling; assistance for students with disabilities; bookstore; campus computer network; career placement assistance; computer lab; computer-assisted instruction; e-mail services; housing assistance; interactive nursing skills videos; Internet; learning resource lab; library services; nursing audiovisuals; placement services for program completers; resume preparation assistance; skills, simulation, or other laboratory; tutoring.

Library Facilities 136,268 volumes (4,000 in health, 2,000 in nursing); 605 periodical subscriptions (114 health-care related).

BACCALAUREATE PROGRAMS

Degree BSN

Available Programs Accelerated RN Baccalaureate; Generic Baccalaureate.

Site Options Canton, OH; Akron, OH.

Study Options Full-time and part-time.

Program Entrance Requirements Minimum overall college GPA of 2.0, transcript of college record, CPR certification, high school foreign language, 3 years high school math, 3 years high school science, high school transcript, immunizations, minimum high school GPA of 2.1, professional liability insurance/malpractice insurance. Transfer students are accepted. **Standardized tests** *Required:* SAT or ACT, TOEFL for international students. **Application** *Deadline:* rolling (freshmen), rolling (transfer). *Notification:* continuous (freshmen). *Application fee:* $25.

Advanced Placement Credit by examination available.

Expenses (2004–05) *Tuition:* full-time $15,100; part-time $500 per contact hour. *Room and board:* $8400; room only: $5200 per academic year. *Required fees:* full-time $408; part-time $17 per credit; part-time $204 per term.

Financial Aid 91% of baccalaureate students in nursing programs received some form of financial aid in 2003–04. *Gift aid (need-based):* Federal Pell, FSEOG, state, private, college/university gift aid from institutional funds. *Loans:* FFEL (Subsidized and Unsubsidized Stafford), Perkins, state, college/university. *Work-Study:* Federal Work-Study, part-time campus jobs. *Application deadline:* Continuous.

Contact Dr. Janis M. Campbell, RN, Chair, Department of Nursing, Walsh University, 2020 East Maple Street, North Canton, OH 44720-3336. *Telephone:* 330-490-7250. *Fax:* 330-490-7206. *E-mail:* jcampbell@walsh.edu.

Wright State University

College of Nursing and Health
Dayton, Ohio

http://www.nursing.wright.edu

Founded in 1964

DEGREES • BSN • MS • MS/MBA

Nursing Program Faculty 60 (30% with doctorates).

Baccalaureate Enrollment 503

Women 91% **Men** 9% **Minority** 8% **International** 2% **Part-time** 29%

Graduate Enrollment 174

Women 96% **Men** 4% **Minority** 4% **International** 1% **Part-time** 74%

Nursing Student Activities Nursing Honor Society, Sigma Theta Tau, Student Nurses' Association, nursing club.

Nursing Student Resources Academic advising; academic or career counseling; assistance for students with disabilities; bookstore; campus computer network; career placement assistance; computer lab; computer-assisted instruction; daycare for children of students; e-mail services; employment services for current students; externships; housing assistance; interactive nursing skills videos; Internet; learning resource lab; library services; nursing audiovisuals; remedial services; resume preparation assistance; skills, simulation, or other laboratory; tutoring.

Library Facilities 695,805 volumes (111,826 in health, 7,646 in nursing); 5,312 periodical subscriptions (1,279 health-care related).

BACCALAUREATE PROGRAMS

Degree BSN

Available Programs Accelerated Baccalaureate for Second Degree; Baccalaureate for Second Degree; Generic Baccalaureate; RN Baccalaureate.

Site Options *Distance Learning:* Celina, OH; Hillsboro, OH; Dayton, OH.

Study Options Full-time and part-time.

Program Entrance Requirements Minimum overall college GPA of 2.5, transcript of college record, written essay, high school transcript, minimum GPA in nursing prerequisites of 2.5, prerequisite course work. Transfer students are accepted. **Standardized tests** *Required:* SAT or ACT, TOEFL for international students. **Application** *Deadline:* rolling (freshmen), rolling (transfer). *Notification:* continuous (freshmen). *Application fee:* $30.

Advanced Placement Credit given for nursing courses completed elsewhere dependent upon specific evaluations.

Expenses (2004–05) *Tuition, state resident:* full-time $6477; part-time $197 per quarter hour. *Tuition, nonresident:* full-time $12,492; part-time $381 per quarter hour. *International tuition:* $12,492 full-time. *Room and board:* $6300; room only: $1300 per academic year. *Required fees:* full-time $750.

Financial Aid 79% of baccalaureate students in nursing programs received some form of financial aid in 2003–04.

Contact Ms. Theresa A. Haghnazarian, Director, Student and Alumni Affairs, College of Nursing and Health, Wright State University, 3640 Colonel Glenn Highway, Dayton, OH 45435. *Telephone:* 937-775-3132. *Fax:* 937-775-4571. *E-mail:* theresa.haghnazarian@wright.edu.

GRADUATE PROGRAMS

Expenses (2004–05) *Tuition, state resident:* full-time $8652; part-time $271 per quarter hour. *Tuition, nonresident:* full-time $14,669; part-time $458 per quarter hour. *International tuition:* $14,669 full-time. *Room and board:* $6300; room only: $1300 per academic year.

Financial Aid 29% of graduate students in nursing programs received some form of financial aid in 2003–04. 15 fellowships with full tuition reimbursements available were awarded; research assistantships, teaching assistantships, Federal Work-Study, institutionally sponsored loans, and unspecified assistantships also available. Aid available to part-time students. *Financial aid application deadline:* 6/1.

Contact Ms. Theresa A. Haghnazarian, Director, Student and Alumni Affairs, College of Nursing and Health, Wright State University, 3640 Colonel Glenn Highway, Dayton, OH 45435. *Telephone:* 937-775-3132. *Fax:* 937-775-4571. *E-mail:* theresa.haghnazarian@wright.edu.

MASTER'S DEGREE PROGRAM

Degrees MS; MS/MBA

Available Programs Master's; Master's for Nurses with Non-Nursing Degrees.

Concentrations Available Health-care administration; nursing administration. *Clinical nurse specialist programs in:* adult health, community health, pediatric, public health, school health. *Nurse practitioner programs in:* acute care, family health, pediatric.

Study Options Full-time and part-time.

Program Entrance Requirements Clinical experience, computer literacy, minimum overall college GPA of 3.0, transcript of college record, written essay, interview, physical assessment course, statistics course, GRE General Test. *Application deadline:* For fall admission, 4/15 (priority date). *Application fee:* $25.

Advanced Placement Credit given for nursing courses completed elsewhere dependent upon specific evaluations.

Degree Requirements 48 total credit hours, thesis or project.

POST-MASTER'S PROGRAM

Areas of Study Nursing education. *Clinical nurse specialist programs in:* school health. *Nurse practitioner programs in:* acute care, family health, pediatric.

CONTINUING EDUCATION PROGRAM

Contact Jay Atwater, Office Assistant, College of Nursing and Health, Wright State University, 3640 Colonel Glenn Highway, Dayton, OH 45435. *Telephone:* 937-775-3577. *Fax:* 937-775-4571. *E-mail:* jay.atwater@wright.edu.

See full description on page 602.

Xavier University

Department of Nursing
Cincinnati, Ohio

Founded in 1831

DEGREES • BSN • MSN • MSN/MBA

Nursing Program Faculty 21 (42% with doctorates).

Baccalaureate Enrollment 120
Women 95% **Men** 5% **Minority** 12% **Part-time** 10%

Graduate Enrollment 66
Women 97% **Men** 3% **Minority** 8% **Part-time** 92%

Nursing Student Activities Sigma Theta Tau.

Nursing Student Resources Academic advising; academic or career counseling; assistance for students with disabilities; bookstore; campus computer network; career placement assistance; computer lab; computer-assisted instruction; e-mail services; employment services for current students; externships; housing assistance; interactive nursing skills videos; Internet; learning resource lab; library services; nursing audiovisuals; paid internships; resume preparation assistance; skills, simulation, or other laboratory; tutoring.

Library Facilities 222,331 volumes (8,900 in health, 1,160 in nursing); 7,756 periodical subscriptions (200 health-care related).

BACCALAUREATE PROGRAMS

Degree BSN

Available Programs Generic Baccalaureate.

Study Options Full-time and part-time.

Program Entrance Requirements Minimum overall college GPA of 2.5, transcript of college record, written essay, high school chemistry, high school foreign language, 3 years high school math, 2 years high school science, high school transcript, minimum high school GPA of 2.7. Transfer students are accepted. **Standardized tests** *Required:* SAT or ACT, TOEFL for international students. **Application** *Deadline:* 2/1 (freshmen), rolling (transfer). *Early decision:* 12/1. *Notification:* 3/15 (freshmen), 1/15 (early action). *Application fee:* $35.

Advanced Placement Credit given for nursing courses completed elsewhere dependent upon specific evaluations.

Expenses (2004–05) *Tuition:* full-time $20,100; part-time $405 per credit hour. *Room and board:* $7690; room only: $4260 per academic year. *Required fees:* full-time $200.

Financial Aid 85% of baccalaureate students in nursing programs received some form of financial aid in 2003–04. *Gift aid (need-based):* Federal Pell, FSEOG, state, private, college/university gift aid from institutional funds. *Loans:* FFEL (Subsidized and Unsubsidized Stafford PLUS), Perkins. *Work-Study:* Federal Work-Study, part-time campus jobs. *Application deadline (priority):* 2/15.

Contact Ms. Marilyn Volk Gomez, Director of Nursing Student Services, Department of Nursing, Xavier University, 3800 Victory Parkway, Cincinnati, OH 45207-7351. *Telephone:* 513-745-4392. *Fax:* 513-745-1087. *E-mail:* gomez@xavier.edu.

GRADUATE PROGRAMS

Expenses (2004–05) *Tuition:* part-time $475 per credit hour.

Financial Aid 30% of graduate students in nursing programs received some form of financial aid in 2003–04. Scholarships, traineeships, and unspecified assistantships available. Aid available to part-time students. *Financial aid application deadline:* 4/1.

Contact Ms. Marilyn Volk Gomez, Director of Nursing Student Services, Department of Nursing, Xavier University, 3800 Victory Parkway, Cincinnati, OH 45207-7351. *Telephone:* 513-745-4392. *Fax:* 513-745-1087. *E-mail:* gomez@xavier.edu.

Xavier University (continued)

MASTER'S DEGREE PROGRAM

Degrees MSN; MSN/MBA

Available Programs Master's; RN to Master's.

Concentrations Available Nursing administration; nursing education.

Study Options Full-time and part-time.

Program Entrance Requirements Minimum overall college GPA of 2.8, transcript of college record, written essay, 3 letters of recommendation, statistics course, GMAT, GRE. *Application deadline:* For fall admission, 8/26 (priority date). Applications are processed on a rolling basis. *Application fee:* $35.

Degree Requirements 36 total credit hours, thesis or project.

Youngstown State University

Department of Nursing
Youngstown, Ohio

Founded in 1908

DEGREES • BSN • MSN

Nursing Program Faculty 22 (18% with doctorates).

Baccalaureate Enrollment 22

Graduate Enrollment 24

Women 75% **Men** 25% **Minority** 13%

Nursing Student Activities Sigma Theta Tau, Student Nurses' Association.

Nursing Student Resources Academic advising; academic or career counseling; assistance for students with disabilities; bookstore; campus computer network; career placement assistance; computer lab; computer-assisted instruction; e-mail services; housing assistance; interactive nursing skills videos; Internet; learning resource lab; library services; nursing audiovisuals; placement services for program completers; resume preparation assistance; skills, simulation, or other laboratory; tutoring.

Library Facilities 991,501 volumes; 2,908 periodical subscriptions.

BACCALAUREATE PROGRAMS

Degree BSN

Site Options Boardman, OH.

Study Options Full-time.

Program Entrance Requirements Minimum overall college GPA of 2.0, transcript of college record, CPR certification, health exam, health insurance, high school biology, high school chemistry, high school foreign language, 3 years high school math, 3 years high school science, high school transcript, immunizations, minimum high school GPA, minimum high school rank, minimum GPA in nursing prerequisites of 2.5, prerequisite course work. Transfer students are accepted. **Standardized tests** *Required:* SAT or ACT, TOEFL for international students. **Application** *Deadline:* 8/15 (freshmen), 8/15 (transfer). *Early decision:* 2/15. *Notification:* continuous (freshmen), 2/15 (early action). *Application fee:* $30.

Advanced Placement Credit by examination available. Credit given for nursing courses completed elsewhere dependent upon specific evaluations.

Financial Aid *Gift aid (need-based):* Federal Pell, FSEOG, state, private, college/university gift aid from institutional funds. *Loans:* FFEL (Subsidized and Unsubsidized Stafford PLUS), Perkins, state, Charles E. Schell Foundation Loans. *Work-Study:* Federal Work-Study, part-time campus jobs. *Application deadline (priority):* 2/15.

Contact Dr. Sharon Phillips, Assistant Professor, Department of Nursing, Youngstown State University, One University Plaza, Youngstown, OH 44555. *Telephone:* 330-941-2328. *Fax:* 330-941-2309. *E-mail:* slphillips@ysu.edu.

GRADUATE PROGRAMS

Financial Aid Federal Work-Study, institutionally sponsored loans, and scholarships available.

Contact Dr. Sharon Shipton, Coordinator, MSN, Department of Nursing, Youngstown State University, One University Plaza, Youngstown, OH 44555. *Telephone:* 330-941-1796. *Fax:* 330-941-2309. *E-mail:* spshipton@ysu.edu.

MASTER'S DEGREE PROGRAM

Degree MSN

Concentrations Available Nurse anesthesia; nursing education.

Study Options Full-time and part-time.

Program Entrance Requirements Clinical experience, computer literacy, transcript of college record, CPR certification, written essay, immunizations, nursing research course, physical assessment course, prerequisite course work, resume, GRE General Test. *Application deadline:* For fall admission, 7/15 (priority date); for spring admission, 12/15 (priority date). Applications are processed on a rolling basis. *Application fee:* $30 ($75 for international students).

Advanced Placement Credit given for nursing courses completed elsewhere dependent upon specific evaluations.

Degree Requirements Thesis or project.

OKLAHOMA

Bacone College

Department of Nursing
Muskogee, Oklahoma

Founded in 1880

DEGREE • BSN

Nursing Program Faculty 8.

Baccalaureate Enrollment 16

Women 100% **Minority** 65%

Nursing Student Activities Student Nurses' Association, nursing club.

Nursing Student Resources Academic advising; bookstore; campus computer network; computer lab; computer-assisted instruction; interactive nursing skills videos; Internet; learning resource lab; library services; nursing audiovisuals; remedial services; skills, simulation, or other laboratory.

Library Facilities 34,564 volumes; 121 periodical subscriptions.

BACCALAUREATE PROGRAMS

Degree BSN

Available Programs Accelerated RN Baccalaureate.

Program Entrance Requirements Transcript of college record, CPR certification, health exam, health insurance, immunizations, 2 letters of recommendation, minimum GPA in nursing prerequisites of 2.5, prerequisite course work, RN licensure. **Standardized tests** *Required:* SAT or ACT, TOEFL for international students. *Recommended:* ACT. **Application** *Deadline:* rolling (freshmen), rolling (transfer). *Notification:* continuous (freshmen). *Application fee:* $25.

Expenses (2003–04) *Tuition:* full-time $9450. *International tuition:* $9450 full-time. *Room and board:* $5700; room only: $3000 per academic year. *Required fees:* full-time $100.

Financial Aid 85% of baccalaureate students in nursing programs received some form of financial aid in 2002–03.

Contact Admissions Officer, Department of Nursing, Bacone College, 2299 Old Bacone Road, Muskogee, OK 74403. *Telephone:* 888-682-5514. *E-mail:* info@bacone.edu.

East Central University

Department of Nursing
Ada, Oklahoma

http://www.ecok.edu/dept/nursing

Founded in 1909

DEGREE • BS

Nursing Program Faculty 17 (29% with doctorates).

Baccalaureate Enrollment 493

Women 86% **Men** 14% **Minority** 44% **International** 1% **Part-time** 14%

Nursing Student Activities Student Nurses' Association, nursing club.

Nursing Student Resources Academic advising; academic or career counseling; assistance for students with disabilities; bookstore; campus computer network; career placement assistance; computer lab; computer-assisted instruction; daycare for children of students; e-mail services; employment services for current students; externships; housing assistance; interactive nursing skills videos; Internet; learning resource lab; library services; nursing audiovisuals; other; placement services for program completers; resume preparation assistance; skills, simulation, or other laboratory; tutoring.

Library Facilities 171,080 volumes; 1,221 periodical subscriptions.

BACCALAUREATE PROGRAMS

Degree BS

Available Programs ADN to Baccalaureate; Generic Baccalaureate.

Site Options *Distance Learning:* Durant, OK; Ardmore, OK; McAlester, OK.

Study Options Full-time and part-time.

Program Entrance Requirements Minimum overall college GPA of 2.5, transcript of college record, CPR certification, health exam, immunizations, professional liability insurance/malpractice insurance, prerequisite course work. Transfer students are accepted. **Standardized tests** *Required:* SAT or ACT, TOEFL for international students. *Recommended:* ACT. **Application** *Application fee:* $20.

Advanced Placement Credit given for nursing courses completed elsewhere dependent upon specific evaluations.

Expenses (2004–05) *Tuition, state resident:* full-time $3000; part-time $92 per credit hour. *Tuition, nonresident:* full-time $9000; part-time $270 per credit hour. *International tuition:* $9000 full-time. *Room and board:* $2500; room only: $1800 per academic year. *Required fees:* full-time $400; part-time $15 per credit; part-time $200 per term.

Financial Aid 63% of baccalaureate students in nursing programs received some form of financial aid in 2003–04. *Gift aid (need-based):* Federal Pell, FSEOG, state, private, college/university gift aid from institutional funds. *Loans:* FFEL (Subsidized and Unsubsidized Stafford PLUS), Perkins, college/university. *Work-Study:* Federal Work-Study, part-time campus jobs. *Application deadline (priority):* 3/1.

Contact Dr. Joseph T. Catalano, Chair, Department of Nursing, East Central University, 1100 East 14th Street, Ada, OK 74820. *Telephone:* 580-310-5434. *Fax:* 580-310-5785. *E-mail:* jcatalan@mailclerk.ecok.edu.

Langston University

School of Nursing and Health Professions
Langston, Oklahoma

http://www.lunet.ed/nurs5.html

Founded in 1897

DEGREE • BSN

Nursing Program Faculty 16 (13% with doctorates).

Nursing Student Activities Student Nurses' Association, nursing club.

Nursing Student Resources Academic advising; academic or career counseling; assistance for students with disabilities; bookstore; campus computer network; career placement assistance; computer lab; computer-assisted instruction; daycare for children of students; e-mail services; housing assistance; interactive nursing skills videos; Internet; learning resource lab; library services; nursing audiovisuals; remedial services; resume preparation assistance; skills, simulation, or other laboratory; tutoring.

Library Facilities 97,565 volumes (35,397 in health, 2,664 in nursing); 1,235 periodical subscriptions (978 health-care related).

BACCALAUREATE PROGRAMS

Degree BSN

Available Programs Generic Baccalaureate; LPN to Baccalaureate; RN Baccalaureate.

Site Options Tulsa, OK.

Study Options Full-time and part-time.

Program Entrance Requirements Minimum overall college GPA of 2.5, transcript of college record, written essay, health exam, immunizations, minimum GPA in nursing prerequisites of 2.5, professional liability insurance/malpractice insurance, prerequisite course work. Transfer students are accepted. **Standardized tests** *Required:* SAT or ACT, TOEFL for international students. ***Placement:*** *Required:* SAT or ACT. **Application** *Deadline:* rolling (freshmen), rolling (transfer).

Advanced Placement Credit by examination available. Credit given for nursing courses completed elsewhere dependent upon specific evaluations.

Expenses (2003–04) *Tuition, state resident:* full-time $1757; part-time $61 per credit hour. *Tuition, nonresident:* full-time $5249; part-time $181 per credit hour. *Required fees:* full-time $798.

Contact Ms. Farretta Hinds, Academic Adviser, School of Nursing and Health Professions, Langston University, 302 University Women Building, Langston, OK 73050. *Telephone:* 405-466-3411. *Fax:* 405-466-2195. *E-mail:* fjhinds@lunet.edu.

Northeastern State University

Department of Nursing
Tahlequah, Oklahoma

http://arapaho.nsuok.edu/~nursing

Founded in 1846

DEGREE • BSN

Nursing Program Faculty 4 (25% with doctorates).

Baccalaureate Enrollment 75

Women 97% **Men** 3% **Minority** 28% **International** 1% **Part-time** 85%

Nursing Student Activities Sigma Theta Tau, Student Nurses' Association.

Nursing Student Resources Academic advising; academic or career counseling; assistance for students with disabilities; bookstore; campus computer network; career placement assistance; computer lab; computer-assisted instruction; e-mail services; employment services for current students; housing assistance; Internet; library services; nursing audiovisuals; placement services for program completers; resume preparation assistance; tutoring.

Library Facilities 424,818 volumes (13,300 in health, 7,200 in nursing); 3,983 periodical subscriptions (200 health-care related).

BACCALAUREATE PROGRAMS

Degree BSN

Available Programs Accelerated RN Baccalaureate; RN Baccalaureate.

Site Options *Distance Learning:* Broken Arrow, OK; Ponca City, OK; Miami, OK.

Program Entrance Requirements Minimum overall college GPA of 2.0, transcript of college record, CPR certification, health exam, immunizations, 3 letters of recommendation, minimum GPA in nursing prerequisites of 2.0, professional liability insurance/malpractice insurance, prerequisite course work, RN licensure. Transfer students are accepted. **Standardized tests** *Required:* ACT, TOEFL for international students. **Application** *Deadline:* 8/5 (freshmen), 8/5 (transfer). *Notification:* continuous (freshmen).

Expenses (2004–05) *Tuition, state resident:* full-time $2625; part-time $88 per credit hour. *Tuition, nonresident:* full-time $7725; part-time $258 per credit hour. *International tuition:* $7725 full-time. *Room and board:* $4620 per academic year. *Required fees:* full-time $900; part-time $30 per credit.

Financial Aid 65% of baccalaureate students in nursing programs received some form of financial aid in 2003–04.

Contact Dr. Joyce A. Van Nostrand, Chair, Department of Health Professions, Department of Nursing, Northeastern State University, PO Box 549, Muskogee, OK 74402-0549. *Telephone:* 918-781-5410. *Fax:* 918-781-5411. *E-mail:* vannostr@nsuok.edu.

Northwestern Oklahoma State University

Division of Nursing
Alva, Oklahoma

http://www.nwosu.edu/nursing

Founded in 1897

DEGREE • BSN

Nursing Program Faculty 10 (10% with doctorates).

Baccalaureate Enrollment 42
Women 95% **Men** 5% **Minority** 5% **International** 2%

Nursing Student Activities Student Nurses' Association.

Nursing Student Resources Academic advising; academic or career counseling; assistance for students with disabilities; bookstore; campus computer network; career placement assistance; computer lab; computer-assisted instruction; e-mail services; housing assistance; Internet; learning resource lab; library services; remedial services; skills, simulation, or other laboratory.

Library Facilities 344,640 volumes; 3,990 periodical subscriptions (59 health-care related).

BACCALAUREATE PROGRAMS

Degree BSN

Site Options *Distance Learning:* Enid, OK; Woodward, OK.

Study Options Full-time and part-time.

Program Entrance Requirements Minimum overall college GPA of 2.5, transcript of college record, CPR certification, health exam, high school transcript, immunizations, 3 letters of recommendation, minimum high school GPA of 2.5, minimum GPA in nursing prerequisites of 2.5, professional liability insurance/malpractice insurance, prerequisite course work. Transfer students are accepted. **Standardized tests** *Required:* SAT or ACT, TOEFL for international students. ***Placement:*** *Required:* SAT or ACT. **Application** *Deadline:* rolling (freshmen), rolling (transfer). *Notification:* continuous (freshmen). *Application fee:* $15.

Advanced Placement Credit by examination available. Credit given for nursing courses completed elsewhere dependent upon specific evaluations.

Expenses (2003–04) *Tuition, state resident:* full-time $1950; part-time $65 per credit hour. *Tuition, nonresident:* full-time $5850; part-time $195 per credit hour. *Room and board:* $2620; room only: $860 per academic year. *Required fees:* full-time $747; part-time $25 per credit.

Financial Aid 74% of baccalaureate students in nursing programs received some form of financial aid in 2002–03. *Gift aid (need-based):* Federal Pell, FSEOG, state, college/university gift aid from institutional funds. *Loans:* FFEL (Subsidized and Unsubsidized Stafford PLUS), Perkins. *Work-Study:* Federal Work-Study, part-time campus jobs. *Application deadline (priority):* 3/1.

Contact Dr. Frankie L. Buechner, Division Director, Division of Nursing, Northwestern Oklahoma State University, 709 Oklahoma Boulevard, Alva, OK 73717-2799. *Telephone:* 580-327-8489. *Fax:* 580-327-8434. *E-mail:* flbuechner@nwosu.edu.

Oklahoma Baptist University

School of Nursing
Shawnee, Oklahoma

Founded in 1910

DEGREE • BSN

Nursing Program Faculty 8 (38% with doctorates).

Baccalaureate Enrollment 109
Women 95% **Men** 5% **Minority** 5% **Part-time** 3%

Nursing Student Activities Sigma Theta Tau, Student Nurses' Association.

Nursing Student Resources Academic advising; academic or career counseling; assistance for students with disabilities; bookstore; campus computer network; computer-assisted instruction; e-mail services; externships; learning resource lab; library services; nursing audiovisuals; resume preparation assistance; skills, simulation, or other laboratory; tutoring.

Library Facilities 230,000 volumes (10,000 in health, 5,500 in nursing); 1,800 periodical subscriptions (60 health-care related).

BACCALAUREATE PROGRAMS

Degree BSN

Available Programs Generic Baccalaureate; LPN to Baccalaureate; RN Baccalaureate.

Study Options Full-time and part-time.

Program Entrance Requirements Minimum overall college GPA of 2.25, transcript of college record, CPR certification, health exam, high school transcript, immunizations, minimum GPA in nursing prerequisites of 2.3, prerequisite course work. Transfer students are accepted. **Standardized tests** *Required:* SAT or ACT, TOEFL for international students. **Application** *Deadline:* rolling (freshmen), 8/1 (transfer). *Notification:* continuous until 9/1 (freshmen). *Application fee:* $25.

Advanced Placement Credit given for nursing courses completed elsewhere dependent upon specific evaluations.

Expenses (2003–04) *Tuition:* full-time $15,268.

Financial Aid 93% of baccalaureate students in nursing programs received some form of financial aid in 2002–03. *Gift aid (need-based):* Federal Pell, FSEOG, state, private, college/university gift aid from institutional funds. *Loans:* FFEL (Subsidized and Unsubsidized Stafford PLUS), Perkins. *Work-Study:* Federal Work-Study, part-time campus jobs. *Application deadline (priority):* 3/1.

Contact Dr. Lana Bolhouse, Dean, School of Nursing, Oklahoma Baptist University, 500 West University, Shawnee, OK 74804. *Telephone:* 405-878-2081. *Fax:* 405-878-2083. *E-mail:* lana_bolhouse@mail.okbu.edu.

Oklahoma City University

Kramer School of Nursing
Oklahoma City, Oklahoma

http://www.okcu.edu ursing

Founded in 1904

DEGREES • BSN • MSN • MSN/MBA

Nursing Program Faculty 16 (19% with doctorates).

Baccalaureate Enrollment 132
Women 76% **Men** 24% **Minority** 45% **International** 9% **Part-time** 6%

Graduate Enrollment 10
Women 90% **Men** 10% **Minority** 30%

Nursing Student Activities Sigma Theta Tau, Student Nurses' Association.

Nursing Student Resources Academic advising; academic or career counseling; assistance for students with disabilities; bookstore; campus computer network; career placement assistance; computer lab; e-mail services; housing assistance; interactive nursing skills videos; Internet; learning resource lab; library services; nursing audiovisuals; skills, simulation, or other laboratory; tutoring.

Library Facilities 440,374 volumes (519 in health, 398 in nursing); 6,017 periodical subscriptions (60 health-care related).

BACCALAUREATE PROGRAMS

Degree BSN

Available Programs ADN to Baccalaureate; Accelerated Baccalaureate for Second Degree; Generic Baccalaureate.

Study Options Full-time.

Program Entrance Requirements Minimum overall college GPA of 3.0, transcript of college record, CPR certification, high school transcript, immunizations, minimum high school GPA of 3.0, minimum GPA in nursing prerequisites of 3.0, professional liability insurance/malpractice insurance, prerequisite course work. Transfer students are accepted. **Standardized**

tests *Required:* SAT or ACT, TOEFL for international students. **Application** *Deadline:* 8/20 (freshmen), rolling (transfer). *Notification:* continuous (freshmen). *Application fee:* $30.

Advanced Placement Credit given for nursing courses completed elsewhere dependent upon specific evaluations.

Expenses (2004–05) *Tuition:* full-time $15,200; part-time $518 per contact hour. *Room and board:* $2975 per academic year. *Required fees:* full-time $750.

Financial Aid 90% of baccalaureate students in nursing programs received some form of financial aid in 2003–04. *Gift aid (need-based):* Federal Pell, FSEOG, state, private, college/university gift aid from institutional funds, United Negro College Fund, Federal Nursing, Native American Grants. *Loans:* Federal Nursing Student Loans, FFEL (Subsidized and Unsubsidized Stafford PLUS), Perkins. *Work-Study:* Federal Work-Study, part-time campus jobs. *Application deadline (priority):* 3/1.

Contact Mrs. Glenda Kirkham, Student Services Assistant, Kramer School of Nursing, Oklahoma City University, 2501 North Blackwelder, Oklahoma City, OK 73106. *Telephone:* 405-208-5901. *Fax:* 405-208-5914. *E-mail:* gkirkham@okcu.edu.

GRADUATE PROGRAMS

Expenses (2004–05) *Tuition:* part-time $604 per contact hour.

Contact Dr. Marvel L. Williamson, Dean and Professor, Kramer School of Nursing, Oklahoma City University, 2501 North Blackwelder, Oklahoma City, OK 73106. *Telephone:* 405-208-5900. *Fax:* 405-208-5914. *E-mail:* mwilliamson@okcu.edu.

MASTER'S DEGREE PROGRAM

Degrees MSN; MSN/MBA

Available Programs Master's.

Study Options Full-time and part-time.

Program Entrance Requirements Minimum overall college GPA of 3.0, transcript of college record.

Degree Requirements 39 total credit hours, thesis or project.

CONTINUING EDUCATION PROGRAM

Contact Dr. Marvel L. Williamson, Dean and Professor, Kramer School of Nursing, Oklahoma City University, 2501 North Blackwelder, Oklahoma City, OK 73106. *Telephone:* 405-208-5900. *Fax:* 405-208-5914. *E-mail:* mwilliamson@okcu.edu.

Oklahoma Panhandle State University

Bachelor of Science in Nursing Program
Goodwell, Oklahoma

http://www.opsu.edu

Founded in 1909

DEGREE • BSN

Nursing Program Faculty 4.

Baccalaureate Enrollment 30
Women 93% **Men** 7% **Minority** 20% **Part-time** 75%

Nursing Student Activities Student Nurses' Association.

Nursing Student Resources Academic advising; academic or career counseling; assistance for students with disabilities; bookstore; library services.

Library Facilities 106,000 volumes; 308 periodical subscriptions.

BACCALAUREATE PROGRAMS

Degree BSN

Available Programs ADN to Baccalaureate.

Program Entrance Requirements Minimum overall college GPA of 2.0, transcript of college record, CPR certification, immunizations, minimum GPA in nursing prerequisites of 2.0, professional liability insurance/malpractice insurance, RN licensure. Transfer students are accepted. **Standardized tests** *Required:* TOEFL for international students. ***Placement:*** *Required:* SAT or ACT. **Application** *Deadline:* rolling (freshmen), rolling (transfer).

Advanced Placement Credit given for nursing courses completed elsewhere dependent upon specific evaluations.

Expenses (2004–05) *Tuition, state resident:* part-time $69 per credit hour. *Tuition, nonresident:* part-time $93 per credit hour.

Financial Aid 50% of baccalaureate students in nursing programs received some form of financial aid in 2003–04.

Contact Lynna Brakhage, RN, Interim Director, Bachelor of Science in Nursing Program, Oklahoma Panhandle State University, PO Box 430, 323 West Eagle Boulevard, Goodwell, OK 73939. *Telephone:* 580-349-1520. *Fax:* 580-349-1529. *E-mail:* nursing@opsu.edu or lynnab@opsu.edu.

Oklahoma Wesleyan University

Division of Nursing
Bartlesville, Oklahoma

http://nursing.okwu.edu

Founded in 1909

DEGREE • BSN

Nursing Program Faculty 31 (35% with doctorates).

Baccalaureate Enrollment 140
Women 96% **Men** 4% **Minority** 23%

Nursing Student Resources Academic advising; academic or career counseling; assistance for students with disabilities; bookstore; campus computer network; computer lab; computer-assisted instruction; interactive nursing skills videos; Internet; learning resource lab; library services; nursing audiovisuals; skills, simulation, or other laboratory.

Library Facilities 124,722 volumes (946 in health, 483 in nursing); 300 periodical subscriptions (40 health-care related).

BACCALAUREATE PROGRAMS

Degree BSN

Available Programs ADN to Baccalaureate; Accelerated RN Baccalaureate; Baccalaureate for Second Degree; Generic Baccalaureate; International Nurse to Baccalaureate; LPN to Baccalaureate; RN Baccalaureate.

Site Options *Distance Learning:* McAlester, OK; Oklahoma City, OK; Tulsa, OK.

Study Options Full-time.

Program Entrance Requirements Minimum overall college GPA of 2.3, transcript of college record, CPR certification, health exam, health insurance, immunizations, 2 letters of recommendation, minimum GPA in nursing prerequisites of 2.75, professional liability insurance/malpractice insurance, prerequisite course work, RN licensure. Transfer students are accepted. **Standardized tests** *Required:* SAT or ACT. *Recommended:* TOEFL for international students. **Application** *Deadline:* rolling (freshmen), rolling (transfer). *Application fee:* $25.

Advanced Placement Credit by examination available. Credit given for nursing courses completed elsewhere dependent upon specific evaluations.

Expenses (2003–04) *Tuition:* full-time $11,550; part-time $425 per credit hour. *International tuition:* $11,550 full-time. *Room and board:* $4600; room only: $1150 per academic year. *Required fees:* full-time $150.

Financial Aid 35% of baccalaureate students in nursing programs received some form of financial aid in 2002–03.

Contact Mrs. Pamela Ann Giles, RN, Chair, Division of Nursing, Oklahoma Wesleyan University, 2201 Silver Lake Road, Bartlesville, OK 74006. *Telephone:* 918-335-6254. *Fax:* 918-335-6204. *E-mail:* pgiles@okwu.edu.

Oral Roberts University

Anna Vaughn School of Nursing
Tulsa, Oklahoma

http://www.oru.edu

Founded in 1963

DEGREE • BSN

Oral Roberts University (continued)

Nursing Program Faculty 13.

Baccalaureate Enrollment 56
Women 96% **Men** 4% **Minority** 14% **International** 2%

Nursing Student Activities Nursing Honor Society, Sigma Theta Tau, Student Nurses' Association.

Nursing Student Resources Academic advising; academic or career counseling; assistance for students with disabilities; bookstore; campus computer network; computer lab; computer-assisted instruction; e-mail services; employment services for current students; externships; housing assistance; interactive nursing skills videos; Internet; learning resource lab; library services; nursing audiovisuals; remedial services; resume preparation assistance; skills, simulation, or other laboratory; tutoring.

Library Facilities 216,691 volumes (8,980 in health, 2,143 in nursing); 600 periodical subscriptions (31,399 health-care related).

BACCALAUREATE PROGRAMS

Degree BSN

Available Programs ADN to Baccalaureate; Generic Baccalaureate.

Study Options Full-time and part-time.

Program Entrance Requirements Minimum overall college GPA of 2.5, transcript of college record, CPR certification, health exam, high school chemistry, 2 years high school math, 2 years high school science, high school transcript, immunizations, minimum high school GPA of 2.5, minimum GPA in nursing prerequisites of 2.5. Transfer students are accepted. **Standardized tests** *Required:* SAT or ACT, TOEFL for international students. **Application** *Deadline:* rolling (freshmen), rolling (transfer). *Early decision:* 9/1. *Notification:* continuous (freshmen), 9/1 (early action). *Application fee:* $35.

Expenses (2004–05) *Tuition:* full-time $14,600; part-time $610 per credit hour. *Room and board:* $6370; room only: $3080 per academic year. *Required fees:* full-time $450; part-time $19 per credit; part-time $225 per term.

Financial Aid 97% of baccalaureate students in nursing programs received some form of financial aid in 2003–04.

Contact Dr. Kenda Jezek, Dean, Anna Vaughn School of Nursing, Oral Roberts University, 7777 South Lewis, Tulsa, OK 74171. *Telephone:* 918-495-6198. *Fax:* 918-495-6020. *E-mail:* kjezek@oru.edu.

Southern Nazarene University
School of Nursing
Bethany, Oklahoma

http://www.snu.edu
Founded in 1899

DEGREES • BS • MS

Nursing Program Faculty 15 (.2% with doctorates).

Baccalaureate Enrollment 200
Women 95% **Men** 5% **Minority** 26% **International** 2%

Graduate Enrollment 15

Nursing Student Activities Sigma Theta Tau, Student Nurses' Association, nursing club.

Nursing Student Resources Academic advising; academic or career counseling; assistance for students with disabilities; bookstore; campus computer network; career placement assistance; computer lab; computer-assisted instruction; e-mail services; employment services for current students; externships; housing assistance; interactive nursing skills videos; Internet; learning resource lab; library services; nursing audiovisuals; placement services for program completers; remedial services; skills, simulation, or other laboratory; tutoring; unpaid internships.

Library Facilities 95,535 volumes; 225 periodical subscriptions.

BACCALAUREATE PROGRAMS

Degree BS

Available Programs Accelerated Baccalaureate; Generic Baccalaureate.

Site Options Tulsa, OK.

Study Options Full-time.

Program Entrance Requirements Transcript of college record, CPR certification, written essay, health exam, health insurance, high school transcript, immunizations, 2 letters of recommendation, minimum high school GPA of 2.75, minimum GPA in nursing prerequisites of 2.75, professional liability insurance/malpractice insurance, prerequisite course work. Transfer students are accepted. **Standardized tests** *Required:* TOEFL for international students. ***Placement:*** *Required:* SAT or ACT. *Recommended:* ACT. **Application** *Deadline:* 8/15 (freshmen), 8/15 (transfer). *Notification:* continuous (freshmen). *Application fee:* $25.

Advanced Placement Credit by examination available. Credit given for nursing courses completed elsewhere dependent upon specific evaluations.

Expenses (2003–04) *Tuition:* full-time $11,310; part-time $377 per credit hour. *International tuition:* $11,310 full-time. *Room and board:* $5048; room only: $2362 per academic year. *Required fees:* full-time $240; part-time $20 per credit.

Financial Aid 80% of baccalaureate students in nursing programs received some form of financial aid in 2002–03.

Contact Dr. Ann Ferguson, Chair, School of Nursing, Southern Nazarene University, 6729 Northwest 39th Expressway, Bethany, OK 73008. *Telephone:* 405-491-6365. *Fax:* 405-717-6264. *E-mail:* aferguso@snu.edu.

GRADUATE PROGRAMS

Expenses (2003–04) *Tuition:* full-time $17,589. *International tuition:* $17,589 full-time.

Financial Aid 85% of graduate students in nursing programs received some form of financial aid in 2002–03.

Contact Dr. Susan Barnes, Coordinator, School of Nursing, Southern Nazarene University, Southern Nazarene University School of Nursing, 6729 Northwest 39th Expressway, Bethany, OK 73008. *Telephone:* 405-491-6663. *Fax:* 405-717-6264. *E-mail:* sbarnes@snu.edu.

MASTER'S DEGREE PROGRAM

Degree MS

Available Programs Accelerated Master's; Master's.

Concentrations Available Nursing education.

Site Options Tulsa, OK.

Study Options Full-time.

Program Entrance Requirements Computer literacy, minimum overall college GPA of 2.75, transcript of college record, interview, 3 letters of recommendation, resume, statistics course.

Degree Requirements 39 total credit hours, thesis or project.

Southwestern Oklahoma State University
Division of Nursing
Weatherford, Oklahoma

http://www.swosu.edu/academic/nurse
Founded in 1901

DEGREE • BSN

Nursing Program Faculty 9 (22% with doctorates).

Baccalaureate Enrollment 57
Women 84% **Men** 16% **Minority** 11% **International** 2%

Nursing Student Activities Nursing Honor Society, Student Nurses' Association, nursing club.

Nursing Student Resources Academic advising; academic or career counseling; assistance for students with disabilities; bookstore; campus computer network; computer lab; computer-assisted instruction; e-mail services; interactive nursing skills videos; Internet; learning resource lab; library services; nursing audiovisuals; remedial services; skills, simulation, or other laboratory; tutoring.

Library Facilities 217,051 volumes; 1,230 periodical subscriptions (284 health-care related).

BACCALAUREATE PROGRAMS

Degree BSN

Site Options *Distance Learning:* Oklahoma City, OK; Altus, OK.

Study Options Full-time.

Program Entrance Requirements Minimum overall college GPA of 2.25, transcript of college record, CPR certification, health exam, high school transcript, immunizations, interview, 3 letters of recommendation, minimum GPA in nursing prerequisites of 2.25, professional liability insurance/malpractice insurance, prerequisite course work. Transfer students are accepted. **Standardized tests** *Required:* ACT, TOEFL for international students. **Application** *Notification:* continuous (freshmen). *Application fee:* $15.

Advanced Placement Credit given for nursing courses completed elsewhere dependent upon specific evaluations.

Expenses (2003–04) *Room and board:* $1455 per academic year.

Financial Aid 50% of baccalaureate students in nursing programs received some form of financial aid in 2002–03.

Contact Ms. Charlene Killgore, Administrative Assistant, Division of Nursing, Southwestern Oklahoma State University, 100 Campus Drive, Weatherford, OK 73096-3098. *Telephone:* 580-774-3261. *Fax:* 580-774-7075. *E-mail:* killgoc@swosu.edu.

University of Central Oklahoma

Department of Nursing
Edmond, Oklahoma

http://nursing.ucok.edu

Founded in 1890

DEGREE • BSN

Nursing Program Faculty 27 (7% with doctorates).

Baccalaureate Enrollment 169

Women 97% **Men** 3% **Minority** 8% **International** 7% **Part-time** 2%

Nursing Student Activities Nursing Honor Society, Sigma Theta Tau, Student Nurses' Association.

Nursing Student Resources Academic advising; academic or career counseling; assistance for students with disabilities; bookstore; campus computer network; career placement assistance; computer lab; computer-assisted instruction; e-mail services; interactive nursing skills videos; Internet; library services; nursing audiovisuals; skills, simulation, or other laboratory.

Library Facilities 254,478 volumes (2,831 in health, 1,733 in nursing); 3,707 periodical subscriptions.

BACCALAUREATE PROGRAMS

Degree BSN

Available Programs Generic Baccalaureate; LPN to Baccalaureate; RN Baccalaureate.

Site Options Oklahoma City, OK.

Study Options Full-time and part-time.

Program Entrance Requirements Minimum overall college GPA of 2.5, transcript of college record, CPR certification, written essay, high school math, immunizations, 3 letters of recommendation, professional liability insurance/malpractice insurance, prerequisite course work. Transfer students are accepted. **Standardized tests** *Required:* SAT or ACT, TOEFL for international students. *Recommended:* ACT. **Application** *Deadline:* rolling (freshmen). *Notification:* continuous until 8/1 (freshmen). *Application fee:* $25.

Advanced Placement Credit given for nursing courses completed elsewhere dependent upon specific evaluations.

Expenses (2004–05) *Tuition, state resident:* full-time $2878; part-time $99 per credit hour. *Tuition, nonresident:* full-time $6669; part-time $230 per credit hour. *International tuition:* $6669 full-time. *Room and board:* $2766 per academic year. *Required fees:* full-time $350.

Financial Aid 35% of baccalaureate students in nursing programs received some form of financial aid in 2003–04.

Contact Vicki Hodges, Administrative Secretary, Department of Nursing, University of Central Oklahoma, 100 North University Drive, Edmond, OK 73034-5209. *Telephone:* 405-974-5000. *E-mail:* vaddison@ucok.edu.

University of Oklahoma Health Sciences Center

College of Nursing
Oklahoma City, Oklahoma

http://nursing.ouhsc.edu/

Founded in 1890

DEGREES • BSN • MS

Nursing Program Faculty 60.

Nursing Student Activities Sigma Theta Tau, Student Nurses' Association.

Nursing Student Resources Academic or career counseling; Internet; library services.

Library Facilities 300,260 volumes; 4,028 periodical subscriptions.

BACCALAUREATE PROGRAMS

Degree BSN

Available Programs Generic Baccalaureate.

Site Options *Distance Learning:* Tulsa, OK; Lawton, OK.

Study Options Full-time and part-time.

Program Entrance Requirements Minimum overall college GPA of 2.5, minimum high school GPA of 2.5, minimum GPA in nursing prerequisites of 2.0, prerequisite course work. Transfer students are accepted. **Standardized tests** *Required:* TOEFL for international students. **Application** *Deadline:* rolling (freshmen). *Notification:* continuous (freshmen). *Application fee:* $40.

Advanced Placement Credit by examination available. Credit given for nursing courses completed elsewhere dependent upon specific evaluations.

Contact Office of Student Affairs, College of Nursing, University of Oklahoma Health Sciences Center, PO Box 26901, 1100 North Stonewall Avenue, Oklahoma City, OK 73190. *Telephone:* 405-271-2125. *Fax:* 405-271-7341.

GRADUATE PROGRAMS

Expenses (2003–04) *Tuition, state resident:* part-time $92 per credit hour. *Tuition, nonresident:* part-time $298 per credit hour. *Required fees:* part-time $14 per credit.

Financial Aid 6 research assistantships (averaging $6,000 per year) were awarded; teaching assistantships, institutionally sponsored loans, scholarships, and traineeships also available.

Contact Office of Student Affairs, College of Nursing, University of Oklahoma Health Sciences Center, PO Box 26901, 1100 North Stonewall Avenue, Oklahoma City, OK 73190. *Telephone:* 405-271-2125. *Fax:* 405-271-7341.

MASTER'S DEGREE PROGRAM

Degree MS

Available Programs Master's; Master's for Non-Nursing College Graduates.

Concentrations Available Health-care administration; nursing education. *Clinical nurse specialist programs in:* acute care, gerontology, parent-child, psychiatric/mental health. *Nurse practitioner programs in:* family health, pediatric.

Site Options Ada, OK. *Distance Learning:* Tulsa, OK; Lawton, OK.

Study Options Full-time and part-time.

Program Entrance Requirements Computer literacy, minimum overall college GPA of 3.0, 3 letters of recommendation, nursing research course, professional liability insurance/malpractice insurance, prerequisite course work, statistics course. *Application deadline:* For fall admission, 6/1; for spring admission, 11/1. Applications are processed on a rolling basis. *Application fee:* $50.

University of Oklahoma Health Sciences Center (continued)

Advanced Placement Credit given for nursing courses completed elsewhere dependent upon specific evaluations.

Degree Requirements Thesis or project, comprehensive exam.

POST-MASTER'S PROGRAM

Areas of Study *Nurse practitioner programs in:* family health, pediatric.

University of Phoenix–Oklahoma City Campus

College of Health and Human Services
Oklahoma City, Oklahoma

Founded in 1976

DEGREES • BSN • MSN • MSN/MBA

Nursing Program Faculty 6.

Baccalaureate Enrollment 1
Women 100% **Minority** 100%

Graduate Enrollment 10
Women 90% **Men** 10% **Minority** 11%

Nursing Student Activities Sigma Theta Tau.

Nursing Student Resources Academic advising; academic or career counseling; computer lab; library services.

Library Facilities 27.1 million volumes; 11,648 periodical subscriptions (1,426 health-care related).

BACCALAUREATE PROGRAMS

Degree BSN

Available Programs ADN to Baccalaureate; Accelerated Baccalaureate.

Site Options Norman, OK.

Study Options Full-time.

Program Entrance Requirements Transcript of college record, immunizations, letters of recommendation. Transfer students are accepted. **Standardized tests** *Required:* TOEFL for international students. **Application** *Deadline:* rolling (freshmen), rolling (transfer). *Application fee:* $85.

Advanced Placement Credit by examination available.

Expenses (2004–05) *Tuition:* full-time $8910; part-time $297 per credit hour. *International tuition:* $8910 full-time. *Required fees:* full-time $110.

Contact Campus College Chair, Nursing, College of Health and Human Services, University of Phoenix–Oklahoma City Campus, 6501 North Broadway Extension, Suite #100, Oklahoma City, OK 73116-8244. *Telephone:* 405-842-8007.

GRADUATE PROGRAMS

Expenses (2004–05) *Tuition:* full-time $9408; part-time $392 per credit hour. *International tuition:* $9408 full-time. *Required fees:* full-time $110.

Financial Aid 7% of graduate students in nursing programs received some form of financial aid in 2003–04.

Contact Campus College Chair, Nursing, College of Health and Human Services, University of Phoenix–Oklahoma City Campus, 6501 North Broadway Extension, Suite #100, Oklahoma City, OK 73116-8244. *Telephone:* 405-842-8007.

MASTER'S DEGREE PROGRAM

Degrees MSN; MSN/MBA

Available Programs Master's.

Concentrations Available Health-care administration; nursing administration; nursing education. *Nurse practitioner programs in:* family health.

Site Options Norman, OK.

Study Options Full-time.

Program Entrance Requirements Clinical experience, computer literacy, transcript of college record.

Degree Requirements 39 total credit hours, thesis or project.

POST-MASTER'S PROGRAM

Areas of Study *Nurse practitioner programs in:* family health.

University of Phoenix–Tulsa Campus

College of Health and Human Services
Tulsa, Oklahoma

Founded in 1998

DEGREES • BSN • MSN • MSN/MBA

Nursing Program Faculty 10 (10% with doctorates).

Graduate Enrollment 1
Women 100%

Nursing Student Activities Sigma Theta Tau.

Nursing Student Resources Academic advising; academic or career counseling; bookstore; computer lab; library services.

Library Facilities 27.1 million volumes; 11,648 periodical subscriptions (1,426 health-care related).

BACCALAUREATE PROGRAMS

Degree BSN

Available Programs ADN to Baccalaureate; Accelerated Baccalaureate.

Study Options Full-time.

Program Entrance Requirements Transcript of college record, immunizations, 1 letter of recommendation. Transfer students are accepted. **Standardized tests** *Required:* TOEFL for international students. **Application** *Deadline:* rolling (freshmen), rolling (transfer). *Application fee:* $85.

Advanced Placement Credit by examination available. Credit given for nursing courses completed elsewhere dependent upon specific evaluations.

Expenses (2004–05) *Tuition:* full-time $8910; part-time $297 per credit hour. *International tuition:* $8910 full-time. *Required fees:* full-time $110.

Contact Campus College Chair, Nursing, College of Health and Human Services, University of Phoenix–Tulsa Campus, 10810 East 45th Street, #103, Tulsa, OK 74146-3801. *Telephone:* 918-622-4877.

GRADUATE PROGRAMS

Expenses (2004–05) *Tuition:* full-time $9408; part-time $392 per credit hour. *International tuition:* $9408 full-time. *Required fees:* full-time $110.

Financial Aid 4% of graduate students in nursing programs received some form of financial aid in 2003–04.

Contact Campus College Chair, Nursing, College of Health and Human Services, University of Phoenix–Tulsa Campus, 10810 East 45th Street, #103, Tulsa, OK 74146-3801. *Telephone:* 918-622-4877.

MASTER'S DEGREE PROGRAM

Degrees MSN; MSN/MBA

Available Programs Master's.

Concentrations Available Health-care administration; nursing administration; nursing education. *Nurse practitioner programs in:* family health.

Study Options Full-time.

Program Entrance Requirements Clinical experience, computer literacy, transcript of college record.

Advanced Placement Credit by examination available. Credit given for nursing courses completed elsewhere dependent upon specific evaluations.

Degree Requirements 39 total credit hours, thesis or project.

POST-MASTER'S PROGRAM

Areas of Study *Nurse practitioner programs in:* family health.

University of Tulsa
School of Nursing
Tulsa, Oklahoma

http://www.cba.utulsa.edu/depts/nursing

Founded in 1894

DEGREE • BSN

Nursing Program Faculty 9 (45% with doctorates).

Baccalaureate Enrollment 65
Women 94% **Men** 6% **Minority** 17% **International** 2% **Part-time** 2%

Nursing Student Activities Sigma Theta Tau, Student Nurses' Association.

Nursing Student Resources Academic advising; academic or career counseling; assistance for students with disabilities; bookstore; campus computer network; career placement assistance; computer lab; computer-assisted instruction; daycare for children of students; e-mail services; externships; housing assistance; interactive nursing skills videos; Internet; learning resource lab; library services; nursing audiovisuals; placement services for program completers; remedial services; resume preparation assistance; skills, simulation, or other laboratory; tutoring.

Library Facilities 940,105 volumes (4,300 in nursing); 6,317 periodical subscriptions (118 health-care related).

BACCALAUREATE PROGRAMS

Degree BSN

Available Programs Generic Baccalaureate; LPN to RN Baccalaureate; RN Baccalaureate.

Study Options Full-time.

Program Entrance Requirements Minimum overall college GPA of 2.5, transcript of college record, CPR certification, written essay, high school transcript, immunizations, minimum GPA in nursing prerequisites. Transfer students are accepted. **Standardized tests** *Required:* SAT or ACT, TOEFL for international students. **Application** *Deadline:* rolling (freshmen), rolling (transfer). *Notification:* continuous (freshmen). *Application fee:* $35.

Advanced Placement Credit by examination available. Credit given for nursing courses completed elsewhere dependent upon specific evaluations.

Expenses (2004–05) *Tuition:* full-time $16,750; part-time $600 per credit hour. *International tuition:* $16,750 full-time. *Room and board:* $5896; room only: $3216 per academic year. *Required fees:* full-time $267.

Financial Aid 90% of baccalaureate students in nursing programs received some form of financial aid in 2003–04. *Gift aid (need-based):* Federal Pell, FSEOG, state, private, college/university gift aid from institutional funds. *Loans:* FFEL (Subsidized and Unsubsidized Stafford PLUS), Perkins, college/university. *Work-Study:* Federal Work-Study, part-time campus jobs. *Application deadline (priority):* 4/1.

Contact Dr. Susan K. Gaston, RN, Director, School of Nursing, University of Tulsa, 600 South College Avenue, Tulsa, OK 74104-3189. *Telephone:* 918-631-3116. *Fax:* 918-631-2068. *E-mail:* susan-gaston@utulsa.edu.

OREGON

Linfield College
School of Nursing
McMinnville, Oregon

http://www.linfield.edu/portland

Founded in 1849

DEGREE • BSN

Nursing Program Faculty 45 (42% with doctorates).

Baccalaureate Enrollment 341
Women 92% **Men** 8% **Minority** 12% **International** 2% **Part-time** 2%

Nursing Student Activities Sigma Theta Tau, Student Nurses' Association, nursing club.

Nursing Student Resources Academic advising; academic or career counseling; bookstore; campus computer network; computer lab; e-mail services; Internet; learning resource lab; library services; nursing audiovisuals; resume preparation assistance; skills, simulation, or other laboratory.

Library Facilities 169,087 volumes (7,201 in health, 1,482 in nursing); 1,278 periodical subscriptions (249 health-care related).

BACCALAUREATE PROGRAMS

Degree BSN

Available Programs Accelerated Baccalaureate for Second Degree; Generic Baccalaureate; RN Baccalaureate.

Site Options Portland, OR.

Study Options Full-time and part-time.

Program Entrance Requirements Minimum overall college GPA of 2.8, transcript of college record, CPR certification, written essay, health exam, immunizations, 1 letter of recommendation, minimum GPA in nursing prerequisites of 2.5, professional liability insurance/malpractice insurance, prerequisite course work. Transfer students are accepted. **Standardized tests** *Required:* SAT or ACT, TOEFL for international students. **Application** *Deadline:* 2/15 (freshmen), 4/15 (transfer). *Early decision:* 11/15. *Notification:* 4/1 (freshmen), 1/15 (early action). *Application fee:* $40.

Advanced Placement Credit given for nursing courses completed elsewhere dependent upon specific evaluations.

Expenses (2004–05) *Tuition:* full-time $21,800; part-time $680 per credit hour. *International tuition:* $21,800 full-time. *Room and board:* room only: $2772 per academic year. *Required fees:* full-time $118.

Financial Aid 97% of baccalaureate students in nursing programs received some form of financial aid in 2003–04. *Gift aid (need-based):* Federal Pell, FSEOG, state, private, college/university gift aid from institutional funds. *Loans:* FFEL (Subsidized and Unsubsidized Stafford PLUS), Perkins, college/university, alternative loans. *Work-Study:* Federal Work-Study, part-time campus jobs. *Application deadline (priority):* 2/1.

Contact Beth A. Woodward, Director, Enrollment Services, School of Nursing, Linfield College, 2255 NW Northrup Street, Portland, OR 97210. *Telephone:* 503-413-8481. *Fax:* 503-413-6283. *E-mail:* bwoodwar@linfield.edu.

CONTINUING EDUCATION PROGRAM

Contact Dr. Beverly Epeneter, Interim Dean, School of Nursing, Linfield College, 2255 NW Northrup Street, Portland, OR 97210. *Telephone:* 503-413-7163. *Fax:* 503-413-6846. *E-mail:* bepenet@linfield.edu.

Oregon Health & Science University
School of Nursing
Portland, Oregon

http://www.ohsu.edu/son

Founded in 1974

DEGREES • BS • MS • MSN/MPH • PHD

Nursing Program Faculty 130 (40% with doctorates).

Baccalaureate Enrollment 637
Minority 12%

Graduate Enrollment 167
Minority 8%

Library Facilities 200,771 volumes (227,344 in health, 7,666 in nursing); 2,110 periodical subscriptions (2,357 health-care related).

BACCALAUREATE PROGRAMS

Degree BS

Oregon Health & Science University (continued)

Available Programs Accelerated Baccalaureate; Generic Baccalaureate; RN Baccalaureate.

Site Options *Distance Learning:* Ashland, OR; La Grande, OR; Klamath Falls, OR.

Study Options Full-time and part-time.

Program Entrance Requirements Minimum overall college GPA of 2.5, transcript of college record, CPR certification, written essay, high school transcript, immunizations, minimum high school GPA of 2.5, prerequisite course work. Transfer students are accepted. **Standardized tests** *Required:* TOEFL for international students. *Required for some:* SAT. **Application** *Application fee:* $60.

Advanced Placement Credit by examination available. Credit given for nursing courses completed elsewhere dependent upon specific evaluations.

Expenses (2003–04) *Tuition, state resident:* full-time $1974; part-time $141 per credit hour. *Tuition, nonresident:* full-time $4592; part-time $328 per credit hour. *Required fees:* full-time $576.

Financial Aid *Gift aid (need-based):* Federal Pell, FSEOG, state, private, college/university gift aid from institutional funds, Health Profession Scholarships. *Loans:* Federal Nursing Student Loans, Federal Direct (Subsidized and Unsubsidized Stafford PLUS), Perkins, state, college/university, alternative loans. *Work-Study:* Federal Work-Study. *Application deadline:* Continuous.

Contact Academic Programs Counselor, School of Nursing, Oregon Health & Science University, 3455 Southwest U.S. Veterans Hospital Road, SN-4N, Portland, OR 97239-2491. *Telephone:* 503-494-7725. *Fax:* 503-494-4350.

GRADUATE PROGRAMS

Expenses (2003–04) *Tuition, state resident:* full-time $3223; part-time $293 per credit hour. *Tuition, nonresident:* full-time $5192; part-time $472 per credit hour. *Required fees:* full-time $296.

Financial Aid 10 fellowships, 42 research assistantships, 8 teaching assistantships were awarded; career-related internships or fieldwork, Federal Work-Study, institutionally sponsored loans, scholarships, and traineeships also available.

Contact Academic Programs Counselor, School of Nursing, Oregon Health & Science University, 3455 Southwest U.S. Veterans Hospital Road, SN-4N, Portland, OR 97239-2491. *Telephone:* 503-494-7725. *Fax:* 503-494-4350.

MASTER'S DEGREE PROGRAM

Degrees MS; MSN/MPH

Concentrations Available Health-care administration; nurse-midwifery; nursing administration. *Clinical nurse specialist programs in:* adult health, cardiovascular, community health, gerontology, medical-surgical, psychiatric/mental health, public health, women's health. *Nurse practitioner programs in:* adult health, family health, gerontology, pediatric, primary care, psychiatric/mental health, women's health.

Site Options *Distance Learning:* Ashland, OR; La Grande, OR; Klamath Falls, OR.

Study Options Full-time and part-time.

Program Entrance Requirements Clinical experience, computer literacy, minimum overall college GPA of 3.0, transcript of college record, CPR certification, written essay, immunizations, 3 letters of recommendation, physical assessment course, resume, statistics course, GRE General Test. *Application deadline:* For fall admission, 1/15 (priority date). Applications are processed on a rolling basis. *Application fee:* $60.

Advanced Placement Credit given for nursing courses completed elsewhere dependent upon specific evaluations.

Degree Requirements 45 total credit hours, thesis or project.

POST-MASTER'S PROGRAM

Areas of Study Nurse-midwifery; nursing education. *Clinical nurse specialist programs in:* adult health, cardiovascular, gerontology, medical-surgical, women's health. *Nurse practitioner programs in:* adult health, family health, gerontology, pediatric, primary care, psychiatric/mental health, women's health.

DOCTORAL DEGREE PROGRAM

Degree PhD

Areas of Study Aging, ethics, faculty preparation, family health, gerontology, health policy, health promotion/disease prevention, health-care systems, human health and illness, illness and transition, nursing policy, nursing research, nursing science, women's health.

Site Options *Distance Learning:* Ashland, OR; La Grande, OR; Klamath Falls, OR.

Program Entrance Requirements 3 letters of recommendation, MSN or equivalent, scholarly papers, statistics course, vita, writing sample, GRE General Test. *Application deadline:* For fall admission, 1/15 (priority date). Applications are processed on a rolling basis. *Application fee:* $60.

Degree Requirements 90 total credit hours, dissertation, oral exam, written exam, residency.

POSTDOCTORAL PROGRAM

Areas of Study Adolescent health, aging, chronic illness, family health, gerontology, health promotion/disease prevention, nursing interventions, nursing research, nursing science, outcomes, self-care, vulnerable population, women's health.

Postdoctoral Program Contact Academic Programs Counselor, School of Nursing, Oregon Health & Science University, 3455 Southwest U.S. Veterans Hospital Road, SN-4N, Portland, OR 97239-2491. *Telephone:* 503-494-7725. *Fax:* 503-494-4350.

CONTINUING EDUCATION PROGRAM

Contact Director of Continuing Education, School of Nursing, Oregon Health & Science University, 3455 Southwest U.S. Veterans Hospital Road, SN-4N (3181), Portland, OR 97239-2491. *Telephone:* 503-494-7725. *Fax:* 503-494-4350.

University of Portland

School of Nursing
Portland, Oregon

http://www.up.edu

Founded in 1901

DEGREES • BSN • MS

Nursing Program Faculty 82 (20% with doctorates).

Baccalaureate Enrollment 470

Women 91% **Men** 9% **Minority** 16% **International** 3% **Part-time** 2%

Graduate Enrollment 25

Women 90% **Men** 10% **Minority** 25% **International** 5% **Part-time** 10%

Nursing Student Activities Sigma Theta Tau, Student Nurses' Association.

Nursing Student Resources Academic advising; academic or career counseling; assistance for students with disabilities; bookstore; campus computer network; career placement assistance; computer lab; computer-assisted instruction; e-mail services; employment services for current students; housing assistance; interactive nursing skills videos; Internet; learning resource lab; library services; nursing audiovisuals; remedial services; resume preparation assistance; skills, simulation, or other laboratory; tutoring.

Library Facilities 350,000 volumes (5,753 in health, 5,753 in nursing); 1,400 periodical subscriptions (184 health-care related).

BACCALAUREATE PROGRAMS

Degree BSN

Available Programs Generic Baccalaureate.

Study Options Full-time and part-time.

Program Entrance Requirements Minimum overall college GPA of 2.5, transcript of college record, CPR certification, written essay, health exam, health insurance, high school transcript, immunizations, 1 letter of recommendation, minimum high school GPA of 2.5, minimum GPA in nursing prerequisites of 2.5, professional liability insurance/malpractice insurance, prerequisite course work. Transfer students are accepted. **Standardized tests** *Required:* SAT or ACT, TOEFL for international students. **Application** *Deadline:* 6/1 (freshmen), 6/1 (transfer). *Notification:* continuous (freshmen). *Application fee:* $50.

Expenses (2004–05) *Tuition:* full-time $23,200; part-time $735 per credit hour. *International tuition:* $23,200 full-time. *Room and board:* $7050 per academic year. *Required fees:* full-time $1270; part-time $35 per credit; part-time $100 per term.

Financial Aid 91% of baccalaureate students in nursing programs received some form of financial aid in 2003–04. *Gift aid (need-based):* Federal Pell, FSEOG, state, private, college/university gift aid from institutional funds. *Loans:* Federal Nursing Student Loans, FFEL (Subsidized and Unsubsidized Stafford PLUS), Perkins, college/university. *Work-Study:* Federal Work-Study, part-time campus jobs. *Application deadline (priority):* 3/1.

Contact Mr. Jim Lyons, Dean of Admissions, School of Nursing, University of Portland, 5000 North Willamette Boulevard, Portland, OR 97203-5798. *Telephone:* 503-943-7147. *E-mail:* admissio@up.edu.

GRADUATE PROGRAMS

Expenses (2004–05) *Tuition:* full-time $23,400; part-time $675 per credit hour. *International tuition:* $23,400 full-time. *Required fees:* full-time $630; part-time $35 per credit; part-time $100 per term.

Financial Aid 85% of graduate students in nursing programs received some form of financial aid in 2003–04. Fellowships, research assistantships, institutionally sponsored loans available. Aid available to part-time students. *Financial aid application deadline:* 3/15.

Contact Mrs. Lynn Miller, Graduate Program Specialist, School of Nursing, University of Portland, 5000 North Willamette Boulevard, Portland, OR 97203-5798. *Telephone:* 503-943-7211. *Fax:* 503-943-7729. *E-mail:* nursing@up.edu.

MASTER'S DEGREE PROGRAM

Degree MS

Available Programs Master's; Master's for Non-Nursing College Graduates; Master's for Nurses with Non-Nursing Degrees.

Concentrations Available Health-care administration; nursing education. *Nurse practitioner programs in:* family health.

Study Options Full-time and part-time.

Program Entrance Requirements Computer literacy, minimum overall college GPA of 3.0, transcript of college record, CPR certification, written essay, immunizations, interview, 2 letters of recommendation, professional liability insurance/malpractice insurance, prerequisite course work, resume, statistics course, GRE General Test. *Application deadline:* Applications are processed on a rolling basis. *Application fee:* $45.

Advanced Placement Credit given for nursing courses completed elsewhere dependent upon specific evaluations.

Degree Requirements 51 total credit hours.

POST-MASTER'S PROGRAM

Areas of Study Nursing education. *Nurse practitioner programs in:* family health.

PENNSYLVANIA

Alvernia College

Nursing
Reading, Pennsylvania

http://www.alvernia.edu

Founded in 1958

DEGREE • BSN

Nursing Program Faculty 8.

Baccalaureate Enrollment 161

Women 98% **Men** 2% **Minority** 10% **International** 3% **Part-time** 20%

Nursing Student Activities Nursing Honor Society, Student Nurses' Association.

Nursing Student Resources Academic advising; academic or career counseling; bookstore; campus computer network; computer lab; computer-assisted instruction; e-mail services; employment services for current students; externships; interactive nursing skills videos; Internet; learning resource lab; library services; nursing audiovisuals; remedial services; skills, simulation, or other laboratory; tutoring.

Library Facilities 89,399 volumes (2,931 in health, 995 in nursing); 378 periodical subscriptions (89 health-care related).

BACCALAUREATE PROGRAMS

Degree BSN

Available Programs Generic Baccalaureate; RN Baccalaureate.

Site Options Pottsville, PA; Reading, PA; Ashland, PA.

Study Options Full-time and part-time.

Program Entrance Requirements Minimum overall college GPA of 2.5, transcript of college record, CPR certification, written essay, health exam, health insurance, high school biology, high school chemistry, 2 years high school math, 2 years high school science, high school transcript, immunizations, 2 letters of recommendation, minimum high school GPA of 2.5, minimum GPA in nursing prerequisites of 2.0. Transfer students are accepted. **Standardized tests** *Required:* SAT or ACT, TOEFL for international students. *Recommended:* SAT. **Application** *Deadline:* rolling (freshmen), rolling (transfer). *Application fee:* $25.

Advanced Placement Credit by examination available. Credit given for nursing courses completed elsewhere dependent upon specific evaluations.

Financial Aid 75% of baccalaureate students in nursing programs received some form of financial aid in 2003–04. *Gift aid (need-based):* Federal Pell, FSEOG, state, private, college/university gift aid from institutional funds. *Loans:* FFEL (Subsidized and Unsubsidized Stafford PLUS), Perkins, college/university, Health Professions Loans. *Work-Study:* Federal Work-Study, part-time campus jobs. *Application deadline:* Continuous.

Contact Mrs. Suzanne Kirk, Nursing Department Chair, Nursing, Alvernia College, 400 Saint Bernardine Street, Reading, PA 19607. *Telephone:* 610-796-8467. *Fax:* 610-796-8464. *E-mail:* suzanne.kirk@alvernia.edu.

CONTINUING EDUCATION PROGRAM

Contact Ms. Noreen Kern, Nursing Outreach Coordinator, Nursing, Alvernia College, 400 Saint Bernardine Street, Reading, PA 19607. *Telephone:* 610-796-5611. *Fax:* 610-796-8464. *E-mail:* noreen.kern@alvernia.edu.

Bloomsburg University of Pennsylvania

Department of Nursing
Bloomsburg, Pennsylvania

http://www.bloomu.edu/academic/nur/

Founded in 1839

DEGREES • BSN • MSN • MSN/MBA

Nursing Program Faculty 24 (50% with doctorates).

Baccalaureate Enrollment 316

Women 94% **Men** 6% **Minority** 3% **Part-time** 10%

Graduate Enrollment 43

Women 95% **Men** 5% **Part-time** 74%

Nursing Student Activities Sigma Theta Tau, Student Nurses' Association, nursing club.

Nursing Student Resources Academic advising; academic or career counseling; assistance for students with disabilities; bookstore; campus computer network; career placement assistance; computer lab; computer-assisted instruction; daycare for children of students; e-mail services; employment services for current students; externships; housing assistance; interactive nursing skills videos; Internet; learning resource lab; library services; nursing audiovisuals; placement services for program completers; remedial services; resume preparation assistance; skills, simulation, or other laboratory; tutoring; unpaid internships.

Bloomsburg University of Pennsylvania (continued)
Library Facilities 408,647 volumes (10,827 in health, 10,827 in nursing); 2,402 periodical subscriptions (78 health-care related).

BACCALAUREATE PROGRAMS

Degree BSN

Available Programs ADN to Baccalaureate; Baccalaureate for Second Degree; Generic Baccalaureate; LPN to RN Baccalaureate; RN Baccalaureate.

Study Options Full-time and part-time.

Program Entrance Requirements Minimum overall college GPA of 2.5, transcript of college record, CPR certification, health exam, health insurance, high school biology, high school chemistry, 2 years high school math, 3 years high school science, high school transcript, immunizations, interview, 3 letters of recommendation, minimum high school GPA of 3.0, minimum high school rank 80%, minimum GPA in nursing prerequisites of 2.5, professional liability insurance/malpractice insurance, prerequisite course work. Transfer students are accepted. **Standardized tests** *Required:* SAT or ACT, TOEFL for international students. **Application** *Deadline:* rolling (freshmen), rolling (transfer). *Early decision:* 11/15. *Notification:* 10/1 (freshmen), 12/1 (out-of-state freshmen), 12/1 (early decision). *Application fee:* $30.

Advanced Placement Credit by examination available. Credit given for nursing courses completed elsewhere dependent upon specific evaluations.

Expenses (2004–05) *Tuition, state resident:* full-time $4810; part-time $200 per credit hour. *Tuition, nonresident:* full-time $12,026; part-time $501 per credit hour. *International tuition:* $12,026 full-time. *Room and board:* $5200; room only: $3012 per academic year. *Required fees:* full-time $1279; part-time $39 per credit; part-time $45 per term.

Financial Aid 76% of baccalaureate students in nursing programs received some form of financial aid in 2003–04.

Contact Dr. Christine Alichnie, Chairperson, Department of Nursing, Bloomsburg University of Pennsylvania, 400 East 2nd Street, MCHS 3109, Bloomsburg, PA 17815. *Telephone:* 570-389-4426. *Fax:* 570-389-5008. *E-mail:* cmalic@bloomu.edu.

GRADUATE PROGRAMS

Expenses (2004–05) *Tuition, state resident:* full-time $5772; part-time $321 per credit hour. *Tuition, nonresident:* full-time $9236; part-time $513 per credit hour. *International tuition:* $9236 full-time. *Room and board:* $5200; room only: $3012 per academic year. *Required fees:* full-time $1318; part-time $40 per credit; part-time $45 per term.

Financial Aid 20% of graduate students in nursing programs received some form of financial aid in 2003–04. Unspecified assistantships available.

Contact Dr. Sharon Haymaker, Coordinator of Graduate Program, Department of Nursing, Bloomsburg University of Pennsylvania, MCHS 3121, Bloomsburg, PA 17815. *Telephone:* 570-389-4602. *Fax:* 570-389-5008. *E-mail:* haymaker@bloomu.edu.

MASTER'S DEGREE PROGRAM

Degrees MSN; MSN/MBA

Available Programs Master's; Master's for Nurses with Non-Nursing Degrees; RN to Master's.

Concentrations Available Nursing administration. *Clinical nurse specialist programs in:* adult health, community health, public health, school health. *Nurse practitioner programs in:* adult health.

Study Options Full-time and part-time.

Program Entrance Requirements Clinical experience, computer literacy, minimum overall college GPA of 3.0, transcript of college record, CPR certification, immunizations, interview, 3 letters of recommendation, nursing research course, physical assessment course, professional liability insurance/malpractice insurance, prerequisite course work, resume, statistics course. *Application deadline:* Applications are processed on a rolling basis. *Application fee:* $30.

Advanced Placement Credit by examination available. Credit given for nursing courses completed elsewhere dependent upon specific evaluations.

Degree Requirements 39 total credit hours, comprehensive exam.

POST-MASTER'S PROGRAM

Areas of Study *Clinical nurse specialist programs in:* school health. *Nurse practitioner programs in:* adult health, family health.

California University of Pennsylvania

Department of Nursing
California, Pennsylvania

http://www.cup.edu/eberly/nursing

Founded in 1852

DEGREE • BSN

Nursing Program Faculty 5 (60% with doctorates).

Baccalaureate Enrollment 121
Women 83% **Men** 17% **Minority** 3% **Part-time** 92%

Nursing Student Activities Sigma Theta Tau.

Nursing Student Resources Academic advising; academic or career counseling; assistance for students with disabilities; bookstore; campus computer network; career placement assistance; computer lab; computer-assisted instruction; daycare for children of students; e-mail services; employment services for current students; Internet; library services; nursing audiovisuals; placement services for program completers; remedial services; resume preparation assistance; tutoring.

Library Facilities 437,160 volumes (3,840 in health, 2,010 in nursing); 881 periodical subscriptions (80 health-care related).

BACCALAUREATE PROGRAMS

Degree BSN

Available Programs RN Baccalaureate.

Site Options West Mifflin, PA. *Distance Learning:* Southpointe, PA.

Study Options Full-time and part-time.

Program Entrance Requirements Minimum overall college GPA of 2.0, transcript of college record, CPR certification, written essay, health exam, health insurance, immunizations, 2 letters of recommendation, professional liability insurance/malpractice insurance, prerequisite course work, RN licensure. Transfer students are accepted. **Standardized tests** *Required:* SAT, TOEFL for international students. *Recommended:* ACT, SAT Subject Tests. **Application** *Deadline:* 8/15 (freshmen), 8/15 (transfer). *Notification:* continuous (freshmen). *Application fee:* $25.

Advanced Placement Credit by examination available. Credit given for nursing courses completed elsewhere dependent upon specific evaluations.

Expenses (2004–05) *Tuition, state resident:* full-time $2405; part-time $200 per credit hour. *Tuition, nonresident:* full-time $3608; part-time $301 per credit hour. *International tuition:* $6013 full-time. *Room and board:* $2689; room only: $1750 per academic year. *Required fees:* full-time $705; part-time $283 per credit.

Financial Aid 80% of baccalaureate students in nursing programs received some form of financial aid in 2003–04.

Contact Dr. Margaret Marcinek, Chairperson, Department of Nursing, California University of Pennsylvania, 250 University Avenue, Box 60, California, PA 15419-1394. *Telephone:* 724-938-5739. *Fax:* 724-938-1612. *E-mail:* marcinek@cup.edu.

Carlow University

Division of Nursing
Pittsburgh, Pennsylvania

http://www.carlow.edu/academic/nursing.html

Founded in 1929

DEGREES • BSN • MSN

Nursing Program Faculty 29 (28% with doctorates).

Baccalaureate Enrollment 258
Women 95% **Men** 5% **Minority** 12% **Part-time** 38%

Graduate Enrollment 83
Women 99% **Men** 1% **Minority** 17% **Part-time** 35%

Nursing Student Activities Nursing Honor Society, Student Nurses' Association.

Nursing Student Resources Academic advising; academic or career counseling; assistance for students with disabilities; bookstore; campus computer network; career placement assistance; computer lab; computer-assisted instruction; daycare for children of students; e-mail services; employment services for current students; externships; housing assistance; Internet; learning resource lab; library services; nursing audiovisuals; other; paid internships; placement services for program completers; remedial services; resume preparation assistance; skills, simulation, or other laboratory; tutoring; unpaid internships.

Library Facilities 81,532 volumes (13,440 in health, 5,190 in nursing); 382 periodical subscriptions (60 health-care related).

BACCALAUREATE PROGRAMS

Degree BSN

Available Programs Accelerated RN Baccalaureate; Baccalaureate for Second Degree; Generic Baccalaureate; LPN to RN Baccalaureate.

Site Options Greensburg, PA; Cranberry Township, PA.

Study Options Full-time and part-time.

Program Entrance Requirements Minimum overall college GPA of 2.5, transcript of college record, CPR certification, health exam, health insurance, high school biology, high school chemistry, 2 years high school math, 2 years high school science, high school transcript, immunizations, interview, minimum high school GPA of 3.0, minimum GPA in nursing prerequisites of 2.0, professional liability insurance/malpractice insurance, prerequisite course work. Transfer students are accepted. **Standardized tests** *Required:* SAT or ACT, TOEFL for international students. **Application** *Deadline:* 4/1 (freshmen), rolling (transfer). *Early decision:* 9/30. *Notification:* continuous (freshmen), 10/30 (early action). *Application fee:* $20.

Advanced Placement Credit by examination available. Credit given for nursing courses completed elsewhere dependent upon specific evaluations.

Expenses (2003–04) *Tuition:* full-time $14,776; part-time $452 per credit hour. *International tuition:* $14,776 full-time. *Room and board:* $6110; room only: $3368 per academic year. *Required fees:* full-time $448; part-time $28 per credit.

Financial Aid 57% of baccalaureate students in nursing programs received some form of financial aid in 2002–03. *Gift aid (need-based):* Federal Pell, FSEOG, state, private, college/university gift aid from institutional funds, Federal Nursing. *Loans:* Federal Nursing Student Loans, FFEL (Subsidized and Unsubsidized Stafford PLUS), Perkins. *Work-Study:* Federal Work-Study. *Application deadline (priority):* 4/1.

Contact Ms. Christine Divine, Director of Admissions, Division of Nursing, Carlow University, Admissions Office, 3333 Fifth Avenue, Pittsburgh, PA 15213. *Telephone:* 412-578-6095. *Fax:* 412-578-6668. *E-mail:* admissions@carlow.edu.

GRADUATE PROGRAMS

Expenses (2003–04) *Tuition:* full-time $4870; part-time $487 per credit hour. *International tuition:* $4870 full-time. *Room and board:* $6110; room only: $3368 per academic year. *Required fees:* full-time $280; part-time $28 per credit.

Financial Aid 57% of graduate students in nursing programs received some form of financial aid in 2002–03. Career-related internships or fieldwork, Federal Work-Study, scholarships, traineeships, and tuition waivers (partial) available. Aid available to part-time students. *Financial aid application deadline:* 4/1.

Contact Susan Shutter, Graduate Admissions Office, Division of Nursing, Carlow University, Office of Graduate Studies, 3333 Fifth Avenue, Pittsburgh, PA 15213. *Telephone:* 412-578-6351. *Fax:* 412-578-6321. *E-mail:* sshutter@carlow.edu.

MASTER'S DEGREE PROGRAM

Degree MSN

Available Programs Accelerated Master's; Master's; RN to Master's.

Concentrations Available Nurse case management; nursing administration. *Clinical nurse specialist programs in:* home health care. *Nurse practitioner programs in:* family health.

Site Options Greensburg, PA; Cranberry Township, PA.

Study Options Full-time and part-time.

Program Entrance Requirements Clinical experience, computer literacy, minimum overall college GPA of 3.0, transcript of college record, written essay, immunizations, interview, 3 letters of recommendation, professional liability insurance/malpractice insurance, prerequisite course work, resume, statistics course, GRE General Test. *Application deadline:* For fall admission, 6/15 (priority date); for spring admission, 11/15 (priority date). Applications are processed on a rolling basis. *Application fee:* $35.

Advanced Placement Credit by examination available. Credit given for nursing courses completed elsewhere dependent upon specific evaluations.

Degree Requirements 56 total credit hours, thesis or project, comprehensive exam.

POST-MASTER'S PROGRAM

Areas of Study Nurse case management. *Clinical nurse specialist programs in:* home health care. *Nurse practitioner programs in:* family health.

CONTINUING EDUCATION PROGRAM

Contact Ms. Susan Shutter, Director of Adult Degree Center, Division of Nursing, Carlow University, 3333 Fifth Avenue, Pittsburgh, PA 15213. *Telephone:* 412-578-6351. *Fax:* 412-578-6321. *E-mail:* sshutter@carlow.edu.

Cedar Crest College

Department of Nursing
Allentown, Pennsylvania

http://www.cedarcrest.edu

Founded in 1867

DEGREE • BS

Nursing Program Faculty 15 (25% with doctorates).

Baccalaureate Enrollment 110

Women 98% **Men** 2% **Minority** 5% **Part-time** 65%

Nursing Student Activities Nursing Honor Society, Sigma Theta Tau, Student Nurses' Association, nursing club.

Nursing Student Resources Academic advising; academic or career counseling; assistance for students with disabilities; bookstore; campus computer network; career placement assistance; computer lab; e-mail services; interactive nursing skills videos; learning resource lab; library services; tutoring.

Library Facilities 133,763 volumes (4,100 in health, 1,250 in nursing); 8,695 periodical subscriptions (82 health-care related).

■ Cedar Crest College offers an undergraduate program in nursing. (Majors in nursing, allied health, and the sciences account for 45% of the College's total student enrollment.) The undergraduate nursing program includes clinical experiences at more than a dozen top-rated health-care facilities within 10 miles of the College, including Pennsylvania's largest teaching hospital. The state-of-the-art Trexler Pavilion for Nursing includes an 8-bed ward for clinical training for nursing students. The program is accredited by the National League for Nursing Accrediting Commission.

BACCALAUREATE PROGRAMS

Degree BS

Available Programs Baccalaureate for Second Degree; Generic Baccalaureate; RN Baccalaureate.

Study Options Full-time and part-time.

Program Entrance Requirements Minimum overall college GPA of 2.5, CPR certification, health exam, health insurance, high school biology, high school chemistry, 3 years high school math, 2 years high school science, high school transcript, immunizations, interview, minimum GPA in nursing prerequisites of 2.5, professional liability insurance/malpractice insurance. Transfer students are accepted. **Standardized tests** *Required:* SAT or ACT, TOEFL for international students. **Application** *Deadline:* rolling (freshmen), rolling (transfer). *Application fee:* $30.

Cedar Crest College (continued)

Advanced Placement Credit by examination available. Credit given for nursing courses completed elsewhere dependent upon specific evaluations.

Expenses (2003–04) *Tuition:* full-time $20,596; part-time $360 per credit hour. *International tuition:* $20,596 full-time. *Room and board:* $7274; room only: $3920 per academic year. *Required fees:* full-time $300.

Financial Aid 92% of baccalaureate students in nursing programs received some form of financial aid in 2002–03.

Contact Dr. Laurie R. Murray, RN, Chairperson and Associate Professor, Department of Nursing, Cedar Crest College, 100 College Drive, Allentown, PA 18104-6196. *Telephone:* 610-606-4606. *Fax:* 610-606-4615. *E-mail:* lrmurray@cedarcrest.edu.

Clarion University of Pennsylvania

School of Nursing
Oil City, Pennsylvania

Founded in 1867

DEGREES • BSN • MSN

Nursing Program Faculty 19 (21% with doctorates).

Baccalaureate Enrollment 85
Women 93% **Men** 7% **Minority** 4% **Part-time** 88%

Graduate Enrollment 59
Women 97% **Men** 3% **Minority** 3% **Part-time** 97%

Nursing Student Activities Sigma Theta Tau, nursing club.

Nursing Student Resources Academic advising; academic or career counseling; assistance for students with disabilities; bookstore; campus computer network; career placement assistance; computer lab; computer-assisted instruction; daycare for children of students; e-mail services; externships; housing assistance; interactive nursing skills videos; Internet; learning resource lab; library services; nursing audiovisuals; placement services for program completers; remedial services; resume preparation assistance; skills, simulation, or other laboratory; tutoring.

Library Facilities 429,800 volumes (12,000 in health, 6,000 in nursing); 750 periodical subscriptions (250 health-care related).

BACCALAUREATE PROGRAMS

Degree BSN

Available Programs ADN to Baccalaureate; RN Baccalaureate.

Site Options *Distance Learning:* Pittsburgh, PA.

Program Entrance Requirements Transfer students are accepted. **Standardized tests** *Required:* SAT or ACT, TOEFL for international students. **Application** *Deadline:* rolling (freshmen), rolling (transfer). *Application fee:* $30.

Expenses (2004–05) *Tuition, state resident:* full-time $4810; part-time $200 per credit hour. *Tuition, nonresident:* full-time $9620; part-time $401 per credit hour. *International tuition:* $9620 full-time. *Required fees:* full-time $581; part-time $45 per credit; part-time $291 per term.

Financial Aid 60% of baccalaureate students in nursing programs received some form of financial aid in 2003–04.

Contact Dr. Mary C. Kavoosi, Director, School of Nursing, Clarion University of Pennsylvania, 1801 West First Street, Oil City, PA 16301. *Telephone:* 814-676-6591 Ext. 1250. *Fax:* 814-676-0251. *E-mail:* mkavoosi@clarion.edu.

GRADUATE PROGRAMS

Expenses (2004–05) *Tuition, state resident:* full-time $5772; part-time $321 per credit hour. *Tuition, nonresident:* full-time $9236; part-time $513 per credit hour. *International tuition:* $9236 full-time. *Required fees:* full-time $677; part-time $57 per credit; part-time $339 per term.

Financial Aid 50% of graduate students in nursing programs received some form of financial aid in 2003–04. 1 research assistantship with full tuition reimbursement available (averaging $4,002 per year) was awarded. *Financial aid application deadline:* 3/1.

Contact Dr. Joyce White, Coordinator, MSN Family Nurse Practitioner Program, School of Nursing, Clarion University of Pennsylvania, Strain Behavioral Science Building, Slippery Rock, PA 16057-1326. *Telephone:* 724-738-2323. *Fax:* 724-738-2881. *E-mail:* joyce.white@sru.edu.

MASTER'S DEGREE PROGRAM

Degree MSN

Available Programs Accelerated RN to Master's; Master's.

Concentrations Available Nursing education. *Nurse practitioner programs in:* family health.

Site Options *Distance Learning:* Slippery Rock, PA; Pittsburgh, PA; Edinboro, PA.

Study Options Full-time and part-time.

Program Entrance Requirements Clinical experience, computer literacy, minimum overall college GPA of 2.7, transcript of college record, CPR certification, written essay, immunizations, interview, 3 letters of recommendation, professional liability insurance/malpractice insurance, statistics course, GRE. *Application deadline:* For fall admission, 7/1; for spring admission, 11/1. *Application fee:* $30.

Advanced Placement Credit given for nursing courses completed elsewhere dependent upon specific evaluations.

Degree Requirements 45 total credit hours, thesis or project, comprehensive exam.

POST-MASTER'S PROGRAM

Areas of Study Nursing education. *Nurse practitioner programs in:* family health.

College Misericordia

Department of Nursing
Dallas, Pennsylvania

http://www.misericordia.edu/nursing

Founded in 1924

DEGREES • BSN • MSN

Nursing Program Faculty 35 (20% with doctorates).

Baccalaureate Enrollment 303
Women 90% **Men** 10% **Minority** 1% **Part-time** 65%

Graduate Enrollment 35
Women 95% **Men** 5% **Minority** 1% **Part-time** 65%

Nursing Student Activities Nursing Honor Society, Sigma Theta Tau, Student Nurses' Association, nursing club.

Nursing Student Resources Academic advising; academic or career counseling; assistance for students with disabilities; bookstore; campus computer network; career placement assistance; computer lab; computer-assisted instruction; e-mail services; employment services for current students; externships; housing assistance; interactive nursing skills videos; Internet; learning resource lab; library services; nursing audiovisuals; paid internships; placement services for program completers; remedial services; resume preparation assistance; skills, simulation, or other laboratory; tutoring.

Library Facilities 90,000 volumes; 575 periodical subscriptions.

BACCALAUREATE PROGRAMS

Degree BSN

Available Programs Accelerated Baccalaureate; Accelerated Baccalaureate for Second Degree; Accelerated RN Baccalaureate; Baccalaureate for Second Degree; Generic Baccalaureate; RN Baccalaureate.

Site Options Nanticoke , PA.

Study Options Full-time and part-time.

Program Entrance Requirements Minimum overall college GPA of 2.5, transcript of college record, high school biology, high school chemistry, 1 year of high school math, high school transcript, letters of recommendation, minimum high school GPA of 2.0, minimum GPA in nursing prerequisites of 3.0, prerequisite course work. Transfer students are accepted. **Standardized tests** *Required:* SAT or ACT, TOEFL for international students. **Application** *Deadline:* rolling (freshmen), rolling (transfer). *Notification:* continuous (freshmen). *Application fee:* $25.

Advanced Placement Credit by examination available. Credit given for nursing courses completed elsewhere dependent upon specific evaluations.

Expenses (2004–05) *Tuition:* full-time $17,160; part-time $395 per credit hour. *Room and board:* $4200; room only: $2200 per academic year. *Required fees:* full-time $700; part-time $150 per term.

Financial Aid 68% of baccalaureate students in nursing programs received some form of financial aid in 2003–04.

Contact Glenn Bozinski, Office of Admissions, Department of Nursing, College Misericordia, 301 Lake Street, Dallas, PA 18612. *Telephone:* 570-674-6434. *E-mail:* gbozinsk@misericordia.edu.

GRADUATE PROGRAMS

Expenses (2004–05) *Tuition:* part-time $495 per credit hour. *Required fees:* part-time $50 per term.

Financial Aid 60% of graduate students in nursing programs received some form of financial aid in 2003–04. Research assistantships, teaching assistantships, career-related internships or fieldwork and traineeships available. Aid available to part-time students. *Financial aid application deadline:* 8/15.

Contact Miss Larree Brown, Adult Education Counselor, Graduate Programs, Department of Nursing, College Misericordia, 301 Lake Street, Dallas, PA 18612. *Telephone:* 570-674-6451. *Fax:* 570-674-8902. *E-mail:* lbrown@misericordia.edu.

MASTER'S DEGREE PROGRAM

Degree MSN

Available Programs Accelerated RN to Master's; Master's; RN to Master's.

Concentrations Available Nursing administration; nursing education. *Clinical nurse specialist programs in:* adult health, community health, maternity-newborn, parent-child. *Nurse practitioner programs in:* family health.

Study Options Part-time.

Program Entrance Requirements Clinical experience, computer literacy, minimum overall college GPA of 3.0, transcript of college record, written essay, 3 letters of recommendation, nursing research course, physical assessment course, professional liability insurance/malpractice insurance, statistics course, GRE General Test or MAT. *Application deadline:* For fall admission, 8/7 (priority date); for spring admission, 1/3. Applications are processed on a rolling basis. *Application fee:* $25.

Advanced Placement Credit given for nursing courses completed elsewhere dependent upon specific evaluations.

Degree Requirements 43 total credit hours, thesis or project.

POST-MASTER'S PROGRAM

Areas of Study *Nurse practitioner programs in:* family health.

DeSales University

Department of Nursing and Health
Center Valley, Pennsylvania

http://www.desales.edu

Founded in 1964

DEGREES • BSN • MSN • MSN/MBA

Nursing Program Faculty 14 (36% with doctorates).

Baccalaureate Enrollment 103
Women 87% **Men** 13% **Minority** 3% **Part-time** 26%

Graduate Enrollment 51
Women 92% **Men** 8% **Minority** 6% **Part-time** 100%

Nursing Student Activities Nursing Honor Society, Sigma Theta Tau, Student Nurses' Association.

Nursing Student Resources Academic advising; academic or career counseling; bookstore; campus computer network; career placement assistance; computer lab; computer-assisted instruction; e-mail services; employment services for current students; externships; interactive nursing skills videos; Internet; learning resource lab; library services; nursing audiovisuals; paid internships; placement services for program completers; remedial services; resume preparation assistance; skills, simulation, or other laboratory; tutoring; unpaid internships.

Library Facilities 138,151 volumes (1,200 in health); 538 periodical subscriptions (100 health-care related).

BACCALAUREATE PROGRAMS

Degree BSN

Available Programs ADN to Baccalaureate; Accelerated RN Baccalaureate; Generic Baccalaureate; RN Baccalaureate.

Study Options Full-time and part-time.

Program Entrance Requirements High school biology, high school chemistry, high school foreign language, 2 years high school math, 3 years high school science, high school transcript, minimum high school GPA of 2.5, minimum high school rank 33%. Transfer students are accepted. **Standardized tests** *Required:* SAT or ACT, TOEFL for international students. **Application** *Deadline:* 8/1 (freshmen), 8/1 (transfer). *Notification:* continuous (freshmen). *Application fee:* $30.

Advanced Placement Credit by examination available. Credit given for nursing courses completed elsewhere dependent upon specific evaluations.

Expenses (2004–05) *Tuition:* full-time $19,000; part-time $665 per credit hour. *International tuition:* $19,000 full-time. *Room and board:* $6810; room only: $3310 per academic year. *Required fees:* full-time $2080; part-time $200 per credit.

Financial Aid 52% of baccalaureate students in nursing programs received some form of financial aid in 2003–04.

Contact Dr. Kerry H. Cheever, Chair, Department of Nursing and Health, DeSales University, 2755 Station Avenue, Center Valley, PA 18034-9568. *Telephone:* 610-282-1100 Ext. 1271. *Fax:* 610-282-2254. *E-mail:* kerry.cheever@desales.edu.

GRADUATE PROGRAMS

Expenses (2004–05) *Tuition:* full-time $14,850; part-time $495 per credit hour. *International tuition:* $14,850 full-time. *Required fees:* full-time $400; part-time $200 per term.

Contact Dr. Carol G. Mest, RN, Director of Graduate Program in Nursing, Department of Nursing and Health, DeSales University, 2755 Station Avenue, Center Valley, PA 18034. *Telephone:* 610-282-1100 Ext. 1271. *Fax:* 610-282-2254. *E-mail:* carol.mest@desales.edu.

MASTER'S DEGREE PROGRAM

Degrees MSN; MSN/MBA

Available Programs Accelerated AD/RN to Master's; Accelerated RN to Master's; Master's; RN to Master's.

Concentrations Available Nursing administration; nursing education. *Clinical nurse specialist programs in:* adult health. *Nurse practitioner programs in:* family health.

Study Options Full-time and part-time.

Program Entrance Requirements Minimum overall college GPA of 3.0, transcript of college record, written essay, interview, 3 letters of recommendation, prerequisite course work, statistics course.

Advanced Placement Credit given for nursing courses completed elsewhere dependent upon specific evaluations.

Degree Requirements 47 total credit hours.

POST-MASTER'S PROGRAM

Areas of Study Nursing education. *Nurse practitioner programs in:* family health.

CONTINUING EDUCATION PROGRAM

Contact Dr. Carol G. Mest, RN, Director of Graduate Program in Nursing, Department of Nursing and Health, DeSales University, 2755 Station Avenue, Center Valley, PA 18034. *Telephone:* 610-282-1100 Ext. 1394. *Fax:* 610-282-2254. *E-mail:* carol.mest@desales.edu.

Drexel University

College of Nursing and Health Professions
Philadelphia, Pennsylvania

http://www.drexel.edu

Founded in 1891

DEGREES • BSN • MSN

Drexel University (continued)

Nursing Program Faculty 40 (33% with doctorates).

Baccalaureate Enrollment 451

Women 80% **Men** 20% **Minority** 30% **International** 2% **Part-time** 35%

Graduate Enrollment 205

Women 85% **Men** 15% **Minority** 10% **Part-time** 80%

Nursing Student Activities Nursing Honor Society, Sigma Theta Tau, Student Nurses' Association.

Nursing Student Resources Academic advising; academic or career counseling; assistance for students with disabilities; bookstore; campus computer network; career placement assistance; computer lab; computer-assisted instruction; e-mail services; housing assistance; interactive nursing skills videos; Internet; learning resource lab; library services; nursing audiovisuals; paid internships; placement services for program completers; remedial services; resume preparation assistance; skills, simulation, or other laboratory; tutoring.

Library Facilities 570,335 volumes (70,000 in health, 15,500 in nursing); 8,321 periodical subscriptions (1,300 health-care related).

BACCALAUREATE PROGRAMS

Degree BSN

Available Programs ADN to Baccalaureate; Accelerated Baccalaureate for Second Degree; RN Baccalaureate.

Site Options *Distance Learning:* Philadelphia, PA.

Study Options Full-time and part-time.

Program Entrance Requirements Transcript of college record, CPR certification, health insurance, high school biology, high school chemistry, 4 years high school math, 2 years high school science, high school transcript, immunizations, 2 letters of recommendation, minimum high school GPA of 3.0, minimum GPA in nursing prerequisites of 2.75. Transfer students are accepted. **Standardized tests** *Required:* SAT or ACT, TOEFL for international students. *Recommended:* SAT. **Application** *Deadline:* 3/1 (freshmen), rolling (transfer). *Notification:* continuous (freshmen). *Application fee:* $50.

Advanced Placement Credit by examination available. Credit given for nursing courses completed elsewhere dependent upon specific evaluations.

Expenses (2004–05) *Tuition:* full-time $21,700; part-time $480 per credit hour. *Required fees:* full-time $1800.

Financial Aid *Gift aid (need-based):* Federal Pell, FSEOG, state, private, college/university gift aid from institutional funds, United Negro College Fund. *Loans:* FFEL (Subsidized and Unsubsidized Stafford PLUS), Perkins, college/university. *Work-Study:* Federal Work-Study. *Application deadline:* 2/15.

Contact Ms. Carolyn Riley, Academic Advisor, College of Nursing and Health Professions, Drexel University, 1515 Race Street, Mail Stop 501, Philadelphia, PA 19102-1192. *Telephone:* 215-762-8347. *Fax:* 215-762-7778. *E-mail:* criley@drexel.edu.

GRADUATE PROGRAMS

Expenses (2004–05) *Tuition:* full-time $24,000; part-time $693 per credit hour. *Required fees:* full-time $100; part-time $45 per credit.

Financial Aid 40% of graduate students in nursing programs received some form of financial aid in 2003–04. Fellowships, research assistantships, teaching assistantships, career-related internships or fieldwork, Federal Work-Study, institutionally sponsored loans, and tuition waivers (partial) available. Aid available to part-time students. *Financial aid application deadline:* 5/1.

Contact Ms. Joyce Segal, Administrative Coordinator, College of Nursing and Health Professions, Drexel University, 1505 Race Street, Mail Stop 501, Philadelphia, PA 19102-1192. *Telephone:* 215-762-1336. *Fax:* 215-762-7778. *E-mail:* joyce.segal@drexel.edu.

MASTER'S DEGREE PROGRAM

Degree MSN

Available Programs Accelerated AD/RN to Master's; Master's; RN to Master's.

Concentrations Available Health-care administration; nurse anesthesia; nursing administration; nursing education. *Clinical nurse specialist programs in:* public health, women's health. *Nurse practitioner programs in:* acute care, family health, psychiatric/mental health.

Site Options *Distance Learning:* Philadelphia, PA.

Study Options Full-time and part-time.

Program Entrance Requirements Clinical experience, computer literacy, minimum overall college GPA of 3.0, transcript of college record, immunizations, interview, 3 letters of recommendation, resume, statistics course. *Application deadline:* Applications are processed on a rolling basis. *Application fee:* $50.

Advanced Placement Credit given for nursing courses completed elsewhere dependent upon specific evaluations.

Degree Requirements 40 total credit hours, thesis or project.

POST-MASTER'S PROGRAM

Areas of Study Health-care administration; nurse anesthesia; nursing administration; nursing education. *Nurse practitioner programs in:* acute care, family health, psychiatric/mental health.

DOCTORAL DEGREE PROGRAM

Program Entrance Requirements GRE General Test. *Application deadline:* Applications are processed on a rolling basis. *Application fee:* $50.

CONTINUING EDUCATION PROGRAM

Contact Prof. Judy Draper, Nurse Planner, Continuing Education, College of Nursing and Health Professions, Drexel University, 245 North 15th Street, Mail Stop 1002, Philadelphia, PA 19102-1192. *Telephone:* 215-762-2650. *Fax:* 215-762-8171. *E-mail:* jdraper@drexel.edu.

See full description on page 476.

Duquesne University
School of Nursing
Pittsburgh, Pennsylvania

http://www.nursing.duq.edu

Founded in 1878

DEGREES • BSN • MSN • MSN/MBA • PHD

Nursing Program Faculty 53 (37% with doctorates).

Baccalaureate Enrollment 366

Women 91% **Men** 9% **Minority** 8% **International** 4% **Part-time** 7%

Graduate Enrollment 150

Women 98% **Men** 2% **Minority** 2% **International** 3% **Part-time** 93%

Nursing Student Activities Nursing Honor Society, Sigma Theta Tau, Student Nurses' Association, nursing club.

Nursing Student Resources Academic advising; academic or career counseling; assistance for students with disabilities; bookstore; campus computer network; career placement assistance; computer lab; computer-assisted instruction; daycare for children of students; e-mail services; employment services for current students; externships; housing assistance; interactive nursing skills videos; Internet; learning resource lab; library services; nursing audiovisuals; paid internships; placement services for program completers; remedial services; resume preparation assistance; skills, simulation, or other laboratory; tutoring; unpaid internships.

Library Facilities 723,919 volumes (27,613 in health, 1,951 in nursing); 1,124 periodical subscriptions (1,779 health-care related).

BACCALAUREATE PROGRAMS

Degree BSN

Available Programs Accelerated Baccalaureate for Second Degree; Accelerated RN Baccalaureate; Generic Baccalaureate; International Nurse to Baccalaureate.

Study Options Full-time and part-time.

Program Entrance Requirements Minimum overall college GPA of 2.5, transcript of college record, written essay, high school biology, high school chemistry, 2 years high school math, 2 years high school science, high school transcript, 1 letter of recommendation, minimum high school GPA of 2.5, minimum high school rank 40%. Transfer students are accepted. **Standardized tests** *Required:* SAT or ACT. *Recommended:* TOEFL for international students. **Application** *Deadline:* 7/1 (freshmen), 7/1 (transfer). *Early decision:* 11/1, 12/1. *Notification:* continuous (freshmen), 12/15 (out-of-state freshmen), 12/15 (early decision), 1/15 (early action). *Application fee:* $50.

Advanced Placement Credit by examination available. Credit given for nursing courses completed elsewhere dependent upon specific evaluations.

Expenses (2004–05) *Tuition:* full-time $19,086; part-time $621 per contact hour. *International tuition:* $19,086 full-time. *Room and board:* $7920 per academic year. *Required fees:* full-time $1667; part-time $65 per credit; part-time $832 per term.

Financial Aid 85% of baccalaureate students in nursing programs received some form of financial aid in 2003–04. *Gift aid (need-based):* Federal Pell, FSEOG, state, private, college/university gift aid from institutional funds. *Loans:* Federal Nursing Student Loans, FFEL (Subsidized and Unsubsidized Stafford PLUS), Perkins, college/university, Health Professions Loans. *Work-Study:* Federal Work-Study. *Application deadline:* 5/1.

Contact Ms. Cherie Remley, Inquiry Manager, School of Nursing, Duquesne University, 600 Forbes Avenue, Pittsburgh, PA 15282-1760. *Telephone:* 412-396-4945. *Fax:* 412-396-6346. *E-mail:* remleyc@duq.edu.

GRADUATE PROGRAMS

Expenses (2004–05) *Tuition:* part-time $670 per contact hour. *Required fees:* part-time $65 per credit.

Financial Aid 30% of graduate students in nursing programs received some form of financial aid in 2003–04. 7 teaching assistantships with partial tuition reimbursements available (averaging $2,200 per year) were awarded; research assistantships, institutionally sponsored loans, scholarships, traineeships, tuition waivers (partial), and unspecified assistantships also available.

Contact Dr. Joan Such Lockhart, Associate Dean, Academic Affairs, School of Nursing, Duquesne University, 542C Fisher Hall, 600 Forbes Avenue, Pittsburgh, PA 15282-1760. *Telephone:* 412-396-6540. *Fax:* 412-396-6346. *E-mail:* lockhart@duq.edu.

MASTER'S DEGREE PROGRAM

Degrees MSN; MSN/MBA

Available Programs Accelerated RN to Master's; Master's.

Concentrations Available Nursing administration; nursing education. *Clinical nurse specialist programs in:* acute care, psychiatric/mental health. *Nurse practitioner programs in:* family health.

Study Options Full-time and part-time.

Program Entrance Requirements Clinical experience, computer literacy, minimum overall college GPA of 3.0, transcript of college record, written essay, interview, 2 letters of recommendation, nursing research course, physical assessment course, prerequisite course work, resume, statistics course, GMAT (MSN/MBA), MAT. *Application deadline:* Applications are processed on a rolling basis. *Application fee:* $62.

Advanced Placement Credit given for nursing courses completed elsewhere dependent upon specific evaluations.

Degree Requirements 40 total credit hours, comprehensive exam.

POST-MASTER'S PROGRAM

Areas of Study Nursing administration; nursing education. *Nurse practitioner programs in:* family health.

DOCTORAL DEGREE PROGRAM

Degree PhD

Available Programs Doctorate.

Areas of Study Nursing research.

Program Entrance Requirements interview by faculty committee, interview, 3 letters of recommendation, MSN or equivalent, scholarly papers, statistics course, vita, writing sample, GRE. *Application deadline:* Applications are processed on a rolling basis. *Application fee:* $62.

Degree Requirements 57 total credit hours, dissertation, oral exam, written exam, residency.

CONTINUING EDUCATION PROGRAM

Contact Ms. Shirley P. Smith, Assistant Professor, School of Nursing, Duquesne University, 600 Forbes Avenue, Pittsburgh, PA 15282-1760. *Telephone:* 412-396-6535. *Fax:* 412-396-6346. *E-mail:* smith1@duq.edu.

See full description on page 480.

Eastern University
Program in Nursing
St. Davids, Pennsylvania

http://www.eastern.edu/academics/

Founded in 1952

DEGREE • BSN

Nursing Program Faculty 6 (50% with doctorates).

Baccalaureate Enrollment 97

Women 98% **Men** 2% **Minority** 25% **International** 7% **Part-time** 10%

Nursing Student Activities Sigma Theta Tau.

Nursing Student Resources Academic advising; academic or career counseling; assistance for students with disabilities; bookstore; campus computer network; career placement assistance; computer lab; computer-assisted instruction; e-mail services; employment services for current students; Internet; learning resource lab; library services; nursing audio-visuals; placement services for program completers; remedial services; resume preparation assistance; skills, simulation, or other laboratory; tutoring; unpaid internships.

Library Facilities 143,815 volumes (5,858 in health, 3,000 in nursing); 1,215 periodical subscriptions (821 health-care related).

BACCALAUREATE PROGRAMS

Degree BSN

Available Programs Accelerated RN Baccalaureate; Baccalaureate for Second Degree.

Site Options Harrisburg, PA; Wynnewood, PA; Phoenixville, PA.

Study Options Full-time.

Program Entrance Requirements Minimum overall college GPA of 2.0, transcript of college record, CPR certification, written essay, health exam, health insurance, high school chemistry, high school transcript, immunizations, interview, 2 letters of recommendation, minimum GPA in nursing prerequisites of 2.5, professional liability insurance/malpractice insurance, prerequisite course work, RN licensure. Transfer students are accepted. **Standardized tests** *Required:* SAT or ACT, TOEFL for international students. **Application** *Deadline:* rolling (freshmen), rolling (transfer). *Notification:* continuous (freshmen). *Application fee:* $25.

Advanced Placement Credit by examination available. Credit given for nursing courses completed elsewhere dependent upon specific evaluations.

Expenses (2004–05) *Tuition:* full-time $11,760; part-time $400 per credit hour. *International tuition:* $11,760 full-time. *Room and board:* $7200 per academic year. *Required fees:* full-time $250; part-time $125 per term.

Financial Aid 30% of baccalaureate students in nursing programs received some form of financial aid in 2003–04.

Contact Mrs. Corinne Latini, RN, RN-BSN Program Advisor, Program in Nursing, Eastern University, 1300 Eagle Road, St. Davids, PA 19087. *Telephone:* 800-732-7669 Ext. 5525. *Fax:* 610-341-1468. *E-mail:* clatini@eastern.edu.

CONTINUING EDUCATION PROGRAM

Contact Mrs. Shelley Robbins, RN, Clinical Lecturer, Program in Nursing, Eastern University, 1300 Eagle Road, St. Davids, PA 19087. *Telephone:* 610-341-5896. *Fax:* 610-225-5016. *E-mail:* srobbin2@eastern.edu.

East Stroudsburg University of Pennsylvania
Department of Nursing
East Stroudsburg, Pennsylvania

http://www3.esu/academics/hshp/nurs/home.asp

Founded in 1893

DEGREE • BS

East Stroudsburg University of Pennsylvania (continued)

Nursing Program Faculty 14 (50% with doctorates).

Baccalaureate Enrollment 154
Women 93% **Men** 7% **Minority** 1%

Nursing Student Activities Nursing Honor Society, Sigma Theta Tau, Student Nurses' Association, nursing club.

Nursing Student Resources Academic advising; academic or career counseling; assistance for students with disabilities; bookstore; campus computer network; career placement assistance; computer lab; computer-assisted instruction; daycare for children of students; e-mail services; employment services for current students; externships; housing assistance; interactive nursing skills videos; Internet; learning resource lab; library services; nursing audiovisuals; other; placement services for program completers; remedial services; resume preparation assistance; skills, simulation, or other laboratory; tutoring; unpaid internships.

Library Facilities 449,107 volumes (16,810 in health, 2,035 in nursing); 1,175 periodical subscriptions (495 health-care related).

BACCALAUREATE PROGRAMS

Degree BS

Available Programs Generic Baccalaureate; LPN to Baccalaureate; RN Baccalaureate.

Study Options Full-time and part-time.

Program Entrance Requirements Minimum overall college GPA of 2.75, transcript of college record, 2 years high school math, 2 years high school science, high school transcript, minimum high school GPA of 3.0, minimum high school rank 75%, minimum GPA in nursing prerequisites of 2.0. Transfer students are accepted. **Standardized tests** *Required:* SAT or ACT, TOEFL for international students. **Application** *Deadline:* 4/1 (freshmen), 5/1 (transfer). *Notification:* continuous until 5/1 (freshmen). *Application fee:* $35.

Advanced Placement Credit by examination available. Credit given for nursing courses completed elsewhere dependent upon specific evaluations.

Expenses (2004–05) *Tuition, state resident:* full-time $4598; part-time $192 per credit hour. *Tuition, nonresident:* full-time $11,496; part-time $479 per credit hour. *Room and board:* $4408 per academic year. *Required fees:* full-time $1281; part-time $54 per credit.

Financial Aid *Gift aid (need-based):* Federal Pell, FSEOG, state, private, college/university gift aid from institutional funds. *Loans:* FFEL (Subsidized and Unsubsidized Stafford PLUS), Perkins, alternative loans. *Work-Study:* Federal Work-Study, part-time campus jobs. *Application deadline:* 3/1.

Contact Dr. Cecile Belisle Champagne, Associate Professor and Chair, Department of Nursing, East Stroudsburg University of Pennsylvania, 200 Prospect Street, East Stroudsburg, PA 18301-2999. *Telephone:* 570-422-3563. *Fax:* 570-422-3848. *E-mail:* cchampagne@po-box.esu.edu.

Edinboro University of Pennsylvania

Department of Nursing
Edinboro, Pennsylvania

http://www.edinboro.edu/cwis/nursing/nursing.html

Founded in 1857

DEGREES • BS • MSN

Nursing Program Faculty 19 (32% with doctorates).

Baccalaureate Enrollment 231
Women 90% **Men** 10% **Minority** 5% **Part-time** 10%

Graduate Enrollment 45
Women 95% **Men** 5% **Minority** 5% **Part-time** 50%

Nursing Student Activities Sigma Theta Tau, Student Nurses' Association.

Nursing Student Resources Academic or career counseling; assistance for students with disabilities; bookstore; campus computer network; career placement assistance; computer lab; computer-assisted instruction; e-mail services; housing assistance; interactive nursing skills videos; Internet; learning resource lab; library services; nursing audiovisuals; remedial services; skills, simulation, or other laboratory; tutoring.

Library Facilities 501,276 volumes; 1,523 periodical subscriptions (105 health-care related).

BACCALAUREATE PROGRAMS

Degree BS

Available Programs ADN to Baccalaureate; Accelerated Baccalaureate for Second Degree; Accelerated LPN to Baccalaureate; Accelerated RN Baccalaureate; Baccalaureate for Second Degree; Generic Baccalaureate; LPN to Baccalaureate; RN Baccalaureate.

Site Options Erie, PA.

Study Options Full-time and part-time.

Program Entrance Requirements Minimum overall college GPA of 2.75, CPR certification, health exam, high school biology, high school chemistry, 1 year of high school math, high school transcript, immunizations, minimum high school rank 40%, minimum GPA in nursing prerequisites of 2.75, professional liability insurance/malpractice insurance, prerequisite course work. Transfer students are accepted. **Standardized tests** *Required:* SAT or ACT, TOEFL for international students. *Required for some:* SAT, ACT. **Application** *Deadline:* rolling (freshmen), rolling (transfer). *Notification:* continuous (freshmen). *Application fee:* $25.

Expenses (2003–04) *Tuition, state resident:* full-time $4598; part-time $192 per credit hour. *Tuition, nonresident:* full-time $6898; part-time $287 per credit hour. *Room and board:* $5342; room only: $3120 per academic year. *Required fees:* full-time $874; part-time $32 per credit; part-time $50 per term.

Contact Mrs. Patricia Louise Nosel, RN, Chair, Department of Nursing, Edinboro University of Pennsylvania, 125 Centennial Hall, Edinboro, PA 16444. *Telephone:* 814-732-1127 Ext. 2900. *Fax:* 814-732-2536. *E-mail:* nosel@edinboro.edu.

GRADUATE PROGRAMS

Expenses (2003–04) *Tuition, state resident:* full-time $5518; part-time $307 per credit hour. *Tuition, nonresident:* full-time $8830; part-time $491 per credit hour. *Room and board:* $5342; room only: $3120 per academic year. *Required fees:* full-time $874; part-time $14 per credit; part-time $25 per term.

Financial Aid Career-related internships or fieldwork, Federal Work-Study, institutionally sponsored loans, scholarships, and unspecified assistantships available.

Contact Director, Graduate Program, Department of Nursing, Edinboro University of Pennsylvania, 135 Centennial Hall, Edinboro, PA 16444. *Telephone:* 814-732-2900. *Fax:* 814-732-2536.

MASTER'S DEGREE PROGRAM

Degree MSN

Available Programs Master's.

Concentrations Available Nursing education. *Nurse practitioner programs in:* family health.

Study Options Full-time and part-time.

Program Entrance Requirements Clinical experience, computer literacy, minimum overall college GPA of 3.0, transcript of college record, CPR certification, written essay, interview, 3 letters of recommendation, nursing research course, professional liability insurance/malpractice insurance, prerequisite course work, resume, statistics course, GRE or MAT. *Application deadline:* Applications are processed on a rolling basis. *Application fee:* $25.

Degree Requirements 45 total credit hours, thesis or project, comprehensive exam.

Gannon University

Villa Maria School of Nursing
Erie, Pennsylvania

Founded in 1925

DEGREES • BSN • MSN

Nursing Program Faculty 12 (25% with doctorates).

Baccalaureate Enrollment 220
Women 88% **Men** 12% **Minority** 4% **Part-time** 5%

Graduate Enrollment 63
Women 73% **Men** 27% **Minority** 6% **Part-time** 35%

Nursing Student Activities Nursing Honor Society, Sigma Theta Tau.

Nursing Student Resources Academic advising; academic or career counseling; assistance for students with disabilities; bookstore; campus computer network; career placement assistance; computer lab; computer-assisted instruction; e-mail services; employment services for current students; externships; housing assistance; interactive nursing skills videos; Internet; learning resource lab; library services; nursing audiovisuals; paid internships; placement services for program completers; remedial services; resume preparation assistance; skills, simulation, or other laboratory; tutoring; unpaid internships.

Library Facilities 270,282 volumes (7,930 in health, 917 in nursing); 6,292 periodical subscriptions (144 health-care related).

BACCALAUREATE PROGRAMS

Degree BSN

Available Programs Generic Baccalaureate; RN Baccalaureate.

Site Options *Distance Learning:* Erie, PA.

Study Options Full-time.

Program Entrance Requirements Minimum overall college GPA of 2.8, CPR certification, health exam, health insurance, high school biology, high school chemistry, high school transcript, immunizations, 1 letter of recommendation, minimum high school GPA of 2.5, minimum high school rank 40%. Transfer students are accepted. **Standardized tests** *Required:* SAT or ACT, TOEFL for international students. **Application** *Deadline:* rolling (freshmen), rolling (transfer). *Application fee:* $25.

Advanced Placement Credit by examination available. Credit given for nursing courses completed elsewhere dependent upon specific evaluations.

Expenses (2004–05) *Tuition:* full-time $9035; part-time $560 per credit hour. *International tuition:* $9035 full-time. *Room and board:* $6770; room only: $3540 per academic year.

Financial Aid 65% of baccalaureate students in nursing programs received some form of financial aid in 2003–04. *Gift aid (need-based):* Federal Pell, FSEOG, state, private, college/university gift aid from institutional funds. *Loans:* Federal Nursing Student Loans, FFEL (Subsidized and Unsubsidized Stafford PLUS), Perkins. *Work-Study:* Federal Work-Study, part-time campus jobs. *Application deadline (priority):* 3/15.

Contact Mrs. Patricia Marshall, RN, Director, BSN Program, Villa Maria School of Nursing, Gannon University, 109 University Square, Erie, PA 16541-0001. *Telephone:* 814-871-5470. *Fax:* 814-871-5662. *E-mail:* marshall001@gannon.edu.

GRADUATE PROGRAMS

Expenses (2004–05) *Tuition:* part-time $557 per credit hour. *Required fees:* part-time $175 per term.

Financial Aid 70% of graduate students in nursing programs received some form of financial aid in 2003–04. Career-related internships or fieldwork and traineeships available. Aid available to part-time students. *Financial aid application deadline:* 7/1.

Contact Dr. Carolynn B. Masters, RN, Director, Villa Maria School of Nursing, Gannon University, 109 University Square, Erie, PA 16541-0001. *Telephone:* 814-871-5463. *Fax:* 814-871-5662. *E-mail:* masters004@gannon.edu.

MASTER'S DEGREE PROGRAM

Degree MSN

Available Programs Master's; RN to Master's.

Concentrations Available Nurse anesthesia; nursing administration; nursing education. *Clinical nurse specialist programs in:* medical-surgical. *Nurse practitioner programs in:* family health.

Site Options *Distance Learning:* Erie, PA.

Study Options Full-time and part-time.

Program Entrance Requirements Clinical experience, minimum overall college GPA of 3.0, transcript of college record, CPR certification, written essay, interview, 4 letters of recommendation, nursing research course, statistics course, GRE General Test, MAT. *Application deadline:* For fall admission, 4/15. *Application fee:* $25.

Advanced Placement Credit given for nursing courses completed elsewhere dependent upon specific evaluations.

Degree Requirements 42 total credit hours, thesis or project.

POST-MASTER'S PROGRAM

Areas of Study Nurse anesthesia; nursing administration. *Clinical nurse specialist programs in:* medical-surgical. *Nurse practitioner programs in:* family health.

See full description on page 490.

Gwynedd-Mercy College
School of Nursing
Gwynedd Valley, Pennsylvania

Founded in 1948

DEGREES • BSN • MSN

Nursing Program Faculty 37 (33% with doctorates).

Baccalaureate Enrollment 100
Women 96% **Men** 4% **Minority** 8% **International** 4% **Part-time** 50%

Graduate Enrollment 45
Women 97% **Men** 3% **Minority** 4% **International** 2% **Part-time** 60%

Nursing Student Activities Sigma Theta Tau, Student Nurses' Association.

Nursing Student Resources Academic advising; bookstore; campus computer network; computer lab; daycare for children of students; interactive nursing skills videos; library services; nursing audiovisuals; resume preparation assistance; skills, simulation, or other laboratory; tutoring.

Library Facilities 99,493 volumes (9,000 in health, 7,688 in nursing); 685 periodical subscriptions (187 health-care related).

■ Gwynedd-Mercy College's (GMC) School of Nursing is one of the finest nursing schools regionally. The program is one of the few articulated nursing programs in the region, allowing students to progress easily from the ASN to BSN to MSN degrees. The program is clinically oriented, placing students in clinical environments in their freshman year. The program offers personal attention, with a student-teacher ratio of 15:1, and 8:1 in the clinical area. In 2002, the NLNAC informed GMC that the associate degree program was approved for continuing accreditation for 8 years, the maximum amount of time that a program can receive.

BACCALAUREATE PROGRAMS

Degree BSN

Available Programs ADN to Baccalaureate; Accelerated RN Baccalaureate; RN Baccalaureate.

Site Options Fort Washington, PA.

Study Options Full-time and part-time.

Program Entrance Requirements Minimum overall college GPA of 2.8, transcript of college record, CPR certification, health exam, health insurance, high school biology, high school chemistry, 2 years high school math, high school transcript, immunizations, letters of recommendation, minimum high school rank 33%, minimum GPA in nursing prerequisites, professional liability insurance/malpractice insurance, RN licensure. Transfer students are accepted. **Standardized tests** *Required:* SAT. *Recommended:* TOEFL for international students. **Application** *Deadline:* rolling (freshmen), 8/20 (transfer). *Notification:* continuous (freshmen). *Application fee:* $25.

Advanced Placement Credit by examination available. Credit given for nursing courses completed elsewhere dependent upon specific evaluations.

Expenses (2004–05) *Tuition:* full-time $17,900; part-time $390 per credit hour. *Room and board:* $8050 per academic year. *Required fees:* full-time $70.

Gwynedd-Mercy College (continued)

Financial Aid 77% of baccalaureate students in nursing programs received some form of financial aid in 2003–04. *Gift aid (need-based):* Federal Pell, FSEOG, state, private, college/university gift aid from institutional funds. *Loans:* Federal Nursing Student Loans, FFEL (Subsidized and Unsubsidized Stafford PLUS), Perkins, alternative loans. *Work-Study:* Federal Work-Study, part-time campus jobs. *Application deadline (priority):* 3/15.

Contact Ms. Kelly Strother, Senior Admissions Counselor, School of Nursing, Gwynedd-Mercy College, PO Box 901, Gwynedd Valley, PA 19437. *Telephone:* 215-646-7300 Ext. 425. *Fax:* 215-641-5556. *E-mail:* strother.k@gmc.edu.

GRADUATE PROGRAMS

Expenses (2004–05) *Tuition:* full-time $4275; part-time $475 per credit hour. *International tuition:* $4275 full-time. *Required fees:* full-time $180; part-time $25 per term.

Financial Aid 40% of graduate students in nursing programs received some form of financial aid in 2003–04. Traineeships available. *Financial aid application deadline:* 8/30.

Contact Dr. Barbara A. Jones, MSN Program Director, School of Nursing, Gwynedd-Mercy College, PO Box 901, 1325 Sumneytown Pike, Gwynedd Valley, PA 19437-0901. *Telephone:* 215-646-7300 Ext. 407. *Fax:* 215-542-5789. *E-mail:* jones.b@gmc.edu.

MASTER'S DEGREE PROGRAM

Degree MSN

Available Programs Master's; RN to Master's.

Concentrations Available *Clinical nurse specialist programs in:* gerontology, oncology, pediatric. *Nurse practitioner programs in:* adult health, pediatric.

Study Options Full-time and part-time.

Program Entrance Requirements Clinical experience, minimum overall college GPA of 3.0, transcript of college record, written essay, immunizations, interview, 2 letters of recommendation, physical assessment course, professional liability insurance/malpractice insurance, statistics course, GRE General Test or MAT. *Application deadline:* For fall admission, 8/1 (priority date); for winter admission, 12/1 (priority date). Applications are processed on a rolling basis. *Application fee:* $25.

Advanced Placement Credit by examination available. Credit given for nursing courses completed elsewhere dependent upon specific evaluations.

Degree Requirements 43 total credit hours.

POST-MASTER'S PROGRAM

Areas of Study *Nurse practitioner programs in:* adult health, pediatric.

CONTINUING EDUCATION PROGRAM

Contact Dr. Patricia Cullen, Director, BSN Program, School of Nursing, Gwynedd-Mercy College, 1325 Sumneytown Pike, PO Box 901, Gwynedd Valley, PA 19437-0901. *Telephone:* 215-646-7300 Ext. 135. *Fax:* 215-641-5564. *E-mail:* cullen.p@gmc.edu.

Holy Family University

School of Nursing and Allied Health Professions
Philadelphia, Pennsylvania

http://www.holyfamily.edu/school_nursing/index.html

Founded in 1954

DEGREES • BSN • MSN

Nursing Program Faculty 40 (28% with doctorates).

Baccalaureate Enrollment 183
Women 90% **Men** 10% **Minority** 25%

Graduate Enrollment 27
Women 97% **Men** 3% **Part-time** 100%

Nursing Student Activities Sigma Theta Tau, Student Nurses' Association.

Nursing Student Resources Academic advising; academic or career counseling; assistance for students with disabilities; bookstore; campus computer network; career placement assistance; computer lab; computer-assisted instruction; daycare for children of students; e-mail services; interactive nursing skills videos; Internet; learning resource lab; library services; nursing audiovisuals; other; resume preparation assistance; skills, simulation, or other laboratory; tutoring.

Library Facilities 126,780 volumes (8,159 in health, 2,177 in nursing); 742 periodical subscriptions (279 health-care related).

BACCALAUREATE PROGRAMS

Degree BSN

Available Programs ADN to Baccalaureate; Accelerated Baccalaureate; Generic Baccalaureate; International Nurse to Baccalaureate; LPN to Baccalaureate; LPN to RN Baccalaureate; RN Baccalaureate.

Site Options Bensalem, PA; Newtown, PA.

Study Options Full-time and part-time.

Program Entrance Requirements Transcript of college record, health exam, high school biology, high school chemistry, high school foreign language, 3 years high school math, 3 years high school science, high school transcript, immunizations, letters of recommendation, minimum high school GPA of 2.5, minimum high school rank 60%, minimum GPA in nursing prerequisites of 2.5. Transfer students are accepted. **Standardized tests** *Required:* SAT or ACT, TOEFL for international students. **Application** *Deadline:* rolling (freshmen), rolling (transfer). *Application fee:* $25.

Expenses (2003–04) *Tuition:* full-time $15,500; part-time $335 per credit hour. *International tuition:* $15,500 full-time.

Financial Aid 85% of baccalaureate students in nursing programs received some form of financial aid in 2002–03. *Gift aid (need-based):* Federal Pell, FSEOG, state, private, college/university gift aid from institutional funds. *Loans:* Federal Nursing Student Loans, FFEL (Subsidized and Unsubsidized Stafford PLUS), Perkins. *Work-Study:* Federal Work-Study, part-time campus jobs. *Application deadline (priority):* 3/1.

Contact Lauren McDermott, Director of Admissions, School of Nursing and Allied Health Professions, Holy Family University, 9701 Frankford Avenue, Philadelphia, PA 19114. *Telephone:* 215-637-3050. *Fax:* 215-281-1022. *E-mail:* lmcdermott@holyfamily.edu.

GRADUATE PROGRAMS

Expenses (2003–04) *Tuition:* part-time $415 per credit hour.

Contact Margaret Wendling, Director of Graduate Admissions, School of Nursing and Allied Health Professions, Holy Family University, 9701 Frankford Avenue, Philadelphia, PA 19114-2094. *Telephone:* 215-637-7203. *Fax:* 215-637-1478. *E-mail:* gradstudy@holyfamily.edu.

MASTER'S DEGREE PROGRAM

Degree MSN

Available Programs Master's.

Concentrations Available Health-care administration; nursing education. *Clinical nurse specialist programs in:* community health.

Site Options Newtown, PA.

Study Options Part-time.

Program Entrance Requirements Transcript of college record, written essay, immunizations, 2 letters of recommendation, nursing research course, professional liability insurance/malpractice insurance, prerequisite course work, resume, statistics course.

Advanced Placement Credit by examination available. Credit given for nursing courses completed elsewhere dependent upon specific evaluations.

Degree Requirements 39 total credit hours, comprehensive exam.

CONTINUING EDUCATION PROGRAM

Contact Ms. Amanda Herz, Director of Admissions and Marketing, Division of Extended Learning, School of Nursing and Allied Health Professions, Holy Family University, 1311 Bristol Pike, Bensalem, PA 19020. *Telephone:* 215-637-7700 Ext. 5002. *Fax:* 215-633-0558. *E-mail:* aherz@holyfamily.edu.

See full description on page 498.

Immaculata University
Department of Nursing
Immaculata, Pennsylvania

http://www.immaculata.edu/nursing/

Founded in 1920

DEGREES • BSN • MSN

Nursing Program Faculty 30 (50% with doctorates).

Nursing Student Activities Nursing Honor Society, Sigma Theta Tau.

Nursing Student Resources E-mail services; library services.

Library Facilities 143,145 volumes; 604 periodical subscriptions (115 health-care related).

BACCALAUREATE PROGRAMS

Degree BSN

Available Programs Accelerated RN Baccalaureate; RN Baccalaureate.

Site Options Abington, PA; Lancaster, PA.

Program Entrance Requirements Minimum overall college GPA of 2.0, transcript of college record, CPR certification, health exam, interview, professional liability insurance/malpractice insurance, prerequisite course work, RN licensure. Transfer students are accepted. **Standardized tests** *Required:* SAT or ACT, TOEFL for international students. *Recommended:* SAT, SAT and SAT Subject Tests or ACT, SAT Subject Tests. **Application** *Deadline:* 8/15 (freshmen), rolling (transfer). *Notification:* 8/15 (freshmen). *Application fee:* $25.

Contact Dr. Janice Cranmer, Chair, Department of Nursing, Immaculata University, 1145 King Road, Immaculata, PA 19345. *Telephone:* 610-647-4400 Ext. 3460. *Fax:* 610-251-1668. *E-mail:* jcranmer@immaculata.edu.

GRADUATE PROGRAMS

Contact Dr. Jean McAleer Klein, Director, MSN Program. *E-mail:* jklein@immaculata.edu.

MASTER'S DEGREE PROGRAM

Degree MSN

Available Programs Master's.

Concentrations Available Nursing administration; nursing education. *Clinical nurse specialist programs in:* psychiatric/mental health.

Study Options Part-time.

Program Entrance Requirements Minimum overall college GPA of 3.0, transcript of college record, interview, 3 letters of recommendation.

CONTINUING EDUCATION PROGRAM

Contact College of Lifelong Learning. *Telephone:* 610-647-4400 Ext. 3239. *E-mail:* srobbins@immaculata.edu.

Indiana University of Pennsylvania
Department of Nursing and Allied Health
Indiana, Pennsylvania

Founded in 1875

DEGREES • BSN • MSN

Nursing Program Faculty 21 (67% with doctorates).

Baccalaureate Enrollment 435
Women 90% **Men** 10% **Minority** 52%

Graduate Enrollment 53
Women 87% **Men** 13% **International** 4% **Part-time** 62%

Nursing Student Activities Nursing Honor Society, Sigma Theta Tau, nursing club.

Nursing Student Resources Academic advising; academic or career counseling; assistance for students with disabilities; bookstore; campus computer network; career placement assistance; computer lab; computer-assisted instruction; e-mail services; employment services for current students; externships; housing assistance; interactive nursing skills videos; Internet; learning resource lab; library services; nursing audiovisuals; remedial services; resume preparation assistance; skills, simulation, or other laboratory; tutoring.

Library Facilities 570,735 volumes (5,758 in health, 3,395 in nursing); 2,626 periodical subscriptions (225 health-care related).

BACCALAUREATE PROGRAMS

Degree BSN

Available Programs Baccalaureate for Second Degree; Generic Baccalaureate; RN Baccalaureate.

Study Options Full-time and part-time.

Program Entrance Requirements 2 Year (s) high school math, high school transcript, minimum high school rank 20%, prerequisite course work. Transfer students are accepted. **Standardized tests** *Required:* SAT or ACT, TOEFL for international students. **Application** *Deadline:* rolling (freshmen), rolling (transfer). *Notification:* 9/1 (freshmen). *Application fee:* $30.

Advanced Placement Credit by examination available. Credit given for nursing courses completed elsewhere dependent upon specific evaluations.

Expenses (2003–04) *Tuition, state resident:* full-time $4378; part-time $182 per credit hour. *Tuition, nonresident:* full-time $10,946; part-time $456 per credit hour. *Room and board:* $4702; room only: $2826 per academic year.

Contact Dr. Rhonda Luckey, Interim Dean of Admissions, Department of Nursing and Allied Health, Indiana University of Pennsylvania, 117 Sutton Hall, Indiana, PA 15705. *E-mail:* admissions-inquiry@iup.edu.

GRADUATE PROGRAMS

Expenses (2003–04) *Tuition, state resident:* full-time $5254; part-time $292 per credit hour. *Tuition, nonresident:* full-time $8408; part-time $467 per credit hour.

Financial Aid 3 research assistantships (averaging $4,740 per year) were awarded; Federal Work-Study also available.

Contact Dr. Michele Gerwick, Department Chair, Department of Nursing and Allied Health, Indiana University of Pennsylvania, 1010 Oakland Avenue, Indiana, PA 15705. *Telephone:* 724-357-2557. *Fax:* 724-357-3267. *E-mail:* mgerwick@iup.edu.

MASTER'S DEGREE PROGRAM

Degree MSN

Available Programs Master's; RN to Master's.

Concentrations Available Nursing administration. *Clinical nurse specialist programs in:* community health.

Site Options Monroeville, PA.

Study Options Full-time and part-time.

Program Entrance Requirements Clinical experience, computer literacy, minimum overall college GPA of 3.0, transcript of college record, written essay, 2 letters of recommendation, nursing research course, professional liability insurance/malpractice insurance, statistics course. *Application deadline:* For fall admission, 7/1 (priority date); for spring admission, 11/1. Applications are processed on a rolling basis. *Application fee:* $30.

Degree Requirements 36 total credit hours, thesis or project.

Kutztown University of Pennsylvania
Department of Nursing
Kutztown, Pennsylvania

http://www.kutztown.edu

Founded in 1866

DEGREE • BSN

Nursing Program Faculty 4 (75% with doctorates).

Baccalaureate Enrollment 122
Women 95% **Men** 5% **Minority** 1% **Part-time** 95%

Kutztown University of Pennsylvania (continued)

Nursing Student Activities Nursing Honor Society, Sigma Theta Tau, Student Nurses' Association.

Nursing Student Resources Academic advising; academic or career counseling; assistance for students with disabilities; bookstore; campus computer network; career placement assistance; computer lab; daycare for children of students; e-mail services; employment services for current students; housing assistance; Internet; library services; nursing audiovisuals; placement services for program completers; remedial services; resume preparation assistance; skills, simulation, or other laboratory.

Library Facilities 500,484 volumes (38,000 in health, 15,000 in nursing); 15,600 periodical subscriptions (108 health-care related).

BACCALAUREATE PROGRAMS

Degree BSN

Available Programs RN Baccalaureate.

Site Options Allentown, PA. *Distance Learning:* Reading, PA.

Study Options Full-time and part-time.

Program Entrance Requirements Transcript of college record, CPR certification, health exam, high school transcript, immunizations, minimum GPA in nursing prerequisites of 2.0, professional liability insurance/malpractice insurance, prerequisite course work, RN licensure. Transfer students are accepted. **Standardized tests** *Required:* SAT or ACT, TOEFL for international students. *Required for some:* SAT Subject Tests. **Application** *Deadline:* 3/1 (freshmen), rolling (transfer). *Notification:* 4/15 (freshmen). *Application fee:* $35.

Advanced Placement Credit by examination available. Credit given for nursing courses completed elsewhere dependent upon specific evaluations.

Expenses (2003–04) *Tuition, state resident:* full-time $2189; part-time $182 per credit hour. *Tuition, nonresident:* full-time $5473; part-time $456 per credit hour. *International tuition:* $5473 full-time.

Contact Dr. Kimberly Anne Johnston, Chairperson, Department of Nursing, Kutztown University of Pennsylvania, 219 Beekey Building, Kutztown, PA 19530. *Telephone:* 610-683-4328. *Fax:* 610-683-4708. *E-mail:* kjohnsto@kutztown.edu.

CONTINUING EDUCATION PROGRAM

Contact Dr. Kimberly Anne Johnston, Chairperson, Department of Nursing, Kutztown University of Pennsylvania, 219 Beekey Education Center, Kutztown University, Kutztown, PA 19530. *Telephone:* 610-683-4328. *Fax:* 610-683-4708. *E-mail:* kjohnsto@kutztown.edu.

La Roche College

Department of Nursing and Nursing Management
Pittsburgh, Pennsylvania

http://www.laroche.edu

Founded in 1963

DEGREES • BSN • MSN

Nursing Program Faculty 11 (45% with doctorates).

Baccalaureate Enrollment 46
Women 89% **Men** 11% **International** 17% **Part-time** 74%

Graduate Enrollment 18
Women 83% **Men** 17% **International** 5% **Part-time** 94%

Nursing Student Activities Sigma Theta Tau.

Nursing Student Resources Academic advising; academic or career counseling; assistance for students with disabilities; bookstore; campus computer network; computer lab; e-mail services; externships; Internet; library services; resume preparation assistance; tutoring.

Library Facilities 108,432 volumes; 601 periodical subscriptions (713 health-care related).

BACCALAUREATE PROGRAMS

Degree BSN

Available Programs Accelerated RN Baccalaureate; RN Baccalaureate.

Site Options Pittsburgh, PA.

Study Options Full-time and part-time.

Program Entrance Requirements Minimum overall college GPA of 2.5, transcript of college record, high school transcript, 2 letters of recommendation, professional liability insurance/malpractice insurance, prerequisite course work, RN licensure. Transfer students are accepted. **Standardized tests** *Required:* SAT or ACT, TOEFL for international students. **Application** *Deadline:* 8/23 (freshmen), rolling (transfer). *Application fee:* $50.

Advanced Placement Credit by examination available. Credit given for nursing courses completed elsewhere dependent upon specific evaluations.

Expenses (2003–04) *Tuition:* full-time $15,220; part-time $465 per credit hour. *International tuition:* $15,220 full-time. *Room and board:* $6474 per academic year. *Required fees:* full-time $100; part-time $7 per credit.

Financial Aid 87% of baccalaureate students in nursing programs received some form of financial aid in 2002–03.

Contact Ms. Renee A. Bowers, Director of Admissions for Graduate and Continuing Education, Department of Nursing and Nursing Management, La Roche College, Office of Admissions for Graduate and Continuing Education, 9000 Babcock Boulevard, Pittsburgh, PA 15237. *Telephone:* 412-536-1262. *Fax:* 412-536-1283. *E-mail:* bowersr1@laroche.edu.

GRADUATE PROGRAMS

Expenses (2003–04) *Tuition:* part-time $485 per credit hour. *Required fees:* full-time $100; part-time $7 per credit.

Contact Ms. Renee A. Bowers, Director of Admissions for Graduate and Continuing Education, Department of Nursing and Nursing Management, La Roche College, Office of Admissions for Graduate and Continuing Education, 9000 Babcock Boulevard, Pittsburgh, PA 15237. *Telephone:* 412-536-1262. *Fax:* 412-536-1283. *E-mail:* bowersr1@laroche.edu.

MASTER'S DEGREE PROGRAM

Degree MSN

Available Programs Master's; RN to Master's.

Concentrations Available Nursing administration. *Clinical nurse specialist programs in:* community health, critical care, gerontology. *Nurse practitioner programs in:* family health.

Study Options Full-time and part-time.

Program Entrance Requirements Clinical experience, minimum overall college GPA of 3.0, transcript of college record, immunizations, interview, 2 letters of recommendation, professional liability insurance/malpractice insurance, resume.

Advanced Placement Credit given for nursing courses completed elsewhere dependent upon specific evaluations.

Degree Requirements 41 total credit hours.

CONTINUING EDUCATION PROGRAM

Contact Ms. Renee A. Bowers, Director of Admissions for Graduate and Continuing Education, Department of Nursing and Nursing Management, La Roche College, Office of Admissions for Graduate and Continuing Education, 9000 Babcock Boulevard, Pittsburgh, PA 15237. *Telephone:* 412-536-1262. *Fax:* 412-536-1283. *E-mail:* bowersr1@laroche.edu.

La Salle University

School of Nursing
Philadelphia, Pennsylvania

http://www.lasalle.edu/academ/nursing

Founded in 1863

DEGREES • BSN • MSN • MSN/MBA

Nursing Program Faculty 45 (32% with doctorates).

Nursing Student Activities Sigma Theta Tau, Student Nurses' Association, nursing club.

Nursing Student Resources Academic advising; academic or career counseling; assistance for students with disabilities; bookstore; campus computer network; career placement assistance; computer lab; computer-assisted instruction; e-mail services; employment services for current students; externships; housing assistance; interactive nursing skills videos; Internet; learning resource lab; library services; nursing audiovisuals; placement services for program completers; remedial services; resume preparation assistance; skills, simulation, or other laboratory; tutoring.

Library Facilities 400,000 volumes (8,350 in nursing); 6,900 periodical subscriptions (310 health-care related).

BACCALAUREATE PROGRAMS

Degree BSN

Available Programs Baccalaureate for Second Degree; Generic Baccalaureate; LPN to Baccalaureate; RN Baccalaureate.

Site Options Newtown, PA.

Study Options Full-time and part-time.

Program Entrance Requirements Minimum overall college GPA of 2.75, transcript of college record, CPR certification, written essay, health exam, health insurance, high school biology, high school chemistry, 3 years high school math, 3 years high school science, high school transcript, immunizations, interview, 2 letters of recommendation, minimum high school GPA of 3.0, minimum high school rank 25%, minimum GPA in nursing prerequisites of 2.75, professional liability insurance/malpractice insurance, prerequisite course work. Transfer students are accepted. **Standardized tests** *Required:* SAT or ACT, TOEFL for international students. **Application** *Deadline:* 8/15 (transfer). *Early decision:* 11/15. *Notification:* continuous (freshmen), 12/15 (early action). *Application fee:* $35.

Advanced Placement Credit by examination available. Credit given for nursing courses completed elsewhere dependent upon specific evaluations.

Expenses (2003–04) *Tuition:* part-time $370 per credit hour. *Required fees:* part-time $75 per term.

Contact Dr. Diane Wieland, Undergraduate Director and Associate Professor, School of Nursing, La Salle University, 1900 West Olney Avenue, Philadelphia, PA 19141. *Telephone:* 215-951-1430. *Fax:* 215-951-1896. *E-mail:* wieland@lasalle.edu.

GRADUATE PROGRAMS

Expenses (2003–04) *Tuition:* part-time $580 per credit hour. *Required fees:* part-time $75 per term.

Contact Dr. Kathleen O. Vito, Director of MSN Program and Associate Professor, School of Nursing, La Salle University, 1900 West Olney Avenue, Philadelphia, PA 19141-1199. *Telephone:* 215-951-1413. *Fax:* 215-951-1896. *E-mail:* vito@lasalle.edu.

MASTER'S DEGREE PROGRAM

Degrees MSN; MSN/MBA

Available Programs Master's; RN to Master's.

Concentrations Available Nurse anesthesia; nursing administration. *Clinical nurse specialist programs in:* adult health, public health. *Nurse practitioner programs in:* adult health, family health.

Site Options Newtown, PA.

Study Options Full-time and part-time.

Program Entrance Requirements Clinical experience, minimum overall college GPA of 3.0, transcript of college record, CPR certification, written essay, immunizations, interview, 2 letters of recommendation, nursing research course, physical assessment course, professional liability insurance/malpractice insurance, resume, statistics course.

Advanced Placement Credit given for nursing courses completed elsewhere dependent upon specific evaluations.

Degree Requirements 41 total credit hours.

POST-MASTER'S PROGRAM

Areas of Study Nurse anesthesia; nursing administration; nursing education. *Clinical nurse specialist programs in:* adult health, public health. *Nurse practitioner programs in:* adult health, family health.

CONTINUING EDUCATION PROGRAM

Contact Dr. Zane Robinson Wolf, Dean and Professor, School of Nursing, La Salle University, 1900 West Olney Avenue, Philadelphia, PA 19141-1199. *Telephone:* 215-951-1432. *Fax:* 215-951-1896. *E-mail:* wolf@lasalle.edu.

Mansfield University of Pennsylvania

Robert Packer Department of Health Sciences
Mansfield, Pennsylvania

http://www.mansfield.edu

Founded in 1857

DEGREES • BSN • MSN

Nursing Program Faculty 13 (40% with doctorates).

Baccalaureate Enrollment 189

Women 95% **Men** 5% **Minority** 5% **International** 1% **Part-time** 10%

Graduate Enrollment 31

Women 100% **Minority** 1% **Part-time** 100%

Nursing Student Activities Student Nurses' Association, nursing club.

Nursing Student Resources Academic advising; academic or career counseling; assistance for students with disabilities; bookstore; campus computer network; career placement assistance; computer lab; daycare for children of students; e-mail services; employment services for current students; housing assistance; Internet; learning resource lab; library services; nursing audiovisuals; remedial services; resume preparation assistance; skills, simulation, or other laboratory; tutoring.

Library Facilities 246,141 volumes (12,000 in health, 2,200 in nursing); 2,948 periodical subscriptions (525 health-care related).

BACCALAUREATE PROGRAMS

Degree BSN

Available Programs Generic Baccalaureate; RN Baccalaureate.

Site Options *Distance Learning:* Sayre, PA.

Study Options Full-time and part-time.

Program Entrance Requirements Minimum overall college GPA of 2.5, transcript of college record, CPR certification, health exam, health insurance, high school biology, high school chemistry, 2 years high school math, 2 years high school science, high school transcript, immunizations, minimum high school GPA of 2.5, minimum high school rank 60%, professional liability insurance/malpractice insurance. Transfer students are accepted. **Standardized tests** *Required:* SAT or ACT, TOEFL for international students. **Application** *Deadline:* rolling (freshmen), rolling (transfer). *Notification:* continuous (freshmen). *Application fee:* $25.

Advanced Placement Credit by examination available. Credit given for nursing courses completed elsewhere dependent upon specific evaluations.

Expenses (2004–05) *Tuition, state resident:* full-time $4598; part-time $192 per credit hour. *Tuition, nonresident:* full-time $11,496; part-time $479 per credit hour. *International tuition:* $11,496 full-time. *Room and board:* $5494; room only: $3432 per academic year. *Required fees:* full-time $1420; part-time $120 per credit; part-time $710 per term.

Financial Aid 85% of baccalaureate students in nursing programs received some form of financial aid in 2003–04. *Gift aid (need-based):* Federal Pell, FSEOG, state, private, college/university gift aid from institutional funds. *Loans:* FFEL (Subsidized and Unsubsidized Stafford PLUS), Perkins, alternative loans. *Work-Study:* Federal Work-Study, part-time campus jobs. *Application deadline (priority):* 3/15.

Contact Admissions Office, Robert Packer Department of Health Sciences, Mansfield University of Pennsylvania, Alumni Hall, Mansfield, PA 16933. *Telephone:* 570-662-4243. *Fax:* 570-662-4121. *E-mail:* admissns@mnsfld.edu.

GRADUATE PROGRAMS

Expenses (2004–05) *Tuition, state resident:* full-time $5518; part-time $307 per credit hour. *Tuition, nonresident:* full-time $8830; part-time $491 per credit hour. *International tuition:* $8830 full-time. *Room and board:* $8870; room only: $3424 per academic year. *Required fees:* full-time $807; part-time $100 per credit; part-time $404 per term.

Financial Aid 50% of graduate students in nursing programs received some form of financial aid in 2003–04.

Contact Dr. Janeen Bartlett Sheehe, Department Chair and Nursing Program Director, Robert Packer Department of Health Sciences, Mansfield University of Pennsylvania, 212C Elliott Hall, Mansfield University, Mansfield, PA 16933. *Telephone:* 570-6624522. *Fax:* 570-6624137. *E-mail:* jsheehe@mansfield.edu.

Mansfield University of Pennsylvania (continued)

MASTER'S DEGREE PROGRAM

Degree MSN

Available Programs Master's.

Concentrations Available Nursing education.

Study Options Part-time.

Program Entrance Requirements Minimum overall college GPA of 3.0, transcript of college record, prerequisite course work.

Degree Requirements 33 total credit hours, thesis or project.

Marywood University

Department of Nursing
Scranton, Pennsylvania

http://www.marywood.edu/uscat/nurs.htm

Founded in 1915

DEGREES • BSN • MSN

Nursing Program Faculty 11 (75% with doctorates).

Baccalaureate Enrollment 89
Women 90% **Men** 10% **Minority** 5% **International** 3% **Part-time** 5%

Graduate Enrollment 8
Women 95% **Men** 5% **Part-time** 90%

Nursing Student Activities Sigma Theta Tau, Student Nurses' Association.

Nursing Student Resources Academic advising; academic or career counseling; assistance for students with disabilities; bookstore; campus computer network; computer lab; daycare for children of students; e-mail services; employment services for current students; interactive nursing skills videos; Internet; learning resource lab; library services; nursing audiovisuals; skills, simulation, or other laboratory; tutoring.

Library Facilities 220,205 volumes (7,400 in health, 3,006 in nursing); 913 periodical subscriptions (750 health-care related).

BACCALAUREATE PROGRAMS

Degree BSN

Available Programs ADN to Baccalaureate; Generic Baccalaureate; LPN to Baccalaureate; RN Baccalaureate.

Study Options Full-time and part-time.

Program Entrance Requirements Transcript of college record, high school biology, high school chemistry, high school transcript, 1 letter of recommendation. Transfer students are accepted. **Standardized tests** *Required:* SAT or ACT, TOEFL for international students. *Recommended:* SAT. **Application** *Deadline:* rolling (freshmen), rolling (transfer). *Notification:* continuous (freshmen). *Application fee:* $30.

Advanced Placement Credit given for nursing courses completed elsewhere dependent upon specific evaluations.

Expenses (2004–05) *Tuition:* full-time $19,600. *International tuition:* $20,600 full-time. *Room and board:* $8582 per academic year. *Required fees:* full-time $545.

Financial Aid 90% of baccalaureate students in nursing programs received some form of financial aid in 2003–04. *Gift aid (need-based):* Federal Pell, FSEOG, state, private, college/university gift aid from institutional funds. *Loans:* FFEL (Subsidized and Unsubsidized Stafford PLUS), Perkins, state, alternative loans. *Work-Study:* Federal Work-Study. *Application deadline:* Continuous.

Contact Dr. Robin Gallagher, Chairperson, Department of Nursing, Marywood University, Center for Natural and Health Science, 2300 Adams Avenue, Scranton, PA 18509. *Telephone:* 570-348-6211 Ext. 2475. *Fax:* 570-961-4761. *E-mail:* gallagher@marywood.edu.

GRADUATE PROGRAMS

Expenses (2004–05) *Tuition:* full-time $11,106; part-time $617 per credit hour. *Room and board:* $8582 per academic year.

Financial Aid 90% of graduate students in nursing programs received some form of financial aid in 2003–04.

Contact Dr. Robin Gallagher, Chairperson, Department of Nursing, Marywood University, Center for Natural and Health Science, 2300 Adams Avenue, Scranton, PA 18509. *Telephone:* 570-348-6211 Ext. 2475. *Fax:* 570-961-4761. *E-mail:* gallagher@marywood.edu.

MASTER'S DEGREE PROGRAM

Degree MSN

Available Programs Master's.

Concentrations Available Nursing administration.

Study Options Full-time and part-time.

Program Entrance Requirements Clinical experience, minimum overall college GPA of 3.0, transcript of college record, written essay, 2 letters of recommendation, nursing research course, physical assessment course, statistics course.

Degree Requirements 39 total credit hours, thesis or project.

Messiah College

Department of Nursing
Grantham, Pennsylvania

http://www.messiah.edu

Founded in 1909

DEGREE • BSN

Nursing Program Faculty 18 (17% with doctorates).

Baccalaureate Enrollment 199
Women 94% **Men** 6% **Minority** 6%

Nursing Student Activities Nursing Honor Society, Sigma Theta Tau, Student Nurses' Association.

Nursing Student Resources Academic advising; academic or career counseling; assistance for students with disabilities; bookstore; campus computer network; career placement assistance; computer lab; computer-assisted instruction; e-mail services; employment services for current students; interactive nursing skills videos; Internet; learning resource lab; library services; nursing audiovisuals; remedial services; resume preparation assistance; skills, simulation, or other laboratory; tutoring.

Library Facilities 290,838 volumes (8,300 in health, 700 in nursing); 5,973 periodical subscriptions (1,040 health-care related).

BACCALAUREATE PROGRAMS

Degree BSN

Available Programs Generic Baccalaureate.

Study Options Full-time and part-time.

Program Entrance Requirements Transcript of college record, CPR certification, written essay, health exam, health insurance, high school foreign language, 2 years high school math, 2 years high school science, high school transcript, immunizations, 2 letters of recommendation, minimum GPA in nursing prerequisites of 2.5, prerequisite course work. Transfer students are accepted. **Standardized tests** *Required:* TOEFL for international students. *Required for some:* SAT or ACT. **Application** *Deadline:* rolling (freshmen). *Early decision:* 10/15, 11/15. *Notification:* continuous (freshmen), 11/1 (out-of-state freshmen), 11/1 (early decision), 12/1 (early action). *Application fee:* $30.

Expenses (2004–05) *Tuition:* full-time $20,120; part-time $840 per credit hour. *International tuition:* $20,120 full-time. *Room and board:* $6840; room only: $3680 per academic year. *Required fees:* full-time $1282.

Financial Aid 93% of baccalaureate students in nursing programs received some form of financial aid in 2003–04.

Contact William Strausbaugh, Dean of Enrollment Management, Department of Nursing, Messiah College, PO Box 3005, One College Avenue, Grantham, PA 17027. *Telephone:* 717-691-6000. *Fax:* 717-796-5374. *E-mail:* strausba@messiah.edu.

Millersville University of Pennsylvania

Department of Nursing
Millersville, Pennsylvania

http://muweb.millersville.edu/~nursing/

Founded in 1855

DEGREES • BSN • MSN

Nursing Program Faculty 10 (70% with doctorates).

Baccalaureate Enrollment 40
Women 95% **Men** 5% **Minority** 18% **Part-time** 80%

Graduate Enrollment 29
Women 86% **Men** 14% **Minority** 3% **Part-time** 100%

Nursing Student Activities Sigma Theta Tau.

Nursing Student Resources Academic advising; assistance for students with disabilities; computer lab; e-mail services; interactive nursing skills videos; Internet; nursing audiovisuals.

Library Facilities 503,145 volumes; 10,861 periodical subscriptions (82 health-care related).

BACCALAUREATE PROGRAMS

Degree BSN

Available Programs RN Baccalaureate.

Study Options Full-time and part-time.

Program Entrance Requirements Transcript of college record, RN licensure. Transfer students are accepted. **Standardized tests** *Required:* SAT or ACT, TOEFL for international students. **Application** *Deadline:* rolling (freshmen), rolling (transfer). *Notification:* continuous (freshmen). *Application fee:* $35.

Expenses (2004–05) *Tuition, state resident:* full-time $11,723; part-time $192 per credit hour. *Tuition, nonresident:* full-time $18,989; part-time $479 per credit hour. *International tuition:* $18,989 full-time. *Room and board:* $5642; room only: $3308 per academic year.

Financial Aid 75% of baccalaureate students in nursing programs received some form of financial aid in 2003–04. *Gift aid (need-based):* Federal Pell, FSEOG, state, private, college/university gift aid from institutional funds, SICO Scholarships. *Loans:* FFEL (Subsidized and Unsubsidized Stafford PLUS), Perkins, college/university. *Work-Study:* Federal Work-Study, part-time campus jobs. *Application deadline:* 3/15.

Contact Dr. Ruth E. Davis, Professor, Department of Nursing, Millersville University of Pennsylvania, Science and Technology Building, Room 119, Millersville, PA 17551-0302. *Telephone:* 717-871-2183. *Fax:* 717-872-3985. *E-mail:* ruth.davis@millersville.edu.

GRADUATE PROGRAMS

Expenses (2004–05) *Tuition, state resident:* full-time $6935; part-time $307 per credit hour. *Tuition, nonresident:* full-time $10,449; part-time $491 per credit hour. *International tuition:* $10,449 full-time. *Room and board:* $5642; room only: $3308 per academic year. *Required fees:* full-time $50; part-time $25 per term.

Financial Aid 5% of graduate students in nursing programs received some form of financial aid in 2003–04. 2 research assistantships with full tuition reimbursements available (averaging $4,000 per year) were awarded; Federal Work-Study, institutionally sponsored loans, and unspecified assistantships also available. Aid available to part-time students. *Financial aid application deadline:* 3/15.

Contact Dr. Barbara F. Haus, RN, Graduate Program Coordinator, Department of Nursing, Millersville University of Pennsylvania, Science and Technology Building, Room 121, PO Box 1002, Millersville, PA 17551-0302. *Telephone:* 717-871-5276. *Fax:* 717-872-3985. *E-mail:* barbara.haus@millersville.edu.

MASTER'S DEGREE PROGRAM

Degree MSN

Available Programs Master's.

Concentrations Available Nurse case management. *Nurse practitioner programs in:* family health.

Study Options Part-time.

Program Entrance Requirements Clinical experience, minimum overall college GPA of 3.0, transcript of college record, interview, 3 letters of recommendation, nursing research course, physical assessment course, resume, statistics course, GRE. *Application deadline:* For fall admission, 3/1; for spring admission, 10/1. Applications are processed on a rolling basis. *Application fee:* $35.

Advanced Placement Credit given for nursing courses completed elsewhere dependent upon specific evaluations.

Degree Requirements 42 total credit hours, thesis or project.

POST-MASTER'S PROGRAM

Areas of Study Nurse case management. *Nurse practitioner programs in:* family health.

CONTINUING EDUCATION PROGRAM

Contact Ms. Bili Mattes, Director, Professional Training and Education, Department of Nursing, Millersville University of Pennsylvania, Office of Professional Training and Education, PO Box 1002, Millersville, PA 17551-0302. *Telephone:* 717-872-3030. *Fax:* 717-871-2022. *E-mail:* bili.mattes@millersville.edu.

Moravian College

St. Luke's School of Nursing
Bethlehem, Pennsylvania

http://www.moravian.edu/academics/departments/nursing

Founded in 1742

DEGREE • BS

Nursing Program Faculty 12 (50% with doctorates).

Baccalaureate Enrollment 128
Women 93% **Men** 7% **Minority** 12% **International** 1% **Part-time** 13%

Nursing Student Activities Nursing Honor Society, Student Nurses' Association.

Nursing Student Resources Academic advising; academic or career counseling; assistance for students with disabilities; bookstore; campus computer network; career placement assistance; computer lab; computer-assisted instruction; e-mail services; employment services for current students; externships; housing assistance; interactive nursing skills videos; Internet; learning resource lab; library services; nursing audiovisuals; paid internships; placement services for program completers; remedial services; resume preparation assistance; skills, simulation, or other laboratory; tutoring.

Library Facilities 256,352 volumes (4,574 in health, 1,819 in nursing); 1,318 periodical subscriptions (262 health-care related).

BACCALAUREATE PROGRAMS

Degree BS

Available Programs Generic Baccalaureate; RN Baccalaureate.

Site Options Bethlehem, PA.

Study Options Full-time and part-time.

Program Entrance Requirements CPR certification, written essay, health exam, health insurance, high school foreign language, 3 years high school math, high school transcript, immunizations, interview, professional liability insurance/malpractice insurance. Transfer students are accepted. **Standardized tests** *Required:* SAT or ACT, TOEFL for international students. **Application** *Deadline:* 2/15 (freshmen), 8/1 (transfer). *Early decision:* 1/15. *Notification:* 3/15 (freshmen), 12/15 (out-of-state freshmen), 12/15 (early decision). *Application fee:* $40.

Advanced Placement Credit by examination available. Credit given for nursing courses completed elsewhere dependent upon specific evaluations.

Expenses (2004–05) *Tuition:* full-time $23,184; part-time $223 per credit hour. *International tuition:* $23,184 full-time. *Room and board:* $7055; room only: $3850 per academic year. *Required fees:* full-time $420; part-time $150 per term.

Moravian College (continued)

Financial Aid 80% of baccalaureate students in nursing programs received some form of financial aid in 2003–04. *Gift aid (need-based):* Federal Pell, FSEOG, state, private, college/university gift aid from institutional funds. *Loans:* FFEL (Subsidized and Unsubsidized Stafford PLUS), Perkins. *Work-Study:* Federal Work-Study, part-time campus jobs. *Application deadline (priority):* 2/15.

Contact Mr. James P. Mackin, Director of Admissions, St. Luke's School of Nursing, Moravian College, 1200 Main Street, Bethlehem, PA 18018. *Telephone:* 800-441-3191. *E-mail:* mejpm01@moravian.edu.

CONTINUING EDUCATION PROGRAM

Contact Dr. Florence Kimball, Dean, St. Luke's School of Nursing, Moravian College, Continuing and Graduate Studies, 1200 Main Street, Bethlehem, PA 18018. *Telephone:* 610-861-1300. *E-mail:* fkimball@moravian.edu.

Mount Aloysius College

Department of Nursing
Cresson, Pennsylvania

http://www.mtaloy.edu

Founded in 1939

DEGREE • BSN

Nursing Program Faculty 4 (25% with doctorates).

Baccalaureate Enrollment 76

Women 90% **Men** 10% **Part-time** 91%

Nursing Student Activities Student Nurses' Association.

Nursing Student Resources Academic advising; academic or career counseling; assistance for students with disabilities; bookstore; campus computer network; career placement assistance; computer lab; computer-assisted instruction; daycare for children of students; e-mail services; externships; housing assistance; interactive nursing skills videos; Internet; learning resource lab; library services; nursing audiovisuals; placement services for program completers; remedial services; resume preparation assistance; skills, simulation, or other laboratory; tutoring; unpaid internships.

Library Facilities 84,174 volumes (6,773 in health, 1,121 in nursing); 279 periodical subscriptions (67 health-care related).

BACCALAUREATE PROGRAMS

Degree BSN

Available Programs ADN to Baccalaureate; Accelerated RN Baccalaureate.

Site Options Johnstown, PA; Altoona, PA.

Study Options Full-time and part-time.

Program Entrance Requirements Transcript of college record, CPR certification, health exam, high school transcript, immunizations, RN licensure. Transfer students are accepted. **Standardized tests** *Required:* SAT or ACT, TOEFL for international students. **Application** *Deadline:* rolling (freshmen), rolling (transfer). *Notification:* continuous (freshmen). *Application fee:* $30.

Advanced Placement Credit by examination available. Credit given for nursing courses completed elsewhere dependent upon specific evaluations.

Expenses (2004–05) *Tuition:* full-time $15,610; part-time $450 per credit hour. *Room and board:* $5960; room only: $2980 per academic year. *Required fees:* full-time $430; part-time $135 per term.

Financial Aid 71% of baccalaureate students in nursing programs received some form of financial aid in 2003–04.

Contact Ms. Rosemary Kehrer, RN, Chairperson, RN-BSN Program, Department of Nursing, Mount Aloysius College, 7373 Admiral Peary Highway, Cresson, PA 16630. *Telephone:* 814-886-6305. *Fax:* 814-886-6374. *E-mail:* rkehrer@mtaloy.edu.

CONTINUING EDUCATION PROGRAM

Contact Dr. Robert E. Breckinridge, Director of the Center for Lifelong Learning, Department of Nursing, Mount Aloysius College, 7373 Admiral Peary Highway, Cresson, PA 16630. *Telephone:* 814-886-6361. *Fax:* 814-886-2978. *E-mail:* rbreckinridge@mtaloy.edu.

Neumann College

Program in Nursing and Health Sciences
Aston, Pennsylvania

Founded in 1965

DEGREES • BS • MS

Nursing Program Faculty 28 (30% with doctorates).

Baccalaureate Enrollment 232

Women 93% **Men** 7% **Minority** 18% **International** 2% **Part-time** 22%

Graduate Enrollment 15

Women 91% **Men** 9% **Minority** 12%

Nursing Student Activities Nursing Honor Society, Sigma Theta Tau, Student Nurses' Association.

Nursing Student Resources Academic advising; academic or career counseling; assistance for students with disabilities; bookstore; campus computer network; career placement assistance; computer lab; computer-assisted instruction; daycare for children of students; e-mail services; employment services for current students; externships; interactive nursing skills videos; Internet; learning resource lab; library services; nursing audiovisuals; remedial services; resume preparation assistance; skills, simulation, or other laboratory; tutoring.

Library Facilities 75,000 volumes (3,956 in health, 1,170 in nursing); 400 periodical subscriptions (155 health-care related).

BACCALAUREATE PROGRAMS

Degree BS

Available Programs Baccalaureate for Second Degree; Generic Baccalaureate; International Nurse to Baccalaureate; RN Baccalaureate.

Study Options Full-time and part-time.

Program Entrance Requirements Minimum overall college GPA of 2.5, transcript of college record, CPR certification, health exam, health insurance, high school biology, high school chemistry, high school foreign language, 2 years high school math, 3 years high school science, high school transcript, immunizations, minimum GPA in nursing prerequisites of 2.5, professional liability insurance/malpractice insurance, prerequisite course work. Transfer students are accepted. **Standardized tests** *Required:* SAT or ACT, TOEFL for international students. **Application** *Deadline:* 4/1 (freshmen), rolling (transfer). *Notification:* continuous (freshmen). *Application fee:* $35.

Advanced Placement Credit by examination available. Credit given for nursing courses completed elsewhere dependent upon specific evaluations.

Expenses (2004–05) *Tuition:* full-time $16,590; part-time $380 per credit hour. *International tuition:* $16,590 full-time. *Room and board:* $7540; room only: $4600 per academic year. *Required fees:* full-time $700; part-time $50 per term.

Financial Aid 95% of baccalaureate students in nursing programs received some form of financial aid in 2003–04.

Contact Mrs. Dana Hutchinson, Admissions Counselor, Program in Nursing and Health Sciences, Neumann College, One Neumann Drive, Aston, PA 19014-1298. *Telephone:* 800-963-8626 Ext. 4571. *Fax:* 610-558-5652. *E-mail:* nursediv@neumann.edu.

GRADUATE PROGRAMS

Expenses (2004–05) *Tuition:* part-time $460 per credit hour.

Financial Aid 40% of graduate students in nursing programs received some form of financial aid in 2003–04. Available to part-time students. *Application deadline:* 3/15.

Contact Mrs. Louise Bank, Admissions Counselor, Program in Nursing and Health Sciences, Neumann College, One Neumann Drive, Aston, PA 19014-1298. *Telephone:* 800-963-8626 Ext. 5613. *Fax:* 610-558-5652. *E-mail:* nursediv@neumann.edu.

MASTER'S DEGREE PROGRAM

Degree MS

Available Programs Master's; RN to Master's.

Concentrations Available Nursing education. *Clinical nurse specialist programs in:* gerontology. *Nurse practitioner programs in:* gerontology.

Study Options Full-time and part-time.

Program Entrance Requirements Minimum overall college GPA of 3.0, transcript of college record, CPR certification, immunizations, interview, 3 letters of recommendation, nursing research course, physical assessment course, professional liability insurance/malpractice insurance, statistics course, GRE or MAT. *Application deadline:* Applications are processed on a rolling basis. *Application fee:* $50.

Advanced Placement Credit by examination available. Credit given for nursing courses completed elsewhere dependent upon specific evaluations.

Degree Requirements 45 total credit hours.

POST-MASTER'S PROGRAM

Areas of Study Nursing education. *Clinical nurse specialist programs in:* gerontology. *Nurse practitioner programs in:* gerontology.

Pennsylvania College of Technology

School of Health Sciences
Williamsport, Pennsylvania

Founded in 1965

DEGREE • BSN

Nursing Program Faculty 37 (5% with doctorates).

Baccalaureate Enrollment 12
Women 100% **International** 1% **Part-time** 92%

Nursing Student Activities Student Nurses' Association.

Nursing Student Resources Academic advising; academic or career counseling; assistance for students with disabilities; bookstore; campus computer network; career placement assistance; computer lab; computer-assisted instruction; daycare for children of students; e-mail services; employment services for current students; externships; housing assistance; interactive nursing skills videos; Internet; learning resource lab; library services; nursing audiovisuals; placement services for program completers; remedial services; resume preparation assistance; skills, simulation, or other laboratory; tutoring.

Library Facilities 96,281 volumes; 9,118 periodical subscriptions.

BACCALAUREATE PROGRAMS

Degree BSN

Available Programs RN Baccalaureate.

Site Options *Distance Learning:* Williamsport, PA.

Program Entrance Requirements Transfer students are accepted. **Standardized tests** *Required:* TOEFL for international students. *Required for some:* SAT. **Application** *Deadline:* 7/1 (freshmen), 7/1 (out-of-state freshmen), rolling (transfer). *Early decision:* 7/1. *Application fee:* $50.

Expenses (2004–05) *Tuition, state resident:* part-time $316 per credit hour. *Tuition, nonresident:* part-time $375 per credit hour. *Required fees:* part-time $60 per credit.

Financial Aid 92% of baccalaureate students in nursing programs received some form of financial aid in 2003–04. *Gift aid (need-based):* Federal Pell, FSEOG, state, private, college/university gift aid from institutional funds. *Loans:* FFEL (Subsidized and Unsubsidized Stafford PLUS). *Work-Study:* Federal Work-Study, part-time campus jobs. *Application deadline (priority):* 4/1.

Contact Pamela L. Starcher, Director of Nursing, School of Health Sciences, Pennsylvania College of Technology, One College Avenue, Williamsport, PA 17701. *Telephone:* 800-367-9222 Ext. 4525. *E-mail:* pstarche@pct.edu.

The Pennsylvania State University University Park Campus

School of Nursing
State College, University Park, Pennsylvania

http://www.hhdev.psu.edu/nurs

Founded in 1855

DEGREES • BS • MS • PHD

Nursing Program Faculty 105 (25% with doctorates).

Baccalaureate Enrollment 748
Women 95% **Men** 5% **Minority** 10% **International** 1% **Part-time** 33%

Graduate Enrollment 40
Women 99% **Men** 1% **Minority** 1% **Part-time** 63%

Nursing Student Activities Sigma Theta Tau, Student Nurses' Association.

Nursing Student Resources Academic advising; academic or career counseling; assistance for students with disabilities; bookstore; campus computer network; career placement assistance; computer lab; computer-assisted instruction; daycare for children of students; e-mail services; employment services for current students; externships; housing assistance; interactive nursing skills videos; Internet; learning resource lab; library services; nursing audiovisuals; paid internships; remedial services; resume preparation assistance; skills, simulation, or other laboratory; tutoring.

Library Facilities 3.1 million volumes (244,000 in health); 36,856 periodical subscriptions (3,500 health-care related).

BACCALAUREATE PROGRAMS

Degree BS

Available Programs Generic Baccalaureate; RN Baccalaureate.

Site Options *Distance Learning:* Altoona, PA; Uniontown, PA; Hershey, PA.

Study Options Full-time.

Program Entrance Requirements Minimum overall college GPA of 3.0, transcript of college record, health exam, high school foreign language, 3 years high school math, 3 years high school science, high school transcript, immunizations. Transfer students are accepted. **Standardized tests** *Required:* SAT or ACT, TOEFL for international students. **Application** *Deadline:* rolling (freshmen), rolling (transfer). *Notification:* continuous (freshmen). *Application fee:* $50.

Advanced Placement Credit given for nursing courses completed elsewhere dependent upon specific evaluations.

Expenses (2004–05) *Tuition, state resident:* full-time $10,408; part-time $399 per credit hour. *Tuition, nonresident:* full-time $20,336; part-time $612 per credit hour. *Room and board:* $6230; room only: $3250 per academic year. *Required fees:* full-time $2750; part-time $375 per term.

Financial Aid 71% of baccalaureate students in nursing programs received some form of financial aid in 2003–04. *Gift aid (need-based):* Federal Pell, FSEOG, state, private, college/university gift aid from institutional funds. *Loans:* FFEL (Subsidized and Unsubsidized Stafford PLUS), Perkins, college/university, alternative loans. *Work-Study:* Federal Work-Study, part-time campus jobs. *Application deadline:* Continuous.

Contact Dr. Raymonde Brown, Professor in Charge of Undergraduate Programs, School of Nursing, The Pennsylvania State University University Park Campus, 210 Health and Human Development East, University Park, PA 16802. *Telephone:* 814-863-3510. *Fax:* 814-863-2925. *E-mail:* rab16@psu.edu.

GRADUATE PROGRAMS

Expenses (2004–05) *Tuition, state resident:* full-time $11,348; part-time $473 per credit hour. *Tuition, nonresident:* full-time $21,498; part-time $896 per credit hour. *Room and board:* $4180; room only: $1200 per academic year. *Required fees:* full-time $448; part-time $224 per term.

Financial Aid 25% of graduate students in nursing programs received some form of financial aid in 2003–04.

Contact Dr. Carol A. Smith, Professor in Charge of Graduate Programs and Outreach, School of Nursing, The Pennsylvania State University University Park Campus, 203 Health and Human Development East, University Park, PA 16802. *Telephone:* 814-863-2211. *Fax:* 814-863-4778. *E-mail:* cas35@psu.edu.

MASTER'S DEGREE PROGRAM

Degree MS

Available Programs Master's; RN to Master's.

Concentrations Available *Clinical nurse specialist programs in:* adult health, community health, gerontology. *Nurse practitioner programs in:* family health, neonatal health.

Site Options *Distance Learning:* Hershey, PA.

Study Options Full-time and part-time.

The Pennsylvania State University University Park Campus (continued)

Program Entrance Requirements Computer literacy, minimum overall college GPA of 3.0, transcript of college record, CPR certification, immunizations, 2 letters of recommendation, physical assessment course, professional liability insurance/malpractice insurance, statistics course.

Advanced Placement Credit given for nursing courses completed elsewhere dependent upon specific evaluations.

Degree Requirements 47 total credit hours, thesis or project.

POST-MASTER'S PROGRAM

Areas of Study *Nurse practitioner programs in:* family health, neonatal health.

DOCTORAL DEGREE PROGRAM

Degree PhD

Available Programs Doctorate.

Areas of Study Bio-behavioral research, gerontology, individualized study, nursing research, nursing science.

Site Options *Distance Learning:* Hershey, PA.

Program Entrance Requirements Minimum overall college GPA of 3.5, interview by faculty committee, interview, 3 letters of recommendation, MSN or equivalent, writing sample.

Degree Requirements 58 total credit hours, dissertation, oral exam, written exam, residency.

POSTDOCTORAL PROGRAM

Areas of Study Gerontology.

Postdoctoral Program Contact Dr. Carol A. Smith, Professor in Charge of Graduate Programs and Outreach, School of Nursing, The Pennsylvania State University University Park Campus, 203 Health and Human Development East, University Park, PA 16802. *Telephone:* 814-863-2211. *Fax:* 814-863-4788. *E-mail:* cas35@psu.edu.

CONTINUING EDUCATION PROGRAM

Contact Dr. Carol A. Smith, Professor in Charge of Graduate Programs and Outreach, School of Nursing, The Pennsylvania State University University Park Campus, 203 Health and Human Development East, University Park, PA 16802. *Telephone:* 814-863-2211. *Fax:* 814-863-4788. *E-mail:* cas35@psu.edu.

Saint Francis University
Department of Nursing
Loretto, Pennsylvania

http://www.francis.edu/academic/Undergraduate/Nursing/Nursinghome.shtml

Founded in 1847

DEGREE • BSN

Nursing Program Faculty 6.

Nursing Student Activities Student Nurses' Association, nursing club.

Nursing Student Resources Academic advising; academic or career counseling; assistance for students with disabilities; bookstore; campus computer network; career placement assistance; computer lab; computer-assisted instruction; e-mail services; employment services for current students; externships; interactive nursing skills videos; Internet; learning resource lab; library services; nursing audiovisuals; resume preparation assistance; skills, simulation, or other laboratory; tutoring.

Library Facilities 118,333 volumes (120,000 in nursing); 7,202 periodical subscriptions.

BACCALAUREATE PROGRAMS

Degree BSN

Available Programs Generic Baccalaureate; RN Baccalaureate.

Study Options Full-time and part-time.

Program Entrance Requirements Transcript of college record, high school biology, high school chemistry, 2 years high school math, 2 years high school science, high school transcript, minimum high school GPA of 3.0, minimum high school rank 50%, minimum GPA in nursing prerequisites of 2.0, prerequisite course work. Transfer students are accepted. **Standardized tests** *Required:* SAT or ACT, TOEFL for international students. **Application** *Deadline:* rolling (freshmen), rolling (transfer). *Application fee:* $30.

Advanced Placement Credit by examination available. Credit given for nursing courses completed elsewhere dependent upon specific evaluations.

Contact Dr. Jean M. Samii, RN, Chairperson, Department of Nursing, Saint Francis University, PO Box 600, 117 Evergreen Drive, 103 Schwab Hall, Loretto, PA 15940-0600. *Telephone:* 814-472-3027. *Fax:* 814-472-3849. *E-mail:* jsamii@francis.edu.

Slippery Rock University of Pennsylvania
Department of Nursing
Slippery Rock, Pennsylvania

http://www.sru.edu/depts/chhs/Nursing/nursing.htm

Founded in 1889

DEGREES • BSN • MSN

Nursing Program Faculty 6 (66% with doctorates).

Nursing Student Activities Sigma Theta Tau.

Nursing Student Resources Computer lab; e-mail services; Internet.

Library Facilities 512,424 volumes (19,604 in health, 1,396 in nursing); 11,987 periodical subscriptions (165 health-care related).

BACCALAUREATE PROGRAMS

Degree BSN

Site Options *Distance Learning:* Cranberry, PA; Wexford, PA.

Study Options Full-time and part-time.

Program Entrance Requirements Minimum overall college GPA of 2.5, transcript of college record, health exam, immunizations, interview, professional liability insurance/malpractice insurance. Transfer students are accepted. **Standardized tests** *Required:* SAT or ACT, TOEFL for international students. **Application** *Notification:* continuous (freshmen). *Application fee:* $25.

Advanced Placement Credit by examination available. Credit given for nursing courses completed elsewhere dependent upon specific evaluations.

Contact Dr. Kathleen Kellinger, Chairperson, Department of Nursing, Slippery Rock University of Pennsylvania, 119 Behavioral Science Building, Slippery Rock, PA 16057. *Telephone:* 724-738-2326. *Fax:* 724-738-2509. *E-mail:* kathleen.kellinger@sru.edu.

GRADUATE PROGRAMS

Financial Aid Teaching assistantships (averaging $3,500 per year); institutionally sponsored loans, scholarships, traineeships, and unspecified assistantships also available.

Contact Dr. Joyce White, Director and Coordinator, Department of Nursing, Slippery Rock University of Pennsylvania, 115A Behavioral Science Building, Slippery Rock, PA 16057. *Telephone:* 724-738-2323. *Fax:* 724-738-2881. *E-mail:* joyce.white@sru.edu.

MASTER'S DEGREE PROGRAM

Degree MSN

Concentrations Available Nursing education. *Nurse practitioner programs in:* family health.

Site Options *Distance Learning:* Cranberry, PA; Wexford, PA.

Study Options Full-time and part-time.

Program Entrance Requirements Clinical experience, computer literacy, minimum overall college GPA of 2.75, transcript of college record, CPR certification, written essay, immunizations, interview, 3 letters of recommendation, professional liability insurance/malpractice insurance, statistics course. *Application deadline:* For fall admission, 7/1 (priority date); for spring admission, 11/1 (priority date). Applications are processed on a rolling basis. *Application fee:* $30.

Advanced Placement Credit by examination available. Credit given for nursing courses completed elsewhere dependent upon specific evaluations.

Degree Requirements 45 total credit hours, thesis or project, comprehensive exam.

Temple University

Department of Nursing
Philadelphia, Pennsylvania

http://www.temple.edu/nursing

Founded in 1884

DEGREES • BSN • MSN

Nursing Program Faculty 37 (50% with doctorates).

Baccalaureate Enrollment 350
Women 89% **Men** 11% **Minority** 49% **Part-time** 62%

Graduate Enrollment 68
Women 85% **Men** 15% **Minority** 16% **Part-time** 50%

Nursing Student Activities Sigma Theta Tau, Student Nurses' Association.

Nursing Student Resources Academic advising; academic or career counseling; assistance for students with disabilities; bookstore; campus computer network; career placement assistance; computer lab; computer-assisted instruction; e-mail services; externships; housing assistance; interactive nursing skills videos; Internet; learning resource lab; library services; nursing audiovisuals; remedial services; resume preparation assistance; skills, simulation, or other laboratory; tutoring.

Library Facilities 3.3 million volumes (60,374 in health, 1,350 in nursing); 20,980 periodical subscriptions (1,350 health-care related).

BACCALAUREATE PROGRAMS

Degree BSN

Available Programs Accelerated Baccalaureate for Second Degree; Generic Baccalaureate; RN Baccalaureate.

Site Options Ambler, PA; Philadelphia, PA; Bethlehem, PA.

Study Options Full-time.

Program Entrance Requirements Minimum overall college GPA of 3.0, transcript of college record, CPR certification, written essay, health exam, health insurance, high school biology, high school chemistry, high school foreign language, 3 years high school math, 3 years high school science, high school transcript, immunizations, interview, minimum high school GPA of 2.0, minimum GPA in nursing prerequisites of 3.0, prerequisite course work. Transfer students are accepted. **Standardized tests** *Required:* SAT or ACT, TOEFL for international students. **Application** *Deadline:* 4/1 (freshmen), 6/15 (transfer). *Notification:* continuous (freshmen). *Application fee:* $35.

Advanced Placement Credit given for nursing courses completed elsewhere dependent upon specific evaluations.

Expenses (2004–05) *Tuition, state resident:* full-time $10,418; part-time $390 per credit hour. *Tuition, nonresident:* full-time $18,578; part-time $644 per credit hour. *Required fees:* full-time $300.

Financial Aid 70% of baccalaureate students in nursing programs received some form of financial aid in 2003–04.

Contact Ms. Bonita Silverman, Associate Professor, Department of Nursing, Temple University, 3307 North Broad Street, Philadelphia, PA 19140. *Telephone:* 215-707-4629. *Fax:* 215-707-1599. *E-mail:* bonita.silverman@temple.edu.

GRADUATE PROGRAMS

Expenses (2004–05) *Tuition, state resident:* part-time $474 per credit hour. *Tuition, nonresident:* part-time $692 per credit hour. *Required fees:* part-time $250 per credit.

Financial Aid 100% of graduate students in nursing programs received some form of financial aid in 2003–04. 1 teaching assistantship with full tuition reimbursement available (averaging $10,650 per year) was awarded; career-related internships or fieldwork, institutionally sponsored loans, and traineeships also available. Aid available to part-time students.

Contact Dr. Jane M. Kurz, Director of Graduate Studies, Department of Nursing, Temple University, 3307 North Broad Street, Philadelphia, PA 19140. *Telephone:* 215-707-5017. *Fax:* 215-707-1599. *E-mail:* jkurz@temple.edu.

MASTER'S DEGREE PROGRAM

Degree MSN

Available Programs Master's.

Concentrations Available *Clinical nurse specialist programs in:* maternity-newborn, psychiatric/mental health. *Nurse practitioner programs in:* adult health, pediatric.

Site Options Philadelphia, PA.

Study Options Full-time and part-time.

Program Entrance Requirements Clinical experience, minimum overall college GPA of 3.0, transcript of college record, CPR certification, written essay, immunizations, interview, 2 letters of recommendation, nursing research course, physical assessment course, professional liability insurance/malpractice insurance, statistics course, GRE General Test. *Application deadline:* For fall admission, 2/15 (priority date). *Application fee:* $40.

Advanced Placement Credit given for nursing courses completed elsewhere dependent upon specific evaluations.

Degree Requirements 36 total credit hours.

POST-MASTER'S PROGRAM

Areas of Study *Clinical nurse specialist programs in:* maternity-newborn, psychiatric/mental health. *Nurse practitioner programs in:* adult health, pediatric.

Thomas Jefferson University

Department of Nursing
Philadelphia, Pennsylvania

http://www.tju.edu

Founded in 1824

DEGREES • BSN • MSN

Nursing Program Faculty 38 (42% with doctorates).

Baccalaureate Enrollment 230
Women 80% **Men** 20% **Minority** 30% **Part-time** 41%

Graduate Enrollment 111
Women 95% **Men** 5% **Minority** 10% **Part-time** 50%

Nursing Student Activities Nursing Honor Society, Sigma Theta Tau, Student Nurses' Association.

Nursing Student Resources Academic advising; academic or career counseling; assistance for students with disabilities; bookstore; campus computer network; career placement assistance; computer lab; computer-assisted instruction; e-mail services; Internet; learning resource lab; library services; nursing audiovisuals; remedial services; resume preparation assistance; skills, simulation, or other laboratory.

Library Facilities 170,000 volumes (146,000 in health, 4,700 in nursing); 2,290 periodical subscriptions (2,100 health-care related).

BACCALAUREATE PROGRAMS

Degree BSN

Available Programs Accelerated Baccalaureate; Accelerated Baccalaureate for Second Degree; Accelerated RN Baccalaureate; Baccalaureate for Second Degree; Generic Baccalaureate; RN Baccalaureate.

Site Options *Distance Learning:* Philadelphia, PA; Atlantic City, NJ.

Study Options Full-time and part-time.

Thomas Jefferson University (continued)

Program Entrance Requirements Minimum overall college GPA of 2.9, transcript of college record, CPR certification, written essay, high school transcript, 2 letters of recommendation, prerequisite course work. Transfer students are accepted. **Standardized tests** *Required:* TOEFL for international students. *Recommended:* SAT or ACT. **Application** *Deadline:* rolling (freshmen), rolling (transfer). *Notification:* continuous (freshmen). *Application fee:* $50.

Advanced Placement Credit by examination available. Credit given for nursing courses completed elsewhere dependent upon specific evaluations.

Financial Aid 60% of baccalaureate students in nursing programs received some form of financial aid in 2003–04. *Gift aid (need-based):* Federal Pell, FSEOG, state, private, college/university gift aid from institutional funds, Scholarships for Disadvantaged Students (SDS). *Loans:* Federal Nursing Student Loans, FFEL (Subsidized and Unsubsidized Stafford PLUS), Perkins, college/university. *Work-Study:* Federal Work-Study. *Application deadline (priority):* 4/1.

Contact Dr. Anne M. McGinley, RN, Director of the Undergraduate Programs, Department of Nursing, Thomas Jefferson University, 130 South Ninth Street, Philadelphia, PA 19107. *Telephone:* 215-503-8104. *Fax:* 215-503-0376. *E-mail:* anne.mcginley@jefferson.edu.

GRADUATE PROGRAMS

Financial Aid 75% of graduate students in nursing programs received some form of financial aid in 2003–04.

Contact Dr. Mary E. Bowen, RN, Vice Chair and Director of Graduate Programs, Department of Nursing, Thomas Jefferson University, 130 South Ninth Street, Suite 1200, Philadelphia, PA 19107. *Telephone:* 215-503-6057. *Fax:* 215-932-1468. *E-mail:* mary.bowen@jefferson.edu.

MASTER'S DEGREE PROGRAM

Degree MSN

Available Programs Accelerated Master's; Accelerated RN to Master's; Master's; Master's for Non-Nursing College Graduates; Master's for Nurses with Non-Nursing Degrees; RN to Master's.

Concentrations Available Nursing informatics. *Clinical nurse specialist programs in:* acute care, adult health, community health, critical care, home health care, medical-surgical, oncology, pediatric, public health. *Nurse practitioner programs in:* acute care, adult health, family health, neonatal health, oncology, pediatric.

Site Options *Distance Learning:* Philadelphia, PA.

Study Options Full-time and part-time.

Program Entrance Requirements Clinical experience, computer literacy, minimum overall college GPA of 3.0, transcript of college record, CPR certification, written essay, interview, 3 letters of recommendation, nursing research course, physical assessment course, professional liability insurance/malpractice insurance, resume, statistics course.

Advanced Placement Credit given for nursing courses completed elsewhere dependent upon specific evaluations.

Degree Requirements 36 total credit hours.

POST-MASTER'S PROGRAM

Areas of Study Nursing informatics. *Nurse practitioner programs in:* acute care, adult health, family health, neonatal health, oncology, pediatric.

CONTINUING EDUCATION PROGRAM

Contact Dr. Mary E. Bowen, RN, Vice Chair and Director of Graduate Programs, Department of Nursing, Thomas Jefferson University, 130 South Ninth Street, 1200 Edison Building, Philadelphia, PA 19107. *Telephone:* 215-503-6057. *Fax:* 215-503-0376. *E-mail:* mary.bowen@jefferson.edu.

See full description on page 544.

University of Pennsylvania

School of Nursing
Philadelphia, Pennsylvania

http://www.nursing.upenn.edu

Founded in 1740

DEGREES • BSN • MSN • MSN/MBA • MSN/MPH • MSN/PHD

Nursing Program Faculty 220 (32% with doctorates).

Baccalaureate Enrollment 492

Women 92% **Men** 8% **Minority** 34% **International** 2% **Part-time** 5%

Graduate Enrollment 364

Women 96% **Men** 4% **Minority** 23% **International** 5% **Part-time** 55%

Nursing Student Activities Nursing Honor Society, Sigma Theta Tau, Student Nurses' Association.

Nursing Student Resources Academic advising; academic or career counseling; assistance for students with disabilities; bookstore; campus computer network; career placement assistance; computer lab; computer-assisted instruction; daycare for children of students; e-mail services; employment services for current students; externships; housing assistance; interactive nursing skills videos; Internet; learning resource lab; library services; nursing audiovisuals; other; paid internships; placement services for program completers; remedial services; resume preparation assistance; skills, simulation, or other laboratory; tutoring; unpaid internships.

Library Facilities 5.4 million volumes (196,474 in health); 39,426 periodical subscriptions (3,607 health-care related).

BACCALAUREATE PROGRAMS

Degree BSN

Available Programs ADN to Baccalaureate; Accelerated Baccalaureate; Accelerated Baccalaureate for Second Degree; Accelerated RN Baccalaureate; Baccalaureate for Second Degree; Generic Baccalaureate; RN Baccalaureate.

Study Options Full-time and part-time.

Program Entrance Requirements Minimum overall college GPA of 3.0, transcript of college record, written essay, health exam, health insurance, high school biology, high school chemistry, high school foreign language, 4 years high school math, 4 years high school science, high school transcript, immunizations, interview, 2 letters of recommendation, minimum high school GPA of 3.0, minimum high school rank 10%. Transfer students are accepted. **Standardized tests** *Required:* SAT and SAT Subject Tests or ACT, SAT II Writing Tests, TOEFL for international students. **Application** *Deadline:* 1/1 (freshmen), 3/15 (transfer). *Early decision:* 11/1. *Notification:* 4/1 (freshmen), 12/15 (out-of-state freshmen), 12/15 (early decision). *Application fee:* $70.

Advanced Placement Credit by examination available. Credit given for nursing courses completed elsewhere dependent upon specific evaluations.

Expenses (2004–05) *Tuition:* full-time $27,544; part-time $3518 per course. *International tuition:* $27,544 full-time. *Room and board:* $8918; room only: $5336 per academic year. *Required fees:* full-time $3172; part-time $370 per credit; part-time $1586 per term.

Financial Aid 96% of baccalaureate students in nursing programs received some form of financial aid in 2003–04. *Gift aid (need-based):* Federal Pell, FSEOG, state, private, college/university gift aid from institutional funds. *Loans:* Federal Nursing Student Loans, FFEL (Subsidized and Unsubsidized Stafford PLUS), Perkins, college/university, supplemental third-party loans (guaranteed by institution). *Work-Study:* Federal Work-Study. *Application deadline (priority):* 2/15.

Contact Ms. Marianne J. Smith, Associate Director of Undergraduate Enrollment Management, School of Nursing, University of Pennsylvania, 420 Guardian Drive, Philadelphia, PA 19104-6096. *Telephone:* 215-898-4416. *Fax:* 215-573-8439. *E-mail:* smithmar@nursing.upenn.edu.

GRADUATE PROGRAMS

Expenses (2004–05) *Tuition:* full-time $26,973; part-time $3392 per course. *International tuition:* $26,973 full-time. *Room and board:* $12,570; room only: $8988 per academic year. *Required fees:* full-time $1966; part-time $289 per credit; part-time $983 per term.

Financial Aid 75% of graduate students in nursing programs received some form of financial aid in 2003–04. Fellowships, research assistantships, teaching assistantships, career-related internships or fieldwork, Federal Work-Study, and institutionally sponsored loans available. Aid available to part-time students. *Financial aid application deadline:* 12/15.

Contact Carol Ladden, Assistant Dean, Admissions and Financial Aid, School of Nursing, University of Pennsylvania, 420 Guardian Drive, Philadelphia, PA 19104-6096. *Telephone:* 215-898-4271. *Fax:* 215-573-8439. *E-mail:* ladden@nursing.upenn.edu.

MASTER'S DEGREE PROGRAM

Degrees MSN; MSN/MBA; MSN/MPH; MSN/PhD

Available Programs Accelerated AD/RN to Master's; Accelerated Master's for Non-Nursing College Graduates; Accelerated RN to Master's; Master's.

Concentrations Available Health-care administration; nurse anesthesia; nurse-midwifery; nursing administration; nursing informatics. *Clinical nurse specialist programs in:* acute care, oncology, perinatal, psychiatric/mental health, public health. *Nurse practitioner programs in:* acute care, adult health, community health, family health, gerontology, neonatal health, occupational health, oncology, pediatric, primary care, women's health.

Site Options *Distance Learning:* Memphis, TN.

Study Options Full-time and part-time.

Program Entrance Requirements Clinical experience, computer literacy, minimum overall college GPA of 3.0, transcript of college record, CPR certification, written essay, immunizations, interview, 2 letters of recommendation, physical assessment course, prerequisite course work, resume, statistics course, GMAT (MBA/MSN), GRE General Test. *Application deadline:* For fall admission, 2/15 (priority date). Applications are processed on a rolling basis. *Application fee:* $70.

Advanced Placement Credit given for nursing courses completed elsewhere dependent upon specific evaluations.

Degree Requirements 36 total credit hours.

POST-MASTER'S PROGRAM

Areas of Study Health-care administration; nurse anesthesia; nurse-midwifery; nursing administration; nursing education; nursing informatics. *Clinical nurse specialist programs in:* acute care, oncology, perinatal, psychiatric/mental health, public health. *Nurse practitioner programs in:* acute care, adult health, community health, family health, gerontology, neonatal health, occupational health, oncology, pediatric, primary care, women's health.

DOCTORAL DEGREE PROGRAM

Degree PhD

Available Programs Doctorate; Post-Baccalaureate Doctorate.

Areas of Study Addiction/substance abuse, aging, bio-behavioral research, biology of health and illness, clinical practice, community health, critical care, ethics, faculty preparation, family health, gerontology, health policy, health promotion/disease prevention, health-care systems, human health and illness, illness and transition, individualized study, information systems, maternity-newborn, neuro-behavior, nursing administration, nursing education, nursing policy, nursing research, nursing science, oncology, urban health, women's health.

Program Entrance Requirements interview by faculty committee, interview, 3 letters of recommendation, MSN or equivalent, statistics course, vita, writing sample, GMAT (MBA/PhD), GRE General Test. *Application deadline:* For fall admission, 2/15 (priority date). Applications are processed on a rolling basis. *Application fee:* $70.

Degree Requirements 39 total credit hours, dissertation, oral exam, written exam, residency.

POSTDOCTORAL PROGRAM

Areas of Study Adolescent health, aging, cancer care, chronic illness, community health, family health, gerontology, health promotion/disease prevention, individualized study, nursing informatics, nursing interventions, nursing research, nursing science, outcomes, self-care, vulnerable population, women's health.

Postdoctoral Program Contact Dr. Susan Gennaro, Director of Doctoral and Post-Doctoral Studies, School of Nursing, University of Pennsylvania, 420 Guardian Drive, Philadelphia, PA 19104-6096. *Telephone:* 215-898-1844. *Fax:* 215-573-6659. *E-mail:* gennaro@nursing.upenn.edu.

CONTINUING EDUCATION PROGRAM

Contact Dr. Kathleen G. Burke, Director, Center for Professional Development, School of Nursing, University of Pennsylvania, 420 Guardian Drive, Philadelphia, PA 19104-6096. *Telephone:* 215-898-4522. *Fax:* 215-573-9103. *E-mail:* burkekg@nursing.upenn.edu.

See full description on page 568.

University of Pittsburgh
School of Nursing
Pittsburgh, Pennsylvania

http://www.nursing.pitt.edu

Founded in 1787

DEGREES • BSN • MSN • PHD

Nursing Program Faculty 99 (21% with doctorates).

Baccalaureate Enrollment 451
Women 90% **Men** 10% **Minority** 7% **International** 1% **Part-time** 9%

Graduate Enrollment 325
Women 81% **Men** 19% **Minority** 6% **International** 2% **Part-time** 57%

Nursing Student Activities Sigma Theta Tau, Student Nurses' Association.

Nursing Student Resources Academic advising; academic or career counseling; assistance for students with disabilities; bookstore; campus computer network; career placement assistance; computer lab; computer-assisted instruction; daycare for children of students; e-mail services; employment services for current students; externships; housing assistance; interactive nursing skills videos; Internet; learning resource lab; library services; nursing audiovisuals; paid internships; placement services for program completers; remedial services; resume preparation assistance; skills, simulation, or other laboratory; tutoring.

Library Facilities 4.6 million volumes (429,581 in health); 3,767 periodical subscriptions (3,800 health-care related).

BACCALAUREATE PROGRAMS

Degree BSN

Available Programs ADN to Baccalaureate; Accelerated Baccalaureate for Second Degree; Generic Baccalaureate; RN Baccalaureate.

Site Options *Distance Learning:* Bradford, PA; Johnstown, PA.

Study Options Full-time.

Program Entrance Requirements Minimum overall college GPA of 3.3, transcript of college record, health exam, health insurance, high school chemistry, 4 years high school math, 3 years high school science, high school transcript, immunizations, 2 letters of recommendation, minimum high school GPA of 3.3. Transfer students are accepted. **Standardized tests** *Required:* SAT or ACT, TOEFL for international students. **Application** *Deadline:* rolling (freshmen), rolling (transfer). *Notification:* continuous (freshmen). *Application fee:* $35.

Advanced Placement Credit by examination available. Credit given for nursing courses completed elsewhere dependent upon specific evaluations.

Expenses (2004–05) *Tuition, state resident:* full-time $6374; part-time $455 per credit hour. *Tuition, nonresident:* full-time $12,392; part-time $885 per credit hour. *International tuition:* $12,392 full-time. *Room and board:* $3800; room only: $2300 per academic year. *Required fees:* full-time $724; part-time $241 per credit; part-time $362 per term.

Financial Aid 70% of baccalaureate students in nursing programs received some form of financial aid in 2003–04. *Gift aid (need-based):* Federal Pell, FSEOG, state, college/university gift aid from institutional funds. *Loans:* Federal Nursing Student Loans, FFEL (Subsidized and Unsubsidized Stafford PLUS), Perkins. *Work-Study:* Federal Work-Study. *Application deadline (priority):* 3/1.

Contact Ms. Rosanna Gartley, Coordinator of Recruitment, School of Nursing, University of Pittsburgh, 239 Victoria Building, 3500 Victoria Street, Pittsburgh, PA 15261. *Telephone:* 412-624-4586. *Fax:* 412-624-2409. *E-mail:* rgartley@pitt.edu.

GRADUATE PROGRAMS

Expenses (2004–05) *Tuition, state resident:* full-time $7299; part-time $599 per credit hour. *Tuition, nonresident:* full-time $10,031; part-time $823 per credit hour. *International tuition:* $10,031 full-time. *Required fees:* full-time $724; part-time $227 per credit; part-time $362 per term.

Financial Aid 70% of graduate students in nursing programs received some form of financial aid in 2003–04. 33 research assistantships with full and partial tuition reimbursements available (averaging $7,538 per year), 10 teaching assistantships with full and partial tuition reimbursements

University of Pittsburgh (continued)
available (averaging $7,474 per year) were awarded; career-related internships or fieldwork, Federal Work-Study, institutionally sponsored loans, scholarships, traineeships, tuition waivers (partial), and unspecified assistantships also available. Aid available to part-time students.

Contact Ms. Rosanna Gartley, Coordinator of Recruitment, School of Nursing, University of Pittsburgh, 239 Victoria Building, 3500 Victoria Street, Pittsburgh, PA 15261. *Telephone:* 412-624-4586. *Fax:* 412-624-2409. *E-mail:* gartley@pitt.edu.

MASTER'S DEGREE PROGRAM

Degree MSN

Available Programs Master's; Master's for Nurses with Non-Nursing Degrees; RN to Master's.

Concentrations Available Nurse anesthesia; nursing administration; nursing education; nursing informatics; nursing research. *Clinical nurse specialist programs in:* medical-surgical, psychiatric/mental health. *Nurse practitioner programs in:* acute care, adult health, family health, pediatric, psychiatric/mental health.

Site Options *Distance Learning:* Bradford, PA; Johnstown, PA.

Study Options Full-time and part-time.

Program Entrance Requirements Clinical experience, minimum overall college GPA of 3.0, transcript of college record, written essay, immunizations, interview, 3 letters of recommendation, professional liability insurance/malpractice insurance, prerequisite course work, resume, statistics course, GRE or MAT. *Application deadline:* Applications are processed on a rolling basis. *Application fee:* $40.

Advanced Placement Credit by examination available. Credit given for nursing courses completed elsewhere dependent upon specific evaluations.

Degree Requirements 52 total credit hours, comprehensive exam.

POST-MASTER'S PROGRAM

Areas of Study Health-care administration; health-care genetics; nursing education; nursing informatics. *Nurse practitioner programs in:* acute care, adult health, pediatric, psychiatric/mental health.

DOCTORAL DEGREE PROGRAM

Degree PhD

Available Programs Doctorate; Post-Baccalaureate Doctorate.

Areas of Study Aging, bio-behavioral research, critical care, human health and illness, nursing research, nursing science, women's health.

Program Entrance Requirements Minimum overall college GPA of 3.5, interview by faculty committee, 3 letters of recommendation, MSN or equivalent, statistics course, vita, writing sample, GRE. *Application deadline:* Applications are processed on a rolling basis. *Application fee:* $40.

Degree Requirements 64 total credit hours, dissertation, oral exam, written exam.

POSTDOCTORAL PROGRAM

Areas of Study Chronic illness, individualized study.

Postdoctoral Program Contact Dr. Judith A. Erlen, Doctoral Program Coordinator and Associate Director of Center for Research in Chronic Disorders, School of Nursing, University of Pittsburgh, 3500 Victoria Street, Pittsburgh, PA 15261. *Telephone:* 412-624-1905. *Fax:* 412-624-8521. *E-mail:* jae001@pitt.edu.

CONTINUING EDUCATION PROGRAM

Contact Gerri Maurer, School of Nursing, University of Pittsburgh, 225 Victoria Building, 3500 Victoria Street, Pittsburgh, PA 15261. *Telephone:* 412-624-7865. *Fax:* 412-624-2401. *E-mail:* gmm23@pitt.edu.

See full description on page 572.

University of Pittsburgh at Bradford

Department of Nursing
Bradford, Pennsylvania

Founded in 1963

DEGREE • BSN

Nursing Program Faculty 3 (66% with doctorates).

Baccalaureate Enrollment 12
Women 90% **Men** 10%

Nursing Student Activities Nursing club.

Nursing Student Resources Academic advising; academic or career counseling; assistance for students with disabilities; bookstore; campus computer network; career placement assistance; computer lab; computer-assisted instruction; e-mail services; employment services for current students; externships; housing assistance; Internet; learning resource lab; library services; nursing audiovisuals; remedial services; resume preparation assistance; skills, simulation, or other laboratory; tutoring; unpaid internships.

Library Facilities 88,969 volumes; 342 periodical subscriptions (50 health-care related).

BACCALAUREATE PROGRAMS

Degree BSN

Available Programs ADN to Baccalaureate; RN Baccalaureate.

Study Options Full-time and part-time.

Program Entrance Requirements Transcript of college record, CPR certification, health exam, health insurance, immunizations, minimum GPA in nursing prerequisites of 2.5, professional liability insurance/malpractice insurance, prerequisite course work, RN licensure. Transfer students are accepted. **Standardized tests** *Required:* SAT or ACT, TOEFL for international students. **Application** *Deadline:* rolling (freshmen), rolling (transfer). *Application fee:* $35.

Advanced Placement Credit by examination available.

Financial Aid 75% of baccalaureate students in nursing programs received some form of financial aid in 2003–04.

Contact Department of Nursing Admissions, Department of Nursing, University of Pittsburgh at Bradford, 300 Campus Drive, Bradford, PA 16701. *Telephone:* 800-872-1787.

The University of Scranton

Department of Nursing
Scranton, Pennsylvania

Founded in 1888

DEGREES • BS • MS

Nursing Program Faculty 30 (85% with doctorates).

Baccalaureate Enrollment 214
Women 93% **Men** 7% **Minority** 6% **Part-time** 7%

Graduate Enrollment 48
Women 82% **Men** 18% **Minority** 4% **Part-time** 30%

Nursing Student Activities Nursing Honor Society, Sigma Theta Tau, Student Nurses' Association, nursing club.

Nursing Student Resources Academic advising; academic or career counseling; bookstore; campus computer network; career placement assistance; computer lab; computer-assisted instruction; e-mail services; interactive nursing skills videos; Internet; learning resource lab; library services; nursing audiovisuals; placement services for program completers; remedial services; resume preparation assistance; skills, simulation, or other laboratory; tutoring.

Library Facilities 465,871 volumes (28,400 in health, 8,484 in nursing); 1,714 periodical subscriptions (106 health-care related).

BACCALAUREATE PROGRAMS

Degree BS

Available Programs ADN to Baccalaureate; Accelerated LPN to Baccalaureate; Baccalaureate for Second Degree; Generic Baccalaureate; LPN to RN Baccalaureate; RN Baccalaureate.

Study Options Full-time and part-time.

Program Entrance Requirements Minimum overall college GPA of 2.5, transcript of college record, written essay, health exam, health insurance, high school biology, high school chemistry, high school foreign language, 3 years high school math, 3 years high school science, high school transcript, immunizations, minimum high school rank 30%. Transfer students are accepted. **Standardized tests** *Required:* SAT or ACT, TOEFL for international students. **Application** *Deadline:* 3/1 (freshmen). *Early decision:* 11/15. *Notification:* continuous until 5/1 (freshmen), 12/15 (early action). *Application fee:* $40.

Advanced Placement Credit by examination available. Credit given for nursing courses completed elsewhere dependent upon specific evaluations.

Expenses (2003–04) *Tuition:* full-time $21,208; part-time $494 per credit hour. *Room and board:* $9039; room only: $5312 per academic year. *Required fees:* full-time $200.

Financial Aid 80% of baccalaureate students in nursing programs received some form of financial aid in 2002–03. *Gift aid (need-based):* Federal Pell, FSEOG, state, private, college/university gift aid from institutional funds. *Loans:* Federal Nursing Student Loans, FFEL (Subsidized and Unsubsidized Stafford PLUS), Perkins. *Work-Study:* Federal Work-Study, part-time campus jobs. *Application deadline (priority):* 2/15.

Contact Dr. Patricia Harrington, Chairperson, Department of Nursing, The University of Scranton, McGurrin Hall, Scranton, PA 18510-4595. *Telephone:* 570-941-7673. *Fax:* 570-941-7903. *E-mail:* harringtonp1@scranton.edu.

GRADUATE PROGRAMS

Expenses (2003–04) *Tuition:* full-time $11,080; part-time $590 per credit hour. *Required fees:* full-time $120.

Financial Aid 90% of graduate students in nursing programs received some form of financial aid in 2002–03. 2 teaching assistantships (averaging $4,725 per year) were awarded. *Financial aid application deadline:* 3/1.

Contact Dr. Mary Jane Hanson, Director, Graduate Nursing Program, Department of Nursing, The University of Scranton, McGurrin Hall, Scranton, PA 18510. *Telephone:* 570-941-4060. *Fax:* 570-941-7093. *E-mail:* hansonm2@scranton.edu.

MASTER'S DEGREE PROGRAM

Degree MS

Available Programs Accelerated AD/RN to Master's; Accelerated Master's; Accelerated RN to Master's; Master's; RN to Master's.

Concentrations Available Nurse anesthesia. *Clinical nurse specialist programs in:* adult health. *Nurse practitioner programs in:* family health.

Study Options Full-time and part-time.

Program Entrance Requirements Clinical experience, minimum overall college GPA of 3.0, transcript of college record, CPR certification, written essay, immunizations, interview, 3 letters of recommendation, nursing research course, physical assessment course, professional liability insurance/malpractice insurance, prerequisite course work, statistics course. *Application deadline:* Applications are processed on a rolling basis. *Application fee:* $50.

Advanced Placement Credit given for nursing courses completed elsewhere dependent upon specific evaluations.

Degree Requirements 46 total credit hours, comprehensive exam.

POST-MASTER'S PROGRAM

Areas of Study Nurse anesthesia. *Clinical nurse specialist programs in:* adult health. *Nurse practitioner programs in:* family health.

Villanova University

College of Nursing
Villanova, Pennsylvania

http://www.nursing.villanova.edu/

Founded in 1842

DEGREES • BSN • MSN • PHD

Nursing Program Faculty 56 (76% with doctorates).

Baccalaureate Enrollment 513
Women 94% **Men** 6% **Minority** 11% **International** 5% **Part-time** 1%

Graduate Enrollment 167
Women 87% **Men** 13% **Minority** 11% **International** 18% **Part-time** 78%

Nursing Student Activities Nursing Honor Society, Sigma Theta Tau, Student Nurses' Association, nursing club.

Nursing Student Resources Academic advising; academic or career counseling; assistance for students with disabilities; bookstore; campus computer network; career placement assistance; computer lab; computer-assisted instruction; e-mail services; employment services for current students; externships; housing assistance; interactive nursing skills videos; Internet; learning resource lab; library services; nursing audiovisuals; resume preparation assistance; skills, simulation, or other laboratory; tutoring.

Library Facilities 900,248 volumes; 10,800 periodical subscriptions (334 health-care related).

BACCALAUREATE PROGRAMS

Degree BSN

Available Programs ADN to Baccalaureate; Accelerated Baccalaureate for Second Degree; Baccalaureate for Second Degree; Generic Baccalaureate; International Nurse to Baccalaureate; RN Baccalaureate.

Study Options Full-time and part-time.

Program Entrance Requirements Transcript of college record, written essay, health exam, health insurance, high school biology, high school chemistry, high school foreign language, 3 years high school math, 3 years high school science, high school transcript, immunizations, minimum high school GPA of 3.0. Transfer students are accepted. **Standardized tests** *Required:* SAT or ACT, TOEFL for international students. **Application** *Deadline:* 1/7 (freshmen), 7/15 (transfer). *Early decision:* 11/1. *Notification:* 4/1 (freshmen), 12/20 (early action). *Application fee:* $70.

Advanced Placement Credit by examination available. Credit given for nursing courses completed elsewhere dependent upon specific evaluations.

Expenses (2004–05) *Tuition:* full-time $27,350; part-time $1140 per credit hour. *International tuition:* $27,350 full-time. *Room and board:* $8610; room only: $4470 per academic year. *Required fees:* full-time $550; part-time $300 per term.

Financial Aid 70% of baccalaureate students in nursing programs received some form of financial aid in 2003–04.

Contact Dr. M. Frances Keen, Assistant Dean and Director, Undergraduate Program, College of Nursing, Villanova University, 800 Lancaster Avenue, Villanova, PA 19085-1690. *Telephone:* 610-519-4926. *Fax:* 610-519-7650. *E-mail:* frances.keen@villanova.edu.

GRADUATE PROGRAMS

Expenses (2004–05) *Tuition:* full-time $5040; part-time $580 per credit hour. *International tuition:* $5040 full-time.

Financial Aid 37% of graduate students in nursing programs received some form of financial aid in 2003–04. Teaching assistantships with full tuition reimbursements available (averaging $10,265 per year); institutionally sponsored loans, scholarships, traineeships, and tuition waivers (full) also available. *Financial aid application deadline:* 3/1.

Contact Dr. Marguerite K. Schlag, Assistant Dean and Director, Graduate Program, College of Nursing, Villanova University, 800 Lancaster Avenue, Villanova, PA 19085-1690. *Telephone:* 610-519-4934. *Fax:* 610-519-7997. *E-mail:* marguerite.schlag@villanova.edu.

MASTER'S DEGREE PROGRAM

Degree MSN

Available Programs Master's.

Concentrations Available Health-care administration; nurse anesthesia; nurse case management; nursing education. *Nurse practitioner programs in:* adult health, gerontology, pediatric.

Study Options Full-time and part-time.

Program Entrance Requirements Clinical experience, minimum overall college GPA of 3.0, transcript of college record, written essay, 3 letters of recommendation, physical assessment course, resume, statistics course, GRE or MAT. *Application deadline:* For fall admission, 7/1 (priority date); for spring admission, 12/1 (priority date). Applications are processed on a rolling basis. *Application fee:* $25.

Degree Requirements 45 total credit hours, thesis or project.

POST-MASTER'S PROGRAM

Areas of Study Nurse anesthesia; nurse case management; nursing education. *Nurse practitioner programs in:* adult health, gerontology, pediatric.

Villanova University (continued)

DOCTORAL DEGREE PROGRAM

Degree PhD

Available Programs Doctorate.

Areas of Study Faculty preparation, nursing education, nursing research.

Program Entrance Requirements Clinical experience, minimum overall college GPA of 3.5, interview, 3 letters of recommendation, MSN or equivalent, scholarly papers, vita, writing sample, GRE. *Application deadline:* For fall admission, 7/1 (priority date); for spring admission, 12/1 (priority date). Applications are processed on a rolling basis. *Application fee:* $25.

Degree Requirements 51 total credit hours, dissertation, oral exam, written exam.

CONTINUING EDUCATION PROGRAM

Contact Dr. Lynore DeSilets, Assistant Dean and Director, Continuing Education, College of Nursing, Villanova University, 800 Lancaster Avenue, Villanova, PA 19085-1690. *Telephone:* 610-519-4931. *Fax:* 610-519-6780. *E-mail:* lyn.desilets@villanova.edu.

See full description on page 590.

Waynesburg College
Department of Nursing
Waynesburg, Pennsylvania

http://www.waynesburg.edu

Founded in 1849

DEGREES • BSN • MSN • MSN/MBA

Nursing Program Faculty 47 (13% with doctorates).

Baccalaureate Enrollment 228
Women 85% **Men** 15% **Minority** 4%

Graduate Enrollment 120
Women 90% **Men** 10% **Minority** 5% **Part-time** 100%

Nursing Student Activities Sigma Theta Tau, Student Nurses' Association.

Nursing Student Resources Academic advising; academic or career counseling; assistance for students with disabilities; bookstore; campus computer network; career placement assistance; computer lab; computer-assisted instruction; e-mail services; employment services for current students; externships; Internet; learning resource lab; library services; nursing audiovisuals; paid internships; placement services for program completers; remedial services; resume preparation assistance; skills, simulation, or other laboratory; tutoring.

Library Facilities 100,000 volumes (4,500 in nursing); 1,189 periodical subscriptions (46 health-care related).

BACCALAUREATE PROGRAMS

Degree BSN

Available Programs Accelerated Baccalaureate for Second Degree; Accelerated RN Baccalaureate; Generic Baccalaureate; LPN to Baccalaureate.

Site Options Canonsburg, PA; Monroeville, PA; Wexford, PA.

Study Options Full-time.

Program Entrance Requirements Minimum overall college GPA of 3.0, transcript of college record, CPR certification, health exam, high school biology, high school chemistry, 2 years high school math, 2 years high school science, high school transcript, immunizations, minimum high school GPA of 3.0, minimum GPA in nursing prerequisites of 3.0, professional liability insurance/malpractice insurance, prerequisite course work. Transfer students are accepted. **Standardized tests** *Required:* SAT or ACT, TOEFL for international students. **Application** *Deadline:* rolling (freshmen), rolling (transfer). *Notification:* continuous (freshmen). *Application fee:* $20.

Advanced Placement Credit by examination available. Credit given for nursing courses completed elsewhere dependent upon specific evaluations.

Expenses (2004–05) *Tuition:* full-time $14,200; part-time $595 per credit hour. *International tuition:* $14,200 full-time. *Room and board:* $5800; room only: $2960 per academic year. *Required fees:* full-time $380.

Financial Aid 90% of baccalaureate students in nursing programs received some form of financial aid in 2003–04. *Gift aid (need-based):* Federal Pell, FSEOG, state, private, college/university gift aid from institutional funds. *Loans:* Federal Nursing Student Loans, FFEL (Subsidized and Unsubsidized Stafford PLUS), Perkins, college/university, alternative loans. *Work-Study:* Federal Work-Study, part-time campus jobs. *Application deadline (priority):* 3/15.

Contact Dr. Nancy Mosser, Director and Chair, Department of Nursing, Waynesburg College, 203 Stewart Science Hall, Waynesburg, PA 15370-1222. *Telephone:* 724-852-3356. *Fax:* 724-852-3220. *E-mail:* nmosser@waynesburg.edu.

GRADUATE PROGRAMS

Expenses (2004–05) *Tuition:* part-time $420 per credit hour.

Financial Aid 40% of graduate students in nursing programs received some form of financial aid in 2003–04.

Contact Dr. Lynette Jack, Director of Accelerated Health Programs, Department of Nursing, Waynesburg College, 1001 Corporate Drive, Canonsburg, PA 15317. *Telephone:* 724-743-2256. *Fax:* 724-743-4425. *E-mail:* ljack@waynesburg.edu.

MASTER'S DEGREE PROGRAM

Degrees MSN; MSN/MBA

Available Programs Accelerated Master's; Accelerated Master's for Nurses with Non-Nursing Degrees; Accelerated RN to Master's.

Concentrations Available Nursing administration; nursing education.

Site Options Canonsburg, PA; Monroeville, PA; Wexford, PA.

Study Options Part-time.

Program Entrance Requirements Clinical experience, computer literacy, minimum overall college GPA of 3.0, transcript of college record, 2 letters of recommendation, resume.

Degree Requirements 36 total credit hours, thesis or project.

West Chester University of Pennsylvania
Department of Nursing
West Chester, Pennsylvania

http://health-sciences.wcupa.edu/nursing

Founded in 1871

DEGREES • BSN • MSN

Nursing Program Faculty 20 (30% with doctorates).

Baccalaureate Enrollment 332
Women 91.9% **Men** 8.1% **Minority** 12% **International** .3% **Part-time** 20.1%

Graduate Enrollment 39
Women 91.3% **Men** 8.7% **Part-time** 84.6%

Nursing Student Activities Nursing Honor Society, Sigma Theta Tau, Student Nurses' Association.

Nursing Student Resources Academic advising; academic or career counseling; assistance for students with disabilities; bookstore; campus computer network; career placement assistance; computer lab; computer-assisted instruction; daycare for children of students; e-mail services; employment services for current students; externships; housing assistance; interactive nursing skills videos; Internet; learning resource lab; library services; nursing audiovisuals; remedial services; resume preparation assistance; skills, simulation, or other laboratory; tutoring.

Library Facilities 744,976 volumes (88 in nursing); 4,593 periodical subscriptions (173 health-care related).

BACCALAUREATE PROGRAMS

Degree BSN

Available Programs Accelerated RN Baccalaureate; Generic Baccalaureate.

Study Options Full-time and part-time.

Program Entrance Requirements Minimum overall college GPA, transcript of college record, written essay, health exam, health insurance, high school biology, high school chemistry, 2 years high school math, 2 years high school science, high school transcript, immunizations, minimum high school GPA, minimum high school rank, minimum GPA in nursing prerequisites. Transfer students are accepted. **Standardized tests** *Required:* SAT or ACT, TOEFL for international students. **Application** *Deadline:* rolling (freshmen), rolling (transfer). *Notification:* continuous (freshmen). *Application fee:* $35.

Advanced Placement Credit given for nursing courses completed elsewhere dependent upon specific evaluations.

Expenses (2004–05) *Tuition, state resident:* full-time $5300; part-time $192 per credit hour. *Tuition, nonresident:* full-time $11,500; part-time $479 per credit hour. *Room and board:* $5932; room only: $3908 per academic year. *Required fees:* full-time $1068; part-time $44 per credit.

Financial Aid *Gift aid (need-based):* Federal Pell, FSEOG, state, college/university gift aid from institutional funds. *Loans:* Federal Nursing Student Loans, FFEL (Subsidized and Unsubsidized Stafford PLUS), Perkins. *Work-Study:* Federal Work-Study, part-time campus jobs. *Application deadline (priority):* 3/1.

Contact Ann C. Stowe, Chairperson, Department of Nursing, West Chester University of Pennsylvania, 100 South Church Street, West Chester, PA 19383. *Telephone:* 610-436-2219. *Fax:* 610-436-3083. *E-mail:* astowe@wcupa.edu.

GRADUATE PROGRAMS

Expenses (2004–05) *Tuition, state resident:* full-time $5254; part-time $292 per credit hour. *Tuition, nonresident:* full-time $8408; part-time $467 per credit hour. *Required fees:* full-time $866; part-time $48 per credit.

Financial Aid 1 research assistantship (averaging $5,000 per year) was awarded; unspecified assistantships also available.

Contact Dr. Janet S. Hickman, Graduate Program Coordinator, Department of Nursing, West Chester University of Pennsylvania, South New Street, Sturzebecker Health Sciences Center, West Chester, PA 19383. *Telephone:* 610-436-2258. *Fax:* 610-436-3083. *E-mail:* jhickman@wcupa.edu.

MASTER'S DEGREE PROGRAM

Degree MSN

Available Programs Master's.

Concentrations Available *Clinical nurse specialist programs in:* community health.

Study Options Full-time and part-time.

Program Entrance Requirements Clinical experience, minimum overall college GPA of 2.5, transcript of college record, interview, 3 letters of recommendation, physical assessment course, professional liability insurance/malpractice insurance, resume, statistics course, GRE General Test or MAT. *Application deadline:* For fall admission, 4/15 (priority date); for spring admission, 10/15. Applications are processed on a rolling basis. *Application fee:* $35.

Advanced Placement Credit given for nursing courses completed elsewhere dependent upon specific evaluations.

Degree Requirements 39 total credit hours, thesis or project.

Widener University

School of Nursing
Chester, Pennsylvania

http://www.widener.edu

Founded in 1821

DEGREES • BSN • DN SC • MSN

Nursing Program Faculty 45 (48% with doctorates).

Baccalaureate Enrollment 419
Women 91% **Men** 9% **Minority** 28% **Part-time** 22%

Graduate Enrollment 129
Women 97% **Men** 3% **Minority** 19% **International** 1% **Part-time** 71%

Nursing Student Activities Sigma Theta Tau, Student Nurses' Association.

Nursing Student Resources Academic advising; academic or career counseling; assistance for students with disabilities; bookstore; campus computer network; career placement assistance; computer lab; computer-assisted instruction; e-mail services; employment services for current students; housing assistance; interactive nursing skills videos; Internet; learning resource lab; library services; nursing audiovisuals; placement services for program completers; remedial services; resume preparation assistance; skills, simulation, or other laboratory; tutoring.

Library Facilities 238,349 volumes (18,135 in health, 12,162 in nursing); 1,974 periodical subscriptions (254 health-care related).

BACCALAUREATE PROGRAMS

Degree BSN

Available Programs ADN to Baccalaureate; Baccalaureate for Second Degree; Generic Baccalaureate; RN Baccalaureate.

Study Options Full-time and part-time.

Program Entrance Requirements Minimum overall college GPA of 2.75, transcript of college record, written essay, health exam, health insurance, high school biology, high school chemistry, high school foreign language, 3 years high school math, 3 years high school science, high school transcript, immunizations, 2 letters of recommendation, minimum GPA in nursing prerequisites of 2.5. Transfer students are accepted. **Standardized tests** *Required:* SAT or ACT, TOEFL for international students. **Application** *Deadline:* rolling (freshmen), rolling (transfer). *Early decision:* 12/1. *Notification:* continuous (freshmen), 12/15 (early action). *Application fee:* $35.

Advanced Placement Credit by examination available. Credit given for nursing courses completed elsewhere dependent upon specific evaluations.

Expenses (2004–05) *Tuition:* full-time $22,800; part-time $760 per credit hour. *International tuition:* $22,800 full-time. *Room and board:* $4400 per academic year. *Required fees:* full-time $200; part-time $100 per term.

Financial Aid 90% of baccalaureate students in nursing programs received some form of financial aid in 2003–04. *Gift aid (need-based):* Federal Pell, FSEOG, state, private, college/university gift aid from institutional funds. *Loans:* FFEL (Subsidized and Unsubsidized Stafford PLUS), Perkins. *Work-Study:* Federal Work-Study. *Application deadline (priority):* 2/15.

Contact Dr. Jane Brennan, Assistant Dean, Undergraduate Program, School of Nursing, Widener University, One University Place, Chester, PA 19013-5892. *Telephone:* 610-499-4211. *Fax:* 610-499-4216. *E-mail:* jane.m.brennan@widener.edu.

GRADUATE PROGRAMS

Expenses (2004–05) *Tuition:* part-time $600 per credit hour. *Required fees:* full-time $200; part-time $100 per term.

Financial Aid 60% of graduate students in nursing programs received some form of financial aid in 2003–04. Career-related internships or fieldwork, Federal Work-Study, and traineeships available. Aid available to part-time students. *Financial aid application deadline:* 4/1.

Contact Dr. Mary Walker, Assistant Dean for Graduate Studies, School of Nursing, Widener University, One University Place, Chester, PA 19013-5892. *Telephone:* 610-499-4208. *Fax:* 610-499-4216. *E-mail:* mary.b.walker@widener.edu.

MASTER'S DEGREE PROGRAM

Degree MSN

Available Programs Accelerated Master's; Master's; RN to Master's.

Concentrations Available Nursing education. *Clinical nurse specialist programs in:* adult health, community health, critical care, psychiatric/mental health. *Nurse practitioner programs in:* family health.

Site Options Harrisburg, PA.

Study Options Full-time and part-time.

Widener University (continued)

Program Entrance Requirements Clinical experience, computer literacy, minimum overall college GPA of 3.0, transcript of college record, CPR certification, immunizations, interview, 2 letters of recommendation, nursing research course, physical assessment course, professional liability insurance/malpractice insurance, prerequisite course work, resume, statistics course, GRE General Test. *Application deadline:* For fall admission, 7/1; for winter admission, 3/1; for spring admission, 11/1. Applications are processed on a rolling basis. *Application fee:* $25 ($300 for international students).

Advanced Placement Credit given for nursing courses completed elsewhere dependent upon specific evaluations.

Degree Requirements 38 total credit hours.

POST-MASTER'S PROGRAM

Areas of Study Nursing education. *Clinical nurse specialist programs in:* adult health, community health, critical care, psychiatric/mental health. *Nurse practitioner programs in:* family health.

DOCTORAL DEGREE PROGRAM

Degree DN Sc

Available Programs Doctorate.

Areas of Study Nursing education.

Program Entrance Requirements Minimum overall college GPA of 3.5, interview, 2 letters of recommendation, MSN or equivalent, statistics course, vita, writing sample, GRE General Test. *Application deadline:* For fall admission, 7/1; for winter admission, 3/1; for spring admission, 11/1. Applications are processed on a rolling basis. *Application fee:* $25 ($300 for international students).

Degree Requirements 63 total credit hours, dissertation, written exam.

See full description on page 600.

Wilkes University

Department of Nursing
Wilkes-Barre, Pennsylvania

http://www.wilkes.edu

Founded in 1933

DEGREES • BS • MS

Nursing Program Faculty 17 (40% with doctorates).

Baccalaureate Enrollment 140
Women 85% **Men** 15% **Minority** 5% **Part-time** 39%

Graduate Enrollment 35
Women 84% **Men** 16%

Nursing Student Activities Sigma Theta Tau, Student Nurses' Association, nursing club.

Nursing Student Resources Academic advising; academic or career counseling; assistance for students with disabilities; bookstore; campus computer network; career placement assistance; computer lab; computer-assisted instruction; daycare for children of students; e-mail services; employment services for current students; externships; housing assistance; interactive nursing skills videos; Internet; learning resource lab; library services; nursing audiovisuals; paid internships; placement services for program completers; remedial services; resume preparation assistance; skills, simulation, or other laboratory; tutoring; unpaid internships.

Library Facilities 236,942 volumes (13,450 in health, 13,000 in nursing); 848 periodical subscriptions (70 health-care related).

BACCALAUREATE PROGRAMS

Degree BS

Available Programs ADN to Baccalaureate; Accelerated Baccalaureate for Second Degree; Accelerated LPN to Baccalaureate; Accelerated RN Baccalaureate; Generic Baccalaureate; LPN to RN Baccalaureate; RN Baccalaureate.

Site Options Scranton, PA; Hazleton, PA.

Study Options Full-time and part-time.

Program Entrance Requirements Minimum overall college GPA of 2.0, transcript of college record, CPR certification, health exam, health insurance, high school biology, high school chemistry, high school foreign language, high school math, high school science, high school transcript, immunizations, minimum high school GPA, professional liability insurance/malpractice insurance, prerequisite course work. Transfer students are accepted. **Standardized tests** *Required:* SAT or ACT, TOEFL for international students. **Application** *Deadline:* rolling (freshmen), rolling (transfer). *Notification:* continuous until 8/30 (freshmen). *Application fee:* $35.

Advanced Placement Credit by examination available. Credit given for nursing courses completed elsewhere dependent upon specific evaluations.

Expenses (2003–04) *Tuition:* full-time $18,660; part-time $515 per credit hour. *Room and board:* room only: $5620 per academic year. *Required fees:* full-time $1250; part-time $20 per credit.

Financial Aid 80% of baccalaureate students in nursing programs received some form of financial aid in 2002–03. *Gift aid (need-based):* Federal Pell, FSEOG, state, private, college/university gift aid from institutional funds. *Loans:* Federal Nursing Student Loans, FFEL (Subsidized and Unsubsidized Stafford PLUS), Perkins, state, college/university, Gulf Oil Loan Fund, Rulison Evans Loan Fund. *Work-Study:* Federal Work-Study, part-time campus jobs. *Application deadline (priority):* 3/1.

Contact Dr. Mary Ann Tamone Merrigan, RN, Chairperson, Department of Nursing, Wilkes University, 109 South Franklin Street, Wilkes-Barre, PA 18766. *Telephone:* 570-408-4074. *Fax:* 570-408-7807. *E-mail:* merrigan@wilkes.edu.

GRADUATE PROGRAMS

Expenses (2003–04) *Tuition:* part-time $650 per credit hour. *Required fees:* part-time $100 per credit.

Financial Aid 50% of graduate students in nursing programs received some form of financial aid in 2002–03.

Contact Dr. Sharon Telban, Director of Gerontology, Department of Nursing, Wilkes University, 109 South Franklin Street, Wilkes-Barre, PA 18766. *Telephone:* 570-408-4076. *Fax:* 570-408-7807. *E-mail:* telban@wilkes.edu.

MASTER'S DEGREE PROGRAM

Degree MS

Available Programs Accelerated AD/RN to Master's; Accelerated RN to Master's; Master's; Master's for Non-Nursing College Graduates; RN to Master's.

Concentrations Available Nursing administration. *Clinical nurse specialist programs in:* gerontology, psychiatric/mental health.

Site Options Scranton, PA.

Study Options Full-time and part-time.

Program Entrance Requirements Clinical experience, minimum overall college GPA of 3.0, transcript of college record, CPR certification, immunizations, interview, 3 letters of recommendation, nursing research course, physical assessment course, professional liability insurance/malpractice insurance, statistics course.

Advanced Placement Credit given for nursing courses completed elsewhere dependent upon specific evaluations.

Degree Requirements 36 total credit hours, thesis or project.

POST-MASTER'S PROGRAM

Areas of Study Nursing administration. *Clinical nurse specialist programs in:* gerontology, psychiatric/mental health.

CONTINUING EDUCATION PROGRAM

Contact Margaret Steele, Chairperson, Center for Continued Learning, Department of Nursing, Wilkes University, Max Roth Center, 2nd Floor, Wilkes University, Wilkes-Barre, PA 18766. *Telephone:* 570-408-4763. *E-mail:* steele@wilkes.edu.

York College of Pennsylvania

Department of Nursing
York, Pennsylvania

http://www.ycp.edu/nursing/index.html

Founded in 1787

DEGREES • BS • MS

Nursing Program Faculty 34 (41% with doctorates).
Baccalaureate Enrollment 576
Women 94% **Men** 6% **Minority** 4% **Part-time** 36%
Graduate Enrollment 58
Women 98% **Men** 2% **Minority** 1% **International** 1% **Part-time** 100%

Nursing Student Activities Sigma Theta Tau, Student Nurses' Association.

Nursing Student Resources Academic advising; academic or career counseling; assistance for students with disabilities; bookstore; campus computer network; career placement assistance; computer lab; computer-assisted instruction; e-mail services; employment services for current students; externships; housing assistance; interactive nursing skills videos; Internet; learning resource lab; library services; nursing audiovisuals; paid internships; placement services for program completers; remedial services; resume preparation assistance; skills, simulation, or other laboratory; tutoring.

Library Facilities 300,000 volumes (6,681 in health, 1,226 in nursing); 1,400 periodical subscriptions (80 health-care related).

BACCALAUREATE PROGRAMS

Degree BS

Available Programs Generic Baccalaureate; LPN to RN Baccalaureate; RN Baccalaureate.

Site Options *Distance Learning:* Harrisburg, PA; Hanover, PA; Chambersburg, PA.

Study Options Full-time and part-time.

Program Entrance Requirements Minimum overall college GPA of 2.8, transcript of college record, CPR certification, written essay, health exam, health insurance, high school biology, high school chemistry, 1 year of high school math, high school science, high school transcript, immunizations, 2 letters of recommendation, minimum high school rank 40%, minimum GPA in nursing prerequisites of 2.8, professional liability insurance/malpractice insurance, prerequisite course work. Transfer students are accepted. **Standardized tests** *Required:* SAT or ACT, TOEFL for international students. **Application** *Deadline:* 8/1 (freshmen), rolling (transfer). *Notification:* continuous (freshmen). *Application fee:* $30.

Advanced Placement Credit by examination available. Credit given for nursing courses completed elsewhere dependent upon specific evaluations.

Expenses (2004–05) *Tuition:* full-time $8600; part-time $260 per credit hour. *Room and board:* $6250; room only: $3475 per academic year. *Required fees:* full-time $584; part-time $325 per term.

Financial Aid 76% of baccalaureate students in nursing programs received some form of financial aid in 2003–04. *Gift aid (need-based):* Federal Pell, FSEOG, state, private, college/university gift aid from institutional funds. *Loans:* Federal Nursing Student Loans, Federal Direct (Subsidized and Unsubsidized Stafford PLUS), FFEL (Subsidized and Unsubsidized Stafford PLUS), Perkins, college/university. *Work-Study:* Federal Work-Study, part-time campus jobs. *Application deadline (priority):* 3/1.

Contact Dr. Jacquelin H. Harrington, RN, Chairperson, Department of Nursing, York College of Pennsylvania, York, PA 17405-7199. *Telephone:* 717-815-1420. *Fax:* 717-849-1651. *E-mail:* jharring@ycp.edu.

GRADUATE PROGRAMS

Expenses (2004–05) *Tuition:* part-time $390 per credit hour. *Required fees:* part-time $220 per term.

Contact Dr. Lynn Warner, RN, Coordinator, Department of Nursing, York College of Pennsylvania, York, PA 17405-7199. *Telephone:* 717-815-1212. *Fax:* 717-849-1651.

MASTER'S DEGREE PROGRAM

Degree MS

Available Programs Master's; RN to Master's.

Concentrations Available Nurse anesthesia; nurse case management; nurse-midwifery; nursing administration; nursing education. *Clinical nurse specialist programs in:* adult health.

Site Options *Distance Learning:* Harrisburg, PA; Hanover, PA; Chambersburg, PA.

Study Options Part-time.

Program Entrance Requirements Clinical experience, computer literacy, minimum overall college GPA of 3.0, transcript of college record, CPR certification, written essay, immunizations, 2 letters of recommendation, nursing research course, physical assessment course, professional liability insurance/malpractice insurance, resume, statistics course.

Advanced Placement Credit given for nursing courses completed elsewhere dependent upon specific evaluations.

Degree Requirements 41 total credit hours, thesis or project.

PUERTO RICO

Inter American University of Puerto Rico, Metropolitan Campus

Carmen Torres de Tiburcio School of Nursing
San Juan, Puerto Rico

http://www.metro.inter.edu/progacad/enfe/nursing/index.html
Founded in 1960

DEGREE • BSN

Nursing Program Faculty 26 (27% with doctorates).
Baccalaureate Enrollment 312
Women 57% **Men** 43%

Nursing Student Activities Student Nurses' Association.

Nursing Student Resources Academic advising; academic or career counseling; assistance for students with disabilities; bookstore; campus computer network; career placement assistance; computer lab; computer-assisted instruction; daycare for children of students; e-mail services; employment services for current students; externships; interactive nursing skills videos; Internet; learning resource lab; library services; nursing audiovisuals; paid internships; placement services for program completers; remedial services; skills, simulation, or other laboratory; tutoring.

Library Facilities 113,200 volumes (36,000 in health, 21,759 in nursing); 2,771 periodical subscriptions (2,090 health-care related).

BACCALAUREATE PROGRAMS

Degree BSN

Available Programs ADN to Baccalaureate; Accelerated Baccalaureate; Generic Baccalaureate.

Study Options Full-time and part-time.

Program Entrance Requirements Minimum overall college GPA of 2.0, transcript of college record, CPR certification, health exam, health insurance, high school transcript, immunizations, 2 letters of recommendation, minimum high school rank 4%, minimum GPA in nursing prerequisites of 2. Transfer students are accepted. **Standardized tests** *Required for some:* SAT. ***Placement:*** *Required for some:* SAT. **Application** *Deadline:* 5/15 (freshmen), 5/15 (transfer).

Advanced Placement Credit by examination available. Credit given for nursing courses completed elsewhere dependent upon specific evaluations.

Expenses (2003–04) *Tuition:* full-time $4290; part-time $1170 per credit hour. *Required fees:* full-time $416; part-time $127 per credit; part-time $208 per term.

Contact Dra. Aurea E. Ayala, DNS, Director, Carmen Torres de Tiburcio School of Nursing, Inter American University of Puerto Rico, Metropolitan Campus, PO Box 191293, San Juan, PR 00919-1293. *Telephone:* 787-763-3066. *Fax:* 787-250-1242 Ext. 2159. *E-mail:* angtorr@inter.edu.

Pontifical Catholic University of Puerto Rico

Department of Nursing
Ponce, Puerto Rico

http://www.pucpr.edu/catalogo/espanol/ciencias/dep_enf.htm

Founded in 1948

DEGREE • BSN

Library Facilities 1,499 volumes in nursing; 58,185 periodical subscriptions.

BACCALAUREATE PROGRAMS

Degree BSN

Available Programs Generic Baccalaureate.

Program Entrance Requirements Minimum overall college GPA of 2.0, CPR certification, health exam, health insurance, immunizations, interview, letters of recommendation, minimum high school GPA of 2.5, prerequisite course work. **Standardized tests** *Required:* SAT. **Application** *Deadline:* 3/15 (freshmen), 3/15 (transfer). *Notification:* continuous (freshmen). *Application fee:* $15.

Contact Prof. Alma Albizu, Coordinator, Department of Nursing, Pontifical Catholic University of Puerto Rico, Avenue Las Americas, Station 6, Ponce, PR 00732. *Telephone:* 787-841-2000 Ext. 1604.

Universidad Adventista de las Antillas

Department of Nursing
Mayagüez, Puerto Rico

Founded in 1957

DEGREE • BSN

Nursing Program Faculty 9 (22% with doctorates).

Baccalaureate Enrollment 232
Women 78% **Men** 22% **Minority** 100% **International** 4% **Part-time** 9%

Nursing Student Activities Nursing club.

Nursing Student Resources Academic advising; academic or career counseling; campus computer network; computer lab; computer-assisted instruction; e-mail services; employment services for current students; housing assistance; interactive nursing skills videos; Internet; learning resource lab; library services; nursing audiovisuals; remedial services; skills, simulation, or other laboratory; tutoring.

Library Facilities 86,465 volumes (4,360 in health, 3,827 in nursing); 452 periodical subscriptions (70 health-care related).

BACCALAUREATE PROGRAMS

Degree BSN

Available Programs Generic Baccalaureate; RN Baccalaureate.

Study Options Full-time.

Program Entrance Requirements Minimum overall college GPA of 2.3, transcript of college record, health exam, health insurance, high school transcript, immunizations, interview, 2 letters of recommendation, minimum high school GPA of 2.5. Transfer students are accepted. **Standardized tests** *Recommended:* SAT or ACT, PAA. **Application** *Application fee:* $20.

Advanced Placement Credit given for nursing courses completed elsewhere dependent upon specific evaluations.

Expenses (2004–05) *Tuition:* full-time $4760. *International tuition:* $4760 full-time. *Room and board:* $2600; room only: $800 per academic year. *Required fees:* full-time $1700.

Financial Aid 85% of baccalaureate students in nursing programs received some form of financial aid in 2003–04.

Contact Mrs. Maria L. Cruz, Director, Department of Nursing, Universidad Adventista de las Antillas, PO Box 118, Mayaguez, PR 00681-0118. *Telephone:* 787-834-9595 Ext. 2209. *Fax:* 787-834-9597. *E-mail:* ycancel@uaa.edu.

CONTINUING EDUCATION PROGRAM

Contact Dr. Lourdes Mendez, RN, Continuing Education Coordinator, Department of Nursing, Universidad Adventista de las Antillas, PO Box 118, Mayaguez, PR 00681-0118. *Telephone:* 787-834-9595 Ext. 2301. *Fax:* 787-834-9597. *E-mail:* lmendez@uaa.edu.

Universidad Metropolitana

Department of Nursing
Río Piedras, Puerto Rico

http://www.suagm.edu/umet/umet_new_web/escuelas/ciencias_tecnologia/ciencias_tecnologia.htm

Founded in 1980

DEGREE • BSN

Library Facilities 5,438 volumes in health; 110 periodical subscriptions health-care related.

BACCALAUREATE PROGRAMS

Degree BSN

Program Entrance Requirements **Standardized tests** *Required:* PAA. **Application** *Deadline:* 7/30 (freshmen), 7/30 (transfer). *Application fee:* $15.

Contact Mayra Pedroza, Associate Dean, Department of Nursing, Universidad Metropolitana, PO Box 21150, San Juan, PR 00928-1150. *Telephone:* 787-766-1717 Ext. 6422. *Fax:* 787-769-7663. *E-mail:* um_mpedroza@suagm.edu.

University of Puerto Rico at Arecibo

Department of Nursing
Arecibo, Puerto Rico

http://upra.edu/asuntosacademicos/enfermeria/menu_enfe.htm

Founded in 1967

DEGREE • BSN

Nursing Program Faculty 21.

Library Facilities 65,000 volumes; 3,660 periodical subscriptions.

BACCALAUREATE PROGRAMS

Degree BSN

Available Programs Generic Baccalaureate.

Program Entrance Requirements **Standardized tests** *Required:* SAT Subject Tests, PAA or SAT I, CEEB. ***Placement:*** *Required:* SAT Subject Tests. **Application** *Deadline:* 12/8 (freshmen), 2/18 (transfer). *Notification:* 3/18 (freshmen).

Contact Coordinator. *Telephone:* 787-878-2830. *Fax:* 787-880-4972.

University of Puerto Rico at Humacao

Department of Nursing
Humacao, Puerto Rico

http://cuhwww.upr.clu.edu/~enfe/

Founded in 1962

DEGREE • BS

Nursing Program Faculty 16 (12% with doctorates).
Nursing Student Activities Student Nurses' Association.
Nursing Student Resources Skills, simulation, or other laboratory.
Library Facilities 64,557 volumes; 2,526 periodical subscriptions.

BACCALAUREATE PROGRAMS

Degree BS
Available Programs Generic Baccalaureate.
Study Options Full-time and part-time.
Program Entrance Requirements Minimum overall college GPA, transcript of college record, health exam, health insurance, high school transcript, immunizations, minimum high school GPA of 2.0, minimum GPA in nursing prerequisites of 2.5. Transfer students are accepted. **Standardized tests** *Required:* CEEB for Puerto Rican applicants, PAA and 3 achievement tests. *Required for some:* SAT, SAT Subject Tests. **Application** *Deadline:* 11/15 (freshmen), 2/15 (transfer). *Notification:* continuous until 4/15 (freshmen). *Application fee:* $15.
Advanced Placement Credit by examination available. Credit given for nursing courses completed elsewhere dependent upon specific evaluations.
Contact Dra. Francisca Rodriguez, Director, Department of Nursing, University of Puerto Rico at Humacao, Humacao, PR 00791. *Telephone:* 787-850-9346. *Fax:* 787-850-9411. *E-mail:* f_rodriguez@webmail.uprh.edu.

University of Puerto Rico, Mayagüez Campus

Department of Nursing
Mayagüez, Puerto Rico

http://www.uprm.edu/enfe/
Founded in 1911

DEGREE • BSN

Nursing Program Faculty 21 (10% with doctorates).
Nursing Student Activities Nursing Honor Society, Sigma Theta Tau, Student Nurses' Association.
Nursing Student Resources Academic advising; academic or career counseling; assistance for students with disabilities; bookstore; campus computer network; career placement assistance; computer lab; computer-assisted instruction; e-mail services; employment services for current students; interactive nursing skills videos; Internet; learning resource lab; library services; nursing audiovisuals; paid internships; placement services for program completers; remedial services; resume preparation assistance; skills, simulation, or other laboratory; tutoring.
Library Facilities 921,392 volumes; 590,716 periodical subscriptions (68 health-care related).

BACCALAUREATE PROGRAMS

Degree BSN
Available Programs Generic Baccalaureate.
Study Options Full-time.
Program Entrance Requirements High school transcript, immunizations. Transfer students are accepted. **Standardized tests** *Required:* SAT, SAT Subject Tests, PEAU. **Application** *Deadline:* 12/15 (freshmen), 2/15 (transfer). *Early decision:* 12/15. *Notification:* 3/15 (freshmen), 12/15 (early action). *Application fee:* $15.
Advanced Placement Credit by examination available.
Contact Director, Department of Nursing, University of Puerto Rico, Mayagüez Campus, PO Box 9015, Mayaguez, PR 00681. *Telephone:* 787-263-3482. *Fax:* 787-832-3875.

CONTINUING EDUCATION PROGRAM

Contact Assistant Professor, Department of Nursing, University of Puerto Rico, Mayagüez Campus, PO Box 9015, College Station, Mayaguez, PR 00681-5000. *Telephone:* 787-265-3842. *Fax:* 787-832-3875.

University of Puerto Rico, Medical Sciences Campus

School of Nursing
San Juan, Puerto Rico

Founded in 1950

DEGREES • BSN • MSN

Nursing Program Faculty 37 (25% with doctorates).
Baccalaureate Enrollment 241
Women 85% **Men** 15% **Part-time** 12%
Graduate Enrollment 158
Women 79% **Men** 21% **Part-time** 6%
Nursing Student Activities Sigma Theta Tau, Student Nurses' Association.
Nursing Student Resources Academic advising; academic or career counseling; assistance for students with disabilities; computer lab; computer-assisted instruction; e-mail services; employment services for current students; interactive nursing skills videos; Internet; library services; nursing audiovisuals; skills, simulation, or other laboratory; tutoring.
Library Facilities 46,679 volumes (7,830 in health, 1,143 in nursing); 1,432 periodical subscriptions (1,215 health-care related).

BACCALAUREATE PROGRAMS

Degree BSN
Available Programs ADN to Baccalaureate; Generic Baccalaureate.
Study Options Full-time and part-time.
Program Entrance Requirements Minimum overall college GPA of 2.0, transcript of college record, health exam, immunizations, interview, minimum high school GPA of 2.0, prerequisite course work. Transfer students are accepted. ***Placement:*** *Required:* SAT. **Application** *Deadline:* 2/18 (transfer). *Application fee:* $15.
Expenses (2004–05) *Tuition, state resident:* full-time $1080; part-time $30 per credit hour. *Tuition, nonresident:* full-time $4630; part-time $386 per credit hour. *International tuition:* $2400 full-time.
Financial Aid 75% of baccalaureate students in nursing programs received some form of financial aid in 2003–04. *Gift aid (need-based):* Federal Pell, FSEOG, state, college/university gift aid from institutional funds, Department of Health and Human Services Scholarships. *Loans:* Perkins, alternative loans. *Work-Study:* Federal Work-Study. *Application deadline:* 5/15.
Contact Dr. Enid Meléndez, Director, BSN Department, School of Nursing, University of Puerto Rico, Medical Sciences Campus, PO Box 365067, San Juan, PR 00936-5067. *Telephone:* 787-758-2525 Ext. 1984. *Fax:* 787-281-0721.

GRADUATE PROGRAMS

Expenses (2004–05) *Tuition, state resident:* full-time $2325; part-time $75 per credit hour. *Tuition, nonresident:* full-time $2825. *International tuition:* $3500 full-time.
Financial Aid 80% of graduate students in nursing programs received some form of financial aid in 2003–04. 8 research assistantships with full tuition reimbursements available (averaging $28,000 per year), 8 teaching assistantships with full tuition reimbursements available (averaging $28,000 per year) were awarded; Federal Work-Study, scholarships, traineeships, tuition waivers (full), and unspecified assistantships also available. *Financial aid application deadline:* 6/30.
Contact Dra. María Declet, Acting Director, MSN Department, School of Nursing, University of Puerto Rico, Medical Sciences Campus, PO Box 365067, San Juan, PR 00936-5067. *Telephone:* 787-758-2525 Ext. 3105. *Fax:* 787-281-0721.

MASTER'S DEGREE PROGRAM

Degree MSN
Available Programs Master's.
Concentrations Available Nurse anesthesia; nursing administration; nursing education. *Clinical nurse specialist programs in:* adult health, community health, critical care, gerontology, maternity-newborn, pediatric, psychiatric/mental health.

University of Puerto Rico, Medical Sciences Campus (continued)

Site Options Mayaguez, PR.

Study Options Full-time and part-time.

Program Entrance Requirements Clinical experience, minimum overall college GPA of 2.5, transcript of college record, immunizations, interview, resume, statistics course, GRE or PAEG. *Application deadline:* For fall admission, 3/31 (priority date). *Application fee:* $25.

Degree Requirements 48 total credit hours, thesis or project.

CONTINUING EDUCATION PROGRAM

Contact Ms. Litza Rivera, Director, School of Nursing, University of Puerto Rico, Medical Sciences Campus, DECEP, PO Box 365067, San Juan, PR 00936-5067. *Telephone:* 787-758-2525 Ext. 2102. *Fax:* 787-281-0721. *E-mail:* lrivera@rcm.upr.edu.

University of the Sacred Heart

Program in Nursing
San Juan, Puerto Rico

Founded in 1935

DEGREES • BSN • MSN

Nursing Student Resources Skills, simulation, or other laboratory.

Library Facilities 1,525 periodical subscriptions.

BACCALAUREATE PROGRAMS

Degree BSN

Available Programs Generic Baccalaureate.

Program Entrance Requirements Standardized tests *Required:* PAA, CEEB. **Application** *Deadline:* 6/30 (freshmen), 6/30 (transfer). *Application fee:* $15.

Contact Department of Natural Science, Program in Nursing, University of the Sacred Heart, PO Box 12383, Loiza Station, Santurce, PR 00914-0383. *Telephone:* 787-728-1515. *Fax:* 787-727-1250.

GRADUATE PROGRAMS

Contact Prof. Pura Julia Cruz, Coordinator, Program in Nursing, University of the Sacred Heart, PO Box 12383, Loiza Station, Santurce, PR 00914-0383. *Telephone:* 787-728-1515 Ext. 2427. *Fax:* 787-727-1250. *E-mail:* pcruz@sagrado.edu.

MASTER'S DEGREE PROGRAM

Degree MSN

Available Programs Master's.

Concentrations Available *Nurse practitioner programs in:* occupational health.

Degree Requirements 37 total credit hours.

RHODE ISLAND

Rhode Island College

Department of Nursing
Providence, Rhode Island

http://www.ric.edu/nursing

Founded in 1854

DEGREE • BS

Nursing Program Faculty 37 (43% with doctorates).

Baccalaureate Enrollment 289
Women 91% **Men** 9% **Minority** 22% **Part-time** 28%

Nursing Student Activities Sigma Theta Tau, Student Nurses' Association, nursing club.

Nursing Student Resources Academic advising; academic or career counseling; assistance for students with disabilities; bookstore; campus computer network; career placement assistance; computer lab; computer-assisted instruction; e-mail services; employment services for current students; housing assistance; interactive nursing skills videos; Internet; learning resource lab; library services; nursing audiovisuals; paid internships; remedial services; resume preparation assistance; skills, simulation, or other laboratory; tutoring.

Library Facilities 639,489 volumes (574 in nursing); 1,192 periodical subscriptions (63 health-care related).

BACCALAUREATE PROGRAMS

Degree BS

Available Programs Baccalaureate for Second Degree; Generic Baccalaureate; RN Baccalaureate.

Site Options Providence, RI.

Study Options Full-time and part-time.

Program Entrance Requirements Minimum overall college GPA of 2.5, CPR certification, health exam, high school biology, high school chemistry, high school foreign language, 4 years high school math, 2 years high school science, high school transcript, immunizations, letters of recommendation, minimum GPA in nursing prerequisites of 2.5, prerequisite course work. Transfer students are accepted. **Standardized tests** *Required:* SAT or ACT, TOEFL for international students. **Application** *Deadline:* 5/1 (freshmen), 6/1 (transfer). *Notification:* continuous (freshmen). *Application fee:* $35.

Advanced Placement Credit given for nursing courses completed elsewhere dependent upon specific evaluations.

Expenses (2004–05) *Tuition, state resident:* full-time $3300; part-time $144 per credit hour. *Tuition, nonresident:* full-time $9500; part-time $400 per credit hour. *Room and board:* $6130; room only: $3250 per academic year. *Required fees:* full-time $785; part-time $21 per credit; part-time $50 per term.

Financial Aid 60% of baccalaureate students in nursing programs received some form of financial aid in 2003–04. *Gift aid (need-based):* Federal Pell, FSEOG, state, private, college/university gift aid from institutional funds. *Loans:* FFEL (Subsidized and Unsubsidized Stafford PLUS), Perkins, state. *Work-Study:* Federal Work-Study. *Application deadline (priority):* 3/1.

Contact Dr. Jane Williams, Chair, Department of Nursing, Rhode Island College, 600 Mount Pleasant Avenue, Providence, RI 02908-1991. *Telephone:* 401-456-8014. *Fax:* 401-456-8206. *E-mail:* jwilliams@ric.edu.

Salve Regina University

Department of Nursing
Newport, Rhode Island

http://www.salve.edu/departments/nur/index.cfm

Founded in 1934

DEGREE • BS

Nursing Program Faculty 20 (50% with doctorates).

Baccalaureate Enrollment 235
Women 97% **Men** 3% **Minority** 7% **Part-time** 23%

Nursing Student Activities Student Nurses' Association.

Nursing Student Resources Academic advising; academic or career counseling; assistance for students with disabilities; bookstore; campus computer network; career placement assistance; computer lab; computer-assisted instruction; e-mail services; housing assistance; interactive nursing skills videos; Internet; learning resource lab; library services; nursing audiovisuals; paid internships; resume preparation assistance; skills, simulation, or other laboratory; tutoring; unpaid internships.

Library Facilities 139,161 volumes (6,882 in health, 1,081 in nursing); 1,221 periodical subscriptions (76 health-care related).

BACCALAUREATE PROGRAMS

Degree BS

Available Programs Generic Baccalaureate; RN Baccalaureate.

Site Options Providence, RI; Warwick, RI. *Distance Learning:* Newport, RI.

Study Options Full-time and part-time.

Program Entrance Requirements Minimum overall college GPA of 2.7, transcript of college record, CPR certification, written essay, health exam, health insurance, high school biology, high school chemistry, high school foreign language, 4 years high school math, 4 years high school science, high school transcript, immunizations, 2 letters of recommendation, minimum GPA in nursing prerequisites of 2.0, professional liability insurance/malpractice insurance, prerequisite course work. Transfer students are accepted. **Standardized tests** *Required:* SAT or ACT, TOEFL for international students. **Application** *Deadline:* 3/1 (freshmen), rolling (transfer). *Early decision:* 11/1. *Notification:* continuous (freshmen), 12/15 (early action). *Application fee:* $40.

Advanced Placement Credit by examination available.

Expenses (2004–05) *Tuition:* full-time $21,750; part-time $725 per credit hour. *International tuition:* $21,750 full-time. *Room and board:* $9000 per academic year. *Required fees:* full-time $450; part-time $40 per term.

Financial Aid 75% of baccalaureate students in nursing programs received some form of financial aid in 2003–04. *Gift aid (need-based):* Federal Pell, FSEOG, state, private, college/university gift aid from institutional funds. *Loans:* Federal Nursing Student Loans, FFEL (Subsidized and Unsubsidized Stafford PLUS), Perkins, college/university, alternative loans. *Work-Study:* Federal Work-Study, part-time campus jobs. *Application deadline (priority):* 3/1.

Contact Mrs. Laura E. McPhie Oliveira, Vice President for Enrollment Services/Dean of Admissions, Department of Nursing, Salve Regina University, 100 Ochre Point Avenue, Newport, RI 02840-4192. *Telephone:* 888-467-2583. *Fax:* 401-848-2823. *E-mail:* sruadmis@salve.edu.

CONTINUING EDUCATION PROGRAM

Contact Mr. Charles H. Reed, Director of Continuing Education Program, Department of Nursing, Salve Regina University, Extension Study/Continuing Education Office, Newport, RI 02840-4192. *Telephone:* 800-637-0002. *Fax:* 401-341-2931. *E-mail:* sruexten@salve.edu.

University of Rhode Island
College of Nursing
Kingston, Rhode Island

http://www.uri.edu/nursing

Founded in 1892

DEGREES • BS • MS • PHD

Nursing Program Faculty 47 (32% with doctorates).

Baccalaureate Enrollment 404

Women 87% **Men** 13% **Minority** 24% **International** 1% **Part-time** 10%

Graduate Enrollment 110

Women 95% **Men** 5% **Minority** 5% **International** 6% **Part-time** 75%

Nursing Student Activities Sigma Theta Tau, Student Nurses' Association.

Nursing Student Resources Academic advising; academic or career counseling; assistance for students with disabilities; bookstore; campus computer network; career placement assistance; computer lab; computer-assisted instruction; e-mail services; externships; housing assistance; interactive nursing skills videos; Internet; learning resource lab; library services; nursing audiovisuals; remedial services; resume preparation assistance; skills, simulation, or other laboratory; tutoring.

Library Facilities 1.2 million volumes; 7,926 periodical subscriptions.

BACCALAUREATE PROGRAMS

Degree BS

Available Programs ADN to Baccalaureate; Generic Baccalaureate; RN Baccalaureate.

Site Options Providence, RI.

Study Options Full-time and part-time.

Program Entrance Requirements Minimum overall college GPA of 2.5, transcript of college record, CPR certification, written essay, health exam, health insurance, high school foreign language, 3 years high school math, 2 years high school science, high school transcript, immunizations, 2 letters of recommendation, minimum high school rank 30%, minimum GPA in nursing prerequisites of 2.2. Transfer students are accepted. **Standardized tests** *Required:* SAT or ACT, TOEFL for international students. **Application** *Deadline:* 2/1 (freshmen), 5/1 (transfer). *Early decision:* 12/15. *Notification:* continuous (freshmen), 1/15 (early action). *Application fee:* $50.

Advanced Placement Credit given for nursing courses completed elsewhere dependent upon specific evaluations.

Expenses (2004–05) *Tuition, state resident:* full-time $4680; part-time $195 per credit hour. *Tuition, nonresident:* full-time $16,266; part-time $678 per credit hour. *International tuition:* $16,266 full-time. *Room and board:* $7500 per academic year. *Required fees:* full-time $3206; part-time $62 per credit.

Financial Aid 70% of baccalaureate students in nursing programs received some form of financial aid in 2003–04. *Gift aid (need-based):* Federal Pell, FSEOG, state, private, college/university gift aid from institutional funds. *Loans:* Federal Nursing Student Loans, Federal Direct (Subsidized and Unsubsidized Stafford PLUS), Perkins, state, college/university. *Work-Study:* Federal Work-Study, part-time campus jobs. *Application deadline (priority):* 3/1.

Contact Undergraduate Admissions Office, College of Nursing, University of Rhode Island, Newman Hall, 14 Upper College Road, Kingston, RI 02881. *Telephone:* 401-874-7100.

GRADUATE PROGRAMS

Expenses (2004–05) *Tuition, state resident:* full-time $4894; part-time $272 per credit hour. *Tuition, nonresident:* full-time $14,180; part-time $788 per credit hour. *International tuition:* $14,180 full-time. *Required fees:* full-time $2978; part-time $62 per credit.

Financial Aid 50% of graduate students in nursing programs received some form of financial aid in 2003–04.

Contact Dr. Donna Schwartz-Barcott, Director of Graduate Programs, College of Nursing, University of Rhode Island, White Hall, Kingston, RI 02881. *Telephone:* 401-874-2766. *Fax:* 401-874-2061. *E-mail:* dsb@uri.edu.

MASTER'S DEGREE PROGRAM

Degree MS

Available Programs Master's; RN to Master's.

Concentrations Available Nurse-midwifery; nursing administration; nursing education. *Clinical nurse specialist programs in:* gerontology, psychiatric/mental health. *Nurse practitioner programs in:* family health.

Site Options Providence, RI.

Study Options Full-time and part-time.

Program Entrance Requirements Clinical experience, minimum overall college GPA of 3.0, transcript of college record, written essay, immunizations, 3 letters of recommendation, nursing research course, professional liability insurance/malpractice insurance, resume, statistics course. *Application deadline:* For fall admission, 4/15. *Application fee:* $35.

Degree Requirements 41 total credit hours, thesis or project, comprehensive exam.

POST-MASTER'S PROGRAM

Areas of Study Nurse-midwifery; nursing administration; nursing education. *Clinical nurse specialist programs in:* gerontology, psychiatric/mental health. *Nurse practitioner programs in:* family health.

DOCTORAL DEGREE PROGRAM

Degree PhD

Available Programs Doctorate.

Areas of Study Nursing research, nursing science.

Program Entrance Requirements Clinical experience, minimum overall college GPA of 3.0, interview by faculty committee, 3 letters of recommendation, MSN or equivalent, scholarly papers, statistics course, vita, writing sample. *Application deadline:* For fall admission, 4/15. *Application fee:* $35.

Degree Requirements 61 total credit hours, dissertation, oral exam, written exam, residency.

SOUTH CAROLINA

Charleston Southern University
Wingo School of Nursing
Charleston, South Carolina

http://www.csuniv.edu
Founded in 1964
DEGREE • BSN

Nursing Program Faculty 11 (18% with doctorates).

Baccalaureate Enrollment 75
Women 90% **Men** 10% **Minority** 25%

Nursing Student Activities Sigma Theta Tau, Student Nurses' Association.

Nursing Student Resources Academic advising; academic or career counseling; assistance for students with disabilities; bookstore; campus computer network; career placement assistance; computer lab; computer-assisted instruction; e-mail services; interactive nursing skills videos; Internet; learning resource lab; library services; nursing audiovisuals; resume preparation assistance; skills, simulation, or other laboratory; tutoring.

Library Facilities 192,600 volumes (2,400 in health, 250 in nursing); 1,111 periodical subscriptions (55 health-care related).

BACCALAUREATE PROGRAMS

Degree BSN

Available Programs ADN to Baccalaureate; Generic Baccalaureate; RN Baccalaureate.

Study Options Full-time.

Program Entrance Requirements Minimum overall college GPA of 2.0, transcript of college record, CPR certification, written essay, health exam, health insurance, immunizations, minimum GPA in nursing prerequisites of 2.5, professional liability insurance/malpractice insurance, prerequisite course work. Transfer students are accepted. **Standardized tests** *Required:* SAT or ACT. **Application** *Deadline:* rolling (freshmen), rolling (transfer). *Notification:* continuous (freshmen). *Application fee:* $30.

Advanced Placement Credit given for nursing courses completed elsewhere dependent upon specific evaluations.

Expenses (2004–05) *Tuition:* full-time $15,292; part-time $247 per credit hour. *International tuition:* $15,292 full-time. *Room and board:* $5878 per academic year. *Required fees:* part-time $499 per term.

Financial Aid 90% of baccalaureate students in nursing programs received some form of financial aid in 2003–04.

Contact Dr. Marian M. Larisey, RN, Dean, Wingo School of Nursing, Charleston Southern University, PO Box 118087, 9200 University Boulevard, Charleston, SC 29423-8087. *Telephone:* 843-863-7075. *Fax:* 843-863-7540. *E-mail:* mlarisey@csuniv.edu.

Clemson University
School of Nursing
Clemson, South Carolina

http://www.hehd.clemson.edu/nursing
Founded in 1889
DEGREES • BS • MS

Nursing Program Faculty 24 (71% with doctorates).

Baccalaureate Enrollment 405

Graduate Enrollment 101

Nursing Student Activities Nursing Honor Society, Sigma Theta Tau, Student Nurses' Association, nursing club.

Nursing Student Resources Academic advising; academic or career counseling; assistance for students with disabilities; bookstore; campus computer network; career placement assistance; computer lab; computer-assisted instruction; e-mail services; employment services for current students; externships; housing assistance; interactive nursing skills videos; Internet; learning resource lab; library services; nursing audiovisuals; other; remedial services; resume preparation assistance; skills, simulation, or other laboratory; tutoring; unpaid internships.

Library Facilities 1.2 million volumes (29,800 in health, 5,548 in nursing); 5,587 periodical subscriptions (877 health-care related).

BACCALAUREATE PROGRAMS

Degree BS

Available Programs Generic Baccalaureate; RN Baccalaureate.

Site Options *Distance Learning:* Greenville, SC.

Study Options Full-time and part-time.

Program Entrance Requirements Minimum overall college GPA of 2.5, transcript of college record, CPR certification, health insurance, high school biology, high school chemistry, 3 years high school math, 3 years high school science, high school transcript, immunizations, minimum high school GPA of 2.5, professional liability insurance/malpractice insurance, prerequisite course work. Transfer students are accepted. **Standardized tests** *Required:* SAT or ACT, TOEFL for international students. **Application** *Deadline:* 5/1 (freshmen), 8/1 (transfer). *Early decision:* 12/1. *Notification:* continuous (freshmen), 2/15 (early action). *Application fee:* $50.

Advanced Placement Credit by examination available. Credit given for nursing courses completed elsewhere dependent upon specific evaluations.

Expenses (2004–05) *Tuition, state resident:* full-time $6958; part-time $288 per credit hour. *Tuition, nonresident:* full-time $14,556; part-time $600 per credit hour. *International tuition:* $14,556 full-time. *Room and board:* $1936; room only: $1035 per academic year. *Required fees:* full-time $1030.

Financial Aid 90% of baccalaureate students in nursing programs received some form of financial aid in 2003–04. *Gift aid (need-based):* Federal Pell, FSEOG, state, private, college/university gift aid from institutional funds, Federal Nursing. *Loans:* FFEL (Subsidized and Unsubsidized Stafford PLUS), Perkins, state, college/university. *Work-Study:* Federal Work-Study, part-time campus jobs. *Application deadline (priority):* 4/1.

Contact Mr. Robert S. Barkley, Director of Admissions, School of Nursing, Clemson University, 106 Sikes Hall, Clemson, SC 29634. *Telephone:* 864-656-5463. *Fax:* 864-656-2464. *E-mail:* rbrtbkl@clemson.edu.

GRADUATE PROGRAMS

Financial Aid Fellowships, research assistantships, teaching assistantships, career-related internships or fieldwork and traineeships available.

Contact Mrs. Lynne McGuirt, Student Services Coordinator, School of Nursing, Clemson University, University Center of Greenville, PO Box 5616, Greenville, SC 29606-5616. *Telephone:* 864-250-8881. *Fax:* 864-250-6711. *E-mail:* lgm@clemson.edu.

MASTER'S DEGREE PROGRAM

Degree MS

Available Programs Master's; RN to Master's.

Concentrations Available Nursing administration; nursing education. *Clinical nurse specialist programs in:* adult health, gerontology, maternity-newborn, pediatric. *Nurse practitioner programs in:* adult health, family health, gerontology.

Site Options *Distance Learning:* Greenville, SC.

Study Options Full-time and part-time.

Program Entrance Requirements Clinical experience, computer literacy, minimum overall college GPA of 3.0, transcript of college record, CPR certification, written essay, 2 letters of recommendation, nursing research course, physical assessment course, professional liability insurance/malpractice insurance, prerequisite course work, statistics course, GRE General Test. *Application deadline:* For fall admission, 6/1; for spring admission, 12/1. *Application fee:* $50.

Advanced Placement Credit by examination available. Credit given for nursing courses completed elsewhere dependent upon specific evaluations.

Degree Requirements 45 total credit hours, thesis or project, comprehensive exam.

POST-MASTER'S PROGRAM

Areas of Study Nursing administration; nursing education. *Nurse practitioner programs in:* family health, gerontology.

CONTINUING EDUCATION PROGRAM

Contact Ms. Olivia Shanahan, Director of Continuing Education, School of Nursing, Clemson University, Edwards Hall, Clemson, SC 29634-0748. *Telephone:* 864-656-3078. *Fax:* 864-656-1877. *E-mail:* olivia@clemson.edu.

Lander University

School of Nursing
Greenwood, South Carolina

http://www.lander.edu/nursing/

Founded in 1872

DEGREE • BSN

Nursing Program Faculty 15 (13% with doctorates).

Baccalaureate Enrollment 251

Women 95% **Men** 5% **Minority** 17% **Part-time** 18%

Nursing Student Activities Sigma Theta Tau, Student Nurses' Association.

Nursing Student Resources Academic advising; academic or career counseling; assistance for students with disabilities; bookstore; campus computer network; career placement assistance; computer lab; computer-assisted instruction; e-mail services; externships; housing assistance; interactive nursing skills videos; Internet; learning resource lab; library services; nursing audiovisuals; resume preparation assistance; skills, simulation, or other laboratory.

Library Facilities 175,366 volumes (5,743 in health, 5,447 in nursing); 763 periodical subscriptions (53 health-care related).

BACCALAUREATE PROGRAMS

Degree BSN

Available Programs Accelerated Baccalaureate; Accelerated Baccalaureate for Second Degree; Accelerated RN Baccalaureate; Baccalaureate for Second Degree; Generic Baccalaureate; RN Baccalaureate.

Study Options Full-time and part-time.

Program Entrance Requirements Minimum overall college GPA of 2.6, transcript of college record, CPR certification, health exam, health insurance, immunizations, professional liability insurance/malpractice insurance, prerequisite course work. Transfer students are accepted. **Standardized tests** *Required:* SAT or ACT, TOEFL for international students. **Application** *Deadline:* 8/1 (freshmen), rolling (transfer). *Notification:* continuous (freshmen). *Application fee:* $35.

Advanced Placement Credit given for nursing courses completed elsewhere dependent upon specific evaluations.

Expenses (2004–05) *Tuition, state resident:* full-time $5856; part-time $244 per credit hour. *Tuition, nonresident:* full-time $12,024; part-time $501 per credit hour. *International tuition:* $12,024 full-time. *Room and board:* $5176; room only: $3172 per academic year. *Required fees:* full-time $160.

Financial Aid 60% of baccalaureate students in nursing programs received some form of financial aid in 2003–04.

Contact Mr. Jonathan T. Reece, Director of Admissions, School of Nursing, Lander University, 320 Stanley Avenue, Greenwood, SC 29649-2099. *Telephone:* 864-388-8307. *Fax:* 864-388-8125. *E-mail:* jreece@lander.edu.

Medical University of South Carolina

College of Nursing
Charleston, South Carolina

http://www.musc.edu/Nursing

Founded in 1824

DEGREES • BSN • MSN • PHD

Nursing Program Faculty 67 (40% with doctorates).

Baccalaureate Enrollment 192

Women 85% **Men** 15% **Minority** 9% **International** 1% **Part-time** 17%

Graduate Enrollment 152

Women 90% **Men** 10% **Minority** 8% **Part-time** 45%

Nursing Student Activities Sigma Theta Tau, Student Nurses' Association.

Nursing Student Resources Academic advising; academic or career counseling; bookstore; campus computer network; career placement assistance; computer lab; computer-assisted instruction; e-mail services; interactive nursing skills videos; Internet; learning resource lab; library services; nursing audiovisuals; remedial services; resume preparation assistance; skills, simulation, or other laboratory; tutoring.

Library Facilities 225,061 volumes; 3,746 periodical subscriptions.

BACCALAUREATE PROGRAMS

Degree BSN

Available Programs ADN to Baccalaureate; Accelerated Baccalaureate; RN Baccalaureate.

Study Options Full-time.

Program Entrance Requirements Transcript of college record, written essay, 3 letters of recommendation, prerequisite course work. Transfer students are accepted. **Standardized tests** *Required:* TOEFL for international students. **Application** *Deadline:* 2/1 (freshmen), 8/25 (transfer). *Application fee:* $75.

Advanced Placement Credit by examination available.

Financial Aid 66% of baccalaureate students in nursing programs received some form of financial aid in 2003–04.

Contact Ms. Carolyn Page, Director of Student Services, College of Nursing, Medical University of South Carolina, 99 Jonathan Lucas Street, PO Box 250160, Charleston, SC 29425. *Telephone:* 843-792-8515. *Fax:* 843-792-9258. *E-mail:* pagecf@musc.edu.

GRADUATE PROGRAMS

Financial Aid 51% of graduate students in nursing programs received some form of financial aid in 2003–04. Federal Work-Study and scholarships available. Aid available to part-time students. *Financial aid application deadline:* 3/15.

Contact Office of Student Services, College of Nursing, Medical University of South Carolina, 99 Jonathan Lucas Street, PO Box 250160, Charleston, SC 29425. *Telephone:* 843-792-8515. *Fax:* 843-792-8515.

MASTER'S DEGREE PROGRAM

Degree MSN

Available Programs Accelerated Master's; Accelerated Master's for Nurses with Non-Nursing Degrees; Accelerated RN to Master's; Master's; RN to Master's.

Concentrations Available Nurse-midwifery; nursing administration; nursing education. *Clinical nurse specialist programs in:* adult health, gerontology, parent-child, psychiatric/mental health. *Nurse practitioner programs in:* adult health, family health, gerontology, neonatal health, pediatric, psychiatric/mental health.

Study Options Full-time and part-time.

Program Entrance Requirements Minimum overall college GPA of 3.0, transcript of college record, written essay, interview, 3 letters of recommendation, physical assessment course, prerequisite course work, resume, statistics course, GRE General Test. *Application deadline:* For fall admission, 8/1; for spring admission, 9/15. *Application fee:* $65.

Advanced Placement Credit given for nursing courses completed elsewhere dependent upon specific evaluations.

Degree Requirements 60 total credit hours.

POST-MASTER'S PROGRAM

Areas of Study Nurse-midwifery; nursing administration; nursing education. *Clinical nurse specialist programs in:* adult health, gerontology, parent-child, psychiatric/mental health. *Nurse practitioner programs in:* adult health, family health, gerontology, pediatric, psychiatric/mental health.

DOCTORAL DEGREE PROGRAM

Degree PhD

Available Programs Doctorate; Post-Baccalaureate Doctorate.

Medical University of South Carolina (continued)

Areas of Study Individualized study.

Program Entrance Requirements Minimum overall college GPA of 3.5, interview by faculty committee, interview, 3 letters of recommendation, MSN or equivalent, scholarly papers, statistics course, vita, writing sample. *Application deadline:* For fall admission, 8/1; for spring admission, 9/15. *Application fee:* $65.

Degree Requirements 62 total credit hours, dissertation, oral exam, written exam.

CONTINUING EDUCATION PROGRAM

Contact Carol McDougall, Continuing Education Center, College of Nursing, Medical University of South Carolina, 99 Jonathan Lucas Street, PO Box 260160, Charleston, SC 29425. *Telephone:* 843-792-3682. *E-mail:* mcdougac@musc.edu.

South Carolina State University
Department of Nursing
Orangeburg, South Carolina

Founded in 1896

DEGREE • BSN

Library Facilities 273,264 volumes; 1,346 periodical subscriptions.

BACCALAUREATE PROGRAMS

Degree BSN

Available Programs Generic Baccalaureate; RN Baccalaureate.

Program Entrance Requirements Minimum overall college GPA of 2.8, immunizations, minimum high school GPA of 2.8. **Standardized tests** *Required:* SAT or ACT, TOEFL for international students. *Recommended:* SAT Subject Tests. **Application** *Deadline:* 7/31 (freshmen), 7/31 (transfer). *Notification:* continuous (freshmen). *Application fee:* $25.

Contact Department of Health Sciences, Department of Nursing, South Carolina State University, 300 College Street, NE, Orangeburg, SC 29117. *Telephone:* 803-536-7063. *Fax:* 803-536-8593.

University of South Carolina
College of Nursing
Columbia, South Carolina

http://www.sc.edu/nursing

Founded in 1801

DEGREES • BSN • MSN • MSN/MPH • PHD

Nursing Program Faculty 59 (34% with doctorates).

Baccalaureate Enrollment 809
Women 93% **Men** 7% **Minority** 26% **Part-time** 11%

Graduate Enrollment 121
Women 95% **Men** 5% **Minority** 15% **Part-time** 61%

Nursing Student Activities Sigma Theta Tau, Student Nurses' Association.

Nursing Student Resources Academic advising; academic or career counseling; assistance for students with disabilities; bookstore; campus computer network; career placement assistance; computer lab; computer-assisted instruction; daycare for children of students; e-mail services; housing assistance; interactive nursing skills videos; Internet; learning resource lab; library services; nursing audiovisuals; remedial services; resume preparation assistance; skills, simulation, or other laboratory; tutoring.

Library Facilities 3.4 million volumes (30,763 in health, 3,125 in nursing); 22,744 periodical subscriptions (443 health-care related).

BACCALAUREATE PROGRAMS

Degree BSN

Available Programs Generic Baccalaureate; RN Baccalaureate.

Study Options Full-time.

Program Entrance Requirements Minimum overall college GPA of 2.75, transcript of college record, high school foreign language, high school math, high school science, high school transcript, immunizations, minimum high school GPA. Transfer students are accepted. **Standardized tests** *Required:* SAT or ACT, TOEFL for international students. **Application** *Deadline:* 12/1 (freshmen), 6/1 (transfer). *Notification:* continuous until 10/1 (freshmen). *Application fee:* $40.

Advanced Placement Credit given for nursing courses completed elsewhere dependent upon specific evaluations.

Expenses (2004–05) *Tuition, state resident:* full-time $7270; part-time $361 per credit hour. *Tuition, nonresident:* full-time $18,658; part-time $890 per credit hour. *International tuition:* $18,658 full-time. *Room and board:* $5590 per academic year. *Required fees:* full-time $464; part-time $10 per credit.

Financial Aid 87% of baccalaureate students in nursing programs received some form of financial aid in 2003–04.

Contact Ms. Gail S. Vereen, Director of Recruitment and Undergraduate Advisement, College of Nursing, University of South Carolina, 1601 Greene Street, Williams Brice Building, Columbia, SC 29208. *Telephone:* 803-777-2526. *Fax:* 803-777-0616. *E-mail:* gsveree@nrwpo.nurs.sc.edu.

GRADUATE PROGRAMS

Expenses (2004–05) *Tuition, state resident:* full-time $8186; part-time $405 per credit hour. *Tuition, nonresident:* full-time $16,726; part-time $821 per credit hour. *International tuition:* $16,726 full-time. *Room and board:* room only: $700 per academic year. *Required fees:* part-time $10 per credit.

Financial Aid 68% of graduate students in nursing programs received some form of financial aid in 2003–04. 3 research assistantships with partial tuition reimbursements available (averaging $1,698 per year), 4 teaching assistantships with partial tuition reimbursements available (averaging $3,275 per year) were awarded; scholarships, traineeships, and unspecified assistantships also available. *Financial aid application deadline:* 4/1.

Contact Ms. Cheryl Nelson-Jackson, Graduate Programs Student Service Coordinator, College of Nursing, University of South Carolina, 1601 Greene Street, Williams Brice Building, Columbia, SC 29208. *Telephone:* 803-777-3754. *Fax:* 803-777-0616. *E-mail:* cheryl.nelsonjackson@sc.edu.

MASTER'S DEGREE PROGRAM

Degrees MSN; MSN/MPH

Available Programs Master's.

Concentrations Available Nursing administration; nursing education. *Clinical nurse specialist programs in:* acute care, community health, psychiatric/mental health, public health. *Nurse practitioner programs in:* acute care, adult health, family health, pediatric, psychiatric/mental health, women's health.

Study Options Full-time and part-time.

Program Entrance Requirements Minimum overall college GPA of 2.75, transcript of college record, written essay, immunizations, 2 letters of recommendation, GRE General Test, MAT. *Application deadline:* For fall admission, 7/1; for winter admission, 5/1; for spring admission, 11/15. Applications are processed on a rolling basis. *Application fee:* $40.

Advanced Placement Credit given for nursing courses completed elsewhere dependent upon specific evaluations.

Degree Requirements 45 total credit hours, thesis or project.

POST-MASTER'S PROGRAM

Areas of Study *Nurse practitioner programs in:* acute care, adult health, family health, pediatric, psychiatric/mental health, women's health.

DOCTORAL DEGREE PROGRAM

Degree PhD

Available Programs Doctorate; Post-Baccalaureate Doctorate.

Areas of Study Individualized study.

Program Entrance Requirements Minimum overall college GPA of 3.5, interview by faculty committee, 3 letters of recommendation, scholarly papers, vita, writing sample, GRE General Test. *Application deadline:* For fall admission, 7/1; for winter admission, 5/1; for spring admission, 11/15. Applications are processed on a rolling basis. *Application fee:* $40.

Degree Requirements 61 total credit hours, dissertation, oral exam, written exam, residency.

University of South Carolina Aiken

School of Nursing
Aiken, South Carolina

http://www.usca.edu/nursing/

Founded in 1961

DEGREE • BSN

Nursing Student Activities Student Nurses' Association.

Library Facilities 165,459 volumes; 745 periodical subscriptions.

BACCALAUREATE PROGRAMS

Degree BSN

Program Entrance Requirements Standardized tests *Required:* SAT or ACT, TOEFL for international students. **Application** *Deadline:* 8/1 (freshmen), 8/1 (transfer). *Notification:* continuous (freshmen). *Application fee:* $35.

Contact Dr. Trudy Groves, RN, Head and BSN Program Director, School of Nursing, University of South Carolina Aiken, 471 University Parkway, Aiken, SC 29801. *Telephone:* 803-648-6851. *Fax:* 803-641-3362. *E-mail:* trudyg@aiken.sc.edu.

University of South Carolina Upstate

Mary Black School of Nursing
Spartanburg, South Carolina

http://www.uscs.edu/academics/mbsn/

Founded in 1967

DEGREE • BSN

Nursing Program Faculty 45 (16% with doctorates).

Baccalaureate Enrollment 212
Women 86% **Men** 14% **Minority** 27% **Part-time** 37%

Nursing Student Activities Nursing Honor Society, Sigma Theta Tau, Student Nurses' Association.

Nursing Student Resources Academic advising; academic or career counseling; assistance for students with disabilities; bookstore; campus computer network; computer lab; computer-assisted instruction; daycare for children of students; e-mail services; externships; interactive nursing skills videos; Internet; learning resource lab; library services; nursing audiovisuals; resume preparation assistance; skills, simulation, or other laboratory; tutoring.

Library Facilities 156,558 volumes (214,998 in health, 23,359 in nursing); 3,151 periodical subscriptions.

BACCALAUREATE PROGRAMS

Degree BSN

Available Programs Accelerated RN Baccalaureate; Generic Baccalaureate.

Study Options Full-time.

Program Entrance Requirements Transcript of college record, minimum GPA in nursing prerequisites of 2.5, prerequisite course work. Transfer students are accepted. **Standardized tests** *Required:* SAT or ACT, TOEFL for international students. **Application** *Notification:* continuous (freshmen). *Application fee:* $35.

Advanced Placement Credit by examination available. Credit given for nursing courses completed elsewhere dependent upon specific evaluations.

Expenses (2003–04) *Tuition, state resident:* full-time $5310; part-time $233 per credit hour. *Tuition, nonresident:* full-time $10,936; part-time $481 per credit hour. *Room and board:* $4940; room only: $2900 per academic year. *Required fees:* full-time $392; part-time $196 per term.

Financial Aid *Gift aid (need-based):* Federal Pell, FSEOG, state, private, college/university gift aid from institutional funds. *Loans:* FFEL (Subsidized and Unsubsidized Stafford PLUS), Perkins, state. *Work-Study:* Federal Work-Study, part-time campus jobs. *Application deadline (priority):* 3/1.

Contact Dr. Angie Davis, Associate Dean, Mary Black School of Nursing, University of South Carolina Upstate, 800 University Way, University of South Carolina Spartanburg, Spartanburg, SC 29303. *Telephone:* 888-551-3858. *Fax:* 864-503-5411. *E-mail:* adavis@uscs.edu.

SOUTH DAKOTA

Augustana College

Department of Nursing
Sioux Falls, South Dakota

http://www.augie.edu

Founded in 1860

DEGREES • BA • MA

Nursing Program Faculty 17 (29% with doctorates).

Baccalaureate Enrollment 206
Women 89% **Men** 11% **Part-time** 1%

Graduate Enrollment 20
Women 99% **Men** 1% **Minority** 1% **Part-time** 100%

Nursing Student Activities Sigma Theta Tau, Student Nurses' Association.

Nursing Student Resources Academic advising; academic or career counseling; assistance for students with disabilities; bookstore; campus computer network; career placement assistance; computer lab; computer-assisted instruction; daycare for children of students; e-mail services; employment services for current students; housing assistance; interactive nursing skills videos; Internet; learning resource lab; library services; nursing audiovisuals; remedial services; resume preparation assistance; skills, simulation, or other laboratory; tutoring; unpaid internships.

Library Facilities 279,918 volumes (6,106 in health, 816 in nursing); 595 periodical subscriptions (61 health-care related).

BACCALAUREATE PROGRAMS

Degree BA

Available Programs Generic Baccalaureate; RN Baccalaureate.

Study Options Full-time.

Program Entrance Requirements Minimum overall college GPA of 2.7, transcript of college record, written essay, health exam, high school transcript, immunizations, 2 letters of recommendation, minimum high school GPA of 3.0, minimum high school rank 50%, minimum GPA in nursing prerequisites of 2.7. Transfer students are accepted. **Standardized tests** *Required:* SAT or ACT, TOEFL for international students. **Application** *Deadline:* 8/1 (freshmen), rolling (transfer). *Notification:* continuous (freshmen).

Advanced Placement Credit given for nursing courses completed elsewhere dependent upon specific evaluations.

Expenses (2004–05) *Tuition:* full-time $17,764; part-time $260 per credit hour. *International tuition:* $17,764 full-time. *Room and board:* $5269; room only: $2600 per academic year. *Required fees:* full-time $490; part-time $108 per term.

Financial Aid 100% of baccalaureate students in nursing programs received some form of financial aid in 2003–04.

Contact Dr. Margot L. Nelson, Professor and Chair, Department of Nursing, Augustana College, 2001 South Summit Avenue, Sioux Falls, SD 57197. *Telephone:* 605-274-4729. *Fax:* 605-274-4723. *E-mail:* margot_nelson@augie.edu.

Augustana College (continued)

GRADUATE PROGRAMS

Expenses (2004–05) *Tuition:* part-time $314 per credit hour.

Contact Dr. Mary Brendtro, Professor of Nursing, Department of Nursing, Augustana College, 2001 South Summit Avenue, Sioux Falls, SD 57197. *Telephone:* 605-274-4725. *Fax:* 605-274-4723. *E-mail:* mary_brendtro@augie.edu.

MASTER'S DEGREE PROGRAM

Degree MA

Available Programs Master's.

Concentrations Available *Clinical nurse specialist programs in:* community health, public health.

Site Options *Distance Learning:* Aberdeen, SD.

Study Options Part-time.

Program Entrance Requirements Clinical experience, minimum overall college GPA of 3.0, transcript of college record, written essay, immunizations, interview, 3 letters of recommendation, professional liability insurance/malpractice insurance, resume, statistics course.

Advanced Placement Credit given for nursing courses completed elsewhere dependent upon specific evaluations.

Degree Requirements 38 total credit hours, thesis or project.

Mount Marty College

Nursing Program
Yankton, South Dakota

http://www.mtmc.edu

Founded in 1936

DEGREE • BSC PN

Nursing Program Faculty 16 (13% with doctorates).

Baccalaureate Enrollment 106

Women 92% **Men** 8% **Minority** 7% **International** 2% **Part-time** 1%

Nursing Student Activities Student Nurses' Association, nursing club.

Nursing Student Resources Academic advising; academic or career counseling; assistance for students with disabilities; bookstore; campus computer network; career placement assistance; computer lab; computer-assisted instruction; daycare for children of students; e-mail services; employment services for current students; externships; housing assistance; interactive nursing skills videos; Internet; learning resource lab; library services; nursing audiovisuals; paid internships; placement services for program completers; remedial services; resume preparation assistance; skills, simulation, or other laboratory; tutoring.

Library Facilities 76,571 volumes (8,700 in health, 5,300 in nursing); 424 periodical subscriptions (92 health-care related).

BACCALAUREATE PROGRAMS

Degree BSc PN

Available Programs ADN to Baccalaureate; Generic Baccalaureate; International Nurse to Baccalaureate; LPN to Baccalaureate; LPN to RN Baccalaureate; RN Baccalaureate.

Site Options Watertown, SD.

Study Options Full-time and part-time.

Program Entrance Requirements Minimum overall college GPA of 2.7, transcript of college record, CPR certification, health exam, health insurance, high school transcript, immunizations, minimum GPA in nursing prerequisites of 2.0, prerequisite course work. Transfer students are accepted. **Standardized tests** *Required:* SAT or ACT, TOEFL for international students. *Recommended:* ACT. **Application** *Deadline:* rolling (freshmen), rolling (transfer). *Notification:* continuous (freshmen). *Application fee:* $35.

Advanced Placement Credit given for nursing courses completed elsewhere dependent upon specific evaluations.

Expenses (2004–05) *Tuition:* full-time $13,256; part-time $360 per credit hour. *International tuition:* $13,256 full-time. *Room and board:* $4764 per academic year. *Required fees:* full-time $2017; part-time $499.50 per credit; part-time $35 per term.

Financial Aid 97% of baccalaureate students in nursing programs received some form of financial aid in 2003–04.

Contact Dr. Ruth A. Pakieser, Chair and Director, Division of Nursing, Nursing Program, Mount Marty College, 1105 West 8th Street, Yankton, SD 57078-3724. *Telephone:* 605-668-1594. *Fax:* 605-668-1607. *E-mail:* rpakieser@mtmc.edu.

Presentation College

Department of Nursing
Aberdeen, South Dakota

http://www.presentation.edu

Founded in 1951

DEGREE • BSN

Nursing Program Faculty 21 (14% with doctorates).

Baccalaureate Enrollment 149

Women 96% **Men** 4% **Minority** 4% **Part-time** 28%

Nursing Student Activities Sigma Theta Tau, Student Nurses' Association, nursing club.

Nursing Student Resources Academic advising; academic or career counseling; assistance for students with disabilities; bookstore; campus computer network; career placement assistance; computer lab; computer-assisted instruction; e-mail services; interactive nursing skills videos; Internet; learning resource lab; library services; nursing audiovisuals; placement services for program completers; remedial services; skills, simulation, or other laboratory; tutoring.

Library Facilities 40,000 volumes (378 in health, 353 in nursing); 430 periodical subscriptions (2,172 health-care related).

BACCALAUREATE PROGRAMS

Degree BSN

Available Programs ADN to Baccalaureate; Baccalaureate for Second Degree; Generic Baccalaureate; LPN to Baccalaureate; RN Baccalaureate.

Site Options *Distance Learning:* Wahpeton, ND; Sioux Falls, SD; Fairmont, MN.

Study Options Full-time and part-time.

Program Entrance Requirements Minimum overall college GPA of 2.5, transcript of college record, written essay, high school biology, high school chemistry, 2 years high school math, high school transcript, immunizations, interview, 2 letters of recommendation, minimum high school GPA of 2.0, minimum GPA in nursing prerequisites of 2.5, prerequisite course work. Transfer students are accepted. **Standardized tests** *Required:* TOEFL for international students, ACT ASSET. *Recommended:* ACT. *Required for some:* ACT. **Application** *Deadline:* rolling (freshmen), rolling (transfer).

Advanced Placement Credit given for nursing courses completed elsewhere dependent upon specific evaluations.

Expenses (2004–05) *Tuition:* full-time $10,400; part-time $365 per credit hour. *International tuition:* $10,400 full-time. *Room and board:* $4550; room only: $3800 per academic year. *Required fees:* full-time $350.

Financial Aid 91% of baccalaureate students in nursing programs received some form of financial aid in 2003–04.

Contact Ms. JoEllen Lindner, Dean of Admissions, Department of Nursing, Presentation College, 1500 North Main Street, Aberdeen, SD 57401. *Telephone:* 605-229-8492. *Fax:* 605-229-8489. *E-mail:* lindnerjo@presentation.edu.

South Dakota State University

College of Nursing
Brookings, South Dakota

http://www.sdstate.org/Academics/CollegeofNursing/

Founded in 1881

DEGREES • BS • MS

Nursing Program Faculty 78 (24% with doctorates).

Baccalaureate Enrollment 392
Women 88% **Men** 12% **Minority** 2%

Graduate Enrollment 102
Women 95% **Men** 5% **Part-time** 95%

Nursing Student Activities Sigma Theta Tau, Student Nurses' Association, nursing club.

Nursing Student Resources Academic advising; academic or career counseling; assistance for students with disabilities; bookstore; campus computer network; career placement assistance; computer lab; computer-assisted instruction; daycare for children of students; e-mail services; employment services for current students; externships; interactive nursing skills videos; Internet; learning resource lab; library services; nursing audiovisuals; paid internships; placement services for program completers; remedial services; resume preparation assistance; skills, simulation, or other laboratory; tutoring.

Library Facilities 555,523 volumes; 6,023 periodical subscriptions (182 health-care related).

BACCALAUREATE PROGRAMS

Degree BS

Available Programs Accelerated Baccalaureate; Generic Baccalaureate; RN Baccalaureate.

Site Options *Distance Learning:* Rapid City, SD; Sioux Falls, SD.

Study Options Full-time.

Program Entrance Requirements Minimum overall college GPA of 2.5, transcript of college record, CPR certification, written essay, health exam, health insurance, immunizations, 3 letters of recommendation, minimum GPA in nursing prerequisites of 2.5, professional liability insurance/malpractice insurance, prerequisite course work. Transfer students are accepted. **Standardized tests** *Required:* ACT, TOEFL for international students. **Application** *Deadline:* rolling (freshmen), rolling (transfer). *Application fee:* $20.

Advanced Placement Credit given for nursing courses completed elsewhere dependent upon specific evaluations.

Expenses (2003–04) *Tuition, state resident:* full-time $2307; part-time $72 per credit hour. *Tuition, nonresident:* full-time $7333; part-time $229 per credit hour. *International tuition:* $7333 full-time. *Room and board:* $1877; room only: $931 per academic year. *Required fees:* full-time $3166; part-time $87 per credit; part-time $397 per term.

Financial Aid 58% of baccalaureate students in nursing programs received some form of financial aid in 2002–03. *Gift aid (need-based):* Federal Pell, FSEOG, private, college/university gift aid from institutional funds, United Negro College Fund, Federal Nursing. *Loans:* Federal Nursing Student Loans, FFEL (Subsidized and Unsubsidized Stafford PLUS), Perkins, college/university, alternative loans. *Work-Study:* Federal Work-Study, part-time campus jobs. *Application deadline (priority):* 3/7.

Contact Dr. Gloria P. Craig, Department Head, Nursing Student Services, College of Nursing, South Dakota State University, Box 2275, Rotunda Lane, NFA 255, Brookings, SD 57007-0098. *Telephone:* 605-688-4106. *Fax:* 605-688-6073. *E-mail:* gloria_craig@sdstate.edu.

GRADUATE PROGRAMS

Expenses (2003–04) *Tuition, state resident:* full-time $2407; part-time $109 per credit hour. *Tuition, nonresident:* full-time $7094; part-time $322 per credit hour. *International tuition:* $7094 full-time. *Required fees:* part-time $87 per credit; part-time $970 per term.

Financial Aid 43% of graduate students in nursing programs received some form of financial aid in 2002–03. Fellowships, research assistantships, teaching assistantships, Federal Work-Study available.

Contact Dr. Penny Powers, Department Head, College of Nursing, South Dakota State University, Box 2275, Rotunda Lane, NFA 217, Brookings, SD 57007-0098. *Telephone:* 605-688-4114. *Fax:* 605-688-5827. *E-mail:* penny_powers@sdstate.edu.

MASTER'S DEGREE PROGRAM

Degree MS

Available Programs Master's; RN to Master's.

Concentrations Available Nursing administration; nursing education. *Nurse practitioner programs in:* neonatal health, primary care, psychiatric/mental health.

Site Options *Distance Learning:* Rapid City, SD; Sioux Falls, SD.

Study Options Full-time and part-time.

Program Entrance Requirements Clinical experience, minimum overall college GPA of 3.0, transcript of college record, written essay, 3 letters of recommendation. *Application deadline:* Applications are processed on a rolling basis. *Application fee:* $15.

Advanced Placement Credit given for nursing courses completed elsewhere dependent upon specific evaluations.

Degree Requirements 53 total credit hours, thesis or project, comprehensive exam.

POST-MASTER'S PROGRAM

Areas of Study *Nurse practitioner programs in:* primary care.

CONTINUING EDUCATION PROGRAM

Contact Dr. Gloria P. Craig, Coordinator, Continuing Nursing Education, College of Nursing, South Dakota State University, Box 2275, Rotunda Lane, NFA 135, Brookings, SD 57007-0098. *Telephone:* 605-688-5745. *Fax:* 605-688-6679. *E-mail:* Gloria_Craig@sdstate.edu.

TENNESSEE

Aquinas College
Department of Nursing
Nashville, Tennessee

http://www.aquinas-tn.edu/nursing/index.htm

Founded in 1961

DEGREE • BSN

Nursing Student Resources Library services.

Library Facilities 45,762 volumes; 301 periodical subscriptions.

BACCALAUREATE PROGRAMS

Degree BSN

Available Programs RN Baccalaureate.

Program Entrance Requirements Interview, 2 letters of recommendation, RN licensure. **Standardized tests** *Required:* SAT or ACT, TOEFL for international students. **Application** *Deadline:* rolling (freshmen), rolling (transfer). *Notification:* continuous (freshmen). *Application fee:* $10.

Advanced Placement Credit given for nursing courses completed elsewhere dependent upon specific evaluations.

Contact Dr. Linda Watlington, RN to BSN Program Director, Department of Nursing, Aquinas College, 4210 Harding Road, Nashville, TN 37205. *Telephone:* 615-222-4038. *E-mail:* admissions@aquinas-tn.edu.

Austin Peay State University
School of Nursing
Clarksville, Tennessee

http://www.apsu.edu/nursing01

Founded in 1927

DEGREE • BSN

Nursing Student Activities Nursing Honor Society, Sigma Theta Tau, Student Nurses' Association.

Austin Peay State University (continued)

Nursing Student Resources Computer lab; computer-assisted instruction; interactive nursing skills videos; nursing audiovisuals; skills, simulation, or other laboratory.

Library Facilities 400,000 volumes (8,249 in health, 1,111 in nursing); 1,754 periodical subscriptions (146 health-care related).

BACCALAUREATE PROGRAMS

Degree BSN

Available Programs Generic Baccalaureate; RN Baccalaureate.

Study Options Full-time.

Program Entrance Requirements Minimum overall college GPA of 2.8, transcript of college record, CPR certification, health insurance, high school transcript, immunizations, minimum GPA in nursing prerequisites of 2.8. Transfer students are accepted. **Standardized tests** *Required:* TOEFL for international students. *Required for some:* SAT or ACT. ***Placement:*** *Required for some:* SAT, ACT. **Application** *Deadline:* 8/29 (freshmen), rolling (transfer). *Notification:* continuous (freshmen). *Application fee:* $15.

Contact Dr. Kathy Martin, RN, Director, School of Nursing, Austin Peay State University, PO Box 4658, Clarksville, TN 37044. *Telephone:* 931-221-7710. *Fax:* 931-221-7388. *E-mail:* martinkl@apsu.edu.

Baptist College of Health Sciences

Nursing Division
Memphis, Tennessee

Founded in 1994

DEGREE • BSN

Nursing Program Faculty 25.

Baccalaureate Enrollment 63

BACCALAUREATE PROGRAMS

Degree BSN

Available Programs Generic Baccalaureate; LPN to Baccalaureate; RN Baccalaureate.

Study Options Full-time and part-time.

Program Entrance Requirements Minimum overall college GPA of 2.5, CPR certification, health exam, health insurance, 2 years high school math, 2 years high school science, high school transcript, immunizations, 3 letters of recommendation, minimum high school GPA of 2.75. Transfer students are accepted. **Standardized tests** *Required:* ACT. **Application** *Deadline:* 6/1 (freshmen), 6/1 (transfer). *Application fee:* $25.

Expenses (2003–04) *Tuition:* part-time $150 per credit hour. *Required fees:* part-time $10 per credit.

Contact Cynthia Davis, Manager of Admissions and Retention, Nursing Division, Baptist College of Health Sciences, 1003 Monroe, Memphis, TN 38104. *Telephone:* 901-572-2465. *Fax:* 901-572-2461. *E-mail:* cynthia.davis@bchs.edu.

Belmont University

School of Nursing
Nashville, Tennessee

http://www.belmont.edu/nursing

Founded in 1951

DEGREES • BSN • MSN

Nursing Program Faculty 32 (16% with doctorates).

Baccalaureate Enrollment 247

Women 91% **Men** 9% **Minority** 6% **International** 1% **Part-time** 8%

Graduate Enrollment 7

Women 100% **Minority** 14% **Part-time** 14%

Nursing Student Activities Nursing Honor Society, Sigma Theta Tau, Student Nurses' Association.

Nursing Student Resources Academic advising; academic or career counseling; bookstore; campus computer network; career placement assistance; computer lab; computer-assisted instruction; e-mail services; employment services for current students; externships; housing assistance; interactive nursing skills videos; Internet; learning resource lab; library services; nursing audiovisuals; placement services for program completers; remedial services; resume preparation assistance; skills, simulation, or other laboratory; tutoring.

Library Facilities 184,835 volumes (5,390 in health, 987 in nursing); 1,311 periodical subscriptions (270 health-care related).

BACCALAUREATE PROGRAMS

Degree BSN

Available Programs ADN to Baccalaureate; Accelerated Baccalaureate; Accelerated Baccalaureate for Second Degree; Baccalaureate for Second Degree; Generic Baccalaureate; LPN to RN Baccalaureate; RN Baccalaureate.

Study Options Full-time and part-time.

Program Entrance Requirements Minimum overall college GPA of 2.5, transcript of college record, CPR certification, written essay, health exam, health insurance, high school biology, high school chemistry, 3 years high school math, 3 years high school science, high school transcript, immunizations, 1 letter of recommendation, minimum high school GPA of 2.5, minimum GPA in nursing prerequisites of 3.0. Transfer students are accepted. **Standardized tests** *Required:* SAT or ACT, TOEFL for international students. **Application** *Deadline:* 5/1 (freshmen), 5/1 (transfer). *Notification:* continuous (freshmen). *Application fee:* $35.

Advanced Placement Credit by examination available. Credit given for nursing courses completed elsewhere dependent upon specific evaluations.

Expenses (2004–05) *Tuition:* full-time $7680; part-time $585 per credit hour. *Room and board:* $3040; room only: $1475 per academic year. *Required fees:* full-time $430; part-time $290 per credit.

Financial Aid 75% of baccalaureate students in nursing programs received some form of financial aid in 2003–04.

Contact Mrs. Cathy Hendon, Admissions Coordinator, School of Nursing, Belmont University, 1900 Belmont Boulevard, Nashville, TN 37212-3757. *Telephone:* 615-460-6107. *Fax:* 615-460-6125. *E-mail:* hendonc@mail.belmont.edu.

GRADUATE PROGRAMS

Expenses (2004–05) *Tuition:* part-time $675 per credit hour. *Required fees:* full-time $200; part-time $100 per credit.

Financial Aid 95% of graduate students in nursing programs received some form of financial aid in 2003–04. Scholarships and traineeships available. *Financial aid application deadline:* 3/1.

Contact Dr. Leslie Higgins, Director, Graduate Program, School of Nursing, Belmont University, 1900 Belmont Boulevard, Nashville, TN 37212-3757. *Telephone:* 615-460-6027. *Fax:* 615-460-5644. *E-mail:* higginsl@mail.belmont.edu.

MASTER'S DEGREE PROGRAM

Degree MSN

Available Programs Master's.

Concentrations Available *Nurse practitioner programs in:* family health.

Study Options Full-time and part-time.

Program Entrance Requirements Clinical experience, minimum overall college GPA of 3.0, transcript of college record, CPR certification, written essay, immunizations, interview, 2 letters of recommendation, resume, GRE. *Application deadline:* For fall admission, 2/15 (priority date); for spring admission, 10/15 (priority date). Applications are processed on a rolling basis. *Application fee:* $50.

Degree Requirements 41 total credit hours, comprehensive exam.

POST-MASTER'S PROGRAM

Areas of Study *Nurse practitioner programs in:* family health.

Carson-Newman College

Department of Nursing
Jefferson City, Tennessee

Founded in 1851

DEGREES • BSN • MSN

Nursing Program Faculty 11 (42% with doctorates).

Baccalaureate Enrollment 154
Women 93% **Men** 7% **Minority** 1% **Part-time** 1%

Graduate Enrollment 20
Women 95% **Men** 5% **Minority** 5% **International** 10% **Part-time** 57%

Nursing Student Activities Sigma Theta Tau, Student Nurses' Association, nursing club.

Nursing Student Resources Academic advising; academic or career counseling; assistance for students with disabilities; bookstore; campus computer network; career placement assistance; computer lab; computer-assisted instruction; e-mail services; employment services for current students; externships; housing assistance; interactive nursing skills videos; Internet; learning resource lab; placement services for program completers; remedial services; resume preparation assistance; skills, simulation, or other laboratory; tutoring; unpaid internships.

Library Facilities 218,371 volumes (1,800 in health); 3,966 periodical subscriptions (180 health-care related).

BACCALAUREATE PROGRAMS

Degree BSN

Available Programs Accelerated Baccalaureate; Generic Baccalaureate; RN Baccalaureate.

Study Options Full-time.

Program Entrance Requirements Minimum overall college GPA of 2.5, transcript of college record, high school transcript, minimum GPA in nursing prerequisites of 2.5, prerequisite course work. Transfer students are accepted. **Standardized tests** *Required:* SAT or ACT, TOEFL for international students. **Application** *Deadline:* 8/1 (freshmen), 8/1 (transfer). *Notification:* continuous (freshmen). *Application fee:* $25.

Advanced Placement Credit given for nursing courses completed elsewhere dependent upon specific evaluations.

Expenses (2004–05) *Tuition:* full-time $6850; part-time $565 per credit hour. *International tuition:* $6850 full-time. *Room and board:* $6000; room only: $3000 per academic year. *Required fees:* full-time $1000.

Financial Aid 90% of baccalaureate students in nursing programs received some form of financial aid in 2003–04. *Gift aid (need-based):* Federal Pell, FSEOG, state, private, college/university gift aid from institutional funds. *Loans:* FFEL (Subsidized and Unsubsidized Stafford PLUS), Perkins, state, college/university, alternative loans. *Work-Study:* Federal Work-Study, part-time campus jobs. *Application deadline (priority):* 4/1.

Contact Dr. Angela F. Wood, RN, Chair, Undergraduate Studies in Nursing, Department of Nursing, Carson-Newman College, 1646 Russell Avenue, Jefferson City, TN 37760. *Telephone:* 865-471-3442. *Fax:* 865-471-4574. *E-mail:* awood@cn.edu.

GRADUATE PROGRAMS

Expenses (2004–05) *Tuition:* full-time $7650; part-time $425 per credit hour. *International tuition:* $7650 full-time. *Required fees:* full-time $200.

Contact Dr. Cynthia Huff, RN, Chair, Graduate Studies in Nursing, Department of Nursing, Carson-Newman College, C-NC Box 71883, 1646 Russell Avenue, Jefferson City, TN 37760. *Telephone:* 865-471-3429. *Fax:* 865-471-4574. *E-mail:* chuff@cn.edu.

MASTER'S DEGREE PROGRAM

Degree MSN

Available Programs Master's.

Concentrations Available Nursing education. *Nurse practitioner programs in:* family health.

Study Options Full-time and part-time.

Program Entrance Requirements Minimum overall college GPA of 3.0, transcript of college record, written essay, 3 letters of recommendation. *Application deadline:* For fall admission, 7/15 (priority date). Applications are processed on a rolling basis. *Application fee:* $50.

Advanced Placement Credit given for nursing courses completed elsewhere dependent upon specific evaluations.

Degree Requirements 45 total credit hours, thesis or project, comprehensive exam.

POST-MASTER'S PROGRAM

Areas of Study Nursing education. *Nurse practitioner programs in:* family health.

Cumberland University
Rudy School of Nursing and Health Professions
Lebanon, Tennessee

http://www.cumberland.edu/academics/nursing/index.html

Founded in 1842

DEGREE • BSN

Nursing Program Faculty 10 (33% with doctorates).

Baccalaureate Enrollment 110
Women 90% **Men** 10% **Minority** 5%

Nursing Student Activities Nursing Honor Society, Student Nurses' Association.

Nursing Student Resources Academic advising; academic or career counseling; assistance for students with disabilities; bookstore; campus computer network; career placement assistance; computer lab; e-mail services; housing assistance; interactive nursing skills videos; Internet; learning resource lab; library services; nursing audiovisuals; resume preparation assistance; skills, simulation, or other laboratory; tutoring.

Library Facilities 50,000 volumes; 130 periodical subscriptions.

BACCALAUREATE PROGRAMS

Degree BSN

Available Programs Baccalaureate for Second Degree; Generic Baccalaureate; LPN to Baccalaureate; RN Baccalaureate.

Study Options Full-time and part-time.

Program Entrance Requirements Minimum GPA in nursing prerequisites of 2.5. Transfer students are accepted. **Standardized tests** *Required:* ACT, SAT or ACT, TOEFL for international students. *Recommended:* SAT. **Application** *Deadline:* rolling (freshmen), rolling (transfer). *Notification:* continuous (freshmen). *Application fee:* $25.

Advanced Placement Credit given for nursing courses completed elsewhere dependent upon specific evaluations.

Financial Aid 100% of baccalaureate students in nursing programs received some form of financial aid in 2002–03.

Contact Ms. Alice Johnson-Davis, Interim Chair and Assistant Professor, Rudy School of Nursing and Health Professions, Cumberland University, One Cumberland Square, Lebanon, TN 37087-3554. *Telephone:* 615-444-2562 Ext. 1037. *Fax:* 615-444-2569. *E-mail:* nursing@cumberland.edu.

East Tennessee State University
College of Nursing
Johnson City, Tennessee

http://www.etsu.edu/etsu.con

Founded in 1911

DEGREES • BSN • DSN • MSN

Nursing Program Faculty 78 (35% with doctorates).

Baccalaureate Enrollment 433
Women 89% **Men** 11% **Minority** 6% **Part-time** 25%

Graduate Enrollment 91
Women 87% **Men** 13% **Minority** 9% **Part-time** 53%

Nursing Student Activities Sigma Theta Tau, Student Nurses' Association.

Nursing Student Resources Academic advising; academic or career counseling; assistance for students with disabilities; bookstore; campus computer network; career placement assistance; computer lab; computer-assisted instruction; daycare for children of students; e-mail services; employment services for current students; externships; housing assistance; interactive nursing skills videos; Internet; learning resource lab; library services; nursing audiovisuals; remedial services; resume preparation assistance; skills, simulation, or other laboratory; tutoring.

Library Facilities 1.1 million volumes (8,026 in health, 1,556 in nursing); 3,714 periodical subscriptions (199 health-care related).

East Tennessee State University (continued)

BACCALAUREATE PROGRAMS

Degree BSN

Available Programs ADN to Baccalaureate; Accelerated Baccalaureate for Second Degree; Accelerated RN Baccalaureate; Generic Baccalaureate; LPN to Baccalaureate.

Site Options Knoxville, TN; Cleveland, TN. *Distance Learning:* Morristown, TN.

Study Options Full-time and part-time.

Program Entrance Requirements Minimum overall college GPA of 2.6, transcript of college record, prerequisite course work. Transfer students are accepted. **Standardized tests** *Required:* SAT or ACT, TOEFL for international students. **Application** *Notification:* continuous (freshmen). *Application fee:* $15.

Advanced Placement Credit given for nursing courses completed elsewhere dependent upon specific evaluations.

Financial Aid *Gift aid (need-based):* Federal Pell, FSEOG, state, private, college/university gift aid from institutional funds, Federal Nursing. *Loans:* FFEL (Subsidized and Unsubsidized Stafford PLUS), Perkins, college/university. *Work-Study:* Federal Work-Study, part-time campus jobs. *Application deadline (priority):* 4/15.

Contact Mr. Scott Crowder-Vaughn, Advisor, College of Nursing, East Tennessee State University, Office of Student Services, PO Box 70617, Johnson City, TN 37614-0617. *Telephone:* 423-439-4578. *Fax:* 423-439-4522. *E-mail:* admitnur@.etsu.edu.

GRADUATE PROGRAMS

Financial Aid 6 research assistantships (averaging $5,500 per year), 4 teaching assistantships (averaging $5,500 per year) were awarded; career-related internships or fieldwork, traineeships, and unspecified assistantships also available.

Contact Ms. Amy Bower, Coordinator, College of Nursing, East Tennessee State University, Office of Student Services, PO Box 70617, Johnson City, TN 37614-0617. *Telephone:* 423-439-4531. *Fax:* 423-439-4522. *E-mail:* bowera@etsu.edu.

MASTER'S DEGREE PROGRAM

Degree MSN

Available Programs Master's.

Concentrations Available Nursing administration; nursing education. *Nurse practitioner programs in:* adult health, family health, gerontology, psychiatric/mental health.

Study Options Full-time and part-time.

Program Entrance Requirements Minimum overall college GPA of 3.0, transcript of college record, written essay, 3 letters of recommendation, GRE General Test. *Application deadline:* For fall admission, 1/15 (priority date). Applications are processed on a rolling basis. *Application fee:* $25 ($35 for international students).

Advanced Placement Credit given for nursing courses completed elsewhere dependent upon specific evaluations.

Degree Requirements 48 total credit hours, comprehensive exam.

POST-MASTER'S PROGRAM

Areas of Study Health-care administration. *Nurse practitioner programs in:* adult health, family health, gerontology, psychiatric/mental health.

DOCTORAL DEGREE PROGRAM

Degree DSN

Available Programs Doctorate.

Areas of Study Advanced practice nursing, individualized study, nursing administration, nursing education.

Program Entrance Requirements Clinical experience, minimum overall college GPA of 3.0, interview by faculty committee, 3 letters of recommendation, MSN or equivalent, statistics course, vita, writing sample. *Application deadline:* For fall admission, 1/15 (priority date). Applications are processed on a rolling basis. *Application fee:* $25 ($35 for international students).

Degree Requirements 62 total credit hours, dissertation, residency.

King College

School of Nursing
Bristol, Tennessee

Founded in 1867

DEGREE • BSN

Nursing Program Faculty 6 (16% with doctorates).

Baccalaureate Enrollment 95
Women 96% **Men** 4% **Minority** 1% **Part-time** 3%

Nursing Student Activities Student Nurses' Association.

Nursing Student Resources Academic advising; academic or career counseling; bookstore; campus computer network; career placement assistance; computer lab; e-mail services; employment services for current students; externships; housing assistance; interactive nursing skills videos; Internet; learning resource lab; library services; nursing audiovisuals; placement services for program completers; remedial services; resume preparation assistance; skills, simulation, or other laboratory; tutoring.

Library Facilities 80,888 volumes; 1,539 periodical subscriptions.

BACCALAUREATE PROGRAMS

Degree BSN

Available Programs Accelerated RN Baccalaureate; Generic Baccalaureate.

Study Options Full-time and part-time.

Program Entrance Requirements Minimum overall college GPA of 2.0, transcript of college record, CPR certification, written essay, health exam, health insurance, high school biology, high school chemistry, 2 years high school math, 2 years high school science, high school transcript, immunizations, 2 letters of recommendation, minimum high school GPA of 2.4, minimum high school rank 25%, minimum GPA in nursing prerequisites of 2.5, professional liability insurance/malpractice insurance, RN licensure. Transfer students are accepted. **Standardized tests** *Required:* SAT or ACT. *Recommended:* TOEFL for international students. **Application** *Deadline:* rolling (freshmen), rolling (transfer). *Notification:* continuous (freshmen). *Application fee:* $20.

Advanced Placement Credit given for nursing courses completed elsewhere dependent upon specific evaluations.

Expenses (2004–05) *Tuition:* full-time $15,986; part-time $500 per credit hour. *International tuition:* $15,986 full-time. *Room and board:* $5460; room only: $2700 per academic year. *Required fees:* full-time $1404; part-time $115 per term.

Financial Aid 90% of baccalaureate students in nursing programs received some form of financial aid in 2003–04. *Gift aid (need-based):* Federal Pell, FSEOG, state, private, college/university gift aid from institutional funds. *Loans:* FFEL (Subsidized and Unsubsidized Stafford PLUS), Perkins, college/university. *Work-Study:* Federal Work-Study, part-time campus jobs. *Application deadline:* Continuous.

Contact Dr. Johanne A. Quinn, Professor and Director, School of Nursing, School of Nursing, King College, 1350 King College Road, Bristol, TN 37620. *Telephone:* 423-652-4748. *Fax:* 423-652-4833. *E-mail:* jaquinn@king.edu.

Lincoln Memorial University

Department of Nursing
Harrogate, Tennessee

http://www.lmunet.edu/academics/undergrad/nursing/

Founded in 1897

DEGREE • BSN

Nursing Program Faculty 7 (57% with doctorates).

Nursing Student Activities Student Nurses' Association.

Nursing Student Resources Academic advising; academic or career counseling; bookstore; campus computer network; career placement assistance; computer lab; e-mail services; externships; interactive nursing skills videos; Internet; learning resource lab; library services; nursing audiovisuals; other; placement services for program completers; skills, simulation, or other laboratory; tutoring.

Library Facilities 145,537 volumes (1,230 in health, 630 in nursing); 251 periodical subscriptions (36 health-care related).

BACCALAUREATE PROGRAMS

Degree BSN

Available Programs RN Baccalaureate.

Site Options Knoxville, TN.

Program Entrance Requirements Minimum overall college GPA of 2.25, transcript of college record, CPR certification, immunizations, 3 letters of recommendation, professional liability insurance/malpractice insurance, prerequisite course work, RN licensure. Transfer students are accepted. **Standardized tests** *Required:* SAT or ACT, TOEFL for international students. **Application** *Deadline:* rolling (freshmen), rolling (transfer). *Application fee:* $25.

Advanced Placement Credit given for nursing courses completed elsewhere dependent upon specific evaluations.

Contact Admissions, Department of Nursing, Lincoln Memorial University, Cumberland Gap Parkway, Harrogate, TN 37752. *Telephone:* 423-869-3611. *Fax:* 423-869-6444. *E-mail:* admissions@lmunet.edu.

Middle Tennessee State University
School of Nursing
Murfreesboro, Tennessee

http://www.mtsu.edu/~nursing/

Founded in 1911

DEGREE • BSN

Nursing Student Activities Sigma Theta Tau, Student Nurses' Association.

Library Facilities 748,888 volumes; 4,144 periodical subscriptions.

BACCALAUREATE PROGRAMS

Degree BSN

Available Programs Generic Baccalaureate; RN Baccalaureate.

Program Entrance Requirements Minimum overall college GPA of 2.50, transcript of college record, minimum GPA in nursing prerequisites of 2.50, prerequisite course work. Transfer students are accepted. **Standardized tests** *Required:* SAT or ACT, TOEFL for international students. **Application** *Deadline:* 7/1 (freshmen), 7/1 (transfer). *Notification:* continuous (freshmen). *Application fee:* $25.

Advanced Placement Credit by examination available. Credit given for nursing courses completed elsewhere dependent upon specific evaluations.

Contact Dr. Pamela G. Holder, RN, Director, School of Nursing, Middle Tennessee State University, PO Box 81, 1301 East Main Street, Murfreesboro, TN 37132-0001. *Telephone:* 615-898-2437. *Fax:* 615-898-5441. *E-mail:* pgholder@mtsu.edu.

CONTINUING EDUCATION PROGRAM

Contact Continuing Studies and Public Service Office, School of Nursing, Middle Tennessee State University, Murfreesboro, TN 37132. *Telephone:* 615-898-2462. *Fax:* 615-898-3593. *E-mail:* learn@mtsu.edu.

Southern Adventist University
School of Nursing
Collegedale, Tennessee

Founded in 1892

DEGREES • BS • MSN • MSN/MBA

Nursing Program Faculty 17 (35% with doctorates).

Baccalaureate Enrollment 350
Women 80% **Men** 20%

Graduate Enrollment 30
Women 98% **Men** 2%

Nursing Student Activities Sigma Theta Tau.

Nursing Student Resources Academic advising; academic or career counseling; assistance for students with disabilities; bookstore; campus computer network; computer lab; computer-assisted instruction; e-mail services; employment services for current students; housing assistance; interactive nursing skills videos; Internet; learning resource lab; library services; nursing audiovisuals; remedial services; resume preparation assistance; skills, simulation, or other laboratory; tutoring.

Library Facilities 139,200 volumes (335 in nursing); 10,479 periodical subscriptions (174 health-care related).

BACCALAUREATE PROGRAMS

Degree BS

Available Programs ADN to Baccalaureate.

Study Options Full-time and part-time.

Program Entrance Requirements Minimum overall college GPA of 2.8, transcript of college record, CPR certification, health exam, high school chemistry, high school transcript, immunizations, 2 letters of recommendation, minimum GPA in nursing prerequisites of 2.8, prerequisite course work. Transfer students are accepted. **Standardized tests** *Required:* SAT and SAT Subject Tests or ACT, TOEFL for international students. **Application** *Deadline:* rolling (freshmen), rolling (transfer). *Notification:* continuous (freshmen). *Application fee:* $25.

Advanced Placement Credit given for nursing courses completed elsewhere dependent upon specific evaluations.

Expenses (2003–04) *Tuition:* full-time $12,400; part-time $525 per contact hour. *Room and board:* $4280; room only: $2289 per academic year. *Required fees:* full-time $1500.

Financial Aid 80% of baccalaureate students in nursing programs received some form of financial aid in 2002–03. *Gift aid (need-based):* Federal Pell, FSEOG, state, private, college/university gift aid from institutional funds. *Loans:* Federal Nursing Student Loans, FFEL (Subsidized and Unsubsidized Stafford PLUS), Perkins, college/university. *Work-Study:* Federal Work-Study, part-time campus jobs. *Application deadline (priority):* 3/31.

Contact Mrs. Linda Marlowe, Admissions and Progressions Coordinator, School of Nursing, Southern Adventist University, PO Box 370, Collegedale, TN 37315-0370. *Telephone:* 423-238-2941. *Fax:* 423-238-3004. *E-mail:* lmarlowe@southern.edu.

GRADUATE PROGRAMS

Contact Mrs. Linda Marlowe, Admissions and Progression Coordinator, School of Nursing, Southern Adventist University, PO Box 370, Collegedale, TN 37315-0370. *Telephone:* 423-238-2940. *Fax:* 423-238-3004. *E-mail:* lmarlowe@southern.edu.

MASTER'S DEGREE PROGRAM

Degrees MSN; MSN/MBA

Available Programs Accelerated RN to Master's; Master's.

Concentrations Available Nursing education. *Nurse practitioner programs in:* adult health, family health.

Study Options Full-time and part-time.

Program Entrance Requirements Clinical experience, minimum overall college GPA of 3.0, transcript of college record, CPR certification, written essay, immunizations, interview, 2 letters of recommendation, prerequisite course work.

Advanced Placement Credit given for nursing courses completed elsewhere dependent upon specific evaluations.

Degree Requirements 51 total credit hours, thesis or project.

CONTINUING EDUCATION PROGRAM

Contact Mrs. Linda Marlowe, Admissions and Progression Coordinator, School of Nursing, Southern Adventist University, PO Box 370, Collegedale, TN 37315-0370. *Telephone:* 423-238-2940. *Fax:* 423-238-3004. *E-mail:* lmarlowe@southern.edu.

Tennessee State University
School of Nursing
Nashville, Tennessee

http://www.tnstate.edu/nurs
Founded in 1912

DEGREES • BSN • MSN

Nursing Program Faculty 37 (50% with doctorates).

Baccalaureate Enrollment 100
Women 95% **Men** 5% **Minority** 75% **International** 1%

Graduate Enrollment 17
Women 97% **Men** 3% **Minority** 85% **International** 2% **Part-time** 20%

Nursing Student Activities Nursing Honor Society, Sigma Theta Tau, Student Nurses' Association.

Nursing Student Resources Academic advising; academic or career counseling; assistance for students with disabilities; bookstore; campus computer network; computer lab; e-mail services; interactive nursing skills videos; Internet; learning resource lab; library services; nursing audiovisuals; tutoring.

Library Facilities 580,650 volumes (50,000 in health, 25,000 in nursing); 300 periodical subscriptions health-care related.

BACCALAUREATE PROGRAMS

Degree BSN

Available Programs Generic Baccalaureate; RN Baccalaureate.

Site Options *Distance Learning:* Nashville, TN.

Study Options Full-time and part-time.

Program Entrance Requirements Minimum overall college GPA of 2.5, transcript of college record, CPR certification, health exam, health insurance, immunizations, minimum GPA in nursing prerequisites of 2.5, professional liability insurance/malpractice insurance, prerequisite course work. Transfer students are accepted. **Standardized tests** *Required:* SAT or ACT, TOEFL for international students. **Application** *Deadline:* 8/1 (freshmen), 8/1 (transfer). *Notification:* continuous until 8/15 (freshmen). *Application fee:* $15.

Financial Aid 60% of baccalaureate students in nursing programs received some form of financial aid in 2002–03. *Gift aid (need-based):* Federal Pell, FSEOG, state, private, college/university gift aid from institutional funds. *Loans:* Federal Direct (Subsidized and Unsubsidized Stafford), FFEL (Subsidized and Unsubsidized Stafford PLUS), Perkins, college/university. *Work-Study:* Federal Work-Study, part-time campus jobs. *Application deadline (priority):* 4/1.

Contact Dr. Yvonne N. Stringfield, RN, BSN Program Director, School of Nursing, Tennessee State University, 3500 John A. Merritt Boulevard, Box 9590, Nashville, TN 37209-1561. *Telephone:* 615-963-7615. *Fax:* 615-963-5593. *E-mail:* ystringfield@tnstate.edu.

GRADUATE PROGRAMS

Financial Aid 75% of graduate students in nursing programs received some form of financial aid in 2002–03. 2 teaching assistantships (averaging $5,924 per year) were awarded.

Contact Dr. Barbara E. Brown, MSN Program Director, School of Nursing, Tennessee State University, 3500 John A. Merritt Boulevard, Box 9590, Nashville, TN 37209-1561. *Telephone:* 615-963-5261. *Fax:* 615-963-7614. *E-mail:* bbrown@tnstate.edu.

MASTER'S DEGREE PROGRAM

Degree MSN

Concentrations Available *Nurse practitioner programs in:* family health.

Study Options Full-time and part-time.

Program Entrance Requirements Clinical experience, computer literacy, minimum overall college GPA of 3.0, transcript of college record, CPR certification, written essay, immunizations, interview, 2 letters of recommendation, physical assessment course, professional liability insurance/malpractice insurance, resume, statistics course, GRE General Test or MAT. *Application deadline:* Applications are processed on a rolling basis. *Application fee:* $15.

Advanced Placement Credit given for nursing courses completed elsewhere dependent upon specific evaluations.

Degree Requirements 43 total credit hours, comprehensive exam.

POST-MASTER'S PROGRAM

Areas of Study *Nurse practitioner programs in:* family health.

CONTINUING EDUCATION PROGRAM

Contact Dr. Mary Ella Graham, RN, Dean, School of Nursing, Tennessee State University, 3500 John A. Merritt Boulevard, Box 9590, Nashville, TN 37209-1561. *Telephone:* 615-963-5254. *Fax:* 615-963-5049. *E-mail:* mgraham1@tnstate.edu.

Tennessee Technological University
School of Nursing
Cookeville, Tennessee

http://www.tntech.edu/www/acad/nursing/
Founded in 1915

DEGREES • BSN • M SC N • MSN

Nursing Program Faculty 19 (16% with doctorates).

Baccalaureate Enrollment 96
Women 89% **Men** 11% **Minority** 1% **Part-time** 6%

Graduate Enrollment 5
Women 100% **Part-time** 100%

Nursing Student Activities Sigma Theta Tau, Student Nurses' Association.

Nursing Student Resources Academic advising; academic or career counseling; assistance for students with disabilities; bookstore; campus computer network; career placement assistance; computer lab; computer-assisted instruction; daycare for children of students; e-mail services; employment services for current students; externships; housing assistance; Internet; learning resource lab; library services; nursing audiovisuals; paid internships; placement services for program completers; remedial services; resume preparation assistance; skills, simulation, or other laboratory; tutoring; unpaid internships.

Library Facilities 640,056 volumes (312,892 in health, 11,893 in nursing); 4,847 periodical subscriptions (96 health-care related).

BACCALAUREATE PROGRAMS

Degree BSN

Available Programs Generic Baccalaureate; RN Baccalaureate.

Study Options Full-time.

Program Entrance Requirements Minimum overall college GPA of 2.5, transcript of college record, CPR certification, health exam, health insurance, high school biology, high school chemistry, high school foreign language, 3 years high school math, 2 years high school science, high school transcript, immunizations, minimum GPA in nursing prerequisites of 2.0, professional liability insurance/malpractice insurance, prerequisite course work. Transfer students are accepted. **Standardized tests** *Required:* SAT or ACT, TOEFL for international students. *Recommended:* ACT. **Application** *Deadline:* 8/1 (freshmen), 8/1 (transfer). *Notification:* continuous (freshmen). *Application fee:* $15.

Advanced Placement Credit given for nursing courses completed elsewhere dependent upon specific evaluations.

Expenses (2004–05) *Tuition, state resident:* full-time $1999; part-time $189 per credit hour. *Tuition, nonresident:* full-time $6243; part-time $557 per credit hour. *Room and board:* $4275; room only: $2735 per academic year. *Required fees:* full-time $838; part-time $416 per term.

Financial Aid 85% of baccalaureate students in nursing programs received some form of financial aid in 2003–04. *Gift aid (need-based):* Federal Pell, FSEOG, state, private, college/university gift aid from institutional funds, United Negro College Fund. *Loans:* Federal Direct (Subsidized and Unsubsidized Stafford), FFEL, Perkins, college/university. *Work-Study:* Federal Work-Study, part-time campus jobs. *Application deadline (priority):* 3/15.

Contact Ms. Becky L. Hull, Academic Advisor, School of Nursing, Tennessee Technological University, PO Box 5001, 805 Quadrangle, Cookeville, TN 38505-0001. *Telephone:* 931-372-3203. *Fax:* 931-372-6244. *E-mail:* nursing@tntech.edu.

GRADUATE PROGRAMS

Expenses (2004–05) *Tuition, state resident:* part-time $297 per credit hour. *Tuition, nonresident:* part-time $665 per credit hour. *Room and board:* room only: $3150 per academic year.

Contact Dr. Marilyn J. Musacchio, Dean and Professor, School of Nursing, Tennessee Technological University, PO Box 5001, 80 West 8th Street, Cookeville, TN 38505-0001. *Telephone:* 931-372-3213. *Fax:* 931-372-6533. *E-mail:* mmusacchio@tntech.edu.

MASTER'S DEGREE PROGRAM

Degrees M Sc N; MSN

Available Programs Master's.

Concentrations Available Nursing education. *Nurse practitioner programs in:* family health.

Study Options Full-time and part-time.

Program Entrance Requirements Computer literacy, transcript of college record, CPR certification, immunizations, 3 letters of recommendation, professional liability insurance/malpractice insurance, resume.

Advanced Placement Credit given for nursing courses completed elsewhere dependent upon specific evaluations.

Degree Requirements 44 total credit hours, thesis or project.

Tennessee Wesleyan College

Fort Sanders Nursing Department
Knoxville, Tennessee

http://www.twcnet.edu/academics/nursing

Founded in 1857

DEGREE • BSN

Nursing Program Faculty 12 (33% with doctorates).

Baccalaureate Enrollment 85

Women 91% **Men** 9% **Minority** 1% **Part-time** 4%

Nursing Student Activities Nursing Honor Society, Student Nurses' Association.

Nursing Student Resources Academic advising; bookstore; computer lab; Internet; library services; nursing audiovisuals; skills, simulation, or other laboratory.

Library Facilities 79,328 volumes (6,000 in health, 4,000 in nursing); 825 periodical subscriptions (175 health-care related).

BACCALAUREATE PROGRAMS

Degree BSN

Available Programs ADN to Baccalaureate; Generic Baccalaureate; RN Baccalaureate.

Site Options Knoxville, TN.

Study Options Full-time and part-time.

Program Entrance Requirements Minimum overall college GPA of 2.7, transcript of college record, CPR certification, written essay, health exam, high school transcript, immunizations, interview, prerequisite course work. Transfer students are accepted. **Standardized tests** *Required:* SAT or ACT. *Recommended:* TOEFL for international students. **Application** *Deadline:* rolling (freshmen), rolling (transfer). *Notification:* continuous (freshmen). *Application fee:* $25.

Advanced Placement Credit given for nursing courses completed elsewhere dependent upon specific evaluations.

Expenses (2004–05) *Tuition:* full-time $13,200; part-time $550 per credit hour.

Financial Aid 92% of baccalaureate students in nursing programs received some form of financial aid in 2003–04.

Contact Fort Sanders Nursing Department, Tennessee Wesleyan College, 9821 Cogdill Road, Suite 2, Knoxville, TN 37932. *Telephone:* 865-777-5100. *Fax:* 865-777-5114.

Union University

School of Nursing
Jackson, Tennessee

http://www.uu.edu/academics/son/

Founded in 1823

DEGREES • BSN • MSN

Nursing Program Faculty 20 (40% with doctorates).

Baccalaureate Enrollment 252

Women 91% **Men** 9% **Minority** 23% **International** 2% **Part-time** 46%

Graduate Enrollment 37

Women 100% **Minority** 50% **Part-time** 16%

Nursing Student Activities Nursing Honor Society, Sigma Theta Tau, Student Nurses' Association.

Nursing Student Resources Academic advising; academic or career counseling; assistance for students with disabilities; bookstore; campus computer network; career placement assistance; computer-assisted instruction; e-mail services; employment services for current students; housing assistance; Internet; library services; nursing audiovisuals; resume preparation assistance; skills, simulation, or other laboratory; tutoring.

Library Facilities 135,877 volumes (6,005 in nursing); 4,655 periodical subscriptions (1,284 health-care related).

BACCALAUREATE PROGRAMS

Degree BSN

Available Programs Accelerated Baccalaureate for Second Degree; Generic Baccalaureate; LPN to Baccalaureate; RN Baccalaureate.

Site Options Germantown, TN.

Study Options Full-time.

Program Entrance Requirements Minimum overall college GPA of 2.5, transcript of college record, CPR certification, health exam, immunizations, minimum GPA in nursing prerequisites of 2.5, prerequisite course work. Transfer students are accepted. **Standardized tests** *Required:* SAT or ACT, TOEFL for international students. *Recommended:* SAT Subject Tests. **Application** *Deadline:* rolling (freshmen), rolling (transfer). *Early decision:* 12/1. *Notification:* continuous until 8/1 (freshmen), 12/15 (early action). *Application fee:* $25.

Advanced Placement Credit by examination available. Credit given for nursing courses completed elsewhere dependent upon specific evaluations.

Expenses (2004–05) *Tuition:* full-time $14,850; part-time $495 per credit hour. *International tuition:* $14,850 full-time. *Room and board:* $2600; room only: $1550 per academic year. *Required fees:* full-time $1500; part-time $175 per credit; part-time $275 per term.

Financial Aid 70% of baccalaureate students in nursing programs received some form of financial aid in 2003–04. *Gift aid (need-based):* Federal Pell, FSEOG, state, private, college/university gift aid from institutional funds. *Loans:* FFEL (Subsidized and Unsubsidized Stafford PLUS), Perkins, college/university, alternative loans. *Work-Study:* Federal Work-Study, part-time campus jobs. *Application deadline (priority):* 1/15.

Contact Paula Karnes, Administrative Assistant, School of Nursing, Union University, 1050 Union University Drive, Jackson, TN 38305. *Telephone:* 731-661-5200. *Fax:* 731-661-5504. *E-mail:* pkarnes@uu.edu.

GRADUATE PROGRAMS

Expenses (2004–05) *Tuition:* full-time $10,890; part-time $330 per credit hour. *International tuition:* $10,890 full-time. *Room and board:* $2600; room only: $1550 per academic year. *Required fees:* full-time $130.

Financial Aid 100% of graduate students in nursing programs received some form of financial aid in 2003–04. Traineeships available.

Contact Dr. Nancy Dayton, Director of the Master of Science in Nursing Program, School of Nursing, Union University, 1050 Union University Drive, Jackson, TN 38305. *Telephone:* 901-759-0029 Ext. 105. *Fax:* 731-661-5504. *E-mail:* ndayton@uu.edu.

Union University (continued)

MASTER'S DEGREE PROGRAM

Degree MSN

Available Programs Master's.

Concentrations Available Nursing administration; nursing education.

Site Options Germantown, TN.

Study Options Full-time and part-time.

Program Entrance Requirements Transcript of college record, CPR certification, immunizations, interview, 3 letters of recommendation, professional liability insurance/malpractice insurance, statistics course, GRE. *Application deadline:* For fall admission, 8/1 (priority date). Applications are processed on a rolling basis. *Application fee:* $25.

Advanced Placement Credit given for nursing courses completed elsewhere dependent upon specific evaluations.

Degree Requirements 38 total credit hours, thesis or project.

CONTINUING EDUCATION PROGRAM

Contact Joyce M. Henderson, Associate Professor, School of Nursing, Union University, 1050 Union University Drive, Jackson, TN 38305. *Telephone:* 731-661-5236. *Fax:* 731-661-5504. *E-mail:* jhenders@uu.edu.

The University of Memphis

Loewenberg School of Nursing
Memphis, Tennessee

http://www.nursing.memphis.edu

Founded in 1912

DEGREES • BSN • MSN

Nursing Program Faculty 49 (47% with doctorates).

Baccalaureate Enrollment 348

Women 80% **Men** 20% **Minority** 28% **International** 1% **Part-time** 10%

Graduate Enrollment 110

Women 80% **Men** 20% **Minority** 30%

Nursing Student Activities Sigma Theta Tau, Student Nurses' Association.

Nursing Student Resources Academic advising; academic or career counseling; assistance for students with disabilities; bookstore; campus computer network; career placement assistance; computer lab; computer-assisted instruction; daycare for children of students; e-mail services; externships; housing assistance; interactive nursing skills videos; Internet; learning resource lab; library services; nursing audiovisuals; paid internships; remedial services; resume preparation assistance; skills, simulation, or other laboratory; tutoring.

Library Facilities 1.1 million volumes (74,513 in health); 15,643 periodical subscriptions (878 health-care related).

BACCALAUREATE PROGRAMS

Degree BSN

Available Programs ADN to Baccalaureate; Accelerated Baccalaureate; Accelerated Baccalaureate for Second Degree; Accelerated RN Baccalaureate; Baccalaureate for Second Degree; Generic Baccalaureate; LPN to Baccalaureate; RN Baccalaureate.

Site Options *Distance Learning:* Jackson, TN.

Study Options Full-time and part-time.

Program Entrance Requirements Minimum overall college GPA of 2.5, transcript of college record, CPR certification, health exam, high school biology, high school chemistry, high school foreign language, 3 years high school math, 2 years high school science, high school transcript, immunizations, minimum high school GPA of 3.0, minimum GPA in nursing prerequisites of 2.4, prerequisite course work. Transfer students are accepted. **Standardized tests** *Required:* SAT or ACT, TOEFL for international students. **Application** *Deadline:* 8/1 (freshmen), 8/1 (transfer). *Notification:* continuous (freshmen). *Application fee:* $15.

Advanced Placement Credit by examination available. Credit given for nursing courses completed elsewhere dependent upon specific evaluations.

Financial Aid 53% of baccalaureate students in nursing programs received some form of financial aid in 2003–04.

Contact Ms. Sheila Hall, Assistant Dean for Student Affairs, Loewenberg School of Nursing, The University of Memphis, 105 Newport Hall, Memphis, TN 38152. *Telephone:* 901-678-2003. *Fax:* 901-678-4906. *E-mail:* shall@memphis.edu.

GRADUATE PROGRAMS

Expenses (2004–05) *Tuition, state resident:* full-time $5450; part-time $297 per credit hour. *Tuition, nonresident:* full-time $14,174; part-time $661 per credit hour. *Room and board:* $8592; room only: $4440 per academic year.

Contact Dr. Robert Koch, RN, Director of Graduate Program, Loewenberg School of Nursing, The University of Memphis, 203 Newport Hall, Memphis, TN 38152. *Telephone:* 901-678-2003. *Fax:* 901-678-4906. *E-mail:* rakoch@memphis.edu.

MASTER'S DEGREE PROGRAM

Degree MSN

Available Programs Accelerated Master's for Nurses with Non-Nursing Degrees; Master's; Master's for Non-Nursing College Graduates; Master's for Nurses with Non-Nursing Degrees.

Concentrations Available Nursing administration; nursing education. *Nurse practitioner programs in:* family health.

Site Options *Distance Learning:* Jackson, TN.

Study Options Full-time and part-time.

Program Entrance Requirements Minimum overall college GPA of 2.8, CPR certification, immunizations, 3 letters of recommendation, professional liability insurance/malpractice insurance.

Advanced Placement Credit given for nursing courses completed elsewhere dependent upon specific evaluations.

Degree Requirements 45 total credit hours, comprehensive exam.

The University of Tennessee

College of Nursing
Knoxville, Tennessee

http://www.nightingale.con.utk.edu

Founded in 1794

DEGREES • BSN • MSN • PHD

Nursing Program Faculty 50 (56% with doctorates).

Baccalaureate Enrollment 249

Women 90% **Men** 10% **Minority** 7% **International** 1% **Part-time** 8%

Graduate Enrollment 151

Women 85% **Men** 15% **Minority** 3% **International** 1% **Part-time** 27%

Nursing Student Activities Sigma Theta Tau, Student Nurses' Association.

Nursing Student Resources Academic advising; academic or career counseling; assistance for students with disabilities; bookstore; campus computer network; computer lab; computer-assisted instruction; e-mail services; employment services for current students; externships; interactive nursing skills videos; Internet; learning resource lab; library services; nursing audiovisuals; remedial services; skills, simulation, or other laboratory; tutoring.

Library Facilities 24.4 million volumes (59,214 in health, 3,711 in nursing); 17,628 periodical subscriptions (572 health-care related).

BACCALAUREATE PROGRAMS

Degree BSN

Available Programs Accelerated RN Baccalaureate; Generic Baccalaureate.

Study Options Full-time and part-time.

Program Entrance Requirements Minimum overall college GPA of 2.5, transcript of college record, CPR certification, health exam, health insurance, immunizations, professional liability insurance/malpractice insurance, prerequisite course work. Transfer students are accepted. **Standardized tests** *Required:* SAT or ACT, TOEFL for international students.

Application *Deadline:* 2/1 (freshmen), 6/1 (transfer). *Early decision:* 11/1. *Notification:* continuous (freshmen), 1/15 (early action). *Application fee:* $25.

Advanced Placement Credit by examination available. Credit given for nursing courses completed elsewhere dependent upon specific evaluations.

Expenses (2004–05) *Tuition, state resident:* full-time $4086; part-time $171 per credit hour. *Tuition, nonresident:* full-time $13,866; part-time $568 per credit hour. *International tuition:* $13,866 full-time. *Room and board:* $9592; room only: $4080 per academic year. *Required fees:* full-time $662; part-time $29 per credit.

Financial Aid 50% of baccalaureate students in nursing programs received some form of financial aid in 2003–04. *Gift aid (need-based):* Federal Pell, FSEOG, state, private, college/university gift aid from institutional funds, Federal Nursing. *Loans:* FFEL (Subsidized and Unsubsidized Stafford PLUS), Perkins, college/university. *Work-Study:* Federal Work-Study, part-time campus jobs. *Application deadline (priority):* 3/1.

Contact Director, Student Services, College of Nursing, The University of Tennessee, 1200 Volunteer Boulevard, Knoxville, TN 37996-4180. *Telephone:* 865-974-7606. *Fax:* 865-974-3569. *E-mail:* bbarret@utk.edu.

GRADUATE PROGRAMS

Expenses (2004–05) *Tuition, state resident:* full-time $4714; part-time $262 per credit hour. *Tuition, nonresident:* full-time $15,754; part-time $792 per credit hour. *International tuition:* $15,754 full-time. *Room and board:* room only: $4800 per academic year. *Required fees:* full-time $642; part-time $46 per credit.

Financial Aid 75% of graduate students in nursing programs received some form of financial aid in 2003–04. 3 fellowships, 1 research assistantship were awarded; teaching assistantships, Federal Work-Study, institutionally sponsored loans, and unspecified assistantships also available. *Financial aid application deadline:* 2/1.

Contact Dr. Sandra L. McGuire, Chair, Masters Program, College of Nursing, The University of Tennessee, 1200 Volunteer Boulevard, Knoxville, TN 37996-4180. *Telephone:* 865-974-4151. *Fax:* 865-974-3569. *E-mail:* smcguire@utk.edu.

MASTER'S DEGREE PROGRAM

Degree MSN

Available Programs Accelerated Master's for Nurses with Non-Nursing Degrees; Accelerated RN to Master's; Master's; Master's for Non-Nursing College Graduates; Master's for Nurses with Non-Nursing Degrees; RN to Master's.

Concentrations Available Nurse anesthesia; nursing administration. *Clinical nurse specialist programs in:* adult health, gerontology, maternity-newborn, pediatric, perinatal, psychiatric/mental health, women's health. *Nurse practitioner programs in:* family health, gerontology, neonatal health, pediatric, primary care, psychiatric/mental health, women's health.

Study Options Full-time.

Program Entrance Requirements Minimum overall college GPA of 3.0, transcript of college record, CPR certification, written essay, immunizations, 3 letters of recommendation, nursing research course, physical assessment course, professional liability insurance/malpractice insurance, prerequisite course work, statistics course, GRE General Test. *Application deadline:* For fall admission, 2/1 (priority date). Applications are processed on a rolling basis. *Application fee:* $35.

Advanced Placement Credit by examination available. Credit given for nursing courses completed elsewhere dependent upon specific evaluations.

Degree Requirements 41 total credit hours, thesis or project, comprehensive exam.

POST-MASTER'S PROGRAM

Areas of Study Nurse anesthesia; nursing administration; nursing education. *Clinical nurse specialist programs in:* adult health, gerontology, maternity-newborn, pediatric, perinatal, psychiatric/mental health, women's health. *Nurse practitioner programs in:* family health, gerontology, neonatal health, pediatric, psychiatric/mental health, women's health.

DOCTORAL DEGREE PROGRAM

Degree PhD

Available Programs Doctorate; Post-Baccalaureate Doctorate.

Areas of Study Bio-behavioral research, biology of health and illness, family health, health promotion/disease prevention, human health and illness, individualized study, neuro-behavior, nursing administration, nursing education, nursing research, nursing science, women's health.

Program Entrance Requirements Minimum overall college GPA of 3.0, interview by faculty committee, interview, 3 letters of recommendation, writing sample, GRE General Test. *Application deadline:* For fall admission, 2/1 (priority date). Applications are processed on a rolling basis. *Application fee:* $35.

Degree Requirements 67 total credit hours, dissertation, oral exam, written exam, residency.

CONTINUING EDUCATION PROGRAM

Contact Dr. Maureen Nalle, Coordinator, Continuing Education, College of Nursing, The University of Tennessee, 1200 Volunteer Boulevard, Knoxville, TN 37996-4180. *Telephone:* 865-974-7598. *Fax:* 865-974-3569. *E-mail:* mnalle@utk.edu.

The University of Tennessee at Chattanooga

School of Nursing
Chattanooga, Tennessee

http://www.utc.edu/~utcnurse/index.htm

Founded in 1886

DEGREES • BSN • MSN

Nursing Program Faculty 25 (65% with doctorates).

Baccalaureate Enrollment 350
Women 85% **Men** 15% **Minority** 12% **Part-time** 5%

Graduate Enrollment 70
Women 60% **Men** 40% **Minority** 20% **Part-time** 30%

Nursing Student Activities Sigma Theta Tau, Student Nurses' Association.

Nursing Student Resources Academic advising; academic or career counseling; assistance for students with disabilities; bookstore; campus computer network; computer lab; e-mail services; interactive nursing skills videos; Internet; learning resource lab; nursing audiovisuals; skills, simulation, or other laboratory.

Library Facilities 491,179 volumes (19,370 in health, 3,100 in nursing); 1,847 periodical subscriptions (200 health-care related).

BACCALAUREATE PROGRAMS

Degree BSN

Available Programs ADN to Baccalaureate; Baccalaureate for Second Degree; Generic Baccalaureate.

Study Options Full-time.

Program Entrance Requirements Minimum overall college GPA of 2.5, transcript of college record, CPR certification, health exam, health insurance, high school foreign language, 3 years high school math, high school transcript, immunizations, 2 letters of recommendation, minimum high school GPA of 2.0, minimum GPA in nursing prerequisites of 2.5, professional liability insurance/malpractice insurance, prerequisite course work. Transfer students are accepted. **Standardized tests** *Required:* SAT or ACT, TOEFL for international students. **Application** *Notification:* continuous (freshmen). *Application fee:* $25.

Advanced Placement Credit by examination available. Credit given for nursing courses completed elsewhere dependent upon specific evaluations.

Expenses (2004–05) *Tuition, state resident:* full-time $4050; part-time $170 per credit hour. *Tuition, nonresident:* full-time $13,300; part-time $515 per credit hour. *Room and board:* room only: $1700 per academic year. *Required fees:* full-time $125.

Financial Aid 60% of baccalaureate students in nursing programs received some form of financial aid in 2003–04.

Contact Dr. Katherine Russell Lindgren, RN, Director, School of Nursing, School of Nursing, The University of Tennessee at Chattanooga, 615 McCallie Avenue, Department 1051, Chattanooga, TN 37403-2598. *Telephone:* 423-425-4750. *Fax:* 423-425-4668. *E-mail:* Kay-Lindgren@utc.edu.

The University of Tennessee at Chattanooga (continued)

GRADUATE PROGRAMS

Expenses (2004–05) *Tuition, state resident:* full-time $4725; part-time $250 per credit hour. *Tuition, nonresident:* full-time $13,000; part-time $715 per credit hour. *Room and board:* room only: $1700 per academic year. *Required fees:* full-time $150.

Financial Aid 70% of graduate students in nursing programs received some form of financial aid in 2003–04. *Application deadline:* 4/1.

Contact Dr. Katherine Russell Lindgren, RN, Coordinator, School of Nursing, The University of Tennessee at Chattanooga, 615 McCallie Avenue, Department 1051, Chattanooga, TN 37403-2598. *Telephone:* 423-425-4750. *Fax:* 423-425-4668. *E-mail:* Kay-Lindgren@utc.edu.

MASTER'S DEGREE PROGRAM

Degree MSN

Available Programs Master's.

Concentrations Available Nurse anesthesia. *Nurse practitioner programs in:* family health.

Site Options Tupelo, MS.

Study Options Full-time and part-time.

Program Entrance Requirements Clinical experience, computer literacy, minimum overall college GPA of 3.0, transcript of college record, CPR certification, written essay, immunizations, interview, 3 letters of recommendation, nursing research course, physical assessment course, resume, statistics course, GRE General Test. *Application deadline:* For fall admission, 8/1 (priority date); for spring admission, 12/1 (priority date). Applications are processed on a rolling basis. *Application fee:* $25.

Advanced Placement Credit given for nursing courses completed elsewhere dependent upon specific evaluations.

Degree Requirements 50 total credit hours, thesis or project.

POST-MASTER'S PROGRAM

Areas of Study Nurse anesthesia. *Nurse practitioner programs in:* family health.

CONTINUING EDUCATION PROGRAM

Contact Dr. Katherine Russell Lindgren, RN, Acting Director, School of Nursing, The University of Tennessee at Chattanooga, 615 McCallie Avenue, Department 1051, Chattanooga, TN 37403-2598. *Telephone:* 423-425-4750. *Fax:* 423-425-4668. *E-mail:* Kay-Lindgren@utc.edu.

The University of Tennessee at Martin

Department of Nursing
Martin, Tennessee

http://www.utm.edu

Founded in 1900

DEGREE • BSN

Nursing Program Faculty 14 (14% with doctorates).

Baccalaureate Enrollment 176

Women 93% **Men** 7% **Minority** 10% **Part-time** 19%

Nursing Student Activities Nursing Honor Society, Sigma Theta Tau, Student Nurses' Association, nursing club.

Nursing Student Resources Academic advising; academic or career counseling; assistance for students with disabilities; bookstore; campus computer network; career placement assistance; computer lab; computer-assisted instruction; daycare for children of students; e-mail services; employment services for current students; housing assistance; interactive nursing skills videos; Internet; learning resource lab; library services; nursing audiovisuals; resume preparation assistance; skills, simulation, or other laboratory; tutoring.

Library Facilities 621,025 volumes (4,945 in health, 1,440 in nursing); 1,994 periodical subscriptions (8,326 health-care related).

BACCALAUREATE PROGRAMS

Degree BSN

Available Programs ADN to Baccalaureate; Accelerated RN Baccalaureate; Generic Baccalaureate; LPN to RN Baccalaureate.

Site Options Jackson, TN.

Study Options Full-time.

Program Entrance Requirements Minimum overall college GPA of 2.0, transcript of college record, CPR certification, health exam, health insurance, high school biology, high school chemistry, high school foreign language, 3 years high school math, 2 years high school science, high school transcript, immunizations, interview, minimum high school GPA of 2.8, minimum GPA in nursing prerequisites of 2.0, professional liability insurance/malpractice insurance, prerequisite course work. Transfer students are accepted. **Standardized tests** *Required:* SAT or ACT, TOEFL for international students. **Application** *Deadline:* rolling (freshmen), rolling (transfer). *Notification:* continuous until 8/1 (freshmen). *Application fee:* $25.

Advanced Placement Credit by examination available. Credit given for nursing courses completed elsewhere dependent upon specific evaluations.

Expenses (2004–05) *Tuition, state resident:* full-time $3412; part-time $176 per credit hour. *Tuition, nonresident:* full-time $8254; part-time $520 per credit hour. *Room and board:* $1960 per academic year. *Required fees:* full-time $900.

Financial Aid 79% of baccalaureate students in nursing programs received some form of financial aid in 2003–04. *Gift aid (need-based):* Federal Pell, FSEOG, state, private. *Loans:* FFEL (Subsidized and Unsubsidized Stafford PLUS), Perkins. *Work-Study:* Federal Work-Study. *Application deadline (priority):* 3/1.

Contact Mrs. Brenda W. Campbell, Program Resource Specialist, Department of Nursing, The University of Tennessee at Martin, Gooch Hall 136J, Martin, TN 38238. *Telephone:* 731-881-7138. *Fax:* 731-881-7939. *E-mail:* brendac@utm.edu.

CONTINUING EDUCATION PROGRAM

Contact Dr. Nancy A. Warren, Professor and Chair, Department of Nursing, The University of Tennessee at Martin, Gooch Hall 136H, Martin, TN 38238. *Telephone:* 731-881-7140. *Fax:* 731-881-7140. *E-mail:* nwarren@utm.edu.

The University of Tennessee Health Science Center

College of Nursing
Memphis, Tennessee

http://www.utmem.edu/nursing

Founded in 1911

DEGREES • BSN • MSN • PHD

Nursing Program Faculty 30 (100% with doctorates).

Graduate Enrollment 164

Women 85% **Men** 15% **Minority** 22%

Nursing Student Activities Sigma Theta Tau, Student Nurses' Association.

Nursing Student Resources Academic advising; academic or career counseling; assistance for students with disabilities; bookstore; campus computer network; computer lab; computer-assisted instruction; e-mail services; Internet; learning resource lab; library services; nursing audiovisuals; paid internships; remedial services; skills, simulation, or other laboratory; tutoring.

Library Facilities 165,200 volumes (194,185 in health, 2,746 in nursing); 1,784 periodical subscriptions (1,852 health-care related).

BACCALAUREATE PROGRAMS

Degree BSN

Available Programs ADN to Baccalaureate; Accelerated Baccalaureate; Accelerated Baccalaureate for Second Degree; Accelerated RN Baccalaureate; Baccalaureate for Second Degree; Generic Baccalaureate; RN Baccalaureate.

Site Options *Distance Learning:* Memphis, TN.

Study Options Full-time.

Program Entrance Requirements Minimum overall college GPA of 3.0, transcript of college record, CPR certification, written essay, health insurance, high school transcript, immunizations, 3 letters of recommendation, minimum GPA in nursing prerequisites of 3.0, prerequisite course work, RN licensure. Transfer students are accepted. **Application** *Application fee:* $25.

Advanced Placement Credit given for nursing courses completed elsewhere dependent upon specific evaluations.

Expenses (2004–05) *Tuition, state resident:* full-time $6840. *Tuition, nonresident:* full-time $22,720.

Financial Aid *Gift aid (need-based):* Federal Pell, FSEOG, state, private, college/university gift aid from institutional funds, Department of Health and Human Services Scholarships. *Loans:* Federal Nursing Student Loans, FFEL (Subsidized and Unsubsidized Stafford PLUS), Perkins, college/university, Federal Health Professions Student Loans, alternative loans. *Work-Study:* Federal Work-Study. *Application deadline (priority):* 2/28.

Contact Mr. Ron Patterson, Assistant Director, Admissions, College of Nursing, The University of Tennessee Health Science Center, 877 Madison Avenue, Suite 637, Memphis, TN 38163. *Telephone:* 901-448-1769. *Fax:* 901-448-4121. *E-mail:* rpatte10@utmem.edu.

GRADUATE PROGRAMS

Expenses (2004–05) *Tuition, state resident:* full-time $7482. *Tuition, nonresident:* full-time $17,642.

Financial Aid 52% of graduate students in nursing programs received some form of financial aid in 2003–04. Fellowships with partial tuition reimbursements available, teaching assistantships, Federal Work-Study, institutionally sponsored loans, scholarships, and traineeships available. Aid available to part-time students. *Financial aid application deadline:* 2/28.

Contact Dr. Carolyn Graff, Assistant Dean, Student Affairs, College of Nursing, The University of Tennessee Health Science Center, 877 Madison Avenue, Suite 637, Memphis, TN 38163. *Telephone:* 901-448-6139. *Fax:* 901-448-4121. *E-mail:* cgraff@utmem.edu.

MASTER'S DEGREE PROGRAM

Degree MSN

Available Programs Master's; RN to Master's.

Concentrations Available Nurse anesthesia; nursing administration. *Clinical nurse specialist programs in:* acute care, critical care, psychiatric/mental health. *Nurse practitioner programs in:* acute care, family health, neonatal health, primary care, psychiatric/mental health.

Site Options *Distance Learning:* Memphis, TN.

Study Options Full-time.

Program Entrance Requirements Clinical experience, computer literacy, minimum overall college GPA of 3.0, transcript of college record, CPR certification, written essay, immunizations, interview, 3 letters of recommendation, professional liability insurance/malpractice insurance, prerequisite course work, GRE General Test. *Application deadline:* For fall admission, 2/1; for winter admission, 9/1. *Application fee:* $50.

Degree Requirements 46 total credit hours.

POST-MASTER'S PROGRAM

Areas of Study Nurse anesthesia; nurse-midwifery; nursing administration. *Clinical nurse specialist programs in:* acute care, critical care, psychiatric/mental health, public health. *Nurse practitioner programs in:* acute care, family health, neonatal health, primary care, psychiatric/mental health.

DOCTORAL DEGREE PROGRAM

Degree PhD

Available Programs Doctorate.

Areas of Study Clinical practice, critical care, health promotion/disease prevention, human health and illness, nursing research, nursing science.

Site Options *Distance Learning:* Memphis, TN.

Program Entrance Requirements Clinical experience, minimum overall college GPA of 3.0, interview by faculty committee, 3 letters of recommendation, MSN or equivalent, writing sample. *Application deadline:* For fall admission, 2/1; for winter admission, 9/1. *Application fee:* $50.

Degree Requirements 60 total credit hours, dissertation.

CONTINUING EDUCATION PROGRAM

Contact Dr. Cynthia Russell, Director, Distributive Programs, College of Nursing, The University of Tennessee Health Science Center, 877 Madison Avenue, Suite 645, Memphis, TN 38163. *Telephone:* 901-448-6424. *Fax:* 901-448-4121. *E-mail:* crussell@utmem.edu.

Vanderbilt University
School of Nursing
Nashville, Tennessee

http://www.mc.vanderbilt.edu/nursing/

Founded in 1873

DEGREES • MSN • MSN/MBA • PHD

Nursing Program Faculty 145 (20% with doctorates).

Graduate Enrollment 456

Women 91% **Men** 9% **Minority** 12% **International** 1% **Part-time** 10%

Nursing Student Activities Sigma Theta Tau.

Nursing Student Resources Academic advising; assistance for students with disabilities; bookstore; campus computer network; career placement assistance; computer lab; computer-assisted instruction; daycare for children of students; e-mail services; housing assistance; Internet; library services; nursing audiovisuals; remedial services; resume preparation assistance; skills, simulation, or other laboratory.

Library Facilities 1.8 million volumes (210,000 in health); 26,885 periodical subscriptions (2,810 health-care related).

■ Vanderbilt University School of Nursing (VUSN) offers a Master of Science in Nursing (MSN) program with multiple-entry options: entry with a non-nursing degree or as a college senior, with an associate degree in nursing, with a diploma in nursing, or with a baccalaureate degree in nursing. VUSN considers the present educational status of each student and incorporates it into an accelerated and highly specialized program that meets individual learning needs. There is even an entry option for students who already have an MSN degree but who want a role change or role expansion. At Vanderbilt, faculty members are committed to the tradition of enhancing the quality of health-care delivery. VUSN's vast selection of nursing specialties allows the School of Nursing to shape the careers of advanced practice nurses today in order to create professional excellence in the health-care leaders of tomorrow.

GRADUATE PROGRAMS

Expenses (2004–05) *Tuition:* full-time $31,590; part-time $810 per quarter hour. *Required fees:* full-time $900.

Financial Aid 94% of graduate students in nursing programs received some form of financial aid in 2003–04. Federal Work-Study, institutionally sponsored loans, and traineeships available. Aid available to part-time students. *Financial aid application deadline:* 3/15.

Contact Ms. Karen Stevens, Director of Student Recruitment, School of Nursing, Vanderbilt University, 229C Godchaux Hall, Nashville, TN 37240. *Telephone:* 615-322-3800. *Fax:* 615-343-0333. *E-mail:* karen.stevens@vanderbilt.edu.

MASTER'S DEGREE PROGRAM

Degrees MSN; MSN/MBA

Available Programs Accelerated AD/RN to Master's; Accelerated Master's; Accelerated Master's for Non-Nursing College Graduates; Accelerated Master's for Nurses with Non-Nursing Degrees; Accelerated RN to Master's.

Concentrations Available Health-care administration; nurse-midwifery; nursing administration; nursing informatics. *Clinical nurse specialist programs in:* acute care, cardiovascular, gerontology, maternity-newborn, pediatric, women's health. *Nurse practitioner programs in:* acute care, adult health, family health, gerontology, neonatal health, pediatric, psychiatric/mental health, women's health.

Vanderbilt University (continued)
Site Options *Distance Learning:* Nashville, TN.

Study Options Full-time and part-time.

Program Entrance Requirements Computer literacy, minimum overall college GPA of 3.0, transcript of college record, CPR certification, written essay, immunizations, 3 letters of recommendation, physical assessment course, prerequisite course work, statistics course, GRE. *Application deadline:* For fall admission, 12/1 (priority date). *Application fee:* $50.

Advanced Placement Credit by examination available. Credit given for nursing courses completed elsewhere dependent upon specific evaluations.

Degree Requirements 39 total credit hours.

POST-MASTER'S PROGRAM

Areas of Study Health-care administration; nurse-midwifery; nursing administration; nursing informatics. *Clinical nurse specialist programs in:* acute care, cardiovascular, gerontology, maternity-newborn, pediatric, women's health. *Nurse practitioner programs in:* acute care, adult health, family health, gerontology, neonatal health, pediatric, psychiatric/mental health, women's health.

DOCTORAL DEGREE PROGRAM

Degree PhD

Available Programs Doctorate.

Areas of Study Addiction/substance abuse, advanced practice nursing, aging, bio-behavioral research, biology of health and illness, community health, critical care, family health, gerontology, health policy, health promotion/disease prevention, health-care systems, human health and illness, illness and transition, information systems, maternity-newborn, nursing administration, nursing policy, nursing research, nursing science, oncology, women's health.

Program Entrance Requirements interview by faculty committee, interview, 3 letters of recommendation, MSN or equivalent, statistics course, vita, writing sample, GRE General Test. *Application deadline:* For fall admission, 12/1 (priority date). *Application fee:* $50.

Degree Requirements 72 total credit hours, dissertation, oral exam, written exam, residency.

POSTDOCTORAL PROGRAM

Areas of Study Individualized study.

Postdoctoral Program Contact Ms. Melanie Lutenbacher, PhD, Director, School of Nursing, Vanderbilt University, Vanderbilt University School of Nursing, 226 Godchaux Hall, Nashville, TN 37240. *Telephone:* 615-343-8977. *Fax:* 615-343-0333. *E-mail:* melanie.lutenbacher@vanderbilt.edu.

CONTINUING EDUCATION PROGRAM

Contact Ms. Ginny Moore, Director of Lifelong Learning, School of Nursing, Vanderbilt University, School of Nursing, 461 21st Avenue, South, Nashville, TN 37240. *Telephone:* 615-343-8493. *Fax:* 615-322-8816. *E-mail:* ginny.moore@vanderbilt.edu.

See full description on page 588.

TEXAS

Abilene Christian University
Abilene Intercollegiate School of Nursing
Abilene, Texas

See description of programs under Abilene Intercollegiate School of Nursing (Abilene, Texas).

Abilene Intercollegiate School of Nursing
Abilene Intercollegiate School of Nursing
Abilene, Texas

http://www.aisn.edu/

DEGREES • BSN • MSN

Nursing Program Faculty 15 (33% with doctorates).

Baccalaureate Enrollment 130
Women 92% **Men** 8% **Minority** 10% **International** 4%

Graduate Enrollment 20
Women 75% **Men** 25% **Minority** 10%

Nursing Student Activities Nursing Honor Society, Sigma Theta Tau, Student Nurses' Association.

Nursing Student Resources Academic advising; academic or career counseling; assistance for students with disabilities; bookstore; campus computer network; career placement assistance; computer lab; computer-assisted instruction; e-mail services; employment services for current students; externships; interactive nursing skills videos; Internet; learning resource lab; library services; nursing audiovisuals; remedial services; resume preparation assistance; skills, simulation, or other laboratory; tutoring.

Library Facilities 9,147 volumes in health, 1,295 volumes in nursing; 156 periodical subscriptions health-care related.

BACCALAUREATE PROGRAMS

Degree BSN

Available Programs Generic Baccalaureate; RN Baccalaureate.

Study Options Full-time.

Program Entrance Requirements Minimum overall college GPA of 2.75, transcript of college record, CPR certification, written essay, health exam, health insurance, immunizations, interview, 3 letters of recommendation, minimum GPA in nursing prerequisites of 3.0, professional liability insurance/malpractice insurance, prerequisite course work. Transfer students are accepted.

Advanced Placement Credit by examination available. Credit given for nursing courses completed elsewhere dependent upon specific evaluations.

Expenses (2004–05) *Tuition:* full-time $23,000; part-time $385 per credit hour. *International tuition:* $23,000 full-time.

Financial Aid 80% of baccalaureate students in nursing programs received some form of financial aid in 2003–04.

Contact Mr. Brent Wallace, Academic Advisor/Director of Marketing, Abilene Intercollegiate School of Nursing, 2149 Hickory Street, Abilene, TX 79601. *Telephone:* 325-672-2441. *Fax:* 325-672-5026. *E-mail:* aisnadv@abilene.com.

GRADUATE PROGRAMS

Expenses (2004–05) *Tuition:* part-time $425 per credit hour.

Financial Aid 50% of graduate students in nursing programs received some form of financial aid in 2003–04.

Contact Dr. Amy Roberts, Director of the Graduate Program, Abilene Intercollegiate School of Nursing, 2149 Hickory Street, Abilene, TX 79601. *Telephone:* 325-672-2441. *Fax:* 325-672-5026. *E-mail:* aroberts@hsutx.edu.

MASTER'S DEGREE PROGRAM

Degree MSN

Available Programs Master's.

Concentrations Available Nursing administration; nursing education. *Nurse practitioner programs in:* family health.

Site Options *Distance Learning:* North Wales, PA.

Study Options Full-time and part-time.

Program Entrance Requirements Clinical experience, minimum overall college GPA of 3.5, transcript of college record, CPR certification, written essay, immunizations, interview, 3 letters of recommendation, physical assessment course, professional liability insurance/malpractice insurance, resume, statistics course.

Advanced Placement Credit given for nursing courses completed elsewhere dependent upon specific evaluations.

Degree Requirements 49 total credit hours, thesis or project.

POST-MASTER'S PROGRAM

Areas of Study *Nurse practitioner programs in:* family health.

CONTINUING EDUCATION PROGRAM

Contact Dr. Janet K. Noles, Dean and Associate Professor, Abilene Intercollegiate School of Nursing, 2149 Hickory Street, Abilene, TX 79601. *Telephone:* 325-672-2441 Ext. 17. *Fax:* 325-672-5026. *E-mail:* jnoles@hsutx.edu.

Angelo State University

Department of Nursing
San Angelo, Texas

http://www.angelo.edu/dept/nur/

Founded in 1928

DEGREES • BSN • MSN

Nursing Program Faculty 20 (35% with doctorates).

Baccalaureate Enrollment 70
Women 87% **Men** 13% **Minority** 10% **Part-time** 71%

Graduate Enrollment 23
Women 74% **Men** 26% **Minority** 22% **Part-time** 39%

Nursing Student Activities Student Nurses' Association.

Nursing Student Resources Academic advising; academic or career counseling; bookstore; campus computer network; computer lab; computer-assisted instruction; e-mail services; housing assistance; interactive nursing skills videos; Internet; learning resource lab; library services; nursing audiovisuals; skills, simulation, or other laboratory; tutoring.

Library Facilities 481,826 volumes (7,560 in health, 762 in nursing); 1,628 periodical subscriptions (390 health-care related).

BACCALAUREATE PROGRAMS

Degree BSN

Available Programs RN Baccalaureate.

Study Options Full-time and part-time.

Program Entrance Requirements Minimum overall college GPA of 2.5, transcript of college record, CPR certification, immunizations, 3 letters of recommendation. Transfer students are accepted. **Standardized tests** *Required:* SAT or ACT, TOEFL for international students. **Application** *Deadline:* 8/1 (freshmen), 8/1 (transfer). *Notification:* continuous (freshmen). *Application fee:* $20.

Expenses (2003–04) *Tuition, state resident:* full-time $2500; part-time $174 per contact hour. *Tuition, nonresident:* full-time $7600; part-time $358 per contact hour. *Room and board:* $4500 per academic year. *Required fees:* full-time $30.

Financial Aid 15% of baccalaureate students in nursing programs received some form of financial aid in 2002–03.

Contact Dr. Molly Allison, Level Director, BSN Program, Department of Nursing, Angelo State University, PO Box 10902, San Angelo, TX 76909. *Telephone:* 915-942-2224 Ext. 259. *Fax:* 915-942-2236. *E-mail:* molly.allison@angelo.edu.

GRADUATE PROGRAMS

Financial Aid 15% of graduate students in nursing programs received some form of financial aid in 2002–03. Fellowships with full and partial tuition reimbursements available, career-related internships or fieldwork, Federal Work-Study, and scholarships available. Aid available to part-time students. *Financial aid application deadline:* 8/1.

Contact Dr. Susan Wilkinson, Graduate Adviser, MSN Program, Department of Nursing, Angelo State University, PO Box 10902, San Angelo, TX 76909. *Telephone:* 915-942-2224. *Fax:* 915-942-2236. *E-mail:* susan.wilkinson@angelo.edu.

MASTER'S DEGREE PROGRAM

Degree MSN

Available Programs Master's.

Concentrations Available Nursing education. *Clinical nurse specialist programs in:* adult health, medical-surgical.

Study Options Full-time and part-time.

Program Entrance Requirements Computer literacy, minimum overall college GPA of 3.0, transcript of college record, 2 letters of recommendation, physical assessment course, statistics course, GRE General Test. *Application deadline:* For fall admission, 7/15 (priority date); for spring admission, 12/8. Applications are processed on a rolling basis. *Application fee:* $25 ($50 for international students).

Advanced Placement Credit given for nursing courses completed elsewhere dependent upon specific evaluations.

Degree Requirements 46 total credit hours, comprehensive exam.

Baylor University

Louise Herrington School of Nursing of Baylor University
Dallas, Texas

http://www.baylor.edu/Nursing

Founded in 1845

DEGREES • BSN • MSN

Nursing Program Faculty 45 (40% with doctorates).

Baccalaureate Enrollment 269
Women 82% **Men** 18% **Minority** 22%

Graduate Enrollment 47
Women 87% **Men** 13% **Minority** 6% **International** 2% **Part-time** 50%

Nursing Student Activities Sigma Theta Tau, Student Nurses' Association.

Nursing Student Resources Academic advising; campus computer network; computer lab; e-mail services; housing assistance; interactive nursing skills videos; Internet; learning resource lab; library services; nursing audiovisuals; skills, simulation, or other laboratory.

Library Facilities 2.3 million volumes (6,000 in health, 5,000 in nursing); 8,429 periodical subscriptions (106 health-care related).

■ Baylor University's Louise Herrington School of Nursing offers BSN and MSN programs in a caring, Christian environment. Low student-teacher ratios allow participatory classroom learning. Clinical instruction is enhanced through access to premier health-care facilities and strong collaboration with health-care providers. Graduates of the BSN program perform well on NCLEX-RN examinations. Graduate programs include advanced nursing leadership, family nurse practitioner (FNP), and neonatal nurse practitioner (NNP). Graduates of the FNP and NNP perform well on national certification examinations. Detailed information about programs can be found on the Web at http://www.baylor.edu/Nursing.

BACCALAUREATE PROGRAMS

Degree BSN

Available Programs Generic Baccalaureate.

Study Options Full-time.

Program Entrance Requirements Minimum overall college GPA of 2.75, transcript of college record, CPR certification, written essay, health exam, immunizations, 3 letters of recommendation, minimum GPA in nursing prerequisites of 2.75, prerequisite course work. Transfer students are accepted. **Standardized tests** *Required:* SAT or ACT, TOEFL for international students. **Application** *Deadline:* rolling (freshmen), rolling (transfer). *Notification:* continuous (freshmen). *Application fee:* $35.

Baylor University (continued)

Advanced Placement Credit given for nursing courses completed elsewhere dependent upon specific evaluations.

Expenses (2004–05) *Tuition:* full-time $17,900; part-time $8950 per semester. *Room and board:* $3336; room only: $3100 per academic year. *Required fees:* full-time $1980.

Financial Aid 91% of baccalaureate students in nursing programs received some form of financial aid in 2003–04.

Contact Miss Tina Sims, Academic Advisor, Louise Herrington School of Nursing of Baylor University, Baylor University, 3700 Worth Street, Dallas, TX 75246. *Telephone:* 214-214-4151. *Fax:* 214-820-3835. *E-mail:* Tina_Sims@baylor.edu.

GRADUATE PROGRAMS

Expenses (2004–05) *Tuition:* full-time $17,900; part-time $8950 per semester. *International tuition:* $19,000 full-time. *Required fees:* full-time $1980.

Financial Aid 100% of graduate students in nursing programs received some form of financial aid in 2003–04.

Contact Dr. Pauline Johnson, Director, Graduate Program, Louise Herrington School of Nursing of Baylor University, Baylor University, 3700 Worth Street, Dallas, TX 75246. *Telephone:* 214-820-3361. *Fax:* 214-820-4770. *E-mail:* pauline_johnson@baylor.edu.

MASTER'S DEGREE PROGRAM

Degree MSN

Available Programs Master's; RN to Master's.

Concentrations Available Nursing administration. *Nurse practitioner programs in:* family health, neonatal health.

Site Options *Distance Learning:* Waco, TX.

Study Options Full-time and part-time.

Program Entrance Requirements Clinical experience, minimum overall college GPA of 3.0, transcript of college record, CPR certification, written essay, immunizations, 3 letters of recommendation, prerequisite course work, statistics course, GRE General Test. *Application deadline:* For fall admission, 8/1; for spring admission, 12/1. Applications are processed on a rolling basis. *Application fee:* $25.

Advanced Placement Credit given for nursing courses completed elsewhere dependent upon specific evaluations.

Degree Requirements 45 total credit hours.

POST-MASTER'S PROGRAM

Areas of Study *Nurse practitioner programs in:* family health, neonatal health.

East Texas Baptist University
Department of Nursing
Marshall, Texas

http://www.etbu.edu

Founded in 1912

DEGREE • BSN

Nursing Program Faculty 5.

Baccalaureate Enrollment 47
Women 90% **Men** 10% **Minority** 22%

Nursing Student Activities Student Nurses' Association, nursing club.

Nursing Student Resources Academic advising; academic or career counseling; assistance for students with disabilities; bookstore; campus computer network; career placement assistance; computer lab; computer-assisted instruction; e-mail services; housing assistance; interactive nursing skills videos; Internet; learning resource lab; library services; nursing audiovisuals; placement services for program completers; remedial services; resume preparation assistance; skills, simulation, or other laboratory; tutoring.

Library Facilities 116,895 volumes (568 in health, 291 in nursing); 668 periodical subscriptions (2,100 health-care related).

BACCALAUREATE PROGRAMS

Degree BSN

Available Programs Generic Baccalaureate; RN Baccalaureate.

Study Options Full-time and part-time.

Program Entrance Requirements Minimum overall college GPA of 2.8, transcript of college record, CPR certification, written essay, health exam, health insurance, immunizations, interview, 2 letters of recommendation, minimum GPA in nursing prerequisites of 2.8, professional liability insurance/malpractice insurance, prerequisite course work. Transfer students are accepted. **Standardized tests** *Required:* SAT or ACT, TOEFL for international students. **Application** *Deadline:* rolling (freshmen), rolling (transfer). *Notification:* continuous (freshmen). *Application fee:* $25.

Expenses (2004–05) *Tuition:* full-time $6000; part-time $300 per credit hour. *International tuition:* $6000 full-time. *Room and board:* $2500; room only: $1500 per academic year. *Required fees:* full-time $800; part-time $200 per term.

Financial Aid 99% of baccalaureate students in nursing programs received some form of financial aid in 2003–04. *Gift aid (need-based):* Federal Pell, FSEOG, state, private, college/university gift aid from institutional funds. *Loans:* FFEL (Subsidized and Unsubsidized Stafford PLUS), Perkins, state, college/university. *Work-Study:* Federal Work-Study, part-time campus jobs. *Application deadline (priority):* 6/1.

Contact Dr. Carolyn Harvey, Dean, Department of Nursing, East Texas Baptist University, 1209 North Grove Street, Marshall, TX 75670-1498. *Telephone:* 903-923-2210. *Fax:* 903-938-9225. *E-mail:* charvey@etbu.edu.

CONTINUING EDUCATION PROGRAM

Contact Dr. Carolyn Harvey, Dean, Department of Nursing, East Texas Baptist University, 1209 North Grove Street, Marshall, TX 75670-1498. *Telephone:* 903-923-2210. *Fax:* 903-938-9225. *E-mail:* charvey@etbu.edu.

Hardin-Simmons University
Abilene Intercollegiate School of Nursing
Abilene, Texas

See description of programs under Abilene Intercollegiate School of Nursing (Abilene, Texas).

Houston Baptist University
College of Nursing
Houston, Texas

Founded in 1960

DEGREE • BSN

Nursing Program Faculty 23 (6% with doctorates).

Baccalaureate Enrollment 60
Women 90% **Men** 10% **Minority** 20% **International** 10%

Nursing Student Activities Nursing Honor Society, Sigma Theta Tau, Student Nurses' Association.

Nursing Student Resources Academic advising; academic or career counseling; assistance for students with disabilities; bookstore; career placement assistance; computer lab; e-mail services; employment services for current students; externships; housing assistance; interactive nursing skills videos; Internet; learning resource lab; library services; nursing audiovisuals; paid internships; placement services for program completers; remedial services; resume preparation assistance; skills, simulation, or other laboratory; tutoring; unpaid internships.

Library Facilities 209,366 volumes (4,276 in health, 1,200 in nursing); 21,000 periodical subscriptions (117 health-care related).

BACCALAUREATE PROGRAMS

Degree BSN

Site Options Houston, TX.

Study Options Full-time.

Program Entrance Requirements Minimum overall college GPA of 2.5, minimum GPA in nursing prerequisites of 2.5. Transfer students are accepted. **Standardized tests** *Required:* SAT or ACT, TOEFL for international students. **Application** *Deadline:* rolling (freshmen), rolling (transfer). *Notification:* continuous (freshmen). *Application fee:* $25.

Advanced Placement Credit by examination available.

Expenses (2003–04) *Tuition:* part-time $370 per credit hour.

Financial Aid 60% of baccalaureate students in nursing programs received some form of financial aid in 2002–03.

Contact Dr. Nancy Yuill, Dean, College of Nursing, Houston Baptist University, 7502 Fondren Street, Houston, TX 77074. *Telephone:* 281-649-3300. *Fax:* 281-649-3340. *E-mail:* nyuill@hbu.edu.

Lamar University
Department of Nursing
Beaumont, Texas

http://dept.lamar.edu/nursing/

Founded in 1923

DEGREES • BSN • MSN

Nursing Program Faculty 32 (22% with doctorates).

Baccalaureate Enrollment 216
Women 82% **Men** 18% **Minority** 30% **International** 1% **Part-time** 1%

Graduate Enrollment 17
Women 58% **Men** 42% **Minority** 25% **Part-time** 83%

Nursing Student Activities Sigma Theta Tau, Student Nurses' Association.

Nursing Student Resources Academic advising; academic or career counseling; assistance for students with disabilities; bookstore; campus computer network; career placement assistance; computer lab; computer-assisted instruction; daycare for children of students; e-mail services; employment services for current students; housing assistance; interactive nursing skills videos; Internet; learning resource lab; library services; nursing audiovisuals; placement services for program completers; remedial services; resume preparation assistance; skills, simulation, or other laboratory; tutoring; unpaid internships.

Library Facilities 698,285 volumes (6,825 in health, 1,800 in nursing); 2,900 periodical subscriptions (199 health-care related).

BACCALAUREATE PROGRAMS

Degree BSN

Available Programs ADN to Baccalaureate; Generic Baccalaureate; RN Baccalaureate.

Study Options Full-time.

Program Entrance Requirements Minimum overall college GPA of 2.0, transcript of college record, CPR certification, immunizations, minimum GPA in nursing prerequisites of 2.0, professional liability insurance/malpractice insurance, prerequisite course work. Transfer students are accepted. **Standardized tests** *Required:* SAT or ACT, TOEFL for international students. *Required for some:* SAT Subject Tests. **Application** *Deadline:* 8/1 (freshmen), 8/1 (transfer). *Notification:* continuous (freshmen).

Advanced Placement Credit given for nursing courses completed elsewhere dependent upon specific evaluations.

Expenses (2004–05) *Tuition, state resident:* full-time $108; part-time $108 per credit hour. *Tuition, nonresident:* full-time $366; part-time $366 per credit hour. *International tuition:* $686 full-time. *Room and board:* $2552; room only: $1725 per academic year. *Required fees:* full-time $1345; part-time $135 per credit; part-time $426 per term.

Financial Aid 80% of baccalaureate students in nursing programs received some form of financial aid in 2003–04. *Gift aid (need-based):* Federal Pell, FSEOG, state, college/university gift aid from institutional funds. *Loans:* FFEL (Subsidized and Unsubsidized Stafford PLUS), Perkins, state, college/university. *Work-Study:* Federal Work-Study, part-time campus jobs. *Application deadline (priority):* 4/1.

Contact Ms. Christina Gushanas, Advisor, Department of Nursing, Lamar University, PO Box 10081, Beaumont, TX 77710. *Telephone:* 409-880-8868. *Fax:* 409-880-7736. *E-mail:* gushanascm@hal.lamar.edu.

GRADUATE PROGRAMS

Expenses (2004–05) *Tuition, state resident:* full-time $2961; part-time $542 per course. *Tuition, nonresident:* full-time $7641; part-time $1316 per course. *Room and board:* room only: $3400 per academic year.

Financial Aid 8% of graduate students in nursing programs received some form of financial aid in 2003–04.

Contact Dr. Nancy Bume, Director of Graduate Nursing Studies, Department of Nursing, Lamar University, PO Box 10081, Beaumont, TX 77710. *Telephone:* 409-880-7720. *Fax:* 409-880-8698. *E-mail:* nancy.blume@lamar.edu.

MASTER'S DEGREE PROGRAM

Degree MSN

Available Programs Master's.

Concentrations Available Health-care administration; nursing education.

Study Options Full-time and part-time.

Program Entrance Requirements Computer literacy, minimum overall college GPA of 3.0, transcript of college record, immunizations, professional liability insurance/malpractice insurance, prerequisite course work, statistics course.

Advanced Placement Credit given for nursing courses completed elsewhere dependent upon specific evaluations.

Degree Requirements 37 total credit hours, thesis or project, comprehensive exam.

CONTINUING EDUCATION PROGRAM

Contact Cindy Stinson, RN, Coordinator of Continuing Education, Department of Nursing, Lamar University, PO Box 10081, Beaumont, TX 77710. *Telephone:* 409-880-8831. *Fax:* 409-880-1865. *E-mail:* stinsonca@hal.lamar.edu.

Lubbock Christian University
Department of Nursing
Lubbock, Texas

Founded in 1957

DEGREE • BSN

Nursing Program Faculty 5 (40% with doctorates).

Library Facilities 113,556 volumes; 545 periodical subscriptions.

BACCALAUREATE PROGRAMS

Degree BSN

Available Programs RN Baccalaureate.

Study Options Part-time.

Program Entrance Requirements Minimum overall college GPA of 2.5, transcript of college record, CPR certification, health exam, immunizations, interview, 2 letters of recommendation, minimum high school GPA, minimum GPA in nursing prerequisites of 2.5, professional liability insurance/malpractice insurance, prerequisite course work, RN licensure. Transfer students are accepted. **Standardized tests** *Required:* SAT or ACT, TOEFL for international students. **Application** *Deadline:* 8/1 (freshmen), rolling (transfer). *Notification:* continuous (freshmen). *Application fee:* $20.

Contact Dr. Beverly Byers, Chair, Department of Nursing, Lubbock Christian University, 5601 West 19th Street, Lubbock, TX 79407. *E-mail:* nursing@lcu.edu.

McMurry University
Abilene Intercollegiate School of Nursing
Abilene, Texas

See description of programs under Abilene Intercollegiate School of Nursing (Abilene, Texas).

Midwestern State University
Nursing Program
Wichita Falls, Texas

Founded in 1922

DEGREES • BSN • MSN

Nursing Program Faculty 16 (22% with doctorates).

Baccalaureate Enrollment 250
Women 90% **Men** 10% **Minority** 25% **Part-time** 1%

Graduate Enrollment 42
Women 80% **Men** 20% **Minority** 83% **International** 13% **Part-time** 70%

Nursing Student Resources Housing assistance.

Library Facilities 484,106 volumes; 1,582 periodical subscriptions.

BACCALAUREATE PROGRAMS

Degree BSN

Available Programs Generic Baccalaureate; RN Baccalaureate.

Study Options Full-time and part-time.

Program Entrance Requirements Transcript of college record, CPR certification, health exam, health insurance, high school transcript, immunizations, minimum GPA in nursing prerequisites of 2.75, professional liability insurance/malpractice insurance, prerequisite course work. Transfer students are accepted. **Standardized tests** *Required:* SAT or ACT, TOEFL for international students. **Application** *Deadline:* 8/7 (freshmen), 8/7 (transfer). *Notification:* continuous until 8/31 (freshmen). *Application fee:* $25.

Advanced Placement Credit by examination available. Credit given for nursing courses completed elsewhere dependent upon specific evaluations.

Expenses (2003–04) *Tuition, state resident:* part-time $159 per credit hour. *Tuition, nonresident:* part-time $377 per credit hour.

Financial Aid 66% of baccalaureate students in nursing programs received some form of financial aid in 2002–03. *Gift aid (need-based):* Federal Pell, FSEOG, state, private, college/university gift aid from institutional funds. *Loans:* FFEL (Subsidized and Unsubsidized Stafford PLUS), Perkins, state, college/university. *Work-Study:* Federal Work-Study, part-time campus jobs. *Application deadline (priority):* 5/1.

Contact Dr. Deborah Ruth Garrison, Chair, Nursing Program, Midwestern State University, 3410 Taft Boulevard, Wichita Falls, TX 76308. *Telephone:* 940-397-4599. *Fax:* 940-397-4513. *E-mail:* deborah.garrison@mwsu.edu.

GRADUATE PROGRAMS

Expenses (2003–04) *Tuition, state resident:* part-time $169 per credit hour. *Tuition, nonresident:* part-time $387 per credit hour.

Financial Aid 100% of graduate students in nursing programs received some form of financial aid in 2002–03. Career-related internships or fieldwork, Federal Work-Study, institutionally sponsored loans, scholarships, and unspecified assistantships available. Aid available to part-time students. *Financial aid application deadline:* 5/1.

Contact Dr. Deborah Ruth Garrison, Chair, Nursing Program, Midwestern State University, 3410 Taft Boulevard, Wichita Falls, TX 76308. *Telephone:* 940-397-4599. *Fax:* 940-397-4513. *E-mail:* deborah.garrison@mwsu.edu.

MASTER'S DEGREE PROGRAM

Degree MSN

Concentrations Available Health-care administration; nursing administration; nursing education. *Nurse practitioner programs in:* family health.

Study Options Full-time and part-time.

Program Entrance Requirements Clinical experience, minimum overall college GPA of 3.0, transcript of college record, immunizations, interview, 3 letters of recommendation, physical assessment course, statistics course, GRE General Test. *Application deadline:* For fall admission, 7/1; for spring admission, 11/1. Applications are processed on a rolling basis. *Application fee:* $35 ($50 for international students).

Degree Requirements 36 total credit hours, thesis or project.

POST-MASTER'S PROGRAM

Areas of Study Nursing education. *Nurse practitioner programs in:* family health.

CONTINUING EDUCATION PROGRAM

Contact Betty Bowles, Coordinator, Professional Outreach Center, Nursing Program, Midwestern State University, 3410 Taft Boulevard, Wichita Falls, TX 76308. *Telephone:* 940-397-4048. *Fax:* 940-397-4513. *E-mail:* betty.bowles@mwsu.edu.

Prairie View A&M University
College of Nursing
Houston, Texas

http://acad.pvamu.edu/content/nursing/

Founded in 1878

DEGREES • BSN • MSN

Nursing Program Faculty 40.

Nursing Student Activities Nursing Honor Society, Sigma Theta Tau, Student Nurses' Association, nursing club.

Nursing Student Resources Academic advising; bookstore; campus computer network; computer lab; e-mail services; learning resource lab; nursing audiovisuals; skills, simulation, or other laboratory.

Library Facilities 347,477 volumes (109 in nursing); 25,911 periodical subscriptions.

BACCALAUREATE PROGRAMS

Degree BSN

Available Programs Generic Baccalaureate; RN Baccalaureate.

Site Options *Distance Learning:* Huntsville, TX; Woodlands, TX; College Station, TX.

Study Options Full-time and part-time.

Program Entrance Requirements Minimum overall college GPA of 2.5, transcript of college record, CPR certification, health exam, immunizations, minimum GPA in nursing prerequisites of 2.0, professional liability insurance/malpractice insurance, prerequisite course work. Transfer students are accepted. **Standardized tests** *Required:* SAT or ACT, TOEFL for international students. **Application** *Deadline:* 6/1 (freshmen), 6/1 (transfer). *Notification:* continuous (freshmen). *Application fee:* $25.

Advanced Placement Credit given for nursing courses completed elsewhere dependent upon specific evaluations.

Contact Dr. Elsa Tansey, Director, College of Nursing, Prairie View A&M University, 1801 Main Street, Suite 801, Houston, TX 77002. *Telephone:* 713-797-7023. *Fax:* 713-797-7013. *E-mail:* elsa_tansey@pvamu.edu.

GRADUATE PROGRAMS

Financial Aid Career-related internships or fieldwork, Federal Work-Study, institutionally sponsored loans, scholarships, and traineeships available.

Contact Dr. Chloe Gaines, Director, College of Nursing, Prairie View A&M University, 1801 Main Street, Suite 1002, Houston, TX 77002. *Telephone:* 713-797-7003. *Fax:* 713-797-7012. *E-mail:* chloe_gaines@pvamu.edu.

MASTER'S DEGREE PROGRAM

Degree MSN

Available Programs Master's.

Concentrations Available *Nurse practitioner programs in:* family health.

Study Options Full-time and part-time.

Program Entrance Requirements Clinical experience, minimum overall college GPA of 2.75, transcript of college record, 3 letters of recommendation, physical assessment course, prerequisite course work, resume, statistics course, MAT or GRE. *Application deadline:* For fall admission, 4/1 (priority date); for spring admission, 7/1 (priority date). Applications are processed on a rolling basis. *Application fee:* $50.

Advanced Placement Credit by examination available. Credit given for nursing courses completed elsewhere dependent upon specific evaluations.

Degree Requirements 53 total credit hours.

Southwestern Adventist University

Department of Nursing
Keene, Texas

Founded in 1894

DEGREE • BS

Nursing Program Faculty 12 (25% with doctorates).

Baccalaureate Enrollment 23
Women 83% **Men** 17% **Minority** 56% **International** 17% **Part-time** 25%

Nursing Student Activities Nursing Honor Society, Sigma Theta Tau.

Nursing Student Resources Academic advising; academic or career counseling; assistance for students with disabilities; bookstore; campus computer network; computer lab; computer-assisted instruction; e-mail services; interactive nursing skills videos; Internet; learning resource lab; library services; nursing audiovisuals; remedial services; skills, simulation, or other laboratory; tutoring.

Library Facilities 108,481 volumes (6,575 in nursing); 457 periodical subscriptions (60 health-care related).

BACCALAUREATE PROGRAMS

Degree BS

Available Programs ADN to Baccalaureate; RN Baccalaureate.

Program Entrance Requirements Transfer students are accepted. **Standardized tests** *Required:* SAT or ACT, TOEFL for international students. **Application** *Deadline:* 8/31 (freshmen), 8/31 (transfer). *Notification:* 9/1 (freshmen).

Expenses (2003–04) *Tuition:* part-time $420 per credit hour. *Room and board:* $5300; room only: $2160 per academic year. *Required fees:* part-time $100 per term.

Financial Aid 60% of baccalaureate students in nursing programs received some form of financial aid in 2002–03. *Gift aid (need-based):* Federal Pell, FSEOG, state, private, college/university gift aid from institutional funds. *Loans:* FFEL (Subsidized and Unsubsidized Stafford PLUS), Perkins, state. *Work-Study:* Federal Work-Study, part-time campus jobs. *Application deadline (priority):* 4/1.

Contact Dr. Penny Moore, RN, Chair, Baccalaureate Faculty and Curriculum, Department of Nursing, Southwestern Adventist University, Keene, TX 76059. *Telephone:* 817-645-3921 Ext. 519. *Fax:* 817-556-4713. *E-mail:* moorep@swau.edu.

CONTINUING EDUCATION PROGRAM

Contact Dr. Penny Moore, RN, Chair, Department of Nursing, Southwestern Adventist University, PO Box 567, Keene, TX 76059. *Telephone:* 817-645-3921 Ext. 235. *Fax:* 817-556-4774. *E-mail:* moorep@swau.edu.

Stephen F. Austin State University

Division of Nursing
Nacogdoches, Texas

http://www.fp.sfasu.edu/nursing/

Founded in 1923

DEGREE • BSN

Nursing Program Faculty 19 (16% with doctorates).

Baccalaureate Enrollment 128
Women 96% **Men** 4% **Minority** 1%

Nursing Student Activities Sigma Theta Tau, Student Nurses' Association.

Nursing Student Resources Academic advising; academic or career counseling; bookstore; computer lab; computer-assisted instruction; e-mail services; interactive nursing skills videos; Internet; library services; nursing audiovisuals; skills, simulation, or other laboratory; tutoring.

Library Facilities 2,791 periodical subscriptions.

BACCALAUREATE PROGRAMS

Degree BSN

Available Programs RN Baccalaureate.

Site Options Lufkin, TX.

Study Options Full-time.

Program Entrance Requirements Minimum overall college GPA of 2.75, transcript of college record, CPR certification, health insurance, high school transcript, immunizations, minimum GPA in nursing prerequisites of 2.5, professional liability insurance/malpractice insurance, prerequisite course work. Transfer students are accepted. **Standardized tests** *Required:* SAT or ACT, TOEFL for international students. **Application** *Deadline:* rolling (freshmen). *Notification:* continuous (freshmen). *Application fee:* $25.

Advanced Placement Credit given for nursing courses completed elsewhere dependent upon specific evaluations.

Expenses (2004–05) *Tuition, state resident:* full-time $3032; part-time $48 per credit hour. *Tuition, nonresident:* full-time $8696; part-time $282 per credit hour. *International tuition:* $14,500 full-time. *Room and board:* $2382 per academic year. *Required fees:* full-time $50.

Contact Dr. Glenda C. Walker, Director, Division of Nursing, Stephen F. Austin State University, SFA Box 6156, Nacogdoches, TX 75962. *Telephone:* 936-468-3604. *Fax:* 936-468-1696.

Tarleton State University

Department of Nursing
Stephenville, Texas

http://www.tarleton.edu/~nursing

Founded in 1899

DEGREE • BSN

Nursing Program Faculty 14 (21% with doctorates).

Baccalaureate Enrollment 212
Women 94% **Men** 6% **Minority** 5% **Part-time** 25%

Nursing Student Activities Nursing Honor Society, Student Nurses' Association.

Nursing Student Resources Academic advising; academic or career counseling; assistance for students with disabilities; bookstore; computer lab; computer-assisted instruction; daycare for children of students; e-mail services; employment services for current students; externships; learning resource lab; library services; nursing audiovisuals; remedial services; resume preparation assistance; skills, simulation, or other laboratory; tutoring; unpaid internships.

Library Facilities 320,302 volumes; 1,150 periodical subscriptions.

BACCALAUREATE PROGRAMS

Degree BSN

Available Programs ADN to Baccalaureate; Generic Baccalaureate; LPN to Baccalaureate.

Site Options *Distance Learning:* Brownwood, TX; Killeen, TX.

Study Options Full-time and part-time.

Program Entrance Requirements Transcript of college record, CPR certification, written essay, health exam, high school transcript, immunizations, 3 letters of recommendation, minimum GPA in nursing prerequisites of 2.5, professional liability insurance/malpractice insurance, prerequisite course work. Transfer students are accepted. **Standardized tests** *Required:* SAT or ACT, TOEFL for international students. **Application** *Deadline:* 6/1 (freshmen), 6/1 (transfer). *Early decision:* 11/30. *Application fee:* $25.

Tarleton State University (continued)

Advanced Placement Credit by examination available. Credit given for nursing courses completed elsewhere dependent upon specific evaluations.

Expenses (2003–04) *Tuition, state resident:* full-time $2225. *Tuition, nonresident:* full-time $8125. *Room and board:* $4774; room only: $2780 per academic year. *Required fees:* full-time $900.

Financial Aid 62% of baccalaureate students in nursing programs received some form of financial aid in 2002–03. *Gift aid (need-based):* Federal Pell, FSEOG, state, private, college/university gift aid from institutional funds. *Loans:* FFEL (Subsidized and Unsubsidized Stafford PLUS), college/university. *Work-Study:* Federal Work-Study, part-time campus jobs. *Application deadline (priority):* 6/1.

Contact Department of Nursing, Department of Nursing, Tarleton State University, Box T-0500, Stephenville, TX 76402. *Telephone:* 254-968-9139. *Fax:* 254-968-9716. *E-mail:* skinner@tarleton.edu.

CONTINUING EDUCATION PROGRAM

Contact Ms. Dokagari (Dok) Woods, Coordinator of Nursing Professional Development, Department of Nursing, Tarleton State University, Tarleton State University, Box T-0500, Stephenville, TX 76042. *Telephone:* 325-649-8058. *Fax:* 325-649-8959. *E-mail:* woods@tarleton.edu.

Texas A&M International University

Canseco School of Nursing
Laredo, Texas

Founded in 1969

DEGREES • BSN • MSN

Nursing Program Faculty 18 (20% with doctorates).

Baccalaureate Enrollment 243
Women 70% **Men** 30% **Minority** 98% **International** 1% **Part-time** 25%

Graduate Enrollment 18

Nursing Student Activities Nursing Honor Society, Student Nurses' Association.

Nursing Student Resources Academic advising; academic or career counseling; assistance for students with disabilities; bookstore; campus computer network; career placement assistance; computer lab; computer-assisted instruction; daycare for children of students; e-mail services; employment services for current students; externships; housing assistance; interactive nursing skills videos; Internet; learning resource lab; library services; nursing audiovisuals; paid internships; placement services for program completers; remedial services; resume preparation assistance; skills, simulation, or other laboratory; tutoring.

Library Facilities 166,951 volumes (8,500 in nursing); 8,492 periodical subscriptions (80 health-care related).

BACCALAUREATE PROGRAMS

Degree BSN

Available Programs Generic Baccalaureate; RN Baccalaureate.

Study Options Full-time.

Program Entrance Requirements Minimum overall college GPA of 2.5, transcript of college record, written essay, health exam, immunizations, 2 letters of recommendation, minimum GPA in nursing prerequisites of 2.5, prerequisite course work. Transfer students are accepted. **Standardized tests** *Required:* SAT or ACT, TOEFL for international students. **Application** *Deadline:* 7/1 (freshmen), 7/1 (transfer). *Notification:* 7/15 (freshmen).

Advanced Placement Credit given for nursing courses completed elsewhere dependent upon specific evaluations.

Expenses (2004–05) *Tuition, state resident:* full-time $2256; part-time $94 per contact hour. *Tuition, nonresident:* full-time $8448; part-time $352 per contact hour. *International tuition:* $8448 full-time. *Room and board:* $4500; room only: $3500 per academic year. *Required fees:* full-time $475.

Financial Aid 85% of baccalaureate students in nursing programs received some form of financial aid in 2003–04.

Contact Dr. Susan Scoville Baker, RN, Director, Canseco School of Nursing, Texas A&M International University, 5201 University Boulevard, Laredo, TX 78041-1900. *Telephone:* 956-326-2450. *Fax:* 956-326-2449. *E-mail:* sbaker@tamiu.edu.

GRADUATE PROGRAMS

Expenses (2004–05) *Tuition, state resident:* full-time $2256; part-time $94 per contact hour. *Tuition, nonresident:* full-time $8448; part-time $352 per contact hour. *International tuition:* $8448 full-time. *Room and board:* $4500; room only: $3500 per academic year. *Required fees:* full-time $475.

Financial Aid 85% of graduate students in nursing programs received some form of financial aid in 2003–04.

Contact Dr. Susan Scoville Baker, Director, Canseco School of Nursing, Texas A&M International University, 5201 University Boulevard, Laredo, TX 78041-1900. *Telephone:* 956-326-2450. *Fax:* 956-326-2449. *E-mail:* sbaker@tamiu.edu.

MASTER'S DEGREE PROGRAM

Degree MSN

Available Programs Master's; Master's for Nurses with Non-Nursing Degrees.

Concentrations Available *Nurse practitioner programs in:* family health.

Study Options Full-time and part-time.

Program Entrance Requirements Clinical experience, minimum overall college GPA of 3.0, transcript of college record, CPR certification, written essay, immunizations, interview, 2 letters of recommendation.

Advanced Placement Credit given for nursing courses completed elsewhere dependent upon specific evaluations.

Degree Requirements 45 total credit hours.

CONTINUING EDUCATION PROGRAM

Contact Natalie Burkhalter, RN, Associate Professor, Canseco School of Nursing, Texas A&M International University, 5201 University Bouelvard, Laredo, TX 78041-1900. *Telephone:* 956-326-2450. *Fax:* 956-326-2449. *E-mail:* natalie@tamiu.edu.

Texas A&M University–Corpus Christi

School of Nursing and Health Sciences
Corpus Christi, Texas

http://www.sci.tamucc.edu/nursing/

Founded in 1947

DEGREES • BSN • MSN

Nursing Program Faculty 45 (65% with doctorates).

Baccalaureate Enrollment 211
Women 82% **Men** 18% **Minority** 40% **International** 1% **Part-time** 31%

Graduate Enrollment 191
Women 80% **Men** 20% **Minority** 48% **Part-time** 98%

Nursing Student Activities Sigma Theta Tau, Student Nurses' Association.

Nursing Student Resources Academic advising; academic or career counseling; assistance for students with disabilities; bookstore; campus computer network; career placement assistance; computer lab; computer-assisted instruction; e-mail services; employment services for current students; housing assistance; interactive nursing skills videos; Internet; learning resource lab; library services; nursing audiovisuals; placement services for program completers; remedial services; resume preparation assistance; skills, simulation, or other laboratory; tutoring.

Library Facilities 731,586 volumes (500 in health, 350 in nursing); 1,901 periodical subscriptions (100 health-care related).

BACCALAUREATE PROGRAMS

Degree BSN

Available Programs ADN to Baccalaureate; Accelerated Baccalaureate for Second Degree; Baccalaureate for Second Degree; Generic Baccalaureate; RN Baccalaureate.

Site Options *Distance Learning:* Victoria, TX.

Study Options Full-time and part-time.

Program Entrance Requirements Minimum overall college GPA of 3.0, transcript of college record, CPR certification, immunizations, professional liability insurance/malpractice insurance, prerequisite course work. Transfer students are accepted. **Standardized tests** *Required:* SAT or ACT, TOEFL for international students. **Application** *Deadline:* 7/1 (freshmen). *Application fee:* $20.

Advanced Placement Credit given for nursing courses completed elsewhere dependent upon specific evaluations.

Expenses (2004–05) *Tuition, state resident:* full-time $3312; part-time $92 per contact hour. *Tuition, nonresident:* full-time $11,801; part-time $328 per contact hour. *International tuition:* $11,801 full-time. *Room and board:* room only: $4560 per academic year. *Required fees:* full-time $1220; part-time $150 per credit; part-time $659 per term.

Financial Aid 70% of baccalaureate students in nursing programs received some form of financial aid in 2003–04.

Contact Dr. Bunny D. Forgione, Associate Dean, School of Nursing and Health Sciences, Texas A&M University–Corpus Christi, 6300 Ocean Drive, Corpus Christi, TX 78412. *Telephone:* 361-825-2740. *Fax:* 361-825-2484. *E-mail:* forgione@falcon.tamucc.edu.

GRADUATE PROGRAMS

Expenses (2004–05) *Tuition, state resident:* full-time $2196; part-time $122 per contact hour. *Tuition, nonresident:* full-time $6840; part-time $380 per contact hour. *International tuition:* $6840 full-time. *Room and board:* room only: $4560 per academic year. *Required fees:* full-time $1140; part-time $174 per credit; part-time $380 per term.

Financial Aid 50% of graduate students in nursing programs received some form of financial aid in 2003–04.

Contact Dr. Eve Layman, RN, Graduate Coordinator, School of Nursing and Health Sciences, Texas A&M University–Corpus Christi, 6300 Ocean Drive, FC164, Corpus Christi, TX 78412. *Telephone:* 361-825-3781. *Fax:* 361-825-2484. *E-mail:* eve.layman@mail.tamucc.edu.

MASTER'S DEGREE PROGRAM

Degree MSN

Available Programs Accelerated AD/RN to Master's; Accelerated Master's for Nurses with Non-Nursing Degrees; Master's.

Concentrations Available Nursing administration. *Clinical nurse specialist programs in:* acute care, pediatric. *Nurse practitioner programs in:* family health.

Site Options *Distance Learning:* Temple, TX; Victoria, TX; Laredo, TX.

Study Options Full-time and part-time.

Program Entrance Requirements Minimum overall college GPA of 3.0, transcript of college record, CPR certification, immunizations, nursing research course, professional liability insurance/malpractice insurance, statistics course.

Advanced Placement Credit by examination available. Credit given for nursing courses completed elsewhere dependent upon specific evaluations.

Degree Requirements 45 total credit hours.

POST-MASTER'S PROGRAM

Areas of Study Nursing administration; nursing education. *Clinical nurse specialist programs in:* acute care, pediatric. *Nurse practitioner programs in:* family health.

CONTINUING EDUCATION PROGRAM

Contact Ms. Petra Martinez, Chair of Continuing Education Committee, School of Nursing and Health Sciences, Texas A&M University–Corpus Christi, 6300 Ocean Drive, ST 316, Corpus Christi, TX 78412. *Telephone:* 361-825-2353. *Fax:* 361-825-3491. *E-mail:* petra.martinez@mail.tamucc.edu.

Texas A&M University–Texarkana

Nursing Department
Texarkana, Texas

Founded in 1971

DEGREE • BSN

Library Facilities 125,991 volumes; 5,709 periodical subscriptions.

BACCALAUREATE PROGRAMS

Degree BSN

Available Programs RN Baccalaureate.

Program Entrance Requirements Transcript of college record, health insurance, immunizations, 2 letters of recommendation, minimum high school GPA of 2.0, minimum GPA in nursing prerequisites of 2.0, professional liability insurance/malpractice insurance, RN licensure. **Standardized tests** *Required:* TOEFL for international students. **Application** *Deadline:* rolling (transfer).

Contact Admissions, Nursing Department, Texas A&M University–Texarkana, 2600 North Robison Road, Texarkana, TX 75501. *Telephone:* 903-223-3069. *Fax:* 903-223-3140. *E-mail:* admissions@tamut.edu.

Texas Christian University

Harris School of Nursing
Fort Worth, Texas

Founded in 1873

DEGREES • BSN • MSN

Nursing Program Faculty 30 (57% with doctorates).

Baccalaureate Enrollment 480

Women 94% **Men** 6% **Minority** 18% **International** 8% **Part-time** 5%

Nursing Student Activities Sigma Theta Tau, Student Nurses' Association.

Nursing Student Resources Academic advising; academic or career counseling; assistance for students with disabilities; bookstore; campus computer network; career placement assistance; computer lab; computer-assisted instruction; e-mail services; externships; interactive nursing skills videos; Internet; learning resource lab; library services; nursing audiovisuals; other; resume preparation assistance; skills, simulation, or other laboratory; tutoring.

Library Facilities 1.3 million volumes (16,505 in health, 3,063 in nursing); 6,229 periodical subscriptions (180 health-care related).

BACCALAUREATE PROGRAMS

Degree BSN

Available Programs Accelerated Baccalaureate; Accelerated Baccalaureate for Second Degree; Generic Baccalaureate.

Site Options *Distance Learning:* Fort Worth, TX.

Study Options Full-time and part-time.

Program Entrance Requirements Minimum overall college GPA of 2.5, transcript of college record, CPR certification, written essay, high school foreign language, 2 years high school math, 2 years high school science, high school transcript, immunizations, minimum high school GPA of 3.0, minimum GPA in nursing prerequisites of 2.5, prerequisite course work. Transfer students are accepted. **Standardized tests** *Required:* SAT or ACT, TOEFL for international students. **Application** *Deadline:* 2/15 (freshmen), 4/15 (transfer). *Early decision:* 11/15. *Notification:* 4/1 (freshmen), 1/1 (early action). *Application fee:* $40.

Advanced Placement Credit by examination available. Credit given for nursing courses completed elsewhere dependent upon specific evaluations.

Financial Aid 60% of baccalaureate students in nursing programs received some form of financial aid in 2003–04.

Contact Mrs. Zoranna Williams, Coordinator of Recruitment and Retention, Harris School of Nursing, Texas Christian University, 2800 West Bowie, Box 298620, Fort Worth, TX 76129. *Telephone:* 817-257-7650. *Fax:* 817-257-7944. *E-mail:* z.williams@tcu.edu.

GRADUATE PROGRAMS

Financial Aid 60% of graduate students in nursing programs received some form of financial aid in 2003–04.

Contact Ms. Kathleen M. Baldwin, Director of Graduate Studies, Harris School of Nursing, Texas Christian University, 2800 West Bowie, Box 298620, Fort Worth, TX 76129. *Telephone:* 817-257-7650 Ext. 6748. *Fax:* 817-257-7944. *E-mail:* k.baldwin@tcu.edu.

Texas Christian University (continued)

MASTER'S DEGREE PROGRAM

Degree MSN

Available Programs Master's; RN to Master's.

Concentrations Available *Clinical nurse specialist programs in:* adult health, medical-surgical.

Site Options *Distance Learning:* Fort Worth, TX.

Study Options Full-time and part-time.

Program Entrance Requirements Clinical experience, minimum overall college GPA of 3.0, transcript of college record, CPR certification, written essay, 3 letters of recommendation, resume.

Degree Requirements 38 total credit hours, thesis or project.

CONTINUING EDUCATION PROGRAM

Contact Dr. Linda Curry, Faculty Relations Committee, Harris School of Nursing, Texas Christian University, TCU Box 298620, Fort Worth, TX 76129. *Telephone:* 817-257-7650 Ext. 7496. *Fax:* 817-257-7944.

Texas Tech University Health Sciences Center

School of Nursing
Lubbock, Texas

http://www.ttunursing.com

Founded in 1969

DEGREES • BSN • MSN • MSN/MBA

Nursing Program Faculty 42 (43% with doctorates).

Nursing Student Activities Nursing Honor Society, Sigma Theta Tau, Student Nurses' Association.

Library Facilities 252,355 volumes in health, 8,800 volumes in nursing; 2,324 periodical subscriptions health-care related.

BACCALAUREATE PROGRAMS

Degree BSN

Available Programs Generic Baccalaureate.

Site Options *Distance Learning:* Odessa, TX; Kerrville, TX.

Study Options Full-time.

Program Entrance Requirements Minimum overall college GPA of 2.5, transcript of college record, health insurance, immunizations, prerequisite course work. Transfer students are accepted.

Advanced Placement Credit given for nursing courses completed elsewhere dependent upon specific evaluations.

Contact Undergraduate Program, School of Nursing, Texas Tech University Health Sciences Center, 3601 4th Street, MS 8331, Lubbock, TX 79430. *Telephone:* 806-743-2737. *Fax:* 806-743-1697.

GRADUATE PROGRAMS

Financial Aid Institutionally sponsored loans, scholarships, and traineeships available.

Contact Dr. Barbara Ann Johnston, Associate Dean for Graduate Programs, School of Nursing, Texas Tech University Health Sciences Center, 3601 4th Street, Lubbock, TX 79430. *Telephone:* 806-743-3055. *Fax:* 806-743-1622. *E-mail:* Barbara.Johnston@ttuhsc.edu.

MASTER'S DEGREE PROGRAM

Degrees MSN; MSN/MBA

Available Programs Master's.

Concentrations Available Nursing administration; nursing education. *Nurse practitioner programs in:* acute care, family health, gerontology, pediatric.

Site Options *Distance Learning:* Odessa, TX; Tyler, TX.

Study Options Full-time and part-time.

Program Entrance Requirements Clinical experience, computer literacy, minimum overall college GPA of 3.0, transcript of college record, CPR certification, written essay, immunizations, 3 letters of recommendation, nursing research course, statistics course, GRE General Test or MAT. *Application deadline:* For fall admission, 7/15 (priority date); for spring admission, 11/15 (priority date). Applications are processed on a rolling basis. *Application fee:* $40.

Advanced Placement Credit given for nursing courses completed elsewhere dependent upon specific evaluations.

Degree Requirements Thesis or project.

POST-MASTER'S PROGRAM

Areas of Study *Nurse practitioner programs in:* acute care, family health, gerontology, pediatric.

CONTINUING EDUCATION PROGRAM

Contact Ms. Shelley Burson, Director of Continuing Nursing Education, School of Nursing, Texas Tech University Health Sciences Center, 3601 4th Street, Lubbock, TX 79430. *Telephone:* 806-743-2734. *Fax:* 806-743-1198. *E-mail:* shelley.burson@ttuhsc.edu.

Texas Woman's University

College of Nursing
Denton, Texas

Founded in 1901

DEGREES • BS • MS • MSN/MHA • PHD

Nursing Program Faculty 117 (54% with doctorates).

Baccalaureate Enrollment 699
Women 95% **Men** 5% **Minority** 40% **International** 2% **Part-time** 21%

Graduate Enrollment 314
Women 94% **Men** 6% **Minority** 33% **International** 1%

Nursing Student Activities Sigma Theta Tau, Student Nurses' Association.

Nursing Student Resources Academic advising; academic or career counseling; assistance for students with disabilities; bookstore; campus computer network; career placement assistance; computer lab; computer-assisted instruction; e-mail services; employment services for current students; Internet; learning resource lab; library services; nursing audiovisuals; placement services for program completers; remedial services; skills, simulation, or other laboratory.

Library Facilities 572,500 volumes (250,000 in health, 26,463 in nursing); 2,537 periodical subscriptions (2,644 health-care related).

BACCALAUREATE PROGRAMS

Degree BS

Available Programs Baccalaureate for Second Degree; Generic Baccalaureate; RN Baccalaureate.

Site Options Dallas, TX. *Distance Learning:* Houston, TX.

Study Options Full-time and part-time.

Program Entrance Requirements Transcript of college record, CPR certification, high school transcript, immunizations, minimum GPA in nursing prerequisites of 3.0, professional liability insurance/malpractice insurance, prerequisite course work. Transfer students are accepted. **Standardized tests** *Required:* SAT or ACT, TOEFL for international students. **Application** *Deadline:* 7/15 (freshmen), 7/15 (transfer). *Notification:* continuous until 8/15 (freshmen). *Application fee:* $30.

Advanced Placement Credit given for nursing courses completed elsewhere dependent upon specific evaluations.

Financial Aid 55% of baccalaureate students in nursing programs received some form of financial aid in 2002–03. *Gift aid (need-based):* Federal Pell, FSEOG, state, private, college/university gift aid from institutional funds. *Loans:* Federal Nursing Student Loans, FFEL (Subsidized and Unsubsidized Stafford PLUS), Perkins, state, college/university, alternative loans. *Work-Study:* Federal Work-Study, part-time campus jobs. *Application deadline (priority):* 4/1.

Contact Dr. Gloria Byrd, BS Program Coordinator, College of Nursing, Texas Woman's University, 1810 Inwood Road, Dallas, TX 75235-7299. *Telephone:* 214-689-6519. *Fax:* 214-689-6539. *E-mail:* gbyrd@twu.edu.

GRADUATE PROGRAMS

Financial Aid 30% of graduate students in nursing programs received some form of financial aid in 2002–03. 7 research assistantships (averaging $9,261 per year), 4 teaching assistantships (averaging $9,261 per year) were awarded; career-related internships or fieldwork, Federal Work-Study, institutionally sponsored loans, scholarships, traineeships, and unspecified assistantships also available. Aid available to part-time students. *Financial aid application deadline:* 3/1.

Contact Ms. Patricia Jones, MS Program Coordinator, College of Nursing, Texas Woman's University, Texas Woman's University College of Nursing, PO Box 425498, Denton, TX 76204-4598. *Telephone:* 940-898-2418. *E-mail:* pjones@twu.edu.

MASTER'S DEGREE PROGRAM

Degrees MS; MSN/MHA

Available Programs Master's; RN to Master's.

Concentrations Available Nursing administration. *Clinical nurse specialist programs in:* adult health, community health, pediatric, women's health. *Nurse practitioner programs in:* adult health, family health, pediatric, women's health.

Site Options Dallas, TX. *Distance Learning:* Houston, TX.

Study Options Full-time and part-time.

Program Entrance Requirements Clinical experience, minimum overall college GPA of 3.0, transcript of college record, CPR certification, immunizations, professional liability insurance/malpractice insurance, statistics course. *Application deadline:* Applications are processed on a rolling basis. *Application fee:* $30 ($50 for international students).

Advanced Placement Credit given for nursing courses completed elsewhere dependent upon specific evaluations.

Degree Requirements 48 total credit hours, thesis or project.

POST-MASTER'S PROGRAM

Areas of Study *Nurse practitioner programs in:* adult health, family health, pediatric, women's health.

DOCTORAL DEGREE PROGRAM

Degree PhD

Available Programs Doctorate.

Areas of Study Nursing research, nursing science, women's health.

Site Options *Distance Learning:* Houston, TX.

Program Entrance Requirements Minimum overall college GPA of 3.5, 2 letters of recommendation, MSN or equivalent, statistics course, vita. *Application deadline:* Applications are processed on a rolling basis. *Application fee:* $30 ($50 for international students).

Degree Requirements 60 total credit hours, dissertation, oral exam, written exam.

University of Mary Hardin-Baylor

College of Nursing
Belton, Texas

Founded in 1845

DEGREE • BSN

Nursing Program Faculty 16 (56% with doctorates).

Baccalaureate Enrollment 213
Women 95% **Men** 5% **Minority** 18% **International** 1% **Part-time** 1%

Nursing Student Activities Sigma Theta Tau, Student Nurses' Association, nursing club.

Nursing Student Resources Academic advising; academic or career counseling; assistance for students with disabilities; bookstore; campus computer network; career placement assistance; computer lab; e-mail services; employment services for current students; housing assistance; Internet; learning resource lab; library services; nursing audiovisuals; placement services for program completers; remedial services; resume preparation assistance; skills, simulation, or other laboratory; tutoring.

Library Facilities 153,120 volumes (7,233 in health, 5,925 in nursing); 1,541 periodical subscriptions (120 health-care related).

BACCALAUREATE PROGRAMS

Degree BSN

Available Programs Baccalaureate for Second Degree; Generic Baccalaureate; RN Baccalaureate.

Study Options Full-time and part-time.

Program Entrance Requirements Minimum overall college GPA of 2.0, transcript of college record, CPR certification, written essay, health exam, health insurance, high school transcript, immunizations, interview, minimum high school rank 50%, minimum GPA in nursing prerequisites of 2.75, professional liability insurance/malpractice insurance, prerequisite course work. Transfer students are accepted. **Standardized tests** *Required:* SAT or ACT. *Recommended:* TOEFL for international students. **Application** *Deadline:* rolling (freshmen), rolling (transfer). *Notification:* continuous (freshmen). *Application fee:* $35.

Advanced Placement Credit given for nursing courses completed elsewhere dependent upon specific evaluations.

Expenses (2004–05) *Tuition:* full-time $11,400; part-time $380 per credit hour. *International tuition:* $11,400 full-time. *Room and board:* $4000 per academic year. *Required fees:* full-time $1280.

Financial Aid 89% of baccalaureate students in nursing programs received some form of financial aid in 2003–04.

Contact Dr. Linda Pehl, Dean, College of Nursing, University of Mary Hardin-Baylor, Box 8015, 900 College Street, Belton, TX 76513-2599. *Telephone:* 254-295-4665. *Fax:* 254-295-4141. *E-mail:* lpehl@umhb.edu.

CONTINUING EDUCATION PROGRAM

Contact Ms. Peggy Craik, RN, Program Administrator, College of Nursing, University of Mary Hardin-Baylor, Box 8015, 900 College Street, Belton, TX 76513-2599. *Telephone:* 254-295-4668. *Fax:* 254-295-4141. *E-mail:* pcraik@umhb.edu.

The University of Texas at Arlington

School of Nursing
Arlington, Texas

http://www.uta.edu/nursing

Founded in 1895

DEGREES • BSN • MSN • MSN/MBA • MSN/MPH • PHD

Nursing Program Faculty 83 (49% with doctorates).

Baccalaureate Enrollment 512
Women 90% **Men** 10% **Minority** 28% **International** 7% **Part-time** 31%

Graduate Enrollment 282
Women 90% **Men** 10% **Minority** 19% **Part-time** 86%

Nursing Student Activities Nursing Honor Society, Sigma Theta Tau, Student Nurses' Association, nursing club.

Nursing Student Resources Academic advising; assistance for students with disabilities; campus computer network; computer lab; e-mail services; externships; interactive nursing skills videos; Internet; learning resource lab; nursing audiovisuals; skills, simulation, or other laboratory.

Library Facilities 1.1 million volumes (35,500 in health, 23,000 in nursing); 3,977 periodical subscriptions (508 health-care related).

BACCALAUREATE PROGRAMS

Degree BSN

Available Programs Generic Baccalaureate; RN Baccalaureate.

Site Options *Distance Learning:* Paris , TX; Waco , TX; Sherman , TX.

Study Options Full-time and part-time.

The University of Texas at Arlington (continued)

Program Entrance Requirements Minimum overall college GPA of 2.5, transcript of college record, CPR certification, written essay, immunizations, interview, minimum GPA in nursing prerequisites, professional liability insurance/malpractice insurance, prerequisite course work. Transfer students are accepted. **Standardized tests** *Required:* SAT or ACT, TOEFL for international students. **Application** *Deadline:* 6/1 (freshmen), rolling (transfer). *Notification:* continuous (freshmen). *Application fee:* $35.

Expenses (2004–05) *Tuition, state resident:* full-time $5300. *Tuition, nonresident:* full-time $14,360. *International tuition:* $14,490 full-time. *Room and board:* $4850; room only: $2130 per academic year. *Required fees:* full-time $1600; part-time $58 per credit; part-time $650 per term.

Financial Aid 35% of baccalaureate students in nursing programs received some form of financial aid in 2003–04. *Gift aid (need-based):* Federal Pell, FSEOG, state, private, college/university gift aid from institutional funds. *Loans:* FFEL (Subsidized and Unsubsidized Stafford PLUS), Perkins, state, college/university. *Work-Study:* Federal Work-Study. *Application deadline (priority):* 5/15.

Contact Ms. Jean Ashwill, RN, Director, Undergraduate Student Services, School of Nursing, The University of Texas at Arlington, 411 South Nedderman Drive, Box 19407, Arlington, TX 76019-0407. *Telephone:* 817-272-2776. *Fax:* 817-272-5006. *E-mail:* nursing@uta.edu.

GRADUATE PROGRAMS

Expenses (2004–05) *Tuition, state resident:* part-time $179 per credit hour. *Tuition, nonresident:* part-time $494 per credit hour. *Room and board:* $4850; room only: $2130 per academic year. *Required fees:* full-time $2214; part-time $59 per credit; part-time $147 per term.

Financial Aid 20% of graduate students in nursing programs received some form of financial aid in 2003–04. 24 fellowships with partial tuition reimbursements available (averaging $3,000 per year), 6 research assistantships (averaging $7,992 per year), 7 teaching assistantships (averaging $10,080 per year) were awarded; career-related internships or fieldwork and traineeships also available. *Financial aid application deadline:* 6/1.

Contact Dr. Susan K. Grove, Associate Dean and Director of Graduate Studies, School of Nursing, The University of Texas at Arlington, 411 South Nedderman Drive, Box 19407, Arlington, TX 76019-0407. *Telephone:* 817-272-7086. *Fax:* 817-272-5006. *E-mail:* grove@uta.edu.

MASTER'S DEGREE PROGRAM

Degrees MSN; MSN/MBA; MSN/MPH

Available Programs Master's.

Concentrations Available Health-care administration; nursing administration. *Nurse practitioner programs in:* acute care, adult health, family health, gerontology, pediatric, psychiatric/mental health.

Study Options Full-time and part-time.

Program Entrance Requirements Computer literacy, minimum overall college GPA of 3.0, transcript of college record, CPR certification, written essay, immunizations, 3 letters of recommendation, physical assessment course, professional liability insurance/malpractice insurance, statistics course, GRE General Test. *Application deadline:* For fall admission, 6/16. Applications are processed on a rolling basis. *Application fee:* $35 ($50 for international students).

Degree Requirements 48 total credit hours, thesis or project, comprehensive exam.

POST-MASTER'S PROGRAM

Areas of Study Nursing education. *Nurse practitioner programs in:* acute care, adult health, family health, gerontology, pediatric, psychiatric/mental health.

DOCTORAL DEGREE PROGRAM

Degree PhD

Available Programs Doctorate.

Areas of Study Faculty preparation, nursing education, nursing research.

Program Entrance Requirements Minimum overall college GPA of 3.0, interview, 3 letters of recommendation, MSN or equivalent, statistics course, GRE General Test. *Application deadline:* For fall admission, 6/16. Applications are processed on a rolling basis. *Application fee:* $35 ($50 for international students).

Degree Requirements 58 total credit hours, dissertation, residency.

CONTINUING EDUCATION PROGRAM

Contact Tanya Truitt, RN, Director of Continuing Nursing Education, School of Nursing, The University of Texas at Arlington, 411 South Nedderman Drive, Box 19407, Arlington, TX 76019-0407. *Telephone:* 817-272-2778. *Fax:* 817-272-5006. *E-mail:* truitt@uta.edu.

The University of Texas at Austin
School of Nursing
Austin, Texas

http://www.utexas.edu/nursing

Founded in 1883

DEGREES • BSN • MSN • MSN/MBA • PHD

Nursing Program Faculty 73 (62% with doctorates).

Baccalaureate Enrollment 701
Women 90.5% **Men** 9.5% **Minority** 33% **International** 1% **Part-time** 13%

Graduate Enrollment 222
Women 88% **Men** 12% **Minority** 27% **International** 9% **Part-time** 24%

Nursing Student Activities Nursing Honor Society, Sigma Theta Tau, Student Nurses' Association, nursing club.

Nursing Student Resources Academic advising; academic or career counseling; assistance for students with disabilities; bookstore; campus computer network; career placement assistance; computer lab; computer-assisted instruction; daycare for children of students; e-mail services; employment services for current students; externships; housing assistance; interactive nursing skills videos; Internet; learning resource lab; library services; nursing audiovisuals; other; paid internships; placement services for program completers; remedial services; resume preparation assistance; skills, simulation, or other laboratory; tutoring; unpaid internships.

Library Facilities 100,000 volumes in health, 80,000 volumes in nursing; 504 periodical subscriptions health-care related.

BACCALAUREATE PROGRAMS

Degree BSN

Available Programs Generic Baccalaureate; RN Baccalaureate.

Study Options Full-time.

Program Entrance Requirements Minimum overall college GPA of 2.5, transcript of college record, CPR certification, written essay, 3 years high school math, 2 years high school science, high school transcript, immunizations, 3 letters of recommendation, minimum GPA in nursing prerequisites of 2.5, professional liability insurance/malpractice insurance, prerequisite course work. Transfer students are accepted. **Standardized tests** *Required:* SAT or ACT, TOEFL for international students. ***Placement:*** *Required for some:* SAT Subject Tests. **Application** *Deadline:* 2/1 (freshmen), 3/1 (transfer). *Notification:* continuous (freshmen). *Application fee:* $50.

Advanced Placement Credit by examination available. Credit given for nursing courses completed elsewhere dependent upon specific evaluations.

Expenses (2003–04) *Tuition, state resident:* full-time $3120. *Tuition, nonresident:* full-time $10,240. *International tuition:* $10,240 full-time. *Room and board:* $7088 per academic year. *Required fees:* full-time $2030; part-time $1015 per term.

Financial Aid 54% of baccalaureate students in nursing programs received some form of financial aid in 2002–03. *Gift aid (need-based):* Federal Pell, FSEOG, state, private, college/university gift aid from institutional funds, Federal Nursing. *Loans:* FFEL (Subsidized and Unsubsidized Stafford PLUS), Perkins, state. *Work-Study:* Federal Work-Study, part-time campus jobs. *Application deadline (priority):* 4/1.

Contact Student Affairs Office, School of Nursing, The University of Texas at Austin, 1700 Red River Street, Austin, TX 78701-1412. *Telephone:* 512-232-4780. *Fax:* 512-232-4777. *E-mail:* nuugrad@uts.cc.utexas.edu.

GRADUATE PROGRAMS

Expenses (2003–04) *Tuition, state resident:* full-time $2842. *Tuition, nonresident:* full-time $7132. *International tuition:* $7132 full-time. *Room and board:* $7088 per academic year. *Required fees:* full-time $1622; part-time $805 per term.

Financial Aid 4 fellowships, 5 research assistantships, 18 teaching assistantships were awarded; scholarships and traineeships also available.

Contact Graduate Student Affairs, School of Nursing, The University of Texas at Austin, Graduate Student Affairs, 1700 Red River Street, Austin, TX 78701-1499. *Telephone:* 512-471-7927. *Fax:* 512-232-4777. *E-mail:* nugrad@uts.cc.utexas.edu.

MASTER'S DEGREE PROGRAM

Degrees MSN; MSN/MBA

Available Programs Master's; Master's for Non-Nursing College Graduates; Master's for Nurses with Non-Nursing Degrees.

Concentrations Available Nursing administration. *Clinical nurse specialist programs in:* adult health, community health, medical-surgical, public health. *Nurse practitioner programs in:* family health, pediatric.

Study Options Full-time and part-time.

Program Entrance Requirements Clinical experience, minimum overall college GPA of 3.0, transcript of college record, CPR certification, written essay, immunizations, interview, 3 letters of recommendation, physical assessment course, professional liability insurance/malpractice insurance, prerequisite course work, resume, statistics course, GRE General Test. *Application deadline:* For fall admission, 12/1. *Application fee:* $50 ($75 for international students).

Advanced Placement Credit given for nursing courses completed elsewhere dependent upon specific evaluations.

Degree Requirements 48 total credit hours.

POST-MASTER'S PROGRAM

Areas of Study *Nurse practitioner programs in:* family health, pediatric.

DOCTORAL DEGREE PROGRAM

Degree PhD

Available Programs Doctorate.

Areas of Study Aging, community health, faculty preparation, gerontology, health promotion/disease prevention, health-care systems, human health and illness, illness and transition, maternity-newborn, nursing administration, nursing research, women's health.

Program Entrance Requirements Minimum overall college GPA of 3.0, interview, 3 letters of recommendation, MSN or equivalent, statistics course, vita, GRE General Test. *Application deadline:* For fall admission, 12/1. *Application fee:* $50 ($75 for international students).

Degree Requirements 64 total credit hours, dissertation, oral exam, written exam, residency.

POSTDOCTORAL PROGRAM

Areas of Study Women's health.

Postdoctoral Program Contact Dr. Lorraine Walker, Assistant Dean for Graduate Programs, School of Nursing, The University of Texas at Austin, 1700 Red River Street, Austin, TX 78701. *Telephone:* 512-232-4751. *Fax:* 512-232-4777. *E-mail:* lwalker@mail.nur.utexas.edu.

The University of Texas at Brownsville

Department of Nursing
Brownsville, Texas

http://www.ntmain.utb.edu/sbs/nursing_dept.html

Founded in 1973

DEGREES • BSN • MS

Nursing Program Faculty 25 (12% with doctorates).

Baccalaureate Enrollment 39
Women 75% **Men** 25%

Graduate Enrollment 7
Women 90% **Men** 10%

Nursing Student Resources Academic advising; academic or career counseling; assistance for students with disabilities; bookstore; campus computer network; computer lab; daycare for children of students; e-mail services; employment services for current students; housing assistance; interactive nursing skills videos; learning resource lab; library services; nursing audiovisuals; skills, simulation, or other laboratory; tutoring.

Library Facilities 174,660 volumes; 4,447 periodical subscriptions.

BACCALAUREATE PROGRAMS

Degree BSN

Available Programs ADN to Baccalaureate.

Site Options *Distance Learning:* Harlingen, TX; Weslaco, TX.

Study Options Full-time and part-time.

Program Entrance Requirements Minimum overall college GPA of 2.0, transcript of college record, CPR certification, high school transcript, immunizations, minimum GPA in nursing prerequisites of 2.5, professional liability insurance/malpractice insurance, prerequisite course work, RN licensure. Transfer students are accepted. **Standardized tests** *Recommended:* TOEFL for international students. ***Placement:*** *Required:* THEA. **Application** *Deadline:* 7/10 (freshmen), 8/1 (transfer).

Advanced Placement Credit given for nursing courses completed elsewhere dependent upon specific evaluations.

Financial Aid 15% of baccalaureate students in nursing programs received some form of financial aid in 2002–03.

Contact Dr. Katherine B. Dougherty, Director RN to BSN Program, Department of Nursing, The University of Texas at Brownsville, 80 Fort Brown, Brownsville, TX 78520. *Telephone:* 956-544-5071. *Fax:* 956-544-8881. *E-mail:* kdougherty@utb.edu.

GRADUATE PROGRAMS

Contact Dr. Ava Miller, Interim Director of Masters Program, Department of Nursing, The University of Texas at Brownsville, 80 Fort Brown, Brownsville, TX 78520. *Telephone:* 956-554-5071. *Fax:* 956-554-5100. *E-mail:* amiller@utb.edu.

MASTER'S DEGREE PROGRAM

Degree MS

Concentrations Available *Clinical nurse specialist programs in:* public health.

Program Entrance Requirements Minimum overall college GPA of 3.0, transcript of college record, immunizations, interview, 2 letters of recommendation, statistics course.

Degree Requirements Thesis or project.

The University of Texas at El Paso

School of Nursing
El Paso, Texas

http://chs.utep.edu/nursing

Founded in 1913

DEGREES • BSN • DSN • MSN

Nursing Program Faculty 42 (33% with doctorates).

Baccalaureate Enrollment 330
Women 75% **Men** 25% **Minority** 71%

Graduate Enrollment 117
Women 80% **Men** 20% **Minority** 73% **International** 1% **Part-time** 97%

Nursing Student Activities Nursing Honor Society, Sigma Theta Tau, Student Nurses' Association.

Nursing Student Resources Academic advising; academic or career counseling; assistance for students with disabilities; bookstore; campus computer network; computer lab; computer-assisted instruction; e-mail services; interactive nursing skills videos; Internet; learning resource lab; library services; nursing audiovisuals; remedial services; skills, simulation, or other laboratory; tutoring.

Library Facilities 961,247 volumes (25,000 in nursing); 3,005 periodical subscriptions.

BACCALAUREATE PROGRAMS

Degree BSN

Available Programs ADN to Baccalaureate; Generic Baccalaureate.

The University of Texas at El Paso (continued)

Study Options Full-time and part-time.

Program Entrance Requirements Minimum overall college GPA of 2.5, CPR certification, health exam, health insurance, high school biology, high school chemistry, high school math, high school science, high school transcript, immunizations, minimum GPA in nursing prerequisites of 2.5, professional liability insurance/malpractice insurance, prerequisite course work. Transfer students are accepted. **Standardized tests** *Required:* TOEFL for international students. *Required for some:* SAT or ACT, PAA. **Application** *Deadline:* 7/31 (freshmen), 7/31 (transfer).

Advanced Placement Credit by examination available. Credit given for nursing courses completed elsewhere dependent upon specific evaluations.

Financial Aid *Gift aid (need-based):* Federal Pell, FSEOG, state, college/university gift aid from institutional funds, Federal Nursing. *Loans:* Federal Nursing Student Loans, FFEL (Subsidized and Unsubsidized Stafford PLUS), Perkins, state, college/university. *Work-Study:* Federal Work-Study, part-time campus jobs. *Application deadline (priority):* 3/15.

Contact School of Nursing, School of Nursing, The University of Texas at El Paso, 1101 North Campbell Street, El Paso, TX 79902. *Telephone:* 915-747-8217. *Fax:* 915-747-7207.

GRADUATE PROGRAMS

Financial Aid Research assistantships (averaging $18,825 per year), teaching assistantships (averaging $18,000 per year) were awarded; fellowships, career-related internships or fieldwork, Federal Work-Study, institutionally sponsored loans, scholarships, and tuition waivers (partial) also available.

Contact Dr. Dorothy Stuppy, Graduate Advisor, School of Nursing, The University of Texas at El Paso, 1101 North Campbell Street, El Paso, TX 79902. *Telephone:* 915-747-7246. *Fax:* 915-747-7207. *E-mail:* dstuppy@utep.edu.

MASTER'S DEGREE PROGRAM

Degree MSN

Available Programs Master's; RN to Master's.

Concentrations Available Nursing administration; nursing education. *Nurse practitioner programs in:* family health, women's health.

Site Options *Distance Learning:* El Paso, TX.

Study Options Full-time and part-time.

Program Entrance Requirements Clinical experience, minimum overall college GPA of 3.0, transcript of college record, CPR certification, written essay, immunizations, interview, nursing research course, professional liability insurance/malpractice insurance, resume, GRE General Test or MAT. *Application deadline:* For fall admission, 7/1; for spring admission, 11/1. Applications are processed on a rolling basis. *Application fee:* $15 ($65 for international students).

Advanced Placement Credit given for nursing courses completed elsewhere dependent upon specific evaluations.

Degree Requirements Thesis or project, comprehensive exam.

POST-MASTER'S PROGRAM

Areas of Study Nursing education. *Nurse practitioner programs in:* family health, women's health.

DOCTORAL DEGREE PROGRAM

Degree DSN

Site Options *Distance Learning:* Houston, TX.

Program Entrance Requirements Minimum overall college GPA of 3.0, MSN or equivalent. *Application deadline:* For fall admission, 7/1; for spring admission, 11/1. Applications are processed on a rolling basis. *Application fee:* $15 ($65 for international students).

Degree Requirements 65 total credit hours, dissertation.

CONTINUING EDUCATION PROGRAM

Contact Ms. Elizabeth Richardson, Professional Development for the Health Sciences, School of Nursing, The University of Texas at El Paso, 1101 North Campbell Street, El Paso, TX 79902. *Telephone:* 915-747-7269. *Fax:* 915-747-7207. *E-mail:* erichardson@utep.edu.

The University of Texas at Tyler
Program in Nursing
Tyler, Texas

http://www.uttyler.edu/nursing

Founded in 1971

DEGREES • BSN • DNS • MSN • MSN/MBA

Nursing Program Faculty 41 (30% with doctorates).

Baccalaureate Enrollment 450

Women 70% **Men** 30% **Minority** 5% **International** 1% **Part-time** 15%

Graduate Enrollment 150

Women 87% **Men** 13% **Minority** 4% **Part-time** 80%

Nursing Student Activities Nursing Honor Society, Sigma Theta Tau, Student Nurses' Association, nursing club.

Nursing Student Resources Academic advising; academic or career counseling; assistance for students with disabilities; bookstore; campus computer network; career placement assistance; computer lab; computer-assisted instruction; e-mail services; employment services for current students; externships; interactive nursing skills videos; Internet; learning resource lab; library services; nursing audiovisuals; remedial services; resume preparation assistance; skills, simulation, or other laboratory; tutoring.

Library Facilities 216,622 volumes (11,000 in health, 5,500 in nursing); 929 periodical subscriptions (150 health-care related).

BACCALAUREATE PROGRAMS

Degree BSN

Available Programs ADN to Baccalaureate; Accelerated RN Baccalaureate; Generic Baccalaureate; International Nurse to Baccalaureate; LPN to Baccalaureate; LPN to RN Baccalaureate; RN Baccalaureate.

Site Options *Distance Learning:* Longview, TX; Palastine, TX.

Study Options Full-time and part-time.

Program Entrance Requirements Minimum overall college GPA of 2.75, transcript of college record, CPR certification, immunizations, minimum GPA in nursing prerequisites of 2.75, professional liability insurance/malpractice insurance, prerequisite course work. Transfer students are accepted. **Standardized tests** *Required:* SAT or ACT, TOEFL for international students. **Application** *Notification:* continuous (freshmen).

Advanced Placement Credit given for nursing courses completed elsewhere dependent upon specific evaluations.

Expenses (2004–05) *Tuition, state resident:* full-time $4042; part-time $135 per credit hour. *Tuition, nonresident:* full-time $12,264; part-time $409 per credit hour. *International tuition:* $12,264 full-time. *Room and board:* room only: $5085 per academic year. *Required fees:* full-time $2600; part-time $170 per credit; part-time $222 per term.

Financial Aid 70% of baccalaureate students in nursing programs received some form of financial aid in 2003–04. *Gift aid (need-based):* Federal Pell, FSEOG, state, private, college/university gift aid from institutional funds, Texas Grant, Teach for Texas Conditional Prog, Institutional Grants (Education Affordability Prog). *Loans:* FFEL (Subsidized and Unsubsidized Stafford PLUS), state. *Work-Study:* Federal Work-Study, part-time campus jobs. *Application deadline (priority):* 4/1.

Contact Andrea Liner, Coordinator, Marketing and Advising, Program in Nursing, The University of Texas at Tyler, 3900 University Boulevard, Tyler, TX 75799. *Telephone:* 903-565-5534. *Fax:* 903-565-5533. *E-mail:* Andrea_Liner@uttyler.edu.

GRADUATE PROGRAMS

Expenses (2004–05) *Tuition, state resident:* full-time $2600; part-time $145 per credit hour. *Tuition, nonresident:* full-time $8272; part-time $460 per credit hour. *International tuition:* $8272 full-time. *Room and board:* room only: $5085 per academic year. *Required fees:* full-time $1912; part-time $106 per credit; part-time $956 per term.

Financial Aid 60% of graduate students in nursing programs received some form of financial aid in 2003–04. 12 fellowships (averaging $1,800 per year), 3 research assistantships (averaging $2,200 per year) were awarded; institutionally sponsored loans also available. *Financial aid application deadline:* 8/1.

Contact Dr. Susan Yarbrough, Assistant Dean of Graduate Studies, Program in Nursing, The University of Texas at Tyler, 3900 University Boulevard, Tyler, TX 75799. *Telephone:* 903-566-7220. *Fax:* 903-565-5533. *E-mail:* syarbrough@mail.uttyl.edu.

MASTER'S DEGREE PROGRAM

Degrees MSN; MSN/MBA

Available Programs Accelerated AD/RN to Master's; Master's; RN to Master's.

Concentrations Available Nursing administration; nursing education. *Nurse practitioner programs in:* acute care, adult health, family health, gerontology, pediatric, women's health.

Site Options *Distance Learning:* Longview, TX; Palastine, TX.

Study Options Full-time and part-time.

Program Entrance Requirements Computer literacy, minimum overall college GPA of 2.75, transcript of college record, CPR certification, immunizations, 4 letters of recommendation, nursing research course, professional liability insurance/malpractice insurance, prerequisite course work, resume, statistics course, GRE General Test or MAT, GMAT. *Application deadline:* For fall admission, 3/1 (priority date); for spring admission, 10/1 (priority date). Applications are processed on a rolling basis.

Advanced Placement Credit given for nursing courses completed elsewhere dependent upon specific evaluations.

Degree Requirements 36 total credit hours, thesis or project, comprehensive exam.

POST-MASTER'S PROGRAM

Areas of Study Nursing administration; nursing education. *Nurse practitioner programs in:* acute care, adult health, family health, gerontology, pediatric, women's health.

DOCTORAL DEGREE PROGRAM

Degree DNS

Available Programs Doctorate.

Areas of Study Nursing science.

Site Options *Distance Learning:* Longview, TX; Palastine, TX.

Program Entrance Requirements Minimum overall college GPA of 3.0, interview by faculty committee, 3 letters of recommendation, MSN or equivalent, scholarly papers, statistics course, vita. *Application deadline:* For fall admission, 3/1 (priority date); for spring admission, 10/1 (priority date). Applications are processed on a rolling basis.

Degree Requirements 65 total credit hours, dissertation, written exam.

CONTINUING EDUCATION PROGRAM

Contact Pamela Martin, RN, Assistant Dean of Undergraduate Studies, Program in Nursing, The University of Texas at Tyler, 3900 University Boulevard, Tyler, TX 75799. *Telephone:* 903-566-7320. *Fax:* 903-565-5533. *E-mail:* pmartin@mail.uttyl.edu.

The University of Texas Health Science Center at Houston

School of Nursing
Houston, Texas

http://son.uth.tmc.edu/

Founded in 1972

DEGREES • BSN • DSN • MSN • MSN/MPH

Nursing Program Faculty 79 (72% with doctorates).

Baccalaureate Enrollment 305
Women 85% **Men** 15% **Minority** 43% **International** 2% **Part-time** 10%

Graduate Enrollment 456
Women 75% **Men** 25% **Minority** 36% **International** 3% **Part-time** 46%

Nursing Student Activities Nursing Honor Society, Sigma Theta Tau, Student Nurses' Association.

Nursing Student Resources Academic advising; academic or career counseling; assistance for students with disabilities; bookstore; campus computer network; computer lab; computer-assisted instruction; daycare for children of students; e-mail services; employment services for current students; externships; interactive nursing skills videos; learning resource lab; library services; nursing audiovisuals; skills, simulation, or other laboratory; tutoring.

Library Facilities 339,062 volumes; 5,581 periodical subscriptions.

BACCALAUREATE PROGRAMS

Degree BSN

Available Programs ADN to Baccalaureate; Accelerated Baccalaureate for Second Degree; Accelerated RN Baccalaureate; Baccalaureate for Second Degree; Generic Baccalaureate.

Site Options *Distance Learning:* Katy, TX; Richmond, TX.

Study Options Full-time.

Program Entrance Requirements Minimum overall college GPA of 2.75, transcript of college record, CPR certification, immunizations, interview, minimum GPA in nursing prerequisites of 3.0, prerequisite course work. Transfer students are accepted. **Standardized tests** *Required:* TOEFL for international students. **Application** *Deadline:* 12/31 (transfer). *Application fee:* $30.

Advanced Placement Credit by examination available.

Expenses (2004–05) *Tuition, state resident:* full-time $4560; part-time $116 per credit hour. *Tuition, nonresident:* full-time $12,320; part-time $308 per credit hour. *International tuition:* $12,320 full-time. *Room and board:* room only: $6000 per academic year. *Required fees:* full-time $1698.

Financial Aid 95% of baccalaureate students in nursing programs received some form of financial aid in 2003–04.

Contact Ms. Laurie G. Rutherford, Coordinator of Admissions, School of Nursing, The University of Texas Health Science Center at Houston, 6901 Bertner St. Suite 220, Houston, TX 77030. *Telephone:* 800-232-8876. *Fax:* 713-500-2007. *E-mail:* Laurie.G.Rutherford@uth.tmc.edu.

GRADUATE PROGRAMS

Expenses (2004–05) *Tuition, state resident:* full-time $3132; part-time $116 per credit hour. *Tuition, nonresident:* full-time $8316; part-time $308 per credit hour. *International tuition:* $8316 full-time. *Room and board:* room only: $6000 per academic year. *Required fees:* full-time $1777.

Financial Aid 95% of graduate students in nursing programs received some form of financial aid in 2003–04. Research assistantships with tuition reimbursements available, teaching assistantships with tuition reimbursements available, institutionally sponsored loans, scholarships, traineeships, and tuition waivers (full) available. Aid available to part-time students.

Contact Admissions, School of Nursing, The University of Texas Health Science Center at Houston, 1100 Holcombe Boulevard, Houston, TX 77030. *Telephone:* 800-232-8876. *Fax:* 713-500-2007. *E-mail:* admissions@uth.tmc.edu.

MASTER'S DEGREE PROGRAM

Degrees MSN; MSN/MPH

Available Programs Accelerated AD/RN to Master's; Master's.

Concentrations Available Nurse anesthesia; nurse case management; nursing administration; nursing education. *Clinical nurse specialist programs in:* acute care, adult health, gerontology, oncology, psychiatric/mental health, women's health. *Nurse practitioner programs in:* acute care, adult health, family health, gerontology, neonatal health, oncology, pediatric, psychiatric/mental health, women's health.

Study Options Full-time and part-time.

Program Entrance Requirements Clinical experience, minimum overall college GPA of 3.5, transcript of college record, CPR certification, immunizations, interview, 3 letters of recommendation, prerequisite course work, resume, statistics course, GRE or MAT. *Application deadline:* For fall admission, 5/1 (priority date). Applications are processed on a rolling basis. *Application fee:* $10.

Degree Requirements 49 total credit hours, thesis or project.

POST-MASTER'S PROGRAM

Areas of Study *Clinical nurse specialist programs in:* acute care, adult health, gerontology, oncology, psychiatric/mental health, women's health. *Nurse practitioner programs in:* acute care, adult health, family health, gerontology, neonatal health, oncology, pediatric, psychiatric/mental health, women's health.

The University of Texas Health Science Center at Houston (continued)

DOCTORAL DEGREE PROGRAM

Degree DSN

Available Programs Doctorate.

Areas of Study Addiction/substance abuse, advanced practice nursing, aging, bio-behavioral research, biology of health and illness, clinical practice, community health, critical care, ethics, faculty preparation, family health, gerontology, health policy, health promotion/disease prevention, health-care systems, human health and illness, illness and transition, individualized study, maternity-newborn, neuro-behavior, nurse case management, nursing administration, nursing education, nursing policy, nursing research, nursing science, oncology, urban health, women's health.

Program Entrance Requirements Minimum overall college GPA of 3.5, interview by faculty committee, 3 letters of recommendation, MSN or equivalent, vita, writing sample, GRE. *Application deadline:* For fall admission, 5/1 (priority date). Applications are processed on a rolling basis. *Application fee:* $10.

Degree Requirements 65 total credit hours, dissertation.

CONTINUING EDUCATION PROGRAM

Contact Gloria Spencer, RN, Coordinator for Continuing Education, School of Nursing, The University of Texas Health Science Center at Houston, 6901 Bertner St. Suite 846, Houston, TX 77030. *Telephone:* 713-500-2023. *Fax:* 713-500-2026. *E-mail:* gloria.m.spencer@uth.tmc.edu.

The University of Texas Health Science Center at San Antonio

School of Nursing
San Antonio, Texas

http://www.nursing.uthscsa.edu

Founded in 1976

DEGREES • BSN • MSN • MSN/MPH • PHD

Nursing Program Faculty 83 (50% with doctorates).

Baccalaureate Enrollment 675
Women 80% **Men** 20% **Minority** 45% **Part-time** 15%

Graduate Enrollment 150
Women 85% **Men** 15% **Minority** 15% **Part-time** 75%

Nursing Student Activities Nursing Honor Society, Sigma Theta Tau, Student Nurses' Association.

Nursing Student Resources Academic advising; assistance for students with disabilities; bookstore; campus computer network; computer lab; computer-assisted instruction; e-mail services; interactive nursing skills videos; Internet; learning resource lab; library services; nursing audiovisuals; remedial services; skills, simulation, or other laboratory; tutoring.

Library Facilities 192,576 volumes (205,641 in health, 2,056 in nursing); 2,501 periodical subscriptions (250 health-care related).

BACCALAUREATE PROGRAMS

Degree BSN

Available Programs ADN to Baccalaureate; Generic Baccalaureate; LPN to Baccalaureate; LPN to RN Baccalaureate; RN Baccalaureate.

Study Options Full-time and part-time.

Program Entrance Requirements Minimum overall college GPA of 2.0, transcript of college record, CPR certification, health insurance, immunizations, minimum GPA in nursing prerequisites of 2.3, professional liability insurance/malpractice insurance, prerequisite course work. Transfer students are accepted. **Standardized tests** *Required for some:* SAT or ACT, THEA. **Application** *Application fee:* $50.

Advanced Placement Credit by examination available. Credit given for nursing courses completed elsewhere dependent upon specific evaluations.

Expenses (2004–05) *Tuition, area resident:* full-time $1440; part-time $48 per credit hour. *Tuition, state resident:* part-time $48 per credit hour. *Tuition, nonresident:* full-time $9180; part-time $306 per credit hour. *International tuition:* $306 full-time. *Required fees:* full-time $950.

Financial Aid 80% of baccalaureate students in nursing programs received some form of financial aid in 2003–04.

Contact Dr. Brenda Jackson, Associate Dean for Undergraduate Studies, School of Nursing, The University of Texas Health Science Center at San Antonio, 7703 Floyd Curl Drive, Mail Code 7945, San Antonio, TX 78229-3900. *Telephone:* 210-567-5810. *Fax:* 210-567-3813. *E-mail:* jacksonbg@uthscsa.edu.

GRADUATE PROGRAMS

Expenses (2004–05) *Tuition, state resident:* full-time $1920; part-time $48 per credit hour. *Tuition, nonresident:* full-time $2769; part-time $306 per credit hour. *International tuition:* $2769 full-time. *Required fees:* full-time $2258.

Financial Aid 40% of graduate students in nursing programs received some form of financial aid in 2003–04. Research assistantships, teaching assistantships, institutionally sponsored loans available. *Financial aid application deadline:* 4/1.

Contact Dr. Beverly Robinson, Associate Dean for Graduate Nursing Program, School of Nursing, The University of Texas Health Science Center at San Antonio, 7703 Floyd Curl Drive, Mail Code 7945, San Antonio, TX 78229-3900. *Telephone:* 210-567-5815. *E-mail:* robinsonb@uthscsa.edu.

MASTER'S DEGREE PROGRAM

Degrees MSN; MSN/MPH

Available Programs Master's; RN to Master's.

Concentrations Available Nursing administration; nursing education; nursing informatics. *Clinical nurse specialist programs in:* acute care, critical care, medical-surgical, psychiatric/mental health. *Nurse practitioner programs in:* family health, gerontology, pediatric, psychiatric/mental health.

Study Options Full-time and part-time.

Program Entrance Requirements Clinical experience, computer literacy, minimum overall college GPA of 3.0, transcript of college record, CPR certification, immunizations, 4 letters of recommendation, professional liability insurance/malpractice insurance, prerequisite course work, statistics course, GRE General Test, MAT. *Application deadline:* For fall admission, 4/1; for spring admission, 10/1. *Application fee:* $15.

Advanced Placement Credit given for nursing courses completed elsewhere dependent upon specific evaluations.

Degree Requirements 40 total credit hours, thesis or project.

POST-MASTER'S PROGRAM

Areas of Study *Nurse practitioner programs in:* family health, gerontology, pediatric.

DOCTORAL DEGREE PROGRAM

Degree PhD

Available Programs Doctorate; Post-Baccalaureate Doctorate.

Areas of Study Clinical practice, community health, nursing research.

Site Options *Distance Learning:* Lubbock, TX; Corpus Christi, TX; Edinburg, TX.

Program Entrance Requirements Minimum overall college GPA of 3.0, interview by faculty committee, interview, 4 letters of recommendation, statistics course. *Application deadline:* For fall admission, 4/1; for spring admission, 10/1. *Application fee:* $15.

Degree Requirements 55 total credit hours, dissertation, oral exam, written exam.

CONTINUING EDUCATION PROGRAM

Contact Rosalie Tierney-Gumaer, Director of Nursing Continuing Education, School of Nursing, The University of Texas Health Science Center at San Antonio, 7703 Floyd Curl Drive, San Antonio, TX 78284. *Telephone:* 210-567-5850. *Fax:* 210-567-5909. *E-mail:* tierneyguma@uthsca.edu.

The University of Texas Medical Branch

School of Nursing
Galveston, Texas

http://www.son.utmb.edu

Founded in 1891

DEGREES • BSN • MSN • PHD

Nursing Program Faculty 64 (68% with doctorates).
Baccalaureate Enrollment 400
Women 86% **Men** 14% **Minority** 32% **International** 2% **Part-time** 43%
Graduate Enrollment 174
Women 88% **Men** 12% **Minority** 20% **International** 1% **Part-time** 63%
Nursing Student Activities Sigma Theta Tau, Student Nurses' Association.

Nursing Student Resources Academic advising; academic or career counseling; assistance for students with disabilities; bookstore; campus computer network; career placement assistance; computer lab; computer-assisted instruction; e-mail services; employment services for current students; interactive nursing skills videos; Internet; learning resource lab; library services; nursing audiovisuals; resume preparation assistance; skills, simulation, or other laboratory; tutoring.

Library Facilities 248,370 volumes (255,594 in health, 11,422 in nursing); 1,980 periodical subscriptions (4,587 health-care related).

BACCALAUREATE PROGRAMS

Degree BSN

Available Programs Accelerated Baccalaureate for Second Degree; Generic Baccalaureate; RN Baccalaureate.

Study Options Full-time and part-time.

Program Entrance Requirements Minimum overall college GPA of 2.0, transcript of college record, CPR certification, written essay, health exam, immunizations, 3 letters of recommendation, minimum GPA in nursing prerequisites of 2.75, professional liability insurance/malpractice insurance, prerequisite course work. Transfer students are accepted. **Standardized tests** *Required:* TOEFL for international students. **Application** *Application fee:* $25.

Advanced Placement Credit given for nursing courses completed elsewhere dependent upon specific evaluations.

Expenses (2004–05) *Tuition, state resident:* full-time $2640; part-time $88 per credit hour. *Tuition, nonresident:* full-time $10,380; part-time $346 per credit hour. *International tuition:* $10,380 full-time. *Room and board:* room only: $2160 per academic year. *Required fees:* full-time $570; part-time $16 per credit; part-time $87 per term.

Financial Aid 50% of baccalaureate students in nursing programs received some form of financial aid in 2003–04. *Gift aid (need-based):* Federal Pell, FSEOG, state, private, college/university gift aid from institutional funds. *Loans:* Federal Nursing Student Loans, Federal Direct (Subsidized and Unsubsidized Stafford PLUS), Perkins, state, college/university. *Work-Study:* Federal Work-Study. *Application deadline:* Continuous.

Contact Dr. Virginia Brooke, Associate Professor and Director of Baccalaureate Programs, School of Nursing, The University of Texas Medical Branch, 301 University Boulevard, Galveston, TX 77555-1029. *Telephone:* 409-772-8594. *Fax:* 409-747-1508. *E-mail:* vbrooke@utmb.edu.

GRADUATE PROGRAMS

Expenses (2004–05) *Tuition, state resident:* full-time $2640; part-time $88 per credit hour. *Tuition, nonresident:* full-time $10,380; part-time $346 per credit hour. *International tuition:* $10,380 full-time. *Room and board:* room only: $2160 per academic year. *Required fees:* full-time $570; part-time $16 per credit; part-time $87 per term.

Financial Aid 25% of graduate students in nursing programs received some form of financial aid in 2003–04.

Contact Ms. Christelle O. Bray, Associate Professor/Masters Program Director and Coordinator of Distance Education, School of Nursing, The University of Texas Medical Branch, 301 University Boulevard, Galveston, TX 77555-1029. *Telephone:* 409-772-8310. *Fax:* 409-772-3770. *E-mail:* cbray@utmb.edu.

MASTER'S DEGREE PROGRAM

Degree MSN

Available Programs Master's.

Concentrations Available Nurse-midwifery. *Nurse practitioner programs in:* acute care, adult health, family health, gerontology, neonatal health, pediatric, primary care, psychiatric/mental health, women's health.

Site Options *Distance Learning:* Nacogdoches, TX.

Study Options Full-time and part-time.

Program Entrance Requirements Clinical experience, computer literacy, minimum overall college GPA of 3.0, transcript of college record, CPR certification, written essay, immunizations, interview, 3 letters of recommendation, statistics course.

Advanced Placement Credit given for nursing courses completed elsewhere dependent upon specific evaluations.

Degree Requirements 39 total credit hours.

POST-MASTER'S PROGRAM

Areas of Study Nurse-midwifery. *Nurse practitioner programs in:* acute care, adult health, family health, gerontology, neonatal health, pediatric, primary care, psychiatric/mental health, women's health.

DOCTORAL DEGREE PROGRAM

Degree PhD

Available Programs Doctorate.

Areas of Study Aging, health promotion/disease prevention, human health and illness, nursing research.

Site Options *Distance Learning:* Nacogdoches, TX.

Program Entrance Requirements Minimum overall college GPA of 3.0, interview by faculty committee, interview, 3 letters of recommendation, MSN or equivalent, statistics course, vita, writing sample.

Degree Requirements 64 total credit hours, dissertation, oral exam, written exam, residency.

CONTINUING EDUCATION PROGRAM

Contact Ms. Phyllis Waters, RN, Director of Continuing Education, School of Nursing, The University of Texas Medical Branch, 524 Jennie Sealy Hospital, 301 University Boulevard, Galveston, TX 77555-1132. *Telephone:* 409-772-2000. *Fax:* 409-747-1531. *E-mail:* pwaters@utmb.edu.

The University of Texas–Pan American

Department of Nursing
Edinburg, Texas

http://www.panam.edu

Founded in 1927

DEGREES • BSN • MSN

Nursing Program Faculty 26 (31% with doctorates).
Baccalaureate Enrollment 145
Women 78% **Men** 22% **Minority** 85% **Part-time** 20%
Graduate Enrollment 60
Women 75% **Men** 25% **Minority** 85% **International** 5% **Part-time** 85%
Nursing Student Activities Sigma Theta Tau, Student Nurses' Association.

Nursing Student Resources Academic advising; academic or career counseling; assistance for students with disabilities; bookstore; campus computer network; career placement assistance; computer lab; computer-assisted instruction; e-mail services; employment services for current students; housing assistance; interactive nursing skills videos; Internet; learning resource lab; library services; nursing audiovisuals; paid internships; remedial services; skills, simulation, or other laboratory; tutoring.

Library Facilities 572,162 volumes (230 in health); 8,135 periodical subscriptions.

BACCALAUREATE PROGRAMS

Degree BSN

Available Programs Generic Baccalaureate; RN Baccalaureate.

Study Options Full-time.

Program Entrance Requirements Transcript of college record, CPR certification, health exam, minimum GPA in nursing prerequisites of 2.5, prerequisite course work. Transfer students are accepted. **Standardized tests** *Required:* SAT or ACT, TOEFL for international students. **Application** *Deadline:* 8/10 (freshmen), 8/10 (transfer). *Notification:* continuous (freshmen).

The University of Texas–Pan American (continued)

Expenses (2003–04) *Tuition, state resident:* full-time $2983; part-time $644 per semester. *Tuition, nonresident:* full-time $10,063; part-time $2060 per semester. *International tuition:* $10,063 full-time. *Room and board:* $2800; room only: $1800 per academic year. *Required fees:* full-time $644; part-time $218 per credit.

Financial Aid 95% of baccalaureate students in nursing programs received some form of financial aid in 2002–03.

Contact Dr. Sandy M. Sanchez, BSN Program Coordinator, Department of Nursing, The University of Texas–Pan American, 1201 West University Drive, Edinburg, TX 78539. *Telephone:* 956-381-3491. *Fax:* 956-381-2875. *E-mail:* ssanchez@panam.edu.

GRADUATE PROGRAMS

Expenses (2003–04) *Tuition, state resident:* full-time $2240; part-time $173 per contact hour. *Tuition, nonresident:* full-time $6120; part-time $409 per contact hour. *International tuition:* $6120 full-time. *Room and board:* $6036; room only: $4036 per academic year. *Required fees:* full-time $573; part-time $27 per credit; part-time $237 per term.

Financial Aid 50% of graduate students in nursing programs received some form of financial aid in 2002–03. Scholarships available. Aid available to part-time students.

Contact Dr. Barbara Tucker, MSN Coordinator, Department of Nursing, The University of Texas–Pan American, 1201 West University Drive, Edinburg, TX 78539. *Telephone:* 956-381-3491 Ext. 3493. *Fax:* 956-381-2875. *E-mail:* btucker@panam.edu.

MASTER'S DEGREE PROGRAM

Degree MSN

Available Programs Master's.

Concentrations Available *Clinical nurse specialist programs in:* adult health. *Nurse practitioner programs in:* family health, pediatric.

Study Options Full-time and part-time.

Program Entrance Requirements Minimum overall college GPA of 3.0, transcript of college record. *Application deadline:* Applications are processed on a rolling basis. *Application fee:* $35.

Advanced Placement Credit given for nursing courses completed elsewhere dependent upon specific evaluations.

Degree Requirements 43 total credit hours, thesis or project.

POST-MASTER'S PROGRAM

Areas of Study *Nurse practitioner programs in:* pediatric.

University of the Incarnate Word

Program in Nursing
San Antonio, Texas

Founded in 1881

DEGREES • BSN • MSN • MSN/MBA

Nursing Program Faculty 25 (57% with doctorates).

Baccalaureate Enrollment 129
Women 88% **Men** 12% **Minority** 57%

Graduate Enrollment 59
Women 83% **Men** 17% **Minority** 59% **Part-time** 76%

Nursing Student Activities Nursing Honor Society, Sigma Theta Tau, Student Nurses' Association.

Nursing Student Resources Academic advising; academic or career counseling; assistance for students with disabilities; bookstore; campus computer network; career placement assistance; computer lab; computer-assisted instruction; e-mail services; employment services for current students; externships; housing assistance; interactive nursing skills videos; Internet; learning resource lab; library services; nursing audiovisuals; paid internships; placement services for program completers; remedial services; resume preparation assistance; skills, simulation, or other laboratory; tutoring; unpaid internships.

Library Facilities 257,651 volumes (6,000 in health, 6,000 in nursing); 19,100 periodical subscriptions (3,048 health-care related).

BACCALAUREATE PROGRAMS

Degree BSN

Available Programs ADN to Baccalaureate; Generic Baccalaureate.

Study Options Full-time.

Program Entrance Requirements Minimum overall college GPA of 2.5, transcript of college record, CPR certification, health exam, health insurance, immunizations, minimum GPA in nursing prerequisites of 2.5, professional liability insurance/malpractice insurance, prerequisite course work. Transfer students are accepted. **Standardized tests** *Required:* SAT or ACT, TOEFL for international students. **Application** *Deadline:* rolling (freshmen), rolling (transfer). *Application fee:* $20.

Advanced Placement Credit given for nursing courses completed elsewhere dependent upon specific evaluations.

Expenses (2004–05) *Tuition:* full-time $15,600; part-time $495 per credit hour. *International tuition:* $15,600 full-time. *Room and board:* $1795 per academic year. *Required fees:* full-time $900; part-time $700 per term.

Financial Aid 90% of baccalaureate students in nursing programs received some form of financial aid in 2003–04. *Gift aid (need-based):* Federal Pell, FSEOG, state, private, college/university gift aid from institutional funds, United Negro College Fund, Federal Nursing. *Loans:* Federal Nursing Student Loans, FFEL (Subsidized and Unsubsidized Stafford PLUS), Perkins, state, alternative loans. *Work-Study:* Federal Work-Study, part-time campus jobs. *Application deadline:* Continuous.

Contact Office of Admissions, Program in Nursing, University of the Incarnate Word, 4301 Broadway, San Antonio, TX 78209. *Telephone:* 210-829-6005.

GRADUATE PROGRAMS

Expenses (2004–05) *Tuition:* part-time $520 per credit hour. *Room and board:* $2290 per academic year. *Required fees:* part-time $49 per credit.

Financial Aid 75% of graduate students in nursing programs received some form of financial aid in 2003–04. Traineeships available. Aid available to part-time students. *Financial aid application deadline:* 3/1.

Contact Dr. Sandra Strickland, Chair of Graduate Program, Program in Nursing, University of the Incarnate Word, 4301 Broadway, San Antonio, TX 78209. *Telephone:* 210-829-3988. *Fax:* 210-829-3174. *E-mail:* strickla@universe.uiwtx.edu.

MASTER'S DEGREE PROGRAM

Degrees MSN; MSN/MBA

Available Programs Master's.

Concentrations Available *Clinical nurse specialist programs in:* adult health.

Study Options Full-time and part-time.

Program Entrance Requirements Clinical experience, minimum overall college GPA of 2.5, transcript of college record, immunizations, 3 letters of recommendation, physical assessment course, professional liability insurance/malpractice insurance, statistics course, GRE General Test. *Application deadline:* For fall admission, 8/15 (priority date); for spring admission, 12/31. Applications are processed on a rolling basis. *Application fee:* $20.

Advanced Placement Credit given for nursing courses completed elsewhere dependent upon specific evaluations.

Degree Requirements 36 total credit hours, thesis or project.

West Texas A&M University

Division of Nursing
Canyon, Texas

http://www.wtamu.edu/nursing

Founded in 1909

DEGREES • BSN • MSN

Nursing Program Faculty 27 (26% with doctorates).

Baccalaureate Enrollment 410
Women 86% **Men** 14% **Minority** 23% **International** 1% **Part-time** 16%

Graduate Enrollment 51
Women 92% **Men** 8% **Minority** 24% **International** 2% **Part-time** 71%

Nursing Student Activities Sigma Theta Tau, Student Nurses' Association.

Nursing Student Resources Academic advising; academic or career counseling; assistance for students with disabilities; bookstore; campus computer network; career placement assistance; computer lab; computer-assisted instruction; daycare for children of students; e-mail services; employment services for current students; housing assistance; interactive nursing skills videos; Internet; learning resource lab; library services; nursing audiovisuals; placement services for program completers; remedial services; resume preparation assistance; skills, simulation, or other laboratory; tutoring.

Library Facilities 1.1 million volumes (16,000 in health, 8,000 in nursing); 5,464 periodical subscriptions (64 health-care related).

BACCALAUREATE PROGRAMS

Degree BSN

Available Programs ADN to Baccalaureate; Generic Baccalaureate; LPN to Baccalaureate.

Study Options Full-time and part-time.

Program Entrance Requirements Minimum overall college GPA of 2.5, transcript of college record, CPR certification, 1 year of high school math, high school transcript, immunizations, minimum GPA in nursing prerequisites of 2.0, prerequisite course work. Transfer students are accepted. **Standardized tests** *Required:* SAT or ACT, TOEFL for international students. **Application** *Deadline:* rolling (freshmen), rolling (transfer). *Notification:* continuous (freshmen). *Application fee:* $25.

Advanced Placement Credit given for nursing courses completed elsewhere dependent upon specific evaluations.

Expenses (2004–05) *Tuition, state resident:* full-time $2580; part-time $86 per credit hour. *Tuition, nonresident:* full-time $11,640; part-time $388 per credit hour. *International tuition:* $11,640 full-time. *Room and board:* $4256; room only: $1990 per academic year. *Required fees:* full-time $932; part-time $142 per credit.

Financial Aid 75% of baccalaureate students in nursing programs received some form of financial aid in 2003–04.

Contact Ms. Lynda Robinson, Admissions Counselor, Division of Nursing, West Texas A&M University, Box 60969, Canyon, TX 79016-0001. *Telephone:* 806-651-2661. *Fax:* 806-651-2632. *E-mail:* lrobinson@mail.wtamu.edu.

GRADUATE PROGRAMS

Expenses (2004–05) *Tuition, state resident:* full-time $1152; part-time $96 per credit hour. *Tuition, nonresident:* full-time $4776; part-time $398 per credit hour. *International tuition:* $4776 full-time. *Room and board:* $4256; room only: $1990 per academic year. *Required fees:* full-time $544; part-time $142 per credit.

Financial Aid 20% of graduate students in nursing programs received some form of financial aid in 2003–04. 1 teaching assistantship with partial tuition reimbursement available (averaging $6,750 per year) was awarded; career-related internships or fieldwork, Federal Work-Study, institutionally sponsored loans, scholarships, and tuition waivers (partial) also available. Aid available to part-time students.

Contact Ms. Lynda Robinson, Admissions Counselor, Division of Nursing, West Texas A&M University, Box 60969, Canyon, TX 79016-0001. *Telephone:* 806-651-2661. *Fax:* 806-651-2632. *E-mail:* lrobinson@mail.wtamu.edu.

MASTER'S DEGREE PROGRAM

Degree MSN

Available Programs Master's.

Concentrations Available Nursing administration; nursing education. *Nurse practitioner programs in:* family health.

Study Options Full-time and part-time.

Program Entrance Requirements Clinical experience, computer literacy, minimum overall college GPA of 3.0, transcript of college record, CPR certification, immunizations, nursing research course, professional liability insurance/malpractice insurance, prerequisite course work, statistics course, GRE General Test. *Application deadline:* Applications are processed on a rolling basis. *Application fee:* $25 ($75 for international students).

Degree Requirements 39 total credit hours, thesis or project.

POST-MASTER'S PROGRAM

Areas of Study *Nurse practitioner programs in:* family health.

UTAH

Brigham Young University
College of Nursing
Provo, Utah

http://nursing.byu.edu
Founded in 1875

DEGREES • BS • MS

Nursing Program Faculty 49 (45% with doctorates).

Baccalaureate Enrollment 283
Women 91% **Men** 9% **Minority** 5% **International** 3% **Part-time** 12%

Graduate Enrollment 24
Women 95% **Men** 5% **Minority** 2% **Part-time** 1%

Nursing Student Activities Nursing Honor Society, Sigma Theta Tau, Student Nurses' Association.

Nursing Student Resources Academic advising; academic or career counseling; assistance for students with disabilities; bookstore; campus computer network; career placement assistance; computer lab; computer-assisted instruction; e-mail services; employment services for current students; housing assistance; interactive nursing skills videos; Internet; learning resource lab; library services; nursing audiovisuals; other; paid internships; resume preparation assistance; skills, simulation, or other laboratory; tutoring.

Library Facilities 3.5 million volumes (24,471 in health, 3,482 in nursing); 27,161 periodical subscriptions (131 health-care related).

BACCALAUREATE PROGRAMS

Degree BS

Available Programs Generic Baccalaureate.

Study Options Full-time and part-time.

Program Entrance Requirements Transcript of college record, CPR certification, written essay, health exam, health insurance, immunizations, 2 letters of recommendation, minimum GPA in nursing prerequisites of 3.0, professional liability insurance/malpractice insurance, prerequisite course work. Transfer students are accepted. **Standardized tests** *Required:* ACT, TOEFL for international students. *Required for some:* SAT or ACT. **Application** *Deadline:* 2/15 (freshmen), 3/15 (transfer). *Notification:* continuous (freshmen). *Application fee:* $30.

Advanced Placement Credit given for nursing courses completed elsewhere dependent upon specific evaluations.

Expenses (2004–05) *Tuition:* full-time $4920; part-time $168 per credit hour. *Room and board:* $6000; room only: $4800 per academic year.

Financial Aid 65% of baccalaureate students in nursing programs received some form of financial aid in 2003–04. *Gift aid (need-based):* Federal Pell, state, private, college/university gift aid from institutional funds. *Loans:* FFEL (Subsidized and Unsubsidized Stafford PLUS), college/university. *Work-Study:* part-time campus jobs. *Application deadline:* Continuous.

Contact Ms. Linda T. Stevens, Advisement Center Supervisor, College of Nursing, Brigham Young University, 550 SWKT, Provo, UT 84602. *Telephone:* 801-422-7211. *Fax:* 801-422-0536. *E-mail:* linda_stevens@byu.edu.

GRADUATE PROGRAMS

Expenses (2004–05) *Tuition:* full-time $6210; part-time $230 per credit hour. *International tuition:* $6210 full-time.

Brigham Young University (continued)

Financial Aid 90% of graduate students in nursing programs received some form of financial aid in 2003–04. Research assistantships with full and partial tuition reimbursements available (averaging $10,000 per year), teaching assistantships with full and partial tuition reimbursements available (averaging $10,000 per year) were awarded; institutionally sponsored loans, scholarships, tuition waivers (full), and unspecified assistantships also available. Aid available to part-time students. *Financial aid application deadline:* 2/1.

Contact Denise Gibbons Davis, Research Center and Graduate Program Secretary, College of Nursing, Brigham Young University, 400 SWKT, PO Box 25426, Provo, UT 84602-5426. *Telephone:* 801-422-4142. *Fax:* 801-422-0536. *E-mail:* denise_gibbons@byu.edu.

MASTER'S DEGREE PROGRAM

Degree MS

Available Programs Master's.

Concentrations Available *Nurse practitioner programs in:* family health.

Study Options Full-time and part-time.

Program Entrance Requirements Clinical experience, minimum overall college GPA of 3.0, transcript of college record, CPR certification, written essay, immunizations, interview, 3 letters of recommendation, prerequisite course work, resume, statistics course, GRE. *Application deadline:* For spring admission, 12/1. Applications are processed on a rolling basis. *Application fee:* $50.

Advanced Placement Credit given for nursing courses completed elsewhere dependent upon specific evaluations.

Degree Requirements 50 total credit hours, thesis or project.

POST-MASTER'S PROGRAM

Areas of Study *Nurse practitioner programs in:* family health.

University of Phoenix–Utah Campus

College of Health and Human Services
Salt Lake City, Utah

Founded in 1984

DEGREES • BSN • MSN • MSN/MBA

Nursing Program Faculty 11.

Baccalaureate Enrollment 27
Women 85% **Men** 15% **Minority** 17%

Graduate Enrollment 11
Women 82% **Men** 18%

Nursing Student Activities Sigma Theta Tau.

Nursing Student Resources Academic advising; academic or career counseling; bookstore; computer lab; library services.

Library Facilities 27.1 million volumes; 11,648 periodical subscriptions (1,426 health-care related).

BACCALAUREATE PROGRAMS

Degree BSN

Available Programs ADN to Baccalaureate; Accelerated RN Baccalaureate.

Site Options Ogden, UT; Provo, UT.

Study Options Full-time.

Program Entrance Requirements 1 letter of recommendation. Transfer students are accepted. **Standardized tests** *Required:* TOEFL for international students. **Application** *Deadline:* rolling (freshmen), rolling (transfer). *Application fee:* $85.

Advanced Placement Credit by examination available.

Expenses (2004–05) *Tuition:* full-time $9540; part-time $318 per credit hour. *Required fees:* full-time $110.

Financial Aid 2% of baccalaureate students in nursing programs received some form of financial aid in 2003–04.

Contact Campus College Chair, Nursing, College of Health and Human Services, University of Phoenix–Utah Campus, 5573 South Green Street, Salt Lake City, UT 84123-4617. *Telephone:* 801-263-1444.

GRADUATE PROGRAMS

Expenses (2004–05) *Tuition:* full-time $8688; part-time $362 per credit hour. *International tuition:* $8688 full-time. *Required fees:* full-time $110.

Financial Aid 1% of graduate students in nursing programs received some form of financial aid in 2003–04.

Contact Campus College Chair, Nursing, College of Health and Human Services, University of Phoenix–Utah Campus, 5573 South Green Street, Salt Lake City, UT 84123-4617. *Telephone:* 801-263-1444.

MASTER'S DEGREE PROGRAM

Degrees MSN; MSN/MBA

Available Programs Master's.

Concentrations Available Health-care administration; nursing administration; nursing education. *Nurse practitioner programs in:* family health.

Site Options Ogden, UT; Provo, UT.

Study Options Full-time.

Program Entrance Requirements Clinical experience, computer literacy, minimum overall college GPA of 2.5, transcript of college record.

Degree Requirements 39 total credit hours, thesis or project.

POST-MASTER'S PROGRAM

Areas of Study *Nurse practitioner programs in:* family health.

University of Utah

College of Nursing
Salt Lake City, Utah

http://www.nurs.utah.edu

Founded in 1850

DEGREES • BS • MS • PHD

Nursing Program Faculty 83 (47% with doctorates).

Baccalaureate Enrollment 342
Women 87% **Men** 13% **Minority** 9% **International** 1% **Part-time** 16%

Graduate Enrollment 200
Women 88% **Men** 12% **Minority** 88% **International** 9% **Part-time** 58%

Nursing Student Activities Sigma Theta Tau, Student Nurses' Association.

Nursing Student Resources Academic advising; academic or career counseling; assistance for students with disabilities; bookstore; campus computer network; computer lab; computer-assisted instruction; e-mail services; externships; interactive nursing skills videos; Internet; learning resource lab; library services; nursing audiovisuals; paid internships; resume preparation assistance; skills, simulation, or other laboratory; unpaid internships.

Library Facilities 3 million volumes (22,000 in health, 8,000 in nursing); 33,517 periodical subscriptions (2,050 health-care related).

BACCALAUREATE PROGRAMS

Degree BS

Available Programs Generic Baccalaureate; RN Baccalaureate.

Study Options Full-time.

Program Entrance Requirements Minimum overall college GPA of 2.8, transcript of college record, CPR certification, written essay, health exam, immunizations, 3 letters of recommendation, minimum GPA in nursing prerequisites of 2.8, professional liability insurance/malpractice insurance, prerequisite course work. Transfer students are accepted. **Standardized tests** *Required:* SAT or ACT, TOEFL for international students. *Recommended:* ACT. **Application** *Deadline:* 4/1 (freshmen), 4/1 (transfer). *Application fee:* $35.

Advanced Placement Credit by examination available. Credit given for nursing courses completed elsewhere dependent upon specific evaluations.

Expenses (2003–04) *Tuition, state resident:* full-time $3100; part-time $962 per semester. *Tuition, nonresident:* full-time $9600; part-time $2900 per semester. *International tuition:* $9600 full-time. *Room and board:* $6000; room only: $4000 per academic year. *Required fees:* full-time $100.

Financial Aid 50% of baccalaureate students in nursing programs received some form of financial aid in 2002–03. *Gift aid (need-based):* Federal Pell, FSEOG, state, private, college/university gift aid from institutional funds. *Loans:* Federal Nursing Student Loans, FFEL (Subsidized and Unsubsidized Stafford PLUS), Perkins, college/university, alternative loans. *Work-Study:* Federal Work-Study. *Application deadline (priority):* 3/15.

Contact Kaelyn Fife, Manager Student Affairs, College of Nursing, University of Utah, 10 South 2000, Salt Lake City, UT 84112-5880. *Telephone:* 801-581-3414. *Fax:* 801-581-4642. *E-mail:* kaelyn.fife@nurs.utah.edu.

GRADUATE PROGRAMS

Expenses (2003–04) *Tuition, state resident:* full-time $4300; part-time $1775 per semester. *Tuition, nonresident:* full-time $10,150; part-time $4000 per semester. *International tuition:* $10,150 full-time. *Room and board:* $6000; room only: $4000 per academic year.

Financial Aid 60% of graduate students in nursing programs received some form of financial aid in 2002–03. Fellowships, research assistantships, teaching assistantships, scholarships available. *Financial aid application deadline:* 2/15.

Contact Ms. Kaelyn Fife, Manager Student Affairs, College of Nursing, University of Utah, 10 South 2000, Salt Lake City, UT 84112-5880. *Telephone:* 801-581-3414. *Fax:* 801-581-4642. *E-mail:* kaelyn.fife@nurs.utah.edu.

MASTER'S DEGREE PROGRAM

Degree MS

Concentrations Available Nurse-midwifery; nursing administration; nursing education; nursing informatics. *Clinical nurse specialist programs in:* acute care, adult health, community health, oncology. *Nurse practitioner programs in:* acute care, adult health, family health, gerontology, neonatal health, oncology, pediatric, psychiatric/mental health, women's health.

Study Options Full-time and part-time.

Program Entrance Requirements Computer literacy, minimum overall college GPA of 3.0, transcript of college record, CPR certification, written essay, immunizations, 3 letters of recommendation, professional liability insurance/malpractice insurance, resume, statistics course, GRE General Test. *Application deadline:* For fall admission, 2/15 (priority date). *Application fee:* $45 ($60 for international students).

Advanced Placement Credit given for nursing courses completed elsewhere dependent upon specific evaluations.

Degree Requirements 35 total credit hours, thesis or project, comprehensive exam.

POST-MASTER'S PROGRAM

Areas of Study *Clinical nurse specialist programs in:* acute care, adult health, community health, oncology. *Nurse practitioner programs in:* acute care, adult health, family health, gerontology, neonatal health, oncology, pediatric, psychiatric/mental health, women's health.

DOCTORAL DEGREE PROGRAM

Degree PhD

Available Programs Doctorate.

Areas of Study Aging, clinical practice, faculty preparation, gerontology, health promotion/disease prevention, health-care systems, individualized study, information systems, nursing administration, nursing education, nursing policy, nursing research, oncology, women's health.

Program Entrance Requirements Minimum overall college GPA of 3.3, interview by faculty committee, interview, 3 letters of recommendation, MSN or equivalent, vita, writing sample, GRE General Test. *Application deadline:* For fall admission, 2/15 (priority date). *Application fee:* $45 ($60 for international students).

Degree Requirements 80 total credit hours, dissertation, oral exam, residency.

POSTDOCTORAL PROGRAM

Areas of Study Gerontology, information systems, nursing informatics, nursing interventions, outcomes.

Postdoctoral Program Contact Dr. Susan Beck, Associate Dean for Research, College of Nursing, University of Utah, 10 South 2000 East, Salt Lake City, UT 84112-5880. *Telephone:* 801-585-9609. *Fax:* 801-581-4642. *E-mail:* susan.beck@nurs.utah.edu.

Utah Valley State College
Department of Nursing
Orem, Utah

http://www.uvsc.edu/nurs/

Founded in 1941

DEGREE • BSN

Nursing Program Faculty 22 (22% with doctorates).

Nursing Student Activities Student Nurses' Association.

Nursing Student Resources Academic advising; academic or career counseling; assistance for students with disabilities; bookstore; campus computer network; career placement assistance; computer lab; daycare for children of students; e-mail services; employment services for current students; interactive nursing skills videos; Internet; learning resource lab; library services; nursing audiovisuals; resume preparation assistance; skills, simulation, or other laboratory; tutoring; unpaid internships.

Library Facilities 173,000 volumes; 6,000 periodical subscriptions.

BACCALAUREATE PROGRAMS

Degree BSN

Available Programs RN Baccalaureate.

Study Options Part-time.

Program Entrance Requirements CPR certification, health exam, health insurance, immunizations, prerequisite course work, RN licensure. Transfer students are accepted. **Standardized tests** *Required:* TOEFL for international students. ***Placement:*** *Required:* SAT I, ACT, or in-house tests. **Application** *Deadline:* rolling (freshmen), rolling (transfer). *Notification:* continuous (freshmen). *Application fee:* $30.

Advanced Placement Credit by examination available.

Expenses (2004–05) *Tuition, state resident:* full-time $1186; part-time $174 per credit hour. *Tuition, nonresident:* full-time $4151; part-time $609 per credit hour. *International tuition:* $4151 full-time. *Required fees:* full-time $416; part-time $40 per credit; part-time $208 per term.

Financial Aid 10% of baccalaureate students in nursing programs received some form of financial aid in 2003–04. *Gift aid (need-based):* Federal Pell, FSEOG, state, private, college/university gift aid from institutional funds. *Loans:* FFEL (Subsidized and Unsubsidized Stafford PLUS), Perkins, college/university. *Work-Study:* Federal Work-Study. *Application deadline (priority):* 6/1.

Contact Mrs. Lynnae Marsing, Acedemic Advisor, Department of Nursing, Utah Valley State College, Department of Nursing, MS 172, 800 West University Parkway, Orem, UT 84058. *Telephone:* 801-863-8199. *Fax:* 801-863-6093. *E-mail:* marsinly@uvsc.edu.

Weber State University
Program in Nursing
Ogden, Utah

Founded in 1889

DEGREE • BSN

Nursing Program Faculty 42 (5% with doctorates).

Baccalaureate Enrollment 140

Women 85% **Men** 15% **Minority** 4% **International** 1% **Part-time** 7%

Nursing Student Activities Sigma Theta Tau, Student Nurses' Association.

Nursing Student Resources Academic advising; academic or career counseling; assistance for students with disabilities; bookstore; campus computer network; career placement assistance; computer lab; computer-assisted instruction; daycare for children of students; e-mail services;

Weber State University (continued)
employment services for current students; housing assistance; interactive nursing skills videos; Internet; learning resource lab; library services; nursing audiovisuals; resume preparation assistance; skills, simulation, or other laboratory; tutoring; unpaid internships.

Library Facilities 734,487 volumes (800 in health, 800 in nursing); 120 periodical subscriptions health-care related.

BACCALAUREATE PROGRAMS

Degree BSN

Available Programs ADN to Baccalaureate.

Site Options *Distance Learning:* Logan, UT; St. George, UT; Payson, UT.

Study Options Full-time and part-time.

Program Entrance Requirements Minimum overall college GPA of 3.0, transcript of college record, written essay, 3 letters of recommendation, minimum GPA in nursing prerequisites of 2.0, prerequisite course work, RN licensure. Transfer students are accepted. **Standardized tests** *Recommended:* TOEFL for international students. ***Placement:*** *Required:* SAT or ACT. **Application** *Deadline:* 8/22 (freshmen), rolling (transfer). *Notification:* continuous (freshmen). *Application fee:* $30.

Advanced Placement Credit by examination available. Credit given for nursing courses completed elsewhere dependent upon specific evaluations.

Expenses (2003–04) *Tuition, state resident:* full-time $2364. *Tuition, nonresident:* full-time $7092. *International tuition:* $7092 full-time. *Required fees:* full-time $515.

Financial Aid 4% of baccalaureate students in nursing programs received some form of financial aid in 2002–03.

Contact Doug Watson, Academic Admissions Advisor, Program in Nursing, Weber State University, 3907 University Circle, Ogden, UT 84408-3907. *Telephone:* 801-626-6128. *Fax:* 801-626-6382. *E-mail:* dwatson@weber.edu.

Westminster College

St. Mark's-Westminster School of Nursing and Health Sciences
Salt Lake City, Utah

http://www.westminstercollege.edu

Founded in 1875

DEGREES • BSN • MSN

Nursing Program Faculty 22 (14% with doctorates).

Baccalaureate Enrollment 157

Graduate Enrollment 15

Women 84% **Men** 16%

Nursing Student Activities Sigma Theta Tau, Student Nurses' Association, nursing club.

Nursing Student Resources Academic advising; academic or career counseling; assistance for students with disabilities; bookstore; campus computer network; career placement assistance; computer lab; computer-assisted instruction; e-mail services; employment services for current students; housing assistance; interactive nursing skills videos; Internet; learning resource lab; library services; nursing audiovisuals; placement services for program completers; remedial services; resume preparation assistance; skills, simulation, or other laboratory; tutoring.

Library Facilities 119,410 volumes; 689 periodical subscriptions.

BACCALAUREATE PROGRAMS

Degree BSN

Available Programs Baccalaureate for Second Degree; Generic Baccalaureate; RN Baccalaureate.

Study Options Full-time.

Program Entrance Requirements Transcript of college record, written essay, 3 letters of recommendation, minimum GPA in nursing prerequisites of 2.5, prerequisite course work. Transfer students are accepted. **Standardized tests** *Required:* SAT or ACT, TOEFL for international students. **Application** *Deadline:* 4/15 (freshmen), rolling (transfer). *Notification:* 10/1 (freshmen). *Application fee:* $40.

Expenses (2003–04) *Tuition:* full-time $16,704. *Room and board:* $5960 per academic year. *Required fees:* full-time $290.

Financial Aid 95% of baccalaureate students in nursing programs received some form of financial aid in 2002–03. *Gift aid (need-based):* Federal Pell, FSEOG, state, private, college/university gift aid from institutional funds, United Negro College Fund, Federal Nursing. *Loans:* FFEL (Subsidized and Unsubsidized Stafford PLUS), Perkins. *Work-Study:* Federal Work-Study, part-time campus jobs. *Application deadline (priority):* 4/15.

Contact Department of Nursing, St. Mark's-Westminster School of Nursing and Health Sciences, Westminster College, 1840 South 1300 East, Salt Lake City, UT 84105. *Telephone:* 801-832-2150. *Fax:* 801-832-3110.

GRADUATE PROGRAMS

Expenses (2003–04) *Tuition:* part-time $696 per credit hour.

Financial Aid Scholarships and tuition remissions available.

Contact Department of Nursing, St. Mark's-Westminster School of Nursing and Health Sciences, Westminster College, 1840 South 1300 East, Salt Lake City, UT 84105. *Telephone:* 801-832-2150. *Fax:* 801-832-3110.

MASTER'S DEGREE PROGRAM

Degree MSN

Available Programs Master's.

Concentrations Available Nursing education. *Nurse practitioner programs in:* family health.

Program Entrance Requirements Transcript of college record, written essay, 3 letters of recommendation, resume. *Application deadline:* For fall admission, 3/1 (priority date). Applications are processed on a rolling basis. *Application fee:* $30.

Advanced Placement Credit given for nursing courses completed elsewhere dependent upon specific evaluations.

Degree Requirements 42 total credit hours, thesis or project.

POST-MASTER'S PROGRAM

Areas of Study *Nurse practitioner programs in:* family health.

See full description on page 598.

VERMONT

Norwich University

Division of Nursing
Northfield, Vermont

http://www.norwich.edu/acad/nursing

Founded in 1819

DEGREE • BSN

Nursing Program Faculty 8 (10% with doctorates).

Baccalaureate Enrollment 90

Women 90% **Men** 10% **Minority** 10% **Part-time** 20%

Nursing Student Activities Student Nurses' Association, nursing club.

Nursing Student Resources Academic advising; academic or career counseling; assistance for students with disabilities; bookstore; campus computer network; career placement assistance; computer lab; e-mail services; employment services for current students; externships; housing assistance; interactive nursing skills videos; Internet; learning resource lab; library services; nursing audiovisuals; placement services for program completers; remedial services; resume preparation assistance; skills, simulation, or other laboratory; tutoring; unpaid internships.

Library Facilities 280,000 volumes; 904 periodical subscriptions.

BACCALAUREATE PROGRAMS

Degree BSN

Available Programs ADN to Baccalaureate; Generic Baccalaureate; RN Baccalaureate.

Site Options Rutland, VT.

Study Options Full-time and part-time.

Program Entrance Requirements Minimum overall college GPA of 2.5, transcript of college record, CPR certification, written essay, health exam, health insurance, high school biology, high school chemistry, 2 years high school math, 2 years high school science, high school transcript, immunizations, interview, 2 letters of recommendation, minimum GPA in nursing prerequisites of 2.5. Transfer students are accepted. **Standardized tests** *Required:* SAT or ACT, TOEFL for international students. *Recommended:* SAT Subject Tests. **Application** *Deadline:* rolling (freshmen), rolling (transfer). *Early decision:* 11/15. *Notification:* continuous (freshmen), 12/15 (out-of-state freshmen), 12/15 (early decision). *Application fee:* $35.

Advanced Placement Credit given for nursing courses completed elsewhere dependent upon specific evaluations.

Expenses (2003–04) *Tuition:* full-time $17,630; part-time $8815 per semester. *Room and board:* $6720 per academic year. *Required fees:* full-time $2150; part-time $530 per term.

Financial Aid 90% of baccalaureate students in nursing programs received some form of financial aid in 2002–03. *Gift aid (need-based):* Federal Pell, FSEOG, state, private, college/university gift aid from institutional funds. *Loans:* FFEL (Subsidized and Unsubsidized Stafford PLUS), Perkins, college/university. *Work-Study:* Federal Work-Study. *Application deadline (priority):* 3/1.

Contact Rose Myers, Admissions Office, Division of Nursing, Norwich University, 158 Harmon Drive, Northfield, VT 05663. *Telephone:* 802-485-2008. *Fax:* 802-485-2032. *E-mail:* nuadm@norwich.edu.

Southern Vermont College

Department of Nursing
Bennington, Vermont

http://www.svc.edu/academics/divisions/nursing.html

Founded in 1926

DEGREE • BSN

Nursing Program Faculty 6.

Library Facilities 26,000 volumes; 250 periodical subscriptions.

BACCALAUREATE PROGRAMS

Degree BSN

Available Programs ADN to Baccalaureate; RN Baccalaureate.

Program Entrance Requirements **Standardized tests** *Required:* SAT or ACT, TOEFL for international students. **Application** *Deadline:* rolling (freshmen), rolling (transfer). *Notification:* continuous (freshmen). *Application fee:* $30.

Advanced Placement Credit by examination available.

Expenses (2003–04) *Tuition:* full-time $11,996; part-time $295 per credit hour. *Room and board:* $3115; room only: $1450 per academic year.

Contact Holly S. Madison, Chair, Department of Nursing, Southern Vermont College, 982 Mansion Drive, Bennington, VT 05201. *Telephone:* 802-447-4656. *Fax:* 802-447-4652.

University of Vermont

Department of Nursing
Burlington, Vermont

Founded in 1791

DEGREES • BS • MS

Nursing Program Faculty 34 (41% with doctorates).

Baccalaureate Enrollment 345
Women 92% **Men** 8% **Minority** 3% **Part-time** 5%

Graduate Enrollment 45
Women 100% **Minority** 4% **Part-time** 66%

Nursing Student Activities Nursing Honor Society, Sigma Theta Tau, Student Nurses' Association.

Nursing Student Resources Academic advising; academic or career counseling; assistance for students with disabilities; bookstore; campus computer network; computer lab; computer-assisted instruction; e-mail services; employment services for current students; interactive nursing skills videos; Internet; learning resource lab; library services; nursing audiovisuals; remedial services; resume preparation assistance; skills, simulation, or other laboratory; tutoring.

Library Facilities 2.4 million volumes (1,250 in health, 1,250 in nursing); 20,216 periodical subscriptions (1,492 health-care related).

■ The University of Vermont offers generic baccalaureate, RN-BS-MS, and master's programs in nursing. The generic baccalaureate program prepares students for the practice of professional nursing. The RN-BS-MS accelerated program is designed for RNs with an associate degree or diploma in nursing. The master's program prepares RNs for advanced practice nursing in the areas of community health or primary care (adult or family nurse practitioner). Students completing the master's program are eligible for specialty certification. Nurses with a bachelor's degree in a field other than nursing are eligible to apply to the master's program through a bridge process.

BACCALAUREATE PROGRAMS

Degree BS

Available Programs Accelerated RN Baccalaureate; Generic Baccalaureate; RN Baccalaureate.

Study Options Full-time and part-time.

Program Entrance Requirements Minimum overall college GPA of 2.0, transcript of college record, written essay, high school biology, high school chemistry, high school foreign language, 3 years high school math, 2 years high school science, high school transcript, immunizations, letters of recommendation, minimum GPA in nursing prerequisites of 2.0. Transfer students are accepted. **Standardized tests** *Required:* SAT or ACT, TOEFL for international students. **Application** *Deadline:* 1/15 (freshmen), 4/1 (transfer). *Early decision:* 11/1. *Notification:* 3/31 (freshmen), 12/15 (early action). *Application fee:* $45.

Advanced Placement Credit by examination available. Credit given for nursing courses completed elsewhere dependent upon specific evaluations.

Expenses (2004–05) *Tuition, state resident:* full-time $9088; part-time $379 per credit hour. *Tuition, nonresident:* full-time $22,728; part-time $947 per credit hour. *Room and board:* $7016 per academic year. *Required fees:* full-time $1138.

Financial Aid 86% of baccalaureate students in nursing programs received some form of financial aid in 2003–04.

Contact Ms. Tacy Lincoln, Director of Student Services, Department of Nursing, University of Vermont, Rowell Building, Room 106, Burlington, VT 05405-0068. *Telephone:* 802-656-0968. *E-mail:* Tacy.Lincoln@uvm.edu.

GRADUATE PROGRAMS

Expenses (2004–05) *Tuition, state resident:* full-time $3411; part-time $379 per credit hour. *Tuition, nonresident:* full-time $8523; part-time $947 per credit hour. *Required fees:* full-time $568; part-time $34 per credit.

Financial Aid 28% of graduate students in nursing programs received some form of financial aid in 2003–04. *Application deadline:* 3/1.

Contact Dr. Gregg E Newschwander, Chair, Department of Nursing, Department of Nursing, University of Vermont, 106 Carrigan Drive, 216 Rowell Building, Burlington, VT 05405-0068. *Telephone:* 802-656-3051. *Fax:* 802-656-8306. *E-mail:* newsch@uvm.edu.

MASTER'S DEGREE PROGRAM

Degree MS

University of Vermont (continued)

Available Programs Master's; Master's for Nurses with Non-Nursing Degrees; RN to Master's.

Concentrations Available *Clinical nurse specialist programs in:* adult health, community health, public health. *Nurse practitioner programs in:* adult health, family health.

Study Options Full-time and part-time.

Program Entrance Requirements Minimum overall college GPA of 3.0, transcript of college record, written essay, 3 letters of recommendation, physical assessment course, statistics course, GRE General Test. *Application deadline:* For fall admission, 4/1 (priority date). Applications are processed on a rolling basis. *Application fee:* $25.

Advanced Placement Credit by examination available. Credit given for nursing courses completed elsewhere dependent upon specific evaluations.

Degree Requirements 57 total credit hours, thesis or project, comprehensive exam.

POST-MASTER'S PROGRAM

Areas of Study *Nurse practitioner programs in:* adult health, family health.

VIRGIN ISLANDS

University of the Virgin Islands

Division of Nursing
Saint Thomas, Virgin Islands

Founded in 1962

DEGREE • BS

Nursing Program Faculty 10 (50% with doctorates).

Baccalaureate Enrollment 48
Women 96% **Men** 4% **Minority** 96% **International** 2% **Part-time** 6%

Nursing Student Activities Student Nurses' Association.

Nursing Student Resources Academic advising; assistance for students with disabilities; bookstore; campus computer network; computer lab; computer-assisted instruction; e-mail services; housing assistance; interactive nursing skills videos; Internet; learning resource lab; library services; nursing audiovisuals; paid internships; skills, simulation, or other laboratory; tutoring.

Library Facilities 106,361 volumes (94,469 in health, 567 in nursing); 136,790 periodical subscriptions (10 health-care related).

BACCALAUREATE PROGRAMS

Degree BS

Available Programs Generic Baccalaureate; RN Baccalaureate.

Site Options St. Thomas, VI.

Study Options Full-time and part-time.

Program Entrance Requirements Minimum overall college GPA of 2.0, CPR certification, health exam, 2 years high school math, high school transcript, immunizations, minimum GPA in nursing prerequisites of 2.0, professional liability insurance/malpractice insurance, prerequisite course work. Transfer students are accepted. **Standardized tests** *Required:* SAT or ACT, TOEFL for international students. **Application** *Deadline:* 4/30 (freshmen), 4/30 (transfer). *Notification:* continuous (freshmen). *Application fee:* $25.

Advanced Placement Credit given for nursing courses completed elsewhere dependent upon specific evaluations.

Expenses (2004–05) *Tuition, state resident:* full-time $3000; part-time $100 per credit hour. *Tuition, nonresident:* full-time $4500; part-time $300 per credit hour. *International tuition:* $4500 full-time. *Room and board:* $4875; room only: $2200 per academic year. *Required fees:* full-time $353; part-time $278 per credit.

Financial Aid 85% of baccalaureate students in nursing programs received some form of financial aid in 2003–04.

Contact Dr. Gloria B. Callwood, Chair, Division of Nursing, University of the Virgin Islands, 2 John Brewer's Bay, St. Thomas, VI 00802-9990. *Telephone:* 340-693-1291. *Fax:* 340-693-1285. *E-mail:* gcallwo@uvi.edu.

CONTINUING EDUCATION PROGRAM

Contact Dr. Gloria B. Callwood, Chair, Division of Nursing, University of the Virgin Islands, 2 John Brewer's Bay, St. Thomas, VI 00802-9990. *Telephone:* 340-693-1291. *Fax:* 340-693-1285. *E-mail:* gcallwo@uvi.edu.

VIRGINIA

Eastern Mennonite University

Department of Nursing
Harrisonburg, Virginia

Founded in 1917

DEGREE • BSN

Nursing Program Faculty 10 (20% with doctorates).

Baccalaureate Enrollment 126
Women 93% **Men** 7% **Minority** 3% **International** 7%

Nursing Student Activities Sigma Theta Tau, Student Nurses' Association.

Nursing Student Resources Academic advising; academic or career counseling; assistance for students with disabilities; bookstore; campus computer network; career placement assistance; computer lab; computer-assisted instruction; e-mail services; employment services for current students; externships; housing assistance; interactive nursing skills videos; Internet; learning resource lab; library services; nursing audiovisuals; placement services for program completers; remedial services; resume preparation assistance; skills, simulation, or other laboratory; tutoring.

Library Facilities 163,932 volumes (1,256 in health, 926 in nursing); 1,112 periodical subscriptions (33 health-care related).

BACCALAUREATE PROGRAMS

Degree BSN

Available Programs ADN to Baccalaureate; Baccalaureate for Second Degree; Generic Baccalaureate; LPN to Baccalaureate.

Site Options Lancaster , PA.

Study Options Full-time and part-time.

Program Entrance Requirements Minimum overall college GPA of 2.6, transcript of college record, CPR certification, written essay, health exam, health insurance, high school chemistry, high school transcript, immunizations, 3 letters of recommendation, minimum high school GPA of 2.0, minimum GPA in nursing prerequisites of 2.6, professional liability insurance/malpractice insurance, prerequisite course work. Transfer students are accepted. **Standardized tests** *Required:* SAT or ACT, TOEFL for international students. **Application** *Deadline:* 8/15 (freshmen), 8/15 (transfer). *Notification:* continuous (freshmen). *Application fee:* $25.

Advanced Placement Credit given for nursing courses completed elsewhere dependent upon specific evaluations.

Expenses (2004–05) *Tuition:* full-time $18,220; part-time $760 per contact hour. *International tuition:* $18,220 full-time. *Required fees:* full-time $200.

Financial Aid 95% of baccalaureate students in nursing programs received some form of financial aid in 2003–04. *Gift aid (need-based):* Federal Pell, FSEOG, state, private, college/university gift aid from institutional funds. *Loans:* Federal Nursing Student Loans, FFEL (Subsidized and Unsubsidized Stafford PLUS), Perkins, state. *Work-Study:* Federal Work-Study, part-time campus jobs. *Application deadline (priority):* 4/15.

Contact Mr. Lawrence W. Miller, Director of Admissions, Department of Nursing, Eastern Mennonite University, 1200 Park Road, Harrisonburg, VA 22802. *Telephone:* 800-368-2665. *Fax:* 540-432-4444. *E-mail:* millerlw@emu.edu.

George Mason University
College of Nursing and Health Science
Fairfax, Virginia

http://cnhs.gmu.edu/

Founded in 1957

DEGREES • BSN • MSN • MSN/MBA • PHD

Nursing Program Faculty 39.

Nursing Student Activities Nursing Honor Society, Sigma Theta Tau, Student Nurses' Association.

Nursing Student Resources E-mail services; skills, simulation, or other laboratory.

Library Facilities 1.5 million volumes (16,172 in nursing); 27,708 periodical subscriptions (200 health-care related).

BACCALAUREATE PROGRAMS

Degree BSN

Available Programs Accelerated Baccalaureate for Second Degree; Accelerated LPN to Baccalaureate; Accelerated RN Baccalaureate; Generic Baccalaureate.

Study Options Full-time and part-time.

Program Entrance Requirements Minimum overall college GPA of 3.0, CPR certification, health exam, health insurance, immunizations, minimum GPA in nursing prerequisites, prerequisite course work. Transfer students are accepted. **Standardized tests** *Required:* SAT or ACT, TOEFL for international students. **Application** *Deadline:* 1/15 (freshmen), 3/15 (transfer). *Notification:* 4/1 (freshmen). *Application fee:* $40.

Contact Dr. Christena Langley, Assistant Dean, Undergraduate Programs and Community Liaison, College of Nursing and Health Science, George Mason University, Mailstop 3C4, 4400 University Drive, Fairfax, VA 22030-4444. *Telephone:* 703-993-1904. *Fax:* 703-993-3606. *E-mail:* clangley@gmu.edu.

GRADUATE PROGRAMS

Financial Aid Fellowships, research assistantships, teaching assistantships, tuition waivers (partial) available.

Contact Dr. Teresa Panniers, Assistant Dean for Graduate Programs, College of Nursing and Health Science, George Mason University, Mailstop 3C4, 4400 University Drive, Fairfax, VA 22030-4444. *Telephone:* 703-993-1947. *Fax:* 703-993-1949. *E-mail:* tpanniers@gmu.edu.

MASTER'S DEGREE PROGRAM

Degrees MSN; MSN/MBA

Available Programs Master's; RN to Master's.

Concentrations Available Nursing administration. *Nurse practitioner programs in:* adult health, family health, gerontology, primary care.

Study Options Full-time and part-time.

Program Entrance Requirements Clinical experience, minimum overall college GPA of 3.0, CPR certification, written essay, immunizations, 3 letters of recommendation, physical assessment course, statistics course. *Application deadline:* For fall admission, 5/1; for spring admission, 11/1. *Application fee:* $60.

POST-MASTER'S PROGRAM

Areas of Study Nursing administration; nursing education.

DOCTORAL DEGREE PROGRAM

Degree PhD

Available Programs Doctorate.

Areas of Study Nursing administration.

Program Entrance Requirements Clinical experience, minimum overall college GPA of 3.25, interview, 3 letters of recommendation, MSN or equivalent, statistics course, writing sample, MAT. *Application deadline:* For fall admission, 5/1; for spring admission, 11/1. *Application fee:* $60.

Degree Requirements 60 total credit hours, dissertation, oral exam, written exam.

POSTDOCTORAL PROGRAM

Postdoctoral Program Contact Mr. Jean Sorrell, Coordinator, College of Nursing and Health Science, George Mason University, Mailstop 3C4, 4400 University Drive, Fairfax, VA 22030-4444. *Telephone:* 703-993-1944. *Fax:* 703-993-1942. *E-mail:* jsorrell@gmu.edu.

CONTINUING EDUCATION PROGRAM

Contact Beverly T. Boyd, RN, Director, Office of Professional Development, College of Nursing and Health Science, George Mason University, Mailstop 3C4, 4400 University Drive, Fairfax, VA 22030-4444. *Telephone:* 703-993-1910. *Fax:* 703-993-3612. *E-mail:* bboyd@gmu.edu.

Hampton University
Department of Nursing
Hampton, Virginia

http://www.hamptonu.edu/nursing/Index.htm

Founded in 1868

DEGREES • BS • MS • PHD

Nursing Program Faculty 35 (51% with doctorates).

Baccalaureate Enrollment 388

Women 91% **Men** 9% **Minority** 97% **International** 3% **Part-time** 3%

Graduate Enrollment 72

Women 86% **Men** 14% **Minority** 58% **Part-time** 35%

Nursing Student Activities Nursing Honor Society, Sigma Theta Tau, Student Nurses' Association.

Nursing Student Resources Academic advising; bookstore; computer lab; e-mail services; interactive nursing skills videos; Internet; library services; tutoring.

Library Facilities 336,092 volumes (4,000 in health, 2,000 in nursing); 1,414 periodical subscriptions (500 health-care related).

BACCALAUREATE PROGRAMS

Degree BS

Available Programs ADN to Baccalaureate; Accelerated Baccalaureate; Accelerated RN Baccalaureate; Baccalaureate for Second Degree; Generic Baccalaureate; LPN to Baccalaureate; LPN to RN Baccalaureate; RN Baccalaureate.

Site Options Virginia Beach, VA.

Study Options Full-time and part-time.

Program Entrance Requirements Minimum overall college GPA of 2.3, transcript of college record, CPR certification, written essay, health exam, health insurance, high school biology, high school chemistry, 3 years high school math, 2 years high school science, high school transcript, immunizations, 2 letters of recommendation, minimum high school GPA of 2.0, minimum high school rank 50%, minimum GPA in nursing prerequisites of 2.0, professional liability insurance/malpractice insurance. Transfer students are accepted. **Standardized tests** *Required:* SAT or ACT, TOEFL for international students. **Application** *Deadline:* 3/1 (freshmen), 3/1 (transfer). *Notification:* continuous until 7/31 (freshmen). *Application fee:* $25.

Advanced Placement Credit by examination available. Credit given for nursing courses completed elsewhere dependent upon specific evaluations.

Expenses (2003–04) *Tuition:* full-time $12,864; part-time $290 per credit hour. *International tuition:* $12,864 full-time. *Room and board:* $18,982; room only: $300 per academic year.

Financial Aid 93% of baccalaureate students in nursing programs received some form of financial aid in 2002–03.

Hampton University (continued)

Contact Mrs. Johnnie Bunch, Chairperson, Department of Undergraduate Nursing Education, Department of Nursing, Hampton University, Freeman Hall, Hampton, VA 23668. *Telephone:* 757-727-5251. *Fax:* 757-727-5423. *E-mail:* nursing@hamptonu.edu.

GRADUATE PROGRAMS

Expenses (2003–04) *Tuition:* full-time $9990; part-time $275 per credit hour. *Room and board:* $29,140; room only: $1000 per academic year.

Financial Aid 90% of graduate students in nursing programs received some form of financial aid in 2002–03. Fellowships, research assistantships, teaching assistantships, career-related internships or fieldwork, Federal Work-Study, institutionally sponsored loans, and scholarships available. Aid available to part-time students. *Financial aid application deadline:* 5/1.

Contact Dr. Arlene Montgomery, Chairperson, Department of Graduate Nursing Education, Department of Nursing, Hampton University, Freeman Hall, Hampton, VA 23668. *Telephone:* 757-727-5251. *Fax:* 757-727-5423.

MASTER'S DEGREE PROGRAM

Degree MS

Available Programs Master's.

Concentrations Available Nursing administration; nursing education. *Clinical nurse specialist programs in:* adult health, community health, psychiatric/mental health. *Nurse practitioner programs in:* family health, gerontology, pediatric, women's health.

Study Options Full-time and part-time.

Program Entrance Requirements Clinical experience, minimum overall college GPA of 2.5, transcript of college record, CPR certification, immunizations, interview, 2 letters of recommendation, nursing research course, physical assessment course, professional liability insurance/malpractice insurance, prerequisite course work, resume, statistics course, GRE General Test. *Application deadline:* For fall admission, 6/1 (priority date); for spring admission, 11/1. Applications are processed on a rolling basis. *Application fee:* $25.

Advanced Placement Credit given for nursing courses completed elsewhere dependent upon specific evaluations.

Degree Requirements 45 total credit hours, thesis or project, comprehensive exam.

POST-MASTER'S PROGRAM

Areas of Study *Nurse practitioner programs in:* family health.

DOCTORAL DEGREE PROGRAM

Degree PhD

Available Programs Doctorate.

Areas of Study Family health.

Program Entrance Requirements Clinical experience, minimum overall college GPA of 3.5, interview, 2 letters of recommendation, MSN or equivalent, scholarly papers, statistics course, vita, writing sample. *Application deadline:* For fall admission, 6/1 (priority date); for spring admission, 11/1. Applications are processed on a rolling basis. *Application fee:* $25.

Degree Requirements 48 total credit hours, dissertation, oral exam, written exam, residency.

James Madison University
Department of Nursing
Harrisonburg, Virginia

http://www.nursing.jmu.edu

Founded in 1908

DEGREES • BSN • MSN

Nursing Program Faculty 18 (33% with doctorates).

Baccalaureate Enrollment 362
Women 96% **Men** 4% **Minority** 4% **Part-time** 1%

Graduate Enrollment 11

Nursing Student Activities Nursing Honor Society, Sigma Theta Tau, Student Nurses' Association.

Nursing Student Resources Academic advising; academic or career counseling; assistance for students with disabilities; bookstore; campus computer network; career placement assistance; computer lab; computer-assisted instruction; e-mail services; employment services for current students; externships; interactive nursing skills videos; Internet; learning resource lab; library services; nursing audiovisuals; paid internships; remedial services; resume preparation assistance; skills, simulation, or other laboratory; unpaid internships.

Library Facilities 67,716 volumes in health, 12,054 volumes in nursing; 565 periodical subscriptions health-care related.

BACCALAUREATE PROGRAMS

Degree BSN

Available Programs Generic Baccalaureate.

Site Options Staunton, VA; Waynesboro, VA; Charlottesville, VA.

Study Options Full-time and part-time.

Program Entrance Requirements Minimum overall college GPA of 2.7, transcript of college record, CPR certification, written essay, health exam, health insurance, immunizations, minimum GPA in nursing prerequisites of 2.0, prerequisite course work. Transfer students are accepted. **Standardized tests** *Required:* SAT or ACT, TOEFL for international students. **Application** *Deadline:* 1/15 (freshmen), 3/1 (transfer). *Early decision:* 11/1. *Notification:* 4/1 (freshmen), 1/15 (early action). *Application fee:* $40.

Expenses (2004–05) *Tuition, state resident:* full-time $5476; part-time $1990 per term. *Tuition, nonresident:* full-time $14,420; part-time $5270 per term. *International tuition:* $14,420 full-time. *Room and board:* $5880; room only: $3661 per academic year. *Required fees:* full-time $275.

Financial Aid 35% of baccalaureate students in nursing programs received some form of financial aid in 2003–04.

Contact Ms. Karen A. McMillen, Administrative Office Specialist II, Department of Nursing, James Madison University, 701 Carrier Drive, MSC 4305, Harrisonburg, VA 22807. *Telephone:* 540-568-6314. *Fax:* 540-568-7896. *E-mail:* mcmillka@jmu.edu.

GRADUATE PROGRAMS

Expenses (2004–05) *Tuition, state resident:* full-time $2712; part-time $226 per credit hour. *Tuition, nonresident:* full-time $7920; part-time $660 per credit hour. *International tuition:* $7920 full-time. *Room and board:* $5880; room only: $3166 per academic year.

Contact Ms. Karen A. McMillen, Administrative Office Specialist II, Department of Nursing, James Madison University, 701 Carrier Drive, MSC 4305, Harrisonburg, VA 22807. *Telephone:* 540-568-6314. *Fax:* 540-568-7896. *E-mail:* mcmillka@jmu.edu.

MASTER'S DEGREE PROGRAM

Degree MSN

Available Programs Master's; RN to Master's.

Concentrations Available Nursing education. *Nurse practitioner programs in:* gerontology.

Study Options Full-time and part-time.

Program Entrance Requirements Clinical experience, computer literacy, minimum overall college GPA of 2.0, transcript of college record, CPR certification, written essay, immunizations, 2 letters of recommendation, physical assessment course, prerequisite course work, resume, statistics course.

Degree Requirements 47 total credit hours, thesis or project.

POST-MASTER'S PROGRAM

Areas of Study Nursing education.

Jefferson College of Health Sciences
Nursing Education Program
Roanoke, Virginia

http://www.jchs.edu

Founded in 1982

DEGREES • BSN • MSN

Nursing Program Faculty 18 (11% with doctorates).

Baccalaureate Enrollment 70
Women 90% **Men** 10% **Minority** 10% **Part-time** 90%

Nursing Student Activities Nursing Honor Society, Student Nurses' Association.

Nursing Student Resources Academic advising; academic or career counseling; assistance for students with disabilities; bookstore; campus computer network; computer lab; computer-assisted instruction; e-mail services; externships; housing assistance; interactive nursing skills videos; Internet; learning resource lab; library services; nursing audiovisuals; skills, simulation, or other laboratory; tutoring.

Library Facilities 10,533 volumes (4,910 in health, 804 in nursing); 376 periodical subscriptions (274 health-care related).

BACCALAUREATE PROGRAMS

Degree BSN

Available Programs ADN to Baccalaureate.

Site Options *Distance Learning:* Roanoke, VA.

Study Options Full-time and part-time.

Program Entrance Requirements Transcript of college record, CPR certification, health insurance, immunizations, prerequisite course work, RN licensure. Transfer students are accepted. **Standardized tests** *Required:* TOEFL for international students. *Recommended:* SAT. *Required for some:* SAT or ACT, ACT ASSET. **Application** *Deadline:* 7/31 (freshmen). *Early decision:* 10/15. *Notification:* continuous until 7/31 (freshmen), 12/1 (out-of-state freshmen), 12/1 (early decision). *Application fee:* $50.

Advanced Placement Credit by examination available. Credit given for nursing courses completed elsewhere dependent upon specific evaluations.

Expenses (2004–05) *Tuition:* full-time $12,000; part-time $275 per credit hour.

Financial Aid 90% of baccalaureate students in nursing programs received some form of financial aid in 2003–04. *Gift aid (need-based):* Federal Pell, FSEOG, state, private, college/university gift aid from institutional funds. *Loans:* FFEL (Subsidized and Unsubsidized Stafford PLUS), alternative loans. *Work-Study:* Federal Work-Study. *Application deadline:* Continuous.

Contact Dr. Lisa Allison-Jones, Nursing Department Chair, Nursing Education Program, Jefferson College of Health Sciences, PO Box 13186, Roanoke, VA 24031-3186. *Telephone:* 540-224-6970. *Fax:* 540-224-4785. *E-mail:* lallisonjones@jchs.edu.

GRADUATE PROGRAMS

Contact Dr. Lisa Allison-Jones, Nursing Department Chair, Nursing Education Program, Jefferson College of Health Sciences, 920 South Jefferson Street, PO Box 13186, Roanoke, VA 24031-3186. *Telephone:* 540-224-6970. *Fax:* 540-224-4785. *E-mail:* lallisonjones@jchs.edu.

MASTER'S DEGREE PROGRAM

Degree MSN

Available Programs Master's; Master's for Nurses with Non-Nursing Degrees.

Concentrations Available Nursing administration; nursing education.

Site Options *Distance Learning:* Roanoke, VA.

Study Options Full-time and part-time.

Program Entrance Requirements Clinical experience, computer literacy, transcript of college record, 2 letters of recommendation, nursing research course, resume, statistics course.

Degree Requirements 37 total credit hours, thesis or project.

CONTINUING EDUCATION PROGRAM

Contact Ms. Bridget Moore, Associate Dean for Program Development and Extended Learning, Nursing Education Program, Jefferson College of Health Sciences, PO Box 13186, Roanoke, VA 24031-3186. *Telephone:* 540-224-4676. *E-mail:* bhmoore@jchs.edu.

Liberty University

Department of Nursing
Lynchburg, Virginia

http://www.liberty.edu

Founded in 1971

DEGREES • BSN • MSN

Nursing Program Faculty 16 (38% with doctorates).

Baccalaureate Enrollment 236
Women 85% **Men** 15% **Minority** 4% **International** 10% **Part-time** 6%

Graduate Enrollment 20
Women 90% **Men** 10% **Part-time** 60%

Nursing Student Activities Student Nurses' Association.

Nursing Student Resources Academic advising; academic or career counseling; assistance for students with disabilities; bookstore; campus computer network; computer lab; e-mail services; interactive nursing skills videos; Internet; learning resource lab; library services; nursing audiovisuals; resume preparation assistance; skills, simulation, or other laboratory; tutoring.

Library Facilities 199,150 volumes (3,632 in health, 3,000 in nursing); 12,426 periodical subscriptions (46 health-care related).

BACCALAUREATE PROGRAMS

Degree BSN

Available Programs Generic Baccalaureate; RN Baccalaureate.

Study Options Full-time and part-time.

Program Entrance Requirements Minimum overall college GPA of 3.0, transcript of college record, CPR certification, written essay, immunizations, 2 letters of recommendation, professional liability insurance/malpractice insurance, prerequisite course work. Transfer students are accepted. **Standardized tests** *Required:* SAT or ACT, TOEFL for international students. *Required for some:* ACT. **Application** *Deadline:* 6/30 (freshmen). *Notification:* continuous until 8/15 (freshmen). *Application fee:* $35.

Advanced Placement Credit given for nursing courses completed elsewhere dependent upon specific evaluations.

Expenses (2004–05) *Tuition:* full-time $12,600; part-time $325 per credit hour. *Room and board:* $5400 per academic year. *Required fees:* full-time $425.

Financial Aid 75% of baccalaureate students in nursing programs received some form of financial aid in 2003–04.

Contact Dr. Deanna Britt, Chair, Department of Nursing, Liberty University, 1971 University Boulevard, Lynchburg, VA 24502. *Telephone:* 804-582-2519. *Fax:* 804-582-7035. *E-mail:* dbritt@liberty.edu.

GRADUATE PROGRAMS

Expenses (2004–05) *Tuition:* part-time $300 per credit hour.

Contact Dr. Hila Spear, Director of Master Program, Department of Nursing, Liberty University, Lynchburg, VA 24502. *Telephone:* 804-582-2519. *E-mail:* hspear@liberty.edu.

MASTER'S DEGREE PROGRAM

Degree MSN

Available Programs Master's.

Concentrations Available *Clinical nurse specialist programs in:* acute care, community health.

Study Options Full-time and part-time.

Program Entrance Requirements Clinical experience, minimum overall college GPA of 3.0, transcript of college record, CPR certification, written essay, immunizations, interview, 3 letters of recommendation, nursing research course, physical assessment course, prerequisite course work, resume, statistics course.

Degree Requirements 36 total credit hours, thesis or project.

Lynchburg College

School of Health Sciences and Human Performance
Lynchburg, Virginia

http://www.lynchburg.edu/schools/NRSG.htm

Founded in 1903

DEGREE • BS

Nursing Program Faculty 9 (33% with doctorates).

Lynchburg College (continued)

Baccalaureate Enrollment 150

Women 85% **Men** 15% **Minority** 10% **International** 2%

Nursing Student Activities Sigma Theta Tau, Student Nurses' Association.

Nursing Student Resources Academic advising; academic or career counseling; assistance for students with disabilities; bookstore; campus computer network; computer lab; computer-assisted instruction; e-mail services; employment services for current students; externships; Internet; learning resource lab; library services; nursing audiovisuals; resume preparation assistance; skills, simulation, or other laboratory; tutoring; unpaid internships.

Library Facilities 287,601 volumes (6,259 in health, 1,881 in nursing); 636 periodical subscriptions (65 health-care related).

BACCALAUREATE PROGRAMS

Degree BS

Available Programs Generic Baccalaureate.

Study Options Full-time and part-time.

Program Entrance Requirements Minimum overall college GPA of 2.0, transcript of college record, CPR certification, written essay, health exam, health insurance, high school biology, high school chemistry, high school foreign language, 3 years high school math, 3 years high school science, high school transcript, immunizations, 1 letter of recommendation, minimum GPA in nursing prerequisites of 2.5, prerequisite course work. Transfer students are accepted. **Standardized tests** *Required:* SAT or ACT, TOEFL for international students. **Application** *Deadline:* rolling (freshmen), rolling (transfer). *Early decision:* 11/15. *Notification:* continuous (freshmen), 12/15 (out-of-state freshmen), 12/15 (early decision). *Application fee:* $30.

Advanced Placement Credit given for nursing courses completed elsewhere dependent upon specific evaluations.

Expenses (2004–05) *Tuition:* full-time $22,640; part-time $325 per credit hour. *International tuition:* $22,640 full-time. *Room and board:* $5000; room only: $2900 per academic year.

Financial Aid 97% of baccalaureate students in nursing programs received some form of financial aid in 2003–04. *Gift aid (need-based):* Federal Pell, FSEOG, state, college/university gift aid from institutional funds. *Loans:* FFEL (Subsidized and Unsubsidized Stafford PLUS), Perkins. *Work-Study:* Federal Work-Study, part-time campus jobs. *Application deadline (priority):* 3/1.

Contact Linda L. Andrews, Dean for the School of Health Sciences and Human Performance, School of Health Sciences and Human Performance, Lynchburg College, McMillan Nursing Building, 1501 Lakeside Drive, Lynchburg, VA 24501-3199. *Telephone:* 434-544-8324. *Fax:* 434-544-8323. *E-mail:* andrews@lynchburg.edu.

Marymount University

School of Health Professions
Arlington, Virginia

http://www.marymount.edu

Founded in 1950

DEGREES • BSN • MSN

Nursing Program Faculty 18 (55% with doctorates).

Baccalaureate Enrollment 91

Women 93% **Men** 7% **Minority** 56% **International** 4% **Part-time** 22%

Graduate Enrollment 44

Women 77% **Men** 23% **Minority** 43% **International** 6% **Part-time** 79%

Nursing Student Activities Sigma Theta Tau, Student Nurses' Association.

Nursing Student Resources Academic advising; academic or career counseling; assistance for students with disabilities; bookstore; campus computer network; career placement assistance; computer lab; computer-assisted instruction; e-mail services; externships; interactive nursing skills videos; Internet; learning resource lab; library services; nursing audiovisuals; paid internships; remedial services; resume preparation assistance; skills, simulation, or other laboratory; tutoring; unpaid internships.

Library Facilities 187,097 volumes (10,000 in health, 1,044 in nursing); 1,048 periodical subscriptions (219 health-care related).

■ Marymount University is a comprehensive, coeducational Catholic university in Arlington, Virginia, minutes from Washington, DC. The School of Health Professions offers nursing programs at the undergraduate and graduate levels. The Bachelor of Science in Nursing (BSN) program is a four-year course of study that combines a liberal arts core with nursing education. The freshman and sophomore curriculum includes general required courses along with science and introductory nursing classes; junior- and senior-year courses are focused on nursing classes with extensive clinical experiences. A special, time-shortened program is available for students who have a previous baccalaureate degree. The graduate nursing program offers Master of Science in Nursing (MSN) degrees and certificates in critical-care nursing, family nurse practitioner, and nursing education. The School of Health Professions also offers an undergraduate degree in health sciences with either a health promotion or a pre–physical therapy concentration, a master's degree program in health promotion management, and a doctorate in physical therapy.

BACCALAUREATE PROGRAMS

Degree BSN

Available Programs ADN to Baccalaureate; Accelerated Baccalaureate; Accelerated Baccalaureate for Second Degree; Accelerated LPN to Baccalaureate; Accelerated RN Baccalaureate; Baccalaureate for Second Degree; Generic Baccalaureate; LPN to Baccalaureate; LPN to RN Baccalaureate; RN Baccalaureate.

Site Options Arlington, VA.

Study Options Full-time and part-time.

Program Entrance Requirements Minimum overall college GPA of 2.0, health exam, health insurance, high school transcript, 2 letters of recommendation, minimum high school GPA of 2.5. Transfer students are accepted. **Standardized tests** *Required:* SAT or ACT, TOEFL for international students. **Application** *Deadline:* rolling (freshmen), rolling (transfer). *Notification:* continuous (freshmen). *Application fee:* $35.

Advanced Placement Credit by examination available. Credit given for nursing courses completed elsewhere dependent upon specific evaluations.

Expenses (2004–05) *Tuition:* full-time $16,952; part-time $549 per credit hour. *International tuition:* $16,952 full-time. *Room and board:* $7520 per academic year. *Required fees:* full-time $1000.

Financial Aid 75% of baccalaureate students in nursing programs received some form of financial aid in 2003–04.

Contact Dr. Liane M. Summerfield, Associate Dean, School of Health Professions, Marymount University, 2807 North Glebe Road, Arlington, VA 22207-4299. *Telephone:* 703-284-1627. *Fax:* 703-284-3819. *E-mail:* liane.summerfield@marymount.edu.

GRADUATE PROGRAMS

Expenses (2004–05) *Tuition:* part-time $526 per credit hour. *Required fees:* part-time $6 per credit.

Financial Aid 28% of graduate students in nursing programs received some form of financial aid in 2003–04. Research assistantships with full tuition reimbursements available, career-related internships or fieldwork and scholarships available. Aid available to part-time students.

Contact Ms. Francesca Reed, Coordinator, Graduate Admissions, School of Health Professions, Marymount University, 2807 North Glebe Road, Arlington, VA 22207-4299. *Telephone:* 703-284-5906. *E-mail:* francesca.reed@marymount.edu.

MASTER'S DEGREE PROGRAM

Degree MSN

Available Programs Master's; RN to Master's.

Concentrations Available Nursing education. *Clinical nurse specialist programs in:* critical care. *Nurse practitioner programs in:* family health.

Site Options Arlington, VA.

Study Options Full-time and part-time.

Program Entrance Requirements Minimum overall college GPA of 3.0, transcript of college record, CPR certification, immunizations, interview, 2 letters of recommendation, professional liability insurance/ malpractice insurance, resume, statistics course. *Application deadline:* Applications are processed on a rolling basis. *Application fee:* $35.

Advanced Placement Credit given for nursing courses completed elsewhere dependent upon specific evaluations.

Degree Requirements 40 total credit hours, comprehensive exam.

POST-MASTER'S PROGRAM

Areas of Study Nursing education. *Clinical nurse specialist programs in:* critical care. *Nurse practitioner programs in:* family health.

Norfolk State University

Department of Nursing
Norfolk, Virginia

http://www.nsu.edu/schools/sciencetech/nursing/

Founded in 1935

DEGREE • BSN

Library Facilities 378,323 volumes; 124,460 periodical subscriptions.

BACCALAUREATE PROGRAMS

Degree BSN

Available Programs Accelerated Baccalaureate for Second Degree; Accelerated LPN to Baccalaureate; Baccalaureate for Second Degree; RN Baccalaureate.

Program Entrance Requirements Minimum overall college GPA of 2.0, transcript of college record, CPR certification, health exam, minimum GPA in nursing prerequisites of 2.0, professional liability insurance/ malpractice insurance, prerequisite course work, RN licensure. Transfer students are accepted. **Standardized tests** *Required:* SAT or ACT, TOEFL for international students. **Application** *Deadline:* 7/15 (freshmen), 7/15 (transfer). *Application fee:* $25.

Contact Department Head, Department of Nursing, Norfolk State University, 700 Park Avenue, Norfolk, VA 23504. *Telephone:* 757-823-9013. *Fax:* 757-823-8241.

Old Dominion University

Department of Nursing
Norfolk, Virginia

http://www.odu.edu/nursson

Founded in 1930

DEGREES • BSN • MSN

Nursing Program Faculty 27 (29% with doctorates).

Baccalaureate Enrollment 598

Women 93% **Men** 7% **Minority** 16% **Part-time** 62%

Graduate Enrollment 173

Women 87% **Men** 13% **Minority** 12% **Part-time** 51%

Nursing Student Activities Sigma Theta Tau, Student Nurses' Association.

Nursing Student Resources Academic advising; bookstore; campus computer network; computer lab; computer-assisted instruction; e-mail services; Internet; learning resource lab; library services; nursing audiovisuals; skills, simulation, or other laboratory; tutoring.

Library Facilities 985,801 volumes (3,745 in health, 2,850 in nursing); 10,579 periodical subscriptions (155 health-care related).

BACCALAUREATE PROGRAMS

Degree BSN

Available Programs Accelerated Baccalaureate; Generic Baccalaureate; RN Baccalaureate.

Site Options *Distance Learning:* Olympia, WA; Yavapai, AZ; Athens, GA.

Study Options Full-time.

Program Entrance Requirements Transcript of college record, minimum GPA in nursing prerequisites of 3.0, prerequisite course work. Transfer students are accepted. **Standardized tests** *Required:* SAT or ACT, TOEFL for international students. **Application** *Deadline:* 3/15 (freshmen), 5/1 (transfer). *Early decision:* 12/15. *Notification:* continuous (freshmen), 1/15 (early action). *Application fee:* $40.

Expenses (2004–05) *Tuition, state resident:* part-time $170 per credit hour. *Tuition, nonresident:* part-time $484 per credit hour. *Room and board:* $5802; room only: $3342 per academic year. *Required fees:* full-time $168; part-time $84 per term.

Financial Aid 48% of baccalaureate students in nursing programs received some form of financial aid in 2003–04. *Gift aid (need-based):* Federal Pell, FSEOG, state, private, college/university gift aid from institutional funds, United Negro College Fund, Federal Nursing. *Loans:* Federal Direct (Subsidized and Unsubsidized Stafford PLUS), Perkins. *Work-Study:* Federal Work-Study. *Application deadline:* 3/15 (priority: 2/15).

Contact Ms. Phyllis D. Barham, Chief Academic Advisor, Department of Nursing, Old Dominion University, Norfolk, VA 23529-0500. *Telephone:* 757-683-5245. *Fax:* 757-683-5253. *E-mail:* pbarham@odu.edu.

GRADUATE PROGRAMS

Expenses (2004–05) *Tuition, area resident:* part-time $246 per credit hour. *Tuition, state resident:* part-time $284 per credit hour. *Tuition, nonresident:* part-time $631 per credit hour. *International tuition:* $18,200 full-time. *Required fees:* part-time $250 per term.

Financial Aid 41% of graduate students in nursing programs received some form of financial aid in 2003–04.

Contact Dr. Laurel Garzon, Graduate Program Director, Department of Nursing, Old Dominion University, School of Nursing, Hughes Hall Room 2091, Norfolk, VA 23529-0500. *Telephone:* 757-683-4298. *Fax:* 757-683-5253. *E-mail:* lgarzon@odu.edu.

MASTER'S DEGREE PROGRAM

Degree MSN

Available Programs Master's; RN to Master's.

Concentrations Available Health-care administration; nurse anesthesia; nurse-midwifery; nursing administration; nursing education. *Clinical nurse specialist programs in:* parent-child. *Nurse practitioner programs in:* family health, pediatric, women's health.

Site Options *Distance Learning:* Olympia, WA; Yavapai, AZ; Athens, GA.

Study Options Full-time and part-time.

Program Entrance Requirements Clinical experience, computer literacy, minimum overall college GPA of 3.0, transcript of college record, CPR certification, written essay, immunizations, interview, 3 letters of recommendation, physical assessment course, statistics course.

Advanced Placement Credit given for nursing courses completed elsewhere dependent upon specific evaluations.

Degree Requirements 47 total credit hours, comprehensive exam.

POST-MASTER'S PROGRAM

Areas of Study Health-care administration; nurse anesthesia; nurse-midwifery; nursing administration; nursing education. *Clinical nurse specialist programs in:* parent-child. *Nurse practitioner programs in:* family health, pediatric, women's health.

CONTINUING EDUCATION PROGRAM

Contact Mrs. Kimberly Curry-Lourenco, Lecturer, Department of Nursing, Old Dominion University, School of Nursing, 2066 Hughes Hall, Norfolk, VA 23529-0500. *Telephone:* 757-683-5261. *Fax:* 757-683-5253. *E-mail:* kcurrylo@odu.edu.

Radford University

School of Nursing
Radford, Virginia

http://www.radford.edu/nurs-web

Founded in 1910

DEGREES • BSN • MSN

Radford University (continued)

Nursing Program Faculty 40 (40% with doctorates).

Baccalaureate Enrollment 143
Women 90% **Men** 10% **Minority** 15% **International** 3%

Graduate Enrollment 44
Women 90% **Men** 10% **Minority** 15% **Part-time** 20%

Nursing Student Activities Nursing Honor Society, Sigma Theta Tau, Student Nurses' Association.

Nursing Student Resources Academic advising; academic or career counseling; assistance for students with disabilities; bookstore; campus computer network; career placement assistance; computer lab; computer-assisted instruction; e-mail services; employment services for current students; externships; housing assistance; interactive nursing skills videos; Internet; learning resource lab; library services; nursing audiovisuals; resume preparation assistance; skills, simulation, or other laboratory; unpaid internships.

Library Facilities 395,643 volumes; 4,162 periodical subscriptions.

BACCALAUREATE PROGRAMS

Degree BSN

Available Programs Generic Baccalaureate; RN Baccalaureate.

Site Options *Distance Learning:* Roanoke, VA.

Study Options Full-time.

Program Entrance Requirements Minimum overall college GPA of 2.5, transcript of college record, CPR certification, written essay, health exam, health insurance, high school biology, high school chemistry, high school transcript, immunizations, minimum GPA in nursing prerequisites of 2.5, prerequisite course work. Transfer students are accepted. **Standardized tests** *Required:* SAT or ACT, TOEFL for international students. **Application** *Deadline:* 4/1 (freshmen), 6/1 (transfer). *Notification:* continuous until 6/1 (freshmen). *Application fee:* $35.

Advanced Placement Credit given for nursing courses completed elsewhere dependent upon specific evaluations.

Expenses (2004–05) *Tuition, state resident:* full-time $12,000; part-time $198 per credit hour. *Tuition, nonresident:* full-time $20,000; part-time $490 per credit hour. *Room and board:* $2900; room only: $1577 per academic year.

Financial Aid 50% of baccalaureate students in nursing programs received some form of financial aid in 2003–04. *Gift aid (need-based):* Federal Pell, FSEOG, state, private, college/university gift aid from institutional funds. *Loans:* Federal Nursing Student Loans, FFEL (Subsidized and Unsubsidized Stafford PLUS), Perkins, state, college/university. *Work-Study:* Federal Work-Study, part-time campus jobs. *Application deadline (priority):* 3/1.

Contact Dr. Marcella Griggs, Director, School of Nursing, Radford University, Box 6964, RU Station, Waldron Hall, Room 305, Radford, VA 24142. *Telephone:* 540-831-7700. *Fax:* 540-831-7716. *E-mail:* nurs-web@radford.edu.

GRADUATE PROGRAMS

Expenses (2004–05) *Tuition, state resident:* full-time $4100; part-time $226 per credit hour. *Tuition, nonresident:* full-time $7500; part-time $417 per credit hour. *Room and board:* $2900; room only: $1577 per academic year.

Financial Aid 90% of graduate students in nursing programs received some form of financial aid in 2003–04. 5 fellowships with tuition reimbursements available (averaging $4,604 per year) were awarded; research assistantships, teaching assistantships with tuition reimbursements available, career-related internships or fieldwork, Federal Work-Study, institutionally sponsored loans, and scholarships also available. *Financial aid application deadline:* 2/1.

Contact Dr. Karolyn Givens, Graduate Program Coordinator, School of Nursing, Radford University, Box 6964, RU Station, Waldron Hall, Radford, VA 24142. *Telephone:* 540-831-7700. *Fax:* 540-831-7716. *E-mail:* nurs-web@radford.edu.

MASTER'S DEGREE PROGRAM

Degree MSN

Available Programs Accelerated RN to Master's; Master's.

Concentrations Available Nurse-midwifery. *Clinical nurse specialist programs in:* adult health, gerontology. *Nurse practitioner programs in:* family health.

Study Options Full-time and part-time.

Program Entrance Requirements Clinical experience, computer literacy, minimum overall college GPA of 3.0, transcript of college record, CPR certification, written essay, immunizations, interview, 3 letters of recommendation, nursing research course, physical assessment course, professional liability insurance/malpractice insurance, prerequisite course work, resume, statistics course, GMAT, GRE General Test, MAT, or NTE. *Application deadline:* For fall admission, 2/1 (priority date); for spring admission, 10/1. Applications are processed on a rolling basis. *Application fee:* $25.

Advanced Placement Credit given for nursing courses completed elsewhere dependent upon specific evaluations.

Degree Requirements 34 total credit hours, thesis or project, comprehensive exam.

Shenandoah University
Division of Nursing
Winchester, Virginia

http://www.su.edu/nursing/index.html

Founded in 1875

DEGREES • BSN • MSN

Nursing Program Faculty 18 (80% with doctorates).

Baccalaureate Enrollment 190
Women 97% **Men** 3% **Minority** 10% **International** 3% **Part-time** 15%

Graduate Enrollment 29
Women 97% **Men** 3% **Minority** 10% **Part-time** 50%

Nursing Student Activities Nursing Honor Society, Student Nurses' Association.

Nursing Student Resources Academic advising; academic or career counseling; assistance for students with disabilities; bookstore; campus computer network; computer lab; daycare for children of students; e-mail services; interactive nursing skills videos; Internet; learning resource lab; library services; nursing audiovisuals; resume preparation assistance; skills, simulation, or other laboratory.

Library Facilities 123,628 volumes (500 in health, 200 in nursing); 11,000 periodical subscriptions (250 health-care related).

BACCALAUREATE PROGRAMS

Degree BSN

Available Programs ADN to Baccalaureate; Accelerated Baccalaureate for Second Degree; Generic Baccalaureate; LPN to Baccalaureate; LPN to RN Baccalaureate; RN Baccalaureate.

Site Options Leesburg, VA.

Study Options Full-time and part-time.

Program Entrance Requirements Minimum overall college GPA of 2.5, transcript of college record, CPR certification, health exam, health insurance, high school biology, high school chemistry, 2 years high school math, high school transcript, immunizations, minimum high school GPA of 2.5, minimum GPA in nursing prerequisites of 2.0, prerequisite course work. Transfer students are accepted. **Standardized tests** *Required:* SAT or ACT, TOEFL for international students. **Application** *Deadline:* rolling (freshmen). *Application fee:* $30.

Advanced Placement Credit by examination available. Credit given for nursing courses completed elsewhere dependent upon specific evaluations.

Expenses (2004–05) *Tuition:* full-time $19,090; part-time $585 per credit hour.

Financial Aid 80% of baccalaureate students in nursing programs received some form of financial aid in 2003–04.

Contact Dr. Sheila Sparks Ralph, Director, Division of Nursing, Shenandoah University, 1460 University Drive, Winchester, VA 22601. *Telephone:* 540-678-4381. *Fax:* 540-665-5519. *E-mail:* ssparks@su.edu.

GRADUATE PROGRAMS

Expenses (2004–05) *Tuition:* part-time $585 per credit hour.

Financial Aid 85% of graduate students in nursing programs received some form of financial aid in 2003–04. 2 teaching assistantships with partial tuition reimbursements available (averaging $10,088 per year) were awarded; institutionally sponsored loans and scholarships also available. Aid available to part-time students. *Financial aid application deadline:* 3/15.

Contact Dr. Patricia Krauskopf, Coordinator, FNP Graduate Program, Division of Nursing, Shenandoah University, 1775 North Sector Court, Winchester, VA 22601. *Telephone:* 540-665-5512. *Fax:* 540-665-5519. *E-mail:* pkrausk@su.edu.

MASTER'S DEGREE PROGRAM

Degree MSN

Available Programs Master's; RN to Master's.

Concentrations Available Nurse case management; nurse-midwifery. *Nurse practitioner programs in:* family health, psychiatric/mental health.

Study Options Full-time and part-time.

Program Entrance Requirements Clinical experience, computer literacy, minimum overall college GPA of 2.8, transcript of college record, CPR certification, immunizations, interview, 3 letters of recommendation, physical assessment course, professional liability insurance/malpractice insurance, prerequisite course work, resume, statistics course, GRE General Test. *Application deadline:* For fall admission, 6/15 (priority date). Applications are processed on a rolling basis. *Application fee:* $30.

Advanced Placement Credit given for nursing courses completed elsewhere dependent upon specific evaluations.

Degree Requirements 37 total credit hours, thesis or project.

POST-MASTER'S PROGRAM

Areas of Study Nurse-midwifery. *Nurse practitioner programs in:* family health, psychiatric/mental health.

CONTINUING EDUCATION PROGRAM

Contact Dr. R.T. Good, Dean, School of Continuing Education, Division of Nursing, Shenandoah University, 1460 University Drive, Winchester, VA 22601. *Telephone:* 540-665-4584. *E-mail:* rtgood@su.edu.

University of Virginia

School of Nursing
Charlottesville, Virginia

http://www.nursing.virginia.edu

Founded in 1819

DEGREES • BSN • MSN • MSN/HSM • MSN/MA • MSN/MBA • MSN/PHD

Nursing Program Faculty 60 (55% with doctorates).

Baccalaureate Enrollment 325

Women 95% **Men** 5% **Minority** 14% **International** 1% **Part-time** 5%

Graduate Enrollment 170

Women 93% **Men** 7% **Minority** 12% **International** 2% **Part-time** 48%

Nursing Student Activities Sigma Theta Tau, Student Nurses' Association, nursing club.

Nursing Student Resources Academic advising; academic or career counseling; assistance for students with disabilities; bookstore; campus computer network; career placement assistance; computer lab; computer-assisted instruction; e-mail services; housing assistance; interactive nursing skills videos; Internet; learning resource lab; library services; nursing audiovisuals; placement services for program completers; remedial services; resume preparation assistance; skills, simulation, or other laboratory; tutoring.

Library Facilities 4.9 million volumes (180,000 in health); 53,015 periodical subscriptions.

BACCALAUREATE PROGRAMS

Degree BSN

Available Programs ADN to Baccalaureate; Generic Baccalaureate; RN Baccalaureate.

Study Options Full-time.

Program Entrance Requirements Transcript of college record, written essay, health insurance, high school biology, high school chemistry, high school foreign language, 2 years high school math, 1 year of high school science, high school transcript, immunizations, 1 letter of recommendation, minimum GPA in nursing prerequisites of 2.0. Transfer students are accepted. **Standardized tests** *Required:* SAT and SAT Subject Tests or ACT, SAT II Writing Tests, TOEFL for international students, students are required to take two SAT tests of their choice. **Application** *Deadline:* 1/2 (freshmen), 3/1 (transfer). *Early decision:* 11/1. *Notification:* 4/1 (freshmen), 12/1 (out-of-state freshmen), 12/1 (early decision). *Application fee:* $40.

Advanced Placement Credit by examination available.

Expenses (2004–05) *Tuition, state resident:* full-time $6553. *Tuition, nonresident:* full-time $22,755. *International tuition:* $22,755 full-time. *Room and board:* $5591 per academic year. *Required fees:* full-time $102.

Financial Aid 25% of baccalaureate students in nursing programs received some form of financial aid in 2003–04.

Contact Dr. Theresa J. Carroll, Assistant Dean for Undergraduate Student Services, School of Nursing, University of Virginia, McLeod Hall, PO Box 800782, Charlottesville, VA 22908. *Telephone:* 888-283-8703. *Fax:* 434-924-0528. *E-mail:* nur-osa@virginia.edu.

GRADUATE PROGRAMS

Expenses (2004–05) *Tuition, state resident:* full-time $9255. *Tuition, nonresident:* full-time $20,255. *International tuition:* $20,255 full-time. *Required fees:* full-time $102.

Financial Aid 90% of graduate students in nursing programs received some form of financial aid in 2003–04. Fellowships, research assistantships, teaching assistantships, Federal Work-Study and scholarships available. *Financial aid application deadline:* 3/1.

Contact Mr. Clay D. Hysell, Assistant Dean for Graduate Student Services, School of Nursing, University of Virginia, McLeod Hall, PO Box 800782, Charlottesville, VA 22908. *Telephone:* 888-283-8703. *Fax:* 434-982-0528. *E-mail:* nur-osa@virginia.edu.

MASTER'S DEGREE PROGRAM

Degrees MSN; MSN/HSM; MSN/MA; MSN/MBA; MSN/PhD

Available Programs Accelerated Master's for Non-Nursing College Graduates; Master's.

Concentrations Available Health-care administration; nursing administration. *Clinical nurse specialist programs in:* acute care, community health, psychiatric/mental health, public health. *Nurse practitioner programs in:* acute care, community health, family health, gerontology, pediatric, primary care, psychiatric/mental health.

Study Options Full-time and part-time.

Program Entrance Requirements Minimum overall college GPA of 3.0, transcript of college record, written essay, 3 letters of recommendation, physical assessment course, resume, statistics course, GRE General Test, MAT. *Application deadline:* For fall and spring admission, 4/1; for winter admission, 11/15. Applications are processed on a rolling basis. *Application fee:* $40.

Advanced Placement Credit given for nursing courses completed elsewhere dependent upon specific evaluations.

POST-MASTER'S PROGRAM

Areas of Study Health-care administration; nursing administration. *Clinical nurse specialist programs in:* acute care, community health, psychiatric/mental health, public health. *Nurse practitioner programs in:* acute care, family health, gerontology, pediatric, primary care, psychiatric/mental health.

DOCTORAL DEGREE PROGRAM

Degree PhD

Available Programs Doctorate; Post-Baccalaureate Doctorate.

Areas of Study Advanced practice nursing, aging, community health, critical care, ethics, faculty preparation, family health, gerontology, health policy, health promotion/disease prevention, health-care systems, information systems, maternity-newborn, nursing administration, nursing education, nursing policy, nursing research, nursing science, oncology, women's health.

University of Virginia (continued)

Program Entrance Requirements Minimum overall college GPA of 3.0, interview by faculty committee, interview, 3 letters of recommendation, scholarly papers, statistics course, vita, writing sample, GRE General Test. *Application deadline:* For fall and spring admission, 4/1; for winter admission, 11/15. Applications are processed on a rolling basis. *Application fee:* $40.

Degree Requirements 69 total credit hours, dissertation, oral exam, written exam, residency.

POSTDOCTORAL PROGRAM

Areas of Study Cancer care, chronic illness, community health, family health, gerontology, nursing research, vulnerable population.

Postdoctoral Program Contact Mr. Clay D. Hysell, Assistant Dean for Graduate Student Services, School of Nursing, University of Virginia, McLeod Hall, PO Box 800782, Charlottesville, VA 22908. *Telephone:* 434-924-0141. *Fax:* 434-924-0528. *E-mail:* cdh6n@virginia.edu.

The University of Virginia's College at Wise

Department of Nursing
Wise, Virginia

http://www.wise.virginia.edu/nursing

Founded in 1954

DEGREE • BSN

Nursing Program Faculty 3 (33% with doctorates).

Baccalaureate Enrollment 36

Women 80% **Men** 20% **Minority** 5% **International** 5% **Part-time** 50%

Nursing Student Resources Academic advising; academic or career counseling; assistance for students with disabilities; bookstore; campus computer network; computer lab; computer-assisted instruction; e-mail services; employment services for current students; externships; housing assistance; interactive nursing skills videos; Internet; learning resource lab; library services; nursing audiovisuals; skills, simulation, or other laboratory; tutoring.

Library Facilities 95,861 volumes (2,192 in health, 540 in nursing); 1,029 periodical subscriptions (126 health-care related).

BACCALAUREATE PROGRAMS

Degree BSN

Available Programs Generic Baccalaureate; RN Baccalaureate.

Site Options Abingdon, VA.

Study Options Full-time and part-time.

Program Entrance Requirements Minimum overall college GPA of 2.0, transcript of college record, CPR certification, health exam, health insurance, immunizations, 3 letters of recommendation, minimum GPA in nursing prerequisites of 2.3, professional liability insurance/malpractice insurance, prerequisite course work. Transfer students are accepted. **Standardized tests** *Required:* SAT or ACT, TOEFL for international students. **Application** *Deadline:* 8/1 (freshmen), 8/15 (transfer). *Early decision:* 2/1. *Notification:* continuous until 8/20 (freshmen), 2/15 (early action). *Application fee:* $25.

Advanced Placement Credit by examination available. Credit given for nursing courses completed elsewhere dependent upon specific evaluations.

Expenses (2003–04) *Tuition, state resident:* full-time $2530; part-time $108 per credit hour. *Tuition, nonresident:* full-time $11,400; part-time $475 per credit hour. *Room and board:* $8500; room only: $6000 per academic year. *Required fees:* full-time $2000; part-time $25 per credit.

Financial Aid 78% of baccalaureate students in nursing programs received some form of financial aid in 2002–03. *Gift aid (need-based):* Federal Pell, FSEOG, state, private, college/university gift aid from institutional funds. *Loans:* FFEL (Subsidized and Unsubsidized Stafford PLUS), Perkins, state, college/university. *Work-Study:* Federal Work-Study. *Application deadline (priority):* 4/1.

Contact Dr. Angela S. Wilson, Associate Professor and Department Chair, Department of Nursing, The University of Virginia's College at Wise, The University of Virginia's College at Wise, One College Avenue, Wise, VA 24293-4400. *Telephone:* 276-328-0275. *Fax:* 276-376-4608. *E-mail:* asw5u@uvawise.edu.

Virginia Commonwealth University

School of Nursing
Richmond, Virginia

http://www.nursing.vcu.edu

Founded in 1838

DEGREES • BS • MS • MS/MPH • PHD

Nursing Program Faculty 84 (51% with doctorates).

Baccalaureate Enrollment 579

Women 92% **Men** 8% **Minority** 28% **Part-time** 55%

Graduate Enrollment 259

Women 93% **Men** 7% **Minority** 16% **International** 3% **Part-time** 49%

Nursing Student Activities Sigma Theta Tau, Student Nurses' Association.

Nursing Student Resources Academic advising; academic or career counseling; assistance for students with disabilities; bookstore; campus computer network; career placement assistance; computer lab; computer-assisted instruction; daycare for children of students; e-mail services; employment services for current students; externships; housing assistance; interactive nursing skills videos; Internet; learning resource lab; library services; nursing audiovisuals; paid internships; remedial services; resume preparation assistance; skills, simulation, or other laboratory; tutoring.

Library Facilities 1.8 million volumes (352,500 in health, 5,982 in nursing); 12,973 periodical subscriptions (4,026 health-care related).

BACCALAUREATE PROGRAMS

Degree BS

Available Programs ADN to Baccalaureate; Accelerated Baccalaureate for Second Degree; Generic Baccalaureate.

Site Options Salem, VA; Newport News, VA; Norfolk, VA.

Study Options Full-time.

Program Entrance Requirements Minimum overall college GPA of 2.5, transcript of college record, CPR certification, written essay, health exam, high school foreign language, 3 years high school math, 2 years high school science, high school transcript, immunizations, 3 letters of recommendation, minimum high school GPA of 2.5, prerequisite course work. Transfer students are accepted. **Standardized tests** *Required:* SAT or ACT, TOEFL for international students. **Application** *Deadline:* 2/1 (freshmen). *Notification:* continuous until 4/1 (freshmen). *Application fee:* $30.

Advanced Placement Credit by examination available. Credit given for nursing courses completed elsewhere dependent upon specific evaluations.

Expenses (2004–05) *Tuition, area resident:* full-time $3780; part-time $158 per credit hour. *Tuition, state resident:* full-time $3780; part-time $158 per unit. *Tuition, nonresident:* full-time $15,904; part-time $663 per term. *International tuition:* $15,904 full-time. *Room and board:* $7000; room only: $3400 per academic year. *Required fees:* full-time $1304.

Financial Aid 70% of baccalaureate students in nursing programs received some form of financial aid in 2003–04. *Gift aid (need-based):* Federal Pell, FSEOG, state, private, college/university gift aid from institutional funds, United Negro College Fund, Federal Nursing. *Loans:* Federal Nursing Student Loans, Federal Direct (Subsidized and Unsubsidized Stafford PLUS), Perkins, state, college/university. *Work-Study:* Federal Work-Study. *Application deadline (priority):* 2/1.

Contact Ms. Susan L. Lipp, Director of Enrollment and Student Services, School of Nursing, Virginia Commonwealth University, 1220 East Broad Street, PO Box 567, Richmond, VA 23298-0567. *Telephone:* 804-828-5171 Ext. 13. *Fax:* 804-828-7743. *E-mail:* slipp@vcu.edu.

GRADUATE PROGRAMS

Expenses (2004–05) *Tuition, state resident:* full-time $6066; part-time $337 per credit hour. *Tuition, nonresident:* full-time $15,904; part-time $663 per semester. *International tuition:* $15,904 full-time. *Room and board:* $7000; room only: $3500 per academic year. *Required fees:* full-time $1304.

Financial Aid 60% of graduate students in nursing programs received some form of financial aid in 2003–04. Fellowships, research assistantships, teaching assistantships, career-related internships or fieldwork and institutionally sponsored loans available.

Contact Ms. Susan L. Lipp, RN, Director of Enrollment and Student Services, School of Nursing, Virginia Commonwealth University, 1220 East Broad Street, PO Box 567, Richmond, VA 23298-0567. *Telephone:* 804-828-5171 Ext. 13. *Fax:* 804-828-7743. *E-mail:* slipp@vcu.edu.

MASTER'S DEGREE PROGRAM

Degrees MS; MS/MPH

Available Programs Accelerated Master's for Non-Nursing College Graduates; Accelerated Master's for Nurses with Non-Nursing Degrees; Master's; RN to Master's.

Concentrations Available Nursing administration. *Clinical nurse specialist programs in:* acute care, community health, psychiatric/mental health. *Nurse practitioner programs in:* acute care, adult health, family health, pediatric, primary care, psychiatric/mental health, women's health.

Study Options Full-time and part-time.

Program Entrance Requirements Computer literacy, minimum overall college GPA of 3.0, transcript of college record, CPR certification, written essay, immunizations, 3 letters of recommendation, nursing research course, physical assessment course, prerequisite course work, statistics course, GRE General Test. *Application deadline:* For fall admission, 2/1 (priority date). *Application fee:* $30.

Advanced Placement Credit given for nursing courses completed elsewhere dependent upon specific evaluations.

Degree Requirements 57 total credit hours.

POST-MASTER'S PROGRAM

Areas of Study Nursing administration. *Clinical nurse specialist programs in:* acute care, psychiatric/mental health. *Nurse practitioner programs in:* acute care, adult health, family health, pediatric, primary care, psychiatric/mental health, women's health.

DOCTORAL DEGREE PROGRAM

Degree PhD

Available Programs Doctorate; Post-Baccalaureate Doctorate.

Areas of Study Bio-behavioral clinical, healing, immunocompetence, risk and resilience.

Program Entrance Requirements Minimum overall college GPA of 3.0, interview by faculty committee, interview, 3 letters of recommendation, MSN or equivalent, statistics course, vita, writing sample, GRE General Test. *Application deadline:* For fall admission, 2/1 (priority date). *Application fee:* $30.

Degree Requirements 63 total credit hours, dissertation, written exam, residency.

See full description on page 592.

WASHINGTON

Eastern Washington University
Intercollegiate Center of Nursing/Washington State University
Cheney, Washington

See description of programs under
Intercollegiate Center of Nursing/Washington State University (Spokane, Washington).

Gonzaga University
Department of Nursing
Spokane, Washington

http://www.gonzaga.edu/nursing

Founded in 1887

DEGREES • BSN • MSN

Nursing Program Faculty 24 (50% with doctorates).

Baccalaureate Enrollment 40
Women 86% **Men** 14% **Minority** 7% **Part-time** 50%

Graduate Enrollment 180
Women 94% **Men** 6% **Minority** 94% **International** 7%

Nursing Student Activities Sigma Theta Tau.

Nursing Student Resources Academic advising; assistance for students with disabilities; bookstore; computer lab; Internet; library services.

Library Facilities 228,622 volumes (35,000 in health, 950 in nursing); 1,435 periodical subscriptions (206 health-care related).

BACCALAUREATE PROGRAMS

Degree BSN

Available Programs ADN to Baccalaureate; RN Baccalaureate.

Program Entrance Requirements Transfer students are accepted. **Standardized tests** *Required:* SAT or ACT, TOEFL for international students. **Application** *Deadline:* 2/1 (freshmen), 6/1 (transfer). *Early decision:* 11/15. *Notification:* 3/15 (freshmen), 1/15 (early action). *Application fee:* $45.

Financial Aid 80% of baccalaureate students in nursing programs received some form of financial aid in 2003–04. *Gift aid (need-based):* Federal Pell, FSEOG, state, private, college/university gift aid from institutional funds, United Negro College Fund, Federal Nursing. *Loans:* Federal Nursing Student Loans, FFEL (Subsidized and Unsubsidized Stafford PLUS), Perkins, state, college/university. *Work-Study:* Federal Work-Study, part-time campus jobs. *Application deadline (priority):* 2/1.

Contact Ms. Jane Tiedt, RN, Community Liaison, Department of Nursing, Gonzaga University, 502 East Boone Avenue, Spokane, WA 99258-0038. *Telephone:* 509-323-6643. *Fax:* 509-323-5827. *E-mail:* tiedt@gu.gonzaga.edu.

GRADUATE PROGRAMS

Financial Aid 75% of graduate students in nursing programs received some form of financial aid in 2003–04. *Application deadline:* 3/1.

Contact Ms. Jane Tiedt, RN, Community Liaison, Department of Nursing, Gonzaga University, 502 East Boone Avenue, Spokane, WA 99258-0038. *Telephone:* 509-323-6643. *Fax:* 509-323-5827. *E-mail:* tiedt@gu.gonzaga.edu.

Gonzaga University (continued)

MASTER'S DEGREE PROGRAM

Degree MSN

Available Programs Accelerated RN to Master's; Master's for Nurses with Non-Nursing Degrees; RN to Master's.

Concentrations Available Health-care administration; nurse case management; nursing administration; nursing education. *Clinical nurse specialist programs in:* adult health, critical care, gerontology, medical-surgical, psychiatric/mental health. *Nurse practitioner programs in:* family health, primary care, psychiatric/mental health.

Study Options Full-time and part-time.

Program Entrance Requirements Clinical experience, computer literacy, minimum overall college GPA of 3.0, transcript of college record, written essay, immunizations, 2 letters of recommendation, nursing research course, resume, statistics course, MAT. *Application deadline:* For fall admission, 7/20 (priority date); for spring admission, 11/1. Applications are processed on a rolling basis. *Application fee:* $40.

Advanced Placement Credit given for nursing courses completed elsewhere dependent upon specific evaluations.

Degree Requirements 48 total credit hours, thesis or project.

POST-MASTER'S PROGRAM

Areas of Study Health-care administration; nursing administration; nursing education. *Clinical nurse specialist programs in:* adult health, critical care, gerontology, medical-surgical, psychiatric/mental health. *Nurse practitioner programs in:* family health, primary care, psychiatric/mental health.

CONTINUING EDUCATION PROGRAM

Contact Ms. Angela Ruff, RN, Continuing Education Coordinator, Department of Nursing, Gonzaga University, 502 East Boone Avenue, Spokane, WA 99258-0038. *Telephone:* 509-323-3572. *Fax:* 509-323-5827. *E-mail:* ruff@gu.gonzaga.edu.

Intercollegiate College of Nursing/ Washington State University

Intercollegiate College of Nursing/Washington State University
Spokane, Washington

http://www.nursing.wsu.edu

DEGREES • BSN • MN

Nursing Program Faculty 101 (31% with doctorates).

Baccalaureate Enrollment 556
Women 89% **Men** 11% **Minority** 11% **Part-time** 20%

Graduate Enrollment 174
Women 91% **Men** 9% **Minority** 7% **Part-time** 72%

Nursing Student Activities Sigma Theta Tau, Student Nurses' Association, nursing club.

Nursing Student Resources Academic advising; academic or career counseling; assistance for students with disabilities; bookstore; campus computer network; computer lab; computer-assisted instruction; e-mail services; interactive nursing skills videos; Internet; learning resource lab; library services; nursing audiovisuals; remedial services; resume preparation assistance; skills, simulation, or other laboratory; tutoring; unpaid internships.

Library Facilities 10,000 volumes in health, 10,000 volumes in nursing; 280 periodical subscriptions health-care related.

BACCALAUREATE PROGRAMS

Degree BSN

Available Programs Generic Baccalaureate; RN Baccalaureate.

Site Options *Distance Learning:* Richland, WA; Vancouver, WA; Yakima, WA.

Study Options Full-time and part-time.

Program Entrance Requirements Minimum overall college GPA of 2.5, transcript of college record, CPR certification, immunizations, minimum GPA in nursing prerequisites of 2.5, prerequisite course work. Transfer students are accepted.

Advanced Placement Credit given for nursing courses completed elsewhere dependent upon specific evaluations.

Expenses (2004–05) *Tuition, state resident:* full-time $5154; part-time $258 per credit hour. *Tuition, nonresident:* full-time $13,572; part-time $679 per credit hour. *International tuition:* $13,572 full-time. *Required fees:* full-time $900; part-time $450 per term.

Contact Ms. Diane Kleweno, Undergraduate Program Coordinator, Intercollegiate College of Nursing/Washington State University, 2917 West Fort George Wright Drive, Spokane, WA 99224-5291. *Telephone:* 509-324-7338. *Fax:* 509-324-7336. *E-mail:* kleweno@wsu.edu.

GRADUATE PROGRAMS

Expenses (2004–05) *Tuition, state resident:* full-time $7428; part-time $371 per credit hour. *Tuition, nonresident:* full-time $17,832; part-time $892 per credit hour. *International tuition:* $17,832 full-time. *Required fees:* full-time $500.

Contact Ms. Margaret Ruby, Administrative Assistant for Academic Affairs, Intercollegiate College of Nursing/Washington State University, 2917 West Fort George Wright Drive, Spokane, WA 99224-5291. *Telephone:* 509-324-7334. *Fax:* 509-324-7336. *E-mail:* mruby@wsu.edu.

MASTER'S DEGREE PROGRAM

Degree MN

Available Programs Accelerated RN to Master's; Master's; Master's for Nurses with Non-Nursing Degrees.

Concentrations Available Nursing administration; nursing education. *Clinical nurse specialist programs in:* community health, school health. *Nurse practitioner programs in:* family health, psychiatric/mental health.

Site Options *Distance Learning:* Richland, WA; Vancouver, WA; Yakima, WA.

Study Options Full-time and part-time.

Program Entrance Requirements Clinical experience, computer literacy, minimum overall college GPA of 3.0, transcript of college record, CPR certification, written essay, immunizations, 3 letters of recommendation, physical assessment course, prerequisite course work, statistics course.

Advanced Placement Credit given for nursing courses completed elsewhere dependent upon specific evaluations.

Degree Requirements 45 total credit hours, thesis or project.

POST-MASTER'S PROGRAM

Areas of Study *Nurse practitioner programs in:* family health, psychiatric/mental health.

CONTINUING EDUCATION PROGRAM

Contact Ms. Carol Johns, Coordinator of Professional Development, Intercollegiate College of Nursing/Washington State University, 2917 West Fort George Wright Drive, Spokane, WA 99224-5291. *Telephone:* 509-324-7354. *Fax:* 509-324-7341. *E-mail:* cjohns@wsu.edu.

Northwest University

The Mark and Huldah Buntain School of Nursing
Kirkland, Washington

http://www.northwestu.edu/

Founded in 1934

DEGREE • BS

Nursing Program Faculty 15 (20% with doctorates).

Baccalaureate Enrollment 65
Women 94% **Men** 6% **Minority** 18%

Nursing Student Resources Academic advising; academic or career counseling; assistance for students with disabilities; bookstore; campus computer network; computer lab; computer-assisted instruction; e-mail services; employment services for current students; housing assistance; interactive nursing skills videos; Internet; learning resource lab; library services; nursing audiovisuals; remedial services; resume preparation assistance; skills, simulation, or other laboratory; tutoring; unpaid internships.

Library Facilities 141,427 volumes (1,684 in health, 310 in nursing); 905 periodical subscriptions (680 health-care related).

BACCALAUREATE PROGRAMS

Degree BS

Available Programs Generic Baccalaureate.

Study Options Full-time.

Program Entrance Requirements Minimum overall college GPA of 3.0, transcript of college record, CPR certification, written essay, health exam, health insurance, high school transcript, immunizations, 2 letters of recommendation, minimum GPA in nursing prerequisites of 3.0, prerequisite course work. Transfer students are accepted. **Standardized tests** *Required:* SAT or ACT, TOEFL for international students. **Application** *Deadline:* 8/1 (freshmen), 8/1 (transfer). *Early decision:* 11/15. *Notification:* continuous (freshmen), 12/1 (early action). *Application fee:* $30.

Expenses (2004–05) *Tuition:* full-time $14,200; part-time $420 per credit hour. *International tuition:* $14,200 full-time. *Room and board:* $6450; room only: $3430 per academic year. *Required fees:* full-time $3259.

Financial Aid 85% of baccalaureate students in nursing programs received some form of financial aid in 2003–04. *Gift aid (need-based):* Federal Pell, FSEOG, state, private, college/university gift aid from institutional funds. *Loans:* FFEL (Subsidized and Unsubsidized Stafford PLUS), Perkins, state, alternative loans. *Work-Study:* Federal Work-Study, part-time campus jobs. *Application deadline (priority):* 3/1.

Contact Dr. Carl Christensen, Dean, The Mark and Huldah Buntain School of Nursing, Northwest University, 5520 108th Avenue, NE, PO Box 579, Kirkland, WA 98083. *Telephone:* 800-669-3781 Ext. 7822. *Fax:* 425-889-7822. *E-mail:* nursing@northwestu.edu.

Pacific Lutheran University
School of Nursing
Tacoma, Washington

http://www.plu.edu/~nurs/

Founded in 1890

DEGREES • BSN • MSN

Nursing Program Faculty 23 (40% with doctorates).

Baccalaureate Enrollment 230
Women 93% **Men** 7% **Minority** 25% **International** 2%

Graduate Enrollment 58
Women 97% **Men** 3% **Minority** 19% **Part-time** 5%

Nursing Student Activities Nursing Honor Society, Sigma Theta Tau, Student Nurses' Association, nursing club.

Nursing Student Resources Academic advising; academic or career counseling; assistance for students with disabilities; bookstore; campus computer network; career placement assistance; computer lab; computer-assisted instruction; e-mail services; employment services for current students; housing assistance; interactive nursing skills videos; Internet; learning resource lab; library services; nursing audiovisuals; paid internships; remedial services; resume preparation assistance; skills, simulation, or other laboratory; tutoring; unpaid internships.

Library Facilities 340,842 volumes (11,300 in health, 5,930 in nursing); 3,370 periodical subscriptions (142 health-care related).

BACCALAUREATE PROGRAMS

Degree BSN

Available Programs ADN to Baccalaureate; Generic Baccalaureate; LPN to Baccalaureate.

Study Options Full-time and part-time.

Program Entrance Requirements Minimum overall college GPA of 3.0, transcript of college record, CPR certification, written essay, health exam, health insurance, 2 years high school math, high school transcript, immunizations, 2 letters of recommendation, minimum GPA in nursing prerequisites of 2.75, professional liability insurance/malpractice insurance, prerequisite course work. Transfer students are accepted. **Standardized tests** *Required:* SAT or ACT, TOEFL for international students. **Application** *Deadline:* rolling (freshmen), rolling (transfer). *Notification:* continuous (freshmen). *Application fee:* $40.

Advanced Placement Credit by examination available. Credit given for nursing courses completed elsewhere dependent upon specific evaluations.

Expenses (2004–05) *Tuition:* full-time $20,790; part-time $648 per credit hour. *International tuition:* $20,790 full-time. *Room and board:* $6410; room only: $4000 per academic year. *Required fees:* full-time $200; part-time $100 per term.

Financial Aid 82% of baccalaureate students in nursing programs received some form of financial aid in 2003–04.

Contact Audrey Cox, Admissions Coordinator, School of Nursing, Pacific Lutheran University, Tacoma, WA 98447-0029. *Telephone:* 253-535-7672. *Fax:* 253-535-7590. *E-mail:* coxae@plu.edu.

GRADUATE PROGRAMS

Expenses (2004–05) *Tuition:* part-time $648 per credit hour. *Room and board:* $6410; room only: $4000 per academic year. *Required fees:* full-time $200; part-time $100 per term.

Financial Aid 100% of graduate students in nursing programs received some form of financial aid in 2003–04. Research assistantships, Federal Work-Study, scholarships, and unspecified assistantships available. *Financial aid application deadline:* 3/1.

Contact Ms. Emily Mize, Graduate Admissions Coordinator, School of Nursing, Pacific Lutheran University, Tacoma, WA 98447-0029. *Telephone:* 253-535-8264. *Fax:* 253-535-7590. *E-mail:* mizeeb@plu.edu.

MASTER'S DEGREE PROGRAM

Degree MSN

Available Programs Accelerated Master's; Master's; Master's for Non-Nursing College Graduates; Master's for Nurses with Non-Nursing Degrees; RN to Master's.

Concentrations Available Health-care administration; nurse case management; nursing administration; nursing education; nursing informatics. *Clinical nurse specialist programs in:* acute care, adult health, medical-surgical. *Nurse practitioner programs in:* family health.

Study Options Full-time and part-time.

Program Entrance Requirements Clinical experience, computer literacy, minimum overall college GPA of 3.0, transcript of college record, CPR certification, written essay, immunizations, interview, 2 letters of recommendation, nursing research course, professional liability insurance/malpractice insurance, prerequisite course work, resume, statistics course, GRE General Test. *Application deadline:* For fall admission, 4/1 (priority date). Applications are processed on a rolling basis. *Application fee:* $35.

Advanced Placement Credit by examination available. Credit given for nursing courses completed elsewhere dependent upon specific evaluations.

Degree Requirements 36 total credit hours, thesis or project.

CONTINUING EDUCATION PROGRAM

Contact Dr. Patsy Maloney, Director, Continuing Nursing Education, School of Nursing, Pacific Lutheran University, Tacoma, WA 98447-0029. *Telephone:* 253-535-7682. *Fax:* 253-535-7590. *E-mail:* malonepl@plu.edu.

Seattle Pacific University
School of Health Sciences
Seattle, Washington

Founded in 1891

DEGREES • BSN • MN/MBA • MSN

Nursing Program Faculty 25 (36% with doctorates).

Seattle Pacific University (continued)

Baccalaureate Enrollment 175
Women 92% **Men** 8% **Minority** 11% **Part-time** 41%

Graduate Enrollment 32
Women 91% **Men** 9% **Minority** 14% **International** 2% **Part-time** 26%

Nursing Student Activities Nursing Honor Society, Sigma Theta Tau, Student Nurses' Association, nursing club.

Nursing Student Resources Academic advising; academic or career counseling; assistance for students with disabilities; bookstore; campus computer network; career placement assistance; computer lab; computer-assisted instruction; e-mail services; employment services for current students; housing assistance; Internet; learning resource lab; library services; nursing audiovisuals; placement services for program completers; remedial services; skills, simulation, or other laboratory; tutoring.

Library Facilities 191,807 volumes (9,500 in health, 2,000 in nursing); 1,230 periodical subscriptions (178 health-care related).

BACCALAUREATE PROGRAMS

Degree BSN

Available Programs Generic Baccalaureate; RN Baccalaureate.

Site Options Bellingham, WA; Seattle, WA; Mt. Vernon, WA.

Study Options Full-time.

Program Entrance Requirements Transcript of college record, written essay, 1 letter of recommendation, minimum GPA in nursing prerequisites of 2.75. Transfer students are accepted. **Standardized tests** *Required:* SAT or ACT, TOEFL for international students. *Recommended:* SAT. **Application** *Deadline:* 6/1 (freshmen), 8/1 (transfer). *Early decision:* 12/1. *Notification:* continuous (freshmen), 2/15 (early action). *Application fee:* $45.

Advanced Placement Credit given for nursing courses completed elsewhere dependent upon specific evaluations.

Expenses (2004–05) *Tuition:* full-time $20,139; part-time $560 per credit hour. *Room and board:* $7368; room only: $3951 per academic year. *Required fees:* full-time $1605.

Financial Aid 84% of baccalaureate students in nursing programs received some form of financial aid in 2003–04.

Contact Dr. Emily Hitchens, Associate Dean, School of Health Sciences, Seattle Pacific University, Marston Hall, #320, 3307 Third Avenue West, Seattle, WA 98119-1997. *Telephone:* 206-281-2964. *Fax:* 206-281-2767. *E-mail:* hitchens@spu.edu.

GRADUATE PROGRAMS

Expenses (2004–05) *Tuition:* part-time $430 per credit hour.

Financial Aid 45% of graduate students in nursing programs received some form of financial aid in 2003–04. 2 teaching assistantships were awarded; career-related internships or fieldwork and traineeships also available.

Contact Prof. Marilyn Moorehouse, Graduate Admissions Counselor, School of Health Sciences, Seattle Pacific University, Marston Hall, 3307 Third Avenue West, Suite 106, Seattle, WA 98119-1922. *Telephone:* 206-281-2888. *Fax:* 206-281-2649. *E-mail:* moorhm@spu.edu.

MASTER'S DEGREE PROGRAM

Degrees MN/MBA; MSN

Available Programs Master's.

Concentrations Available Nursing administration; nursing education. *Clinical nurse specialist programs in:* adult health, cardiovascular, community health, critical care, family health, gerontology, home health care, maternity-newborn, medical-surgical, occupational health, oncology, parent-child, pediatric, perinatal, psychiatric/mental health, public health, rehabilitation, school health, women's health. *Nurse practitioner programs in:* adult health, family health, gerontology.

Study Options Full-time and part-time.

Program Entrance Requirements Computer literacy, minimum overall college GPA of 3.0, transcript of college record, CPR certification, written essay, immunizations, interview, 3 letters of recommendation, nursing research course, physical assessment course, professional liability insurance/malpractice insurance, prerequisite course work, statistics course, GRE General Test. *Application deadline:* For fall admission, 9/1 (priority date). Applications are processed on a rolling basis. *Application fee:* $50.

Degree Requirements 52 total credit hours, thesis or project.

POST-MASTER'S PROGRAM

Areas of Study Nursing education. *Nurse practitioner programs in:* adult health, family health, gerontology.

Seattle University
College of Nursing
Seattle, Washington

http://www.seattleu.edu/nurs

Founded in 1891

DEGREES • BSN • MSN

Nursing Program Faculty 51 (46% with doctorates).

Baccalaureate Enrollment 378
Women 91% **Men** 9% **Minority** 40% **International** 1% **Part-time** 5%

Graduate Enrollment 57
Women 86% **Men** 14% **Minority** 32% **International** 2% **Part-time** 18%

Nursing Student Activities Sigma Theta Tau, Student Nurses' Association.

Nursing Student Resources Academic advising; academic or career counseling; assistance for students with disabilities; bookstore; campus computer network; career placement assistance; computer lab; computer-assisted instruction; e-mail services; housing assistance; interactive nursing skills videos; Internet; learning resource lab; library services; nursing audiovisuals; remedial services; resume preparation assistance; skills, simulation, or other laboratory.

Library Facilities 141,478 volumes (9,534 in health); 2,701 periodical subscriptions (132 health-care related).

BACCALAUREATE PROGRAMS

Degree BSN

Available Programs Baccalaureate for Second Degree; Generic Baccalaureate.

Study Options Full-time and part-time.

Program Entrance Requirements Minimum overall college GPA of 2.75, transcript of college record, written essay, high school chemistry, 3 years high school math, 2 years high school science, high school transcript, 2 letters of recommendation, minimum high school GPA of 2.75, minimum high school rank 50%, minimum GPA in nursing prerequisites of 2.75, prerequisite course work. Transfer students are accepted. **Standardized tests** *Required:* SAT or ACT, TOEFL for international students. **Application** *Deadline:* 7/1 (freshmen), 8/1 (transfer). *Notification:* continuous (freshmen). *Application fee:* $45.

Advanced Placement Credit given for nursing courses completed elsewhere dependent upon specific evaluations.

Expenses (2004–05) *Tuition:* full-time $21,285; part-time $473 per credit hour. *Room and board:* $6138; room only: $4653 per academic year. *Required fees:* full-time $450.

Financial Aid 87% of baccalaureate students in nursing programs received some form of financial aid in 2003–04. *Gift aid (need-based):* Federal Pell, FSEOG, state, private, college/university gift aid from institutional funds. *Loans:* Federal Nursing Student Loans, Federal Direct (Subsidized and Unsubsidized Stafford PLUS), Perkins, alternative loans. *Work-Study:* Federal Work-Study, part-time campus jobs. *Application deadline (priority):* 2/1.

Contact Rita Tower, Pre-major Advisor, College of Nursing, Seattle University, 900 Broadway, Seattle, WA 98122. *Telephone:* 206-296-2242. *Fax:* 206-296-5544. *E-mail:* rstower@seattleu.edu.

GRADUATE PROGRAMS

Expenses (2004–05) *Tuition:* full-time $14,000; part-time $449 per credit hour. *Required fees:* full-time $220.

Financial Aid 81% of graduate students in nursing programs received some form of financial aid in 2003–04. Fellowships, research assistantships, career-related internships or fieldwork and Federal Work-Study available. Aid available to part-time students.

Contact Dr. Kathryn Anderson, Graduate Program Director, College of Nursing, Seattle University, 900 Broadway, Seattle, WA 98122-4340. *Telephone:* 206-296-5666. *Fax:* 206-296-5544. *E-mail:* kathryna@seattleu.edu.

MASTER'S DEGREE PROGRAM

Degree MSN

Available Programs Accelerated Master's for Nurses with Non-Nursing Degrees; Master's.

Concentrations Available *Clinical nurse specialist programs in:* community health. *Nurse practitioner programs in:* family health, psychiatric/mental health.

Study Options Full-time and part-time.

Program Entrance Requirements Clinical experience, minimum overall college GPA of 3.0, transcript of college record, CPR certification, written essay, immunizations, interview, 2 letters of recommendation, professional liability insurance/malpractice insurance, resume, statistics course, GRE General Test. *Application deadline:* For fall admission, 7/1. *Application fee:* $55.

Advanced Placement Credit given for nursing courses completed elsewhere dependent upon specific evaluations.

Degree Requirements 63 total credit hours, thesis or project.

POST-MASTER'S PROGRAM

Areas of Study *Nurse practitioner programs in:* family health, psychiatric/mental health.

University of Washington
School of Nursing
Seattle, Washington

Founded in 1861

DEGREES • BSN • MN • MN/MPH • MSN/MHA • PHD

Nursing Program Faculty 156 (98% with doctorates).

Baccalaureate Enrollment 405
Women 81.5% **Men** 18.5% **Minority** 26% **Part-time** 45%

Graduate Enrollment 395
Women 91% **Men** 9% **Minority** 12% **International** 9% **Part-time** 57%

Nursing Student Activities Sigma Theta Tau, Student Nurses' Association.

Nursing Student Resources Academic advising; bookstore; campus computer network; computer-assisted instruction; e-mail services; employment services for current students; interactive nursing skills videos; Internet; learning resource lab; library services.

Library Facilities 5.8 million volumes (123,098 in health); 50,245 periodical subscriptions (4,000 health-care related).

BACCALAUREATE PROGRAMS

Degree BSN

Available Programs Generic Baccalaureate; RN Baccalaureate.

Site Options Tacoma, WA; Bothell, WA.

Study Options Full-time.

Program Entrance Requirements Minimum overall college GPA of 2.0, transcript of college record, CPR certification, written essay, immunizations, 1 letter of recommendation, minimum GPA in nursing prerequisites of 2.0, prerequisite course work. Transfer students are accepted. **Standardized tests** *Required:* SAT or ACT, TOEFL for international students. **Application** *Deadline:* 1/15 (freshmen), 2/15 (transfer). *Notification:* continuous until 4/15 (freshmen). *Application fee:* $37.

Expenses (2004–05) *Tuition, state resident:* full-time $1762. *Tuition, nonresident:* full-time $5972. *International tuition:* $5972 full-time.

Financial Aid 65% of baccalaureate students in nursing programs received some form of financial aid in 2003–04.

Contact Ms. Carolyn A. Chow, Director of Admissions and Multicultural Student Affairs, School of Nursing, University of Washington, Health Sciences Building, Box 357260, Seattle, WA 98195. *Telephone:* 206-543-8736. *Fax:* 206-685-1613. *E-mail:* egg@u.washington.edu.

GRADUATE PROGRAMS

Expenses (2004–05) *Tuition, state resident:* full-time $8310; part-time $371 per credit hour. *Tuition, nonresident:* full-time $17,590; part-time $829 per credit hour.

Financial Aid 75% of graduate students in nursing programs received some form of financial aid in 2003–04. Fellowships with full tuition reimbursements available, research assistantships with partial tuition reimbursements available, teaching assistantships with partial tuition reimbursements available, Federal Work-Study, institutionally sponsored loans, scholarships, and traineeships available. *Financial aid application deadline:* 2/28.

Contact Ms. Carolyn A. Chow, Director of Admissions and Multicultural Student Affairs, School of Nursing, University of Washington, Health Sciences Building, Box 357260, Seattle, WA 98195. *Telephone:* 206-543-8736. *Fax:* 206-685-1613. *E-mail:* egg@u.washington.edu.

MASTER'S DEGREE PROGRAM

Degrees MN; MN/MPH; MSN/MHA

Available Programs Master's; Master's for Non-Nursing College Graduates; Master's for Nurses with Non-Nursing Degrees.

Concentrations Available Nurse-midwifery; nursing administration; nursing education. *Clinical nurse specialist programs in:* acute care, cardiovascular, community health, critical care, gerontology, home health care, maternity-newborn, medical-surgical, occupational health, oncology, pediatric, perinatal, psychiatric/mental health, women's health. *Nurse practitioner programs in:* acute care, adult health, family health, gerontology, neonatal health, pediatric, primary care, psychiatric/mental health, women's health.

Site Options Tacoma, WA; Bothell, WA. *Distance Learning:* Port Angeles, WA.

Study Options Full-time and part-time.

Program Entrance Requirements Minimum overall college GPA of 3.0, transcript of college record, CPR certification, written essay, immunizations, 3 letters of recommendation, resume, statistics course, GRE. *Application deadline:* For fall admission, 2/1. *Application fee:* $50.

Degree Requirements 38 total credit hours, thesis or project.

POST-MASTER'S PROGRAM

Areas of Study *Clinical nurse specialist programs in:* acute care, cardiovascular, community health, critical care, gerontology, home health care, maternity-newborn, medical-surgical, occupational health, oncology, pediatric, perinatal, psychiatric/mental health, women's health. *Nurse practitioner programs in:* acute care, adult health, family health, gerontology, neonatal health, pediatric, primary care, psychiatric/mental health, women's health.

DOCTORAL DEGREE PROGRAM

Degree PhD

Available Programs Doctorate for Nurses with Non-Nursing Degrees; Post-Baccalaureate Doctorate.

Areas of Study Individualized study, nursing science.

Program Entrance Requirements Minimum overall college GPA of 3.0, 3 letters of recommendation, scholarly papers, statistics course, writing sample, GRE. *Application deadline:* For fall admission, 2/1. *Application fee:* $50.

Degree Requirements 99 total credit hours, dissertation, oral exam, written exam, residency.

POSTDOCTORAL PROGRAM

Postdoctoral Program Contact Office of Academic Programs, School of Nursing, University of Washington, T-310 Health Sciences Building, Box 357260, Seattle, WA 98195. *Telephone:* 206-543-8736. *Fax:* 206-685-1613. *E-mail:* sonapo@u.washington.edu.

CONTINUING EDUCATION PROGRAM

Contact Dr. Ruth Craven, Associate Dean for Educational Outreach, School of Nursing, University of Washington, Box 357260, Seattle, WA 98195. *Telephone:* 206-221-2406. *Fax:* 206-685-1613. *E-mail:* ruthc@u.washington.edu.

Walla Walla College

School of Nursing
College Place, Washington

http://www.wwc.edu/academics/department/nursing

Founded in 1892

DEGREE • BS

Nursing Program Faculty 18 (17% with doctorates).

Baccalaureate Enrollment 125
Women 92% **Men** 8% **Minority** 10% **International** 1% **Part-time** 1%

Nursing Student Activities Nursing Honor Society, nursing club.

Nursing Student Resources Academic advising; assistance for students with disabilities; bookstore; campus computer network; computer lab; e-mail services; Internet; learning resource lab; library services; nursing audiovisuals; resume preparation assistance; skills, simulation, or other laboratory; tutoring.

Library Facilities 178,450 volumes (10,000 in health, 7,000 in nursing); 1,105 periodical subscriptions (450 health-care related).

BACCALAUREATE PROGRAMS

Degree BS

Available Programs ADN to Baccalaureate; Generic Baccalaureate; LPN to Baccalaureate.

Site Options Portland, OR.

Study Options Full-time and part-time.

Program Entrance Requirements Minimum overall college GPA of 2.5, transcript of college record, CPR certification, written essay, health exam, health insurance, 3 years high school math, 2 years high school science, high school transcript, immunizations, 3 letters of recommendation, minimum high school GPA of 2.5, minimum GPA in nursing prerequisites of 2.5, prerequisite course work. Transfer students are accepted. **Standardized tests** *Required:* SAT or ACT, TOEFL for international students. *Recommended:* ACT. **Application** *Deadline:* rolling (freshmen), rolling (transfer). *Notification:* continuous (freshmen). *Application fee:* $40.

Advanced Placement Credit given for nursing courses completed elsewhere dependent upon specific evaluations.

Expenses (2004–05) *Tuition:* full-time $17,655; part-time $462 per quarter hour. *International tuition:* $17,655 full-time. *Room and board:* $4389; room only: $2955 per academic year. *Required fees:* full-time $774; part-time $25 per credit; part-time $58 per term.

Financial Aid 95% of baccalaureate students in nursing programs received some form of financial aid in 2003–04.

Contact Jan Thurnhofer, RN, Student Program Advisor, School of Nursing, Walla Walla College, 10345 Southeast Market Street, Portland, OR 97216. *Telephone:* 503-251-6115 Ext. 7304. *Fax:* 503-251-6249. *E-mail:* thurnja@wwc.edu.

Washington State University

Intercollegiate Center of Nursing/Washington State University
Pullman, Washington

See description of programs under
Intercollegiate Center of Nursing/Washington State University (Spokane, Washington).

Whitworth College

Intercollegiate Center of Nursing/Washington State University
Spokane, Washington

See description of programs under
Intercollegiate Center of Nursing/Washington State University (Spokane, Washington).

WEST VIRGINIA

Alderson-Broaddus College

Department of Nursing
Philippi, West Virginia

Founded in 1871

DEGREE • BSN

Nursing Program Faculty 10.

Baccalaureate Enrollment 208
Women 98% **Men** 2% **Minority** 2% **Part-time** 2%

Nursing Student Activities Student Nurses' Association.

Nursing Student Resources Academic advising; academic or career counseling; assistance for students with disabilities; bookstore; campus computer network; computer lab; computer-assisted instruction; e-mail services; Internet; learning resource lab; library services; nursing audiovisuals; remedial services; resume preparation assistance; skills, simulation, or other laboratory; tutoring.

Library Facilities 100,000 volumes (6,000 in health); 9,000 periodical subscriptions (172 health-care related).

BACCALAUREATE PROGRAMS

Degree BSN

Available Programs Accelerated LPN to Baccalaureate; Accelerated RN Baccalaureate; Generic Baccalaureate; LPN to Baccalaureate; LPN to RN Baccalaureate; RN Baccalaureate.

Site Options Clarksburg, WV.

Study Options Full-time.

Program Entrance Requirements Minimum overall college GPA of 2.0, transcript of college record, CPR certification, health exam, high school transcript, immunizations, minimum GPA in nursing prerequisites of 2.0, professional liability insurance/malpractice insurance, prerequisite course work. Transfer students are accepted. **Standardized tests** *Required:* SAT or ACT, TOEFL for international students. **Application** *Deadline:* rolling (freshmen), rolling (transfer). *Notification:* continuous until 8/31 (freshmen). *Application fee:* $10.

Advanced Placement Credit by examination available. Credit given for nursing courses completed elsewhere dependent upon specific evaluations.

Expenses (2004–05) *Tuition:* full-time $21,335.

Financial Aid 98% of baccalaureate students in nursing programs received some form of financial aid in 2003–04.

Contact Mrs. Threasia L. Witt, RN, Interim Chairperson, Department of Nursing, Alderson-Broaddus College, Box 2003, Philippi, WV 26416. *Telephone:* 304-457-1700 Ext. 285. *Fax:* 304-457-6293. *E-mail:* witttl@mail.ab.edu.

Bluefield State College
Program in Nursing
Bluefield, West Virginia

http://www.bluefieldstate.edu
Founded in 1895

DEGREE • BSN

Nursing Program Faculty 3 (1% with doctorates).

Baccalaureate Enrollment 60
Women 95% **Men** 5% **Minority** 1% **Part-time** 2%

Nursing Student Activities Sigma Theta Tau, Student Nurses' Association.

Nursing Student Resources Academic advising; academic or career counseling; assistance for students with disabilities; bookstore; campus computer network; career placement assistance; computer lab; computer-assisted instruction; e-mail services; interactive nursing skills videos; Internet; learning resource lab; library services; nursing audiovisuals; resume preparation assistance; skills, simulation, or other laboratory; tutoring.

Library Facilities 76,391 volumes (5,649 in health, 1,250 in nursing); 2,453 periodical subscriptions (200 health-care related).

BACCALAUREATE PROGRAMS

Degree BSN

Available Programs RN Baccalaureate.

Study Options Full-time and part-time.

Program Entrance Requirements Minimum overall college GPA of 2.5, transcript of college record, CPR certification, health exam, immunizations, 1 letter of recommendation, prerequisite course work. Transfer students are accepted. **Standardized tests** *Recommended:* SAT or ACT, TOEFL for international students. **Application** *Deadline:* rolling (freshmen), rolling (transfer). *Notification:* continuous (freshmen).

Expenses (2003–04) *Tuition, area resident:* full-time $1403; part-time $117 per credit hour. *Tuition, nonresident:* full-time $3447; part-time $289 per credit hour. *Required fees:* full-time $120.

Financial Aid 62% of baccalaureate students in nursing programs received some form of financial aid in 2002–03.

Contact Ms. Beth Ann Pritchett, Director, Program in Nursing, Bluefield State College, 219 Rock Street, Bluefield, WV 24701. *Telephone:* 304-327-4139. *Fax:* 304-327-4219. *E-mail:* bpritchett@bluefield.wvnet.edu.

Fairmont State University
School of Nursing/Allied Health Adm.
Fairmont, West Virginia

http://www.fscwv.edu
Founded in 1865

DEGREE • BSN

Nursing Program Faculty 3 (33% with doctorates).

Baccalaureate Enrollment 70
Women 97% **Men** 3% **Part-time** 70%

Nursing Student Activities Student Nurses' Association.

Nursing Student Resources Academic advising; academic or career counseling; assistance for students with disabilities; bookstore; campus computer network; computer lab; computer-assisted instruction; e-mail services; housing assistance; interactive nursing skills videos; Internet; learning resource lab; library services; nursing audiovisuals; placement services for program completers; remedial services; resume preparation assistance; skills, simulation, or other laboratory; tutoring.

Library Facilities 276,722 volumes (7,000 in health, 1,100 in nursing); 883 periodical subscriptions (50 health-care related).

BACCALAUREATE PROGRAMS

Degree BSN

Available Programs ADN to Baccalaureate; LPN to RN Baccalaureate; RN Baccalaureate.

Study Options Full-time and part-time.

Program Entrance Requirements Minimum overall college GPA of 2.5, transcript of college record, CPR certification, health exam, high school chemistry, immunizations, 1 letter of recommendation, minimum GPA in nursing prerequisites of 3.0, prerequisite course work, RN licensure. Transfer students are accepted. **Standardized tests** *Required:* SAT or ACT, TOEFL for international students. **Application** *Deadline:* 6/15 (freshmen), 6/15 (transfer).

Advanced Placement Credit by examination available. Credit given for nursing courses completed elsewhere dependent upon specific evaluations.

Expenses (2004–05) *Tuition, state resident:* full-time $1565; part-time $132 per credit hour. *Tuition, nonresident:* full-time $3519; part-time $294 per credit hour. *International tuition:* $3519 full-time. *Room and board:* $2530; room only: $1205 per academic year. *Required fees:* full-time $100.

Financial Aid 80% of baccalaureate students in nursing programs received some form of financial aid in 2003–04. *Gift aid (need-based):* Federal Pell, FSEOG, state, private, college/university gift aid from institutional funds. *Loans:* Federal Direct (Subsidized and Unsubsidized Stafford PLUS), Perkins. *Work-Study:* Federal Work-Study, part-time campus jobs. *Application deadline:* 2/1 (priority: 3/1).

Contact Dr. Mary G. Meighen, Professor, School of Nursing/Allied Health Adm., Fairmont State University, 1201 Locust Avenue, Fairmont, WV 26554. *Telephone:* 304-367-4761. *Fax:* 304-367-4268. *E-mail:* mmeighen@fairmontstate.edu.

CONTINUING EDUCATION PROGRAM

Contact Dr. Mary G. Meighen, Professor, School of Nursing/Allied Health Adm., Fairmont State University, 1201 Locust Avenue, Fairmont, WV 26554. *Telephone:* 304-367-4761. *Fax:* 304-367-4268. *E-mail:* mmeighen@fairmontstate.edu.

Marshall University
College of Nursing and Health Professions
Huntington, West Virginia

http://www.marshall.edu/conhp
Founded in 1837

DEGREES • BSN • MSN

Nursing Program Faculty 35 (23% with doctorates).

Baccalaureate Enrollment 345
Women 80% **Men** 20% **Minority** 5% **Part-time** 35%

Graduate Enrollment 100
Women 90% **Men** 10% **Part-time** 60%

Nursing Student Activities Sigma Theta Tau, Student Nurses' Association, nursing club.

Nursing Student Resources Academic advising; academic or career counseling; assistance for students with disabilities; bookstore; campus computer network; career placement assistance; computer lab; computer-assisted instruction; daycare for children of students; e-mail services; employment services for current students; externships; housing assistance; interactive nursing skills videos; Internet; learning resource lab; library services; nursing audiovisuals; placement services for program completers; remedial services; resume preparation assistance; skills, simulation, or other laboratory; tutoring.

Library Facilities 478,274 volumes (20,200 in health, 6,400 in nursing); 5,314 periodical subscriptions (500 health-care related).

BACCALAUREATE PROGRAMS

Degree BSN

Available Programs Accelerated RN Baccalaureate; Generic Baccalaureate.

Site Options *Distance Learning:* Williamson, WV; South Charleston, WV; Point Pleasant, WV.

Study Options Full-time.

Marshall University (continued)

Program Entrance Requirements Minimum overall college GPA of 2.5, transcript of college record, high school transcript, minimum high school GPA of 2.5. Transfer students are accepted. **Standardized tests** *Required:* SAT or ACT, TOEFL for international students. **Application** *Deadline:* rolling (freshmen), rolling (transfer). *Notification:* continuous (freshmen). *Application fee:* $25.

Advanced Placement Credit given for nursing courses completed elsewhere dependent upon specific evaluations.

Expenses (2004–05) *Tuition, state resident:* full-time $2814; part-time $151 per credit hour. *Tuition, nonresident:* full-time $8142; part-time $414 per credit hour. *International tuition:* $8142 full-time. *Room and board:* $7162; room only: $4480 per academic year. *Required fees:* full-time $450; part-time $11 per credit; part-time $225 per term.

Financial Aid 52% of baccalaureate students in nursing programs received some form of financial aid in 2003–04.

Contact Dr. Sandra Marra, Chairman, Nursing, College of Nursing and Health Professions, Marshall University, One John Marshall Drive, Huntington, WV 25755-9500. *Telephone:* 304-696-2639. *Fax:* 304-696-6739. *E-mail:* Nursing@marshall.edu.

GRADUATE PROGRAMS

Expenses (2004–05) *Tuition, state resident:* full-time $4040; part-time $214 per credit hour. *Tuition, nonresident:* full-time $11,306; part-time $617 per credit hour. *International tuition:* $11,306 full-time. *Room and board:* $8142; room only: $4480 per academic year. *Required fees:* full-time $450; part-time $11 per credit; part-time $225 per term.

Financial Aid 51% of graduate students in nursing programs received some form of financial aid in 2003–04.

Contact Dr. Sandra Marra, Chairman, Nursing, College of Nursing and Health Professions, Marshall University, One John Marshall Drive, Huntington, WV 25755-9500. *Telephone:* 304-696-2639. *Fax:* 304-696-6739. *E-mail:* Nursing@marshall.edu.

MASTER'S DEGREE PROGRAM

Degree MSN

Available Programs Master's.

Concentrations Available Nursing administration; nursing education. *Nurse practitioner programs in:* family health.

Site Options *Distance Learning:* South Charleston, WV.

Study Options Full-time and part-time.

Program Entrance Requirements Minimum overall college GPA of 3.0, transcript of college record, nursing research course, resume, statistics course, GRE General Test.

Advanced Placement Credit given for nursing courses completed elsewhere dependent upon specific evaluations.

Degree Requirements 36 total credit hours, thesis or project.

POST-MASTER'S PROGRAM

Areas of Study Nursing administration; nursing education. *Nurse practitioner programs in:* family health.

Mountain State University
Program in Nursing
Beckley, West Virginia

http://www.mountainstate.edu

Founded in 1933

DEGREES • BSN • MSN

Nursing Program Faculty 16 (13% with doctorates).

Nursing Student Activities Nursing Honor Society, Student Nurses' Association.

Nursing Student Resources Academic advising; academic or career counseling; bookstore; campus computer network; computer lab; computer-assisted instruction; Internet; library services; nursing audiovisuals; resume preparation assistance; skills, simulation, or other laboratory; tutoring.

Library Facilities 93,527 volumes (11,378 in health, 1,217 in nursing); 7,030 periodical subscriptions (1,000 health-care related).

BACCALAUREATE PROGRAMS

Degree BSN

Available Programs ADN to Baccalaureate; Baccalaureate for Second Degree; Generic Baccalaureate; LPN to Baccalaureate; RN Baccalaureate.

Site Options *Distance Learning:* Martinsburg, WV.

Study Options Full-time and part-time.

Program Entrance Requirements Minimum overall college GPA of 2.5, transcript of college record, CPR certification, health exam, health insurance, high school biology, 2 years high school science, high school transcript, immunizations, minimum high school GPA of 2.5. Transfer students are accepted. **Standardized tests** *Required:* TOEFL for international students. *Required for some:* SAT or ACT, SAT Subject Tests. **Application** *Deadline:* rolling (freshmen), rolling (transfer). *Application fee:* $25.

Advanced Placement Credit by examination available. Credit given for nursing courses completed elsewhere dependent upon specific evaluations.

Contact Dr. Patsy Haslam, Senior Academic Officer, Program in Nursing, Mountain State University, PO Box 9003, Beckley, WV 25802-9003. *Telephone:* 304-929-1327. *Fax:* 304-253-0789. *E-mail:* phaslam@mountainstate.edu.

GRADUATE PROGRAMS

Contact Dr. Jessica Sharp, Graduate Program Director, Program in Nursing, Mountain State University, PO Box 9003, Beckley, WV 25802-9003. *Telephone:* 304-929-1425. *E-mail:* jsharp@mountainstate.edu.

MASTER'S DEGREE PROGRAM

Degree MSN

Available Programs Master's.

Concentrations Available Nursing administration; nursing education. *Nurse practitioner programs in:* family health.

Study Options Full-time and part-time.

Program Entrance Requirements Clinical experience, transcript of college record, nursing research course, prerequisite course work, statistics course.

Advanced Placement Credit given for nursing courses completed elsewhere dependent upon specific evaluations.

Degree Requirements 35 total credit hours, thesis or project.

POST-MASTER'S PROGRAM

Areas of Study *Clinical nurse specialist programs in:* family health.

CONTINUING EDUCATION PROGRAM

Contact Dr. Patsy Haslam, Senior Academic Officer, Program in Nursing, Mountain State University, PO Box 9003, Beckley, WV 25802-9003. *Telephone:* 304-929-1327. *Fax:* 304-253-0789. *E-mail:* phaslam@mountainstate.edu.

Shepherd University
Department of Nursing Education
Shepherdstown, West Virginia

http://www.shepherd.edu/nurseweb/

Founded in 1871

DEGREE • BSN

Nursing Program Faculty 7 (43% with doctorates).

Baccalaureate Enrollment 66
Women 92.4% **Men** 7.6% **Minority** 1.5%

Nursing Student Activities Nursing Honor Society, Student Nurses' Association.

Nursing Student Resources Academic advising; academic or career counseling; assistance for students with disabilities; bookstore; campus computer network; career placement assistance; computer lab; computer-assisted instruction; e-mail services; employment services for current students; housing assistance; Internet; learning resource lab; library services; nursing audiovisuals; placement services for program completers; remedial services; resume preparation assistance; skills, simulation, or other laboratory; tutoring.

Library Facilities 183,197 volumes (3,644 in health, 501 in nursing); 918 periodical subscriptions (111 health-care related).

BACCALAUREATE PROGRAMS

Degree BSN

Available Programs ADN to Baccalaureate; Generic Baccalaureate; RN Baccalaureate.

Study Options Full-time.

Program Entrance Requirements Minimum overall college GPA of 2.5, transcript of college record, CPR certification, written essay, health exam, immunizations, interview, minimum GPA in nursing prerequisites of 2.0, prerequisite course work. Transfer students are accepted. **Standardized tests** *Required:* SAT or ACT, TOEFL for international students. **Application** *Deadline:* rolling (freshmen), rolling (transfer). *Early decision:* 11/15. *Notification:* continuous until 8/15 (freshmen), 12/15 (early action). *Application fee:* $35.

Advanced Placement Credit by examination available. Credit given for nursing courses completed elsewhere dependent upon specific evaluations.

Expenses (2004–05) *Tuition, state resident:* full-time $6540; part-time $136 per credit hour. *Tuition, nonresident:* full-time $8030; part-time $334 per credit hour. *Room and board:* $5400; room only: $2700 per academic year. *Required fees:* full-time $330.

Financial Aid 63% of baccalaureate students in nursing programs received some form of financial aid in 2003–04.

Contact Dr. Kathleen B. Gaberson, Professor and Chair, Department of Nursing Education, Department of Nursing Education, Shepherd University, PO Box 3210, Shepherdstown, WV 25443. *Telephone:* 304-876-5341. *Fax:* 304-876-5169. *E-mail:* kgaberso@shepherd.edu.

CONTINUING EDUCATION PROGRAM

Contact Dr. Kathleen B. Gaberson, Professor and Chair, Department of Nursing Education, Department of Nursing Education, Shepherd University, PO Box 3210, Shepherdstown, WV 25443. *Telephone:* 304-876-5341. *Fax:* 304-876-5169. *E-mail:* kgaberso@shepherd.edu.

University of Charleston

Department of Nursing
Charleston, West Virginia

http://www.ucwv.edu/dhs/bsn

Founded in 1888

DEGREE • BSN

Nursing Program Faculty 10 (30% with doctorates).

Baccalaureate Enrollment 103

Women 92% **Men** 8% **Minority** 5% **Part-time** 3%

Nursing Student Activities Sigma Theta Tau, Student Nurses' Association, nursing club.

Nursing Student Resources Academic advising; academic or career counseling; assistance for students with disabilities; bookstore; campus computer network; career placement assistance; computer lab; computer-assisted instruction; e-mail services; employment services for current students; externships; housing assistance; interactive nursing skills videos; Internet; learning resource lab; library services; nursing audiovisuals; paid internships; placement services for program completers; remedial services; resume preparation assistance; skills, simulation, or other laboratory; tutoring; unpaid internships.

Library Facilities 111,264 volumes (3,900 in health, 1,550 in nursing); 2,011 periodical subscriptions (75 health-care related).

BACCALAUREATE PROGRAMS

Degree BSN

Available Programs Generic Baccalaureate.

Study Options Full-time and part-time.

Program Entrance Requirements Minimum overall college GPA of 2.75, transcript of college record, CPR certification, health exam, high school biology, 1 year of high school math, high school transcript, immunizations, minimum high school GPA of 2.75, professional liability insurance/malpractice insurance. Transfer students are accepted. **Standardized tests** *Required:* SAT or ACT, TOEFL for international students. **Application** *Deadline:* rolling (freshmen), rolling (out-of-state freshmen), rolling (transfer). *Notification:* continuous (freshmen), continuous (out-of-state freshmen). *Application fee:* $25.

Advanced Placement Credit given for nursing courses completed elsewhere dependent upon specific evaluations.

Expenses (2004–05) *Tuition:* full-time $20,200; part-time $840 per credit hour. *Room and board:* $4060 per academic year. *Required fees:* full-time $120.

Financial Aid 95% of baccalaureate students in nursing programs received some form of financial aid in 2003–04. *Gift aid (need-based):* Federal Pell, FSEOG, state, private, college/university gift aid from institutional funds, Council of Independent Colleges Tuition Exchange grants, Tuition Exchange Inc. grants. *Loans:* Federal Nursing Student Loans, FFEL (Subsidized and Unsubsidized Stafford PLUS), Perkins, alternative loans. *Work-Study:* Federal Work-Study, part-time campus jobs. *Application deadline (priority):* 3/1.

Contact Director of Admissions, Department of Nursing, University of Charleston, 2300 MacCorkle Avenue, SE, Charleston, WV 25304. *Telephone:* 304-357-4750 Ext. 4750. *Fax:* 304-357-4781. *E-mail:* admissions@uchaswv.edu.

West Liberty State College

Department of Health Sciences
West Liberty, West Virginia

http://www.wlsc.edu/nursing/index.htm

Founded in 1837

DEGREE • BSN

Nursing Program Faculty 10 (30% with doctorates).

Baccalaureate Enrollment 100

Women 85% **Men** 15% **Minority** 3% **International** 1% **Part-time** 24%

Nursing Student Activities Student Nurses' Association.

Nursing Student Resources Academic advising; academic or career counseling; assistance for students with disabilities; bookstore; campus computer network; career placement assistance; computer lab; computer-assisted instruction; externships; housing assistance; interactive nursing skills videos; Internet; learning resource lab; library services; nursing audiovisuals; placement services for program completers; resume preparation assistance; skills, simulation, or other laboratory; tutoring; unpaid internships.

Library Facilities 194,715 volumes (2,500 in health, 750 in nursing); 485 periodical subscriptions (350 health-care related).

BACCALAUREATE PROGRAMS

Degree BSN

Available Programs Accelerated RN Baccalaureate; Generic Baccalaureate.

Site Options *Distance Learning:* Wheeling, WV.

Study Options Full-time and part-time.

West Liberty State College (continued)

Program Entrance Requirements Minimum overall college GPA of 2.5, minimum high school GPA of 3.0, minimum GPA in nursing prerequisites. Transfer students are accepted. **Standardized tests** *Required:* SAT or ACT, TOEFL for international students. **Application** *Notification:* continuous (freshmen).

Advanced Placement Credit by examination available. Credit given for nursing courses completed elsewhere dependent upon specific evaluations.

Expenses (2004–05) *Tuition, state resident:* full-time $3340; part-time $145 per credit hour. *Tuition, nonresident:* full-time $8314; part-time $347 per credit hour. *International tuition:* $8314 full-time. *Room and board:* $6656; room only: $4540 per academic year. *Required fees:* full-time $300; part-time $150 per term.

Financial Aid 65% of baccalaureate students in nursing programs received some form of financial aid in 2003–04.

Contact Dr. Donna J. Lukich, Nursing Program Director/Dean, School of Sciences, Department of Health Sciences, West Liberty State College, PO Box 295, CMC #140, West Liberty, WV 26074. *Telephone:* 304-336-8108. *Fax:* 304-336-5104. *E-mail:* lukichda@wlsc.edu.

West Virginia University

School of Nursing
Morgantown, West Virginia

http://www.hsc.wvu.edu/son/

Founded in 1867

DEGREES • BSN • DSN • MSN

Nursing Program Faculty 74 (45% with doctorates).

Baccalaureate Enrollment 550
Women 94% **Men** 6% **Minority** 5% **International** 2%

Graduate Enrollment 101
Women 93% **Men** 7% **Part-time** 50%

Nursing Student Activities Nursing Honor Society, Sigma Theta Tau, Student Nurses' Association.

Nursing Student Resources Academic advising; academic or career counseling; assistance for students with disabilities; bookstore; campus computer network; career placement assistance; computer lab; computer-assisted instruction; e-mail services; employment services for current students; externships; housing assistance; interactive nursing skills videos; Internet; learning resource lab; library services; nursing audiovisuals; paid internships; remedial services; resume preparation assistance; skills, simulation, or other laboratory; tutoring.

Library Facilities 1.7 million volumes (211,803 in health, 2,663 in nursing); 9,107 periodical subscriptions (1,662 health-care related).

BACCALAUREATE PROGRAMS

Degree BSN

Available Programs Accelerated Baccalaureate for Second Degree; Baccalaureate for Second Degree; Generic Baccalaureate; RN Baccalaureate.

Site Options *Distance Learning:* Glenville, WV; Parkersburg, WV; Charleston, WV.

Study Options Full-time and part-time.

Program Entrance Requirements Minimum overall college GPA of 2.5, transcript of college record, CPR certification, written essay, health insurance, high school biology, high school chemistry, 3 years high school math, 2 years high school science, high school transcript, immunizations, minimum high school GPA of 2.5, minimum GPA in nursing prerequisites of 2.0, prerequisite course work. Transfer students are accepted. **Standardized tests** *Required:* SAT or ACT, TOEFL for international students. **Application** *Deadline:* 8/1 (freshmen), 8/1 (transfer). *Application fee:* $25.

Advanced Placement Credit by examination available. Credit given for nursing courses completed elsewhere dependent upon specific evaluations.

Financial Aid 70% of baccalaureate students in nursing programs received some form of financial aid in 2003–04.

Contact Dr. Betty Shelton, RN, Assistant Dean, Student Services, School of Nursing, West Virginia University, PO Box 9600, 6702 RCB Health Sciences Center, South, Morgantown, WV 26506-9600. *Telephone:* 304-293-6650. *Fax:* 304-293-2784. *E-mail:* bshelton@hsc.wvu.edu.

GRADUATE PROGRAMS

Financial Aid 25% of graduate students in nursing programs received some form of financial aid in 2003–04. 1 teaching assistantship was awarded; institutionally sponsored loans, tuition waivers (full and partial), and graduate administrative assistantships also available. *Financial aid application deadline:* 2/1.

Contact Prof. Mary Jane Smith, Associate Dean, Graduate Academic Affairs, School of Nursing, West Virginia University, PO Box 9640, 6417 RCB Health Sciences Center, South, Morgantown, WV 26506-9600. *Telephone:* 304-293-4298. *Fax:* 304-293-2784. *E-mail:* mjsmith@hsc.wvu.edu.

MASTER'S DEGREE PROGRAM

Degree MSN

Available Programs Master's; RN to Master's.

Concentrations Available *Nurse practitioner programs in:* family health, pediatric, primary care.

Site Options *Distance Learning:* Charleston, WV.

Study Options Full-time and part-time.

Program Entrance Requirements Computer literacy, minimum overall college GPA of 3.0, transcript of college record, CPR certification, written essay, immunizations, 3 letters of recommendation, nursing research course, physical assessment course, resume, statistics course, GRE General Test. *Application deadline:* For fall admission, 6/1. Applications are processed on a rolling basis. *Application fee:* $45.

Advanced Placement Credit by examination available. Credit given for nursing courses completed elsewhere dependent upon specific evaluations.

Degree Requirements 44 total credit hours, thesis or project, comprehensive exam.

POST-MASTER'S PROGRAM

Areas of Study *Nurse practitioner programs in:* family health, pediatric, primary care.

DOCTORAL DEGREE PROGRAM

Degree DSN

Available Programs Doctorate.

Areas of Study Advanced practice nursing, ethics, faculty preparation, family health, health policy, health promotion/disease prevention, health-care systems, human health and illness, illness and transition, nursing education, nursing policy, nursing research, nursing science.

Site Options *Distance Learning:* Charleston, WV.

Program Entrance Requirements Minimum overall college GPA of 3.0, interview by faculty committee, interview, 3 letters of recommendation, MSN or equivalent, scholarly papers, statistics course, vita, writing sample, GRE General Test. *Application deadline:* For fall admission, 6/1. Applications are processed on a rolling basis. *Application fee:* $45.

Degree Requirements 54 total credit hours, dissertation, oral exam, written exam.

West Virginia Wesleyan College

Department of Nursing
Buckhannon, West Virginia

Founded in 1890

DEGREE • BSN

Nursing Program Faculty 6 (50% with doctorates).

Baccalaureate Enrollment 87
Women 91% **Men** 9% **Minority** 4% **International** 1% **Part-time** 30%

Nursing Student Activities Sigma Theta Tau, Student Nurses' Association.

Nursing Student Resources Academic advising; academic or career counseling; assistance for students with disabilities; bookstore; campus computer network; career placement assistance; computer-assisted instruction; e-mail services; employment services for current students; externships; Internet; learning resource lab; library services; nursing audiovisuals; placement services for program completers; remedial services; resume preparation assistance; tutoring.

Library Facilities 91,061 volumes (4,000 in health, 600 in nursing); 2,462 periodical subscriptions (90 health-care related).

BACCALAUREATE PROGRAMS

Degree BSN

Available Programs Generic Baccalaureate; RN Baccalaureate.

Study Options Full-time and part-time.

Program Entrance Requirements Minimum overall college GPA of 2.5, transcript of college record, CPR certification, health exam, health insurance, high school transcript, immunizations, interview, minimum high school GPA of 2.3, minimum GPA in nursing prerequisites of 2.0, prerequisite course work. Transfer students are accepted. **Standardized tests** *Required:* SAT or ACT, TOEFL for international students. *Required for some:* SAT Subject Tests. ***Placement:*** *Required for some:* SAT or ACT. **Application** *Deadline:* 7/1 (freshmen), 7/1 (transfer). *Early decision:* 12/1, 10/1. *Notification:* continuous (freshmen), 1/31 (out-of-state freshmen), 1/31 (early decision), 10/20 (early action). *Application fee:* $35.

Advanced Placement Credit by examination available. Credit given for nursing courses completed elsewhere dependent upon specific evaluations.

Expenses (2003–04) *Tuition:* full-time $17,900; part-time $320 per credit hour. *Room and board:* $4820; room only: $2430 per academic year. *Required fees:* full-time $200.

Financial Aid 90% of baccalaureate students in nursing programs received some form of financial aid in 2002–03.

Contact Mrs. Shauna Lively Aurelio, Chairperson, Department of Nursing, West Virginia Wesleyan College, 59 College Avenue, Buckhannon, WV 26201-2995. *Telephone:* 304-473-8224. *Fax:* 304-473-8435. *E-mail:* aurelio_s@wvwc.edu.

CONTINUING EDUCATION PROGRAM

Contact Ms. Judith McKinney, EdD, Chairperson, Department of Nursing, West Virginia Wesleyan College, 59 College Avenue, Buckhannon, WV 26201. *Telephone:* 304-473-8224. *E-mail:* mckinney@wvwc.edu.

Wheeling Jesuit University

Department of Nursing
Wheeling, West Virginia

http://www.wju.edu/academics/nursing/welcome.asp

Founded in 1954

DEGREES • BSN • MSN

Nursing Program Faculty 9 (50% with doctorates).

Library Facilities 153,590 volumes (5,065 in nursing); 512 periodical subscriptions (90 health-care related).

BACCALAUREATE PROGRAMS

Degree BSN

Study Options Full-time and part-time.

Program Entrance Requirements 2 Year (s) high school math, 1 year of high school science, high school transcript, minimum high school rank 50%. Transfer students are accepted. **Standardized tests** *Required:* SAT or ACT, TOEFL for international students. **Application** *Deadline:* rolling (freshmen), rolling (transfer). *Notification:* continuous (freshmen). *Application fee:* $25.

Advanced Placement Credit by examination available. Credit given for nursing courses completed elsewhere dependent upon specific evaluations.

Expenses (2003–04) *Tuition:* full-time $18,920. *Room and board:* $6000; room only: $2780 per academic year.

Contact Admissions Office, Department of Nursing, Wheeling Jesuit University, 316 Washington Avenue, Wheeling, WV 26003-6233. *Telephone:* 304-243-2359. *Fax:* 304-243-2397.

GRADUATE PROGRAMS

Expenses (2003–04) *Tuition:* part-time $470 per credit hour.

Financial Aid Federal Work-Study, scholarships, and unspecified assistantships available.

Contact Program Contact, Department of Nursing, Wheeling Jesuit University, 316 Washington Avenue, Wheeling, WV 26003-6233. *Telephone:* 304-243-2344. *Fax:* 304-243-2608.

MASTER'S DEGREE PROGRAM

Degree MSN

Available Programs Master's.

Concentrations Available Nursing administration; nursing education. *Nurse practitioner programs in:* family health.

Study Options Full-time and part-time.

Program Entrance Requirements Computer literacy, minimum overall college GPA of 3.0, 3 letters of recommendation, statistics course, GRE General Test. *Application deadline:* For fall admission, 8/1 (priority date); for spring admission, 12/15 (priority date). Applications are processed on a rolling basis. *Application fee:* $25.

Advanced Placement Credit given for nursing courses completed elsewhere dependent upon specific evaluations.

Degree Requirements 42 total credit hours, comprehensive exam.

WISCONSIN

Alverno College

Division of Nursing
Milwaukee, Wisconsin

http://www.alverno.edu

Founded in 1887

DEGREE • BSN

Nursing Program Faculty 25 (12% with doctorates).

Baccalaureate Enrollment 638
Women 100% **Minority** 38% **Part-time** 26%

Nursing Student Activities Student Nurses' Association.

Nursing Student Resources Academic advising; academic or career counseling; assistance for students with disabilities; bookstore; campus computer network; career placement assistance; computer lab; computer-assisted instruction; daycare for children of students; e-mail services; employment services for current students; externships; housing assistance; interactive nursing skills videos; Internet; learning resource lab; library services; nursing audiovisuals; remedial services; resume preparation assistance; skills, simulation, or other laboratory; tutoring; unpaid internships.

Library Facilities 82,416 volumes; 1,382 periodical subscriptions.

BACCALAUREATE PROGRAMS

Degree BSN

Available Programs ADN to Baccalaureate; Baccalaureate for Second Degree; Generic Baccalaureate; LPN to Baccalaureate; RN Baccalaureate.

Study Options Full-time and part-time.

Program Entrance Requirements Transcript of college record, written essay, high school biology, high school chemistry, 3 years high school math, 2 years high school science, high school transcript, minimum high school GPA of 2.0, prerequisite course work. Transfer students are accepted. **Standardized tests** *Required:* TOEFL for international students. *Recommended:* ACT. **Application** *Deadline:* rolling (freshmen), rolling (transfer). *Notification:* continuous (freshmen). *Application fee:* $20.

Alverno College (continued)

Advanced Placement Credit by examination available. Credit given for nursing courses completed elsewhere dependent upon specific evaluations.

Expenses (2004–05) *Tuition:* full-time $14,904; part-time $621 per credit hour. *International tuition:* $14,904 full-time. *Room and board:* $5400 per academic year.

Financial Aid 98% of baccalaureate students in nursing programs received some form of financial aid in 2003–04.

Contact Dr. Judeen A. Schulte, Chairperson and Professor, Division of Nursing, Alverno College, 3400 South 43rd Street, PO Box 343922, Milwaukee, WI 53234-3922. *Telephone:* 414-382-6284. *Fax:* 414-382-6279. *E-mail:* judeen.schulte@alverno.edu.

CONTINUING EDUCATION PROGRAM

Contact Ms. Debra Pass, Director, Professional and Community Education, Division of Nursing, Alverno College, 3400 South 43rd Street, PO Box 343922, Milwaukee, WI 53234-3922. *Telephone:* 414-382-6177. *Fax:* 414-382-6354. *E-mail:* debra.pass@alverno.edu.

Bellin College of Nursing
Nursing Program
Green Bay, Wisconsin

http://www.bcon.edu

Founded in 1909

DEGREES • BSN • MSN

Nursing Program Faculty 19 (16% with doctorates).

Baccalaureate Enrollment 216
Women 94% **Men** 6% **Minority** 3% **Part-time** 16%

Graduate Enrollment 23
Women 92% **Men** 8% **Minority** 8% **Part-time** 100%

Nursing Student Activities Sigma Theta Tau, Student Nurses' Association.

Nursing Student Resources Academic advising; academic or career counseling; career placement assistance; computer lab; computer-assisted instruction; e-mail services; interactive nursing skills videos; Internet; learning resource lab; library services; nursing audiovisuals; resume preparation assistance; skills, simulation, or other laboratory; tutoring.

Library Facilities 7,000 volumes (7,000 in health, 4,000 in nursing); 225 periodical subscriptions (228 health-care related).

BACCALAUREATE PROGRAMS

Degree BSN

Available Programs Accelerated Baccalaureate; Generic Baccalaureate.

Study Options Full-time and part-time.

Program Entrance Requirements Minimum overall college GPA of 2.7, transcript of college record, high school biology, high school chemistry, 3 years high school math, 3 years high school science, high school transcript, interview, 3 letters of recommendation, minimum high school GPA of 3.25, minimum GPA in nursing prerequisites of 2.7. Transfer students are accepted. **Standardized tests** *Required:* ACT. **Application** *Deadline:* rolling (freshmen), rolling (transfer). *Notification:* continuous (freshmen). *Application fee:* $30.

Advanced Placement Credit given for nursing courses completed elsewhere dependent upon specific evaluations.

Expenses (2004–05) *Tuition:* full-time $13,559; part-time $646 per credit hour. *International tuition:* $23,605 full-time. *Required fees:* full-time $291.

Financial Aid 93% of baccalaureate students in nursing programs received some form of financial aid in 2003–04. *Gift aid (need-based):* Federal Pell, FSEOG, state, private, college/university gift aid from institutional funds. *Loans:* FFEL (Subsidized and Unsubsidized Stafford PLUS), college/university. *Work-Study:* Federal Work-Study. *Application deadline (priority):* 3/1.

Contact Dr. Penny Croghan, Director of Admission, Nursing Program, Bellin College of Nursing, 725 South Webster Avenue, Green Bay, WI 54301. *Telephone:* 920-433-5803. *Fax:* 920-433-7416. *E-mail:* pcroghan@bcon.edu.

GRADUATE PROGRAMS

Expenses (2004–05) *Tuition:* part-time $475 per credit hour. *Required fees:* part-time $135 per term.

Financial Aid 61% of graduate students in nursing programs received some form of financial aid in 2003–04.

Contact Dr. Vera Dauffenbach, Interim Director of Graduate Program, Nursing Program, Bellin College of Nursing, 725 South Webster Avenue, PO Box 23400, Green Bay, WI 54305. *Telephone:* 920-433-3409. *Fax:* 920-433-7416. *E-mail:* vkdauffe@bcon.edu.

MASTER'S DEGREE PROGRAM

Degree MSN

Available Programs Master's.

Concentrations Available Nursing administration; nursing education.

Study Options Full-time and part-time.

Program Entrance Requirements Computer literacy, transcript of college record, written essay, interview, 3 letters of recommendation, nursing research course, resume, statistics course.

Advanced Placement Credit given for nursing courses completed elsewhere dependent upon specific evaluations.

Degree Requirements 38 total credit hours, thesis or project.

Cardinal Stritch University
Ruth S. Coleman College of Nursing
Milwaukee, Wisconsin

http://www.stritch.edu/nursing

Founded in 1937

DEGREES • BSN • MSN

Nursing Program Faculty 40 (12% with doctorates).

Baccalaureate Enrollment 50

Graduate Enrollment 25

Nursing Student Resources Academic advising; academic or career counseling; bookstore; campus computer network; career placement assistance; computer lab; e-mail services; employment services for current students; Internet; library services; resume preparation assistance.

Library Facilities 124,897 volumes (119,700 in health, 4,662 in nursing); 667 periodical subscriptions (85 health-care related).

■ Stritch is the only school in Wisconsin to offer the full range of nursing programs, from ADN to MSN. While the ADN is offered in a traditional format, both the accelerated BSN and the semi-accelerated MSN are structured to allow professionals to work full-time while earning their degrees. The ADN prepares students for entry into nursing and offers eligibility to take the NCLEX (Nursing Certificate Licensure Examination). The BSN focuses on giving students a broader knowledge base, leading to greater career opportunities. The MSN has an educational focus for nurses who want to function as nurse educators in various client communities.

BACCALAUREATE PROGRAMS

Degree BSN

Available Programs Accelerated RN Baccalaureate.

Site Options Milwaukee, WI.

Study Options Part-time.

Program Entrance Requirements Minimum overall college GPA of 2.33, transcript of college record, health exam, 2 years high school math, 2 years high school science, high school transcript, minimum high school GPA of 2.33, minimum high school rank 50%, RN licensure. Transfer students are accepted. **Standardized tests** *Required:* SAT or ACT, TOEFL for international students. *Recommended:* ACT. **Application** *Deadline:* rolling (freshmen), rolling (transfer). *Application fee:* $25.

Advanced Placement Credit by examination available. Credit given for nursing courses completed elsewhere dependent upon specific evaluations.

Expenses (2004–05) *Tuition:* part-time $420 per credit hour.

Contact Janet Beitz, BSN Program Contact, Ruth S. Coleman College of Nursing, Cardinal Stritch University, 6801 North Yates Road, Milwaukee, WI 53217-3985. *Telephone:* 414-410-4391. *Fax:* 414-410-4385. *E-mail:* jabeitz@stritch.edu.

GRADUATE PROGRAMS

Expenses (2004–05) *Tuition:* part-time $480 per credit hour.

Contact Ms. Carolyn Marohl, MSN Program Contact, Ruth S. Coleman College of Nursing, Cardinal Stritch University, 6801 North Yates Road, Milwaukee, WI 53217-3985. *Telephone:* 800-347-8822 Ext. 4709. *E-mail:* cjmarohl@stritch.edu.

MASTER'S DEGREE PROGRAM

Degree MSN

Available Programs Accelerated Master's.

Concentrations Available Nursing education.

Study Options Full-time and part-time.

Program Entrance Requirements Minimum overall college GPA of 2.75, transcript of college record, written essay, interview, 3 letters of recommendation, resume.

Advanced Placement Credit by examination available. Credit given for nursing courses completed elsewhere dependent upon specific evaluations.

Degree Requirements 36 total credit hours, thesis or project.

See full description on page 464.

Columbia College of Nursing/ Mount Mary College Nursing Program

Columbia College of Nursing/Mount Mary College Nursing Program
Milwaukee, Wisconsin

http://www.mtmary.edu/nursing.htm

Founded in 2002

DEGREE • BSN

Nursing Program Faculty 17 (32% with doctorates).

Baccalaureate Enrollment 269
Women 99% **Men** 1% **Part-time** 9%

Nursing Student Activities Nursing Honor Society, Sigma Theta Tau, Student Nurses' Association, nursing club.

Nursing Student Resources Academic advising; academic or career counseling; bookstore; campus computer network; career placement assistance; computer lab; computer-assisted instruction; daycare for children of students; e-mail services; employment services for current students; Internet; learning resource lab; library services; nursing audiovisuals; resume preparation assistance; skills, simulation, or other laboratory; tutoring; unpaid internships.

Library Facilities 9,400 volumes in health, 8,000 volumes in nursing; 275 periodical subscriptions health-care related.

■ Columbia College of Nursing has a long and proud history in nursing education, dating back to 1901. Jointly, Columbia College of Nursing and Mount Mary College offer a Bachelor of Science in Nursing (BSN) degree. Within a liberal arts framework, students integrate the latest in nursing instruction with challenging clinical placements, enabling them to meet the challenges of health care today and into the future. The nursing program is approved by the Wisconsin State Board of Nursing and is accredited by the National League for Nursing Accrediting Commission. The nursing program is a member of the American Association of Colleges of Nursing. Financial aid is available. http://www.ccon.edu; http://www.mtmary.edu

BACCALAUREATE PROGRAMS

Degree BSN

Available Programs Generic Baccalaureate.

Site Options Milwaukee, WI.

Study Options Full-time and part-time.

Program Entrance Requirements Minimum overall college GPA of 2.5, transcript of college record, health exam, health insurance, high school biology, high school chemistry, 2 years high school math, 2 years high school science, high school transcript, minimum high school GPA of 2.5, minimum high school rank 40%, minimum GPA in nursing prerequisites of 2.5. Transfer students are accepted.

Advanced Placement Credit by examination available. Credit given for nursing courses completed elsewhere dependent upon specific evaluations.

Expenses (2004–05) *Tuition:* full-time $15,975; part-time $466 per contact hour. *International tuition:* $15,975 full-time. *Room and board:* $5350 per academic year. *Required fees:* full-time $1180; part-time $50 per credit.

Financial Aid 90% of baccalaureate students in nursing programs received some form of financial aid in 2003–04.

Contact Ms. Ronda Bond, Nursing Recruiter, Columbia College of Nursing/Mount Mary College Nursing Program, 2900 North Menomonee River Parkway, Milwaukee, WI 53222. *Telephone:* 414-256-1219 Ext. 193. *Fax:* 414-256-0180. *E-mail:* bondr@mtmary.edu.

See full description on page 470.

Concordia University Wisconsin

Division of Nursing
Mequon, Wisconsin

http://www.cuw.edu

Founded in 1881

DEGREES • BSN • MSN

Nursing Program Faculty 24 (8% with doctorates).

Baccalaureate Enrollment 211
Women 91% **Men** 9% **Minority** 6% **International** 1%

Graduate Enrollment 158
Women 89% **Men** 11% **Minority** 4%

Nursing Student Activities Nursing Honor Society, Student Nurses' Association.

Nursing Student Resources Academic advising; academic or career counseling; assistance for students with disabilities; bookstore; campus computer network; career placement assistance; computer lab; computer-assisted instruction; e-mail services; employment services for current students; externships; interactive nursing skills videos; Internet; learning resource lab; library services; nursing audiovisuals; placement services for program completers; resume preparation assistance; skills, simulation, or other laboratory; tutoring.

Library Facilities 365,314 volumes (3,852 in health, 771 in nursing); 4,440 periodical subscriptions (203 health-care related).

BACCALAUREATE PROGRAMS

Degree BSN

Available Programs ADN to Baccalaureate; Generic Baccalaureate; LPN to Baccalaureate; RN Baccalaureate.

Concordia University Wisconsin (continued)

Study Options Full-time.

Program Entrance Requirements Transcript of college record, CPR certification, health exam, health insurance, high school transcript, immunizations, minimum high school GPA of 2.75, minimum GPA in nursing prerequisites of 2.75. Transfer students are accepted. **Standardized tests** *Required:* ACT, TOEFL for international students. **Application** *Deadline:* 8/15 (freshmen), 8/15 (transfer). *Notification:* continuous until 8/15 (freshmen). *Application fee:* $35.

Advanced Placement Credit given for nursing courses completed elsewhere dependent upon specific evaluations.

Expenses (2004–05) *Tuition:* full-time $16,910; part-time $683 per credit hour. *Room and board:* $6230 per academic year.

Contact Dr. Grace A. Peterson, Chairperson, Division of Nursing, Concordia University Wisconsin, 12800 North Lake Shore Drive, Mequon, WI 53097. *Telephone:* 262-243-4205 Ext. 4205. *Fax:* 262-243-4466. *E-mail:* grace.peterson@cuw.edu.

GRADUATE PROGRAMS

Expenses (2004–05) *Tuition:* part-time $420 per credit hour.

Contact Dr. Ruth Gresley, Director, Graduate Nursing, Division of Nursing, Concordia University Wisconsin, 12800 North Lake Shore Drive, Mequon, WI 53097. *Telephone:* 262-243-4452. *Fax:* 262-243-4506. *E-mail:* ruth.gresley@cuw.edu.

MASTER'S DEGREE PROGRAM

Degree MSN

Available Programs Master's.

Concentrations Available Nursing education. *Nurse practitioner programs in:* family health, gerontology.

Study Options Full-time and part-time.

Program Entrance Requirements Clinical experience, computer literacy, minimum overall college GPA of 3.0, transcript of college record, CPR certification, written essay, immunizations, interview, 2 letters of recommendation, physical assessment course, professional liability insurance/malpractice insurance, resume, statistics course. *Application deadline:* For fall admission, 8/1 (priority date). Applications are processed on a rolling basis. *Application fee:* $35.

Advanced Placement Credit given for nursing courses completed elsewhere dependent upon specific evaluations.

Degree Requirements 44 total credit hours, thesis or project.

CONTINUING EDUCATION PROGRAM

Contact Dr. Grace A. Peterson, Chairperson, Division of Nursing, Concordia University Wisconsin, 12800 North Lake Shore Drive, Mequon, WI 53097. *Telephone:* 262-243-4205 Ext. 4205. *Fax:* 262-243-4466. *E-mail:* grace.peterson@cuw.edu.

Edgewood College

Program in Nursing
Madison, Wisconsin

http://nursing.edgewood.edu

Founded in 1927

DEGREES • BS • MS

Nursing Program Faculty 24 (21% with doctorates).

Baccalaureate Enrollment 177
Women 94% **Men** 6% **Minority** 2% **International** 1% **Part-time** 35%

Graduate Enrollment 38
Women 86% **Men** 14% **Minority** 2% **Part-time** 100%

Nursing Student Activities Sigma Theta Tau, Student Nurses' Association.

Nursing Student Resources Academic advising; academic or career counseling; assistance for students with disabilities; bookstore; campus computer network; career placement assistance; computer lab; computer-assisted instruction; daycare for children of students; e-mail services; employment services for current students; housing assistance; interactive nursing skills videos; Internet; learning resource lab; library services; nursing audiovisuals; resume preparation assistance; skills, simulation, or other laboratory; tutoring.

Library Facilities 90,253 volumes (3,000 in health, 935 in nursing); 447 periodical subscriptions (43 health-care related).

BACCALAUREATE PROGRAMS

Degree BS

Available Programs Baccalaureate for Second Degree; Generic Baccalaureate.

Study Options Full-time and part-time.

Program Entrance Requirements Minimum overall college GPA of 2.5, transcript of college record, CPR certification, written essay, health exam, high school biology, high school chemistry, high school foreign language, high school math, high school transcript, immunizations, minimum high school GPA of 2.5, minimum GPA in nursing prerequisites of 2.5, prerequisite course work. Transfer students are accepted. **Standardized tests** *Required:* SAT or ACT, TOEFL for international students. **Application** *Deadline:* rolling (freshmen), rolling (transfer). *Notification:* continuous (freshmen). *Application fee:* $25.

Advanced Placement Credit given for nursing courses completed elsewhere dependent upon specific evaluations.

Expenses (2004–05) *Tuition:* full-time $16,050; part-time $494 per credit hour. *International tuition:* $16,050 full-time. *Room and board:* $5500; room only: $2700 per academic year. *Required fees:* full-time $1130; part-time $565 per term.

Financial Aid 76% of baccalaureate students in nursing programs received some form of financial aid in 2003–04. *Gift aid (need-based):* Federal Pell, FSEOG, state, private, college/university gift aid from institutional funds. *Loans:* FFEL (Subsidized and Unsubsidized Stafford PLUS), Perkins, state, college/university. *Work-Study:* Federal Work-Study, part-time campus jobs. *Application deadline (priority):* 3/15.

Contact Dr. Mary L. Kelly-Powell, Chairperson and Associate Professor, Program in Nursing, Edgewood College, 1000 Edgewood College Drive, Madison, WI 53711. *Telephone:* 608-663-2292. *Fax:* 608-663-2863. *E-mail:* mkellypowell@edgewood.edu.

GRADUATE PROGRAMS

Expenses (2004–05) *Tuition:* part-time $524 per credit hour.

Financial Aid 10% of graduate students in nursing programs received some form of financial aid in 2003–04.

Contact Dr. Mary L. Kelly-Powell, Chairperson and Associate Professor, Program in Nursing, Edgewood College, 1000 Edgewood College Drive, Madison, WI 53711. *Telephone:* 608-663-2292. *Fax:* 608-663-2863. *E-mail:* mkellypowell@edgewood.edu.

MASTER'S DEGREE PROGRAM

Degree MS

Available Programs Master's.

Concentrations Available Nursing administration; nursing education.

Study Options Part-time.

Program Entrance Requirements Clinical experience, computer literacy, minimum overall college GPA of 3.0, transcript of college record, CPR certification, written essay, immunizations, 2 letters of recommendation, nursing research course, prerequisite course work. *Application deadline:* For fall admission, 8/1 (priority date); for spring admission, 1/10 (priority date). Applications are processed on a rolling basis. *Application fee:* $25.

Advanced Placement Credit given for nursing courses completed elsewhere dependent upon specific evaluations.

Degree Requirements 36 total credit hours.

Marian College of Fond du Lac

Nursing Studies Division
Fond du Lac, Wisconsin

http://www.mariancollege.edu

Founded in 1936

DEGREES • BSN • MSN

Baccalaureate Enrollment 221
Women 95% **Men** 5% **Minority** 1% **Part-time** 7%

Graduate Enrollment 39
Women 97% **Men** 3% **Part-time** 15%

Nursing Student Activities Student Nurses' Association.

Nursing Student Resources Academic advising; academic or career counseling; assistance for students with disabilities; bookstore; career placement assistance; computer lab; daycare for children of students; e-mail services; externships; interactive nursing skills videos; Internet; learning resource lab; library services; nursing audiovisuals.

Library Facilities 90,327 volumes (3,000 in health, 2,500 in nursing); 737 periodical subscriptions (91 health-care related).

BACCALAUREATE PROGRAMS

Degree BSN

Available Programs ADN to Baccalaureate; Generic Baccalaureate.

Site Options Appleton, WI; Beaver Dam, WI. *Distance Learning:* Milwaukee, WI.

Study Options Full-time and part-time.

Program Entrance Requirements Transcript of college record, high school biology, high school chemistry, 3 years high school math, high school science, high school transcript, minimum high school GPA of 2.5. Transfer students are accepted. **Standardized tests** *Required:* SAT or ACT, TOEFL for international students. **Application** *Deadline:* rolling (freshmen), rolling (transfer). *Notification:* continuous until 8/15 (freshmen). *Application fee:* $20.

Advanced Placement Credit given for nursing courses completed elsewhere dependent upon specific evaluations.

Expenses (2003–04) *Tuition:* full-time $14,700; part-time $270 per credit hour. *Room and board:* $5520; room only: $3200 per academic year. *Required fees:* full-time $300; part-time $160 per term.

Financial Aid 98% of baccalaureate students in nursing programs received some form of financial aid in 2002–03.

Contact Nancy Ricketts, Basic Nursing Academic Advisor, Nursing Studies Division, Marian College of Fond du Lac, 45 South National Avenue, Fond du Lac, WI 54935. *Telephone:* 920-923-8732. *Fax:* 920-923-8770. *E-mail:* nricketts@mariancollege.edu.

GRADUATE PROGRAMS

Expenses (2003–04) *Tuition:* full-time $6750; part-time $375 per credit hour. *Required fees:* full-time $200.

Contact Graduate Department, Nursing Studies Division, Marian College of Fond du Lac, 45 South National Avenue, Fond du Lac, WI 54935-4699. *Telephone:* 920-923-8094. *Fax:* 920-923-8094. *E-mail:* admissions@mariancollege.edu.

MASTER'S DEGREE PROGRAM

Degree MSN

Available Programs Master's.

Concentrations Available Nursing education. *Nurse practitioner programs in:* adult health.

Site Options *Distance Learning:* Milwaukee, WI.

Study Options Full-time and part-time.

Program Entrance Requirements Clinical experience, minimum overall college GPA of 3.0, transcript of college record, CPR certification, written essay, immunizations, 3 letters of recommendation, nursing research course, professional liability insurance/malpractice insurance, resume, statistics course.

Advanced Placement Credit given for nursing courses completed elsewhere dependent upon specific evaluations.

Degree Requirements 39 total credit hours, thesis or project.

POST-MASTER'S PROGRAM

Areas of Study Nursing education.

Marquette University
College of Nursing
Milwaukee, Wisconsin

http://www.marquette.edu/nursing

Founded in 1881

DEGREES • BSN • MSN • MSN/MBA • PHD

Nursing Program Faculty 45 (73% with doctorates).

Baccalaureate Enrollment 439
Women 95% **Men** 5% **Minority** 10% **Part-time** 10%

Graduate Enrollment 188
Women 95% **Men** 5% **Minority** 4% **Part-time** 61%

Nursing Student Activities Sigma Theta Tau, Student Nurses' Association.

Nursing Student Resources Academic advising; academic or career counseling; assistance for students with disabilities; bookstore; campus computer network; career placement assistance; computer lab; computer-assisted instruction; daycare for children of students; e-mail services; employment services for current students; externships; housing assistance; interactive nursing skills videos; Internet; learning resource lab; library services; nursing audiovisuals; paid internships; remedial services; resume preparation assistance; skills, simulation, or other laboratory; tutoring.

Library Facilities 1.1 million volumes (58,262 in health, 4,483 in nursing); 5,894 periodical subscriptions (818 health-care related).

BACCALAUREATE PROGRAMS

Degree BSN

Available Programs Generic Baccalaureate; RN Baccalaureate.

Study Options Full-time and part-time.

Program Entrance Requirements Minimum overall college GPA of 2.5, transcript of college record, written essay, high school biology, high school chemistry, 3 years high school math, high school transcript, minimum high school GPA of 2.5, minimum high school rank 25%. Transfer students are accepted. **Standardized tests** *Required:* SAT or ACT, TOEFL for international students. **Application** *Deadline:* 12/1 (freshmen), 12/1 (transfer). *Notification:* 1/15 (freshmen). *Application fee:* $30.

Advanced Placement Credit given for nursing courses completed elsewhere dependent upon specific evaluations.

Expenses (2004–05) *Tuition:* full-time $21,550; part-time $635 per credit hour. *Room and board:* $7070 per academic year. *Required fees:* full-time $520.

Financial Aid 90% of baccalaureate students in nursing programs received some form of financial aid in 2003–04. *Gift aid (need-based):* Federal Pell, FSEOG, state, private, college/university gift aid from institutional funds. *Loans:* Federal Nursing Student Loans, Federal Direct (Subsidized and Unsubsidized Stafford PLUS), Perkins, state, college/university, alternative loans. *Work-Study:* Federal Work-Study, part-time campus jobs. *Application deadline:* Continuous.

Contact Dr. Janet W. Krejci, RN, Associate Dean for Undergraduate Programs, College of Nursing, Marquette University, Clark Hall, PO Box 1881, Milwaukee, WI 53201-1881. *Telephone:* 414-288-3809. *Fax:* 414-288-1597. *E-mail:* janet.krejci@marquette.edu.

GRADUATE PROGRAMS

Expenses (2004–05) *Tuition:* full-time $11,880; part-time $660 per credit hour. *International tuition:* $11,880 full-time. *Room and board:* $6198; room only: $4950 per academic year.

Financial Aid 53% of graduate students in nursing programs received some form of financial aid in 2003–04. 6 research assistantships, 1 teaching assistantship were awarded; career-related internships or fieldwork, Federal Work-Study, institutionally sponsored loans, scholarships, and tuition waivers (full and partial) also available. Aid available to part-time students. *Financial aid application deadline:* 2/15.

Marquette University (continued)

Contact Dr. Judith Fitzgerald Miller, RN, Associate Dean for Graduate Programs & Research, College of Nursing, Marquette University, Clark Hall, PO Box 1881, Milwaukee, WI 53201-1881. *Telephone:* 414-288-3869. *Fax:* 414-288-1597. *E-mail:* judith.miller@marquette.edu.

MASTER'S DEGREE PROGRAM

Degrees MSN; MSN/MBA

Available Programs Accelerated AD/RN to Master's; Accelerated Master's for Non-Nursing College Graduates; Accelerated RN to Master's; Master's; Master's for Non-Nursing College Graduates; Master's for Nurses with Non-Nursing Degrees; RN to Master's.

Concentrations Available Nurse-midwifery; nursing administration. *Clinical nurse specialist programs in:* adult health, gerontology, pediatric. *Nurse practitioner programs in:* acute care, adult health, gerontology, pediatric.

Study Options Full-time and part-time.

Program Entrance Requirements Minimum overall college GPA of 3.0, transcript of college record, written essay, 3 letters of recommendation, nursing research course, physical assessment course, resume, statistics course, GRE General Test. *Application fee:* $40.

Advanced Placement Credit given for nursing courses completed elsewhere dependent upon specific evaluations.

Degree Requirements 42 total credit hours, comprehensive exam.

POST-MASTER'S PROGRAM

Areas of Study Nurse-midwifery; nursing administration. *Clinical nurse specialist programs in:* adult health, gerontology, pediatric. *Nurse practitioner programs in:* acute care, adult health, gerontology, pediatric.

DOCTORAL DEGREE PROGRAM

Degree PhD

Available Programs Doctorate.

Areas of Study Faculty preparation, health promotion/disease prevention, health-care systems, human health and illness, illness and transition, nursing education, nursing research, nursing science.

Program Entrance Requirements Minimum overall college GPA of 3.2, interview, 3 letters of recommendation, MSN or equivalent, statistics course, vita, writing sample. *Application fee:* $40.

Degree Requirements 51 total credit hours, dissertation, oral exam, written exam, residency.

CONTINUING EDUCATION PROGRAM

Contact Dr. Lea Acord, Dean, College of Nursing, Marquette University, Clark Hall, PO Box 1881, Milwaukee, WI 53201-1881. *Telephone:* 414-288-3812. *Fax:* 414-288-1597. *E-mail:* lea.acord@marquette.edu.

See full description on page 516.

Milwaukee School of Engineering

School of Nursing
Milwaukee, Wisconsin

http://www.msoe.edu/nursing

Founded in 1903

DEGREE • BSN

Nursing Program Faculty 9 (39% with doctorates).

Baccalaureate Enrollment 110

Women 90% **Men** 10% **Minority** 20%

Nursing Student Activities Student Nurses' Association.

Nursing Student Resources Academic advising; academic or career counseling; assistance for students with disabilities; bookstore; campus computer network; career placement assistance; computer lab; computer-assisted instruction; e-mail services; externships; housing assistance; interactive nursing skills videos; Internet; learning resource lab; library services; nursing audiovisuals; placement services for program completers; remedial services; resume preparation assistance; skills, simulation, or other laboratory; tutoring.

Library Facilities 59,564 volumes (1,956 in health, 1,126 in nursing); 585 periodical subscriptions (116 health-care related).

BACCALAUREATE PROGRAMS

Degree BSN

Available Programs Generic Baccalaureate; RN Baccalaureate.

Study Options Full-time and part-time.

Program Entrance Requirements Minimum overall college GPA of 2.5, transcript of college record, CPR certification, health exam, health insurance, high school biology, high school chemistry, 3 years high school math, 3 years high school science, high school transcript, immunizations, minimum high school GPA of 2.8, professional liability insurance/malpractice insurance. Transfer students are accepted. **Standardized tests** *Required:* SAT or ACT, TOEFL for international students. **Application** *Deadline:* rolling (freshmen), rolling (transfer). *Notification:* continuous (freshmen). *Application fee:* $25.

Advanced Placement Credit by examination available. Credit given for nursing courses completed elsewhere dependent upon specific evaluations.

Expenses (2004–05) *Tuition:* full-time $23,034; part-time $402 per credit hour. *International tuition:* $23,034 full-time. *Room and board:* $5610; room only: $3600 per academic year. *Required fees:* full-time $1140.

Financial Aid 100% of baccalaureate students in nursing programs received some form of financial aid in 2003–04.

Contact Dr. Debra L. Jenks, RN, Interim Chair, School of Nursing, Milwaukee School of Engineering, 1025 North Broadway Street, Milwaukee, WI 53202-3109. *Telephone:* 414-277-4516. *Fax:* 414-277-4540. *E-mail:* jenks@msoe.edu.

University of Wisconsin–Eau Claire

College of Nursing and Health Sciences
Eau Claire, Wisconsin

http://www.uwec.edu/Nurs/

Founded in 1916

DEGREES • BSN • MSN

Nursing Program Faculty 37 (43% with doctorates).

Baccalaureate Enrollment 645

Women 92% **Men** 8% **Minority** 5% **Part-time** 15%

Graduate Enrollment 61

Women 93% **Men** 7% **Minority** 2% **Part-time** 84%

Nursing Student Activities Sigma Theta Tau, Student Nurses' Association.

Nursing Student Resources Academic advising; academic or career counseling; assistance for students with disabilities; bookstore; campus computer network; career placement assistance; computer lab; computer-assisted instruction; daycare for children of students; e-mail services; employment services for current students; housing assistance; interactive nursing skills videos; Internet; learning resource lab; library services; nursing audiovisuals; placement services for program completers; remedial services; resume preparation assistance; tutoring.

Library Facilities 764,275 volumes (65,000 in nursing); 2,448 periodical subscriptions (2,049 health-care related).

■ The College of Nursing and Health Sciences has an excellent reputation for the high quality of its educational programs and its graduates. The College offers bachelor's and master's degrees in nursing and participates in a statewide Collaborative Nursing Program for registered nurses to earn a BSN. Master's-level options include adult or family health specialization and advanced clinical practice, education, or administration role preparation. Baccalaureate-level students receive clinical experiences in acute-care facilities, community health agencies, schools, home-care agencies, and the College of Nursing and Health Sciences clinic. Through distance technology, bachelor's and some master's courses are available at a satellite in Marshfield, Wisconsin.

BACCALAUREATE PROGRAMS

Degree BSN

Available Programs Generic Baccalaureate; RN Baccalaureate.

Site Options *Distance Learning:* Marshfield, WI.

Study Options Full-time and part-time.

Program Entrance Requirements Minimum overall college GPA of 2.75, transcript of college record, CPR certification, written essay, health exam, high school biology, high school chemistry, high school foreign language, 3 years high school math, 3 years high school science, high school transcript, immunizations, minimum high school GPA of 2.0. Transfer students are accepted. **Standardized tests** *Required:* SAT or ACT, TOEFL for international students. **Application** *Deadline:* rolling (freshmen), 7/1 (transfer). *Notification:* continuous (freshmen). *Application fee:* $35.

Advanced Placement Credit by examination available.

Expenses (2004–05) *Tuition, state resident:* full-time $4864; part-time $203 per credit hour. *Tuition, nonresident:* full-time $14,910; part-time $621 per credit hour. *Room and board:* $4580; room only: $2480 per academic year.

Financial Aid 67% of baccalaureate students in nursing programs received some form of financial aid in 2003–04. *Gift aid (need-based):* Federal Pell, FSEOG, state, private, college/university gift aid from institutional funds, Federal Nursing. *Loans:* Federal Direct (Subsidized and Unsubsidized Stafford PLUS), Perkins, college/university, alternative loans. *Work-Study:* Federal Work-Study, part-time campus jobs. *Application deadline (priority):* 4/15.

Contact Dr. Linda Elaine Wendt, Dean, College of Nursing and Health Sciences, University of Wisconsin–Eau Claire, 105 Garfield Avenue, Eau Claire, WI 54701-4004. *Telephone:* 715-836-5287. *Fax:* 715-836-5925. *E-mail:* wendtle@uwec.edu.

GRADUATE PROGRAMS

Expenses (2004–05) *Tuition, state resident:* full-time $5922; part-time $329 per credit hour. *Tuition, nonresident:* full-time $16,531; part-time $918 per credit hour. *Room and board:* $4580; room only: $2480 per academic year.

Financial Aid 38% of graduate students in nursing programs received some form of financial aid in 2003–04. 3 teaching assistantships (averaging $3,400 per year) were awarded; Federal Work-Study also available. Aid available to part-time students. *Financial aid application deadline:* 3/1.

Contact Dr. Linda Elaine Wendt, Dean, College of Nursing and Health Sciences, University of Wisconsin–Eau Claire, 105 Garfield Avenue, Eau Claire, WI 54702-4004. *Telephone:* 715-836-5287. *Fax:* 715-836-5925. *E-mail:* wendtle@uwec.edu.

MASTER'S DEGREE PROGRAM

Degree MSN

Available Programs Master's; RN to Master's.

Concentrations Available Nursing administration; nursing education. *Clinical nurse specialist programs in:* adult health, family health. *Nurse practitioner programs in:* adult health, family health.

Study Options Full-time and part-time.

Program Entrance Requirements Clinical experience, minimum overall college GPA of 3.0, transcript of college record, written essay, physical assessment course, professional liability insurance/malpractice insurance, statistics course, GRE General Test. *Application deadline:* For fall admission, 2/1 (priority date). Applications are processed on a rolling basis. *Application fee:* $45.

Degree Requirements 36 total credit hours.

CONTINUING EDUCATION PROGRAM

Contact Dr. Douglas A. Pearson, Interim Director of Continuing Education, College of Nursing and Health Sciences, University of Wisconsin–Eau Claire, Eau Claire, WI 54702-4004. *Telephone:* 715-836-3636. *Fax:* 715-836-5263. *E-mail:* pearsoda@uwec.edu.

University of Wisconsin–Green Bay

BSN–LINC Online RN–BSN Program
Green Bay, Wisconsin

http://www.bsnlinc.wisconsin.edu/

Founded in 1968

DEGREE • BSN

Nursing Program Faculty 5 (60% with doctorates).

Baccalaureate Enrollment 168
Women 93% **Men** 7% **Minority** 5% **Part-time** 100%

Nursing Student Activities Sigma Theta Tau, Student Nurses' Association.

Nursing Student Resources Academic advising; academic or career counseling; bookstore; career placement assistance; computer lab; e-mail services; employment services for current students; Internet; learning resource lab; library services; nursing audiovisuals; resume preparation assistance; skills, simulation, or other laboratory.

Library Facilities 333,482 volumes (1,000 in health, 675 in nursing); 5,512 periodical subscriptions (100 health-care related).

BACCALAUREATE PROGRAMS

Degree BSN

Available Programs RN Baccalaureate.

Study Options Full-time and part-time.

Program Entrance Requirements Minimum overall college GPA of 2.5, transcript of college record, prerequisite course work, RN licensure. Transfer students are accepted. **Standardized tests** *Required:* SAT or ACT, TOEFL for international students. **Application** *Notification:* continuous until 8/15 (freshmen). *Application fee:* $35.

Expenses (2004–05) *Tuition, state resident:* part-time $215 per credit hour. *Tuition, nonresident:* part-time $330 per credit hour.

Financial Aid 25% of baccalaureate students in nursing programs received some form of financial aid in 2003–04.

Contact Ms. Stacey Moyer, Advisor, BSN–LINC Online RN–BSN Program, University of Wisconsin–Green Bay, 2420 Nicolet Drive, Green Bay, WI 54311-7001. *Telephone:* 920-465-2934. *Fax:* 920-465-2854. *E-mail:* moyers@uwgb.edu.

University of Wisconsin–Madison

School of Nursing
Madison, Wisconsin

http://www.son.wisc.edu

Founded in 1848

DEGREES • BS • MS • PHD

Nursing Program Faculty 56 (39% with doctorates).

Baccalaureate Enrollment 324
Women 92% **Men** 8% **Minority** 5% **International** 2% **Part-time** 20%

Graduate Enrollment 171
Women 96% **Men** 4% **Minority** 5% **International** 7% **Part-time** 63%

Nursing Student Activities Nursing Honor Society, Sigma Theta Tau, Student Nurses' Association.

Nursing Student Resources Academic advising; academic or career counseling; assistance for students with disabilities; bookstore; campus computer network; career placement assistance; computer lab; computer-assisted instruction; daycare for children of students; e-mail services; externships; housing assistance; interactive nursing skills videos; Internet; learning resource lab; library services; nursing audiovisuals; paid internships; resume preparation assistance; skills, simulation, or other laboratory; tutoring.

Library Facilities 334,378 volumes in health, 8,164 volumes in nursing; 1,483 periodical subscriptions health-care related.

University of Wisconsin–Madison (continued)

BACCALAUREATE PROGRAMS

Degree BS

Available Programs ADN to Baccalaureate; Generic Baccalaureate; RN Baccalaureate.

Site Options *Distance Learning:* LaCrosse, WI.

Study Options Full-time and part-time.

Program Entrance Requirements Minimum overall college GPA of 2.75, transcript of college record, CPR certification, written essay, high school foreign language, 3 years high school math, 3 years high school science, high school transcript, immunizations, minimum GPA in nursing prerequisites of 2.75, prerequisite course work. Transfer students are accepted. **Standardized tests** *Required:* SAT or ACT, TOEFL for international students. **Application** *Deadline:* 2/1 (freshmen), 2/1 (transfer). *Notification:* continuous (freshmen). *Application fee:* $35.

Advanced Placement Credit by examination available. Credit given for nursing courses completed elsewhere dependent upon specific evaluations.

Expenses (2004–05) *Tuition, state resident:* full-time $2933; part-time $246 per credit hour. *Tuition, nonresident:* full-time $9933; part-time $830 per credit hour. *International tuition:* $9933 full-time. *Room and board:* $5700; room only: $4500 per academic year. *Required fees:* full-time $5866; part-time $246 per credit; part-time $2933 per term.

Financial Aid 33% of baccalaureate students in nursing programs received some form of financial aid in 2003–04. *Gift aid (need-based):* Federal Pell, FSEOG, state, private, college/university gift aid from institutional funds. *Loans:* Federal Nursing Student Loans, FFEL (Subsidized and Unsubsidized Stafford PLUS), Perkins, state, college/university. *Work-Study:* Federal Work-Study. *Application deadline:* Continuous.

Contact Jane Schimmel, Academic Advisor, School of Nursing, University of Wisconsin–Madison, 600 Highland Avenue, Room K6/142, Madison, WI 53792-2455. *Telephone:* 608-263-5166. *Fax:* 608-263-5296. *E-mail:* jcschimm@wisc.edu.

GRADUATE PROGRAMS

Expenses (2004–05) *Tuition, state resident:* full-time $8320; part-time $522 per credit hour. *Tuition, nonresident:* full-time $23,590; part-time $1476 per credit hour. *Room and board:* $6940; room only: $6940 per academic year.

Financial Aid 55% of graduate students in nursing programs received some form of financial aid in 2003–04. 15 fellowships with tuition reimbursements available (averaging $17,000 per year), 12 research assistantships with tuition reimbursements available (averaging $17,000 per year), 8 teaching assistantships with tuition reimbursements available (averaging $11,000 per year) were awarded; career-related internships or fieldwork, Federal Work-Study, institutionally sponsored loans, scholarships, traineeships, and unspecified assistantships also available. Aid available to part-time students. *Financial aid application deadline:* 6/1.

Contact Ms. Marcia Voss, Graduate Program Coordinator, School of Nursing, University of Wisconsin–Madison, 600 Highland Avenue, K6/140, Clinical Science Center, Madison, WI 53792-2455. *Telephone:* 608-263-5258. *Fax:* 608-263-5296. *E-mail:* mlvoss@wisc.edu.

MASTER'S DEGREE PROGRAM

Degree MS

Available Programs Accelerated RN to Master's; Master's; Master's for Nurses with Non-Nursing Degrees.

Concentrations Available Nurse case management; nursing education. *Clinical nurse specialist programs in:* adult health, gerontology, medical-surgical, pediatric, perinatal, psychiatric/mental health, women's health. *Nurse practitioner programs in:* acute care, adult health, gerontology, pediatric, psychiatric/mental health, women's health.

Study Options Full-time and part-time.

Program Entrance Requirements Clinical experience, minimum overall college GPA of 3.0, transcript of college record, written essay, immunizations, 3 letters of recommendation, resume, statistics course, GRE General Test. *Application deadline:* For fall admission, 3/1 (priority date); for spring admission, 10/1 (priority date). *Application fee:* $45.

Advanced Placement Credit given for nursing courses completed elsewhere dependent upon specific evaluations.

Degree Requirements 36 total credit hours.

POST-MASTER'S PROGRAM

Areas of Study Nurse case management; nursing education. *Clinical nurse specialist programs in:* adult health, gerontology, medical-surgical, pediatric, perinatal, psychiatric/mental health, women's health. *Nurse practitioner programs in:* acute care, adult health, gerontology, pediatric, psychiatric/mental health, women's health.

DOCTORAL DEGREE PROGRAM

Degree PhD

Available Programs Doctorate; Post-Baccalaureate Doctorate.

Areas of Study Aging, bio-behavioral research, biology of health and illness, community health, faculty preparation, family health, gerontology, health policy, health promotion/disease prevention, human health and illness, information systems, nursing education, nursing research, oncology, women's health.

Program Entrance Requirements Minimum overall college GPA of 3.0, interview, 3 letters of recommendation, scholarly papers, vita, writing sample, GRE General Test. *Application deadline:* For fall admission, 3/1 (priority date); for spring admission, 10/1 (priority date). *Application fee:* $45.

Degree Requirements 60 total credit hours, dissertation, written exam, residency.

POSTDOCTORAL PROGRAM

Areas of Study Adolescent health, aging, cancer care, chronic illness, community health, family health, gerontology, health promotion/disease prevention, individualized study, nursing informatics, nursing interventions, nursing research, vulnerable population, women's health.

Postdoctoral Program Contact Gale Barber, Assistant Dean for Graduate Studies, School of Nursing, University of Wisconsin–Madison, 600 Highland Avenue, Room K6/134, Madison, WI 53792-2455. *Telephone:* 608-263-5172. *Fax:* 608-263-5296. *E-mail:* mgbarber@wisc.edu.

CONTINUING EDUCATION PROGRAM

Contact Ms. Donna Haack, Program Assistant, School of Nursing, University of Wisconsin–Madison, 600 Highland Avenue, H6/158, Clinical Science Center, Madison, WI 53792-2455. *Telephone:* 608-263-5336. *Fax:* 608-263-5332. *E-mail:* dmhaack@wisc.edu.

See full description on page 582.

University of Wisconsin–Milwaukee

College of Nursing
Milwaukee, Wisconsin

http://www.nursing.uwm.edu

Founded in 1956

DEGREES • BSN • MS • MSN/MBA • PHD

Nursing Program Faculty 34 (100% with doctorates).

Baccalaureate Enrollment 1,548 **Women** 88% **Men** 12% **Minority** 14% **International** 2% **Part-time** 54%

Graduate Enrollment 181
Women 93% **Men** 7% **Minority** 11% **International** 7% **Part-time** 72%

Nursing Student Activities Sigma Theta Tau, Student Nurses' Association.

Nursing Student Resources Academic advising; academic or career counseling; campus computer network; computer lab; computer-assisted instruction; e-mail services; interactive nursing skills videos; Internet; learning resource lab; nursing audiovisuals; remedial services; skills, simulation, or other laboratory; tutoring.

Library Facilities 1.4 million volumes (320,089 in health, 178,089 in nursing); 8,240 periodical subscriptions (926 health-care related).

■ The University of Wisconsin–Milwaukee is a Carnegie Foundation–ranked Research Institution. The College of Nursing is nationally recognized for its faculty, programs, and alumni. Students are prepared as nurse leaders at the baccalaureate, master's, and doctoral levels for multiple roles in health care. Faculty members and students are involved in education, research, and service in more than 125 health-care settings. The College supports the Harriet H. Werley Center for Nursing Research and Evaluation, the Center for Cultural Diversity and Health, the Center for Nursing History, and the Nursing Learning Resource Center. The College also has 4 community nursing centers within its Institute for Urban Health Partnerships, which provides national and international leadership in health promotion and primary health care.

BACCALAUREATE PROGRAMS

Degree BSN

Available Programs Accelerated Baccalaureate for Second Degree; Generic Baccalaureate; RN Baccalaureate.

Site Options West Bend, WI; Kenosha, WI.

Study Options Full-time and part-time.

Program Entrance Requirements Minimum overall college GPA of 2.0, transcript of college record, written essay, high school chemistry, high school foreign language, 3 years high school math, 3 years high school science, high school transcript, minimum high school GPA of 2.0, minimum high school rank 50%, minimum GPA in nursing prerequisites of 2.5, prerequisite course work. Transfer students are accepted. **Standardized tests** *Required:* SAT or ACT, TOEFL for international students, ACT for state residents. *Recommended:* SAT. **Application** *Deadline:* 8/1 (freshmen), rolling (transfer). *Notification:* continuous (freshmen). *Application fee:* $35.

Advanced Placement Credit by examination available. Credit given for nursing courses completed elsewhere dependent upon specific evaluations.

Expenses (2004–05) *Tuition, state resident:* full-time $5138; part-time $214 per credit hour. *Tuition, nonresident:* full-time $17,890; part-time $745 per credit hour. *International tuition:* $17,890 full-time. *Room and board:* $5730; room only: $3150 per academic year. *Required fees:* part-time $30 per credit; part-time $348 per term.

Financial Aid 70% of baccalaureate students in nursing programs received some form of financial aid in 2003–04.

Contact Ms. Donna Wier, Senior Advisor, College of Nursing, University of Wisconsin–Milwaukee, Student Affairs, PO Box 413, Milwaukee, WI 53201. *Telephone:* 414-229-5481. *Fax:* 414-229-5554. *E-mail:* ddw@uwm.edu.

GRADUATE PROGRAMS

Expenses (2004–05) *Tuition, state resident:* full-time $7434; part-time $465 per credit hour. *Tuition, nonresident:* full-time $21,800; part-time $1363 per credit hour. *International tuition:* $21,800 full-time. *Room and board:* $5730; room only: $3150 per academic year. *Required fees:* part-time $348 per term.

Financial Aid 52% of graduate students in nursing programs received some form of financial aid in 2003–04. 2 fellowships, 9 teaching assistantships were awarded; research assistantships, career-related internships or fieldwork, Federal Work-Study, and unspecified assistantships also available. Aid available to part-time students. *Financial aid application deadline:* 4/15.

Contact Ms. Ahnalee Brincks, Advisor, College of Nursing, University of Wisconsin–Milwaukee, Student Affairs, PO Box 413, Milwaukee, WI 53201. *Telephone:* 414-229-5473. *Fax:* 414-229-5554. *E-mail:* brincks@uwm.edu.

MASTER'S DEGREE PROGRAM

Degrees MS; MSN/MBA

Available Programs Master's; RN to Master's.

Concentrations Available Health-care administration; nursing education. *Clinical nurse specialist programs in:* adult health, community health, parent-child, psychiatric/mental health, women's health. *Nurse practitioner programs in:* family health.

Site Options Kenosha, WI.

Study Options Full-time and part-time.

Program Entrance Requirements Clinical experience, minimum overall college GPA of 2.75, transcript of college record, written essay, interview, 3 letters of recommendation, statistics course, GRE General Test or MAT. *Application deadline:* For fall admission, 1/1 (priority date); for spring admission, 9/1. Applications are processed on a rolling basis. *Application fee:* $45 ($75 for international students).

Advanced Placement Credit given for nursing courses completed elsewhere dependent upon specific evaluations.

Degree Requirements 46 total credit hours, thesis or project.

POST-MASTER'S PROGRAM

Areas of Study *Nurse practitioner programs in:* family health.

DOCTORAL DEGREE PROGRAM

Degree PhD

Available Programs Doctorate; Post-Baccalaureate Doctorate.

Areas of Study Individualized study, nursing research.

Program Entrance Requirements Minimum overall college GPA of 3.2, interview, 3 letters of recommendation, MSN or equivalent, scholarly papers, vita, writing sample. *Application deadline:* For fall admission, 1/1 (priority date); for spring admission, 9/1. Applications are processed on a rolling basis. *Application fee:* $45 ($75 for international students).

Degree Requirements 49 total credit hours, dissertation, oral exam, written exam, residency.

CONTINUING EDUCATION PROGRAM

Contact Dr. Elizabeth Fayram, Director, Continuing Education, College of Nursing, University of Wisconsin–Milwaukee, PO Box 413, Milwaukee, WI 53201. *Telephone:* 414-229-5617. *Fax:* 414-229-2596. *E-mail:* fayram@csd.uwm.edu.

See full description on page 584.

University of Wisconsin–Oshkosh

College of Nursing
Oshkosh, Wisconsin

http://www.uwosh.edu/con

Founded in 1871

DEGREES • BSN • MSN

Nursing Program Faculty 71 (25% with doctorates).

Baccalaureate Enrollment 1,031 **Women** 93% **Men** 7% **Minority** 5% **Part-time** 9%

Graduate Enrollment 75
Women 93% **Men** 7% **Minority** 94% **Part-time** 53%

Nursing Student Activities Sigma Theta Tau, Student Nurses' Association, nursing club.

Nursing Student Resources Academic advising; academic or career counseling; assistance for students with disabilities; bookstore; campus computer network; career placement assistance; computer lab; computer-assisted instruction; daycare for children of students; e-mail services; employment services for current students; externships; interactive nursing skills videos; Internet; learning resource lab; library services; nursing audiovisuals; paid internships; placement services for program completers; resume preparation assistance; skills, simulation, or other laboratory; tutoring; unpaid internships.

Library Facilities 446,774 volumes; 5,219 periodical subscriptions.

BACCALAUREATE PROGRAMS

Degree BSN

Available Programs Accelerated Baccalaureate; Accelerated Baccalaureate for Second Degree; Baccalaureate for Second Degree; Generic Baccalaureate; RN Baccalaureate.

Site Options *Distance Learning:* Wausau, WI.

Study Options Full-time and part-time.

University of Wisconsin–Oshkosh (continued)

Program Entrance Requirements Minimum overall college GPA of 2.75, transcript of college record, CPR certification, health exam, 3 years high school math, 3 years high school science, immunizations, minimum high school rank 50%, minimum GPA in nursing prerequisites of 2.0, prerequisite course work. Transfer students are accepted. **Standardized tests** *Required:* SAT or ACT, TOEFL for international students, ACT required for state residents. **Application** *Deadline:* 8/1 (freshmen), 8/1 (transfer). *Notification:* continuous (freshmen). *Application fee:* $35.

Advanced Placement Credit by examination available. Credit given for nursing courses completed elsewhere dependent upon specific evaluations.

Expenses (2004–05) *Tuition, state resident:* full-time $4616; part-time $194 per credit hour. *Tuition, nonresident:* full-time $14,662; part-time $612 per credit hour. *International tuition:* $14,662 full-time. *Room and board:* $4420; room only: $2530 per academic year. *Required fees:* full-time $112; part-time $56 per term.

Financial Aid 50% of baccalaureate students in nursing programs received some form of financial aid in 2003–04. *Gift aid (need-based):* Federal Pell, FSEOG, state, private, college/university gift aid from institutional funds, Federal Nursing. *Loans:* Federal Nursing Student Loans, FFEL (Subsidized and Unsubsidized Stafford PLUS), Perkins, state. *Work-Study:* Federal Work-Study, part-time campus jobs. *Application deadline (priority):* 3/15.

Contact Dr. Stephanie Stewart, RN, Director, Undergraduate Program, College of Nursing, University of Wisconsin–Oshkosh, 800 Algoma Boulevard, Oshkosh, WI 54901-8660. *Telephone:* 920-424-1028. *Fax:* 920-424-0123. *E-mail:* stewart@uwosh.edu.

GRADUATE PROGRAMS

Expenses (2004–05) *Tuition, state resident:* full-time $5848; part-time $326 per credit hour. *Tuition, nonresident:* full-time $16,456; part-time $916 per credit hour. *International tuition:* $16,456 full-time. *Room and board:* $2630; room only: $2530 per academic year.

Financial Aid 40% of graduate students in nursing programs received some form of financial aid in 2003–04. Fellowships, research assistantships with partial tuition reimbursements available, institutionally sponsored loans, scholarships, traineeships, tuition waivers (partial), and unspecified assistantships available. *Financial aid application deadline:* 3/15.

Contact Dr. Rosemary Smith, Director, Graduate Program, College of Nursing, University of Wisconsin–Oshkosh, 800 Algoma Boulevard, Oshkosh, WI 54901-8660. *Telephone:* 920-424-2106. *Fax:* 920-424-0123. *E-mail:* smithr@uwosh.edu.

MASTER'S DEGREE PROGRAM

Degree MSN

Available Programs Master's.

Concentrations Available *Nurse practitioner programs in:* adult health, family health.

Study Options Full-time and part-time.

Program Entrance Requirements Clinical experience, computer literacy, minimum overall college GPA of 3.0, transcript of college record, CPR certification, written essay, immunizations, interview, 3 letters of recommendation, physical assessment course, statistics course. *Application deadline:* For fall admission, 12/15. *Application fee:* $45.

Degree Requirements 49 total credit hours, thesis or project.

POST-MASTER'S PROGRAM

Areas of Study *Nurse practitioner programs in:* adult health, family health.

CONTINUING EDUCATION PROGRAM

Contact Ms. Jackie Thompson-Ehlers, RN, Coordinator, Continuing Education, College of Nursing, University of Wisconsin–Oshkosh, 800 Algoma Boulevard, Oshkosh, WI 54901-8660. *Telephone:* 920-424-2129. *Fax:* 920-424-0123. *E-mail:* thomsone@uwosh.edu.

Viterbo University
School of Nursing
La Crosse, Wisconsin

http://www.viterbo.edu

Founded in 1890

DEGREES • BSN • MSN

Nursing Program Faculty 29 (7% with doctorates).

Baccalaureate Enrollment 547

Women 94% **Men** 6% **Minority** 3% **International** 1% **Part-time** 5%

Graduate Enrollment 52

Women 100% **Part-time** 15%

Nursing Student Activities Sigma Theta Tau, Student Nurses' Association.

Nursing Student Resources Academic advising; academic or career counseling; assistance for students with disabilities; bookstore; campus computer network; computer lab; e-mail services; interactive nursing skills videos; Internet; learning resource lab; library services; nursing audiovisuals; resume preparation assistance; skills, simulation, or other laboratory; tutoring.

Library Facilities 92,591 volumes (5,200 in health, 3,398 in nursing); 491 periodical subscriptions (312 health-care related).

BACCALAUREATE PROGRAMS

Degree BSN

Available Programs Generic Baccalaureate; RN Baccalaureate.

Site Options Janesville, WI; Wausau, WI; Reedsburg, WI.

Study Options Full-time and part-time.

Program Entrance Requirements Minimum overall college GPA of 2.5, CPR certification, health exam, high school chemistry, 1 year of high school math, 2 years high school science, high school transcript, immunizations, minimum high school GPA of 2.0, minimum GPA in nursing prerequisites of 2.5, prerequisite course work. Transfer students are accepted. **Standardized tests** *Required:* ACT, TOEFL for international students. **Application** *Deadline:* rolling (freshmen), rolling (transfer). *Notification:* continuous until 8/15 (freshmen). *Application fee:* $25.

Advanced Placement Credit given for nursing courses completed elsewhere dependent upon specific evaluations.

Expenses (2004–05) *Tuition:* full-time $15,570; part-time $455 per credit hour. *Room and board:* $5135; room only: $4500 per academic year. *Required fees:* full-time $300.

Financial Aid 88% of baccalaureate students in nursing programs received some form of financial aid in 2003–04. *Gift aid (need-based):* Federal Pell, FSEOG, state, private, college/university gift aid from institutional funds. *Loans:* Federal Nursing Student Loans, FFEL (Subsidized and Unsubsidized Stafford PLUS), Perkins. *Work-Study:* Federal Work-Study, part-time campus jobs. *Application deadline (priority):* 3/15.

Contact Dr. Roland Nelson, Director of Admission, School of Nursing, Viterbo University, 900 Viterbo Drive, LaCrosse, WI 54601. *Telephone:* 608-796-3010. *Fax:* 608-796-3050. *E-mail:* adm.buzz@viterbo.edu.

GRADUATE PROGRAMS

Expenses (2004–05) *Tuition:* part-time $475 per credit hour.

Financial Aid 33% of graduate students in nursing programs received some form of financial aid in 2003–04.

Contact Dr. Bonnie Nesbitt, Director, School of Nursing, Viterbo University, 900 Viterbo Drive, LaCrosse, WI 54601. *Telephone:* 608-796-3688. *Fax:* 608-796-3668. *E-mail:* bjnesbitt@viterbo.edu.

MASTER'S DEGREE PROGRAM

Degree MSN

Available Programs Master's.

Concentrations Available Health-care administration; nursing education. *Nurse practitioner programs in:* adult health.

Study Options Full-time and part-time.

Program Entrance Requirements Clinical experience, computer literacy, minimum overall college GPA of 3.0, transcript of college record, CPR certification, written essay, immunizations, interview, 3 letters of recommendation, nursing research course, physical assessment course, resume, statistics course.

Advanced Placement Credit given for nursing courses completed elsewhere dependent upon specific evaluations.

Degree Requirements 37 total credit hours, thesis or project.

POST-MASTER'S PROGRAM

Areas of Study Nursing education. *Nurse practitioner programs in:* adult health.

WYOMING

University of Wyoming
Fay W. Whitney School of Nursing
Laramie, Wyoming

http://www.uwyo.edu/nursing

Founded in 1886

DEGREES • BSN • MS

Nursing Program Faculty 31 (45% with doctorates).

Baccalaureate Enrollment 132
Women 90% **Men** 10% **Minority** 9% **Part-time** 45%

Graduate Enrollment 81
Women 93% **Men** 7% **Minority** 4% **Part-time** 82%

Nursing Student Activities Sigma Theta Tau, Student Nurses' Association.

Nursing Student Resources Academic advising; academic or career counseling; assistance for students with disabilities; bookstore; campus computer network; career placement assistance; computer lab; computer-assisted instruction; e-mail services; employment services for current students; externships; housing assistance; interactive nursing skills videos; Internet; learning resource lab; library services; nursing audiovisuals; paid internships; remedial services; resume preparation assistance; skills, simulation, or other laboratory; tutoring; unpaid internships.

Library Facilities 1.3 million volumes (75,025 in health, 2,725 in nursing); 13,256 periodical subscriptions (612 health-care related).

BACCALAUREATE PROGRAMS

Degree BSN

Available Programs Generic Baccalaureate; RN Baccalaureate.

Site Options *Distance Learning:* Laramie, WY.

Study Options Full-time.

Program Entrance Requirements Transcript of college record, CPR certification, written essay, health insurance, high school transcript, immunizations, 1 letter of recommendation, minimum GPA in nursing prerequisites of 2.5, professional liability insurance/malpractice insurance, prerequisite course work, RN licensure. Transfer students are accepted. **Standardized tests** *Required:* TOEFL for international students. *Required for some:* SAT or ACT. **Application** *Deadline:* 8/10 (freshmen), 8/10 (transfer). *Notification:* continuous (freshmen). *Application fee:* $30.

Advanced Placement Credit given for nursing courses completed elsewhere dependent upon specific evaluations.

Financial Aid 93% of baccalaureate students in nursing programs received some form of financial aid in 2003–04. *Gift aid (need-based):* Federal Pell, FSEOG, state, private, college/university gift aid from institutional funds. *Loans:* FFEL (Subsidized and Unsubsidized Stafford PLUS), Perkins, alternative loans. *Work-Study:* Federal Work-Study. *Application deadline (priority):* 2/1.

Contact Ms. Claire Hitchcock, Office Associate, Fay W. Whitney School of Nursing, University of Wyoming, Department 3065, 1000 East University Avenue, Laramie, WY 82071-3065. *Telephone:* 307-766-4291. *Fax:* 307-766-4294. *E-mail:* nurs.inq@uwyo.edu.

GRADUATE PROGRAMS

Financial Aid 72% of graduate students in nursing programs received some form of financial aid in 2003–04. Teaching assistantships with full tuition reimbursements available (averaging $10,062 per year); research assistantships with full tuition reimbursements available, career-related internships or fieldwork, institutionally sponsored loans, scholarships, and traineeships also available. Aid available to part-time students. *Financial aid application deadline:* 3/1.

Contact Ms. Claire Hitchcock, Office Associate, Fay W. Whitney School of Nursing, University of Wyoming, Department 3065, 1000 East University Avenue, Laramie, WY 82071-3065. *Telephone:* 307-766-4291. *Fax:* 307-766-4294. *E-mail:* nurs.inq@uwyo.edu.

MASTER'S DEGREE PROGRAM

Degree MS

Available Programs Master's; Master's for Nurses with Non-Nursing Degrees.

Concentrations Available Nursing education. *Nurse practitioner programs in:* family health.

Site Options *Distance Learning:* Laramie, WY.

Study Options Full-time and part-time.

Program Entrance Requirements Minimum overall college GPA of 3.0, transcript of college record, CPR certification, written essay, immunizations, interview, 3 letters of recommendation, nursing research course, physical assessment course, professional liability insurance/malpractice insurance, resume, statistics course, GRE General Test. *Application deadline:* For fall admission, 11/1 (priority date); for spring admission, 2/1 (priority date). *Application fee:* $70.

Advanced Placement Credit given for nursing courses completed elsewhere dependent upon specific evaluations.

Degree Requirements 52 total credit hours, thesis or project.

POST-MASTER'S PROGRAM

Areas of Study Nursing education. *Nurse practitioner programs in:* family health.

CANADA

ALBERTA

Athabasca University
Centre for Nursing and Health Studies
Athabasca, Alberta

http://www.athabascau.ca/cnhs/

Founded in 1970

DEGREES • BN • MN

Nursing Program Faculty 27 (60% with doctorates).

Baccalaureate Enrollment 1,346

Graduate Enrollment 546

Nursing Student Resources Academic advising; academic or career counseling; assistance for students with disabilities; computer lab; computer-assisted instruction; e-mail services; interactive nursing skills videos; Internet; library services; nursing audiovisuals; tutoring.

Library Facilities 143,000 volumes; 12,000 periodical subscriptions.

BACCALAUREATE PROGRAMS

Degree BN

Available Programs LPN to Baccalaureate; RN Baccalaureate.

Site Options *Distance Learning:* Edmonton, AB; Calgary, AB.

Study Options Full-time and part-time.

Program Entrance Requirements Minimum overall college GPA of 2.5, transcript of college record, CPR certification, high school chemistry, 3 years high school math, 3 years high school science, immunizations, minimum high school GPA of 2.0, minimum GPA in nursing prerequisites of 2.0, RN licensure. Transfer students are accepted. **Application** *Deadline:* rolling (freshmen), rolling (transfer). *Notification:* continuous (freshmen). *Application fee:* CAN$60.

Advanced Placement Credit by examination available. Credit given for nursing courses completed elsewhere dependent upon specific evaluations.

Expenses (2004–05) *Tuition, area resident:* part-time CAN$578 per course. *Tuition, state resident:* part-time CAN$633 per course. *Tuition, nonresident:* part-time CAN$828 per course.

Contact Donna Dunn, Centre Administrative Assistant, Centre for Nursing and Health Studies, Athabasca University, 1 University Drive, Athabasca, AB T9S 3A3. *Telephone:* 800-788-9041 Ext. 6381. *Fax:* 780-675-6468. *E-mail:* donnad@athabascau.ca.

GRADUATE PROGRAMS

Expenses (2004–05) *Tuition, area resident:* part-time CAN$990 per course. *Tuition, state resident:* part-time CAN$1190 per course. *Tuition, nonresident:* part-time CAN$1190 per course.

Contact Donna Dunn, Centre Administrative Assistant, Centre for Nursing and Health Studies, Athabasca University, 1 University Drive, Athabasca, AB T9S 3A3. *Telephone:* 800-788-9041 Ext. 6381. *Fax:* 780-675-6468. *E-mail:* donnad@athabascau.ca.

MASTER'S DEGREE PROGRAM

Degree MN

Available Programs Master's.

Concentrations Available Health-care administration. *Nurse practitioner programs in:* community health, primary care.

Study Options Full-time and part-time.

Program Entrance Requirements Clinical experience, computer literacy, minimum overall college GPA of 3.0, transcript of college record, CPR certification, immunizations, 3 letters of recommendation, nursing research course, prerequisite course work, resume, statistics course.

Advanced Placement Credit given for nursing courses completed elsewhere dependent upon specific evaluations.

Degree Requirements 33 total credit hours, thesis or project, comprehensive exam.

University of Alberta
Faculty of Nursing
Edmonton, Alberta

Founded in 1906

DEGREES • BSCN • MN • PHD

Nursing Program Faculty 122 (57% with doctorates).

Baccalaureate Enrollment 1,192 **Women** 94% **Men** 6% **International** 1% **Part-time** 14%

Graduate Enrollment 206
Women 96% **Men** 4% **International** 4% **Part-time** 69%

Nursing Student Activities Nursing Honor Society, Sigma Theta Tau, Student Nurses' Association.

Nursing Student Resources Academic advising; academic or career counseling; assistance for students with disabilities; bookstore; campus computer network; career placement assistance; computer lab; computer-assisted instruction; daycare for children of students; e-mail services; employment services for current students; housing assistance; interactive nursing skills videos; Internet; learning resource lab; library services; nursing audiovisuals; other; paid internships; remedial services; resume preparation assistance; skills, simulation, or other laboratory; tutoring; unpaid internships.

Library Facilities 9.7 million volumes (234,555 in health, 58,639 in nursing); 1,577 periodical subscriptions health-care related.

BACCALAUREATE PROGRAMS

Degree BScN

Available Programs Baccalaureate for Second Degree; RN Baccalaureate; RPN to Baccalaureate.

Site Options Fort McMurray, AB; Red Deer, AB; Grande Prairie, AB.

Study Options Full-time.

Program Entrance Requirements Minimum overall college GPA of 3.0, transcript of college record, CPR certification, health exam, health insurance, high school biology, high school chemistry, 3 years high school math, 3 years high school science, high school transcript, immunizations, minimum high school GPA of 3.0, minimum high school rank 75%. Transfer students are accepted. **Standardized tests** *Recommended:* SAT, SAT Subject Tests. **Application** *Deadline:* 5/1 (freshmen), 5/1 (transfer). *Notification:* continuous until 9/1 (freshmen). *Application fee:* CAN$100.

Advanced Placement Credit by examination available.

Expenses (2004–05) *Tuition:* full-time CAN$6000; part-time CAN$150 per credit hour. *International tuition:* CAN$12,000 full-time. *Room and board:* CAN$6184; room only: CAN$3104 per academic year. *Required fees:* full-time CAN$631; part-time CAN$135 per term.

Financial Aid 50% of baccalaureate students in nursing programs received some form of financial aid in 2003–04. *Loans:* college/university.

Contact Ian Payne, Student Advisor, Faculty of Nursing, University of Alberta, 3-107 Clinical Sciences Building, Edmonton, AB T6G 2G3. *Telephone:* 780-492-9546. *Fax:* 780-492-4844. *E-mail:* ian.payne@ualberta.ca.

GRADUATE PROGRAMS

Expenses (2004–05) *Tuition, state resident:* full-time CAN$3921; part-time CAN$646 per course. *Tuition, nonresident:* full-time CAN$3921; part-time CAN$646 per course. *International tuition:* CAN$6957 full-time. *Room and board:* room only: CAN$5352 per academic year.

Financial Aid 47% of graduate students in nursing programs received some form of financial aid in 2003–04. 12 fellowships with partial tuition reimbursements available (averaging $23,868 per year), 27 research assistantships with partial tuition reimbursements available (averaging $6,186 per year), 12 teaching assistantships with partial tuition reimbursements available (averaging $2,365 per year) were awarded; institutionally sponsored loans and scholarships also available.

Contact Elaine Carswell, Assistant to Associate Dean. *Telephone:* 780-492-6251. *Fax:* 780-492-6029. *E-mail:* elaine.carswell@ualberta.ca.

MASTER'S DEGREE PROGRAM

Degree MN

Available Programs Master's.

Concentrations Available *Clinical nurse specialist programs in:* acute care, adult health, cardiovascular, community health, critical care, family health, gerontology, maternity-newborn, medical-surgical, occupational health, oncology, parent-child, pediatric, perinatal, psychiatric/mental health, public health, women's health.

Study Options Full-time and part-time.

Program Entrance Requirements Clinical experience, computer literacy, minimum overall college GPA of 3.0, transcript of college record, CPR certification, 3 letters of recommendation, nursing research course, physical assessment course, statistics course. *Application deadline:* For fall admission, 6/1; for winter admission, 10/1; for spring admission, 2/1. Applications are processed on a rolling basis.

Advanced Placement Credit given for nursing courses completed elsewhere dependent upon specific evaluations.

Degree Requirements 33 total credit hours, thesis or project.

POST-MASTER'S PROGRAM

Areas of Study *Clinical nurse specialist programs in:* acute care, adult health, cardiovascular, community health, critical care, family health, gerontology, maternity-newborn, medical-surgical, occupational health, oncology, parent-child, pediatric, perinatal, psychiatric/mental health, public health, women's health.

DOCTORAL DEGREE PROGRAM

Degree PhD

Available Programs Doctorate.

Areas of Study Health policy, nursing education, nursing policy, nursing research.

Program Entrance Requirements Clinical experience, minimum overall college GPA of 3.0, 3 letters of recommendation, MSN or equivalent, scholarly papers, statistics course, vita, writing sample. *Application deadline:* For fall admission, 6/1; for winter admission, 10/1; for spring admission, 2/1. Applications are processed on a rolling basis.

Degree Requirements 36 total credit hours, dissertation, oral exam, written exam, residency.

POSTDOCTORAL PROGRAM

Postdoctoral Program Contact Dr. Phyllis Giovannetti, Associate Dean, Graduate Education, Faculty of Nursing, University of Alberta, Clinical Sciences Building, Third Floor, Edmonton, AB T6G 2G3. *Telephone:* 780-492-6764. *Fax:* 780-492-2551. *E-mail:* phyllis.giovannetti@ualberta.ca.

CONTINUING EDUCATION PROGRAM

Contact Ms. Elaine Carswell, Assistant to Associate Dean, Faculty of Nursing, University of Alberta, Edmonton, AB T6G 2G3. *Telephone:* 780-492-6251. *Fax:* 780-492-6314. *E-mail:* elaine.carswell@ualberta.ca.

University of Calgary
Faculty of Nursing
Calgary, Alberta

http://www.ucalgary.ca/nu

Founded in 1945

DEGREES • BN • MN • PHD

Nursing Program Faculty 50 (85% with doctorates).

Baccalaureate Enrollment 930
Women 90% **Men** 10%

Graduate Enrollment 110
Women 95% **Men** 5% **International** 1% **Part-time** 21%

Nursing Student Activities Student Nurses' Association.

Nursing Student Resources Academic advising; academic or career counseling; assistance for students with disabilities; bookstore; campus computer network; computer lab; computer-assisted instruction; e-mail services; externships; housing assistance; interactive nursing skills videos; Internet; learning resource lab; library services; nursing audiovisuals; resume preparation assistance; skills, simulation, or other laboratory; tutoring.

Library Facilities 2.4 million volumes; 20,237 periodical subscriptions.

BACCALAUREATE PROGRAMS

Degree BN

Available Programs Accelerated Baccalaureate; Accelerated Baccalaureate for Second Degree; Baccalaureate for Second Degree; Generic Baccalaureate; RN Baccalaureate.

Site Options Medicine Hat, AB. *Distance Learning:* Calgary, AB.

Study Options Full-time.

Program Entrance Requirements Minimum overall college GPA of 3.3, transcript of college record, CPR certification, health exam, high school biology, high school chemistry, 3 years high school math, high school transcript, immunizations, minimum high school rank 78%. Transfer students are accepted. **Standardized tests** *Required for some:* SAT, SAT Subject Tests, SAT II Writing Tests. **Application** *Deadline:* 4/1 (freshmen). *Notification:* continuous (freshmen). *Application fee:* CAN$130.

Advanced Placement Credit by examination available. Credit given for nursing courses completed elsewhere dependent upon specific evaluations.

Financial Aid *Loans:* college/university. *Application deadline:* 6/15.

Contact Laura Hampson, Student Advisor, Faculty of Nursing, University of Calgary, 2500 University Drive NW, Calgary, AB T2N 1N4. *Telephone:* 403-220-4636. *Fax:* 403-284-4803. *E-mail:* hampson@ucalgary.ca.

GRADUATE PROGRAMS

Expenses (2003–04) *Tuition, state resident:* full-time CAN$13,641; part-time CAN$581 per course. *Tuition, nonresident:* full-time CAN$13,641; part-time CAN$581 per course. *International tuition:* CAN$27,282 full-time.

Financial Aid 38% of graduate students in nursing programs received some form of financial aid in 2002–03. 13 teaching assistantships (averaging $7,000 per year) were awarded; institutionally sponsored loans and scholarships also available. Aid available to part-time students.

Contact Ms. Jolene Chipiuk, Administrative Assistant, Graduate Programs, Faculty of Nursing, University of Calgary, Faculty of Nursing, University of Calgary, 2500 University Drive NW, Calgary, AB T2N 1N4. *Telephone:* 403-220-6241. *Fax:* 403-284-4803. *E-mail:* jchipiuk@ucalgary.ca.

MASTER'S DEGREE PROGRAM

Degree MN

Available Programs Master's; RN to Master's.

Concentrations Available *Clinical nurse specialist programs in:* acute care, adult health, cardiovascular, community health, critical care, family health, gerontology, maternity-newborn, medical-surgical, parent-child, pediatric, perinatal, psychiatric/mental health, public health, rehabilitation, women's health. *Nurse practitioner programs in:* acute care, adult health, neonatal health.

Study Options Full-time and part-time.

Program Entrance Requirements Clinical experience, computer literacy, minimum overall college GPA of 3.0, transcript of college record, CPR certification, written essay, 3 letters of recommendation, nursing research course, statistics course. *Application deadline:* For fall admission, 2/1. *Application fee:* $60.

Advanced Placement Credit given for nursing courses completed elsewhere dependent upon specific evaluations.

Degree Requirements 30 total credit hours, thesis or project, comprehensive exam.

University of Calgary (continued)

POST-MASTER'S PROGRAM

Areas of Study *Nurse practitioner programs in:* acute care, adult health, neonatal health.

DOCTORAL DEGREE PROGRAM

Degree PhD

Available Programs Doctorate; Doctorate for Nurses with Non-Nursing Degrees.

Areas of Study Advanced practice nursing, aging, clinical practice, community health, critical care, ethics, family health, gerontology, health promotion/disease prevention, health-care systems, human health and illness, illness and transition, individualized study, maternity-newborn, neuro-behavior, nursing research, women's health.

Site Options *Distance Learning:* Calgary, AB.

Program Entrance Requirements Clinical experience, minimum overall college GPA of 3.0, 3 letters of recommendation, MSN or equivalent, scholarly papers, statistics course, vita, writing sample. *Application deadline:* For fall admission, 2/1. *Application fee:* $60.

Degree Requirements Dissertation, oral exam, written exam.

CONTINUING EDUCATION PROGRAM

Contact Christiane Roy, Team Leader, Continuing Education for Nurses, Faculty of Nursing, University of Calgary, 2500 University Drive NW, Calgary, AB T2N 1N4. *Telephone:* 403-220-7630. *E-mail:* croy@ucalgary.ca.

The University of Lethbridge
School of Health Sciences
Lethbridge, Alberta

http://home.uleth.ca/hlsc/

Founded in 1967

DEGREES • BN • M SC

Nursing Program Faculty 30 (20% with doctorates).

Baccalaureate Enrollment 228
Women 91% **Men** 9% **Part-time** 3%

Graduate Enrollment 3
Women 67% **Men** 33%

Nursing Student Activities Nursing club.

Nursing Student Resources Academic advising; academic or career counseling; assistance for students with disabilities; bookstore; campus computer network; computer lab; e-mail services; employment services for current students; housing assistance; interactive nursing skills videos; Internet; learning resource lab; library services; nursing audiovisuals; remedial services; resume preparation assistance; skills, simulation, or other laboratory; tutoring; unpaid internships.

Library Facilities 539,154 volumes (14,743 in health, 2,554 in nursing); 1,614 periodical subscriptions (11,168 health-care related).

BACCALAUREATE PROGRAMS

Degree BN

Available Programs Generic Baccalaureate; RN Baccalaureate.

Site Options Lethbridge, AB.

Study Options Full-time.

Program Entrance Requirements CPR certification, high school biology, high school chemistry, 3 years high school math, 3 years high school science, high school transcript, immunizations, minimum high school rank 70%. Transfer students are accepted. **Standardized tests** *Required for some:* SAT and SAT Subject Tests or ACT, SAT II Writing Tests. **Application** *Deadline:* 8/29 (freshmen), 8/29 (transfer). *Early decision:* 4/1. *Notification:* continuous (freshmen), 4/22 (out-of-state freshmen), 4/22 (early decision). *Application fee:* CAN$60.

Advanced Placement Credit given for nursing courses completed elsewhere dependent upon specific evaluations.

Expenses (2003–04) *Tuition, state resident:* full-time CAN$4499; part-time CAN$475 per course. *Tuition, nonresident:* full-time CAN$4499; part-time CAN$475 per course. *International tuition:* CAN$8467 full-time. *Room and board:* CAN$3246; room only: CAN$1480 per academic year.

Financial Aid *Gift aid (need-based):* private, college/university gift aid from institutional funds. *Loans:* FFEL (Subsidized and Unsubsidized Stafford PLUS). *Application deadline:* Continuous.

Contact Mr. Tom Samuel, Academic Advisor, School of Health Sciences, The University of Lethbridge, 4401 University Drive, Lethbridge, AB T1K 3M4. *Telephone:* 403-329-2649. *Fax:* 403-329-2668. *E-mail:* tom.samuel@uleth.ca.

GRADUATE PROGRAMS

Expenses (2003–04) *Tuition, state resident:* full-time CAN$5358; part-time CAN$539 per course. *Tuition, nonresident:* full-time CAN$5358; part-time CAN$539 per course. *International tuition:* CAN$10,098 full-time. *Room and board:* CAN$3246; room only: CAN$1480 per academic year.

Contact Mr. Tom Samuel, Academic Advisor, School of Health Sciences, The University of Lethbridge, 4401 University Drive, Lethbridge, AB T1K 3M4. *Telephone:* 403-329-2649. *Fax:* 403-329-2668. *E-mail:* tom.samuel@uleth.ca.

MASTER'S DEGREE PROGRAM

Degree M Sc

Available Programs Master's.

Study Options Full-time and part-time.

Program Entrance Requirements Clinical experience, minimum overall college GPA of 3.0, transcript of college record, CPR certification, immunizations, interview.

Advanced Placement Credit given for nursing courses completed elsewhere dependent upon specific evaluations.

Degree Requirements Thesis or project, comprehensive exam.

BRITISH COLUMBIA

British Columbia Institute of Technology
School of Health Sciences
Burnaby, British Columbia

http://www.health.bcit.ca/nursing/

Founded in 1964

DEGREE • BSCN

Nursing Program Faculty 44.

Nursing Student Activities Student Nurses' Association.

Nursing Student Resources Academic advising; academic or career counseling; assistance for students with disabilities; bookstore; campus computer network; computer lab; computer-assisted instruction; housing assistance; interactive nursing skills videos; Internet; learning resource lab; library services; nursing audiovisuals; skills, simulation, or other laboratory; tutoring; unpaid internships.

Library Facilities 169,404 volumes (100 in health, 50 in nursing); 1,080 periodical subscriptions (100 health-care related).

BACCALAUREATE PROGRAMS

Degree BScN

Available Programs Generic Baccalaureate; RPN to Baccalaureate.

Study Options Full-time.

Program Entrance Requirements CPR certification, written essay, high school biology, high school chemistry, high school math, immunizations, interview, 1 letter of recommendation, prerequisite course work. **Application** *Application fee:* CAN$60.

Contact Ms. Loreen Martin, Program Assistant, School of Health Sciences, British Columbia Institute of Technology, 3700 Willingdon Avenue, SE12, Room 418, Burnaby, BC V5G 3H2. *Telephone:* 604-432-8884. *Fax:* 604-436-9590. *E-mail:* loreen_martin@bcit.ca.

CONTINUING EDUCATION PROGRAM

Contact Ms. Roz Cowan, Advisor, School of Health Sciences, British Columbia Institute of Technology, 3700 Willingdon Avenue, SE12, Room 328, Burnaby, BC V5G 3H2. *Telephone:* 604-451-7100. *E-mail:* rosaleen_cowan@bcit.ca.

Kwantlen University College
Faculty of Community and Health Sciences
Surrey, British Columbia

DEGREE • BSN

Nursing Program Faculty 58 (14% with doctorates).

Baccalaureate Enrollment 344
Part-time 14%

Nursing Student Resources Academic advising; academic or career counseling; assistance for students with disabilities; bookstore; campus computer network; career placement assistance; computer lab; computer-assisted instruction; e-mail services; employment services for current students; interactive nursing skills videos; Internet; learning resource lab; library services; nursing audiovisuals; remedial services; resume preparation assistance; skills, simulation, or other laboratory.

BACCALAUREATE PROGRAMS

Degree BSN

Available Programs Generic Baccalaureate; RN Baccalaureate.

Study Options Full-time.

Program Entrance Requirements CPR certification, high school biology, high school chemistry, 2 years high school science, high school transcript, immunizations. Transfer students are accepted. **Application** *Deadline:* 6/30 (freshmen), 5/30 (out-of-state freshmen), 6/30 (transfer). *Early decision:* 2/28. *Notification:* continuous until 6/30 (freshmen), 5/30 (out-of-state freshmen), 3/31 (out-of-state freshmen), 3/31 (early decision). *Application fee:* CAN$40.

Advanced Placement Credit given for nursing courses completed elsewhere dependent upon specific evaluations.

Contact Ms. Kim Jans, Admissions Department, Faculty of Community and Health Sciences, Kwantlen University College, 12666 72nd Avenue, Surrey, BC V3W 2M8. *Telephone:* 604-599-2317. *E-mail:* kim.jans@kwantlen.ca.

Malaspina University-College
Department of Nursing
Nanaimo, British Columbia

http://www.mala.bc.ca/www/discover/health/index.htm

Founded in 1969

DEGREE • BSCN

Nursing Program Faculty 44 (2% with doctorates).

Baccalaureate Enrollment 268

Nursing Student Activities Student Nurses' Association.

Nursing Student Resources Academic advising; academic or career counseling; assistance for students with disabilities; bookstore; campus computer network; computer lab; computer-assisted instruction; daycare for children of students; e-mail services; employment services for current students; housing assistance; interactive nursing skills videos; Internet; learning resource lab; library services; nursing audiovisuals; paid internships; remedial services; resume preparation assistance; skills, simulation, or other laboratory; unpaid internships.

BACCALAUREATE PROGRAMS

Degree BScN

Available Programs Generic Baccalaureate; LPN to Baccalaureate; RN Baccalaureate.

Study Options Full-time.

Program Entrance Requirements CPR certification, health exam, health insurance, high school biology, high school chemistry, high school math, immunizations, minimum GPA in nursing prerequisites, prerequisite course work. Transfer students are accepted. **Application** *Application fee:* CAN$30.

Advanced Placement Credit given for nursing courses completed elsewhere dependent upon specific evaluations.

Contact Jacqueline M. Fournier, Chair of Bachelor of Science in Nursing Programs, Department of Nursing, Malaspina University-College, 900 Fifth Street, Nanaimo, BC V9R 5S5. *Telephone:* 250-740-6260. *Fax:* 250-740-6468. *E-mail:* fournier@mala.bc.ca.

Okanagan University College
Nursing Department
Kelowna, British Columbia

DEGREE • BSN

Nursing Program Faculty 40 (20% with doctorates).

Baccalaureate Enrollment 292
Women 90% **Men** 10%

Nursing Student Resources Academic advising; academic or career counseling; assistance for students with disabilities; bookstore; campus computer network; computer lab; computer-assisted instruction; daycare for children of students; e-mail services; Internet; learning resource lab; library services; nursing audiovisuals; resume preparation assistance; skills, simulation, or other laboratory.

Library Facilities 315,772 volumes; 1,477 periodical subscriptions.

BACCALAUREATE PROGRAMS

Degree BSN

Available Programs Generic Baccalaureate; LPN to RN Baccalaureate; RN Baccalaureate.

Study Options Full-time and part-time.

Program Entrance Requirements Minimum overall college GPA, transcript of college record, CPR certification, health exam, health insurance, high school biology, high school chemistry, high school math, 2 years high school science, high school transcript, immunizations, minimum high school GPA, minimum high school rank 67%, minimum GPA in nursing prerequisites. Transfer students are accepted. **Application** *Deadline:* rolling (freshmen), rolling (transfer). *Notification:* continuous (freshmen). *Application fee:* CAN$20.

Expenses (2003–04) *Tuition, area resident:* full-time CAN$3600; part-time CAN$1000 per semester. *Room and board:* CAN$4500; room only: CAN$3000 per academic year. *Required fees:* full-time CAN$1800.

Financial Aid *Application deadline:* Continuous.

Contact Dr. Joan Bassett-Smith, Director, Nursing Department, Okanagan University College, 3333 College Way, Kelowna, BC V1V 1V7. *Telephone:* 250-762-5445 Ext. 7951. *Fax:* 250-470-6085. *E-mail:* bassettsmith@ouc.bc.ca.

Trinity Western University
Department of Nursing
Langley, British Columbia

Founded in 1962

DEGREE • BSCN

Trinity Western University (continued)
Nursing Program Faculty 10 (20% with doctorates).

Baccalaureate Enrollment 143
Women 91% **Men** 9% **Minority** 7%

Nursing Student Activities Student Nurses' Association.

Nursing Student Resources Academic advising; academic or career counseling; assistance for students with disabilities; bookstore; campus computer network; computer lab; computer-assisted instruction; e-mail services; employment services for current students; housing assistance; interactive nursing skills videos; Internet; learning resource lab; library services; nursing audiovisuals; resume preparation assistance; skills, simulation, or other laboratory.

Library Facilities 190,565 volumes (7,000 in health, 3,050 in nursing); 11,000 periodical subscriptions (134 health-care related).

BACCALAUREATE PROGRAMS

Degree BScN

Available Programs Generic Baccalaureate.

Study Options Full-time.

Program Entrance Requirements Minimum overall college GPA of 2.0, CPR certification, health exam, health insurance, high school biology, high school chemistry, 1 year of high school math, 2 years high school science, high school transcript, immunizations, 2 letters of recommendation, minimum high school GPA of 2.7, minimum GPA in nursing prerequisites of 2.3. Transfer students are accepted. **Standardized tests** *Required for some:* SAT or ACT. **Application** *Deadline:* 6/15 (freshmen), 6/15 (transfer). *Notification:* continuous (freshmen). *Application fee:* $40.

Advanced Placement Credit given for nursing courses completed elsewhere dependent upon specific evaluations.

Expenses (2004–05) *Tuition:* full-time CAN$6000; part-time CAN$395 per credit hour. *Room and board:* CAN$3500; room only: CAN$2000 per academic year. *Required fees:* full-time CAN$500.

Financial Aid 50% of baccalaureate students in nursing programs received some form of financial aid in 2003–04. *Gift aid (need-based):* private, college/university gift aid from institutional funds. *Loans:* FFEL (Subsidized and Unsubsidized Stafford PLUS), federal and provincial loans. *Application deadline (priority):* 2/28.

Contact Ms. Barbara Pesut, Director of Nursing, Department of Nursing, Trinity Western University, 7600 Glover Road, Langley, BC V2Y 1Y1. *Telephone:* 604-888-7511 Ext. 3283. *Fax:* 604-513-2018. *E-mail:* pesut@twu.ca.

University College of the Cariboo

School of Nursing
Kamloops, British Columbia

http://www.cariboo.bc.ca/nursing/index.html
Founded in 1970

DEGREE • BSN

Nursing Program Faculty 56.

Library Facilities 223,300 volumes (7,326 in health, 2,275 in nursing); 920 periodical subscriptions (89 health-care related).

BACCALAUREATE PROGRAMS

Degree BSN

Study Options Full-time and part-time.

Program Entrance Requirements Minimum overall college GPA of 2.7, transcript of college record, CPR certification, health exam, high school biology, high school chemistry, high school foreign language, high school math, high school science, high school transcript, immunizations, interview, 2 letters of recommendation, minimum high school GPA of 2.3, minimum GPA in nursing prerequisites of 2.3. Transfer students are accepted. **Application** *Deadline:* 3/1 (freshmen), 3/1 (transfer). *Notification:* continuous until 3/1 (freshmen). *Application fee:* CAN$25.

Advanced Placement Credit given for nursing courses completed elsewhere dependent upon specific evaluations.

Contact School of Nursing, School of Nursing, University College of the Cariboo, 900 College Drive, PO Box 3010, Kamloops, BC V2C 5N3. *Telephone:* 250-828-5435. *Fax:* 250-828-5450.

CONTINUING EDUCATION PROGRAM

Contact Mme. Inga Thomson Hilton, Continuing Studies, School of Nursing, School of Nursing, University College of the Cariboo, 900 College Drive, PO Box 3010, Kamloops, BC V2C 5N3. *Telephone:* 250-828-5210. *Fax:* 250-371-5510. *E-mail:* thomson@cariboo.bc.ca.

The University of British Columbia

School of Nursing
Vancouver, British Columbia

http://www.nursing.ubc.ca
Founded in 1915

DEGREES • BSN • MSN • PHD

Nursing Program Faculty 51 (50% with doctorates).

Baccalaureate Enrollment 600

Graduate Enrollment 200

Library Facilities 4.7 million volumes; 44,722 periodical subscriptions.

BACCALAUREATE PROGRAMS

Degree BSN

Available Programs Baccalaureate for Second Degree; Generic Baccalaureate; RN Baccalaureate.

Study Options Full-time and part-time.

Program Entrance Requirements Minimum overall college GPA of 3.6, CPR certification, high school biology, high school chemistry, high school foreign language, 3 years high school math, 3 years high school science, high school transcript, immunizations, minimum high school GPA, prerequisite course work. Transfer students are accepted. **Standardized tests** *Recommended:* SAT or ACT. **Application** *Deadline:* 2/28 (freshmen), 2/28 (transfer). *Notification:* continuous until 8/31 (freshmen). *Application fee:* CAN$100.

Advanced Placement Credit given for nursing courses completed elsewhere dependent upon specific evaluations.

Financial Aid 23% of baccalaureate students in nursing programs received some form of financial aid in 2003–04. *Gift aid (need-based):* private, college/university gift aid from institutional funds, provincial scholarships/grants, Federal Canada Study Grants. *Loans:* FFEL (Subsidized and Unsubsidized Stafford PLUS), college/university, Canadian Student Loans, Provincial Student Loans. *Work-Study:* part-time campus jobs. *Application deadline:* 9/15 (priority: 4/15).

Contact Nursing Programs, School of Nursing, The University of British Columbia, T201-2211 Wesbrook Mall, Vancouver, BC V6T 2B5. *Telephone:* 604-822-7420. *Fax:* 604-822-7466. *E-mail:* information@nursing.ubc.ca.

GRADUATE PROGRAMS

Financial Aid 10% of graduate students in nursing programs received some form of financial aid in 2003–04. 4 fellowships (averaging $8,000 per year), 14 research assistantships (averaging $800 per year), 3 teaching assistantships were awarded.

Contact Ann Hilton, MSN Advisor, School of Nursing, The University of British Columbia, T201-2211 Wesbrook Mall, Vancouver, BC V6T 2B5. *Telephone:* 604-822-7498. *Fax:* 604-822-7466. *E-mail:* hilton@nursing.ubc.ca.

MASTER'S DEGREE PROGRAM

Degree MSN

Available Programs Master's.

Concentrations Available *Nurse practitioner programs in:* family health.

Study Options Full-time and part-time.

Program Entrance Requirements Minimum overall college GPA of 3.3, transcript of college record, 3 letters of recommendation, resume. *Application deadline:* For fall admission, 4/30; for spring admission, 1/30. *Application fee:* $65.

Advanced Placement Credit given for nursing courses completed elsewhere dependent upon specific evaluations.

Degree Requirements 33 total credit hours, thesis or project.

DOCTORAL DEGREE PROGRAM

Degree PhD

Available Programs Doctorate.

Areas of Study Nursing research.

Program Entrance Requirements interview, 3 letters of recommendation, MSN or equivalent, statistics course, vita, writing sample. *Application deadline:* For fall admission, 4/30; for spring admission, 1/30. *Application fee:* $65.

Degree Requirements 18 total credit hours, dissertation, oral exam, written exam, residency.

POSTDOCTORAL PROGRAM

Areas of Study Nursing research.

Postdoctoral Program Contact Joy Johnson, PhD Advisor, School of Nursing, The University of British Columbia, T-160-2211 Wesbrook Mall, Vancouver, BC V6T 2B5. *Telephone:* 604-822-7435. *Fax:* 604-822-7869. *E-mail:* joy.johnson@ubc.ca.

CONTINUING EDUCATION PROGRAM

Contact Paula Tognazzini, Instructor, School of Nursing, The University of British Columbia, T201-2211 Wesbrook Mall, Vancouver, BC V6T 2B5. *Fax:* 604-822-7466. *E-mail:* tognazzini@nursing.ubc.ca.

University of Northern British Columbia

Nursing Programme
Prince George, British Columbia

http://www.unbc.ca/nursing/

DEGREE • BSN

Nursing Program Faculty 12 (18% with doctorates).

Nursing Student Activities Student Nurses' Association.

Nursing Student Resources Academic or career counseling; computer lab; e-mail services; Internet; learning resource lab; library services; skills, simulation, or other laboratory.

Library Facilities 617,236 volumes (4,000 in health, 2,000 in nursing); 7,854 periodical subscriptions (300 health-care related).

BACCALAUREATE PROGRAMS

Degree BSN

Available Programs Generic Baccalaureate.

Site Options Prince George, BC.

Study Options Full-time and part-time.

Program Entrance Requirements Minimum overall college GPA of 2.33, transcript of college record, CPR certification, health exam, high school biology, high school chemistry, 1 year of high school math, 4 years high school science, high school transcript, immunizations, minimum high school GPA of 2.3, minimum high school rank 65%, minimum GPA in nursing prerequisites of 2.0, professional liability insurance/malpractice insurance. Transfer students are accepted. **Application** *Deadline:* 3/1 (freshmen), 3/1 (transfer). *Application fee:* CAN$25.

Advanced Placement Credit given for nursing courses completed elsewhere dependent upon specific evaluations.

Contact Acting Chair of Nursing Programme, Nursing Programme, University of Northern British Columbia, 3333 University Way, Prince George, BC V2N 4Z9. *Telephone:* 250-960-6309. *Fax:* 250-960-5744. *E-mail:* norrisp@unbc.ca.

University of Victoria

School of Nursing
Victoria, British Columbia

http://web.uvic.ca/nurs/

Founded in 1963

DEGREES • BSN • MN • PHD

Nursing Program Faculty 21 (95% with doctorates).

Baccalaureate Enrollment 1,100 **Women** 95% **Men** 5% **Part-time** 50%

Nursing Student Activities Student Nurses' Association.

Nursing Student Resources Academic advising; assistance for students with disabilities; bookstore; campus computer network; computer lab; e-mail services; employment services for current students; interactive nursing skills videos; Internet; library services; nursing audiovisuals; remedial services; resume preparation assistance; unpaid internships.

Library Facilities 1.8 million volumes; 14,000 periodical subscriptions.

BACCALAUREATE PROGRAMS

Degree BSN

Site Options Vancouver, BC.

Program Entrance Requirements Minimum overall college GPA of 3.5, transcript of college record, CPR certification, high school transcript, immunizations, prerequisite course work. Transfer students are accepted. **Application** *Deadline:* 4/30 (freshmen), 4/30 (transfer). *Early decision:* 2/28. *Notification:* continuous (freshmen), 5/1 (early action). *Application fee:* CAN$100.

Financial Aid *Gift aid (need-based):* college/university gift aid from institutional funds. *Loans:* Federal Direct (Subsidized and Unsubsidized Stafford PLUS), FFEL (Subsidized and Unsubsidized Stafford PLUS). *Application deadline (priority):* 6/30.

Contact Joan Gillie, Admissions and Liaison Officer, School of Nursing, University of Victoria, PO Box 1700, HSD Building, Room A 402, Victoria, BC V8W 2Y2. *Telephone:* 250-721-7961. *Fax:* 250-721-6231. *E-mail:* jgillie@uvic.ca.

GRADUATE PROGRAMS

Contact Joan Gillie, Admissions Liaison Officer, School of Nursing, University of Victoria, PO Box 1700, Victoria, BC V8W 2Y2. *Telephone:* 250-721-7961. *Fax:* 250-721-6231. *E-mail:* jgillie@uvic.ca.

MASTER'S DEGREE PROGRAM

Degree MN

Available Programs Master's.

Site Options Victoria.

Study Options Full-time and part-time.

Program Entrance Requirements Clinical experience, transcript of college record, letters of recommendation.

Advanced Placement Credit given for nursing courses completed elsewhere dependent upon specific evaluations.

Degree Requirements 18 total credit hours, thesis or project.

DOCTORAL DEGREE PROGRAM

Degree PhD

Program Entrance Requirements Clinical experience, MSN or equivalent.

Degree Requirements Dissertation.

MANITOBA

Brandon University

School of Health Studies
Brandon, Manitoba

http://www.brandonu.ca/academic/health studies

Founded in 1899

DEGREE • BN

Brandon University (continued)

Nursing Program Faculty 16.

Baccalaureate Enrollment 44
Women 100% **Minority** 6% **Part-time** 2%

Nursing Student Activities Student Nurses' Association.

Nursing Student Resources Academic advising; academic or career counseling; assistance for students with disabilities; bookstore; campus computer network; career placement assistance; computer lab; e-mail services; employment services for current students; housing assistance; interactive nursing skills videos; Internet; library services; resume preparation assistance; skills, simulation, or other laboratory; tutoring.

Library Facilities 238,816 volumes; 1,699 periodical subscriptions.

BACCALAUREATE PROGRAMS

Degree BN

Available Programs Baccalaureate for Second Degree; Generic Baccalaureate; LPN to Baccalaureate; RN Baccalaureate.

Study Options Full-time and part-time.

Program Entrance Requirements Minimum overall college GPA of 2.0, CPR certification, immunizations, minimum GPA in nursing prerequisites of 2.0, prerequisite course work. Transfer students are accepted. **Application** *Deadline:* rolling (freshmen), rolling (transfer). *Notification:* continuous until 9/30 (freshmen). *Application fee:* CAN$35.

Advanced Placement Credit given for nursing courses completed elsewhere dependent upon specific evaluations.

Expenses (2004–05) *Tuition, state resident:* full-time CAN$3018; part-time CAN$301 per course. *Tuition, nonresident:* full-time CAN$3018; part-time CAN$301 per course.

Financial Aid *Gift aid (need-based):* college/university gift aid from institutional funds. *Loans:* provincial and federal student loans. *Application deadline (priority):* 6/30.

Contact Ms. Tracey Collyer, Instructional Associate/Student Advisor, School of Health Studies, Brandon University, 270 18th Street, Brandon, MB R7A 6A9. *Telephone:* 204-571-8567. *Fax:* 204-571-8568. *E-mail:* collyert@brandonu.ca.

University of Manitoba
Faculty of Nursing
Winnipeg, Manitoba

http://www.umanitoba.ca/faculties/nursing/
Founded in 1877

DEGREES • BN • MN

Nursing Program Faculty 122 (20% with doctorates).

Baccalaureate Enrollment 1,228 **Women** 89% **Men** 11% **Part-time** 35%

Graduate Enrollment 97
Women 96% **Men** 4% **Part-time** 82%

Nursing Student Activities Nursing Honor Society, Sigma Theta Tau, Student Nurses' Association.

Nursing Student Resources Academic advising; academic or career counseling; assistance for students with disabilities; bookstore; campus computer network; computer lab; daycare for children of students; e-mail services; employment services for current students; housing assistance; interactive nursing skills videos; Internet; learning resource lab; library services; skills, simulation, or other laboratory; unpaid internships.

Library Facilities 1.6 million volumes (137,100 in health, 5,000 in nursing); 12,800 periodical subscriptions (2,208 health-care related).

BACCALAUREATE PROGRAMS

Degree BN

Available Programs Generic Baccalaureate; RN Baccalaureate.

Site Options Brandon, MB; Norway House, MB.

Study Options Full-time and part-time.

Program Entrance Requirements Minimum overall college GPA of 2.0, transcript of college record, CPR certification, high school chemistry, high school math, high school science, high school transcript, immunizations, minimum high school GPA of 2.0, prerequisite course work. Transfer students are accepted. **Application** *Deadline:* 7/1 (freshmen), 7/1 (transfer). *Notification:* continuous (freshmen). *Application fee:* CAN$35.

Advanced Placement Credit given for nursing courses completed elsewhere dependent upon specific evaluations.

Financial Aid *Gift aid (need-based):* state, private, college/university gift aid from institutional funds. *Loans:* Federal Direct (Subsidized and Unsubsidized Stafford PLUS), FFEL (Subsidized and Unsubsidized Stafford PLUS), Perkins, state, college/university, TERI Loans. *Work-Study:* part-time campus jobs. *Application deadline (priority):* 6/30.

Contact Dr. Wanda Chernomas, Associate Dean Undergraduate Program, Faculty of Nursing, University of Manitoba, 277 Helen Glass Centre for Nursing, Winnipeg, MB R3T 2N2. *Telephone:* 204-474-6771. *Fax:* 204-474-7682. *E-mail:* wanda_chernomas@umanitoba.ca.

GRADUATE PROGRAMS

Contact Graduate Program Assistant, Faculty of Nursing, University of Manitoba, Helen Glass Centre for Nursing, Winnipeg, MB R3T 2N2. *Telephone:* 204-474-6216. *Fax:* 204-474-7682. *E-mail:* nursing_grad@umanitoba.ca.

MASTER'S DEGREE PROGRAM

Degree MN

Concentrations Available Nursing administration. *Clinical nurse specialist programs in:* acute care, gerontology, perinatal. *Nurse practitioner programs in:* primary care.

Study Options Full-time and part-time.

Program Entrance Requirements Clinical experience, minimum overall college GPA of 3.0, transcript of college record, written essay, 3 letters of recommendation, nursing research course, resume, statistics course. *Application deadline:* For fall admission, 3/1. *Application fee:* CAN$50.

Advanced Placement Credit given for nursing courses completed elsewhere dependent upon specific evaluations.

Degree Requirements 27 total credit hours, thesis or project, comprehensive exam.

CONTINUING EDUCATION PROGRAM

Contact Dr. Dean Care, Academic Assistant to the Dean, Faculty of Nursing, University of Manitoba, 395 Helen Glass Centre for Nursing, Winnipeg, MB R3T 2N2. *Telephone:* 204-474-9958. *Fax:* 204-474-7682. *E-mail:* dean_care@umanitoba.ca.

NEW BRUNSWICK

Université de Moncton
School of Nursing
Moncton, New Brunswick

Founded in 1963

DEGREES • BSCN • M SC N

Nursing Program Faculty 24 (25% with doctorates).

Baccalaureate Enrollment 570
Women 90% **Men** 10% **International** 1%

Graduate Enrollment 8

Nursing Student Activities Student Nurses' Association.

Nursing Student Resources Academic or career counseling; assistance for students with disabilities; bookstore; campus computer network; career placement assistance; computer lab; computer-assisted instruction; daycare for children of students; e-mail services; externships; housing assistance;

Internet; library services; nursing audiovisuals; placement services for program completers; resume preparation assistance; unpaid internships.

Library Facilities 789,046 volumes; 2,059 periodical subscriptions.

BACCALAUREATE PROGRAMS

Degree BScN

Available Programs RN Baccalaureate.

Site Options Moncton, NB; Edmundston, NB; Bathurst, NB.

Study Options Full-time and part-time.

Program Entrance Requirements Transcript of college record, CPR certification, high school biology, high school chemistry, 12 years high school math, high school science, high school transcript, immunizations, minimum high school rank 65%. Transfer students are accepted. **Application** *Deadline:* 6/1 (freshmen), 2/1 (out-of-state freshmen), 6/1 (transfer). *Notification:* continuous until 9/1 (freshmen), continuous until 8/15 (out-of-state freshmen). *Application fee:* $30.

Advanced Placement Credit given for nursing courses completed elsewhere dependent upon specific evaluations.

Expenses (2003–04) *Tuition, state resident:* full-time CAN$4126; part-time CAN$139 per credit hour. *Tuition, nonresident:* full-time CAN$4126; part-time CAN$139 per credit hour. *International tuition:* CAN$7063 full-time. *Room and board:* CAN$4636; room only: CAN$2360 per academic year.

Financial Aid 20% of baccalaureate students in nursing programs received some form of financial aid in 2002–03. *Gift aid (need-based):* private, college/university gift aid from institutional funds. *Loans:* Federal Direct (Subsidized and Unsubsidized Stafford PLUS), FFEL (Subsidized and Unsubsidized Stafford PLUS), college/university, federal and provincial loan programs. *Work-Study:* part-time campus jobs. *Application deadline:* 2/28.

Contact Yoland Bordeleau, Bureau de Liaison, School of Nursing, Université de Moncton, Pavillon Leopold Taillon, Moncton, NB E1A 3E9. *Telephone:* 506-858-4443. *Fax:* 506-858-4544. *E-mail:* bordely@umoncton.ca.

GRADUATE PROGRAMS

Expenses (2003–04) *Tuition, state resident:* part-time CAN$161 per credit hour. *Tuition, nonresident:* part-time CAN$161 per credit hour. *International tuition:* CAN$11,655 full-time. *Room and board:* CAN$4636; room only: CAN$2360 per academic year. *Required fees:* full-time CAN$7245.

Financial Aid 10% of graduate students in nursing programs received some form of financial aid in 2002–03.

Contact Yoland Bordeleau, Bureau de Liaison, School of Nursing, Université de Moncton, Pavillon Leopold Taillon, Moncton, NB E1A 3E9. *Telephone:* 506-858-4443. *Fax:* 506-858-4544. *E-mail:* bordely@umoncton.ca.

MASTER'S DEGREE PROGRAM

Degree M Sc N

Available Programs Master's; RN to Master's.

Concentrations Available Health-care administration; nurse case management; nursing administration; nursing education. *Clinical nurse specialist programs in:* community health, family health, home health care, occupational health, pediatric, psychiatric/mental health, public health, school health. *Nurse practitioner programs in:* adult health, community health, family health, oncology, primary care.

Site Options Moncton, NB.

Study Options Full-time and part-time.

Program Entrance Requirements Minimum overall college GPA of 3.0, transcript of college record, CPR certification, written essay, 2 letters of recommendation, resume, statistics course.

Advanced Placement Credit given for nursing courses completed elsewhere dependent upon specific evaluations.

Degree Requirements 45 total credit hours, thesis or project.

CONTINUING EDUCATION PROGRAM

Contact Mr. Charles Antoine Leblanc, Adjoint au directeur éducation permanente, School of Nursing, Université de Moncton, Éducation permanente, Moncton, NB E1A 3E9. *Telephone:* 506-858-4121. *E-mail:* leblanca@umoncton.ca.

University of New Brunswick Fredericton

Faculty of Nursing
Fredericton, New Brunswick

http://www.unbf.ca/nursing/

Founded in 1785

DEGREES • BN • MN

Nursing Program Faculty 64 (8% with doctorates).

Baccalaureate Enrollment 526
Women 95% **Men** 5%

Graduate Enrollment 85
Women 99% **Men** 1% **Part-time** 82%

Nursing Student Activities Student Nurses' Association, nursing club.

Nursing Student Resources Academic advising; academic or career counseling; assistance for students with disabilities; bookstore; campus computer network; computer lab; computer-assisted instruction; daycare for children of students; e-mail services; interactive nursing skills videos; Internet; learning resource lab; library services; nursing audiovisuals; resume preparation assistance; skills, simulation, or other laboratory; tutoring.

Library Facilities 1.1 million volumes (12,547 in health, 1,910 in nursing); 4,817 periodical subscriptions (250 health-care related).

BACCALAUREATE PROGRAMS

Degree BN

Available Programs Generic Baccalaureate.

Site Options *Distance Learning:* Moncton, NB; Bathurst, NB.

Study Options Full-time.

Program Entrance Requirements Transcript of college record, CPR certification, written essay, health exam, high school biology, high school chemistry, high school math, high school transcript, immunizations, interview, minimum high school rank 70%, minimum GPA in nursing prerequisites, prerequisite course work. Transfer students are accepted. **Standardized tests** *Required for some:* SAT. **Application** *Deadline:* 3/31 (freshmen), 3/31 (transfer). *Notification:* continuous until 8/31 (freshmen). *Application fee:* CAN$35.

Advanced Placement Credit given for nursing courses completed elsewhere dependent upon specific evaluations.

Financial Aid *Gift aid (need-based):* private, college/university gift aid from institutional funds. *Loans:* Federal Direct (Subsidized and Unsubsidized Stafford PLUS), college/university, federal/provincial loans. *Work-Study:* part-time campus jobs. *Application deadline:* 5/15 (priority: 2/15).

Contact Assistant Dean, Faculty of Nursing, University of New Brunswick Fredericton, PO Box 4400, Fredericton, NB E3B 5A3. *Telephone:* 506-458-7670. *Fax:* 506-447-3374. *E-mail:* dburrell@unb.ca.

GRADUATE PROGRAMS

Contact Graduate Assistant, Faculty of Nursing, University of New Brunswick Fredericton, PO Box 4400, Fredericton, NB E3B 5A3. *Telephone:* 506-451-6844. *Fax:* 506-447-3374. *E-mail:* fperry@unb.ca.

MASTER'S DEGREE PROGRAM

Degree MN

Available Programs Master's.

Concentrations Available Nurse case management; nursing administration; nursing education; nursing informatics. *Clinical nurse specialist programs in:* acute care, adult health, cardiovascular, community health, critical care, family health, gerontology, maternity-newborn, medical-surgical, oncology, parent-child, pediatric, psychiatric/mental health, public health, school health, women's health. *Nurse practitioner programs in:* acute care, adult health, community health, family health, gerontology, neonatal health, pediatric, primary care, psychiatric/mental health, women's health.

Study Options Full-time and part-time.

Program Entrance Requirements Clinical experience, computer literacy, minimum overall college GPA of 3.0, transcript of college record, written essay, 3 letters of recommendation, nursing research course, physical assessment course, professional liability insurance/malpractice insurance, prerequisite course work, statistics course.

University of New Brunswick Fredericton (continued)

Advanced Placement Credit given for nursing courses completed elsewhere dependent upon specific evaluations.

Degree Requirements 27 total credit hours, thesis or project.

CONTINUING EDUCATION PROGRAM

Contact Faculty of Nursing, Faculty of Nursing, University of New Brunswick Fredericton, PO Box 4400, Fredericton, NB E3B 5A3. *Telephone:* 506-453-4642. *Fax:* 506-447-3057. *E-mail:* nursing@unb.ca.

NEWFOUNDLAND AND LABRADOR

Memorial University of Newfoundland

School of Nursing
St. John's, Newfoundland and Labrador

http://www.nurs.mun.ca

Founded in 1925

DEGREES • BN • MN

Nursing Program Faculty 44 (24% with doctorates).

Baccalaureate Enrollment 642
Women 91% **Men** 9% **International** 2% **Part-time** 53%

Graduate Enrollment 92
Women 93% **Men** 7% **Part-time** 84%

Nursing Student Activities Student Nurses' Association.

Nursing Student Resources Academic advising; academic or career counseling; assistance for students with disabilities; bookstore; campus computer network; computer lab; computer-assisted instruction; daycare for children of students; e-mail services; employment services for current students; interactive nursing skills videos; Internet; learning resource lab; library services; nursing audiovisuals; skills, simulation, or other laboratory; tutoring.

Library Facilities 1.2 million volumes (40,000 in health, 5,000 in nursing); 17,000 periodical subscriptions (3,800 health-care related).

BACCALAUREATE PROGRAMS

Degree BN

Available Programs Accelerated Baccalaureate; Generic Baccalaureate; RN Baccalaureate.

Study Options Full-time.

Program Entrance Requirements CPR certification, health exam, high school biology, high school chemistry, high school transcript, immunizations, 2 letters of recommendation. Transfer students are accepted. **Application** *Deadline:* rolling (freshmen), 3/1 (out-of-state freshmen), 3/1 (transfer). *Notification:* continuous (freshmen), continuous (out-of-state freshmen). *Application fee:* CAN$80.

Advanced Placement Credit given for nursing courses completed elsewhere dependent upon specific evaluations.

Expenses (2004–05) *Required fees:* full-time $2550; part-time $255 per credit; part-time $1275 per term.

Financial Aid *Loans:* college/university. *Application deadline:* Continuous.

Contact Ms. June Ellis, Consortium Coordinator, School of Nursing, Memorial University of Newfoundland, St. John's, NF A1B 3R6. *Telephone:* 709-737-6871. *Fax:* 709-737-3890. *E-mail:* junee@mun.ca.

GRADUATE PROGRAMS

Expenses (2004–05) *Required fees:* full-time $1500; part-time $750 per term.

Financial Aid Fellowships, research assistantships, teaching assistantships available.

Contact Dr. Alice Gaudine, Associate Director, Graduate Program and Research, School of Nursing, Memorial University of Newfoundland, Health Science Centre, Prince Philip Parkway, St. John's, NF A1B 3V6. *Telephone:* 709-777-6679. *Fax:* 709-777-7037. *E-mail:* agaudine@mun.ca.

MASTER'S DEGREE PROGRAM

Degree MN

Available Programs Master's.

Concentrations Available *Nurse practitioner programs in:* acute care, pediatric.

Study Options Full-time and part-time.

Program Entrance Requirements Clinical experience, minimum overall college GPA of 3.0, transcript of college record, CPR certification, written essay, 3 letters of recommendation, nursing research course, resume, statistics course. *Application deadline:* For fall admission, 12/31 (priority date). Applications are processed on a rolling basis. *Application fee:* $40.

Degree Requirements 24 total credit hours, thesis or project.

NOVA SCOTIA

Dalhousie University

School of Nursing
Halifax, Nova Scotia

http://www.dal.ca/nursing

Founded in 1818

DEGREES • BSCN • MN • MN/MHSA • PHD

Nursing Program Faculty 56 (28% with doctorates).

Baccalaureate Enrollment 535
Women 90% **Men** 10% **Minority** 2% **Part-time** 2%

Graduate Enrollment 98
Women 97% **Men** 3% **Part-time** 86%

Nursing Student Activities Sigma Theta Tau, Student Nurses' Association.

Nursing Student Resources Academic advising; academic or career counseling; assistance for students with disabilities; bookstore; campus computer network; computer lab; computer-assisted instruction; daycare for children of students; e-mail services; employment services for current students; externships; housing assistance; interactive nursing skills videos; Internet; learning resource lab; library services; nursing audiovisuals; resume preparation assistance; skills, simulation, or other laboratory; tutoring.

Library Facilities 1.7 million volumes; 8,306 periodical subscriptions.

BACCALAUREATE PROGRAMS

Degree BScN

Available Programs Accelerated Baccalaureate; Accelerated Baccalaureate for Second Degree; Baccalaureate for Second Degree; Generic Baccalaureate; RN Baccalaureate.

Site Options Yarmouth, NS.

Study Options Full-time and part-time.

Program Entrance Requirements Minimum overall college GPA of 2.5, transcript of college record, high school biology, high school chemistry, 3 years high school math, high school transcript, immunizations, minimum high school rank 70%, minimum GPA in nursing prerequisites of 2.5, prerequisite course work. Transfer students are accepted. **Standardized tests** *Required:* SAT. **Application** *Deadline:* 6/1 (freshmen), 6/1 (transfer). *Early decision:* 3/15. *Notification:* continuous (freshmen). *Application fee:* CAN$45.

Advanced Placement Credit given for nursing courses completed elsewhere dependent upon specific evaluations.

Financial Aid *Gift aid (need-based):* private, college/university gift aid from institutional funds, Vermont Grants. *Loans:* Federal Direct (Subsidized and Unsubsidized Stafford), FFEL (Subsidized and Unsubsidized Stafford PLUS), college/university, Canadian Loans. *Application deadline:* Continuous.

Contact Ms. Lucille Wittstock, Associate Director, Undergraduate Student Affairs, School of Nursing, Dalhousie University, 5869 University Avenue, Halifax, NS B3H 3J5. *Telephone:* 902-494-2004. *Fax:* 902-494-3487. *E-mail:* lucille.wittstock@dal.ca.

GRADUATE PROGRAMS

Financial Aid 14% of graduate students in nursing programs received some form of financial aid in 2003–04. Fellowships, research assistantships, teaching assistantships available.

Contact Dr. Joan Evans, Associate Director, Graduate Program, School of Nursing, Dalhousie University, 5869 University Avenue, Halifax, NS B3H 3J5. *Telephone:* 902-494-2391. *Fax:* 902-494-3487. *E-mail:* joan.evans@dal.ca.

MASTER'S DEGREE PROGRAM

Degrees MN; MN/MHSA

Available Programs Master's.

Concentrations Available *Clinical nurse specialist programs in:* adult health, community health, family health, maternity-newborn, parent-child, pediatric, psychiatric/mental health, public health. *Nurse practitioner programs in:* acute care, adult health, gerontology, neonatal health, oncology.

Study Options Full-time and part-time.

Program Entrance Requirements Clinical experience, minimum overall college GPA of 3.0, transcript of college record, immunizations, interview, 3 letters of recommendation, nursing research course, prerequisite course work, statistics course, GRE General Test. *Application deadline:* For fall admission, 4/1 (priority date); for winter admission, 10/31. Applications are processed on a rolling basis. *Application fee:* $60.

Degree Requirements 36 total credit hours, thesis or project.

POST-MASTER'S PROGRAM

Areas of Study *Nurse practitioner programs in:* acute care, adult health, gerontology, neonatal health, oncology.

DOCTORAL DEGREE PROGRAM

Degree PhD

Available Programs Doctorate.

Areas of Study Advanced practice nursing, aging, community health, family health, health policy, health promotion/disease prevention, human health and illness, illness and transition, maternity-newborn, nursing policy, nursing research, nursing science, oncology, women's health.

Program Entrance Requirements Clinical experience, minimum overall college GPA of 3.3, interview, 3 letters of recommendation, MSN or equivalent, vita, writing sample. *Application deadline:* For fall admission, 4/1 (priority date); for winter admission, 10/31. Applications are processed on a rolling basis. *Application fee:* $60.

Degree Requirements 27 total credit hours, dissertation, oral exam, written exam, residency.

St. Francis Xavier University

Department of Nursing
Antigonish, Nova Scotia

http://www.stfx.ca

Founded in 1853

DEGREE • BSCN

Nursing Program Faculty 67 (10% with doctorates).

Baccalaureate Enrollment 1,067 **Women** 90% **Men** 10% **Minority** 5% **International** 1% **Part-time** 40%

Nursing Student Activities Student Nurses' Association, nursing club.

Nursing Student Resources Academic advising; academic or career counseling; assistance for students with disabilities; bookstore; campus computer network; career placement assistance; computer lab; computer-assisted instruction; daycare for children of students; e-mail services; employment services for current students; externships; housing assistance; interactive nursing skills videos; Internet; learning resource lab; library services; nursing audiovisuals; other; paid internships; placement services for program completers; remedial services; resume preparation assistance; skills, simulation, or other laboratory; tutoring; unpaid internships.

Library Facilities 632,575 volumes (4,000 in health, 4,000 in nursing); 3,282 periodical subscriptions (1,015 health-care related).

BACCALAUREATE PROGRAMS

Degree BScN

Available Programs Accelerated Baccalaureate; Accelerated Baccalaureate for Second Degree; Accelerated LPN to Baccalaureate; Generic Baccalaureate; RN Baccalaureate.

Site Options Sydney, NS.

Study Options Full-time.

Program Entrance Requirements Transcript of college record, CPR certification, health exam, high school biology, high school chemistry, 2 years high school math, 2 years high school science, high school transcript, immunizations, minimum high school GPA, prerequisite course work. Transfer students are accepted. **Standardized tests** *Recommended:* SAT or ACT, SAT Subject Tests, SAT II Writing Tests. *Required for some:* SAT or ACT, SAT II Writing Tests. **Application** *Deadline:* rolling (freshmen), rolling (transfer). *Notification:* continuous until 8/15 (freshmen). *Application fee:* CAN$40.

Advanced Placement Credit given for nursing courses completed elsewhere dependent upon specific evaluations.

Expenses (2004–05) *Tuition, area resident:* full-time CAN$5310; part-time CAN$188 per credit hour. *Room and board:* CAN$5695 per academic year. *Required fees:* full-time CAN$573.

Financial Aid 95% of baccalaureate students in nursing programs received some form of financial aid in 2003–04. *Gift aid (need-based):* private, college/university gift aid from institutional funds. *Loans:* Federal Direct (Subsidized Stafford PLUS), FFEL (Subsidized Stafford PLUS), college/university. *Application deadline:* Continuous.

Contact Mr. Rob Parker, Manager of Recruitment and Admissions, Department of Nursing, St. Francis Xavier University, PO Box 5000, Antigonish, NS B2G 2W5. *Telephone:* 902-867-5386. *Fax:* 902-867-2329. *E-mail:* rparker@stfx.ca.

CONTINUING EDUCATION PROGRAM

Contact Ms. Patricia MacDonald, RN, Program Director, Distance Nursing Program, Department of Nursing, St. Francis Xavier University, Post-RN BScN Part-Time Distance Program, Antigonish, NS B2G 2W5. *Telephone:* 902-867-5186. *Fax:* 902-867-5154. *E-mail:* pmacdona@stfx.ca.

ONTARIO

Brock University

Department of Nursing
St. Catharines, Ontario

http://www.brocku.ca/nursing/

Founded in 1964

DEGREE • BSCN

Nursing Student Resources Computer-assisted instruction.

Library Facilities 1.6 million volumes; 856,587 periodical subscriptions.

BACCALAUREATE PROGRAMS

Degree BScN

Brock University (continued)

Available Programs Generic Baccalaureate; RN Baccalaureate.

Study Options Full-time and part-time.

Program Entrance Requirements Standardized tests *Recommended:* SAT and SAT Subject Tests or ACT. **Application** *Deadline:* 4/1 (transfer). *Notification:* continuous (freshmen). *Application fee:* CAN$115.

Contact Dr. Linda Ritchie, RN, Chair and Assistant Professor, Department of Nursing, Brock University, 500 Glenridge Avenue, St. Catharines, ON L2S 3A1. *Telephone:* 905-688-5550 Ext. 4781. *E-mail:* lritchie@health.pec.brocku.ca.

Lakehead University
School of Nursing
Thunder Bay, Ontario

http://www.lakeheadu.ca

Founded in 1965

DEGREE • BSN

Nursing Program Faculty 11 (27% with doctorates).

Baccalaureate Enrollment 450

Nursing Student Activities Nursing club.

Nursing Student Resources Academic advising; academic or career counseling; assistance for students with disabilities; bookstore; campus computer network; computer lab; daycare for children of students; e-mail services; interactive nursing skills videos; library services; nursing audiovisuals; skills, simulation, or other laboratory; tutoring.

Library Facilities 719,253 volumes; 2,100 periodical subscriptions.

BACCALAUREATE PROGRAMS

Degree BSN

Available Programs Generic Baccalaureate; RN Baccalaureate.

Study Options Full-time and part-time.

Program Entrance Requirements Transcript of college record, CPR certification, health insurance, high school biology, high school chemistry, 4 years high school math, high school transcript, immunizations. Transfer students are accepted. **Application** *Deadline:* rolling (freshmen), rolling (transfer). *Notification:* continuous until 9/18 (freshmen). *Application fee:* CAN$85.

Advanced Placement Credit given for nursing courses completed elsewhere dependent upon specific evaluations.

Expenses (2003–04) *Tuition, state resident:* full-time CAN$5000. *Tuition, nonresident:* full-time CAN$5000.

Contact Dr. Lorne McDougall, Director, School of Nursing, Lakehead University, 955 Oliver Road, Thunder Bay, ON P7B 5E1. *Telephone:* 807-343-8115. *Fax:* 807-343-8246. *E-mail:* lorne.mcdougall@lakehead.ca.

Laurentian University
School of Nursing
Sudbury, Ontario

Founded in 1960

DEGREE • BSCN

Nursing Program Faculty 20 (20% with doctorates).

Nursing Student Resources Internet.

Library Facilities 696,838 volumes.

BACCALAUREATE PROGRAMS

Degree BScN

Study Options Full-time and part-time.

Program Entrance Requirements CPR certification, health exam, high school biology, high school chemistry, high school transcript, immunizations, prerequisite course work. Transfer students are accepted. **Application** *Deadline:* 2/1 (freshmen), 2/1 (out-of-state freshmen), rolling (transfer). *Application fee:* CAN$50.

Advanced Placement Credit given for nursing courses completed elsewhere dependent upon specific evaluations.

Contact Dr. Ellen Rukholm, Director, School of Nursing, Laurentian University, 935 Ramsey Lake Road, Sudbury, ON P3E 2C6. *Telephone:* 705-675-1151 Ext. 3808. *Fax:* 705-675-4861. *E-mail:* erukholm@nickel.laurentian.ca.

CONTINUING EDUCATION PROGRAM

Contact Dr. Ellen Rukholm, Director, School of Nursing, Laurentian University, 935 Ramsey Lake Road, Sudbury, ON P3E 2C6. *Telephone:* 705-675-1151 Ext. 3808. *Fax:* 705-675-4861. *E-mail:* erukholm@nickel.laurentian.ca.

McMaster University
School of Nursing
Hamilton, Ontario

http://www.fhs.mcmaster.ca/nursing

Founded in 1887

DEGREES • BSCN • M SC • MSN/PHD

Nursing Program Faculty 53 (47% with doctorates).

Baccalaureate Enrollment 548

Women 90% **Men** 10% **Part-time** 20%

Nursing Student Activities Student Nurses' Association.

Nursing Student Resources Academic advising; academic or career counseling; assistance for students with disabilities; bookstore; campus computer network; career placement assistance; computer lab; daycare for children of students; e-mail services; employment services for current students; housing assistance; Internet; learning resource lab; library services; nursing audiovisuals; placement services for program completers; remedial services; resume preparation assistance; skills, simulation, or other laboratory; tutoring.

Library Facilities 1.7 million volumes (150,446 in health); 11,976 periodical subscriptions (89,267 health-care related).

BACCALAUREATE PROGRAMS

Degree BScN

Available Programs Baccalaureate for Second Degree; Generic Baccalaureate; RN Baccalaureate.

Site Options Kitchener, ON.

Study Options Full-time and part-time.

Program Entrance Requirements CPR certification, health exam, high school biology, high school chemistry, 4 years high school math, 4 years high school science, high school transcript, immunizations, minimum high school GPA of 3.0, minimum high school rank 75%. Transfer students are accepted. **Application** *Deadline:* 7/15 (freshmen), 5/1 (out-of-state freshmen), 7/15 (transfer). *Early decision:* 3/1. *Notification:* continuous until 9/1 (freshmen), 6/12 (early action). *Application fee:* CAN$95.

Advanced Placement Credit by examination available. Credit given for nursing courses completed elsewhere dependent upon specific evaluations.

Expenses (2003–04) *Tuition, state resident:* full-time CAN$4767; part-time CAN$134 per unit. *Tuition, nonresident:* full-time CAN$4767; part-time CAN$134 per unit. *International tuition:* CAN$13,185 full-time. *Room and board:* CAN$7000; room only: CAN$3345 per academic year. *Required fees:* full-time CAN$175.

Financial Aid *Gift aid (need-based):* college/university gift aid from institutional funds. *Loans:* FFEL (Subsidized and Unsubsidized Stafford PLUS). *Work-Study:* part-time campus jobs. *Application deadline:* Continuous.

Contact Admissions Coordinator, School of Nursing, McMaster University, Hamilton, ON L8N 3Z5. *Telephone:* 905-525-9140 Ext. 22232. *Fax:* 905-528-4727. *E-mail:* bscnprog@mcmaster.ca.

GRADUATE PROGRAMS

Contact Graduate Program Admissions, School of Nursing, McMaster University, 1200 Main Street, West, Room 3N10, Hamilton, ON L8N 3Z5. *Telephone:* 905-525-9140 Ext. 22982. *Fax:* 905-546-1129.

MASTER'S DEGREE PROGRAM

Degrees M Sc; MSN/PhD

Available Programs Master's.

Concentrations Available *Clinical nurse specialist programs in:* perinatal. *Nurse practitioner programs in:* neonatal health.

Study Options Full-time and part-time.

Program Entrance Requirements Transcript of college record, written essay, 2 letters of recommendation.

Advanced Placement Credit given for nursing courses completed elsewhere dependent upon specific evaluations.

Degree Requirements Thesis or project.

DOCTORAL DEGREE PROGRAM

Degree PhD

Available Programs Doctorate.

Program Entrance Requirements 2 letters of recommendation, MSN or equivalent, vita.

Degree Requirements Dissertation, oral exam.

Nipissing University

Nursing Department
North Bay, Ontario

Founded in 1992

DEGREE • BSCN

Nursing Program Faculty 14 (21% with doctorates).

Baccalaureate Enrollment 138

Women 98% **Men** 2% **Minority** 2% **International** 1% **Part-time** 10%

Nursing Student Activities Student Nurses' Association.

Nursing Student Resources Academic advising; academic or career counseling; assistance for students with disabilities; bookstore; campus computer network; career placement assistance; computer lab; computer-assisted instruction; daycare for children of students; e-mail services; employment services for current students; housing assistance; interactive nursing skills videos; Internet; learning resource lab; library services; nursing audiovisuals; placement services for program completers; remedial services; resume preparation assistance; skills, simulation, or other laboratory; tutoring; unpaid internships.

Library Facilities 180,397 volumes (2,800 in health, 1,820 in nursing); 5,680 periodical subscriptions (2,430 health-care related).

BACCALAUREATE PROGRAMS

Degree BScN

Available Programs Generic Baccalaureate.

Study Options Full-time.

Program Entrance Requirements Minimum overall college GPA of 3.0, transcript of college record, high school biology, high school chemistry, 4 years high school math, high school transcript, immunizations, minimum high school rank 70%. Transfer students are accepted. **Application** *Deadline:* 6/1 (freshmen), 6/1 (transfer). *Notification:* continuous until 6/1 (freshmen). *Application fee:* CAN$40.

Expenses (2004–05) *Tuition, state resident:* full-time CAN$3950; part-time CAN$395 per course. *Tuition, nonresident:* full-time CAN$3950; part-time CAN$395 per course. *International tuition:* CAN$9826 full-time. *Room and board:* room only: CAN$3965 per academic year. *Required fees:* full-time CAN$793; part-time CAN$45 per credit.

Financial Aid 44% of baccalaureate students in nursing programs received some form of financial aid in 2003–04.

Contact Admissions Office. *Telephone:* 705-474-3450 Ext. 4521.

Queen's University at Kingston

School of Nursing
Kingston, Ontario

http://meds.queensu.ca/nursing

Founded in 1841

DEGREES • BNSC • M SC

Nursing Program Faculty 20 (80% with doctorates).

Baccalaureate Enrollment 400

Women 95% **Men** 5%

Graduate Enrollment 25

Nursing Student Activities Student Nurses' Association.

Nursing Student Resources Academic advising; academic or career counseling; assistance for students with disabilities; bookstore; campus computer network; career placement assistance; computer lab; computer-assisted instruction; daycare for children of students; e-mail services; employment services for current students; housing assistance; interactive nursing skills videos; Internet; learning resource lab; library services; nursing audiovisuals; resume preparation assistance; skills, simulation, or other laboratory; tutoring; unpaid internships.

Library Facilities 3.5 million volumes (5,209 in health, 3,652 in nursing); 16,109 periodical subscriptions (1,054 health-care related).

BACCALAUREATE PROGRAMS

Degree BNSc

Available Programs Generic Baccalaureate.

Study Options Full-time.

Program Entrance Requirements CPR certification, high school biology, high school chemistry, high school math, high school science, high school transcript, immunizations, minimum high school GPA, minimum high school rank. Transfer students are accepted. **Standardized tests** *Required:* SAT or ACT. **Application** *Deadline:* 2/25 (freshmen), 5/15 (transfer). *Notification:* continuous until 5/28 (freshmen). *Application fee:* CAN$90.

Financial Aid 42% of baccalaureate students in nursing programs received some form of financial aid in 2003–04. *Gift aid (need-based):* state, private, college/university gift aid from institutional funds. *Loans:* FFEL (Subsidized and Unsubsidized Stafford PLUS), college/university, federal aid provincial loans. *Work-Study:* part-time campus jobs. *Application deadline:* Continuous.

Contact Prof. Susan Laschinger, Chair, Admissions Committee, School of Nursing, Queen's University at Kingston, Cataraqui Building, 92 Barrie Street, Kingston, ON K7L 3N6. *Telephone:* 613-533-6000 Ext. 74743. *Fax:* 613-533-6770. *E-mail:* lasching@post.queensu.ca.

GRADUATE PROGRAMS

Financial Aid 60% of graduate students in nursing programs received some form of financial aid in 2003–04. 25 fellowships (averaging $6,636 per year), 4 research assistantships, 9 teaching assistantships (averaging $2,592 per year) were awarded; institutionally sponsored loans and scholarships also available. *Financial aid application deadline:* 2/1.

Contact Dr. Ann Brown, Graduate Coordinator, School of Nursing, Queen's University at Kingston, Cataraqui Building, 90 Barrie Street, Kingston, ON K7L 3N6. *Telephone:* 613-533-6000 Ext. 74763. *Fax:* 613-533-6770. *E-mail:* browna@post.queensu.ca.

MASTER'S DEGREE PROGRAM

Degree M Sc

Available Programs Master's.

Study Options Full-time.

Program Entrance Requirements Transcript of college record, 2 letters of recommendation, nursing research course, prerequisite course work, statistics course. *Application deadline:* For winter admission, 2/1 (priority date). Applications are processed on a rolling basis. *Application fee:* CAN$70.

Degree Requirements Thesis or project.

Ryerson University
Program in Nursing
Toronto, Ontario

http://www.ryerson.ca/nursing

Founded in 1948

DEGREE • BSCN

Nursing Program Faculty 64 (17% with doctorates).

Baccalaureate Enrollment 1,806 **Women** 92% **Men** 8% **Part-time** 42%

Nursing Student Activities Sigma Theta Tau, Student Nurses' Association, nursing club.

Nursing Student Resources Academic advising; academic or career counseling; assistance for students with disabilities; bookstore; campus computer network; career placement assistance; computer lab; computer-assisted instruction; daycare for children of students; e-mail services; housing assistance; interactive nursing skills videos; Internet; learning resource lab; library services; nursing audiovisuals; remedial services; resume preparation assistance; skills, simulation, or other laboratory; tutoring.

Library Facilities 606,603 volumes (42,000 in health, 6,000 in nursing); 25,675 periodical subscriptions (1,500 health-care related).

BACCALAUREATE PROGRAMS

Degree BScN

Available Programs Accelerated RN Baccalaureate; Generic Baccalaureate; RN Baccalaureate.

Study Options Full-time.

Program Entrance Requirements Transcript of college record, CPR certification, health exam, health insurance, high school biology, high school chemistry, high school math, high school transcript, immunizations, minimum high school rank 75%. Transfer students are accepted. **Application** *Deadline:* 3/1 (transfer). *Notification:* continuous (freshmen). *Application fee:* CAN$95.

Advanced Placement Credit given for nursing courses completed elsewhere dependent upon specific evaluations.

Expenses (2004–05) *Tuition, state resident:* full-time CAN$4757. *Tuition, nonresident:* full-time CAN$4757. *International tuition:* CAN$13,421 full-time. *Room and board:* CAN$7651; room only: CAN$5151 per academic year. *Required fees:* full-time CAN$50.

Financial Aid 44% of baccalaureate students in nursing programs received some form of financial aid in 2003–04. *Gift aid (need-based):* college/university gift aid from institutional funds. *Loans:* Federal Direct (Subsidized and Unsubsidized Stafford). *Application deadline:* 1/15.

Contact Richard Perras, Student Affairs Coordinator, Program in Nursing, Ryerson University, 350 Victoria Street, Room POD-474, Toronto, ON M5B 2K3. *Telephone:* 416-979-5000 Ext. 6318. *Fax:* 416-979-5332. *E-mail:* rperras@ryerson.ca.

CONTINUING EDUCATION PROGRAM

Contact Paula Mastrilli, Program Manager, Nursing Division, Program in Nursing, Ryerson University, 350 Victoria Street, Room POD-476A, Toronto, ON M5B 2K3. *Telephone:* 416-979-5178. *Fax:* 416-979-5277. *E-mail:* pmastril@ryerson.ca.

Trent University
Nursing Program
Peterborough, Ontario

http://www.trentu.ca/nursing/

Founded in 1963

DEGREE • BSCN

Nursing Program Faculty 42 (14% with doctorates).

Baccalaureate Enrollment 399

Nursing Student Activities Student Nurses' Association.

Nursing Student Resources Academic advising; academic or career counseling; assistance for students with disabilities; bookstore; campus computer network; computer lab; computer-assisted instruction; e-mail services; employment services for current students; housing assistance; interactive nursing skills videos; Internet; learning resource lab; library services; nursing audiovisuals; remedial services; resume preparation assistance; skills, simulation, or other laboratory; tutoring.

Library Facilities 579,557 volumes (6,393 in health, 1,281 in nursing); 2,312 periodical subscriptions (360 health-care related).

BACCALAUREATE PROGRAMS

Degree BScN

Available Programs RN Baccalaureate.

Site Options Peterborough, ON.

Study Options Full-time.

Program Entrance Requirements CPR certification, health exam, high school biology, high school chemistry, 4 years high school math, 4 years high school science, high school transcript, minimum high school rank 70%. Transfer students are accepted. **Standardized tests** *Required for some:* SAT or ACT. **Application** *Deadline:* 6/1 (freshmen), 6/1 (transfer). *Application fee:* CAN$95.

Expenses (2004–05) *Tuition, state resident:* full-time CAN$4185. *Tuition, nonresident:* full-time CAN$4185. *International tuition:* CAN$12,978 full-time. *Room and board:* CAN$7566 per academic year. *Required fees:* full-time CAN$1295.

Contact Ms. Carol Weafer-Lloyd, Liaison and Admissions Officer, Nursing Program, Trent University, Trent/Fleming Nursing Program, 1600 Westbank Drive, Peterborough, ON K9J 7B8. *Telephone:* 705-748-1011 Ext. 7809. *Fax:* 705-748-1088. *E-mail:* nursing@trentu.ca.

University of Ottawa
School of Nursing
Ottawa, Ontario

http://www.health.uottawa.ca/sn/

Founded in 1848

DEGREES • BSCN • MSCN • PHD

Nursing Program Faculty 150 (18% with doctorates).

Baccalaureate Enrollment 1,324 **Women** 94% **Men** 6% **Part-time** 21%

Graduate Enrollment 78
Women 99% **Men** 1% **Part-time** 79%

Nursing Student Activities Student Nurses' Association.

Nursing Student Resources Academic advising; academic or career counseling; assistance for students with disabilities; bookstore; campus computer network; computer lab; e-mail services; housing assistance; learning resource lab; library services; skills, simulation, or other laboratory; tutoring.

Library Facilities 2.6 million volumes (54,000 in health, 7,000 in nursing); 9,183 periodical subscriptions (1,050 health-care related).

BACCALAUREATE PROGRAMS

Degree BScN

Available Programs Generic Baccalaureate; RN Baccalaureate.

Site Options *Distance Learning:* Kahnawake, PQ; Montreal , QC.

Study Options Full-time.

Program Entrance Requirements Transcript of college record, CPR certification, high school biology, high school chemistry, high school math, high school transcript, immunizations. Transfer students are accepted. **Application** *Deadline:* 6/30 (freshmen). *Notification:* continuous until 8/30 (freshmen). *Application fee:* CAN$85.

Advanced Placement Credit given for nursing courses completed elsewhere dependent upon specific evaluations.

Expenses (2004–05) *Tuition:* full-time CAN$4163; part-time CAN$165 per credit hour. *International tuition:* CAN$11,750 full-time. *Room and board:* room only: CAN$3528 per academic year. *Required fees:* full-time CAN$413.

Financial Aid *Gift aid (need-based):* state, private, college/university gift aid from institutional funds. *Loans:* provincial and federal loans. *Work-Study:* Federal Work-Study, part-time campus jobs. *Application deadline:* 1/31.

Contact Marguerite Félix, Assistant Director of Generic Baccalaureate Program, School of Nursing, University of Ottawa, 451 Smyth Road, Ottawa, ON K1H 8M5. *Telephone:* 613-562-5800 Ext. 8535. *Fax:* 613-562-5443. *E-mail:* mfelix@uottawa.ca.

GRADUATE PROGRAMS

Expenses (2004–05) *Tuition:* full-time CAN$1845; part-time CAN$200 per credit hour. *International tuition:* CAN$8000 full-time. *Room and board:* room only: CAN$3528 per academic year. *Required fees:* full-time CAN$477.

Financial Aid Fellowships, research assistantships, teaching assistantships, Federal Work-Study available.

Contact Dr. Jean Dunning, PhD, Assistant Director of Graduate Program, School of Nursing, University of Ottawa, 451 Smyth Road, Ottawa, ON K1H 8M5. *Telephone:* 613-562-5800 Ext. 8422. *Fax:* 613-562-5473. *E-mail:* jdunning@uottawa.ca.

MASTER'S DEGREE PROGRAM

Degree M Sc N

Available Programs Master's.

Concentrations Available *Clinical nurse specialist programs in:* acute care, community health. *Nurse practitioner programs in:* primary care.

Site Options *Distance Learning:* Sudbury, ON.

Program Entrance Requirements Clinical experience, minimum overall college GPA of 3.0, transcript of college record, written essay, immunizations, 3 letters of recommendation, nursing research course, physical assessment course, prerequisite course work, statistics course. *Application fee:* $60.

Advanced Placement Credit given for nursing courses completed elsewhere dependent upon specific evaluations.

Degree Requirements 24 total credit hours, thesis or project.

DOCTORAL DEGREE PROGRAM

Degree PhD

Available Programs Doctorate.

Areas of Study Health promotion/disease prevention, health-care systems, information systems, nursing policy, nursing research, nursing science.

Program Entrance Requirements Minimum overall college GPA of 0, 3 letters of recommendation, MSN or equivalent, statistics course, vita, writing sample. *Application fee:* $60.

Degree Requirements 18 total credit hours, dissertation, oral exam, written exam, residency.

University of Toronto
Faculty of Nursing
Toronto, Ontario

http://www.nursing.utoronto.ca/

Founded in 1827

DEGREES • BSCN • MN • MN/MBA • PHD

Nursing Program Faculty 36 (69% with doctorates).

Nursing Student Activities Student Nurses' Association.

Nursing Student Resources Tutoring.

Library Facilities 10.3 million volumes; 53,547 periodical subscriptions.

BACCALAUREATE PROGRAMS

Degree BScN

Available Programs Generic Baccalaureate.

Study Options Full-time.

Program Entrance Requirements Minimum overall college GPA of 3.0, transcript of college record, written essay, 2 letters of recommendation, prerequisite course work. **Standardized tests** *Required for some:* SAT, SAT Subject Tests. **Application** *Deadline:* 3/1 (freshmen), 7/1 (transfer). *Notification:* continuous (freshmen). *Application fee:* CAN$43.

Expenses (2004–05) *Tuition, state resident:* full-time CAN$5616; part-time CAN$936 per course. *Tuition, nonresident:* full-time CAN$5616; part-time CAN$936 per course. *International tuition:* CAN$12,638 full-time. *Room and board:* CAN$7000; room only: CAN$5000 per academic year. *Required fees:* full-time CAN$764; part-time CAN$193 per term.

Financial Aid 50% of baccalaureate students in nursing programs received some form of financial aid in 2003–04. *Work-Study:* Federal Work-Study.

Contact Office of Student Affairs, Faculty of Nursing, University of Toronto, 50 St. George Street, Toronto, ON M5S 3H4. *Telephone:* 416-978-2863. *Fax:* 416-978-8222. *E-mail:* inquiry.nursing@utoronto.ca.

GRADUATE PROGRAMS

Expenses (2004–05) *Tuition, state resident:* full-time CAN$6136; part-time CAN$1841 per course. *Tuition, nonresident:* full-time CAN$6136; part-time CAN$1841 per course. *International tuition:* CAN$13,184 full-time. *Room and board:* CAN$7000; room only: CAN$5000 per academic year. *Required fees:* full-time CAN$734; part-time CAN$160 per term.

Financial Aid 14% of graduate students in nursing programs received some form of financial aid in 2003–04.

Contact Office of Student Affairs, Faculty of Nursing, University of Toronto, 50 St. George Street, Toronto, ON M5S 3H4. *Telephone:* 416-978-2863. *Fax:* 416-978-8222. *E-mail:* inquiry.nursing@utoronto.ca.

MASTER'S DEGREE PROGRAM

Degrees MN; MN/MBA

Available Programs Master's.

Concentrations Available Nursing administration. *Clinical nurse specialist programs in:* critical care, psychiatric/mental health, women's health. *Nurse practitioner programs in:* acute care.

Study Options Full-time and part-time.

Program Entrance Requirements Clinical experience, minimum overall college GPA of 3.0, transcript of college record, written essay, 3 letters of recommendation, resume, statistics course.

Degree Requirements 9 total credit hours.

POST-MASTER'S PROGRAM

Areas of Study *Nurse practitioner programs in:* acute care.

DOCTORAL DEGREE PROGRAM

Degree PhD

Available Programs Doctorate.

Areas of Study Community health, family health, human health and illness, nursing administration, nursing science, women's health.

Program Entrance Requirements Minimum overall college GPA of 3.3, 2 letters of recommendation, MSN or equivalent, scholarly papers, vita, writing sample.

Degree Requirements Dissertation, oral exam.

POSTDOCTORAL PROGRAM

Postdoctoral Program Contact Graduate Department, Faculty of Nursing, University of Toronto, 50 St. George Street, Toronto, ON M5S 3H4. *Telephone:* 416-978-8069.

The University of Western Ontario
School of Nursing
London, Ontario

Founded in 1878

DEGREES • BSCN • M SC N • PHD

Nursing Program Faculty 62 (12% with doctorates).

The University of Western Ontario (continued)
Baccalaureate Enrollment 482
Women 96% **Men** 4% **Part-time** 2%

Graduate Enrollment 43
Women 89% **Men** 11% **Part-time** 39%

Nursing Student Activities Nursing Honor Society, Sigma Theta Tau, Student Nurses' Association.

Nursing Student Resources Academic advising; academic or career counseling; assistance for students with disabilities; bookstore; campus computer network; computer lab; computer-assisted instruction; daycare for children of students; e-mail services; employment services for current students; housing assistance; interactive nursing skills videos; Internet; learning resource lab; library services; nursing audiovisuals; resume preparation assistance; unpaid internships.

Library Facilities 3.1 million volumes (357,263 in health, 40 in nursing); 38,517 periodical subscriptions (250 health-care related).

BACCALAUREATE PROGRAMS

Degree BScN

Available Programs Generic Baccalaureate; RN Baccalaureate.

Study Options Full-time.

Program Entrance Requirements CPR certification, high school biology, high school chemistry, 4 years high school math, high school science, high school transcript, immunizations, minimum high school rank 80%. Transfer students are accepted. **Standardized tests** *Required for some:* SAT. **Application** *Deadline:* 6/1 (freshmen), 5/15 (out-of-state freshmen), 6/1 (transfer). *Application fee:* CAN$100.

Advanced Placement Credit given for nursing courses completed elsewhere dependent upon specific evaluations.

Expenses (2004–05) *Room and board:* CAN$7643 per academic year. *Required fees:* full-time CAN$5039; part-time CAN$956 per credit.

Financial Aid *Gift aid (need-based):* private, college/university gift aid from institutional funds. *Work-Study:* part-time campus jobs. *Application deadline:* Continuous.

Contact Ms. Denice Litzan, Academic Advisor, School of Nursing, The University of Western Ontario, London, ON N6A 5C1. *Telephone:* 519-661-2111 Ext. 86564. *Fax:* 519-850-2514. *E-mail:* dlitzan@uwo.ca.

GRADUATE PROGRAMS

Expenses (2004–05) *Tuition:* full-time CAN$7310; part-time CAN$1096 per term. *International tuition:* CAN$18,095 full-time.

Financial Aid 1% of graduate students in nursing programs received some form of financial aid in 2003–04. 5 research assistantships (averaging $7,500 per year), 10 teaching assistantships (averaging $8,900 per year) were awarded. *Financial aid application deadline:* 4/1.

Contact Ms. Lori Johnson, Graduate Affairs Assistant, School of Nursing, The University of Western Ontario, London, ON N6A 5C1. *Telephone:* 519-661-3409. *Fax:* 519-850-2514. *E-mail:* ljohns24@uwo.ca.

MASTER'S DEGREE PROGRAM

Degree M Sc N

Available Programs Master's.

Concentrations Available Health-care administration; nursing administration; nursing education.

Study Options Full-time and part-time.

Program Entrance Requirements Minimum overall college GPA of 3.5, transcript of college record, CPR certification, written essay, immunizations, interview, 2 letters of recommendation, nursing research course, professional liability insurance/malpractice insurance, prerequisite course work, resume, statistics course. *Application deadline:* For fall admission, 2/1. *Application fee:* $50.

Degree Requirements 7 total credit hours, thesis or project.

DOCTORAL DEGREE PROGRAM

Degree PhD

Available Programs Doctorate.

Areas of Study Addiction/substance abuse, aging, clinical practice, community health, family health, health promotion/disease prevention, health-care systems, human health and illness, individualized study, nursing administration, nursing education, nursing research, nursing science, women's health.

Program Entrance Requirements Clinical experience, minimum overall college GPA of 3.5, interview by faculty committee, interview, 2 letters of recommendation, MSN or equivalent, scholarly papers, statistics course, vita, writing sample. *Application deadline:* For fall admission, 2/1. *Application fee:* $50.

Degree Requirements 4 total credit hours, dissertation.

University of Windsor
School of Nursing
Windsor, Ontario

http://www.uwindsor.ca/nursing
Founded in 1857

DEGREES • BSCN • M SC

Nursing Program Faculty 21 (65% with doctorates).

Baccalaureate Enrollment 584
Women 89% **Men** 11% **Part-time** 10%

Graduate Enrollment 34
Women 97% **Men** 3% **Part-time** 91%

Nursing Student Activities Nursing Honor Society, Student Nurses' Association, nursing club.

Nursing Student Resources Academic advising; academic or career counseling; assistance for students with disabilities; bookstore; campus computer network; computer lab; computer-assisted instruction; daycare for children of students; e-mail services; employment services for current students; externships; housing assistance; interactive nursing skills videos; Internet; learning resource lab; library services; nursing audiovisuals; remedial services; resume preparation assistance; skills, simulation, or other laboratory; tutoring; unpaid internships.

Library Facilities 2.8 million volumes (41,874 in health); 25,458 periodical subscriptions (521 health-care related).

BACCALAUREATE PROGRAMS

Degree BScN

Available Programs Generic Baccalaureate; RN Baccalaureate.

Study Options Full-time and part-time.

Program Entrance Requirements CPR certification, health exam, health insurance, high school biology, high school chemistry, high school math, 4 years high school science, high school transcript, immunizations, minimum high school rank 72%. Transfer students are accepted. **Standardized tests** *Required for some:* SAT, SAT and SAT Subject Tests or ACT. **Application** *Deadline:* rolling (freshmen), 7/1 (out-of-state freshmen), rolling (transfer). *Notification:* continuous until 8/30 (freshmen). *Application fee:* CAN$60.

Advanced Placement Credit given for nursing courses completed elsewhere dependent upon specific evaluations.

Expenses (2004–05) *Room and board:* $5000 per academic year. *Required fees:* full-time $5000; part-time $494 per credit.

Financial Aid *Gift aid (need-based):* college/university gift aid from institutional funds. *Loans:* college/university. *Work-Study:* part-time campus jobs. *Application deadline:* 6/15.

Contact Nursing, School of Nursing, University of Windsor, 401 Sunset Avenue, Windsor, ON N9B 3P4. *Telephone:* 519-253-3000 Ext. 2258. *Fax:* 519-973-7084. *E-mail:* nursing@uwindsor.ca.

GRADUATE PROGRAMS

Contact Dr. Debbie Kane, Graduate Coordinator, School of Nursing, University of Windsor, Faculty of Nursing, 401 Sunset Avenue, Windsor, ON N9B 3P4. *Telephone:* 519-253-3000 Ext. 2268. *Fax:* 519-973-7084. *E-mail:* dkane@uwindsor.ca.

MASTER'S DEGREE PROGRAM

Degree M Sc

Available Programs Master's.

Study Options Full-time and part-time.

Program Entrance Requirements Transcript of college record, written essay, interview, 3 letters of recommendation, nursing research course, physical assessment course, statistics course.

Advanced Placement Credit given for nursing courses completed elsewhere dependent upon specific evaluations.

Degree Requirements 10 total credit hours, thesis or project.

CONTINUING EDUCATION PROGRAM

Contact Program Contact, School of Nursing, University of Windsor, 401 Sunset Avenue, Windsor, ON N9B 3P4. *Telephone:* 519-253-3000. *Fax:* 519-971-3608.

York University

School of Nursing, Atkinson Faculty of Liberal and Profesional Studies
Toronto, Ontario

Founded in 1959

DEGREE • BSCN

Nursing Program Faculty 19 (79% with doctorates).

Baccalaureate Enrollment 850
Women 96% **Men** 4% **Minority** 30% **International** 1% **Part-time** 15%

Nursing Student Resources Academic advising; academic or career counseling; assistance for students with disabilities; bookstore; campus computer network; career placement assistance; computer lab; computer-assisted instruction; daycare for children of students; e-mail services; employment services for current students; housing assistance; interactive nursing skills videos; Internet; learning resource lab; library services; nursing audiovisuals; skills, simulation, or other laboratory; unpaid internships.

Library Facilities 6.1 million volumes; 540,000 periodical subscriptions.

BACCALAUREATE PROGRAMS

Degree BScN

Available Programs Generic Baccalaureate; RN Baccalaureate.

Site Options King City, ON; Barrie, ON; Oshawa, ON.

Study Options Full-time and part-time.

Program Entrance Requirements CPR certification, written essay, health exam, high school biology, high school chemistry, high school math, high school science, high school transcript, immunizations, 1 letter of recommendation, minimum high school GPA, minimum GPA in nursing prerequisites. Transfer students are accepted. **Standardized tests** *Required:* SAT or ACT. **Application** *Deadline:* 2/1 (freshmen), 2/1 (transfer). *Early decision:* 2/1. *Notification:* 6/1 (early action). *Application fee:* CAN$90.

Advanced Placement Credit by examination available. Credit given for nursing courses completed elsewhere dependent upon specific evaluations.

Financial Aid *Gift aid (need-based):* private, college/university gift aid from institutional funds. *Loans:* Federal Direct (Subsidized and Unsubsidized Stafford PLUS), FFEL (Subsidized and Unsubsidized Stafford PLUS), Canadian Student Loans, Ontario Student Loans. *Application deadline:* Continuous.

Contact Dr. Kathleen Macdonald, Director, School of Nursing, Atkinson Faculty of Liberal and Profesional Studies, York University, Atkinson Room 418, 4700 Keele Street, Toronto, ON M3J-1P3. *Telephone:* 416-736-5271 Ext. 66351. *Fax:* 416-736-5714. *E-mail:* kathem@yorku.ca.

CONTINUING EDUCATION PROGRAM

Contact Dr. Janet Jeffrey, Undergraduate Program Director, School of Nursing, Atkinson Faculty of Liberal and Profesional Studies, York University, Atkinson Room 404, 4700 Keele Street, Toronto, ON M3J 1P3. *Telephone:* 416-736-5271. *Fax:* 416-736-5714. *E-mail:* jjeffrey@york.edu.

PRINCE EDWARD ISLAND

University of Prince Edward Island

School of Nursing
Charlottetown, Prince Edward Island

Founded in 1834

DEGREE • BSCN

Nursing Program Faculty 10 (2% with doctorates).

Baccalaureate Enrollment 211
Women 97% **Men** 3% **International** 1%

Nursing Student Activities Nursing Honor Society, Student Nurses' Association, nursing club.

Nursing Student Resources Academic advising; academic or career counseling; assistance for students with disabilities; bookstore; campus computer network; career placement assistance; computer lab; computer-assisted instruction; daycare for children of students; e-mail services; employment services for current students; housing assistance; interactive nursing skills videos; Internet; learning resource lab; library services; nursing audiovisuals; placement services for program completers; remedial services; resume preparation assistance; skills, simulation, or other laboratory; tutoring.

Library Facilities 394,000 volumes; 1,700 periodical subscriptions.

BACCALAUREATE PROGRAMS

Degree BScN

Available Programs Generic Baccalaureate.

Study Options Full-time and part-time.

Program Entrance Requirements Transcript of college record, CPR certification, high school chemistry, high school math, high school science, high school transcript, immunizations, minimum high school GPA of 3.0, minimum high school rank 75%, minimum GPA in nursing prerequisites of 3.0, prerequisite course work. Transfer students are accepted. **Application** *Deadline:* 8/15 (freshmen), 4/1 (out-of-state freshmen), 8/15 (transfer). *Notification:* continuous until 8/31 (freshmen), continuous until 6/30 (out-of-state freshmen). *Application fee:* CAN$35.

Advanced Placement Credit given for nursing courses completed elsewhere dependent upon specific evaluations.

Expenses (2003–04) *Tuition, area resident:* full-time CAN$822; part-time CAN$411 per course. *International tuition:* CAN$1700 full-time. *Room and board:* CAN$6658; room only: CAN$3840 per academic year.

Financial Aid *Gift aid (need-based):* private, college/university gift aid from institutional funds. *Loans:* Federal Direct (Subsidized and Unsubsidized Stafford). *Application deadline:* Continuous.

Contact Mary-Lou Austin, Executive Assistant to the Dean, School of Nursing, University of Prince Edward Island, 550 University Avenue, Charlottetown, PE C1A 4P3. *Telephone:* 902-566-0733. *Fax:* 902-566-0777. *E-mail:* mlaustin@upei.ca.

QUEBEC

McGill University

School of Nursing
Montréal, Quebec

http://www.nursing.mcgill.ca

Founded in 1821

DEGREES • BSCN • M SC • PHD

Nursing Program Faculty 16 (56% with doctorates).

McGill University (continued)

Baccalaureate Enrollment 193
Women 94% **Men** 6% **Minority** 3% **International** 2% **Part-time** 23%

Graduate Enrollment 81
Women 96% **Men** 4% **International** 3% **Part-time** 30%

Nursing Student Activities Student Nurses' Association.

Nursing Student Resources Academic advising; academic or career counseling; assistance for students with disabilities; bookstore; campus computer network; career placement assistance; computer lab; e-mail services; Internet; learning resource lab; library services; nursing audiovisuals; skills, simulation, or other laboratory; tutoring; unpaid internships.

Library Facilities 4.2 million volumes (250,000 in health); 25,673 periodical subscriptions (1,500 health-care related).

BACCALAUREATE PROGRAMS

Degree BScN

Available Programs Generic Baccalaureate; RN Baccalaureate.

Study Options Full-time.

Program Entrance Requirements Minimum overall college GPA of 3.0, transcript of college record, high school chemistry, 4 years high school math, 4 years high school science, high school transcript, minimum high school GPA of 3.3, minimum high school rank 25%. Transfer students are accepted. **Standardized tests** *Required:* SAT and SAT Subject Tests or ACT. **Application** *Deadline:* 1/15 (freshmen), 1/15 (transfer). *Notification:* continuous (freshmen). *Application fee:* CAN$60.

Expenses (2003–04) *Tuition, state resident:* full-time CAN$1668; part-time CAN$56 per credit hour. *Tuition, nonresident:* full-time CAN$4173; part-time CAN$56 per credit hour. *International tuition:* CAN$11,340 full-time. *Required fees:* full-time CAN$1104; part-time CAN$164 per term.

Financial Aid 19% of baccalaureate students in nursing programs received some form of financial aid in 2002–03. *Loans:* FFEL (Subsidized and Unsubsidized Stafford PLUS), college/university, alternative loans. *Work-Study:* part-time campus jobs. *Application deadline:* Continuous.

Contact Ms. Celine Arseneault, Student Affairs Coordinator—Undergraduate Programs, School of Nursing, McGill University, Wilson Hall Bldg.—Room 203, 3506 University Street, Montreal, QC H3A 2A7. *Telephone:* 514-398-3784. *Fax:* 514-398-8455. *E-mail:* celine.arseneault@mcgill.ca.

GRADUATE PROGRAMS

Expenses (2003–04) *Tuition, state resident:* full-time CAN$1668; part-time CAN$834 per semester. *Tuition, nonresident:* full-time CAN$4173; part-time CAN$2087 per semester. *International tuition:* CAN$9468 full-time. *Required fees:* full-time CAN$1196; part-time CAN$624 per term.

Financial Aid Institutionally sponsored loans and scholarships available.

Contact Ms. Anna M. Santandrea, Students Affairs Coordinator, Graduate & Post-Doctoral Studies, School of Nursing, McGill University, McGill University, School of Nursing, 3506 University Street, Montreal, QC H3A 2A7. *Telephone:* 514-398-4151. *Fax:* 514-398-8455. *E-mail:* anna.santandrea@mcgill.ca.

MASTER'S DEGREE PROGRAM

Degree M Sc

Available Programs Master's; Master's for Non-Nursing College Graduates.

Concentrations Available *Clinical nurse specialist programs in:* acute care, adult health, cardiovascular, community health, critical care, family health, gerontology, home health care, maternity-newborn, medical-surgical, oncology, parent-child, pediatric, perinatal, psychiatric/mental health, public health, rehabilitation, women's health. *Nurse practitioner programs in:* pediatric.

Study Options Full-time and part-time.

Program Entrance Requirements Clinical experience, minimum overall college GPA of 3.0, transcript of college record, CPR certification, written essay, immunizations, interview, 3 letters of recommendation, resume, statistics course, GRE General Test. *Application deadline:* For fall admission, 3/1 (priority date). Applications are processed on a rolling basis. *Application fee:* CAN$60.

Degree Requirements 48 total credit hours, thesis or project.

DOCTORAL DEGREE PROGRAM

Degree PhD

Available Programs Doctorate.

Areas of Study Nursing research.

Program Entrance Requirements Minimum overall college GPA of 3.3, interview by faculty committee, interview, 2 letters of recommendation, MSN or equivalent, scholarly papers, statistics course, vita, GRE General Test. *Application deadline:* For fall admission, 3/1 (priority date). Applications are processed on a rolling basis. *Application fee:* CAN$60.

Degree Requirements Dissertation, oral exam, written exam, residency.

POSTDOCTORAL PROGRAM

Postdoctoral Program Contact Dr. C. Celeste Johnston, Associate Director, Research, School of Nursing, McGill University, 3506 University Street, Montreal, QC H3A 2A7. *Telephone:* 514-398-4157. *Fax:* 514-398-8455. *E-mail:* celeste.johnston@mcgill.ca.

Université de Montréal
Faculty of Nursing
Montréal, Quebec

http://www.scinf.umontreal.ca

Founded in 1920

DEGREES • BSCN • M SC • PHD

Nursing Program Faculty 35 (80% with doctorates).

Nursing Student Activities Student Nurses' Association.

Library Facilities 32,536 volumes in health, 32,536 volumes in nursing; 18,330 periodical subscriptions (1,319 health-care related).

BACCALAUREATE PROGRAMS

Degree BScN

Study Options Full-time and part-time.

Program Entrance Requirements Transfer students are accepted. **Application** *Deadline:* 3/1 (freshmen), 3/1 (transfer). *Notification:* 5/15 (freshmen). *Application fee:* CAN$30.

Contact Joelle Bisson De Courval, Assistant to Vice Dean of Studies, Faculty of Nursing, Université de Montréal, CP 6128, Succursale Centre-Ville, Montreal, QC H3C 3J7. *Telephone:* 514-343-6439. *Fax:* 514-343-2306. *E-mail:* bissondj@scinf.umontreal.ca.

GRADUATE PROGRAMS

Financial Aid Fellowships, research assistantships, teaching assistantships, career-related internships or fieldwork, Federal Work-Study, and institutionally sponsored loans available.

Contact Dr. Louise Gagnon, Vice Dean of Studies, Faculty of Nursing, Université de Montréal, CP 6128, Succursale Centre-Ville, Montreal, QC H3C 3J7. *Telephone:* 514-343-6111 Ext. 7098. *Fax:* 514-343-2306. *E-mail:* Louise.Gagnon@umontreal.ca.

MASTER'S DEGREE PROGRAM

Degree M Sc

Study Options Full-time and part-time.

Program Entrance Requirements Transcript of college record, nursing research course, statistics course. *Application deadline:* For fall and spring admission, 2/1 (priority date); for winter admission, 11/1 (priority date). Applications are processed on a rolling basis. *Application fee:* $30.

Degree Requirements 45 total credit hours.

DOCTORAL DEGREE PROGRAM

Degree PhD

Program Entrance Requirements MSN or equivalent. *Application deadline:* For fall and spring admission, 2/1 (priority date); for winter admission, 11/1 (priority date). Applications are processed on a rolling basis. *Application fee:* $30.

Degree Requirements 90 total credit hours, dissertation.

POSTDOCTORAL PROGRAM

Postdoctoral Program Contact Ms. Jacinthe Pepin, Vice Dean of Studies, Faculty of Nursing, Université de Montréal, CP 6128, Succursale Centre-Ville, Montreal, QC H3C 3J7. *Telephone:* 514-343-6178. *Fax:* 514-343-2306. *E-mail:* jacinthe.pepin@umontreal.ca.

Université de Sherbrooke

Department of Nursing
Sherbrooke, Quebec

http://www.usherbrooke.ca/scinf/

Founded in 1954

DEGREES • BSCN • M SC • PHD

Nursing Program Faculty 19 (69% with doctorates).

Baccalaureate Enrollment 471
Women 90% **Men** 10% **Minority** .5% **Part-time** 30%

Graduate Enrollment 30
Women 95% **Men** 5% **Part-time** 50%

Nursing Student Activities Student Nurses' Association.

Nursing Student Resources Academic advising; academic or career counseling; assistance for students with disabilities; bookstore; computer lab; computer-assisted instruction; e-mail services; externships; housing assistance; Internet; learning resource lab; library services; nursing audio-visuals; tutoring.

Library Facilities 1.2 million volumes (40,000 in health, 4,000 in nursing); 5,937 periodical subscriptions (3,000 health-care related).

BACCALAUREATE PROGRAMS

Degree BScN

Available Programs RN Baccalaureate.

Site Options Longueuil, QC.

Study Options Full-time and part-time.

Program Entrance Requirements Transcript of college record, high school chemistry, 4 years high school math, immunizations, professional liability insurance/malpractice insurance, RN licensure. Transfer students are accepted. **Application** *Deadline:* 3/1 (freshmen). *Notification:* continuous until 5/15 (freshmen). *Application fee:* CAN$50.

Advanced Placement Credit given for nursing courses completed elsewhere dependent upon specific evaluations.

Expenses (2004–05) *Room and board:* room only: CAN$1800 per academic year. *Required fees:* full-time CAN$2400; part-time CAN$155 per credit.

Financial Aid *Gift aid (need-based):* state, private, college/university gift aid from institutional funds. *Loans:* state, college/university. *Work-Study:* part-time campus jobs. *Application deadline:* 3/31.

Contact Mrs. Lise R. Talbot, Assistant Dean and Director, Department of Nursing, Université de Sherbrooke, 3001, 12e Avenue Nord, Sherbrooke, QC J1H 5N4. *Telephone:* 819-563-5365. *Fax:* 819-820-6816. *E-mail:* lise.talbot@USherbrooke.ca.

GRADUATE PROGRAMS

Expenses (2004–05) *Room and board:* room only: CAN$1800 per academic year. *Required fees:* full-time CAN$900.

Contact Dr. Frances Gallagher, Coordinator, Department of Nursing, Université de Sherbrooke, 3001, 12e Avenue Nord, Sherbrooke, QC J1H 5N4. *Telephone:* 819-564-5354. *Fax:* 819-820-6816. *E-mail:* Frances.Gallagher@USherbrooke.ca.

MASTER'S DEGREE PROGRAM

Degree M Sc

Available Programs Master's.

Concentrations Available *Clinical nurse specialist programs in:* acute care, community health, family health, gerontology.

Site Options Longueuil, QC.

Study Options Full-time and part-time.

Program Entrance Requirements Transcript of college record, interview, 3 letters of recommendation, nursing research course, professional liability insurance/malpractice insurance, resume.

Degree Requirements 45 total credit hours, thesis or project.

DOCTORAL DEGREE PROGRAM

Degree PhD

Available Programs Doctorate.

Areas of Study Advanced practice nursing, aging, biology of health and illness, clinical practice, community health, critical care, family health, gerontology, health promotion/disease prevention, human health and illness, illness and transition, information systems, maternity-newborn, neuro-behavior, nurse case management, nursing administration, nursing education, nursing policy, nursing research, nursing science, oncology, women's health.

Site Options Longueuil, QC.

Program Entrance Requirements Clinical experience, interview, 3 letters of recommendation, MSN or equivalent, statistics course, vita, writing sample.

Degree Requirements 90 total credit hours, dissertation, oral exam, written exam.

POSTDOCTORAL PROGRAM

Postdoctoral Program Contact Dr. Lise R. Talbot, Assistant Dean and Director, Department of Nursing, Université de Sherbrooke, 3001, 12e Avenue Nord, Sherbrooke, QC J1H 5N4. *Telephone:* 819-564-5365. *Fax:* 819-820-6816. *E-mail:* Lise.Talbot@usherbrooke.ca.

Université du Québec à Chicoutimi

Program in Nursing
Chicoutimi, Quebec

Founded in 1969

DEGREES • BNSC • MSN

Nursing Program Faculty 8 (1% with doctorates).

Baccalaureate Enrollment 600
Women 90% **Men** 10% **Minority** 5% **Part-time** 75%

Graduate Enrollment 30
Women 90% **Men** 10% **Minority** 1% **Part-time** 100%

Nursing Student Activities Student Nurses' Association.

Nursing Student Resources Academic advising; academic or career counseling; assistance for students with disabilities; bookstore; campus computer network; computer lab; computer-assisted instruction; e-mail services; employment services for current students; externships; housing assistance; Internet; learning resource lab; library services; nursing audio-visuals; resume preparation assistance; skills, simulation, or other laboratory; tutoring; unpaid internships.

Library Facilities 689,214 volumes; 5,092 periodical subscriptions.

BACCALAUREATE PROGRAMS

Degree BNSc

Available Programs Accelerated RN Baccalaureate; RN Baccalaureate.

Site Options Alma, PQ. *Distance Learning:* Sept-Iles, PQ; St. Felicien, PQ.

Study Options Full-time and part-time.

Program Entrance Requirements Minimum overall college GPA, health exam, immunizations, interview. Transfer students are accepted. **Application** *Deadline:* 3/1 (freshmen). *Notification:* 5/15 (freshmen).

Advanced Placement Credit given for nursing courses completed elsewhere dependent upon specific evaluations.

Financial Aid *Gift aid (need-based):* private, college/university gift aid from institutional funds. *Loans:* college/university. *Work-Study:* part-time campus jobs.

Contact Mme. Celine L'Esperance, Secretariat, Program in Nursing, Université du Québec à Chicoutimi, 555 Boulevard de l'Universite, Chicoutimi, QC G7H 2B1. *Telephone:* 418-545-5011 Ext. 5315. *Fax:* 418-545-5012.

GRADUATE PROGRAMS

Contact Francoise Courville, Program in Nursing, Université du Québec à Chicoutimi, 555 Boulevard de l'Université, Chicoutimi, QC G7H 2B1. *Telephone:* 418-545-5011 Ext. 2374. *Fax:* 418-545-5012. *E-mail:* francoise_courville@uqac.ca.

Université du Québec à Chicoutimi (continued)

MASTER'S DEGREE PROGRAM

Degree MSN

Available Programs Accelerated RN to Master's; RN to Master's.

Concentrations Available *Clinical nurse specialist programs in:* acute care, adult health, cardiovascular, community health, critical care, family health, gerontology, home health care, maternity-newborn, medical-surgical, occupational health, oncology, parent-child, pediatric, perinatal, psychiatric/mental health, public health, rehabilitation, school health, women's health.

Site Options Alma, PQ. *Distance Learning:* St. Felicien, PQ.

Study Options Part-time.

Program Entrance Requirements Clinical experience, minimum overall college GPA of 3.0, transcript of college record, written essay, interview, 3 letters of recommendation, nursing research course, professional liability insurance/malpractice insurance, statistics course.

Advanced Placement Credit given for nursing courses completed elsewhere dependent upon specific evaluations.

Degree Requirements 45 total credit hours, thesis or project.

Université du Québec à Rimouski

Program in Nursing
Rimouski, Quebec

http://www.uquebec.ca/mscinf/

Founded in 1973

DEGREES • BSCN • M SC N

Nursing Program Faculty 8 (38% with doctorates).

Baccalaureate Enrollment 750
Women 90% **Men** 10% **Part-time** 74%

Graduate Enrollment 13
Women 93% **Men** 7% **Part-time** 100%

Nursing Student Activities Student Nurses' Association.

Nursing Student Resources Academic advising; academic or career counseling; assistance for students with disabilities; bookstore; campus computer network; career placement assistance; computer lab; daycare for children of students; e-mail services; employment services for current students; housing assistance; Internet; learning resource lab; library services; nursing audiovisuals; other; placement services for program completers; resume preparation assistance; skills, simulation, or other laboratory; tutoring.

Library Facilities 263,142 volumes (5,200 in health, 1,100 in nursing); 3,951 periodical subscriptions (1,300 health-care related).

BACCALAUREATE PROGRAMS

Degree BScN

Available Programs RN Baccalaureate.

Site Options Levis, QC.

Study Options Full-time and part-time.

Program Entrance Requirements Transcript of college record, professional liability insurance/malpractice insurance, prerequisite course work. Transfer students are accepted. **Application** *Deadline:* 3/1 (freshmen). *Notification:* 5/15 (freshmen).

Advanced Placement Credit by examination available.

Expenses (2003–04) *Tuition, state resident:* full-time CAN$1884; part-time CAN$208 per course. *Tuition, nonresident:* full-time CAN$4339; part-time CAN$440 per course. *International tuition:* CAN$10,734 full-time. *Room and board:* room only: CAN$2500 per academic year. *Required fees:* part-time CAN$91 per credit; part-time CAN$942 per term.

Financial Aid 8% of baccalaureate students in nursing programs received some form of financial aid in 2002–03. *Loans:* college/university.

Contact Nicole Allard, Directrice, Program in Nursing, Université du Québec à Rimouski, 300 allée des Ursulines, Rimouski, QC G5L 3A1. *Telephone:* 418-723-1986 Ext. 1730. *Fax:* 418-724-1849. *E-mail:* nicole_allard@uqar.qc.ca.

GRADUATE PROGRAMS

Expenses (2003–04) *Tuition, state resident:* full-time CAN$2766; part-time CAN$922 per trimester. *Tuition, nonresident:* full-time CAN$3331; part-time CAN$1110 per trimester. *International tuition:* CAN$14,466 full-time. *Room and board:* room only: CAN$2500 per academic year.

Financial Aid 17% of graduate students in nursing programs received some form of financial aid in 2002–03.

Contact Dr. Nicole Ouellet, Directrice, Program in Nursing, Université du Québec à Rimouski, 300 allée des Ursulines, Rimouski, QC G5H 3K6. *Telephone:* 418-723-1986 Ext. 1874. *Fax:* 418-724-1849. *E-mail:* nicole_ouellet@uqar.qc.ca.

MASTER'S DEGREE PROGRAM

Degree M Sc N

Available Programs Master's.

Concentrations Available *Clinical nurse specialist programs in:* community health, critical care, gerontology, psychiatric/mental health.

Study Options Full-time and part-time.

Program Entrance Requirements Clinical experience, transcript of college record, interview, 3 letters of recommendation, nursing research course, prerequisite course work, statistics course.

Advanced Placement Credit given for nursing courses completed elsewhere dependent upon specific evaluations.

Degree Requirements 45 total credit hours, thesis or project.

CONTINUING EDUCATION PROGRAM

Contact Mme. Huguette Lagacé, Coordonnatrice, Program in Nursing, Université du Québec à Rimouski, 300 allée des Ursulines, Rimouski, QC G5L 3A1. *Telephone:* 418-723-1986 Ext. 1818. *Fax:* 418-724-1525. *E-mail:* formationcontinue@uqar.qc.ca.

Université du Québec à Trois-Rivières

Program in Nursing
Trois-Rivières, Quebec

Founded in 1969

DEGREES • BSN • MSN

Library Facilities 464,338 volumes.

BACCALAUREATE PROGRAMS

Degree BSN

Program Entrance Requirements Transfer students are accepted. **Application** *Deadline:* 3/1 (freshmen). *Notification:* 6/1 (freshmen). *Application fee:* CAN$30.

Contact Dr. Michele Côté, Directrice, Program in Nursing, Université du Québec à Trois-Rivières, Casier Postal 500, Trois Rivieres, QC G9A 5H7. *Telephone:* 819-376-5011 Ext. 3471. *Fax:* 819-376-5218. *E-mail:* michele_cote@uqtr.ca.

GRADUATE PROGRAMS

Contact Lisette Richard, Program Contact, Program in Nursing, Université du Québec à Trois-Rivières, Casier Postal 500, Trois Rivieres, QC G9A 5H7. *Telephone:* 819-376-5011 Ext. 3464. *E-mail:* Lisette_Richard@uqtr.ca.

MASTER'S DEGREE PROGRAM

Degree MSN

Université du Québec en Abitibi-Témiscamingue

Département des sciences sociales et de la santé
Rouyn-Noranda, Quebec

http://www.uqat.uquebec.ca/gestac/prg/7855.asp

Founded in 1983

DEGREE • BN

Nursing Program Faculty 12.
Baccalaureate Enrollment 78
Women 95% **Men** 5% **Part-time** 64%

Nursing Student Resources Academic advising; assistance for students with disabilities; bookstore; campus computer network; computer lab; computer-assisted instruction; housing assistance; Internet; library services; resume preparation assistance; skills, simulation, or other laboratory.

Library Facilities 135,882 volumes (3,239 in health, 715 in nursing); 302 periodical subscriptions (17 health-care related).

BACCALAUREATE PROGRAMS

Degree BN

Program Entrance Requirements Transfer students are accepted. **Application** *Deadline:* rolling (freshmen). *Notification:* 5/15 (freshmen). *Application fee:* CAN$30.

Expenses (2003–04) *Tuition, state resident:* full-time CAN$1858; part-time CAN$221 per course. *Tuition, nonresident:* full-time CAN$1858; part-time CAN$221 per course. *Required fees:* part-time CAN$56 per credit; part-time CAN$929 per term.

Financial Aid 60% of baccalaureate students in nursing programs received some form of financial aid in 2002–03. *Loans:* college/university.

Contact Lyne Fecteau, Professeure, Département des sciences sociales et de la santé, Université du Québec en Abitibi-Témiscamingue, 445 Boulevard de l'Université, Rouyn-Noranda, QC J9X 5E4. *Telephone:* 819-762-0971 Ext. 2370. *Fax:* 819-797-4727. *E-mail:* lyne.fecteau@uqat.ca.

Université du Québec en Outaouais

Département des Sciences Infirmières
Gatineau, Quebec

Founded in 1981

DEGREES • BSCN • M SC N

Nursing Program Faculty 10 (60% with doctorates).
Baccalaureate Enrollment 450
Women 90% **Men** 10% **Minority** 20% **International** 1% **Part-time** 90%
Graduate Enrollment 30
Women 97% **Men** 3% **Minority** 3% **Part-time** 97%

Nursing Student Activities Student Nurses' Association.

Nursing Student Resources Academic advising; academic or career counseling; bookstore; campus computer network; computer lab; daycare for children of students; e-mail services; employment services for current students; externships; housing assistance; Internet; learning resource lab; library services; nursing audiovisuals; placement services for program completers; skills, simulation, or other laboratory.

Library Facilities 230,910 volumes; 12,351 periodical subscriptions.

BACCALAUREATE PROGRAMS

Degree BScN

Available Programs ADN to Baccalaureate; Generic Baccalaureate; RN Baccalaureate.

Site Options St-Jerome, PQ; Laval, PQ; Mont-Laurier, PQ.

Study Options Full-time.

Program Entrance Requirements CPR certification, high school chemistry, immunizations, interview, RN licensure. Transfer students are accepted. **Application** *Deadline:* 3/1 (freshmen). *Notification:* 5/15 (freshmen).

Advanced Placement Credit by examination available. Credit given for nursing courses completed elsewhere dependent upon specific evaluations.

Expenses (2003–04) *Tuition, state resident:* full-time CAN$2340; part-time CAN$336 per course. *Required fees:* full-time CAN$2340; part-time CAN$112 per credit; part-time CAN$1170 per term.

Financial Aid *Loans:* college/university.

Contact Chantal Saint-Pierre, Directrice, Département des Sciences Infirmières, Université du Québec en Outaouais, Office: C-3336, Hull, QC J8X 3X7. *Telephone:* 819-595-3900 Ext. 2345. *Fax:* 819-595-3801. *E-mail:* chantal.st-pierre@uqo.ca.

GRADUATE PROGRAMS

Expenses (2003–04) *Tuition, state resident:* part-time CAN$224 per course. *Tuition, nonresident:* .

Contact Ms. Chantal Saint-Pierre, Directrice, Module des sciences de la sante, Département des Sciences Infirmières, Université du Québec en Outaouais, Office: D-0414, Gatineau, QC J8X 3X7. *Telephone:* 819-595-3900 Ext. 2344. *Fax:* 819-595-3801. *E-mail:* chantal.st-pierre@uqo.ca.

MASTER'S DEGREE PROGRAM

Degree M Sc N

Available Programs Master's.

Concentrations Available *Clinical nurse specialist programs in:* community health, critical care, psychiatric/mental health, rehabilitation.

Study Options Full-time and part-time.

Program Entrance Requirements Computer literacy, 3 letters of recommendation, nursing research course, resume, statistics course.

Advanced Placement Credit given for nursing courses completed elsewhere dependent upon specific evaluations.

Degree Requirements 45 total credit hours, thesis or project.

Université Laval

Faculty of Nursing
Québec, Quebec

http://www.fsi.ulaval.ca

Founded in 1852

DEGREES • BSCN • MSN • PHD

Nursing Program Faculty 25 (64% with doctorates).

Library Facilities 2.8 million volumes (118,994 in health, 3,781 in nursing); 13,928 periodical subscriptions (624 health-care related).

BACCALAUREATE PROGRAMS

Degree BScN

Program Entrance Requirements Transfer students are accepted. **Application** *Deadline:* 3/1 (freshmen), 5/1 (transfer). *Application fee:* CAN$30.

Contact Ms. Lucie Turgeon-Rheault, Program Director, Faculty of Nursing, Université Laval, Sainte-Foy, QC G1K 7P4. *Telephone:* 418-656-2131 Ext. 3388. *Fax:* 418-656-7747. *E-mail:* lucie.turgeon-rheault@fsi.ulaval.ca.

GRADUATE PROGRAMS

Financial Aid Fellowships (averaging $5,000 per year), research assistantships (averaging $6,500 per year), teaching assistantships (averaging $6,500 per year) were awarded; scholarships, traineeships, and tuition waivers (partial) also available.

Contact Faculty of Nursing, Faculty of Nursing, Université Laval, Pavillion Paul-Comtois, Bureau 4106, Sainte-Foy, QC G1K 7P4. *Telephone:* 418-656-3356. *Fax:* 418-656-7304. *E-mail:* fsi@fsi.ulaval.ca.

MASTER'S DEGREE PROGRAM

Degree MSN

Concentrations Available *Nurse practitioner programs in:* community health.

Program Entrance Requirements Clinical experience, 3 letters of recommendation, nursing research course, resume, statistics course, French exam. *Application deadline:* For fall admission, 2/1 (priority date); for winter admission, 11/1 (priority date); for spring admission, 4/1 (priority date). Applications are processed on a rolling basis. *Application fee:* $30.

Degree Requirements 48 total credit hours.

Université Laval (continued)

DOCTORAL DEGREE PROGRAM

Degree PhD

Areas of Study Community health.

CONTINUING EDUCATION PROGRAM

Contact Mariette Blais, Program Contact, Faculty of Nursing, Université Laval, Sainte-Foy, QC G1K 7P4. *Telephone:* 418-656-2131 Ext. 2633. *Fax:* 418-656-7747. *E-mail:* Mariette.Blais@fsi.ulaval.ca.

SASKATCHEWAN

University of Saskatchewan

College of Nursing
Saskatoon, Saskatchewan

http://www.usask.ca/nursing/

Founded in 1907

DEGREES • BSN • MN

Nursing Program Faculty 84 (35% with doctorates).

Baccalaureate Enrollment 1,174 **Women** 93% **Men** 7% **Minority** 5% **Part-time** 17%

Graduate Enrollment 48
Women 94% **Men** 6% **Minority** 2% **Part-time** 62%

Nursing Student Activities Student Nurses' Association.

Nursing Student Resources Academic advising; academic or career counseling; assistance for students with disabilities; bookstore; campus computer network; computer lab; computer-assisted instruction; daycare for children of students; e-mail services; employment services for current students; interactive nursing skills videos; Internet; learning resource lab; library services; nursing audiovisuals; remedial services; resume preparation assistance; skills, simulation, or other laboratory; tutoring.

Library Facilities 1.8 million volumes (120,000 in health, 7,000 in nursing); 16,900 periodical subscriptions (1,000 health-care related).

BACCALAUREATE PROGRAMS

Degree BSN

Available Programs Accelerated Baccalaureate; Accelerated RN Baccalaureate; Generic Baccalaureate; RN Baccalaureate; RPN to Baccalaureate.

Site Options Prince Albert, SK; Regina , SK; Saskatoon , SK.

Study Options Full-time and part-time.

Program Entrance Requirements Transcript of college record, high school biology, high school chemistry, 4 years high school math, 4 years high school science, high school transcript, minimum high school GPA of 2.0. Transfer students are accepted. **Application** *Deadline:* 5/15 (freshmen), 5/15 (transfer). *Early decision:* 5/15. *Notification:* continuous (freshmen). *Application fee:* CAN$75.

Advanced Placement Credit given for nursing courses completed elsewhere dependent upon specific evaluations.

Expenses (2003–04) *Tuition, state resident:* full-time CAN$4680; part-time CAN$156 per credit hour. *Tuition, nonresident:* full-time CAN$4680; part-time CAN$156 per credit hour. *International tuition:* CAN$11,700 full-time. *Room and board:* CAN$4783; room only: CAN$1470 per academic year. *Required fees:* full-time CAN$395; part-time CAN$106 per term.

Financial Aid 80% of baccalaureate students in nursing programs received some form of financial aid in 2002–03. *Gift aid (need-based):* private, college/university gift aid from institutional funds. *Loans:* college/university, Canadian Student Loans, Provincial Loans. *Application deadline:* 4/1.

Contact Ms. Eileen Zagiel, Admissions and Records Secretary, College of Nursing, University of Saskatchewan, 107 Wiggins Road, Saskatoon, SK S7N 5E5. *Telephone:* 306-966-6231. *Fax:* 306-966-6621. *E-mail:* eileen.zagiel@usask.ca.

GRADUATE PROGRAMS

Expenses (2003–04) *Tuition, state resident:* full-time CAN$4830; part-time CAN$161 per credit hour. *Tuition, nonresident:* full-time CAN$4830; part-time CAN$161 per credit hour. *Room and board:* CAN$4783; room only: CAN$1470 per academic year. *Required fees:* full-time CAN$489; part-time CAN$103 per term.

Financial Aid 30% of graduate students in nursing programs received some form of financial aid in 2002–03. Fellowships, research assistantships, teaching assistantships available. *Financial aid application deadline:* 1/31.

Contact Dr. Gail Laing, Chairperson, Graduate Program, College of Nursing, University of Saskatchewan, 107 Wiggins Road, Saskatoon, SK S7N 5E5. *Telephone:* 306-966-6229. *Fax:* 306-966-1745. *E-mail:* gail.laing@sask.usask.ca.

MASTER'S DEGREE PROGRAM

Degree MN

Available Programs Master's.

Concentrations Available *Clinical nurse specialist programs in:* psychiatric/mental health. *Nurse practitioner programs in:* psychiatric/mental health.

Study Options Full-time and part-time.

Program Entrance Requirements Clinical experience, minimum overall college GPA of 2.5, transcript of college record, interview, 3 letters of recommendation, nursing research course, statistics course. *Application deadline:* For fall admission, 7/1 (priority date). Applications are processed on a rolling basis. *Application fee:* $50.

Advanced Placement Credit given for nursing courses completed elsewhere dependent upon specific evaluations.

Degree Requirements 24 total credit hours, thesis or project.

CONTINUING EDUCATION PROGRAM

Contact Prof. Barbara Smith, Director, College of Nursing, University of Saskatchewan, Continuing Nursing Education, Box 60000 RPO, Saskatoon, SK S7N 4J8. *Telephone:* 306-966-6223. *Fax:* 306-866-7673. *E-mail:* smithb@sask.usask.ca.

IN-DEPTH DESCRIPTIONS OF NURSING PROGRAMS

Baker University
School of Nursing
Baldwin City, Kansas

THE UNIVERSITY

Baker University was established in 1858 as the first four-year college in the state of Kansas. With 146 years of tradition, Baker embodies an unusual blend of innovation, tradition, quality, and community. Affiliated with the United Methodist Church, the University is dedicated to excellence in liberal and professional education, to the integration of learning with faith and values, and to the personal development of each community member.

The University attracts the serious student who expects to encounter challenge in the classroom but also enjoys participating in a multitude of extracurricular activities—sports, forensics, radio, the newspaper, theater, music, and departmental and special interest organizations.

THE SCHOOL OF NURSING

The Baker University School of Nursing was established in the Pozez Education Center at Stormont-Vail Health*Care* in Topeka, Kansas, to provide much-needed nursing education for the students in Baker's service region. The School of Nursing offers an academic program leading to a baccalaureate degree. The generic baccalaureate degree program in nursing comprises four full-time semesters of upper-division study after completion of general education requirements. A baccalaureate degree completion program for registered nurses is composed of one year of full-time study or part-time study over several semesters. Students may enter the nursing program during the fall or spring semester.

The mission of Baker University School of Nursing is to prepare nurses for professional practice as providers of general health care for individuals, families, and communities within the global environment. As an institution related to the United Methodist Church, the School embodies the belief that the integration of faith and values into the curriculum promotes the intellectual growth and personal development of each individual. The nurse will have the ability to communicate; think critically; perform clinical skills competently; participate in lifelong education; assume the roles of care provider, manager, and member of a profession; and make ethical decisions based on a sound value system and broad knowledge base.

While course demands are rigorous, the goals of nursing education at Baker are accomplished in a climate of collaboration and cooperation among faculty members and students—a hallmark of the Baker experience. Classes are small and friendly. The teacher-student ratio is approximately 1:8. Baker takes a holistic approach to nursing, teaching the art and science of nursing to those who want to make a critical difference in a profession that is more important today than ever before.

Baker University is accredited by the Higher Learning Commission of the North Central Association of Colleges and Schools and the Kansas State Board of Education. The School of Nursing program is accredited by the Commission on Collegiate Nursing Education and approved by the Kansas State Board of Nursing.

PROGRAMS OF STUDY

Baker University offers two degree tracks in nursing education. Both lead to a Bachelor of Science in Nursing (B.S.N.) degree. One program is for students who have not practiced in the nursing profession. They have attended college for two years either at Baker's College of Arts and Sciences in Baldwin City or elsewhere and are accepted for their final two years of study into Baker's School of Nursing.

The other program is for practicing nurses who wish to complete their four-year degree. This program offers courses at convenient times and addresses topics in a way that is most meaningful to the group.

ACADEMIC FACILITIES

The Pozez Education Center at Stormont-Vail Health*Care* in Topeka, Kansas, provides both administrative offices and excellent educational facilities for the School of Nursing. Large modern classrooms, fully equipped clinical laboratories, and individual study areas provide functional and appealing space. A computer lab is accessible to students for both word processing and interactive tutorial programs in nursing. The Stauffer Health Science Library provides a strong learning resource for both students and faculty members. The library is located on the ground level of the Pozez Education Center.

LOCATION

The main campus of Baker University and home of the College of Arts and Sciences is in Baldwin City, Kansas, a beautiful small community of tree-lined streets and rich tradition that is about 40 miles southwest of Kansas City and 40 miles southeast of Topeka. The historic campus is only a few blocks south of the old Santa Fe Trail, now followed by U.S. Highway 56. It is easily accessible from north or south by U.S. 59 and from east or west by U.S. 56.

The School of Nursing is located in the Pozez Education Center of Stormont-Vail Health*Care* in Topeka. This modern facility provides administrative offices, classrooms, laboratories, and a library.

STUDENT SERVICES

Baker University offers many services to meet individual student needs. These include orientation, career counseling and placement, personal counseling, tutoring, and other academic support services. Academic support resources available to students in the School of Nursing include academic advising, tutoring, counseling, orientation, and testing. In addition, nursing students are encouraged to use, at no cost, the Mabee Health and Fitness Center.

Each student is assigned a faculty adviser upon entering the nursing program. The adviser provides the student with assistance in academic program planning and matters pertaining to academic work and can also provide assistance with study habits and personal adjustment problems.

THE NURSING STUDENT GROUP

There are approximately 125 students enrolled in the undergraduate nursing program. Approximately 90 percent are women and 8 percent are members of minority groups. Virtually all graduates find employment within three months of graduation, and most secure jobs while they are still in school.

COSTS

Tuition for the 2004–05 academic year for full-time students (12–18 credit hours) at Baker University School of Nursing was $10,250 per year. Part-time students paid $300 per credit hour. Full-time students should plan to spend up to $500 per semester for books and supplies.

FINANCIAL AID

Baker University is committed to helping students and parents find resources to finance their university experience. Approximately 95 percent of Baker's undergraduate students receive some form of financial assistance. Financial need is met through a combination of scholarships, grants, and loans. By completing the Free Application for Federal Student Aid (FAFSA), a student is considered for all federal, state, and institutional funds administered by Baker.

APPLYING

Students may be admitted to the nursing program after two years of study in Baker's College of Arts and Sciences or after successful completion of program requirements at other universities.

The Student Affairs Committee selects students from applicants who best meet requirements. All program prerequisites must be completed with a grade of C or higher, with an overall prerequisite cumulative GPA of at least 2.7. Each individual is considered for admission based on the following factors: academic history, prerequisite cumulative GPA, math and science prerequisite GPA, number of prerequisite courses completed, other degrees conferred, and interview with faculty. Applicants who do not meet all School of Nursing admission requirements may be reviewed for further consideration by the Student Affairs Committee upon request by the applicant.

For further information about applying to the College of Arts and Sciences, applicants should refer to *Peterson's Guide to Four-Year Colleges* or to the Baker Web site at http://www.bakeru.edu.

The School of Nursing admits students in both the fall and spring semesters. Baker College of Arts and Sciences students receive priority admission to the nursing school. Interested applicants should contact Debbie Wallace, Student Affairs Specialist, 785-354-5850 or 888-866-4242 (toll-free).

CORRESPONDENCE AND INFORMATION:

Baker University
School of Nursing
Stormont-Vail Health*Care* Campus
1500 Southwest 10th Street
Topeka, Kansas 66604-1351
Telephone: 785-354-5851
800-866-4242 (toll-free)

Debbie Wallace
Student Affairs Specialist
School of Nursing
Telephone: 785-354-5850
888-866-4242 (toll-free)
E-mail: debbie.wallace@stormontvail.org

Chris Claussen
Associate Director of Admissions
Telephone: 785-594-8324
800-873-4282 (toll-free)
E-mail: chris.claussen@bakeru.edu

Casey Wright
Financial Aid Counselor/Student Loan Processor
Telephone: 785-594-8348
800-873-4282 (toll-free)
E-mail: casey.wright@bakeru.edu

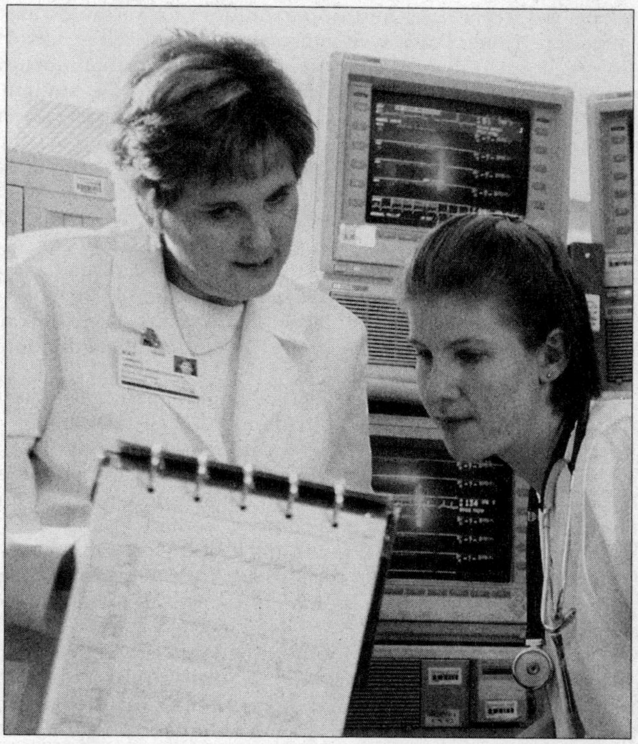

Baker University nursing students are in clinical settings in their first semester of the program.

Blessing-Rieman College of Nursing

Quincy, Illinois

THE COLLEGE

Blessing-Rieman College of Nursing (B-RCN) prides itself on personal attention tailored to each student's needs and the high-quality nursing education it has offered for more than 100 years. The Blessing Hospital School of Nursing, one of the first nursing schools in the state of Illinois, was founded in 1891 to train nurses for area health-care needs. Today, it is a small private college offering a Bachelor of Science in Nursing (B.S.N.) degree conferred jointly with a partner college, either Culver-Stockton College in Canton, Missouri, or Quincy University in Quincy, Illinois. This flexibility offers students many options not available from other programs while providing a high-quality college education and excellent nursing education at a regional medical center.

To learn more about a career in nursing, students should contact the Admissions Department to reserve a space at "Nursing in Action," a half-day program designed to show students the advantages and opportunities of a versatile career in nursing. Nurse Shadow visits are also offered. These involve following a staff nurse in the hospital during a normal morning or afternoon. Campus tours can be arranged at students' convenience by contacting the Admissions Office (phone number listed below).

Blessing-Rieman is accredited by the National League for Nursing Accrediting Commission, the Commission on Collegiate Nursing Education, and the Higher Learning Commission (HLC) of the North Central Association of Colleges and Schools. Students participate in the Student Nurse Organization and act as representatives on College committees. The College offers apartments for upper-level students, a state-of-the-art child-care facility, a fitness center, and 50 percent meal discounts at the hospital cafeteria.

Culver-Stockton College (C-SC) is an independent, private college affiliated with the Christian Church (Disciples of Christ). Chartered in 1853, the scenic campus overlooks the Mississippi River in Canton, Missouri, 20 miles from Quincy, Illinois. The college offers music, theater, intercollegiate and intramural sports, student government, residence and dining halls, numerous clubs and organizations, and Greek life. Faculty members have received state recognition for the quality of their teaching. Culver-Stockton is accredited by HLC and other agencies.

Quincy University (QU), founded by Franciscans in 1860, is an independent institution rooted in the Catholic tradition. Cultural, social, and recreational opportunities include intercollegiate sports, a new fitness center with an indoor pool, fine arts, student government, radio and TV studios, and housing options. QU is accredited by HLC and other agencies.

PROGRAM OF STUDY

Nursing courses are designed to help students acquire the knowledge, skills, and values needed to become professional nurses fully equipped to handle today's practice. Graduates are also prepared for leadership positions or further education in specialty fields. The joint Bachelor of Science in Nursing degree program for new college students is typically four years of study. Students are nursing majors all four years, and nursing classes begin in the freshman year. All freshman classes are provided on the partner campus, and students are required to live on campus. During the sophomore year, students come together for nursing classes on the Blessing-Rieman campus but continue to live on the partner campus. Nursing clinical experiences begin in the sophomore year at Blessing Hospital and other area health-care agencies. In the junior and senior years, students have usually completed most general education courses on the partner campus and may choose to live on the Blessing campus while focusing more on nursing courses and clinicals. Junior-level nursing instruction includes medical-surgical, psychiatric, obstetrical, and pediatric course work and clinicals. Senior nursing courses include community health, acute-care nursing, professionalism, leadership, and research. Blessing-Rieman has separate tracks for LPNs and RNs who wish to complete their B.S.N. degree.

The joint-degree program with Culver-Stockton requires 124 semester hours, including English, speech, physical education, and Christian heritage core courses; computer science, fine arts, social science, and humanities general education courses; natural science, mathematics, psychology, and philosophy support courses; and 61 hours of nursing courses.

The joint-degree program with Quincy University requires 126 semester hours, including English, social sciences, humanities, fine arts, theology, and physical education general education courses; computer science and statistics tool courses; natural science and speech support courses; and 61 hours of nursing courses.

AFFILIATIONS WITH HEALTH-CARE FACILITIES

Blessing-Rieman is located on the campus of Blessing Hospital, a fully accredited major medical facility serving the surrounding 100-mile radius. Students have direct access to clinical areas of the hospital, with College instructors and hospital staff members providing guidance. Nearby clinics, health departments, nursing homes, and other health agencies offer additional clinical experiences.

ACADEMIC FACILITIES

Blessing-Rieman has computer-networked, air-conditioned classrooms and offices. A student lounge and locker room are adjacent to the classrooms. The Blessing Health Professions Library provides an extensive collection of books, journals, and audiovisual teaching materials as well as study areas and a computer lab open to students that provides software, Internet access, online research databases, and other resources. Students on the C-SC and QU campuses also have access to computers and libraries equipped with extensive resources.

Hands-on training in the College Skills Lab is provided prior to clinical experience. After demonstration by the Lab Coordinator, students use actual clinical equipment in a simulated hospital setting to practice nursing skills and clinical decision making. Skills Lab practice allows students to approach actual clinical experiences with confidence.

LOCATION

Blessing-Rieman College of Nursing is located in Quincy, Illinois, a city of around 45,000 people, on the bluff overlooking the Mississippi River in west-central Illinois. The city is known for its history, architecture, arts, and quality of life. The Adams County seat, Quincy has an Amtrak station, regional airport, TV and radio stations, convention center, numerous hotels and restaurants, shopping malls, theaters, and a symphony orchestra, and it is the site of fairs, festivals, and cultural events.

STUDENT SERVICES

One of the greatest benefits of the joint programs in nursing is that throughout their four-year concurrent enrollment, students enjoy all of the services and activities of Blessing-Rieman and the partnering institution as well as those of Blessing Hospital, whose state-of-the-art child-care center and fitness center are available for students.

THE NURSING STUDENT GROUP

Most students receive some form of financial aid. Many students choose to hold part-time jobs, including some who work in the College as Student Assistants. Enrollment varies from 175 to 250 students. Five to 10 percent of the students are men, and about 5 percent are members of minority groups. Of the graduates who seek employment, 100 percent have a position before graduation.

COSTS

According to the College's partnership agreements, tuition and fees for the first two years are set by the partner institutions, and the last two years are set by B-RCN. Approximate tuition for the Culver-Stockton program is $13,200 and the Quincy University program is about $17,140. B-RCN tuition is $8681 for the junior and senior years. Students should check with the Admissions Office for current rates.

FINANCIAL AID

Significant scholarships and financial aid (federal, local, state, and private) are available at each institution, whether need-based and/or for academic achievement. Students should contact the admissions office for further information.

APPLYING

Qualifications for acceptance as a nursing major include a minimum 3.0 high school GPA, graduation in the upper half of the class, and a composite ACT score of at least 22 or an SAT I combined score of at least 920. High school courses must include 4 units of English; at least 2 units of science, including biology and chemistry; 3 units of social science; and 2 units of math, including 1 unit of algebra. Nontraditional students should contact the admissions office for requirements.

CORRESPONDENCE AND INFORMATION:

Blessing-Rieman College of Nursing
Broadway at 11th
Quincy, Illinois 62305-7005
Telephone: 217-228-5520
800-877-9140 Ext. 6961 or 6964 (toll-free)
E-mail: admissions@brcn.edu
World Wide Web: http://www.brcn.edu

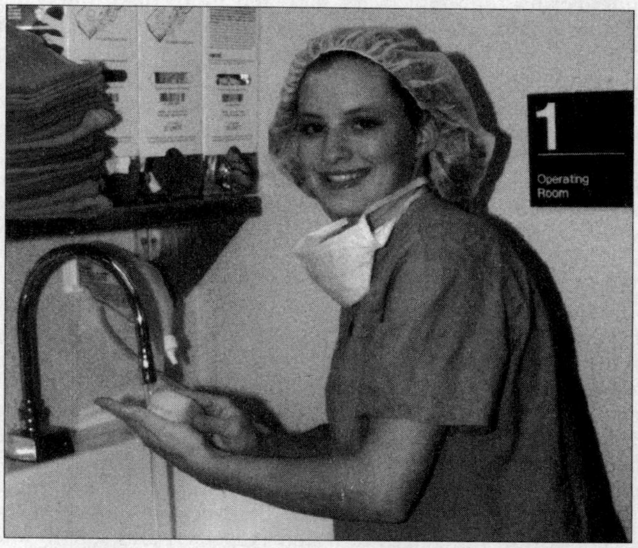

Nursing clinical experiences take place at Blessing Hospital and at other area health-care agencies.

Boston College
William F. Connell School of Nursing
Chestnut Hill, Massachusetts

THE COLLEGE
Boston College is a coeducational university with an average population of 8,900 undergraduate students and 4,700 graduate students who represent every state and more than ninety-nine countries. Founded in 1863, it is one of the oldest Jesuit-affiliated universities in the country and one of the largest private universities in the nation.

The reputation of the university, securely established after more than a century of proven excellence, continues to gain stature. In recent years, surveys undertaken by periodicals such as *Barron's* and *U.S. News & World Report* have consistently ranked Boston College among the top colleges and universities in the nation and as one of the best values in higher education.

THE SCHOOL OF NURSING
Founded in 1947, the Boston College William F. Connell School of Nursing is one of the largest Jesuit schools of nursing. The baccalaureate and master's programs are accredited by the Commission on Collegiate Nursing Education. Currently, the School of Nursing offers baccalaureate, master's, master's entry (for students with a degree in a field other than nursing), or RN/M.S., M.S./M.B.A., M.S./M.A., Ph.D., and continuing education programs. Graduates of the programs are highly successful in clinical, academic, administrative, and research careers in nursing. They are widely respected and sought after for regional, national, and international positions.

The School of Nursing has 44 full-time faculty members teaching and advising in both the undergraduate and graduate programs. They are highly qualified, clinically and academically, and many are certified for advanced clinical practice. More than 90 percent of the tenured and tenure-track faculty members hold an earned doctorate in nursing or in related fields and are actively engaged in research. The faculty is widely published and includes nursing scholars who are recognized as experts and leaders in their fields both nationally and internationally.

PROGRAMS OF STUDY
The baccalaureate program is a full-time, four-year program of study. The thirty-eight-course curriculum that is required for graduation consists of university core requirements; electives; nursing courses, which include simulated and audiovisual laboratory activities on campus; and clinical learning activities in a vast variety of health-care settings. The curriculum is designed to develop students' diagnostic, therapeutic, and ethical reasoning in nursing practice. The graduate is prepared as a generalist able to care for individuals and groups at each developmental level and in various health-care settings. Options are available for baccalaureate students to begin master's-level courses during their undergraduate nursing program.

Undergraduate nursing students may enroll for one semester during their junior or senior year in any number of study-abroad programs sponsored by Boston College or by other U.S. colleges and universities.

The main objective of the master's program is to prepare nurses for advanced practice, including clinical specialist, nurse anesthetist, and nurse practitioner. There are eight areas of specialization: nurse anesthesia, adult, community health, gerontologic, women's, children's, family, and psychiatric–mental health nursing. An Additional Specialty Concentration is available for RNs who have an M.S. in nursing and wish to enhance their educational background in an additional specialty area. Two dual-degree programs are offered: M.S. in nursing/M.B.A. and M.S. in nursing/M.A. in pastoral ministry. In addition, individuals with a non-nursing baccalaureate or higher degree may apply to the M.S. Entry into Nursing Program. The focus in the specialty areas is on human responses to actual or potential health problems. The approach to clients is multifaceted and includes the development of advanced competencies in clinical judgment. Numerous community agencies in and around Boston are used for the clinical practicum of the program. A thesis is optional. Full-time students can complete the program in one to two years, and part-time students may take up to five years.

The Ph.D. program in nursing is the first doctoral program in nursing to be offered at a Jesuit university. The focus of the Ph.D. program is the preparation of scholars for leadership positions in clinical nursing research. Each student is mentored by a faculty member with expertise in the student's area of interest. Core areas of doctoral study are concepts of nursing science, methods of theory development, and qualitative and quantitative research methods needed to extend nursing knowledge. The full-time plan allows the student to take 10 credits of course work per semester for the first two years of study before entering the dissertation phase of the program. The part-time plan allows the student to take 6 to 7 credits of course work per semester for the first three years of study before entering the dissertation phase of the program. Various learning opportunities are available through interdisciplinary colloquia at the university and health-care agencies and clinical research practicums with faculty mentors.

ACADEMIC FACILITIES
A member of the Association of Research Libraries, Boston College's libraries offer a wealth of resources and services to support faculty and student research activities. The book collection consists of more than 2 million volumes, and the nursing holdings have been characterized by nursing leaders as one of the finest collections in the world. A special reference librarian serves as a liaison for all School of Nursing needs. Other nursing resource facilities available to enhance student learning include the Kennedy Audiovisual Center, the Nursing Simulation Laboratory, and a computer lab, all housed within the School of Nursing. The university also offers a wide range of services, such as technical support, audiovisual and computing facilities, and academic and research centers.

LOCATION
Boston College is located in a beautiful suburban setting just minutes from downtown Boston. Boston is a city that offers an outstanding combination of history, culture, and vitality, and it is home to a number of the world's most renowned health-care institutions. Students and faculty members enjoy the unique advantages of metropolitan Boston in addition to the beauty and tranquility of the suburban campus. The scenic grounds and stately Gothic architecture of the 200-acre campus provide an atmosphere conducive to both study and socializing.

STUDENT SERVICES
Health, counseling, and career planning services are available to all graduate and undergraduate students, including programs for African-American, Hispanic, Asian, and Native American

students as well as for international students. A wide variety of recreational and cultural facilities and on- and off-campus housing options are available to students.

THE NURSING STUDENT GROUP

Students at Boston College reflect a diversity of interests and backgrounds. The student body is drawn from every race, religion, and economic background as well as from every state in the Union and numerous countries. Currently, the School of Nursing has approximately 330 undergraduate students, 140 master's students, and 45 doctoral students. The students' ages range from 18 to 50, and many are employed and/or married with children.

COSTS

For 2004–05, undergraduate tuition was $28,940. Room rates averaged $6000, board was approximately $3600, and health, recreation, and activity fees averaged $600. Books, supplies, and other expenses were estimated at $600.

For 2004–05, graduate tuition was $836 per credit hour. Charges for books, fees, supplies, housing, and transportation are additional.

FINANCIAL AID

Boston College offers a variety of scholarships, grants, loans, and employment to assist students in financing their education. The majority of undergraduate students receive some form of financial aid. Financial aid awards are made by the Financial Aid Office to freshmen and transfer students on the basis of academic promise and demonstrated financial need. Notice of such awards made to incoming freshmen and transfer students usually accompanies notification of the students' acceptance by the university. Opportunities include work-study and job referral positions and undergraduate research fellowships.

Graduate students may apply for financial assistance from both the university Financial Aid Office and the School of Nursing. Opportunities include federal traineeships, tuition remission scholarships, university fellowships, and teaching and research assistantships. The university also has competitive minority fellowships for doctoral students.

APPLYING

For the undergraduate program, the type of college-preparatory program viewed as the best foundation for college work usually includes at least 4 units of English, a foreign language, math, social science, and a laboratory science. Students applying to the School of Nursing are required to complete at least 1 unit of chemistry. All applicants must complete the Scholastic Assessment Test (SAT I) and SAT II Subject Tests in writing, mathematics (level I or II), and a third subject of the applicant's choice. In place of the Scholastic Assessment Test, applicants may take American College Testing's ACT Assessment. Qualifying Advanced Placement scores or successful completion of college courses prior to freshman enrollment may help students to place out of core requirements.

Students applying to the undergraduate program are required to submit the Common Application, the Boston College Supplemental Application for Admission, and the appropriate nonrefundable application fee ($60 for domestic applicants and $70 for international applicants) by January 2. It is the candidate's responsibility to ensure that all credentials are sent to and received by the Office of Undergraduate Admissions. Candidates are notified of action taken on their applications between April 1 and 15. Candidates accepted for admission are required to forward an acceptance fee by May 1.

Applicants to the master's program should submit GRE scores, three references, and a personal goal statement. A minimum GPA of 3.0, a transcript from an accredited baccalaureate nursing program, and previous course work in statistics are required. Application deadlines are as follows: for full-time and part-time study for May or September admission, March 15; and for January admission, October 15. January 2 is the deadline for applicants with non-nursing baccalaureate or higher degrees to apply to the Master's Entry into Nursing Program. Applications to the nurse anesthesia program are due September 15 for January enrollment.

Applicants to the doctoral program should submit GRE scores; three references; a career goals statement; evidence of scholarship, including a writing sample; a curriculum vitae; transcripts from an accredited M.S. program in nursing; and previous course work in statistics. An interview is required. The deadline is January 31 of the year of admission. The application fee for each graduate program is $40 and is nonrefundable. International students must also provide TOEFL scores.

CORRESPONDENCE AND INFORMATION

For the undergraduate program:

Director of Undergraduate Admissions
Boston College
Devlin Hall, Room 208
Chestnut Hill, Massachusetts 02467-3812
Telephone: 617-552-3100

Associate Dean, Undergraduate Program
William F. Connell School of Nursing
Boston College
Chestnut Hill, Massachusetts 02467-3812
Telephone: 617-552-4925

For the graduate programs:

Associate Dean, Graduate Programs
William F. Connell School of Nursing
Boston College
Chestnut Hill, Massachusetts 02467-3812
Telephone: 617-552-4928
World Wide Web: http://bc.edu/nursing

Cardinal Stritch University
Ruth S. Coleman College of Nursing
Milwaukee, Wisconsin

THE UNIVERSITY
Cardinal Stritch University is a coeducational university that is rooted in the liberal arts and was established in the Franciscan Catholic tradition. Since its founding in 1937 by the Sisters of St. Francis of Assisi, Stritch has emerged as the largest Franciscan institution of higher education in North America and the second-largest private university in Wisconsin.

With a total population of more than 7,600 students on two campuses and at numerous off-site locations, Stritch's size can be deceiving. While the University provides access to all the resources associated with large universities, it still offers the benefits of personal attention, small class sizes, and one-on-one instruction that are associated with smaller institutions. The University keeps up to date with changes and needs in technology, society, and the workforce, yet it remains committed to maintaining the high-quality, value-centered education that has defined Stritch's history and continues to attract its diverse student population.

THE COLLEGE OF NURSING
Within a framework of Franciscan values, which emphasize compassion and respect for individuals, the Ruth S. Coleman College of Nursing provides educational programs in an open and caring environment at the associate, bachelor's, and master's degree levels. For more than two decades, Stritch's nursing programs have integrated nursing theory and practices to meet the emerging health needs of all clients, with a focus on innovation and flexibility. More than 1,100 graduates of the University's nursing programs can attest to the student-centered learning environment in which faculty members focus primarily on teaching and helping students realize their potential as individuals, professional nurses, and responsible members of the world community.

While the associate degree program is offered in a traditional format, Stritch's nontraditional bachelor's and master's degree programs are geared toward working nurses, with classes meeting just one or two nights per week. In all programs, students are engaged in a variety of clinical experiences with the area's top community health-care agencies and hospitals. As a result, all Stritch nursing graduates achieve job placement within six months of graduation.

PROGRAMS OF STUDY
Cardinal Stritch University is the only school in Wisconsin to offer the full range of nursing degree programs, from the A.D.N. to the M.S.N., with an additional program tailored specifically for Licensed Practical Nurses (LPN).

The basic associate degree program prepares students for entry into nursing practice. Upon completion of the five-semester A.D.N. program, the graduate is eligible to take the National Council Licensure Examination for Registered Nurses (NCLEX-RN) to become a registered nurse. To complete the degree, 70 credit hours are required—38 in nursing and 32 in liberal arts core courses.

The University's LPN to A.D.N. program is designed to give LPNs the opportunity to complete the necessary course work to become a registered nurse in just three semesters. Credits may be granted to incoming students based on prior experiences. The program is aimed at further developing each LPN's abilities to practice nursing using the principles of health promotion, maintenance, and restoration across the life span in a variety of structured client settings. To complete this degree, 70 credit hours are required—38 in nursing and 32 in liberal arts core courses.

With a recently improved curriculum, the five-semester A.D.N. program includes a full range of studies encompassing the entire life cycle (prenatal, pediatrics, adult, geriatrics, and death). The program also features substantial community contact and expanded clinical experiences. Faculty members emphasize theory, problem solving, and critical thinking and offer a broad perspective on the nursing field. The A.D.N. naturally feeds into the B.S.N. completion program for those who choose to continue their education.

The Bachelor of Science in Nursing completion program prepares the A.D.N. or diploma graduate to practice professional nursing with a broad knowledge base. Nurses who are seeking a promotion, increased job choices, management opportunities, or broader nursing knowledge find this two-year, accelerated program to be a flexible complement to their full-time work schedule. With classes meeting just one night per week, nurses gain valuable experience in the field while taking classes toward the B.S.N.

The nontraditional format of the B.S.N. program is based on adult learning principles, with a cohort-group learning format. As a member of a cohort group, students become part of a learning community that encourages and supports professional growth and facilitates social connections among peers as well as the wider nursing and health-care communities. The B.S.N. program's classroom environment encourages open communication, while the curriculum focuses on the health continuum throughout the life span. Students focus on areas of their particular nursing interest and take advantage of faculty and clinical experiences to discover widely diverse learning options. Completion of the program requires 128 credits. Some credits may be earned through credit for prior learning or standardized testing.

Cardinal Stritch University is the only school in the Milwaukee area to offer a semiaccelerated M.S.N. program with an educational focus for working nurses who want to function as nurse educators in a variety of client communities, such as staff development, client teaching, health promotion, and community and nursing education. This unique focus gives graduates more opportunities in existing and expanding practice areas—everything from health-care organizations to businesses.

M.S.N. course theory is carefully merged with practical applications, allowing program participants to identify their individual needs of study and then create final projects that they can present to current and/or prospective employers. Course work and study provide a foundation for doctoral or advanced study. Students in this thirty-month master's program attend classes one to two nights a week for six semesters to complete the requirements for the M.S.N. The curriculum is computer enhanced and delivered in a semimodular cohort-group format. To complete the degree, 36 credit hours are required, with 32 hours of course work and 4 hours of project work.

ACADEMIC FACILITIES
An exceptional resource, the state-of-the-art library is easily accessible and contains a wealth of information necessary to complete in-depth research. Staffed by professional librarians, the library's holdings change daily and currently include nearly 130,000 items in a variety of formats as well as 630 current print periodical subscriptions and access to more than 3,000 in electronic format. The library offers the resources of eight college libraries through its collaborative Southeastern Wisconsin Information Technology Exchange (SWITCH) consortium and Topcat, a combined online public access catalog. The library offers

an array of electronic databases, full-text and other resources, and interactive research services that are available to its community of learners—both on site and from wherever learning is taking place. The library's resources also include a number of laptop computers, which are available for checkout for up to seven days at a time.

The Information Technology department gives students a competitive edge in today's computerized society. There are open computer labs, public spaces with computers and network connections for laptops/personal computers, wireless access to the Internet in public spaces, and discipline-specific computer labs. The student computing areas are equipped with laser products and scanners and house approximately 350 PC and Macintosh computers.

LOCATION

Cardinal Stritch University's 40-acre, parklike main campus is situated in a quiet suburban neighborhood just north of Milwaukee. Downtown Milwaukee is a short 15-minute drive from the campus, while access to Lake Michigan is within several blocks. The campus is conveniently accessible from Interstate 43, which offers a direct, easy route to Mitchell International Airport, the downtown Amtrak train station, and the Greyhound bus depot. The Milwaukee County Transit System provides students with a public transportation option when they are involved in off-campus pursuits. Interstate 43 is also a link to the excitement of downtown, which is home to numerous ethnic and American restaurants, specialty retailers, a mall, art and public museums, several conference and performance centers, and cultural and sports entertainment.

STUDENT SERVICES

Issues related to health, counseling, career planning, and study skills are attended to by professionals in various campus departments. Workout facilities, including a weight room with fitness equipment and an indoor track, are open to all students. The Offices of Multicultural Relations, Vocation Development, and International Programs provide assistance and opportunities for growth to Stritch's diverse student body.

THE NURSING STUDENT GROUP

Many of Stritch's 400 undergraduate and graduate nursing students are professional nurses who are able to work full-time and maintain a full course load at the University. Other nursing students live on campus and concentrate fully on their course work. Overall, the Ruth S. Coleman College of Nursing is a close-knit, diverse community of faculty and staff members and students.

COSTS

Full-time undergraduate tuition for 2004–05 was $15,360 per year (12–17 credits per semester). Room and board were $5280, and various meal plans are available. Part-time undergraduate tuition was $420 per credit. Graduate tuition was $480 per credit. Books are an additional cost.

FINANCIAL AID

A wide range of financial aid options are available, including government-subsidized loan and grant programs, University scholarships, on-campus employment opportunities, and off-campus internships. Approximately 80 percent of full-time students receive financial aid, and the average financial aid package is around $9000. Eligibility for need-based grant and loan programs is determined through filing the Free Application for Federal Student Aid (FAFSA). Candidates for financial aid should complete and mail the FAFSA by March 1.

APPLYING

The University accepts applications on a rolling admission basis. Applicants are notified of the decision two weeks after all records are complete. Each nursing program adheres to the general admission requirements of the University, with the addition of several requirements specific to the A.D.N., B.S.N. completion, or M.S.N. program. Both general and specific admission requirements are listed in detail in the University's undergraduate and graduate catalogs. Transfer students are encouraged to apply and must meet selective criteria determined by the College of Nursing.

CORRESPONDENCE AND INFORMATION:

To learn more about the A.D.N. or B.S.N. program:
Janet Beitz, College of Nursing
Telephone: 414-410-4391 or 800-347-8822 Ext. 4391
E-mail: jabeitz@stritch.edu
or
Office of Undergraduate Admissions
Cardinal Stritch University
6801 North Yates Road
Milwaukee, Wisconsin 53217-3985
Telephone: 414-410-4040
800-347-8822 Ext. 4040 (toll-free)
E-mail: admityou@stritch.edu
World Wide Web: http://www.stritch.edu

For the M.S.N. program:
Carolyn Marohl
Telephone: 414-410-4709 or 800-347-8822 Ext. 4709
E-mail: cjmarohl@stritch.edu
or
Office of Graduate Admissions
Cardinal Stritch University
6801 North Yates Road
Milwaukee, Wisconsin 53217-3985
Telephone: 414-410-4042
800-347-8822 Ext. 4042 (toll-free)
E-mail: gradadm@stritch.edu
World Wide Web: http://www.stritch.edu

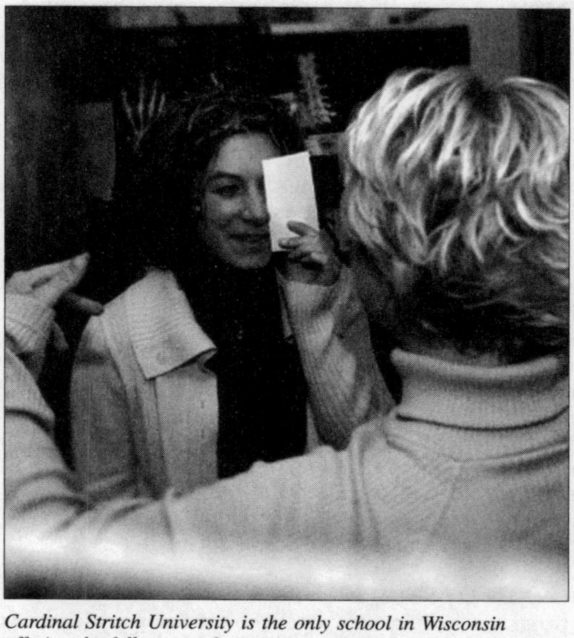

Cardinal Stritch University is the only school in Wisconsin offering the full range of nursing programs, from associate through master's degrees.

Colby-Sawyer College
Department of Nursing
New London, New Hampshire

THE UNIVERSITY

Colby-Sawyer College, founded in 1837 in the New England academy tradition and engaged in higher education since 1928, is an independent, coeducational, residential undergraduate college that offers equal education to women and men. The College provides programs of study that innovatively integrate liberal arts and sciences with professional preparation. Through all of its programs, the College encourages students to realize their full intellectual and personal potential so they may gain understanding about themselves, others, and the forces shaping the rapidly changing and pluralistic world.

Students come from all over the United States and from seven other countries, with 70 percent of the students coming from outside of New Hampshire. Colby-Sawyer has a distinguished faculty dedicated to undergraduate teaching, and a personalized education is ensured by the 12:1 student-faculty ratio and average class size of 19. The College's faculty members are graduates of some of the finest schools and colleges of nursing in the country.

The College is accredited by the New England Association of Schools and Colleges, and professional programs carry the appropriate accreditations. Colby-Sawyer has been recently recognized by *U.S. News & World Report* as one of the top eleven in its category (of almost 100 colleges).

THE DEPARTMENT OF NURSING

The faculty members in the Department of Nursing have diverse and extensive experience in both practice and teaching. They have undergraduate and graduate degrees from Boston College, Northeastern, NYU, Smith, Yale, and the Universities of Texas and California at San Francisco. They have practiced in a variety of renowned settings and have published research, scholarly articles, and books. They serve on editorial and professional advisory boards at the state and national levels.

The Department of Nursing recognizes that nursing education must be responsive to trends in health care and at the same time must be grounded in a core curriculum. In May 2000 and again in May 2002, the Department of Nursing was awarded grant funding by the Helene Fuld Institute in New York, an indication that the Department is held in high esteem for its innovative approach to nursing education. The purpose of the grants has been to develop and implement a new nursing curriculum that integrates the principles of community-based health care along with those of more traditional inpatient care.

The nursing program is accredited by the Commission for Collegiate Nursing Education and approved by the New Hampshire Board of Nursing. The Colby-Sawyer College Honor Society for Nursing is applying for membership in Sigma Theta Tau, an international nursing honor society.

PROGRAMS OF STUDY

The program leading to a Bachelor of Science degree with a major in nursing (B.S.) integrates knowledge from the liberal arts and sciences with professional education. Students are prepared to take the Nursing Certification Licensure Examination (NCLEX) for Registered Nurses, to assume entry-level positions in professional nursing, and to enroll in graduate studies.

In addition to a liberal education, the nursing program includes the core knowledge and skills essential to entry-level nursing practice, the values of the healing professions, and the development of the professional role of the nurse. Nursing courses cover a range of topics and issues relevant to health care across the life span and within the increasingly complex health-care environment. Topics include health assessment and history taking; pharmacology; the pathology of disease process; nursing interventions with elders, adults, and children; reproductive health; mental health and illness; health promotion; health-care policy and research; community and public health; leadership and management; and legal and ethical issues.

Students begin clinical internships in the sophomore year. Throughout the program, they spend 70 percent of their time in inpatient and home care settings and 30 percent of their time in community settings. Students conclude the program with a semester-long preceptorship in the spring of the senior year. During the preceptorship, students work one-on-one with a registered nurse under the guidance of nursing faculty members. Preceptorship settings have included hematology special care, postanesthesia care, emergency department, cardiac intervention, and many others.

In order to prepare students for NCLEX, which is a computer-adapted test, all nursing course exams are taken on computer. Students use software packages to practice exam skills and assess their knowledge throughout the program. In the spring of the senior year, faculty members facilitate an NCLEX review course with senior students.

AFFILIATIONS WITH HEALTH-CARE FACILITIES

The nursing program is enriched by its strong relationships with its clinical affiliates: Dartmouth-Hitchcock Medical Center (DHMC), Lake Sunapee Region Visiting Nurse Association, the Visiting Nurses' Alliance of New Hampshire and Vermont, Concord Hospital, and New London Hospital. In the junior year, students practice with community nurse mentors to assess the health needs of individuals and families in homes, schools, and clinics. In the senior year, students do a yearlong Community Capstone. This initiative is unique among undergraduate nursing programs and is based on the nursing program's relationships with a school-based clinic, an adult living community, and a cancer center. Students work in small teams to assess the health needs of these communities and to implement appropriate interventions, such as health and education programs, policy development, and follow-up care. Each senior class passes on these community initiatives to subsequent classes, so that students' practice has a lasting impact on the community.

ACADEMIC FACILITIES

The College has made a strong commitment to providing students with state-of-the-art technology. In 2000, the College received a grant of $1 million dedicated to the use of technology. The College has standardized on a Windows platform and has deployed Windows-based computers in every department. Campus servers primarily use Windows NT and run the Microsoft Suite. All computers in networked buildings, including the Nursing Lab, have access to the Internet and Intranet.

There are seventeen smart classrooms, ten computer labs, and Internet and network access in every classroom. Nursing courses are posted on Blackboard.com, so students and faculty members may hold online discussions or access the course syllabus, announcements, and assignments at any time. Nursing exams are taken online through Blackboard.com.

The Nursing Laboratory includes a state-of-the-art simulated hospital environment in which students can develop the essential skills for entry-level practice. Equipment includes a head wall unit and high-tech bed with oxygen, suction, an ECG monitor, an electronic vital-signs monitor, a defibrillator, and specialty intravenous pumps. In addition, the Nursing Lab contains a simulated home-care environment. Nursing students also use the critical-care nursing lab at Dartmouth-Hitchcock Medical Center.

The Susan Colgate Cleveland Library/Learning Center holds more than 80,000 volumes and more than 800 journal titles as well as videos, audiocassettes, and CD-ROMs. Computer workstations are available for access to the library's online catalog, electronic databases, and the Internet. The nursing program's Computer Assisted Learning Laboratory is housed in the library. Students have access to interactive CD-ROMs that help them learn about clinical procedures before they practice them in the Nursing Lab and perform them in the hospital. Nursing students also have a networked course package that helps prepare them for NCLEX. Interlibrary loan service provides access to library holdings throughout New England and beyond. Colby-Sawyer College nursing students have access to the Dartmouth Biomedical Library.

The Academic Development Center at James House provides one-on-one peer tutorials. The staff consists of faculty members, peer tutors, and learning specialists who assist students with diagnosed learning differences. The Harrington Center for Career Development assists students with resume preparation, interview skills, and placements for jobs and internships.

LOCATION

Colby-Sawyer's 190-acre campus is located on the crest of a hill in New London, New Hampshire. Its beautiful grounds and stately Georgian architecture create a picturesque and safe environment that is conducive to learning. Colby-Sawyer is located in the heart of the Dartmouth–Lake Sunapee region, a four-season recreational and cultural community known for the natural beauty of its lakes and mountains. Boston is only 1½ hours away and Montreal is 3½ hours away, so students have access to these major cities. The nearby seacoast at Portsmouth and the surrounding lakes, mountains, and state parks provide opportunities for hiking, camping, golf, tennis, canoeing, swimming, ice-skating, and Nordic and Alpine skiing. Arts and cultural opportunities can be found in New London as well as in nearby Concord, the state capital, and Hanover, the home of Dartmouth College.

STUDENT LIFE

Varsity sports for men and women include Alpine ski racing, basketball, riding, soccer, swimming, tennis, and track and field. Women also compete in varsity lacrosse and volleyball, and men compete in baseball.

The Dan and Kathleen Hogan Sports Center contains a large field house with three multipurpose courts, a suspended track, and a six-lane, NCAA-size swimming pool. The Van Cise Fitness Center is furnished with top-flight equipment.

All students are members of the Student Government Association. There are numerous groups that provide students with leadership possibilities outside of the classroom. These include the Campus Activities Board (CAB), the dance club, Cross Cultural Club, Alpha Chi honor society, yearbook, Admissions Key Association, Art Student's League, Film Society, Student Nurses' Association, community service, radio station, drama club, the *Courier* (newspaper), and other clubs and intramural sports.

THE NURSING STUDENT GROUP

The Colby-Sawyer College Student Nurses' Association (SNA) is one of the most active in the state. In addition to a variety of community service projects, SNA members participate in the National Student Nurses' Association conference each year.

COSTS

For 2004–05, the comprehensive fee, which includes tuition, room, board, and fees, was $32,260. Tuition was $23,310, room was $4980, and board was $3970. Approximately $1550 should be allowed for books, supplies, and personal expenses.

FINANCIAL AID

Through its financial aid program, Colby-Sawyer offers assistance to 80 percent of the student body. This aid is made possible through endowment income and scholarships, grant and loan funds, and funds provided through state and federal programs. Students who have achieved success in academics and have special talents as well as those who have demonstrated financial need are offered financial aid.

Each applicant must submit the Free Application for Federal Student Aid (FAFSA) and the Colby-Sawyer Application for Financial Aid by February 15. Candidates for merit awards must also submit the Application for Merit Awards. Financial aid is awarded on an annual basis.

APPLYING

The College recommends that prospective students present at least 15 units of college-preparatory work. The usual program includes 4 years of English, 3 years of mathematics, 2 years of the same foreign language, 3 or more years of social studies, and 2 or more years of a laboratory science. Prospective nursing students should have 3 years of college-preparatory lab science, including biology and chemistry; a minimum SAT I combined score of 1000; and a minimum high school GPA of 2.5. Students who do not meet these criteria may still apply, and their qualifications will be evaluated in the context of their overall performance. Students who wish to transfer into the nursing program should supply copies of course descriptions from the catalogs and/or syllabi of the institution(s) from which they wish to transfer credit.

Colby-Sawyer operates on a rolling admission system. Applications for Early Notification must be submitted by December 15. A completed application includes a high school transcript (including first-quarter grades for the senior year), SAT I or ACT scores, two letters of recommendation (one from a teacher and one from a guidance professional), a personal statement, and a $40 nonrefundable application fee. While an admission interview is not required, every applicant is encouraged to visit Colby-Sawyer for a tour and interview. Interviews often play an important part in the admission file.

CORRESPONDENCE AND INFORMATION:

Office of Admissions
Colby-Sawyer College
100 Main Street
New London, New Hampshire 03257-4648
Telephone: 603-526-3700
800-272-1015 (toll-free)
Fax: 603-526-3452

The College of New Rochelle
School of Nursing
New Rochelle, New York

THE COLLEGE

One of the oldest in Westchester County, the College of New Rochelle was founded in 1904 by Mother Irene Gill, OSU, as the first Catholic college for women in New York State. The College, now independent, established the Graduate School in 1969, the School of New Resources (for adult learners) in 1972, and the School of Nursing in 1976. The School of Arts and Sciences (the seminal unit) continues the tradition of enrolling only women; the other three schools admit both women and men. The College of New Rochelle is chartered by the New York State Board of Regents and is accredited by the Middle States Association of Colleges and Schools.

There are nineteen major buildings, including Leland Castle, a National Historic Site and the first home of the College; the 180,000-volume Mother Irene Gill Library, currently undergoing a multimillion dollar renovation; a chapel; four large residence halls; a Student Service Center; two science buildings; and the Mooney Center, formerly known as the College Center.

Although there have been fundamental changes in the expression of the College's Mission since the late 1960s, the College of New Rochelle has remained faithful to its mission and has responded flexibly to the higher learning needs of the community it serves. From this tradition, the College derives its dedication to the education of women and men in the liberal arts and in professional studies. Building on its original commitment to women, the College also reaches out to those who have not previously had access to higher education. It places particular emphasis on the concept of lifelong learning.

The College is committed to a respect and concern for each individual. It seeks to challenge students to achieve the full development of their individual talents and a greater understanding of themselves. It encourages the examination of values through the creative and responsible use of reason. The College strives to articulate its academic tradition and religious heritage in ways that are consonant with the best contemporary understandings of both. It provides opportunities for spiritual growth in a context of freedom and ecumenism.

Finally, with justice as its guiding principle, the College tries to respond to the needs of society through its education programs and service activities and through fostering the concept of education for service.

THE SCHOOL OF NURSING

In May 1975, the Board of Trustees of the College of New Rochelle approved a proposal to establish a School of Nursing. The curriculum, leading to a Bachelor of Science in Nursing degree, was approved by the New York State Education Department in spring 1976. In fall 1976, the first freshmen were admitted to the program, and in 1980, the first class graduated.

PROGRAMS OF STUDY

The B.S.N. Program for Second Degree Students is open to women and men who hold undergraduate degrees from four-year colleges or universities in an area other than nursing. Five semesters of clinical nursing courses are required after completing all prerequisite courses. Students may begin studies in the fall, spring, or summer semesters and may include prerequisite courses in their individualized plan of study. Opportunities for acceleration in the program are also available.

Programs designed for registered nurses include an RN-B.S.N. and RN-B.S.N.-M.S. option.

In 1983, a Graduate Program in Nursing was established in the School of Nursing, funded for a three-year period by a half-million-dollar federal grant from the Division of Nursing of the Department of Health and Human Services. The Master of Science degree program offered by the School of Nursing is designed to prepare graduates for the roles of advanced-practice nursing (acute-care nurse practitioner, family nurse practitioner, clinical nurse specialist in holistic nursing, and nursing and health-care management). The program is designed to accommodate the needs of part-time or full-time students, with theoretical courses offered in the late afternoon or evening or on weekends. Consistent with the philosophy of the College of New Rochelle, the Graduate Program in Nursing provides small classes and individualized advisement and program planning. Post-master's certificate programs are offered for advanced-practice tracks plus the nurse educator role.

ACADEMIC FACILITIES

The Learning Center for Nursing (LCN) is a multiresource facility for the School. It is composed of five specialized areas. The Nursing Laboratory is designed for the teaching and reinforcement of basic and advanced nursing skills development. Simulating a hospital setting, client-care units are equipped with variable-height beds, overbed tables, bedside cabinets, and medication areas. Each unit has wall-mounted otoscopes, ophthalmoscopes, and blood pressure cuffs. In addition, to facilitate learning in the community clinical practice settings, there are client areas equipped with examination tables. There are several mannequins, models, and simulators that facilitate learning and allow for realistic practice of a wide array of skills. Registered nurses serve as preceptors to students for individualized instruction and mentoring. There is also a computer interactive video system that supports students' skill development.

The Media Laboratory offers a variety of audiovisual resources for self-guided study. Audiovisual equipment includes color television/VCR centers and slide projectors for a media library containing more than 470 videotapes and more than fifty-five slide sets. This area is also equipped with viewing carrels and a 25-inch color television/VCR for group or classroom use.

The Computer Center is the third area where students learn, practice, and apply a variety of computer skills. This area contains multimedia personal computers, IBM or IBM-compatible personal computers, printers, and interactive video systems. The College of New Rochelle School of Nursing has served as a Fuld Institute for Technology in Nursing Education (FITNE) Interactive Demonstration Center for computer-interactive video system technology. A CD-ROM version of the Cumulative Index to Nursing and Allied Health Literature (CINAHL), an easy-to-search index, provides coverage of articles included in more than 550 nursing journals and primary publications. A variety of software is available, including RNCAT (a computerized adaptive testing program simulating NCLEX-RN), computer-assistive instruction software, and popular business applications (word processing, database management, spreadsheet, and graphics).

The fourth area is the Group Instruction Room, which is designed to facilitate independent and small-group study and support research activity. It houses a small library of current textbooks on clinical skills and issues, including a section referenced by the computer-based health-care consulting system.

The Electronic Classroom is equipped with personal computers for both students and faculty members. State-of-the-art computers, printers, a projection boxlight, and scanner are housed here. The goal of the Electronic Classroom is to facilitate group learning through technology using Internet and instructional software.

A Holistic Caring Project offers students techniques and energy work to foster self-care, reduce stress, and promote wellness.

LOCATION

The principal campus of the College of New Rochelle is located on 20 beautiful acres in the southeastern corner of Westchester County, New York, 1 mile west of Long Island Sound and 16 miles north of mid-Manhattan. It is easily accessible by commuter trains and school-sponsored buses. The area contains numerous parks and recreational areas; the Long Island Sound, with its many beaches, is within walking distance; and New York City is a half hour away.

STUDENT SERVICES

The Mentor Connection Program provides professional and leadership development opportunities for undergraduate and graduate students. Mentors consist of alumni, faculty members, administrators, peers, and professional nurses. The mentor-protégé relationship is a developmental process that empowers and nurtures the participants over time. Mutual growth, learning, and sharing occur in an atmosphere of affirmation, collegiality, respect, and support.

THE NURSING STUDENT GROUP

There are 517 students in the programs of the School of Nursing. Of those, 91 are in the graduate program, 212 are in the RN-B.S.N. Completion Program, 137 are in the basic undergraduate program, and 80 are in the second degree program. Ninety-five percent of the students are women, and 60 percent are part-time.

COSTS

Tuition and other changes are set at the minimum for financially responsible operations and are below actual costs. Gifts and grants received through the generosity of alumni, friends, corporations, and foundations play a significant part in reducing this difference. Undergraduate tuition for full-time students (12–16 credits) is $9550. Part-time charges are $643 per credit. Nonmatriculated students also pay $643 per credit. The charge to audit a course is one half the usual tuition per credit hour.

Students enrolled in the RN-B.S.N. Second Degree Programs are billed at the per-credit rates listed above.

Graduate tuition is $530 per credit.

FINANCIAL AID

The Financial Aid Program of the College of New Rochelle fulfills several objectives. The College firmly believes that by providing financial assistance to needy and deserving students of diverse economic and social backgrounds and by rewarding academic achievement, it may best promote and maintain the educational goals that are central to the mission of the institution. The ability to furnish a financial aid package to students who might otherwise be unable to obtain a high-quality education clearly benefits and enriches the College community.

The Office of Financial Aid is dedicated to the service of students. The financial aid staff is trained to provide individual and group counseling to students about their financial responsibilities and available aid programs.

APPLYING

Admission to the B.S.N. program is open to high school graduates, transfer students from two- or four-year colleges or universities, registered nurses who are graduates of diploma or associate degree programs, and college graduates with non-nursing degrees. To be considered for admission, applicants must have taken 16 academic units in secondary school that include three science courses, including a laboratory chemistry and a laboratory biology, and three courses in mathematics (algebra I and II and geometry). A written statement of the candidate's academic and personal qualities should be prepared by the principal or guidance counselor and submitted with the transcript. Applicants are encouraged to submit other information in support of their credentials. SAT I or ACT scores are also required. There is a $20 nonrefundable application fee. In cases of economic hardship, a fee waiver may be requested. Admission requirements for the RN-B.S.N. option include current professional registered nurse licensure and an employer recommendation.

Residents of New York State who do not qualify for regular admission and who come from low-income backgrounds may be considered for the College's Community Leadership Program.

Admission to the graduate program is selective. Criteria for admission include graduation from an accredited baccalaureate nursing program or a nursing program deemed comparable by the World Education Services with a minimum GPA of 3.0; an application, including an essay describing goals for graduate study in nursing; a resume; a personal interview (distance permitting); two letters of recommendation, preferably from a nursing administrator and a faculty member; completion of a basic statistics course (course may be taken concurrently with graduate study); current malpractice insurance; current New York State RN licensure; completion of health requirements; completion of a physical assessment course for clinical majors; at least one year of tertiary-care experience for acute-care nurse practitioner applicants and one year of clinical experience for the family nurse practitioner track and holistic clinical nurse specialist track; and a nonrefundable $30 application fee. Applicants who do not meet the 3.0 GPA requirement for admission may submit a written request to the Graduate Nursing Admissions Committee for a review of their application portfolio.

CORRESPONDENCE AND INFORMATION:

The College of New Rochelle
29 Castle Place
New Rochelle, New York 10805-2339
Telephone: 914-654-5000
E-mail: ddemarest@cnr.edu
World Wide Web: http://www.cnr.edu

Columbia College of Nursing
Mount Mary College
Nursing Program
Milwaukee, Wisconsin

THE COLLEGES

The history of Columbia College of Nursing began more than 100 years ago. In 1901, the school was part of the Knowlton Hospital and Training School. In 1909, the Columbia Hospital Corporation took over Knowlton Hospital and changed the name to the Columbia Hospital School of Nursing. In 1919, both hospital and school moved to their current location on Milwaukee's east side. In 1956, an addition to the original 1919 building was completed, and it serves, in part, as the present-day Columbia College of Nursing building.

Mount Mary College, an urban Catholic college for women sponsored by the School Sisters of Notre Dame, is located on the northwest side of Milwaukee. Mount Mary's roots are deep in the history of Wisconsin. St. Mary's Institute was founded in Prairie du Chien in 1872. In 1913, it extended its educational program to the postsecondary level and was chartered as St. Mary's College, a four-year Catholic college for women, the first in the state to grant degrees. Its academic standards were accepted by the North Central Association of Colleges in 1926. The institution changed its name to Mount Mary College when it moved to its present location in 1929.

The Mount Mary College campus is home to freshman and sophomore nursing students as well as other Mount Mary students. The student residence, Caroline Hall, provides sports and recreational facilities, a student lounge, and the Marian Art Gallery. Notre Dame Hall is the location of administrative offices, classrooms, laboratories, art and music studios, the Walter and Olive Stiemke Memorial Hall and Conference Center, Macintosh computer laboratories, and two chapels. Kostka Hall houses the 800-seat theater, studios for the fashion department, and faculty offices. Dining facilities, the bookstore, post office, the Advising and Career Development Office, and the fitness center and locker rooms are found in Bergstrom Hall.

Minutes away, on Milwaukee's east side, the Columbia College of Nursing campus is home to junior and senior nursing students. In addition to comprehensive, state-of-the-art academic facilities described later, the campus includes the Columbia Residence Hall, the Campus Center, bookstore, fitness center, laundry room, kitchenette, and recreational facilities.

THE INTERCOLLEGIATE NURSING PROGRAM

In fall of 2002, Mount Mary College and the Columbia College of Nursing established a joint Bachelor of Science in Nursing (B.S.N.) degree program. The combination of Columbia College of Nursing's history of excellence with Mount Mary's highly respected liberal arts education offers a program of high-quality preparation for a career in nursing. Within the liberal arts framework, students integrate the most up-to-date nursing instruction with challenging clinical placements. The nursing program is approved by the Wisconsin State Board of Nursing and is accredited by the National League for Nursing Accrediting Commission and the North Central Association of Colleges and Schools Commission on Institutions of Higher Education. Mount Mary College is approved by the State of Wisconsin to confer degrees and by the Wisconsin State Department of Public Instruction for teachers' certificates. The College is fully accredited by the Higher Learning Commission.

PROGRAMS OF STUDY

The Columbia/Mount Mary College nursing program offers multiple formats for students seeking a nursing degree. Columbia College of Nursing and Mount Mary College offer a unique intercollegiate program leading to a Bachelor of Science in Nursing degree. An RN-B.S.N. completion program is also available.

AFFILIATIONS WITH HEALTH-CARE FACILITIES

Affiliations between Columbia College of Nursing and Southeastern Wisconsin community clinical sites further guarantee that students, while experiencing the latest advances in nursing education, also remain on the cutting edge of today's changing health-care environment.

ACADEMIC FACILITIES

On the Mount Mary campus, the Patrick and Beatrice Haggerty Library collection includes more than 110,000 volumes and 500 subscription periodical titles, along with a significant collection of audiovisual materials. Several offices are located in the lower level of Haggerty Library, including the Teacher Education Center, the Academic Resource Center, the Development Office, and Computer Services, which includes three computer labs. Mount Mary College recently constructed a new Science, Technology, and Campus Center. This $7-million, 33,000-square-foot, three-story building is a state-of-the-art facility that includes science, nursing, and occupational therapy labs; classrooms; a cyber café; meeting rooms; a theater/conference area; and student social areas.

The Columbia College of Nursing campus houses newly renovated classrooms with state-of-the-art projection technology and Internet access. The College's Ellen A. Bacon Library hosts a collection of 9,200 professional books, journals, and bound volumes. The Helene Fuld Learning Resource Center affords students 24-hour access to the Columbia–St. Mary's Health System network.

LOCATION

Columbia College of Nursing, located on Milwaukee's east side, is surrounded by residential neighborhoods near Lake Michigan and the University of Wisconsin–Milwaukee. The College is served by most of the city's major bus routes and is near a diverse assortment of shops, restaurants, and entertainment and recreational facilities.

Located on 80 acres on Milwaukee's northwest side, Mount Mary provides a park-like campus featuring stately stone buildings, gorgeous green lawns, and beautiful wooded areas in a residential area of Milwaukee.

STUDENT SERVICES

To broaden their cultural awareness, Columbia College of Nursing and Mount Mary encourage their students to take advantage of a variety of study-abroad opportunities. Accordingly, Mount Mary College sponsors an annual summer study program in Rome. In summer 2001, Mount Mary became the first college in Wisconsin to hold a license to operate a program in Rome. In November 2001, Mount Mary and the Universidad Católica de Santa Maria (UCSM) of Arequipa, Peru, signed a cooperative agreement to promote student exchanges. UCSM is a natural partner: its location in the second-largest city in Peru provides practical learning experiences for virtually all professional programs while providing an ideal site for Spanish language acquisition and cultural immersion. In addition to these study-abroad programs, the College also maintains affiliate relationships with numerous international colleges and universities, including the American College, Dublin; the American Intercontinental University, London and Dubai; Nanzan College, Japan; and Notre Dame College, Kyoto, Japan. In 2000, Mount Mary joined a consortium directed by the Wisconsin Association of Independent Colleges and Universities that enables member institutions to share study-abroad opportunities.

The College sponsors many social activities, including performances by musicians and comedians, dances, and all-campus picnics. These events are sponsored by the Mount Mary Programming and Activities Council (MMPAC), Student Government, Hall Council, and other groups on campus. Other events include films, concerts, and lectures. Students from other colleges are welcome to attend campus events. Through participation in clubs/organizations, students have opportunities to develop leadership skills, collaborate with other clubs/organizations, network, and explore areas of interest. Special and professional interests are served by affiliates of national societies. Physical fitness and an interest in athletics are fostered through various activities, fitness programs, health and dance courses, and intramural and intercollegiate athletics. Mount Mary College is a provisional member of NCAA Division III. The Blue Angels compete in soccer, softball, volleyball, basketball, and tennis.

Athletic facilities include a gymnasium, indoor swimming pool, outdoor soccer field, fitness center, and sand volleyball court. Academic and professional student services are available to all students. Services include tutoring and assistance with tests through the Academic Resource Center; advising, resume writing, and career planning through the Advising and Career Development Office; and personal counseling through the Counseling Center.

COSTS

For the 2004–05 academic year, full-time undergraduate tuition is $15,975 per year, and $466 per credit for part-time undergraduates. There is a $1000 per year nursing program fee for full-time undergraduates, and, for part-time undergraduates, the nursing fee is $50 per credit. Various other fees also apply. Room and board costs average $5270.

FINANCIAL AID

The Financial Aid Office at Mount Mary College develops a financial package on an individual basis for each qualified student. Approximately 90 percent of full-time Columbia/Mount Mary students receive some form of financial assistance. Students filing for financial aid should complete the Free Application for Federal Student Aid (FAFSA). Additional information on numerous merit-based scholarships, grants, and work-study opportunities is available for incoming freshmen as well as transfer students. Students should contact the Enrollment Office for more information.

APPLYING

Candidates for admission are considered on the basis of academic preparation, scholarship, and evidence of the ability to do college work and benefit from it. Fifteen secondary school units are required for students entering directly from high school into the nursing program. The 15 units must consist of 2 in biology; 2 chemistry; 2 algebra; 3 English; 4 history, language, or social science; and 2 electives. Each applicant is reviewed individually. Transfer and nontraditional student admission requirements can be found on the Mount Mary College Web site listed in the Correspondence and Information section. International students must take the Test of English as a Foreign Language (TOEFL). Early acceptance is available at Mount Mary College and advanced placement is honored. Mount Mary has a rolling admission policy. An admission decision is sent as soon as all required materials have been received and reviewed by the Enrollment Office. After notification of acceptance, students wishing to enroll need to submit the $200 tuition deposit. Neither Columbia College of Nursing nor Mount Mary discriminate against any individual for reasons of race, color, religion, age, disability, or national or ethnic origin. The nursing program is open to both men and women.

CORRESPONDENCE AND INFORMATION

Enrollment Office
Mount Mary College
2900 North Menomonee River Parkway
Milwaukee, Wisconsin 53222-4597
Telephone: 414-256-1219
800-321-6265 (toll-free)
World Wide Web: http://www.mtmary.edu

Columbia College of Nursing
2121 East Newport
Milwaukee, Wisconsin 53211
World Wide Web: http://www.ccon.edu

THE FACULTY

Virginia Bastian, Clinical Assistant Professor; M.S., Wisconsin–Milwaukee, 1996; Nurse Practitioner. Child and adolescent health.

Susan Cole, Assistant Professor; M.S, Marquette, 1991. Medical surgical nursing.

Ann Cook, Professor; Ph.D., Wisconsin–Milwaukee, 1995. Community and medical-surgical nursing.

Katherine Dimmock, Professor and Dean; Ed.D., Northern Illinois, 1985; J.D., Indiana–Purdue at Indianapolis, 1998; M.S.N., Indiana University, 1980.

Dorothy Hagemeier, Assistant Professor; M.S.N., Marquette, 1974. Medical-surgical nursing.

Mark Hirschmann, Professor; Ph.D., Purdue, 1986. Psychiatric and mental health nursing, community nursing.

Debra Johnson, Associate Professor; M.S.N., Wisconsin–Madison, 1977. Pediatrics.

Sandra Pasch, Assistant Professor; M.S., Rochester, 1981; M.A., Medical College of Wisconsin, 1999. Psychiatric and mental health nursing; bioethics.

Mary Ross, Clinical Assistant Professor; M.S., Ohio State, 1992; Medical-surgical nursing.

Kimberly Schuster, Clinical Assistant Professor; M.S.N., Northern Illinois, 1985. Medical-surgical nursing, oncology.

Gladys Simandl, Professor; Ph.D., Wisconsin–Milwaukee, 1990. Community nursing.

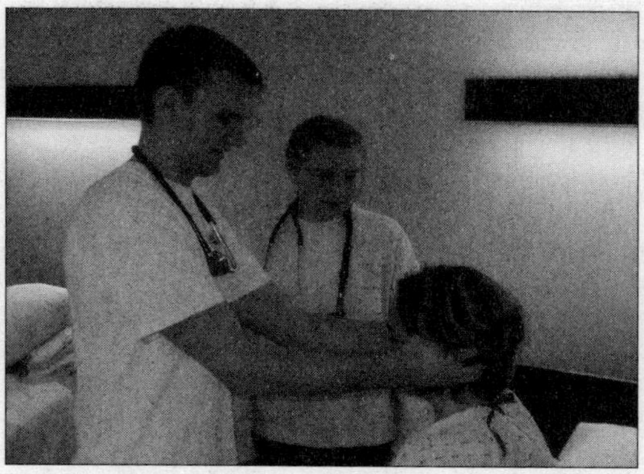

Clinical experiences are an integral part of the Mount Mary College/Columbia College of Nursing program.

Columbia University
School of Nursing
New York, New York

THE UNIVERSITY

By royal charter of King George III of England, Columbia University was founded in 1754 as King's College. It is the oldest institution of higher learning in New York State and the fifth-largest in the nation. A private, nonsectarian institution, Columbia University has, since its inception, addressed the issues of the moment, making important contributions to American life through teaching and research. It is organized into fifteen schools and is associated with more than seventy research and public service institutions and twenty-two scholarly journals. One of its most notable affiliations is with the research-oriented New York–Presbyterian Medical Center. The New York–Presbyterian Hospital, together with the Health Science Division of Columbia University, which includes the Schools of Medicine, Dental and Oral Surgery, Nursing, and Public Health and programs in physical therapy, nutrition, and occupational therapy, constitute the Columbia University Medical Center. Total enrollment is close to 2,500 at the Health Science Campus and nearly 17,500 at the Morningside Campus.

THE SCHOOL OF NURSING

Founded in 1892 as the Presbyterian Hospital School of Nursing, the School first offered the baccalaureate degree when it joined Columbia University. In 1956, it became the first nursing program in the country to award a master's degree in a clinical nursing specialty. Today, the primary focus of the School is to educate advanced practice nurses: nurse practitioners, nurse midwives, and nurse anesthetists. This is done through the academic program at the graduate and advanced certificate levels. The School also offers a research-focused doctoral program (D.N.Sc.) with an emphasis on advanced practice and health outcomes.

The curriculum is focused on preparing professional nurses who think critically, exercise technical competence, and make socially significant contributions to society through theory-based practice. The faculty members endeavor to provide knowledge, to stimulate learning, to define issues, and to serve as resource persons, clinicians, administrators, leaders, and innovators in nursing. A major strength of the School is that the faculty members maintain clinical practices in their advanced roles and incorporate students into these settings. One of these practices, Columbia Advanced Practice Nurse Associates (CAPNA), has gained national exposure as an innovative model of primary-care delivery by advanced practice nurses who are on the primary provider panels of several major managed-care organizations.

In addition to these programs, the School contains four academic centers: the Center for AIDS Research, the Center for Health Policy and Health Services Research, the Center for Evidence-Based Practice, and the World Health Organization Collaborating Center for International Nursing Development in Advanced Practice. Columbia was the first nursing school to be awarded this designation, which makes the School an active participant in international exchange and collaborative research in advanced practice and health services research. It also facilitates the development of international study opportunities for its students.

PROGRAMS OF STUDY

The School of Nursing offers four levels of educational programs. The Entry to Practice (ETP) Program is an accelerated combined-degree program (B.S./M.S.) for non-nurse baccalaureate-prepared graduates, designed to prepare the student for a career as an advanced practice nurse. Academic studies are closely integrated with clinical experience. The prelicensure phase of the program consists of 60 credits, which are completed through full-time study, with a two-month residency. Upon completion, the student is eligible to take the professional nurse licensure examination in any state. In the postlicensure phase, the student follows the curriculum for a clinical specialty, which is described later in this section. Part-time study is available during the postlicensure phase.

The Accelerated Master's Program (AMP) is also a combined-degree program (B.S./M.S.), designed to further the educational and career goals of RNs who have an associate degree in nursing. Phase I consists of 42 credits of course work taken at the School and other undergraduate institutions. This B.S./M.S. program can be completed in five or six semesters.

The Graduate Program, leading to the M.S. degree, affords baccalaureate-prepared nurses the opportunity to increase their knowledge in advanced nursing practice. The School currently offers twelve graduate majors that include anesthesia, acute-care, neonatal, psychiatric–mental health nursing, midwifery, oncology, the primary-care specialties (adult, family, geriatric, and pediatric), women's health, and informatics. The credit requirements range from 45 to 59 and are allocated among core, major, and elective courses. Cross-site curricula are available in selected programs. Joint degrees are available with the Schools of Public Health and Business Administration.

The Advanced Certificate Program allows RNs with a master's degree in nursing to pursue an advanced practice program as a nurse practitioner. The credit requirements range from 22 to 34 credits.

The Doctor of Nursing Science Program is designed to prepare clinical nurse scholars to examine, shape, and refine the health-care delivery system. The program consists of 90 credits beyond the baccalaureate degree. Of these, 45 credits are credits earned at the master's level in a clinical specialist/nurse practitioner program.

AFFILIATIONS WITH HEALTH-CARE FACILITIES

The center of clinical activity at Columbia University Medical Center is the New York Presbyterian Medical Center, which includes a number of world-renowned facilities. Among the most notable are the Neurological Institute, the Eye Institute, Children's Hospital of New York, Sloane Hospital for Women, the Center for Geriatrics and Gerontology, the Organ Transplant Center, and the Center for Health Promotion and Disease

Prevention. In addition, approximately 150 other sites in the tristate area are available for clinical education.

ACADEMIC FACILITIES

The Augustus C. Long Library is the fourth-largest academic medical library in the country and is part of the Columbia University Library system, which encompasses approximately forty libraries and more than 4 million volumes. The Long Library houses more than 400,000 volumes and receives more than 4,500 journals, most of which can be accessed through online computer search programs. The Media and Computer Center contains more than 3,000 audiovisual and computer-assisted instruction programs, including slides, videodiscs, tapes, and a wide variety of personal computer applications. Other services include microfilming, interlibrary loans, study and conference facilities, and photocopying services. The Special Collections Section houses several thousand rare works including the Florence Nightingale Collection, which is featured at exhibitions along with rare holdings of Freud and Webster.

The School of Nursing's Technology Learning Center contains seven patient units, which provide a hands-on environment for developing psychomotor skills, as well as state-of-the-art computer-assisted monitoring equipment that simulates a real clinical environment.

LOCATION

The School of Nursing is part of the Columbia University Medical Center, a 20-acre campus overlooking the Hudson River on Manhattan's Upper West Side. Students can avail themselves of the recreational, cultural, and educational events and entertainment that have made New York City famous.

STUDENT SERVICES

The Office of Student Administrative Services is the hub of all student projects, programs, and services, and it coordinates activities with many other departments. Among the organizations and services provided are housing, dining, health, athletic facilities, a Wellness Program, counseling and advisement, parking, shuttle bus, financial aid, a bookstore, orientation, student records, the Office of Multicultural Affairs, Disability Services, and the International Student Office.

THE NURSING STUDENT GROUP

About 600 students are enrolled each year in the School of Nursing, and they represent a diverse group of nursing professionals. They come from all over the country, but most are from the tristate area.

COSTS

During the 2004–05 academic year, tuition for undergraduates was $907 per credit. For graduate students, tuition ranged from $907 to $1151 per credit. Average housing costs at the Medical Center ranged from $4000 to $6000. Other expenses, including health fees, books, personal expenses, transportation, and uniforms, were estimated at $5000.

FINANCIAL AID

The goal of the School of Nursing financial aid program is to provide as many students as possible with sufficient resources to meet their needs and to distribute funds to eligible students in a fair and equitable manner. Financial aid is met through a combination of scholarships, grants, work, and loans. Students should be able to meet all expenses for the academic year through a combination of these resources.

APPLYING

Admission is based on past academic and professional performance. Admission requirements include an application form with a fee (either printed or online); a typed, double-spaced, one-page personal statement describing professional goals and aspirations; three letters of reference; official transcripts from all postsecondary schools; official GRE scores; a minimum undergraduate grade point average of 3.0; and undergraduate courses in statistics and physical assessment.

Entry-to-Practice candidates (non-nurse college graduates) enroll once per year beginning on or about June 1. Applications are required by November 15 and acceptance decisions are mailed in January. Applications received after November 15 are considered. ETP students must have at least 9 credits of science including anatomy and physiology.

Most applicants may enroll in January, May, or September, and applications are received and decisions made on a rolling-year basis. RN applicants must submit a copy of their current license and registration. Enrollment in some specialties may require a course in physical assessment and a minimum of one year of clinical experience relevant to the chosen clinical major. There are additional admission requirements for the D.N.Sc. and Nurse Anesthesia Program.

CORRESPONDENCE AND INFORMATION

Columbia University School of Nursing
Office of Admissions
630 West 168th Street Box 6
New York, New York 10032
Telephone: 800-899-8895
Fax: 212-305-3680
E-mail: nursing@columbia.edu
World Wide Web: http://www.nursing.hs.columbia.edu

Dominican University of California
School of Arts and Sciences
San Rafael, California

THE UNIVERSITY
Dominican University of California is a coeducational, independent, liberal arts university of Catholic heritage offering more than thirty bachelors and master's degrees. Dominican has a commitment to interdisciplinary study in the humanities, a global perspective, and the involvement of students in their own intellectual, spiritual, ethical, and social development. The University was founded in 1890 by the Dominican Sisters of San Rafael. It was the first Catholic college in the state of California to offer the baccalaureate degree to women. Today, Dominican University derives no direct financial support from the church or the state.

THE SCHOOL
The School of Arts and Sciences strives to support the idea that nursing is a dynamic, interpersonal process based on the premise of individual worth and human dignity and to teach that the goal of nursing is to help individuals, families, and groups achieve and maintain self-care in coping with actual and potential health problems. Nursing is a human service provided when clients' self-care capabilities are inadequate to promote, maintain, and restore health. The Department of Nursing faculty members bring deep understanding and rich backgrounds of both clinical and teaching experience to the program. All full-time faculty members are master's prepared, and the majority are also doctorally prepared or are currently engaged in doctoral work.

PROGRAMS OF STUDY
Dominican University offers a Bachelor of Science in Nursing (B.S.N.) for women and men wishing to enter the field of professional nursing. Registered nurses can also earn a B.S.N. through the University's evening and weekend program. Students complete one year of prerequisite courses before beginning the clinical nursing major in the sophomore year. Clinical experiences in the sophomore, junior, and senior years take place at a variety of affiliated agencies. Throughout the four-year program, lecture classes are held on the Dominican campus. Upon satisfactory completion of the nursing curriculum, students are granted the Bachelor of Science in Nursing degree, are eligible to take the State Board Examination for licensure as a registered nurse (RN), and can obtain a California Public Health Nursing Certificate. Advanced placement is available for transfer students from other nursing programs, registered nurses, licensed vocational nurses, and health-care workers who wish to obtain a baccalaureate degree in nursing. Dominican also offers a Master of Science in Nursing (M.S.N.) program that prepares nurses for advanced practice as clinical nurse specialists in integrated health practices. A 30-unit option is also available for licensed vocational nurses. The nursing program is accredited by the California Board of Registered Nursing and the National League for Nursing Accrediting Commission.

AFFILIATIONS WITH HEALTH-CARE FACILITIES
The Department of Nursing is affiliated with a number of health-care agencies and institutions in the Bay Area, offering students clinical learning opportunities with diverse populations in a wide variety of settings. Agencies include Marin General Hospital; Marin County Health Department; St. Francis Medical Center, San Francisco; and Kaiser Permanente in San Rafael, among others.

ACADEMIC FACILITIES
The Archbishop Alemany Library houses more than 83,000 volumes in open stacks, 3,100 reels of microfilm, 775 videocassettes, 225 audiocassettes and CDs, subscriptions to more than 400 periodicals in print, and another 1,100 volumes in full-text online. More than 1,700 are health and nursing related, with nearly seventy-five periodicals in print dealing with these topics. Reference services, including access to a variety of computerized database and indexes, and multimedia facilities are provided to assist students with their studies and assignments. Nursing students have access to CINAHL, MEDLINE, and PsycINFO and all online health-related information resources. The library also houses the campus computer center.

Within the School itself, the E. L. Wiegand Nursing Laboratory offers students the opportunity to acquire nursing skills in a simulated clinical setting. Computer-assisted instruction and a number of other audiovisual programs are available for student use in this lab.

LOCATION
The University is located on 80 wooded acres in a peaceful residential neighborhood of San Rafael, just 15 minutes north of San Francisco and less than a half hour's drive from Pacific Ocean beaches. Students at the University enjoy the intimacy of a small university while benefiting from easy access to the resources of Marin County and the broader San Francisco Bay Area. Marin offers hills for hiking, redwood forests, and ocean shoreline for walking, and, in general, an unsurpassed lifestyle. In addition, students are only a short distance from San Francisco, which offers world-renowned opera, symphonies, ballet, museums, and championship athletic teams. Dominican is also less than an hour's drive from California's wine country and Silicon Valley.

STUDENT SERVICES
The Office of Student Development coordinates many of the services that support the University's educational mission and the personal, social, physical, spiritual, and professional development of students. Services provided include career services, athletics (NAIA men's and women's basketball, soccer, and tennis and women's volleyball and softball), recreational sports, on-campus housing, campus ministry, the campus health center, counseling services, and student government (ASDC). There are also many student-formed groups and clubs to choose from on campus. The School of Arts and Sciences has an active chapter of the California Nurses Students' Association and a nursing honor society.

THE NURSING STUDENT GROUP
There are approximately 200 students enrolled in the undergraduate nursing programs; of these, 91 percent are women, 48 percent are members of minority groups, and 2 percent are international. There are currently 18 M.S.N. students.

COSTS
The 2003–04 tuition costs for full-time students (12–17 units) were $22,320. Part-time students paid $930 per unit. Room and board were an additional $9400. The tuition reservation deposit was $250, and there was an additional nursing major fee of $400 per semester when taking clinicals. Mandatory health insurance was $518 per year for those without coverage. Additional

expenses for the nursing program included uniforms, books, supplies, a physical examination, annual tuberculosis screening and immunization, and transportation between the University and affiliated clinical agencies.

FINANCIAL AID

The University manages an extensive financial assistance program to ensure that a highly qualified and diverse population is able to matriculate and continue to graduation. The assistance programs take two major forms: scholarships and need-based financial aid. In addition to administering federal and state aid programs, Dominican University also awards a number of scholarships and grants annually from income provided by annual gifts and endowed funds as well as from its own general funds. The Financial Aid Office matches the intentions of the donor to the academic and other qualifications of students with need.

APPLYING

Applicants who are qualified for admission to Dominican University are admitted as nursing majors in the preclinical program. Students are considered for placement in sophomore clinical classes in the fall or spring semesters if the following minimal admission criteria are fulfilled: completion of elementary algebra, completion of all prerequisite courses (inorganic and organic chemistry; human anatomy and physiology; nutrition; introduction to psychology, sociology, or anthropology; and English), and maintenance of an overall GPA of at least 2.5. Advanced placement students can be admitted for either the spring or fall semesters.

CORRESPONDENCE AND INFORMATION:

Office of Admissions
Dominican University of California
50 Acacia Avenue
San Rafael, California 94901-2298
Telephone: 415-485-3204
888-323-6763 (toll-free)
E-mail: enroll@dominican.edu
World Wide Web: http://www.dominican.edu

Dominican University School of Arts and Sciences
Department of Nursing
Telephone: 415-485-3295
E-mail: nursing@dominican.edu

THE FACULTY

Kathleen Beebe, Assistant Professor; Ph.D., RN.
Margaret Fink, Assistant Professor; M.S.N., RN.
Linda Gabriel-Marin, Assistant Professor; M.S.N., RN.
Barbara Ganley, Assistant Professor; Ph.D., RN.
Mary Ann Haeuser, Assistant Professor; M.S.N.
Adrina Lemos, Assistant Professor; M.S.N., RN.
Luanne Linnard-Palmer, Professor; Ed.D., RN.
Ron Morrison, Assistant Professor; M.S., RN.
Dottie Needham, Department Chair; D.N.S., RN.
Ingrid Sheets, Assistant Professor; M.S., RN.

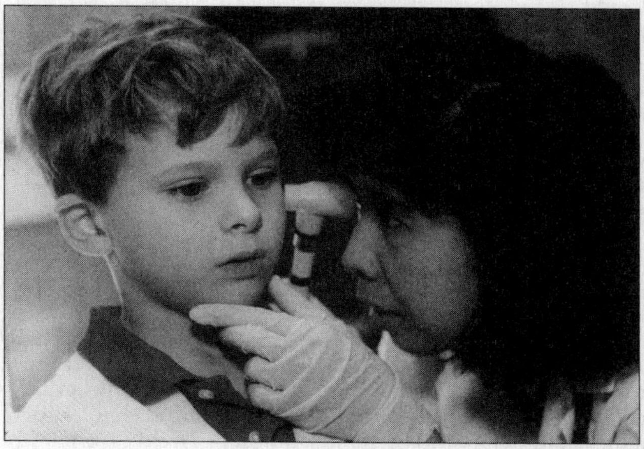

The School of Arts and Sciences at Dominican University of California offers its students a wide variety of clinical experiences.

Drexel University
College of Nursing and Health Professions
Philadelphia, Pennsylvania

THE UNIVERSITY

On July 1, 2002, Drexel University's Board of Trustees unanimously voted to merge the academic programs of Drexel and MCP Hahnemann Universities. With the addition of the nation's largest private medical school, an outstanding college of nursing and health professions, and one of only two schools of public health in Pennsylvania, Drexel University now comprises eleven colleges and schools. This combination of expertise in advanced technology and cooperative education and academic programs in medicine and health-related fields means that students are offered an exceptional set of skills with which to succeed in today's ever-changing world.

THE COLLEGE OF NURSING AND HEALTH PROFESSIONS

Drexel has a 130-year legacy of educating nurses. Hospital-based nursing programs began in 1864 at what was then the Female Medical College of Pennsylvania and in 1890 at the Hahnemann Hospital Training School for Nurses. With the consolidation of Medical College of Pennsylvania and Hahnemann University in 1993, Hahnemann's undergraduate and graduate nursing programs and Medical College of Pennsylvania's nurse anesthesia program were combined into the College of Nursing and Health Professions.

Today, with the merger of MCP Hahnemann with Drexel University, this tradition of health sciences education has taken another step forward. Undergraduate and graduate programs in health professions, nursing, public health, medicine, and biomedical graduate studies stand alongside Drexel's established and renowned programs.

PROGRAMS OF STUDY

Drexel's College of Nursing and Health Professions offers a variety of educational programs that prepare nurses and future nurses for exciting opportunities. Several undergraduate programs are offered. The Bachelor of Science in Nursing (B.S.N.) program is a full-time, five-year program that leads to the B.S.N. The program is one of only a few in the country that offers three paid, six-month cooperative education experiences in the field of nursing in addition to traditional clinical experiences. The Accelerated B.S.N./M.S.N. program allows students to complete both the Bachelor of Science in Nursing and the Master of Science in Nursing degrees in five years. The Accelerated Career Entry (ACE) program is an eleven-month, intensive, full-time B.S.N. program for students who already have bachelor's or graduate degrees in another field. The R.N./B.S.N Completion program, available online or in class, is a B.S.N. completion program for nurses from associate and diploma nursing programs. The R.N./B.S.N./M.S.N. program is an accelerated program designed for graduates of associate degree and diploma nursing programs who are committed to earning the Master of Science in Nursing degree.

The M.S.N. programs prepare nurse practitioners in a variety of specialty areas, such as family care, acute care, pediatric care, perioperative, psychiatric–mental health care, and women's health. (Women's health is offered in collaboration with Planned Parenthood Federation of America.) M.S.N. programs in education, nursing leadership and management, public health, and clinical trials research are also offered. Another exciting option is the VIP-M.S.N. (Versatile Individualized Program), which allows students the opportunity to design their own unique area of concentration. In response to health-care-system needs, innovative M.S.N. tracks are in continuous development.

The M.S.N. in nurse anesthesia is a nationally recognized program that prepares nurses to practice as anesthetists. The R.N./M.S.N. program is for nurses who hold a B.A. or B.S. in an area other than nursing. An M.S.N. Completion program is offered for graduates of certificate nurse practitioner or nurse anesthesia programs. The RNFA is a one-semester course that meets one of the eligibility requirements to become a certified as an RN first assistant. Certificate programs are offered for individuals who have earned an M.S.N. and seek further preparation to qualify for state or national certification. There are certificate programs in education, nursing leadership and management, and clinical trials research.

The B.S.N. program, the Accelerated Career Entry option, the R.N./B.S.N Completion program, and the M.S.N. program are accredited by the National League for Nursing Accrediting Commission and the American Association of Colleges of Nursing. The nurse anesthesia M.S.N. program is accredited by the Council on Accreditation of the Nurse Anesthesia Educational Programs.

ACADEMIC FACILITIES

The Clinical Resource Learning Center (CRLC) provides a simulated environment in which students can safely learn and practice clinical skills. Students practice head-to-toe assessments, invasive as well as noninvasive procedures, and interpersonal skills. Students also have an opportunity learn how to manage real-life emergencies and clinical situations with SIM-MAN®, a simulated patient that can mimic patient signs and symptoms. The CRLC consists of a physical assessment lab, media center and media classroom, nursing therapeutics lab, and two rehabilitation sciences labs.

LOCATION

Drexel University's Center City Hahnemann Campus is spread over more than a city block and includes classrooms, research areas, student lounge and activity areas, and an array of educational and student-life resources. Students have the use of the Student Life Center, which includes a Nautilus-equipped fitness center, and there are lounges throughout the campus that offer video games and television as well as comfortable space to eat and socialize. Intramural sports teams are also available at the Center City Campus.

The 636-bed Hahnemann University Hospital is located on the campus. In 2002, Drexel University merged with MCP Hahnemann University, and the new Center City location name reflects its history as one of Philadelphia's progressive medical institutions. At the Center City Hahnemann Campus, the College of Nursing and Health Profession's Nursing Co-op Program provides eighteen months of co-op education designed to expose students to various career options.

STUDENT SERVICES

Many services are offered to students. These include Academic Enrichment Services (ACT 101), the Center for Student Academic Resources, the Office of International Student Services, the Office of Multicultural Programs and Special Projects, Residential Life and Off-Campus Housing, Student Counseling Center, and Student Disability Services as well as student organizations and government and many activities for students. There is a Health Sciences Campus Bookstore and a chapter of the Student Nurses' Association of Pennsylvania.

THE NURSING STUDENT GROUP

There are approximately 380 undergraduates and 260 graduate students in the nursing programs. About 75 percent are women. Most of the undergraduates attend on a full-time basis, while most graduate students attend part-time.

COSTS

Tuition for the 2003 academic year was $19,900 per year for the B.S.N. Co-op program and $565 per credit for the RN-B.S.N. program. The ACE program cost a total of $22,000.

FINANCIAL AID

Drexel University offers a full program of financial aid in the form of low-interest educational loans, alumni endorsement scholarships, grants, and campus work-study opportunities. Additional financial aid and work programs are available to students who qualify.

APPLYING

Drexel University offers programs for applicants with both nursing and non-nursing backgrounds. Admissions requirements vary by program.

CORRESPONDENCE AND INFORMATION

Drexel University
Office of Admissions
Health Sciences Programs
245 North 15th Street, Mail Stop 472
Philadelphia, Pennsylvania 19102
Telephone: 215-762-8288
800-2DREXEL Ext. 6333 (toll-free)
E-mail: enroll@drexel.edu
World Wide Web: http://www.drexel.edu

THE FACULTY

Undergraduate Faculty

Joyce Bedoian, Clinical Assistant Professor; M.S.N., Pennsylvania; RN.

Barbara Blair, Assistant Professor; M.S.N., Pennsylvania; RN, CS. Huntington's disease, eating disorders, panic disorder.

Renee Byfield, Clinical Assistant Professor; M.S.N., Pace; RN.

Frances Cornelius, Assistant Professor; M.S.N., Wayne State; RN. Environmental health and health literacy; health promotion, health behavior; health risks in cardiovascular health, diabetes, and asthma.

Heyward Michael Dreher, Assistant Professor; D.N.Sc., Widener; RN. Sleep and HIV, nursing interventions for sleep pattern disturbances, innovative teaching pedagogies.

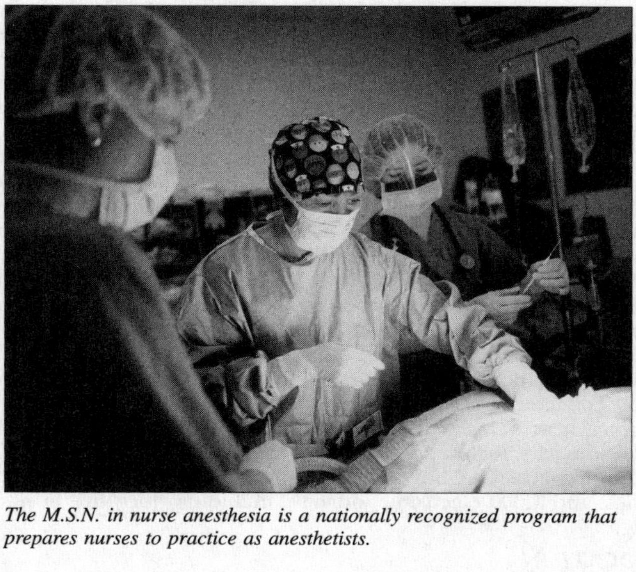

The M.S.N. in nurse anesthesia is a nationally recognized program that prepares nurses to practice as anesthetists.

Anne Ferrari, Assistant Professor; M.S.N., Ed.D., Temple; RN. Fear of falling among community-living adults over 65.

Marcia Gardner, Assistant Professor; M.A., NYU; RN, CPNP, CPN.

Mary Gallagher Gordon, Clinical Assistant Professor; M.S.N., Pennsylvania; RN.

Beulah Hall, Associate Professor; M.S.N., Ed.D., Temple; RN. Depression among the poor.

Katherine Hasson, Clinical Assistant Professor; M.S.N., Villanova; RN.

Karen Henken, Assistant Professor; M.S.N., Pennsylvania; RN.

Lorraine Igo, Assistant Professor; Ed.D., Widener; RN.

Priscilla Killian, Assistant Professor; M.S.N., LaSalle; RN, CS. Stress and its effects on the health of urban minority populations; program treatment and outreach effectiveness in the chronic and persistently mentally ill; the expanding role of the psychiatric nurse practitioner.

Janet Manco, Clinical Assistant Professor; M.S.N., LaSalle; RN.

Faye Pearlman, Clinical Assistant Professor; M.B.A., M.S., Pennsylvania; RN.

Alice Poyss, Associate Professor; Ph.D., Pennsylvania; RN, CRNP, ANP-C, CS. Nutrition, asthma, managed care.

Margaret Schmidt, Clinical Assistant Professor; M.S.N., Hahnemann; RN.

Joanne Schwartz, Assistant Professor; M.S.N., Pennsylvania; RN, CRNP.

Geraldine Sherzer, Adjunct Assistant Professor; M.S.N., Villanova; B.S.N.; RN.

Mary Ellen Smith, Assistant Professor and Director, Undergraduate Program; Ph.D., Duquesne; RN, CS. Social, cultural, and economic determinants of bone marrow donation; psychological impact of bone marrow transplantation among recipients and donors.

Magdeleine Vasso, Clinical Assistant Professor; M.S.N., Widener; RN.

Regina Wright, Clinical Assistant Professor; M.S.N., Pennsylvania; RN, CEN.

Full-Time Graduate Faculty

Elizabeth Blunt, Assistant Professor and Director, Graduate Nursing Program; M.S.N., Pennsylvania; RN, CEN, CRN. Nurse practitioner prescribing practices, online education.

Michael Booth, Nurse Anesthesia Program; M.S.N., Allegheny University of the Health Sciences; RN, CRNA.

Sandra Davis, Acute Care Nurse Practitioner Program; M.S.N., Pennsylvania; RN, CRNP.

Gloria Donnelly, Graduate Program Leadership; Ph.D., Bryn Mawr; RN, FAAN.

William Fehder, Nurse Anesthesia Program; Ph.D., Pennsylvania; RN, CRNA. Psychoneuroimmunology: the role of the neuropeptide Substance P in mediating the effects of anxiety and other forms of stress on immune function.

Patricia Gerrity, Health Promotion/Community; Ph.D., Pennsylvania; RN, FAAN.

Elizabeth Gonzalez, Psychiatric–Mental Health Practitioner Program; Ph.D., NYU; RN, CS. Stress and coping in family caregivers of patients with dementia, minority health, anxiety and depression among medically ill elderly.

Debra McGrath, M.S.N., Pennsylvania; RN, CRNP. Developing continuing nursing information for the World Wide Web.

Barbara K. Rideout, Family Nurse Practitioner Program; M.S.N., Villanova; RN, CS, CRNP.

Albert Rundio, Education, Nursing Leadership and Management Program; Ph.D., Pennsylvania; RN, CRNP.

John Strange, Nurse Anesthesia Program; M.S.N., Columbia; CRNA.

Suzanne Willard, Family Nurse Practitioner Program; M.S.N., Pennsylvania; RN, CRNP.

John Wisniewski, Nurse Anesthesia Program; M.S.N., Allegheny University of the Health Sciences; RN, CRNA.

Duke University
School of Nursing
Durham, North Carolina

THE UNIVERSITY
Since its founding in 1839 as the Union Institute, and later as Trinity College before incorporating in 1924, the basic principles of Duke University have remained constant. Through changing generations of students, the objective has been to encourage individuals to achieve, to the extent of their capacities, an understanding and appreciation of the world in which they live, their relationship to it, their opportunities, and their responsibilities. Today, Duke University has 12,000 students, of whom 5,250 (400 of whom are part-time) are enrolled in the graduate and professional programs, representing nearly every state and many countries.

The School of Medicine, School of Nursing, and Duke Hospital and Health Network are the core institutions of the Duke University Medical Center and Health System, which ranks among the outstanding health-care providers of the world. The opening of Duke Hospital North in 1980 made Duke Hospital, with 1,048 beds, one of the most modern patient-care facilities available anywhere. The mission of the Health System is to be a leader in world health care. This involves maintaining superiority in its four primary functions: excellent patient care, dedication to educational programs, national and international distinction in the quality of research, and service to the region.

THE SCHOOL OF NURSING
Since the founding of the School in 1930, Duke has prepared outstanding clinicians, educators, and researchers and is continuing this tradition. Drawing on the intellectual and clinical resources of both Duke University Medical Center and Duke University, the School offers an Accelerated Bachelor of Science in Nursing degree (for second degree students) and a Master of Science in Nursing degree program that balances education, practice, and research.

Faculty members work closely with students to challenge and nurture them; students not only practice with state-of-the-art science and technology in a great medical center but also have opportunities to work in rural and underserved areas.

PROGRAMS OF STUDY
The School of Nursing offers a 58-credit-hour, full-time, Accelerated Bachelor of Science in Nursing (B.S.N.) degree program in a sixteen-month, intensive format. In addition, a flexible, 39- to 59-credit program leading to the Master of Science in Nursing (M.S.N.) degree is offered. There are also two joint-degree programs: in conjunction with the Fuqua School of Business, a joint M.S.N./M.B.A. degree, and, in conjunction with the Divinity School, a joint M.S.N./Master of Church Ministries degree. The School of Nursing also offers a collaborative arrangement with Meredith College in Raleigh, North Carolina, that facilitates completion of the M.S.N. degree in nursing and health-care leadership at the Duke School of Nursing and the M.B.A. at Meredith College. The School of Nursing also offers a post-master's certificate to students who have already earned an M.S.N. The purpose of the Master of Science in Nursing program is to prepare professional nurses for advanced practice in a clinical speciality, administration, or education. Graduates are prepared as clinical nurse specialists in gerontology, oncology, critical care, pediatrics, or neonatal care; as adult nurse practitioners (with specialization in primary care, acute care, cardiovascular care, or oncology/HIV); as gerontological nurse practitioners, family nurse practitioners, neonatal nurse practitioners, pediatric acute/chronic care nurse practitioners, pediatric nurse practitioners, or combined neonatal-pediatric nurse practitioners with an emphasis on rural health care; as nursing health-care leadership administrators and managers; clinical research managers; nurse anesthetists; advanced practice nurses prepared to serve faith communities; and nurse educators. The clinical research management program, the nursing and health-care leadership program, the nursing education program, the nursing informatics program, and selected nurse practitioner core courses are available online to distance education students. The family nurse practitioner, adult nurse practitioner, and gerontological nurse practitioner programs are also available online. The integration of education, practice, and research is basic to the entire curriculum as well as to the activities of each student, and the program is designed to provide maximum flexibility for full-time or part-time study.

AFFILIATIONS WITH HEALTH-CARE FACILITIES
As one of the leading national and international academic health systems, Duke University Health System has assembled and integrated a comprehensive range of health-care resources providing the very best in patient care, health education, and clinical research. The clinical faculty members of the Duke University School of Nursing number more than 100 and represent all specialties. Clinical faculty members actively participate in nursing education and practice nursing in hospitals and ambulatory settings. Cooperative teaching and clinical facilities, including health departments, retirement centers, and private practices in both urban and rural settings, are available to students mostly within the state of North Carolina. Occasionally, placements are arranged out-of-state or in other countries to accommodate the student's needs.

Nationally recognized centers with which the School of Nursing is affiliated include the Duke Heart Center, the Center for Aging and Human Development, the Comprehensive Cancer Center, the Comprehensive Sickle Cell Center, Alzheimer's Disease Research Center, Duke Hypertension Center, Duke–VA Center for Cerebrovascular Research, Cystic Fibrosis/Chest Center and Clinic, Sleep Disorders Center, the Eye Center, and the Geriatric Research, Education, and Clinical Center.

ACADEMIC FACILITIES
The goal of the Duke Nursing Research Center is to facilitate the conduct of clinical research by the students and faculty and nursing staff members. The center provides support for research through assistance with literature searches, development of research designs, the Institutional Review Board and/or the protection of human subjects consultation, data collection and data management, grant proposal development, and editorial review.

The Duke School of Nursing is a national leader in online education; all of the School's courses are enriched by the use of technology. There is a student computer laboratory containing fifteen computer workstations, and a computing orientation seminar enables students to take full advantage of technology. The School also supports a new Center for Instruction Technology and Distance Learning, the purpose of which is to provide technical support for online education and classroom technology.

The Medical Center Library, located in the Seeley G. Mudd Communications Center and Library Building, provides services and collections necessary to support educational, research, and clinical activities. The library has sizable holdings of nursing books and journals, including 300,000 bound volumes in health, 6,000 bound volumes in nursing, 2,375 health-care-related periodical titles, and 1,000 electronic journals, including thirty-five in nursing.

LOCATION
Durham, a city of 223,000, is about 250 miles south of Washington, D.C. Durham and nearby Raleigh and Chapel Hill constitute the

three points of the Research Triangle, one of the nation's foremost centers of research-oriented industries and government, research, and regulatory agencies.

STUDENT SERVICES

The University has many resources and activities to offer students. These include the Graduate and Professional Student Council, the Women's Center, the Mary Lou Williams Center for Black Culture, and the International House as well as the full programs of the Office of Cultural Affairs, the Duke University Campus Ministry, the Duke University Union, the Office of Student Activities, and recreational clubs.

THE NURSING STUDENT GROUP

Approximately 105 students are enrolled in the accelerated B.S.N. degree program, and 339 students are enrolled in the M.S.N. and post-master's certificate programs. About 12 percent are men, and 13 percent are members of minority groups.

COSTS

Tuition in 2004–05 was $699 per credit hour for graduate nursing courses and $551 per credit hour for undergraduate nursing courses.

FINANCIAL AID

Merit and need-based scholarships, traineeships, and federal/state loan programs are generally available. Approximately 80 percent of School of Nursing students receive some form of financial aid.

APPLYING

Admission requirements for the Accelerated B.S.N. program include a bachelor's degree from an accredited college or university, a minimum 3.0 GPA on a 4.0 scale, three letters of recommendation, GRE or MAT scores, and completion of all required prerequisites. Admission requirements for the graduate program include a bachelor's degree with an upper-division nursing major from an NLNAC- or CCNE-accredited program, a preferred undergraduate scholastic average of 3.0 or better on a 4.0 scale, an introductory course in descriptive and inferential statistics, GRE or MAT scores not more than five years old, and licensure as a registered nurse in North Carolina. An interview is requested; if distance prohibits this, a telephone interview may be arranged. Exceptions to any of the above qualifications are considered on an individual basis.

Duke University does not discriminate on the basis of race, color, national and ethnic origin, handicap, sexual orientation or preference, gender, or age in the administration of educational policies, admission policies, financial aid, employment, or any other University program or activity. It admits qualified students to all the rights, privileges, programs, and activities generally accorded or made available to students.

CORRESPONDENCE AND INFORMATION

Office of Admissions and Student Services
Duke University School of Nursing
Box 3322 Medical Center
Durham, North Carolina 27710
Telephone: 919-684-4248
877-415-3853 (graduate; toll-free)
866-844-5617 Ext. 223 (A-B.S.N.; toll-free)
Fax: 919-668-4693
E-mail: SONAdmissions@mc.duke.edu
World Wide Web: http://www.nursing.duke.edu

THE FACULTY

Ruth Anderson, Associate Professor; Ph.D., Texas at Austin, 1987; RN.

Donald Bailey, Assistant Professor; Ph.D., North Carolina at Chapel Hill, 2002; RN.

Julie V. Barroso, Assistant Professor; Ph.D., Texas at Austin; RN, ANP, CS.

Jane Blood-Siegfried, Assistant Professor; D.N.S., UCLA, 1995; RN, PNP.

Margaret Bowers, Assistant Clinical Professor; M.S.N., Duke, 1990; RN, FNP.

Wanda Bradshaw, Assistant Clinical Professor; M.S.N., Duke, 1996; RN, PNP, NNP.

Debra Brandon, Assistant Professor; Ph.D., North Carolina at Chapel Hill, 2000; RN.

Margaret D. Brekenridge, Consulting Associate Professor; M.S.N., Virginia Commonwealth, 1984; RN, FNP.

Mary T. Champagne, Associate Professor; Ph.D., Texas at Austin, 1981; RN.

Elizabeth Clipp, Professor; Ph.D., Cornell, 1984; RN.

Kirsten Corazzini-Gomez, Assistant Professor; Ph.D., Massachusetts Boston, 2000.

Susan Denman, Assistant Professor; Ph.D., North Carolina at Chapel Hill, 1996; RN, FNP.

Sharron Docherty, Assistant Professor; Ph.D., North Carolina at Chapel Hill, 1999; RN.

Anthony T. Dren, Consulting Professor; Ph.D., Michigan, 1966.

Pamela Edwards, Associate Consulting Professor; M.S.N., Ed.D., North Carolina State, 1989; RN, BC.

Catherine Gilliss, Dean and Vice Chancellor for Nursing Affairs for Duke University Health System; D.N.Sc., Duke, 1971; RN.

Linda K. Goodwin, Assistant Professor; Ph.D., Kansas, 1992; RN.

Mary Hall, Assistant Clinical Professor; M.S.N., Duke, 1994; RN.

Kathleen R. Harden, Clinical Associate Professor; M.S., St. Mary's of Minnesota, 1996; RN, CRNA.

Judith C. Hays, Associate Professor and Division Chief of the Accelerated B.S.N. Program; Ph.D., Yale, 1991; RN.

Cristina Hendrix, Assistant Professor; Ph.D., LSU, 2001; RN.

Elizabeth Hill, Assistant Professor; D.N.Sc., Catholic University, 1993; RN.

Mary C. Karlet, Assistant Clinical Professor and Interim Associate Dean for Academic Affairs; Ph.D., Wayne State, 1992; RN, CRNA.

Marcia S. Lorimer, Assistant Clinical Professor; M.S.N., Virginia, 1988; RN, PNP.

Michelle Martin, Assistant Professor; Ph.D., Case Western Reserve, 2001; RN.

Eleanor S. McConnell, Assistant Research Professor; Ph.D., North Carolina at Chapel Hill, 1995; RN.

Mary Miller-Bell, Adjunct Associate Professor; Pharm.D., North Carolina at Chapel Hill, 1998.

Brenda M. Nevidjon, Associate Clinical Professor; M.S.N., North Carolina at Chapel Hill, 1978; RN.

Judith K. Payne, Assistant Professor; Ph.D., Iowa, 1998; RN, AOCN, CS.

Marva M. Price, Assistant Professor; Dr.P.H., North Carolina at Chapel Hill, 1994; RN, FNP; FAAN.

Carla Rapp, Assistant Professor; Ph.D., Iowa, 1999; RN, CRRN.

Susan Schneider, Assistant Professor; Ph.D., Case Western Reserve, 1998; RN.

Nancy Short, Assistant Professor and Assistant Dean for Evaluation; M.B.A., Dr.P.H., North Carolina at Chapel Hill, 2003; RN.

Steven Talbert, Assistant Professor; Ph.D., Kentucky, 2002; RN.

Lisa J. Thiemann, Assistant Clinical Professor; M.N.A., Mayo School of Health-Related Sciences; RN, CRNA.

J. Frank Titch, Clinical Associate Professor; M.S.N.A., Virginia Commonwealth; RN, CRNA.

Barbara S. Turner, Professor, Associate Dean, Director of Nursing Research, and Division Chief; D.N.Sc., California, San Francisco, 1984; RN; FAAN.

George H. Turner III, Assistant Clinical Professor; M.A., Webster, 1978; RPh.

Kathleen M. Turner, Assistant Clinical Professor and Associate Director of the Accelerated B.S.N. Program; M.S.N., Duke, 1993; RN.

Queen Utley-Smith, Assistant Professor; Ed.D., North Carolina State, 1999; RN.

Ann White, Assistant Clinical Professor; M.S.N., Duke, 1992; RN.

Duquesne University
School of Nursing
Pittsburgh, Pennsylvania

THE UNIVERSITY

Duquesne University, located in Pittsburgh, Pennsylvania, America's renaissance city, is a private coeducational Catholic university with ten schools and an enrollment of more than 10,000 students. Currently, the University is experiencing record-breaking growth, and nearly 100 nations and every state are represented in Duquesne's student body.

With a 125-year-old tradition of scholarship and community service, Duquesne has a well-earned reputation among the top Catholic universities in the United States. Duquesne is committed to providing education for the mind, heart, and spirit. The University offers a wide variety of activities and volunteer opportunities that complement the curriculum and provide a broad, well-balanced, and fully integrated education.

THE SCHOOL OF NURSING

Founded in 1937, the School of Nursing at Duquesne was the first nursing school in Pennsylvania to offer a baccalaureate program in nursing, and it was among the first in the nation to offer an online doctoral program in nursing. Continuing that tradition of innovation, Duquesne's School of Nursing offers a wide variety of online and traditional degree and certificate programs. A leader in nursing education for generations, the School of Nursing at Duquesne maintains the highest standards of clinical competency, academic achievement, and dedication to helping others.

Community service that provides an unmatched educational experience is one of the hallmarks of a nursing education at Duquesne. This commitment to service holds true for the faculty and staff, as well. Members of the School of Nursing's award-winning faculty have been widely recognized for their volunteer work as well as their clinical expertise, research accomplishments, and teaching skills.

Faculty members operate a number of Nurse-Managed Wellness Centers in underserved communities, where nurses and other health-care providers promote health and wellness and monitor chronic medical conditions. The clinics offer students an invaluable clinical learning experience and an ongoing opportunity for community service.

Duquesne's Center for International Nursing offers students a transcultural perspective on health care. Through student/faculty exchange programs, collaborative international research projects, and hands-on training in other countries, the Center provides a range of educational, research, and nursing leadership opportunities for students and faculty members. The center's transcultural experiences are designed to meet not only curricular requirements but also individual student needs at the undergraduate, graduate, and postgraduate levels.

The Center for Health Care Diversity addresses health-care equity and diversity issues in minority populations through community-focused research, nursing education programs, health policy development, and community service.

PROGRAMS OF STUDY

The School of Nursing offers baccalaureate, master's, and doctoral degrees as well as a variety of professional certificates. School of Nursing students may enroll part-time or full-time. The undergraduate program of the School of Nursing leads to the degree of Bachelor of Science in Nursing (B.S.N.). At the undergraduate level, Duquesne offers a four-year B.S.N., the RN-B.S.N./M.S.N., and the Second Degree B.S.N. The B.S.N. program is designed to educate nurse generalists and usually requires four years of full-time study. The curriculum (130 credits) provides students with a strong foundation in the natural, biological, and behavioral sciences, most of which are taken during the first two years of study. Students receive an introduction to the nursing profession at the freshman level and begin clinical experience with clients and families during the sophomore year. The junior and senior years are devoted almost exclusively to clinical experience. Undergraduate minors for nursing students are available in business, psychology, sociology, Spanish, and communication. In addition, the School offers a unique undergraduate focus area in music therapy as well as a business certificate for nursing students.

Pittsburgh is home to a number of world-class medical centers that provide Duquesne nursing students with state-of-the-art clinical experience. Duquesne faculty members teach all professional courses as well as guide and direct the clinical learning experiences.

The Second Degree B.S.N. program allows the non-nurse with a baccalaureate degree to achieve a Bachelor of Science in Nursing degree in twelve months. After all requirements for the B.S.N. degree have been completed, students are eligible to take the state board examination for nursing licensure. The program begins in August and includes three semesters of intensive course work using traditional classroom instruction, creative Web-enhanced seminars for nonclinical courses, and more than 1,000 hours of clinical practice in leading health-care settings. Upon completion of the B.S.N. requirements, students who have maintained a 3.0 QPA may begin M.S.N. course work.

The RN-B.S.N./M.S.N. program is offered entirely online for registered nurses pursuing B.S.N. and M.S.N. degrees. Through transfer credits, CLEP testing, and challenging examinations, this program permits a registered nurse to apply previous learning experience toward the requirements of a B.S.N. degree. After completing the required core curriculum and nursing prerequisites, the B.S.N. program can be completed online and part-time in five semesters. In this program, a B.S.N. is awarded after the completion of 32 nursing credits, 17 of which are master's-level credits. Upon completion of the B.S.N., students have the option of earning an M.S.N. degree at Duquesne, which can be obtained in an additional two years of part-time study. The Miller Analogies Test (MAT), a required admission test for the M.S.N. program, is waived for students with a 3.0 GPA who have met all graduate admissions criteria.

The Online M.S.N. program, which is offered entirely online, is based on the belief that specialization in nursing is gained at the graduate level. This program is designed to meet the current and future needs of nurses who are likely to hold leadership positions. It educates nurses to plan, initiate, effect, and evaluate change; ensure high-quality patient care; and enhance the profession. Working nurses may continue their employment while undertaking this course of study through part-time enrollment, or course work may be undertaken on a full-time basis. Core curriculum courses in this program are available through distance learning options.

Six areas of specialization exist in the M.S.N. program: nursing education (37 credits), nursing administration (39 credits), family nurse practitioner (46 credits), forensic nursing

(36 credits), acute-care clinical nurse specialist (38 credits), and psychiatric–mental health nursing (35 credits).

Post-master's certificates offered online give professional nurses the opportunity to learn skills and acquire information that may not have been offered in graduate programs. Course work in these nondegree programs is designed to prepare nurses for certification through applicable professional organizations. Duquesne offers the following post-master's certificates: nursing administration (15 credits), nursing education (12–16 credits), family nurse practitioner (34 credits), forensic nursing (19 credits), psychiatric–mental health (21 credits), and transcultural/international nursing (12 credits).

The Online Doctor of Philosophy (Ph.D.) degree (57 credits) prepares nurses for a lifetime of intellectual inquiry and creative scholarship. This online program permits students to earn a doctoral degree in nursing using state-of-the-art distance education technology. Online courses are asynchronous, meaning that students can complete their work anytime and anywhere via the Internet. Mandatory fieldwork can be conducted near the student's home. Ph.D. students are required to be on campus for one week each spring during the completion of their required course work (a period that varies from two to four years). During that week, students meet with faculty advisers, attend lectures by visiting professors, participate in seminars for required courses, complete examinations, and participate in program evaluation.

ACADEMIC FACILITIES

Duquesne University's Gumberg Library houses extensive collections of digital research databases and electronic journals, books, and reference works, which are accessible from remote locations. The library's facilities include CD-ROM collections as well as numerous computers and multimedia learning tools. The School of Nursing houses the Nursing Resource Center, which provides students with new, state-of-the-art computerized educational tools and a realistic practice setting for learning clinical skills and procedures.

LOCATION

Duquesne's campus provides a comfortable and secure academic and social atmosphere that is just minutes from downtown Pittsburgh. The scenic, hilltop campus is readily accessible to the city's business, cultural, entertainment, and shopping districts while still offering students the privacy and peaceful atmosphere of a self-contained 43-acre campus. Home to many of the nation's corporations and rated as one of the nation's most livable cities, Pittsburgh combines the best features of urban life with the charm, pace, and personality of small-town living.

STUDENT SERVICES

Duquesne University offers a variety of services that help students achieve their academic and professional goals and grow socially, spiritually, and personally. Support services include student health services, an Office of Freshman Development and Special Student Services, a Career Services Center, an office of Comprehensive Student Advisement, the University Counseling Center, a Learning Skills Center, and Campus Ministry. In addition, an Office of International Programs assists students and scholars from other countries who are pursuing undergraduate and graduate studies at Duquesne.

THE NURSING STUDENT GROUP

The School of Nursing currently has an enrollment of approximately 400 B.S.N. students, of whom 5 percent are enrolled part-time. Ten percent are members of minority groups, and 8 percent are men. Of the nearly 140 M.S.N. students, 95 percent are part-time. The Ph.D. program has more than 50 students. Duquesne's nursing students come from around the United States and the world. In addition to challenging clinical and classroom learning, Duquesne's nursing students are involved in a full range of campus activities, including student government, fraternities, sororities, and social and professional organizations (Alpha Tau Delta, Sigma Theta Tau International Honor Society, Chi Eta Phi, and the Student Nurses Association of Pennsylvania). Nursing students have excelled in many sports at Duquesne, including football, baseball, crew, volleyball, soccer, lacrosse, cross-country, swimming, and diving.

COSTS

For the 2004–05 academic year, undergraduate tuition and fees for full-time students (12–18 credits) were $20,753 per year. Undergraduate room and board per semester were $3910 (double room). Undergraduate tuition and fees were $686 per credit for part-time students. Graduate tuition and fees (part-time or full-time) were $735 per credit. Other estimated undergraduate nursing school expenses each semester include books and supplies, $500; student liability insurance, $25; and uniforms, $120.

FINANCIAL AID

Tuition at Duquesne is among the lowest among private national universities, and competitive financial aid packages make a Duquesne education more affordable. Financial aid includes scholarships, grants, loans, and part-time employment awarded to help students meet the costs of education. Awards, both merit-based and need-based, come through a variety of sources, including programs administered by the federal and state government, private organizations, and the University. Duquesne is constantly developing resources for funding scholarships and providing financial assistance, and the School of Nursing maintains numerous listings of nursing funding sources for undergraduate and graduate nursing education, including federal, state, and private organizations and local hospital discounts. Students must apply for any awards by May 1 of each year.

APPLYING

Students with above-average high school records whose first college of choice is Duquesne may apply for early decision admission. Early decision applications must be submitted on or before November 1 of the student's senior year for consideration for the following fall semester. Early decision acceptance notifications are made by December 15, after which time students have two weeks to submit the required deposit. Admission requirements for the undergraduate and graduate programs are specific for each degree option. Transfer and international applicants must fulfill all undergraduate or graduate admission requirements. A personal or telephone interview with a School of Nursing representative is highly recommended and may be required, depending on the program of study. Interested applicants should contact the School of Nursing or visit the School's Web site for detailed information.

CORRESPONDENCE AND INFORMATION

Duquesne University School of Nursing
600 Forbes Avenue
Pittsburgh, Pennsylvania 15282-1760

Telephone: 412-396-6550 (general information)
412-396-4945 (program inquiries)

Fax: 412-396-6346
E-mail: nursing@duq.edu
World Wide Web: http://www.nursing.duq.edu

D'Youville College
Department of Nursing
Buffalo, New York

THE COLLEGE

D'Youville College is a private, coeducational, liberal arts and professional college offering students a high-quality education in more than thirty undergraduate and graduate degree programs. Founded in 1908 by the Grey Nuns as the first college for women in western New York to offer baccalaureate degrees to women, it was named for their founder, Saint Marguerite D'Youville. The current enrollment is 2,500 men and women. Students learning is facilitated by the low 14:1 student-faculty ratio. The College is committed to helping its students grow not only academically but also in the social and personal areas of their college experience.

THE DEPARTMENT OF NURSING

D'Youville College has been educating and preparing professional nurses for careers since 1942; the first Bachelor of Science in Nursing class graduated in 1946. In 1957, the RN to B.S.N. degree program was initiated, offering a specialized curriculum for the working professional nurse. All programs offered by the nursing department are fully accredited by the Commission on Collegiate Nursing Education (CCNE) and approved by the New York State Education Department.

The nursing faculty members are committed, dedicated educators who pride themselves on providing individual attention. Faculty members, the majority of whom are prepared at the doctorate level, represent diverse backgrounds, both clinically and educationally, providing numerous specialty areas for the students to draw upon.

PROGRAMS OF STUDY

D'Youville College has been growing and attracting students from all over the world since 1908, playing a leadership role in the areas of professional health training. D'Youville offers a four-year Bachelor of Science in Nursing (B.S.N.) degree program, and students interested in pursuing careers in nursing also have the option of completing a dual-degree, five-year sequence to graduate with both a baccalaureate and a master's degree. It is a direct-entry program in which accepted students do not have to reapply or requalify for upper-division courses. The B.S.N. degree program combines a liberal arts foundation with professional nursing course work. Students begin their clinical experiences at area hospitals and health facilities in their sophomore year. Areas of clinical experience include geriatrics, pediatrics, OB/maternity, and medical/surgical nursing. To hone their clinical and research skills, students participate in internships during the summer of their junior year. The two-year RN to B.S.N. degree program includes an RN to B.S.N./M.S. option and an RN to B.S.N./M.S. in community health nursing option, in which RNs complete an additional year of study and graduate with both degrees. Convenient class scheduling provides working nursing professionals with the opportunity to study full-time by attending only two days a week. This alternative scheduling allows students to continue working in their professions while earning their degrees. In 2005, a new nursing flextrack program becomes available for students who want a B.S.N. but have a bachelor's degree in another major.

At the graduate level, nursing programs include Master of Science (M.S.) in community health nursing with concentrations in holistic nursing, hospice and palliative care nursing, nursing management, and nursing education; M.S. in nursing with choice of clinical focus; and Master of Science in family nurse practitioner studies as well as a post-master's certificate in family nurse practitioner studies.

AFFILIATIONS WITH HEALTH-CARE FACILITIES

Specific facilities with which D'Youville has affiliations include Catholic Health System, which encompasses Mercy Hospital of Buffalo and Kenmore Mercy Hospital; Erie County Medical Center; WNY's Level I Trauma and Burn Center; Buffalo Psychiatric Center; Kaleida Health Care System, which comprises Women and Children's Hospital of Buffalo, Buffalo General Hospital, Millard Fillmore Hospital, and the Visiting Nurses Association of Western New York; BryLin Hospital; and the world-renowned Roswell Park Cancer Institute.

ACADEMIC FACILITIES

D'Youville's new, modern Library Resource Center, which was completed in 1999, contains 154,000 volumes, including microtext and software and subscriptions to 870 periodicals and newspapers. The multimillion-dollar Health Science Building houses laboratories, including those for anatomy, organic chemistry, quantitative analysis, and computer science. It also houses classrooms, faculty member offices, and development centers, including one for career development. In addition, there are also an academic center that opened in 2001 and a new apartment residence opening in January 2005.

LOCATION

D'Youville is situated on Buffalo's residential west side. The College is within minutes of many social attractions, including the downtown shopping center, the Kleinhans Music Hall, the Albright-Knox Art Gallery, two museums, and several theaters that offer stage productions. Seasonal changes in the area offer a variety of recreational opportunities. Buffalo is only 90 miles from Toronto and 25 minutes from Niagara Falls.

STUDENT SERVICES

The College offers a full range of student services. The D'Youville Freshman Experience (DFX) is designed to help make the students' first year exciting, fun, and challenging. At orientation, students are assigned a College mentor and register for the FOCUS Freshmen Seminar. There are also activities and leadership opportunities (D'Youville Leads) as well as a peer mentor program coordinated through the Leadership Development Institute. The College also has a Career Services Center, the Learning Center, the Multicultural Affairs Office, and the Personal Counseling Center.

THE NURSING STUDENT GROUP

D'Youville has both traditional and nontraditional students from a variety of ethnic backgrounds in the nursing program, enhancing the educational and social experiences. Nursing organizations on campus include the National Student Nurse Association (NSNA), which is open to all nursing students. Students who excel academically may be invited to join the Society of Nursing, Sigma Theta Tau International.

COSTS

For 2004–05, tuition was $7345 per semester, and room and board cost $3670 per semester. A general College fee is required and is based on credit hours taken. Graduate tuition for

2004–05 was $520 per credit hour. Students in the B.S.N./M.S. programs pay undergraduate tuition.

FINANCIAL AID

All students enrolled in the RN degree-completion program are offered a 50 percent tuition reduction. Ninety percent of D'Youville freshmen receive financial aid. This includes nearly $2 million in grants and scholarships. Grants include Federal Pell Grants and Supplemental Education Opportunity Grants, New York State Tuition Assistance Program, and the Aid for Part-Time Study Program. Federal Work-Study programs, federally insured loans, and flexible payment plans are also available. All applicants are reviewed for academic scholarships at the time of acceptance. Notifications of awards are made. D'Youville's new Instant Scholarship Program offers scholarships with total values up to $45,900 for undergraduate and dual-degree programs.

APPLYING

D'Youville admits students on a rolling admission basis; therefore, applications are reviewed as they are received by the Admissions Office. Undergraduate applicants must submit a completed application along with a $25 processing fee; official high school transcripts or, for transfer students, official transcripts from colleges previously attended; SAT or ACT scores; and letters of recommendation.

Applicants to the master's program must present a baccalaureate degree in nursing from an accredited college or university program; a valid New York state or provincial license to practice nursing; evidence of an undergraduate course in statistics and an undergraduate course in computer science or its equivalent; and evidence of capability to succeed in a graduate program, as shown by an overall undergraduate GPA of at least 3.0 (based on a 4.0 system), an overall undergraduate GPA of at least 2.7 with a 3.0 or better in the upper half of undergraduate work, an overall undergraduate GPA of at least 2.7 with a 3.0 or better in the major field, or a baccalaureate degree in nursing plus a master's degree in another field from an accredited college or university with an overall GPA of at least 3.5. Candidates for the post-master's certificate program in family nurse practitioner studies must have a master's degree in nursing.

CORRESPONDENCE AND INFORMATION

Department of Nursing
D'Youville College
320 Porter Avenue
Buffalo, New York 14201-9985
Telephone: 716-829-7613
Fax: 716-829-8159
E-mail: admissions@dyc.edu
World Wide Web: http://www.dyc.edu

THE FACULTY

Patricia Bahn, M.S., RN. Adult health/nursing admininstration, holistic health/oncology.

Joan Cookfair, Ed.D., RN. Publications and practice centers on community health nursing specialty.

Carol Gutt, Ed.D., RN. Child health/curriculum/wellness.

Dorothy Hoehne, Ph.D., RN. Maternal child nursing/teaching higher education, instructional communications, research and evaluation.

Janet Ihlenfeld, Ph.D., RN. Social support and job satisfaction, pediatric/neonatal critical care, children in the community.

Verna Kieffer, D.N.S., RN. Community wellness, adult health, gerontology, quality of life and quality of care issues.

Edith Malizia, Ed.D., RN. Adult health, education administration.

Pamela Miller, M.S., RN, WHNP.

Karen Piotrowski, M.S., RN. Labor, childbirth.

Bernadette Pursel, M.S. Community health nursing.

Connie Jozwiak Shields, Ph.D., RN, ANP. Adult primary-care nursing.

Judith Stanley, M.S.N., RN. Hospital patient advocacy and education, supervision and administration of home infusion therapy, complementary and alternative-healing modalities (biofeedback, hypnosis, imagery).

Paul Violanti, M.S., RN, PNP, FNP. International medical missions and refugees.

Dawn Williams, M.S., RN. Adult health, medical surgery.

Emory University
Nell Hodgson Woodruff School of Nursing
Atlanta, Georgia

THE UNIVERSITY

Emory University, founded by the Methodist Church in 1836, has 11,781 students and 2,500 faculty members who represent all regions of the United States and about ninety other nations. Emory has nine major academic divisions, numerous centers for advanced study, and a host of prestigious affiliated institutions. The University has a two-year and four-year undergraduate college, a graduate school of arts and sciences, and professional schools of medicine, theology, law, nursing, public health, and business.

THE SCHOOL OF NURSING

The Nell Hodgson Woodruff School of Nursing was founded in 1905 as the Training School for Nurses at Wesley Memorial Hospital in Atlanta. In 1922, the hospital and school of nursing were moved to the Emory University campus and functioned as a diploma school with a three-year hospital program. In 1944, the school became an integral part of Emory University, offering the Bachelor of Science in Nursing degree. The diploma program was offered concurrently until its discontinuation in 1949. The School of Nursing was named the Nell Hodgson Woodruff School of Nursing in 1968 in honor of Mrs. Woodruff, who supported the School of Nursing throughout her lifetime. The School offers undergraduate, graduate, and doctoral nursing education to nearly 300 students.

PROGRAMS OF STUDY

The Bachelor of Science in Nursing (B.S.N.) degree provides a strong academic foundation that focuses on connecting the theoretical basis of nursing with the development of critical-thinking and decision-making skills. The first two years of general education course work (including prerequisites) may be taken at any accredited university or liberal arts college. Specific humanities, social science, science, and elective courses that equal 60 semester hours are required for admission to the B.S.N. program at Emory. During the second year of prerequisite course work, students apply for admission to the School of Nursing. Qualified students are then admitted for the remaining two years of professional study. The four-semester, 60-semester-hour nursing program combines clinical and in-class experiences. The goals of the School of Nursing are to advance nursing knowledge, produce nurse leaders, and design new models of care.

Students who hold a bachelor's degree in another area but are interested in becoming nurses are eligible for the B.S.N. program. Students enroll into the B.S.N. program and complete their nursing studies in four semesters. Emory University also has a B.S.N./M.S.N. Segue Option program for non-nurses interested in becoming nurse practitioners and/or clinical nurse specialists. Students must have a bachelor's degree in some area besides nursing to be eligible. This program provides a seamless course of study through accelerated admission into the B.S.N. program followed by direct entry into the M.S.N. program after receiving RN licensure.

The master's degree programs combine the advantages of outstanding facilities, a well-crafted curriculum, high-quality instruction, a prestigious and far-reaching reputation, and courses that are relevant to today's evolving practice environment. A wealth of clinical venues are available in the Atlanta metropolitan area, and clinical experiences are precisely geared to students' career focuses. Emory offers M.S.N., RN-M.S.N. Bridge, M.S.N.-M.P.H., post-master's, and Ph.D. programs.

Programs of study leading to the Master of Science in Nursing (M.S.N.) include the following specialties: acute/critical care, adult nurse practitioner, adult oncology, emergency nurse practitioner, family nurse-midwife, family nurse practitioner, gerontology, international health, leadership in health care, public-health nursing, nursing administration, nurse-midwifery, pediatrics, women's health nurse practitioner, women's health for graduates of Title X programs, and women's health nurse practitioner/adult health practitioner. Length of the specialty programs ranges from three semesters (one calendar year) to five consecutive semesters of full-time study. Part-time study is available. Students sit for certification as nurse practitioners, clinical nurse specialists, or both. The RN/M.S.N. bridge program provides an opportunity for associate degree or diploma-prepared nurses to obtain the Master of Science in Nursing. Students in the RN/M.S.N. program complete 24 semester hours of bridge course work prior to beginning the specialty curriculum of choice. In addition, a dual M.S.N./Master of Public Health (M.S.N./M.P.H.) is available, and post-master's options are available in all graduate specialty areas.

The Ph.D. in nursing offers flexible specialization options and is a four-year, full-time program. Students accepted to the program receive an annual stipend plus financial support to cover tuition for a maximum of four years.

AFFILIATIONS WITH HEALTH-CARE FACILITIES

The Nell Hodgson Woodruff School of Nursing maintains close ties with the Centers for Disease Control and Prevention (CDC), and the American Cancer Society. The School of Nursing at Emory is also the home of the Lillian Carter Center for International Nursing. Students at Emory have access to more than 200 diverse clinical learning sites.

ACADEMIC FACILITIES

In January 2001, the School of Nursing opened a state-of-the-art facility for nursing study and research. The building unites scholarship and teaching under one roof. The School of Nursing is part of the Robert W. Woodruff Health Sciences Center, a major provider of patient care and a national leader in clinical and research programs. Emory University is a close collaborator with the Carter Center, a nonprofit, nonpartisan public policy institute founded by former President Jimmy Carter and his wife Rosalynn.

LOCATION

Emory University is located 6 miles northeast of downtown Atlanta. Emory is positioned along Clifton Road, which is also the home of the U.S. Centers for Disease Control and Prevention and the American Cancer Society. With top-tier entertainment, cultural attractions, sports, and shopping, Atlanta has something for everyone.

STUDENT SERVICES

Nursing students at Emory enjoy a vibrant campus life. Opportunities for involvement on campus and within the nursing school are abundant. Emory students also have the opportunity to participate in student nursing organizations on the local, state, and national levels.

THE NURSING STUDENT GROUP

During the 2004–05 academic year, the School of Nursing enrolled 195 undergraduate students, 179 graduate students, and 17 doctoral students from across the nation and around the world.

COSTS

In 2004–05, full-time undergraduate tuition was $13,109 per semester. The student activity fee was $71 per semester or $5 per semester hour. The student athletic fee was $105 per semester or $25 for the summer semester.

Full-time graduate tuition was $13,109 per semester or $1092 per semester hour for part-time students (fewer than 12 semester hours). The student activity fee was $71 per semester or $5 per semester hour. The student athletic fee was $75 per semester or $25 for the summer semester.

FINANCIAL AID

Emory University and Nell Hodgson Woodruff School of Nursing are committed to providing a generous package of financial assistance to all who qualify. Currently, 96 percent of undergraduate nursing students and 95 percent of graduate nursing students receive financial assistance.

Students who apply for financial assistance at Emory University are considered for a combination of scholarships, grants, and low-interest loans. Merit-based scholarships are available at both the undergraduate and graduate levels.

APPLYING

All applicants to the School of Nursing are considered on an individual basis. Applications and supporting credentials should be submitted as early as possible in the academic year prior to entrance; however, applications are reviewed as long as class space is available. The School of Nursing selects those applicants who are best qualified academically and personally. After all application materials are received, the Admissions Committee reviews the applicant's credentials and makes the decision to accept, defer, or deny. Final acceptance is contingent upon satisfactory completion of prerequisite course work.

CORRESPONDENCE AND INFORMATION

Office of Admission
School of Nursing
Emory University
1520 Clifton Road
Atlanta, Georgia 30322
Telephone: 404-727-7980
800-222-3879 (toll-free)
Fax: 404-727-8509
E-mail: admit@nursing.emory.edu
World Wide Web: http://www.nursing.emory.edu

THE FACULTY

Sheila Abner, Instructor; Ph.D., Michigan State, 2000. Microbiology.
Corrine Abraham, Associate; M.N., Emory, 1985. Adult health.
Pam Altman, Instructor; M.S.N., Jacksonville, 2004.
Kelly Brewer, Associate; M.S.N., Arkansas, 1992. Adult health.
Holly L. Brown, Associate; M.S.N., Pennsylvania, 1989. Gerontological nursing.
Karen Jo Campbell, Instructor; M.N., Emory, 1991. Child health.
Patricia C. Clark, Assistant Professor; Ph.D., Rochester, 1998. Post-stroke and Alzheimer's disease.
Carolyn Clevenger, Instructor; M.S.N., Emory, 2002.
Jo Ann Dalton, Professor and Honeycutt Chair of Adult and Elder Health and Interim Associate Dean for Academic Affairs; Ed.D., North Carolina State, 1984. Adult education.
Julie Davey, Instructor; M.S.N., Emory, 2001.
Madge M. Donnellan, Clinical Associate Professor; Ph.D., Tennessee, 1988. Family/community nursing.
Elizabeth Downes, Clinical Assistant Professor; M.S.N., Tennessee, 1986. International nursing and health.
Sandra Dunbar, Professor; D.S.N., Alabama at Birmingham, 1982. Adaptation to the stresses of acute and chronic cardiovascular illness.
Sara Edwards, Associate; M.N., Emory, 1994. Midwifery and maternal nursing.
Kate Franzek, Clinical Associate Professor; M.S., Emory, 1999. Nursing and public health.
Sarah B. Freeman, Clinical Professor; Ph.D., Georgia State, 1989. Decision making and ethics.
Mary L. Garvin-Surpris, Associate; M.S., New Rochelle, 1993. Adult health.
Rebecca Gary, Associate; Ph.D., North Carolina at Chapel Hill, 2003.
Maggie P. Gilead, Associate Professor; Ph.D., Emory, 1981. Psychiatric/mental health.
Judy Gretz, Instructor; M.S., Texas Woman's, 1977. Nursing.
Jill Hamilton, Assistant Research Professor; Ph.D., North Carolina at Chapel Hill, 2001.
Leslie Holmes, Associate; M.S.N., Medical University of South Carolina, 1993. Parental response to a child's life-threatening event.
Roberta Kaplow, Clinical Professor; Ph.D., NYU, 1998. Critical care and oncology nursing.
Barbara Kaplan, Associate; M.S.N., Emory, 1992. Nursing education.
Maureen A. Kelley, Clinical Associate Professor and Chair, Family and Community Nursing; Ph.D., Medical College of Georgia, 1993. Midwifery.
Joyce L. King, Clinical Assistant Professor; Ph.D., Emory, 1995. Fat cell metabolism, insulin resistance, leptin production.
James Lawrence, Instructor; M.S.N., Emory, 1998.
Sally T. Lehr, Clinical Assistant Professor; Ph.D., Georgia State, 1981. Psychiatric/mental health.
Maureen O. Lobb, Associate; Ph.D., Georgia State, 1992. Community health nursing.
Kathy Markowski, Associate; M.S.N., DePaul, 1980. Adult health.
Jane E. Mashburn, Clinical Associate Professor; M.N., Emory, 1978. Midwifery.
Kathryn Matthews, Associate; M.S.N., Pennsylvania, 1976. Family/community nursing.
Marcia K. McDonnell, Assistant Professor; D.S.N., Alabama, 1996. HIV/AIDS and women.
Michelle Mott, Instructor; M.S.N., Pennsylvania, 1999.
Joyce P. Murray, Professor; Ed.D., Georgia, 1989. Domestic violence, international nursing education.
Lynda P. Nauright, Professor; Ed.D., Georgia, 1975. Work environment.
Michael W. Neville, Clinical Associate Professor; Doctor of Pharmacy, Georgia, 1992. Pharmacology.
Chris O'Brien, Instructor; M.P.H., Emory, 1989.
Helen S. O'Shea, Professor Emerita; Ph.D., Georgia State, 1980. Adult health.
Kathy Parker, Edith Honeycutt Professor in Nursing; Ph.D., Georgia State, 1990. Sleep in patients with chronic illness.
Quyen Phan, Instructor; M.S.N., Emory, 2004. Leadership in public-health nursing.
Marcene L. Powell, Professor; D.S.W., Utah, 1981. Parenting practices.
Barbara D. Reeves, Clinical Assistant Professor; M.S.N., Vanderbilt, 1979. Family/community nursing.
Bethany D. Robertson, Associate; M.S.N., Emory, 1992. Obstetrics/gynecology ecological nursing.
Martha F. Rogers, Clinical Professor; M.D., Medical College of Georgia, 1976. Pediatrics/international and community nursing.
Deborah A. Ryan, Clinical Associate Professor; M.S.N., Marquette, 1981. Pediatrics.
Marla E. Salmon, Professor and Dean; Sc.D., Johns Hopkins, 1977. Health workforce and health services.
Lynn Sibley, Clinical Associate Professor; Ph.D., Colorado, 1993. Maternal-Child health.
Donna J. Smith, Associate; M.S.N., Emory, 1997. Adult and elder health.
Linda Smith, Instructor; M.Div., Emory, 2004. Theology.
Linda Spencer, Clinical Associate Professor; Ph.D., Georgia State, 1988. Public health nursing.
Debra Stevens, Adjunct Faculty; M.S., Emory, 2001. Leadership in health care.
Ora Strickland, Professor; Ph.D., North Carolina at Greensboro, 1977. Women's health and minority health.
Darla R. Ura, Clinical Associate Professor; M.A., Ball State, 1974. Adherence to HIV medications.
Jeannie Weston, Instructor; M.S., Maryland, 1982. Maternal child nursing.
Lynette Wright, Clinical Associate Professor; M.N., Emory, 1974. Distance learning strategies, human genetics.
Erin M. York, Associate; M.S., Georgia State, 1995. Pediatric nursing.
Weihua Zhang, Associate; Ph.D., Georgia State, 2004. Critical-care nursing.

Excelsior College
Nursing Program
Albany, New York

EXCELSIOR COLLEGE
The World's Largest Educator of Nurses At-A-Distance

THE COLLEGE

Excelsior College, a private institution, was founded in 1971 to make college degrees more accessible to busy, working adults while focusing on its founding philosophy: "What you know is more important than where or how you learned it." Thus, most Excelsior College students are returning to college to complete an education begun elsewhere. Because it has no residency requirement, the College accepts a broad array of prior college-level credit in transfer, including credit earned in classroom and distance courses from Excelsior College and other regionally accredited colleges and universities; proficiency examinations such as Excelsior College Examinations and CLEP; and corporate and military training recognized for the award of college-level credit by the American Council on Education (ACE), Center for Adult Learning and Educational Credentials. A recognized leader in distance education, Excelsior College offers degree programs in nursing, business, liberal arts, technology, and certificates in nursing specialties. With more than 100,000 graduates, the College's associate, baccalaureate, and master's degree programs are accessible worldwide. This enables students to work at their own pace while maintaining a full-time work schedule and family and civic responsibilities.

Since 1977, Excelsior College has been accredited by the Commission on Higher Education of the Middle States Association of Colleges and Schools, 3624 Market Street, Philadelphia, Pennsylvania 19104, 215-662-5606. The Commission on Higher Education is an institutional accrediting agency recognized by the U.S. Secretary of Education and the Council for Higher Education Accreditation (CHEA). All the College's academic programs, including its undergraduate and graduate programs in nursing, are registered (i.e., approved) by the New York State Education Department. The associate, baccalaureate, and master's degree programs in nursing are accredited by the National League for Nursing Accrediting Commission (NLNAC), 61 Broadway, New York, New York 10006, 800-669-1656. The NLNAC is a specialized accrediting agency recognized by the U.S. Secretary of Education.

Excelsior College Examinations are recognized by the American Council on Education (ACE), Center for Adult Learning and Educational Credentials, for the award of college-level credit. Excelsior College Examinations in nursing are the only nursing examinations approved by ACE. This school is a nonprofit corporation authorized by the State of Oregon to offer and confer the academic degrees described herein, following a determination that state academic standards will be satisfied under OAR 583-030. Inquiries concerning the standards or school compliance may be directed to the Oregon Office of Educational Policy and Planning, 255 Capitol Street, NE, Suite 126, Salem, Oregon 97310-1338.

THE NURSING PROGRAM

The Excelsior College Nursing Program began offering the first nontraditional distance nursing programs in the United States in 1975. Today, it has more than 30,000 graduates among its several programs. Representing the largest assessment-based nursing program in the nation, Excelsior College's programs have served as models for the development of other nontraditional programs. Faculty members are selected for their expertise in curriculum development and program evaluation. They represent leaders in nursing education.

At the undergraduate level, Excelsior College offers nursing degree programs leading to an Associate in Science, Associate in Applied Science, and a Bachelor of Science including a B.S. degree in nursing (completion program for RNs). All offered at a distance, its undergraduate programs have been specifically designed to meet the educational needs of qualified individuals with significant background and/or experience in clinically oriented health-care disciplines. The requirements for these programs may be met by completing a series of examinations that measure a student's knowledge of nursing theory and a student's clinical competency. Excelsior College performance (clinical) examinations are administered through a national network of Regional Performance Assessment Centers (RPAC). The Nursing Management Certificate program is made up of five online courses.

At the graduate level, delivered online, Excelsior offers a Master of Science degree in nursing (clinical systems management), an RN-M.S. in nursing program, and a program leading to a Certificate in Health-Care Informatics.

PROGRAMS OF STUDY

The purpose of the Excelsior College associate degree nursing program is to provide an alternative educational approach to earning an associate degree in nursing. The student's qualifications as a learned individual and a competent member of the nursing profession are documented through an objective assessment program in general education and nursing. The program is designed to promote a sense of social responsibility and personal fulfillment by emphasizing the need for students to evaluate their own learning and potential achievements in terms of professional relevance and personal goals, proficiency in the practice of nursing, and a foundation for lifelong learning. The associate degree program is divided into two components: general education (31 semester hours) and nursing (36 semester hours). The general education component is very flexible so that adult students can build the degree to meet their interests and needs. It includes requirements in anatomy, physiology, microbiology, lifespan developmental psychology, sociology, and English composition. Students can meet these requirements through classroom or distance courses from Excelsior College and other regionally accredited colleges or through proficiency examinations. The nursing component comprises seven Excelsior College theory examinations and one performance examination.

The purpose of the bachelor's degree in nursing program is to offer an alternative educational approach to earning a baccalaureate degree in nursing. The student's qualifications as a learned individual and competent member of the nursing profession are documented through an objective assessment program of general and professional education designed to promote an awareness of the human experience and an appreciation for the contributions of people from diverse cultures through the study of liberal arts and sciences; a sense of social responsibility and personal fulfillment by emphasizing the need for individuals to evaluate their own potential and learning achievements in terms of professional relevance and personal goals; proficiency in the practice of professional nursing by providing assessment of baccalaureate-level competencies in the liberal arts and sciences and in nursing; and a foundation for graduate specialization.

The bachelor's degree program is divided into two components: general education (61 semester hours) and nursing (60 semester hours). The general education component is very flexible so that adult students may build the degree to meet their interests and needs. It includes requirements in anatomy, physiology, microbiology, psychology, sociology, statistics, and English composition. Students can meet these requirements through classroom or distance courses from Excelsior College and other regionally accredited colleges or through proficiency examinations. The nursing component comprises three Excelsior College theory examinations and four performance examinations.

To test the clinical competencies of its nursing students, Excelsior College pioneered the creation of rigorous performance examinations. The program is self-paced, and students can take performance examinations at any of four RPACs located in California, Georgia, New York, and Wisconsin.

College courses in nursing and nursing theory examinations may not be accepted for credit if they were completed more than five years prior to enrollment.

The purpose of the online M.S. in nursing degree program is to offer a high-quality educational program in clinical systems management to students at a distance. This degree program is to be the entry for students into the role of the nurse administrator. It is also available as the RN-M.S. degree program for registered nurses, who must complete requirements for both the bachelor's and master's program segments. Engaging in the study of foundational material for advanced nursing roles, the exploration of health-care informatics, and in-depth study of the administrative role, master's-level students in the program earn a total of 44 graduate-level credits through online course work, computer-delivered assessments, and an interactive capstone experience. The health-care informatics portion of the program is a 12-credit curriculum that includes four online courses with interactive components. A health-care informatics certificate program is available as a 17-hour curriculum, 12 of which may be applied toward the online master's degree program.

ACADEMIC FACILITIES

As a distance education program, Excelsior College provides a variety of guided learning services to students, such as study guides, learning modules, online workshops, performance examination workshops, teleconferences, comprehensive online library services, an online bookstore, and computer conference groups facilitated at the College's Electronic Peer Network (EPN), a "virtual student union." The College maintains DistanceLearn, a database of more than 18,000 examinations and courses available from accredited institutions at a distance. Academic advisers and nurse faculty members are available to provide services to students by telephone, fax, computer, and mail.

LOCATION

Because its programs are provided at a distance, the College moves with students whenever and wherever they move. The administrative offices are located in Albany, the capital of New York State. Each year the College holds a formal commencement ceremony to recognize all who have completed a degree that year. Proud of their accomplishment, many students travel great distances to participate in commencement festivities.

THE NURSING STUDENT GROUP

The 1,500 adult students enrolled in the Bachelor of Science in nursing program represent diverse backgrounds in terms of age, ethnicity, nationality, and professional experience. Most are registered nurses. Of the more than 16,000 students enrolled in the associate degree program, most are licensed practical/vocational nurses (LPNs/LVNs). The average student has ten years of health-care experience. Graduates of the College are employed in various health-care settings and are accepted into most graduate programs.

COSTS

Excelsior College charges an $875 (associate degree programs) or $995 (baccalaureate degree programs) fee at enrollment, which covers initial evaluation of a student's existing academic records and academic advisement and program planning services for one year; a $430 (associate) or $495 (baccalaureate) annual fee for each year after the first, which covers the ongoing evaluation of academic records submitted by a student and academic and program planning services for an additional twelve months; and a $480 (associate) or $495 (baccalaureate) fee for a final evaluation and verification of all academic records prior to program completion and graduation. Different fees and fee structures apply to military students, certificate and graduate programs, and to students who choose to pay their Excelsior College enrollment expenses via the College's FACTS Payment Plan. Detailed fee schedules are available in hard copy and on the College's Web site. Additional costs depend on the amount of credit students need to earn and what credit sources they choose. Proficiency examinations are the least expensive mode of earning credit. Students should also figure in costs for books and other learning materials, travel, postage, online resources, and miscellaneous charges and supplies.

FINANCIAL AID

Some financial aid is available, particularly the College's President's Scholarships and aid connected with Veterans Affairs benefits. The College participates in a variety of alternative loan programs. Students seeking financial aid should contact the Excelsior College Financial Aid Office before enrolling.

APPLYING

Students must apply for admission to the Excelsior College School of Nursing and, once accepted, enroll in Excelsior College. The Excelsior College nursing degree programs are specifically designed to serve individuals with significant background or experience in clinically oriented health-care disciplines. Therefore, undergraduate admission to the program is open to registered nurses, licensed practical/vocational nurses, paramedics, military service corpsmen, individuals who hold a degree in a clinically oriented health-care field in which they have had the opportunity to provide direct patient care (i.e., physicians, respiratory therapists, respiratory care practitioners, and physicians' assistants), or individuals who have completed 50 percent or more of the clinical nursing courses in a program leading to RN licensure. Exceptions may be made for individuals who do not meet these qualifications but who can document significant clinical background. Specific admission requirements regarding the RN-M.S. and M.S. programs are detailed in the nursing catalog.

CORRESPONDENCE AND INFORMATION

Admissions Office
Excelsior College
7 Columbia Circle
Albany, New York 12203-5159

Telephone: 518-464-8500
Fax: 518-464-8777
E-mail: admissions@excelsior.edu
World Wide Web: http://www.excelsior.edu

Fairleigh Dickinson University
Henry P. Becton School of Nursing and Allied Health
Teaneck-Hackensack, New Jersey

THE UNIVERSITY

Founded in 1942, Fairleigh Dickinson University (FDU) is an independent nonsectarian institution of higher education offering high-quality, career-oriented undergraduate and graduate programs. Fairleigh Dickinson is one of New Jersey's leading institutions of private higher education, with nearly 100 career-oriented programs at the undergraduate and graduate levels. The University has two campuses in northern New Jersey—Metropolitan Campus in Teaneck and College at Florham in Madison—and the Wroxton College campus in Oxfordshire, England. While the majority of nursing studies courses are offered at the Metropolitan Campus, the RN to B.S.N. to M.S.N. program is also offered at the College at Florham. Nursing students may take non-nursing classes at any of the University's campuses. Clinical site experiences are prearranged at a wide variety of health-care agencies.

THE SCHOOL OF NURSING

Established in 1952, Fairleigh Dickinson's nursing program focuses on preparing individuals who will enhance society and the health-care environment. It does so through course work that prepares graduates to function within a global health-care system. This philosophy reflects the educational tradition that has been the hallmark of the University, long recognized for its career-oriented studies enriched by a liberal arts tradition.

The faculty of the School of Nursing and Allied Health is committed to the belief that a basis of scientific knowledge is essential for professional nursing practice. The program views the professional nurse as an independent and interdependent practitioner who functions as a client advocate, change agent, innovator, planner, leader, and consumer of research. Nursing education at FDU encourages students to understand cultural differences and the relationship between human beings and their environment. The School approaches nursing as a collaborative learning process. Courses reflect a strong commitment to the development of critical thinking, ethical decision making, and cultural competence.

PROGRAMS OF STUDY

The undergraduate program offers three specific study tracks leading to the Bachelor of Science in Nursing (B.S.N.) degree: basic four-year studies, a choice of accelerated one-year (full-time) or two-year (evening) studies for individuals who already hold a baccalaureate degree, and a B.S.N. to M.S.N. program for RNs from diploma or associate degree nursing programs. The basic four-year B.S.N. program is offered during the daytime, although many of the required and elective liberal arts courses for the degree are also available during the evening. The Accelerated B.S.N. program is an intensive, concentrated course of study designed to enable participants to complete their degree in one or two calendar years. Nursing courses for full-time, one-year students are offered during the daytime and evening, starting in mid-May, five days per week; nursing courses for part-time, two-year students are offered during the evening, starting in September, four evenings per week.

Students interested in the RN to B.S.N. to M.S.N. program can enroll at any time during the academic year and take classes on a part-time or full-time basis. Students can choose from evening studies on the Metropolitan Campus or a full-time, one-day-a-week (9 a.m. to 9 p.m.) program at the College at Florham. Two graduate nursing courses are offered in the RN to B.S.N. curriculum as an incentive for students who are pursuing the M.S.N. degree.

The Master of Science in Nursing (M.S.N.) program offers both a clinical and nonclinical track. The clinical track prepares adult nurse practitioners for an educational or administrative role. Nonclinical tracks are offered in education and nursing informatics. An M.S.N. for RNs with non-nursing Bachelor of Science (B.S.) degrees is also available. Special emphasis is given to nursing as a human science, nursing education, and advanced nursing practice. New programs include the M.S.N. in nursing informatics and an M.S.N. for RNs with non-nursing B.S. degrees.

The M.S.N. program consists of 45 to 46 credits, which full-time students can complete in two academic years, including the intervening summer. Graduates of the program are eligible to take the national certification exams of the American Academy of Nurse Practitioners (AANP) and the American Nurses Credentialing Center (ANCC) to become certified nurse practitioners. Nationally certified graduates may also obtain licensure from the New Jersey Board for Prescriptive Practice.

Individuals holding an M.S.N. degree may pursue a post-M.S.N. graduate certificate in nursing education, advanced practice, or nursing administration.

Allied health programs offered by the School are the associate degree in radiography (A.S.), the B.S. in radiologic technology, the B.S. in medical technology, and the B.S. in clinical laboratory science with majors in toxicology, cytotechnology, and medical technology. On the graduate level, the M.S. in medical technology is offered. All programs offer both full-time and part-time study options.

AFFILIATIONS WITH HEALTH-CARE FACILITIES

The School of Nursing and Allied Health has built a strong network of participating clinical agencies to provide excellent and diverse clinical experiences for nursing students. These agencies include American Red Cross, Bergen Crossroads Chapter, Ridgewood; Atlantic Health System; Barnert Hospital, Paterson; Bergen Community Health Care, Inc., Westwood; Bergen Regional Medical Center, Paramus; Beth Israel Medical Center, Newark; Charter Behavioral Health Systems, Summit; Children's Specialized Hospital, Mountainside; Englewood Hospital and Medical Center; Englewood Hospital Home Health and Hospice; Essex Valley Visiting Nurse Association, East Orange; Hackensack University Medical Center; Holy Name Hospital, Teaneck; Home Health Agency of Hackensack Medical Center; Hospice of New Jersey, Wayne; Morristown Memorial Hospital; New Jersey Veterans Administration Hospital, East Orange; New York City Health and Hospital Corporation; Overlook Hospital, Summit; Pascack Valley Hospital, Westwood; St. Barnabus Medical Center, Livingston; St. Clare's Hospital, Dover; St. Joseph's Hospital and Medical Center, Paterson; St. Joseph's Wayne Hospital, Wayne; St. Mary's Hospital, Passaic; Summit Hospital; University of Medicine and Dentistry of New Jersey, Newark; The Valley Hospital, Ridgewood; Valley Home Care, Inc., Paramus; and Visiting Health Services of Passaic Valley and Passaic Valley Hospice, Totowa.

ACADEMIC FACILITIES

The Metropolitan Campus has nearly sixty buildings situated on 88 acres. In addition to the computer and laboratory facilities available at any major institution of higher education, FDU provides state-of-the-art equipment specifically for nursing students. The School of Nursing and Allied Health maintains modern facilities located in Dickinson Hall on the Metropolitan Campus. In its four specialized laboratories, students are taught patient care and a wide variety of nursing skills by the faculty members. The nursing laboratories are equipped with interactive computer programs that enable students to practice and develop their skills independently using the technology frequently found in clinical settings.

LOCATION

The Metropolitan Campus is situated along the east and west banks of the Hackensack River about 10 minutes from New York City. The campus is directly accessible from Route 4 and is 6 miles west of the George Washington Bridge. Easy access to New York City enables students and faculty members to take advantage of the city's financial, cultural, and international activities. The College at Florham is located at the outskirts of Morristown on Route 124, 35 miles from New York City. It is convenient to both the railroad and New Jersey bus transit. The campus is 166 acres of beautifully landscaped property. Originally an estate, its Georgian-style buildings have been adapted to the University's needs.

STUDENT SERVICES

The University community is a total learning environment shared by students and faculty and staff members. To this end, strong support services are provided to enhance both the classroom and extracurricular experiences. Academic and career advisement and library and computer services are complemented by personal counseling, social and cultural activities, and programs that promote cross-cultural understanding. Lectures, seminars, concerts, performances, and special events are frequently offered on both campuses. Each year, the Fairleigh Dickinson University Student Nurses Association sponsors a variety of professional and social activities. Fairleigh Dickinson is home to the Epsilon Ro chapter of Sigma Theta Tau, the international nursing honor society.

THE NURSING STUDENT GROUP

Approximately 300 students are enrolled at the School. Twenty percent of students in the traditional baccalaureate program are men, and more than 50 percent are members of minority groups. In 2003, 100 percent of all School of Nursing and Allied Health graduates passed the National Council Licensure Examination for Registered Nurses.

COSTS

For the 2003–04 academic year, undergraduate full-time tuition (12 to 18 credits per semester) and fees varied by campus: $22,515 at College at Florham in Madison and $20,969 at Metropolitan Campus in Teaneck. The individual undergraduate per-credit rate was $637. Graduate tuition was $700 per credit plus an additional technology fee of $230 for part-time students or $480 for full-time students. Nursing students also pay for nursing lab fees, books, and uniforms. Although costs varied by residence hall and meal plan, typical annual room and board costs in 2003–04 were $4832 for students at the College at Florham and $5232 at the Metropolitan Campus.

FINANCIAL AID

Each year, the University awards more than $27 million from federal, state, and University sources in financial aid to students. In addition to its excellent need-based financial aid awards, the University also recognizes outstanding academic performance through its annually renewable Col. Fairleigh S. Dickinson Scholarships, worth up to $22,000 a year. For information on merit- and need-based financial aid, students should contact the Office of Financial Aid on the Metropolitan Campus at 201-692-2368.

APPLYING

For admission into the basic 128-credit, four-year track leading to the B.S.N. degree, applicants should be graduates of an accredited secondary school, with a record indicating the potential to succeed in college. Applicants should have completed the following high school studies: 4 units of English, 2 units of history, 1 unit of chemistry with lab, 1 unit of biology with lab, and 2 units of college-preparatory mathematics. In addition, 2 units of foreign language and 1 unit of physics are recommended. A minimum of 16 high school academic units is required for admission. A minimum score of 1000 on the SAT I is necessary for admission. November, December, or January test scores are preferred. An interview with the nursing faculty is recommended.

Applicants to the 59-credit accelerated track leading to the B.S.N. degree should have earned a baccalaureate degree from a regionally accredited college or university, with a cumulative GPA of 2.7 or higher (based on a 4.0 scale). The following prerequisites, completed at a college level, are also required for enrollment: human anatomy and physiology (8 credits, with lab), chemistry (4 credits, with lab), microbiology (4 credits, with lab), economics (3 credits), bioethics (3 credits), statistics (3 credits), and a pharmacology course comparable to FDU's course Drugs and the Body (2 credits). An interview with the nursing faculty is also recommended.

To be considered for the M.S.N. program, applicants should be graduates of a National League for Nursing (NLN)–accredited B.S.N. program with an undergraduate cumulative GPA of 3.0 or higher. Proof of registered nurse licensure, two essays showing evidence of suitability for graduate study in nursing, and proficiency in spoken and written English also are required. Undergraduate prerequisites include courses in health assessment, statistics, and nursing research. A personal interview may be necessary on request from the faculty.

Applicants to the post-M.S.N. program should hold an M.S.N. from an accredited college or university and be eligible for licensure in New Jersey. A personal interview may be requested.

Students interested in transferring to FDU's School of Nursing and Allied Health from regionally accredited institutions may be admitted with advanced standing upon presentation of official transcripts to the Office of University Admissions and an interview with a School of Nursing and Allied Health faculty member. To transfer, a student must have grades of C or higher. Students transferring from accredited baccalaureate degree nursing programs may be awarded credit for nursing courses with grades of C+ or higher that are comparable to FDU's courses. A student interview and catalog descriptions and syllabi of previous courses are used to determine comparability.

CORRESPONDENCE AND INFORMATION

Dr. Minerva Guttman
Director, School of Nursing and Allied Health
Fairleigh Dickinson University
1000 River Road, H-DH4-02
Teaneck, New Jersey 07666
Telephone: 201-692-2888 (Nursing and Allied Health)
800-338-8803 (University Admissions, toll-free)

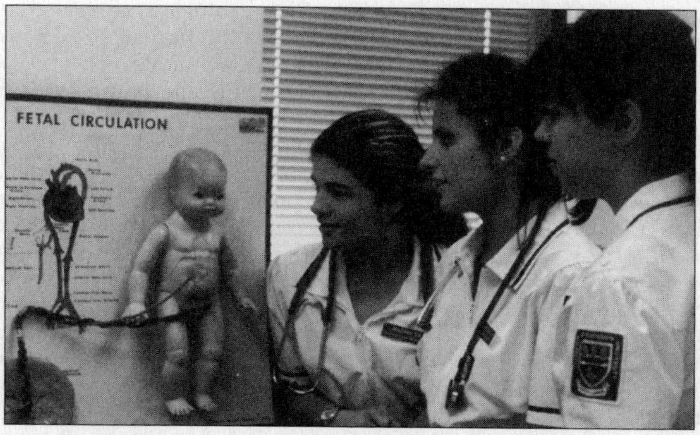

Students examine a student-created learning aid.

Gannon University
Villa Maria School of Nursing
Erie, Pennsylvania

THE UNIVERSITY

A Catholic, diocesan, student-centered university, Gannon University is dedicated to holistic education in the Judeo-Christian tradition. The University faculty and staff members are committed to excellence and continuous improvement in teaching, learning, scholarship, research, and service.

Gannon University is a coeducational institution with 3,400 students, providing a caring environment that fosters inclusiveness and cultural diversity. Gannon's outstanding values-based education combines liberal arts with professional specializations to prepare students for leadership roles in their careers, society, and church. A range of campus organizations and activities encourages academic interests, community service, and moral and spiritual growth. Gannon also offers students a broad program of intramural and intercollegiate athletics.

Gannon offers associate, bachelor's, master's, doctoral, and preprofessional degrees in more than seventy academic majors in sciences, health sciences, engineering, humanities, business, and education.

THE SCHOOL OF NURSING

The Villa Maria School of Nursing offers baccalaureate and master's degree programs. Gannon's community-based nursing curriculum maintains a balanced study of natural and social sciences and the humanities within the context of professional education; fosters creative thinking and effective communication; and promotes caring, respect, and concern for individuals, communities, and society. All programs hold preliminary accreditation by the Commission on Collegiate Nursing Education (CCNE). Gannon's nursing faculty members have graduate preparation in their clinical areas of specializations and are skilled clinical practitioners.

The purpose of the professional nursing program is to prepare students for life as well as for the practice of professional nursing. The community-based baccalaureate program provides competencies, knowledge, values, and roles that prepare professional nurses to provide high-quality care to diverse populations, in and across all environments.

Gannon is able to accommodate an entering baccalaureate class of 60 each year.

PROGRAMS OF STUDY

In the baccalaureate program, the professional nurse's role is integrated in each clinical nursing course. The School prepares high-quality graduates. Freshman students begin the investigation into the profession of nursing with seminar courses. Sophomore students begin clinical course work.

Gannon offers a certification program for school nurses, in cooperation with the School of Education. Requirements include successful completion of the B.S.N. program requirements, successful completion of required additional course work, and licensure in the commonwealth of Pennsylvania.

Options for registered nurses are available, including RN to B.S.N. and RN to M.S.N., offering an articulation path to the B.S.N. or the M.S.N. degree. Students follow a course of study that includes challenge exams, transfer credits, and validation of prior learning by a student-created portfolio. The options focus on nonduplication of previously learned nursing knowledge.

Gannon also offers a graduate program in nursing. The Master of Science in Nursing (M.S.N.) program integrates nursing education, research, and practice and is designed so that the professional nurse can respond to the challenge of unresolved problems in nursing and in health-care systems. Students may choose the Master of Science in Nursing degree program with options in nursing administration, medical-surgical nursing, family nurse practitioner, or nurse anesthesia. The M.S.N. program requires a total of 42 to 48 credit hours depending on the specific option. The curriculum plan includes core courses, 6 credits; research component, 9 credits; specialty area, 18 credits; and cognate/support courses, 6 credits. Each graduate student is expected to complete a research thesis or project. The program may be completed by enrolling full-time or part-time, with the exception of the nurse anesthesia option, which can be completed only by enrolling full-time.

ACADEMIC FACILITIES

The Nash Library currently has more than 250,000 bound volumes. The library subscribes to more than 1,000 periodicals and has book and periodical materials on various forms of microfilms and microcards. The library contains a personal computer lab; a lecture room; a curriculum library; the Founder's Room for fine and rare books; the Cyber Café, containing personal computers, laptop ports, and cappuccino and juice machines; lounges; study rooms; typing rooms; an information-retrieval system; a TV studio; the latest audiovisual and tape equipment; and a multimedia studio classroom. In addition, students may use the facilities and resources of the Erie County Law Library and the Erie County Library. For specialized research projects, an efficient interlibrary loan service is available.

The Zurn Science Center has laboratories for research in biology, anatomy, physics, chemistry, and engineering. The building also houses three computer laboratories, including an IBM PC lab. The A. J. Palumbo Academic Center houses Gannon's Villa Maria School of Nursing and features modern nursing arts labs and classrooms so that students can apply theory to practice. Additional features of the A. J. Palumbo Academic Center include state-of-the-art multimedia tiered classrooms with video teleconferencing capabilities for distance-learning opportunities, additional computer labs, and student study lounges. Other University facilities include a radio station, a theater, the Career Development and Employment Services Center, and the Waldron Campus Center.

All academic buildings at Gannon are wireless.

LOCATION

Erie is Pennsylvania's fourth-largest city and is located in the northwest corner of the state on the shores of Lake Erie. It is approximately 120 miles north of Pittsburgh, Pennsylvania; 90 miles east of Cleveland, Ohio; and 90 miles west of Buffalo, New York. The campus is within 5 miles of Interstates 79 and 90 and 5 miles from Erie International Airport. Erie is also serviced by rail and bus transportation.

STUDENT SERVICES

Gannon prides itself on meeting the personal and professional needs of all students. The Career Development and Employment Services Center for Experiential Education helps students in all stages of career preparation from determining interests and aptitudes to writing a resume and conducting a job search. Counseling Services also provides support for students' personal concerns. Gannon has a math center, a writing center, and an advising center, which students can visit for additional help on assignments.

THE NURSING STUDENT GROUP

There are currently 199 students in the Bachelor of Science in Nursing program and 83 students in the Master of Science in Nursing program. Ninety percent of the B.S.N. graduates are employed in their field, and more than 90 percent of the M.S.N. graduates are employed in the nursing profession.

COSTS

In 2004–05, full-time undergraduate tuition was $8515 per semester or $17,030 per academic year ($18,070 for engineering and health sciences). Tuition for part-time students was $400–$560 per credit hour. Room and board were approximately $3500 per semester. The total cost for the academic year at Gannon, including books and supplies, was between $17,500 and $19,220 for commuting students and $24,490 and $26,210 for resident students, depending on the program of study.

FINANCIAL AID

In order to bring a Gannon education to qualified students who could not otherwise afford it, the University offers an integrated financial aid program of scholarships, grants, loans, and employment. An application for financial aid must be filed with the application for admission. The filing has no effect on the decision of the Admissions Committee. Gannon's financial aid program is open to all full-time students attending classes during the period from August to May. All students seeking aid should file the admission and financial aid applications no later than March 1.

Nursing students wishing to pursue a career in the Army may participate in Gannon's Army ROTC program through the Partnership in Nursing Education (PNE) program. PNE students receive officer training in addition to their required course work and have the opportunity to apply for ROTC scholarships.

APPLYING

To obtain admission into the B.S.N. program, students must have completed work equal to a standard high school curriculum with a minimum of 16 units with a grade of C or better to meet the preprofessional requirements of the State Board of Nursing. Requirements include 4 units of English, 3 units of social studies, 2 units of science in biology and chemistry and labs, and 2 units of college-preparatory math, one of which must be algebra. Additional requirements include a minimum GPA of 2.5 (transfer students must have a 2.8 GPA); a combined SAT I score of 1010 or higher, with a mathematics score of at least 510; and rank in the top 40 percent of the high school class. All applicants are required to submit scores on either the SAT I or ACT, an up-to-date transcript of the high school record showing rank in class (plus a college transcript for transfer applicants), a completed application form, and a nonrefundable $25 application fee.

Requirements for students applying to graduate programs include an introductory statistics course and a research course with a grade of at least a B in both courses, competitive scores on the GRE, three letters of recommendation, RN licensure, and an interview.

CORRESPONDENCE AND INFORMATION

Mr. Christopher Tremblay
Director of Admissions
Gannon University
109 University Square
Erie, Pennsylvania 16541
Telephone: 814-871-7240
800-GANNON-U (toll-free)
Fax: 814-871-5803
E-mail: admissions@gannon.edu
World Wide Web: http://www.gannon.edu

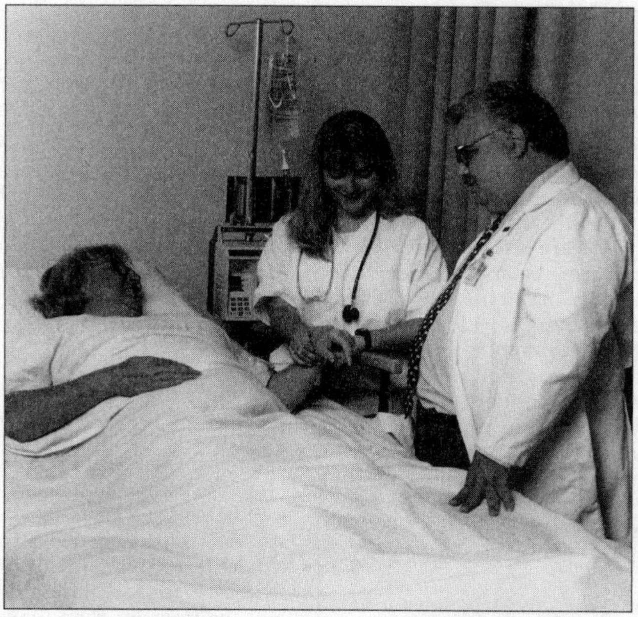

Gannon University nursing students participate in professional clinical rotations offering a variety of specialty areas with patients of different age groups and health conditions.

Georgetown University
School of Nursing and Health Studies
Washington, D.C.

THE UNIVERSITY

Georgetown University was founded in 1789 and is the oldest Catholic, Jesuit institution of higher learning in the United States. Washington, D.C., the nation's capital, is one of the most important cities in the world. Health policy and medical economics decisions are debated daily in many arenas, and decisions are made that shape the delivery of health care in this country and abroad. Cultural and social opportunities are limitless.

The diversity of the student population at Georgetown provides a stimulating environment for student life and study. All fifty states and more than 100 countries are represented by the 12,000 men and women currently enrolled in undergraduate, graduate, and professional programs.

THE SCHOOL OF NURSING AND HEALTH STUDIES

The School, founded in 1903, is conveniently located on the Main Campus next to the Georgetown University Medical Center. The Concentrated Care Center, Georgetown University Hospital, Pasquerilla Healthcare Center, Perinatal Center, and Lombardi Cancer Research Center provide access to an abundant patient population, while their proximity to the John Vinton Dahlgren Medical Library yields an ideal coordination of academic, clinical, and research facilities. This physical and functional relationship among nursing, medical, and academic facilities creates an integrated, comprehensive educational environment unavailable at many other universities.

PROGRAMS OF STUDY

The School of Nursing and Health Studies offers baccalaureate and master's degrees in nursing as well as non-nursing degrees. All nursing programs have been accredited by the National League for Nursing Accrediting Commission. There are two undergraduate majors offered in the School: the traditional Bachelor of Science in Nursing (B.S.N.) degree program and the Bachelor of Science (B.S.) degree program in health studies. An accelerated second-degree B.S.N. program for students with a bachelor's degree in a non-nursing field, an RN–B.S.N./M.S., and a traditional transfer option into the B.S.N. and B.S. in health studies programs are also offered. The nursing and health studies components are a balance between a strong theoretical base and clinical skills. Students study the curative and restorative aspects of health care, as well as health maintenance and health education. Clinical practice culminates in the senior practicum. This practicum is designed to ease the transition of the individual from the role of student to that of graduate health-care professional. Students are permitted to choose an area of concentration based on the various clinical settings available to the School. In keeping with the University's commitment to international work and study, students have opportunities for intercultural clinical experience; to date, these have included work in Appalachia, Guatemala, England, Ireland, and Australia.

The Master of Science degree programs lead to advanced nursing practice in five specialty areas: nurse midwifery, acute-care nurse practitioner, critical-care clinical nurse specialist, family nurse practitioner, and nurse anesthesia. Health systems administration is taught in conjunction with the School of Business and does not require a B.S.N. All bachelor's degrees are welcome. Post-master's options are available in all programs except nurse anesthesia.

AFFILIATIONS WITH HEALTH-CARE FACILITIES

In addition to the Georgetown University Hospital, the School is affiliated with many of the Washington-area health institutions. Some of these include Bethesda Naval Medical Center, National Children's Hospital, U.S. Department of Human Services, Walter Reed Hospital, and Hospice of the District of Columbia, to name only a few.

ACADEMIC FACILITIES

The School's classrooms, faculty, and administration are located in St. Mary's Hall. Students also have classes and laboratories on the main campus and in the medical school. The Medical Center's exciting research, innovative techniques, and sophisticated instrumentation provide an exemplary background for student clinical practice. A special clinical emphasis in home health care is included. There are varied educational resources at Georgetown's three campus libraries: the Lauinger Library, the Riggs Bioethics Library, and the Dahlgren Medical Library.

A simulation center contains five hospital-bed units, storage cabinets for teaching models, and equipment for teaching physical assessment. The center also includes a new METI Human Patient Simulator, which is used by faculty members and students, both undergraduate and graduate, in various courses.

LOCATION

The University is located in historic Georgetown. Students come to the University recognizing the special opportunities, the wealth of experience, and the insights and exposure that life in Washington will provide. Located less than 2 miles from the White House and 3 miles from the Capitol, the University is set high on a bluff overlooking picturesque Georgetown and the Potomac River. The Lauinger Library provides a panoramic view of Washington's skyline, including the Washington Monument, the Lincoln and Jefferson memorials, and the John F. Kennedy Center for the Performing Arts. More than 240 other libraries, museums, and research facilities in the city are open to Georgetown students, including the world-famous Library of Congress, National Archives, Smithsonian Institution, Folger Shakespeare Library, and National Gallery of Art. Most international embassies and federal government agencies have library facilities with staff members who are willing to help students.

STUDENT SERVICES

The Leavey Center serves as a hub of activity for social and academic campus life. The building includes three distinct components: a Conference Center, Guest House, and Student Activities Building. The Leavey Center also contains a 450-seat cafeteria, fast-food shops, a bookstore, the Faculty Club, and the Hoya Restaurant. At Georgetown, athletic activity and physical well-being are integral to the happiness and health of its students, and Yates Field House provides every means necessary to achieve this goal. It is a four-level, 142,300-square-foot structure with facilities for tennis, squash, basketball, racquetball, badminton, handball, swimming, volleyball, weightlifting, and track.

THE NURSING STUDENT GROUP

Approximately 450 undergraduate students are currently enrolled in the nursing and health studies programs. The master's program has approximately 185 students enrolled both full- and part-time.

COSTS

Undergraduate tuition for the 2004–04 academic year was $29,808. Room and board were $10,154 per academic year. Full-time graduate program tuition was $27,528 per academic year. Part-time graduate program tuition was $1147 per credit hour. University housing includes apartments, dormitories, town houses, and college houses. Accommodations are also available in apartments and houses in the Georgetown area surrounding the University. Both the University and the public transportation system provide excellent facilities to meet students' needs.

FINANCIAL AID

In cases of economic need, the University makes every effort to provide financial aid in the form of scholarships, grants, loans, and jobs to enable students to come to Georgetown. The amount of financial assistance given varies with the demonstrated financial need of the applicant. Qualified applicants may be admitted to the U.S. Army or Naval ROTC, which supports a unit on the Georgetown campus. Full-tuition scholarship assistance and subsistence allowances are available. An Air Force unit is available at a neighboring institution.

APPLYING

The School welcomes applications from men and women, without distinction on the basis of race, sex, or religious beliefs. Transfer students and candidates with degrees in fields other than nursing are encouraged to apply. All candidates are required to take the SAT I offered by the College Board or the ACT examination offered by American College Testing.

Graduate school admission requirements include a baccalaureate degree, a minimum undergraduate GPA of 3.0 on a 4.0 scale, RN licensure, three letters of reference, Graduate Record Examinations scores or the Miller Analogies Test scores, completion of an introductory course in statistical methods, and one year's experience as an RN. Those applying for the health systems administration program must have a bachelor's degree, but a nursing major is not required. For a more detailed description of the application process, students should contact the admissions office.

CORRESPONDENCE AND INFORMATION

Office of Undergraduate Admissions
White Gravenor, 101
Georgetown University
37th and O Street, NW
Washington, D.C. 20057
Telephone: 202-687-3600

Office of Graduate Admissions
Intercultural Center, 302
Georgetown University
37th and O Street, NW
Washington, D.C. 20057
Telephone: 202-687-5568

School of Nursing and Health Studies
3700 Reservoir Road, NW
Washington, D.C. 20007
Telephone: 202-687-2781 (undergraduate programs)
202-687-8439 (graduate programs)
Fax: 202-687-5553

Office of Student Financial Services
G-19 Healy Hall, Box 571252
Washington, D.C. 20057
Telephone: 202-687-4547
Fax: 202-687-6542

THE ADMINISTRATION

Better R. Keltner, Dean; Ph.D.; RN, FAAN.

Jean Kelley, Chair, Department of Advanced Practice Nursing; Ph.D.; APRN, BC.

Michael Relf, Chair, Department of Professional Nursing; Ph.D.; RN.

Goshen College
Department of Nursing
Goshen, Indiana

GOSHEN COLLEGE

THE COLLEGE

Goshen College is a four-year liberal arts college owned by and operated as a ministry of the Mennonite Church. Founded in 1894, the College is nationally recognized for its excellent academic program and Christian ideals. The College stresses academic excellence, international education, and personal and spiritual growth. There is a diverse student body of about 1,000 students from thirty-seven states and Puerto Rico, Canada, and thirty other countries. A majority of the classes have 25 or fewer students. The College motto is "Culture for Service."

The College is fully accredited by the North Central Association of Colleges and Schools.

THE DEPARTMENT OF NURSING

The Department of Nursing was founded in 1950. Programs offered are the generic baccalaureate and an accelerated RN baccalaureate.

Goshen College is home to the oldest private baccalaureate nursing program in Indiana. The nursing program recently received ten years of accreditation by the Commission on Collegiate Nursing Education. Clinical experiences in the nursing major include a wide range of hospital and community experiences. The B.S.N.-completion option for RNs allows the student to work while pursuing further education, with classes conducted in the evening hours and individually arranged clinical experiences.

Goshen College's nursing program is highly respected in this country and abroad. Its graduates are known by their ethical standards, personal integrity, Christian commitment, caring attitude, and clinical knowledge. Goshen College is primarily a teaching institution. The faculty members are highly committed to teaching and maintaining up-to-date clinical practice through faculty practice arrangements.

There are approximately 95 students enrolled in the two educational tracks. Students enjoy small class sizes in clinical courses, one-on-one student-faculty relationships, and interactive learning experiences. Students are encouraged to foster personal wellness in a variety of ways, including active participation in sports, music, drama, campus clubs, service, and commitment to a liberal arts education.

The Department's mission statement holds that within the community of faith and learning at Goshen College, the nursing program nurtures students in the process of becoming informed, articulate, sensitive, and responsible professional nurses. Graduates are prepared to engage in lifelong learning and in right relationships with recipients of care and the dynamic environmental system to promote health, healing, and wholeness.

PROGRAMS OF STUDY

The Department is committed to a high-quality program with an emphasis in liberal arts and the discipline of nursing. The nursing program has a basic and a B.S.N. completion track. The program outcomes are the same for students enrolled in either track. Both programs confer the Bachelor of Science in Nursing (B.S.N.) degree.

Graduation requirements for the generic baccalaureate track are completion of 120 credit hours accepted by Goshen College, successful completion of all nursing courses, a cumulative grade point average of 2.5 or higher in college course work, and demonstration of competency. Of the required 120 credit hours, 41 are in supporting courses and 46 are in nursing courses. Nursing students complete the same general education course requirements as students in other majors.

A typical plan of study for this track involves taking chemistry and the physics of life, human anatomy and physiology, general psychology, principles of sociology, and general education the first year. Second-year courses are microbiology, human nutrition, developmental psychology, marriage and family, theories and practice of nursing, nursing skills and physical assessment, and general education. Human pathophysiology, abnormal psychology, pharmacology and drug administration, nursing care of the adult, gerontological nursing, bioethics, nursing care of the expanding family, and nursing care of the child are typical third-year courses. In the fourth year, courses in nursing research, psychiatric/mental health nursing, nursing care in the home, community health nursing, acute-care nursing, leadership in nursing, senior seminar in nursing, and general education are usually taken.

The core requirements in international/intercultural education provide students with an opportunity to learn about the values and assumptions of their own and other cultures. Most students choose to meet this requirement by participating in the unique Study-Service Term (SST). SST requirements may be met by spending fourteen weeks in a developing nation. Groups of about 20 students are led by a Goshen College professor. Students live with host families and study the language and culture of the host country. The SST requirement may also be met by taking 12 hours of SST alternate courses on campus, which must include one in language

The RN to B.S.N. Completion Program allows registered nurses to complete a B.S.N. degree program in about eighteen months. The track is designed to affirm personal and professional strengths. The program is offered in collaboration with the Division of Adult and External Studies (DAES). Each group of RNs progresses through the courses as a cohort group. Classes meet one night a week for 4 hours and vary in length from two to ten weeks. Clinical experiences for specified courses are arranged at other times during the week. There are thirteen courses that provide 40 credit hours, of which 28 are upper-level nursing credits and 12 are general education credits.

ACADEMIC FACILITIES

The campus library has 123,000 volumes (2,023 in health and nursing) and 672 periodical subscriptions (fifty-five health-related). In addition, the library offers individualized reference service, computerized database searching, and computerized catalog capabilities. The College is home to the Mennonite Historical Library and the archives of the Mennonite Church.

Departmental resources include a computer lab, nursing audiovisuals, interactive nursing skills videos, CD-ROM resources, and a learning resource lab.

Computing resources include two large computer labs on campus to which students have access 22 hours a day. Student rooms within residence halls are wired for campus computer network access. Computing Services provides an expanding array of network services and technical support to the campus. Thirteen campus classrooms are wired for computer-generated multimedia presentations.

LOCATION

This residential college is located in Goshen, Indiana, a town of about 24,000 people. Goshen is 120 miles east of Chicago and approximately 40 miles from South Bend airport.

STUDENT SERVICES

Student services and resources include a health clinic, child-care facilities, personal and career counseling, an institutionally sponsored work-study program, job placement, a campus safety program, and special assistance for disabled students.

The College's cabin and meditation garden are available for quiet reflection and contemplation. The Recreation-Fitness Center includes three basketball courts, a swimming pool, a jogging track, racquetball courts, a weight room, classrooms, and an athletic training room.

COSTS

In 2004–05, the comprehensive fee for full-time study is $24,700. This includes $18,200 for tuition, $3300 for room, $2900 for board, and a technology fee of $300. Books and supplies cost approximately $720 and personal expenses, approximately $1000. The summer session cost $940 per course.

FINANCIAL AID

Institutionally sponsored need-based and non-need-based grants and scholarships, institutionally sponsored long-term loans, the Federal Work-Study Program, Federal Supplemental Educational Opportunity Grants, Federal Direct Student Loans, Federal Perkins Loans, and Federal Nursing Student Loans are available sources of financial aid. In 2002–03, 98 percent of undergraduate nursing students received some form of financial aid. Specialized scholarships are available for nursing students who demonstrate leadership abilities, high scholastic standing, financial need, and/or the desire to work in a mission/service setting. All the nursing students who applied for financial aid during the 2002–03 academic year received it.

APPLYING

Students seeking admission to the nursing program must first be admitted to Goshen College. Admission to the nursing major is a separate process that is usually initiated during the second semester of the first year. Admission criteria include essential abilities necessary to learn the professional nurse role and a cumulative GPA of 2.5 or higher.

CORRESPONDENCE AND INFORMATION

Goshen College
Admissions Department
1700 South Main
Goshen, Indiana 46526

Telephone: 800-348-7422 (toll-free)
Fax: 219-535-7609
E-mail: admissions@goshen.edu
World Wide Web: http://www.goshen.edu

THE FACULTY

Vicky S. Kirkton, Director of Nursing and Associate Professor of Nursing; M.S., Ball State, 1983.

Fern L. Brunner, Associate Professor of Nursing; M.S.N., Indiana–Purdue at Indianapolis, 1990.

Evelyn J. Driver, Associate Professor of Nursing; Ph.D., Virginia, 1997.

Mervin R. Helmuth, Associate Professor of Nursing; M.N., Florida, 1970.

Brenda S. Srof, Associate Professor of Nursing; M.S.N., Oral Roberts, 1986; Ph.D. candidate.

Ruth Stotzfus, Assistant Professor of Nursing and Director of Wellness and Health Center; M.S.N., Indiana–Purdue at Indianapolis, 1987.

Frances Weaver-Grill, Associate Professor of Nursing; M.S.N., SUNY at Binghamton, 1986; CFNP.

Gail Weybright, Associate Professor of Nursing; M.S.N., Valparaiso, 1999.

Hawai'i Pacific University
School of Nursing
Kaneohe, Hawai'i

THE UNIVERSITY

Hawai'i Pacific University (HPU) is an independent, coeducational, career-oriented, comprehensive university with a foundation in the liberal arts. Undergraduate and graduate degrees are offered in more than fifty different areas. Hawai'i Pacific prides itself on maintaining small class size and individual attention to students.

Students at HPU come from every state in the union and more than 100 countries around the world. The diversity of the student body stimulates learning about other cultures firsthand, both in and out of the classroom. There is no majority population at HPU. Students are encouraged to examine the values, customs, traditions, and principles of others to gain a clearer understanding of their own perspectives. HPU students develop friendships with students from throughout the United States and the world and make important connections for success in the global community of the twenty-first century.

THE SCHOOL OF NURSING

The School of Nursing began with 36 students in the fall of 1982 as a program designed to facilitate the completion of the baccalaureate degree by registered nurses. In September 1984, the program was expanded to accommodate the educational needs of licensed practical nurses. In the fall of 1987, 24 students were accepted into a newly developed four-year program. The qualities of humanism, caring, and collaboration provide a foundation to the comprehensive study of the art and science of nursing. Students learn in a flexible, multicultural environment and receive high-quality instruction in classrooms consisting of 24 to 32 students and clinical groups consisting of 8 to 10 students.

The education and expertise gained by HPU nursing students allow them to gain experience in the physical, mental, emotional, and spiritual care of clients from varied age groups and multiple ethnic backgrounds.

PROGRAMS OF STUDY

The baccalaureate nursing program offers five pathways toward a Bachelor of Science in Nursing degree. These include a Basic Pathway for the beginning or transfer student with fewer than 45 college credits, a Twenty-Three Month Pathway for transfer students who have at least a 3.0 GPA, an LPN to B.S.N. Pathway for U.S. licensed practical nurses, an RN to B.S.N. Pathway for licensed registered nurses from associate degree or diploma programs, and an International Nurse Pathway for persons who have graduated from a nursing program in another country and are not licensed in the United States.

HPU's graduate nursing program brings together theory and community-based practice in an M.S.N. program that offers the registered nurse the opportunity to advance as either a community clinical nurse specialist (CNS) or family nurse practitioner (FNP). Students interested in gaining a solid foundation in current business and management practice may pursue a joint M.S.N./M.B.A. degree. An RN to M.S.N. Pathway allows registered nurses without baccalaureate degrees in nursing to make the transition into the M.S.N. program. Students entering the RN to M.S.N. Pathway are granted provisional admission status until all prerequisites are completed.

The goal of the School of Nursing at Hawai'i Pacific University is to prepare a liberally educated professional nurse. The professional nurse has the following attributes: he or she synthesizes knowledge from the humanities, the arts, and the natural, behavioral, and nursing sciences to provide competent nursing services within a multicultural society; incorporates the caring ethic as the foundation of nursing practice; develops a commitment to altruistic service valued by society, is sensitive to the diverse needs of vulnerable groups, and has active involvement in health-care delivery policy; and promotes the integration of body, mind, and spirit through utilizing the nursing process, diagnostic and ethical reasoning, and critical thinking to assist the client in achieving mutually determined health goals. The professional nurse also practices autonomously along the continuum of novice to expert through collaboration and consultation as a member of a multidisciplinary health-care team; applies beginning leadership and management knowledge and skills to nursing practice; participates in the research process, evaluates findings for applicability and utilization in nursing practice, and contributes to the body of nursing practice; and continues to pursue knowledge and expertise commensurate with the evolving professional scope of practice.

AFFILIATIONS WITH HEALTH-CARE FACILITIES

The School of Nursing chooses facilities that give students the best experience possible. Within these facilities, the choice of clinical units is made based upon the learning needs of the students. The majority of clinical faculty members are currently actively employed in the clinical specialties and/or facilities where they teach.

ACADEMIC FACILITIES

All nursing lecture and science laboratory classes are held on the suburban and residential windward Hawai'i Loa campus where life revolves around the Amos N. Starr and Juliette Montague Cooke Academic Center (AC). The AC houses faculty and staff offices, classrooms and nursing laboratories, an art gallery, and the Atherton Learning Resources Center, which includes a library with extensive collections in the areas of Asian studies, marine science, and nursing. The Boyd MacNaughton Pacific Resources Room houses the Hawai'iana and Pacific special collections. The Academic Computer Center provides access to both Macintosh and IBM computers. The Learning Assistance Laboratory includes a collection of automated audio, video, and interactive nursing learning resources. In addition, nursing students utilize the resources of the Hawai'i Medical Library, the most comprehensive facility of its type in the state.

LOCATION

With two campuses linked by shuttle, Hawai'i Pacific combines the excitement of an urban, downtown campus with the serenity of the windward Hawai'i Loa campus set in the lush foothills of the Koolau Mountains. The main campus is located in downtown Honolulu, the business and financial center of the Pacific. Eight miles away, situated on 135 acres in Kaneohe, the windward Hawai'i Loa campus is the site of the nursing, environmental science, and marine science programs and a variety of other course offerings. Students may attend some non-nursing classes on either campus. The beautiful weather, for which Hawai'i is famous, allows for unlimited recreational opportunities year-round. The emphasis on a career-related curriculum keeps students focused on their academic goals. The economy in Hawai'i makes cooperative education and internship experiences hard to beat. Students desiring to expand their horizons in preparation for the changing global economy find Hawai'i a working laboratory. The many opportunities available at HPU provide for a healthy combination of school, work, and fun.

STUDENT SERVICES

The University has many services to meet student needs, including a professional staff of advisers who are available throughout the year to assist undergraduate students in advising and counseling matters. Other services include career placement programs; a cooperative education program; international student advising; various student organizations, including the Student Nurses' Association; and numerous honor societies, including Sigma Theta Tau International Nursing Honor Society. A director of student life and a residence life staff are actively involved in all aspects of student life.

HPU competes in NCAA Division II intercollegiate sports. Men's athletic programs include baseball, basketball, cross-country, and tennis. Women's athletics include cross-country, softball, tennis, and volleyball.

The Housing Office at HPU offers many services and options for students. On-campus residence halls with cafeteria service are available on the windward Hawai'i Loa campus, while off-campus apartments are available in the Waikiki area, near the downtown campus, for those seeking more independent living arrangements.

THE NURSING STUDENT GROUP

The students in the School of Nursing are representative of the global community in terms of age, ethnicity, citizenship, gender, and professional experience. Students may attend either full- or part-time, with a substantial number of students choosing to accelerate the completion of their degree by studying during summer sessions. Various nursing courses are offered during summer sessions.

COSTS

Tuition for the 2004–05 academic year was $10,922 for freshmen and sophomores and $15,632 for juniors and seniors. Part-time student tuition was $205 per unit for 1 to 7 credits and $455 per unit for 8 to 11 credits for freshmen and sophomores. For part-time juniors and seniors, the tuition was $651 per unit for 1 to 11 credits. Residence hall room and board were $7928, and off-campus apartments (operated by Cadmus Properties Corporation) rented for between $2900 and $3300 per semester. (There was an additional $500 refundable security deposit required for residence halls and off-campus apartments.)

FINANCIAL AID

The University provides financial aid for qualified students through institutional, state, and federal aid programs. Approximately 40 percent of the University's students receive financial aid. Among the forms of aid available are Federal Perkins Loans, Federal Stafford Student Loans, Guaranteed Parental Loans, Federal Pell Grants, and Federal Supplemental Educational Opportunity Grants. To apply for aid, students must submit the Free Application for Federal Student Aid (FAFSA). The FAFSA may be submitted at any time, but the priority deadline is March 1. Several local health-care agencies award low-interest loans to student nurses, which are forgiven for various lengths of service following successful completion of the NCLEX-RN examination.

APPLYING

Candidates are notified of admission decisions on a rolling basis, usually within two weeks of receipt of application materials. Early entrance and deferred entrance are available. HPU accepts the Common Application form.

CORRESPONDENCE AND INFORMATION

Office of Admissions
Hawai'i Pacific University
1164 Bishop Street, Suite 200
Honolulu, Hawai'i 96813
Telephone: 808-544-0238
866-CALL-HPU (toll-free)
Fax: 808-544-1136
E-mail: admissions@hpu.edu
World Wide Web: http://www.hpu.edu/Petersons

THE FACULTY

Dale Allison, Professor; Ph.D., Pennsylvania; APRN-Rx.
Margaret Anderson, Associate Professor; Ed.D, M.S.N., San Francisco; APRN.
Epifinia Baranda, Assistant Professor; M.S.N., Phoenix; APRN.
Linda Beechinor, Assistant Professor; M.S., Hawai'i; APRN-Rx, BC, FNP.
Patricia Bemis, Assistant Professor; M.S., Hawai'i; RN.
Henny Breen, Assistant Professor; M.S.N., Hawai'i; M.Ed., Toronto; RN.
Patricia Burrell, Associate Professor and Assistant Dean of Nursing for Students; Ph.D., Utah; APRN, BC.
Nita Jane Carrington, Assistant Professor; M.S.N., M.B.A., Portland; RN, ANP.
ReNel Davis, Associate Professor; Ph.D., Colorado; RN.
Laura Dower, Assistant Professor; M.S.N., Hawai'i Pacific, RN.
David J. Dunham, Assistant Professor; M.S., Hawai'i; RN, CRNI.
Hobie Etta Feagai, Assistant Professor; M.S.N., Tennessee, Knoxville; APRN-Rx, BC, FNP.
Janice Haley, Associate Professor; Ph.D., Hawai'i; APRN, CPNP.
Sherry Hester, Assistant Professor; M.S.N., RN, CS, APRN.
Judith Holland, Assistant Professor; Ph.D., Denver; RN.
Marianne Hultgren, Assistant Professor; M.S., Utah; RN.
Linda Humes, Visiting Assistant Professor; M.S.N., Georgia State; APRN, FNP, WOCNC.
Holly Kailani, Associate Professor; M.S., Hawai'i; RN, C, WHNP.
Valerie Kido, Assistant Professor; M.S., Hawai'i; RN.
Betty Kohal, Assistant Professor; M.S.N., Vanderbilt; APRN, BC.
Patricia Lange-Otsuka, Associate Professor; Ed.D., Nova Southeastern; M.S.N., APRN, BC.
Leanne Logan, Assistant Professor; M.S.N., RN, BC.
Peter Look, Assistant Professor; M.S.N., Texas at El Paso; RN.
Michelle Marineau, Assistant Professor; M.S.N., Grand Valley State; APRN-Rx, BC, FNP.
Lila Montambo, Assistant Professor; M.S.N., Michigan; RN.
Mary Iwalani Moore, Assistant Professor; M.S.N., APRN.
Mercy Mott, Assistant Professor; M.S., UCLA; APRN, CNS.
Lynell Rogers, Assistant Professor; M.N., Hawai'i; RN.
Catherine Ryan, Assistant Professor; M.S., Georgetown; RN, CNM.
Dianne Sandy, Assistant Professor; M.S.N., Hawai'i Pacific; RN, FNP.
Patricia Slachta, Associate Professor; Ph.D., Adelphi; APRN, CWOCN, BC.
Frances Spohn, Assistant Professor; M.S., M.P.H., Hawai'i; RN, CHES.
John Stepulis, Assistant Professor; M.S.N., Vanderbilt; RN.
Barbara Tomlinson, Assistant Professor; M.S.N., Florida; B.B.A., RN.
Sharyl Toscano, Assistant Professor; Ph.D., Boston College; RN-CS, FNP.
Jeanine Tweedie, Assistant Professor; M.S.N., Utah; RN.
Carol Winters-Moorhead, Professor and Dean, School of Nursing, Hawai'i Loa Campus; Ph.D., Pittsburgh; RN.

Holy Family University
School of Nursing and Allied Health Professions
Philadelphia, Pennsylvania

Holy Family UNIVERSITY

THE UNIVERSITY

Holy Family University, founded in 1954 by the Congregation of the Sisters of the Holy Family of Nazareth, is a fully accredited, Catholic, private, coeducational, four-year commuter university. It has three locations, one in northeast Philadelphia and two in Bucks County (Bensalem and Newtown), Pennsylvania. The University provides liberal arts and professional programs for more than 2,600 full- and part-time undergraduate and graduate students in day and evening classes. Undergraduate students take a core curriculum of courses in the humanities and social and natural sciences that serve as a basis for broadening ethical and moral values and perspectives. The University provides master's degrees in four areas (counseling psychology, human resources management, nursing, and education) and a variety of nondegree teacher certification programs.

THE SCHOOL OF NURSING

The undergraduate nursing program at Holy Family University, inaugurated in 1971, has been continually accredited by the National League for Nursing or the National League for Nursing Accrediting Commission.

The School of Nursing central office is located in the Nurse Education Building on one of the Northeast Philadelphia locations. The School has 16 full-time faculty members, a part-time learning resource coordinator, and more than 25 part-time faculty members. The student-faculty ratio in clinical courses is usually 8:1, which maintains clinical groups at a size that affords each student valuable learning experiences with appropriate instruction, guidance, and supervision. The nursing school administration consists of a dean, a B.S.N. chair, an M.S.N. chair, and a Student Affairs chair.

The teaching-learning environment focuses on enhancing the student's ability to integrate and use health-related concepts and principles in a contemporary and changing health-care delivery system. Faculty members view their teaching role as facilitators and change agents and provide the needed guidance for the learning process to proceed. The student is expected to assume an active role in the learning experience.

PROGRAMS OF STUDY

The Bachelor of Science in Nursing (B.S.N.) and the Master of Science in Nursing (M.S.N.) degrees are offered. In addition, a school nurse certificate program is provided in collaboration with Eastern University. The baccalaureate nursing program prepares a nursing generalist who possesses the ability to develop selected leadership roles in the delivery of nursing services. The roles of caregiver, client advocate, teacher, and counselor emerge as reasonable expectations for baccalaureate graduates. In addition, the ability to critique and use research appropriately in practice is anticipated. As professional nurses, graduates accept responsibility for their own professional growth and for the advancement of the profession at large.

Students are introduced to the nursing profession during the freshman year in college. Beginning in the second year, clinical courses provide students with the opportunity to apply theory to practice in selected health-care settings. In the third and fourth years, students practice in a variety of health-care settings and in the community. This diversity of hospital and community clinical sites affords students caregiving experiences with clients across the life span who have various cultural, socioeconomic, and religious backgrounds. Small classroom sizes and limited numbers of students in clinical groups are hallmarks for enhanced student learning and interaction.

The B.S.N. program may be completed during the day on a full-time or part-time basis. Part-time students also may attend courses in the evening, with clinical experiences on the weekend.

An accelerated RN-B.S.N. curriculum that encourages registered nurses to continue their education and to pursue the Bachelor of Science in Nursing degree is also offered. Recognizing that registered nurses already have a background in clinical nursing, the University respects the students' prior education in order to prevent unnecessary repetition of nursing courses completed in their initial educational programs. The program includes courses designed specifically for RNs, coupled with a plan to accept direct transfer of 32 nursing credits and additional credits as appropriate.

An LPN/LVN-B.S.N. track curriculum option is also available. Similar to the RN-B.S.N. track, the LPN/LVN track respects the student's prior nursing education and offers the direct transfer of 5 nursing credits and the opportunity to obtain 9 credits through competency validation and to take course challenge examinations for up to an additional 12 credits.

The purpose of the Master of Science in Nursing program is to provide a graduate nursing curriculum that is tailored to address current and future global health-care needs and issues in a variety of health-care settings; to offer students the opportunity to develop expertise and prepare for certification, where it is available, in the specialty areas of community health, nursing education, or nursing administration; and to provide a foundation for doctoral study.

The M.S.N. program provides an interdisciplinary curriculum grounded by professional nursing standards, ethical and moral precepts, and scientific principles. Each concentration requires 39 credit hours distributed among core, concentration, and specialty requirements. The core curriculum provides a strong foundation in nursing theory, research, health policy, ethics, and health promotion; concentration requirements enhance knowledge in areas related to the chosen specialty; and nursing role specialty requirements allow students to focus on developing advanced knowledge, skills, and practical experience in roles related to selected areas of nursing practice.

The M.S.N. program may be completed on a part-time basis, with individualized practica developed to enhance past work experience and areas of interest. A key feature of this program is that a bachelor's degree in nursing is not required for admission. Licensed registered nurses with baccalaureate degrees in related areas may apply. Individuals without a baccalaureate nursing degree must validate equivalent competencies in nursing leadership, research, and community health through examination, course work, or portfolio evaluation.

AFFILIATIONS WITH HEALTH-CARE FACILITIES

All nursing programs maintain affiliations with a wide variety of clinical agencies and are constantly investigating additional settings that will provide effective learning experiences for the students. Large teaching tertiary-care centers, such as St. Christopher's Hospital for Children, Albert Einstein Medical Center, and Friends Hospital in urban Philadelphia, are used, as are community-based institutions such as Nazareth Hospital and St. Mary Medical Center.

Clinical experiences in the community include hospice care, clinics, home care, and generalized service provided by the health department. Nursing care in the community is integrated into each of the clinical courses and provides students with an understanding of nursing's role within the changing health-care delivery system.

ACADEMIC FACILITIES

The nursing programs have their own learning resource center located in the Nursing Education Building. The center includes a clinical skills laboratory with an advanced skills component, a computer lab, and an audiovisual resources center. This learning resources center has its own coordinator, and the facility is available to students for independent study and for the practice of nursing skills.

LOCATION

The University's three locations are easily accessible from Philadelphia, Montgomery, and Bucks Counties in Pennsylvania and Burlington, Camden, Gloucester, Hunterdon, and Mercer Counties in New Jersey.

The northeast Philadelphia campus of 47 acres is located in a safe residential section close to the Philadelphia–Bucks County line and just a mile from two exits of Interstate 95 (Academy and Woodhaven). It can be reached easily by automobile or by public and rail transportation. It is ½ mile from Amtrak's major northeast rail line, which also carries commuter traffic between Trenton, New Jersey, and Philadelphia.

In nearby Bensalem Township, Bucks County, Holy Family opened its new Woodhaven site, housing the Extended Learning Division and serving as the headquarters for accelerated programs. This site on Bristol Pike is at the Woodhaven exit of I-95.

Holy Family's picturesque Newtown location on 155 acres in Bucks County is also accessible via I-95 off Route 332 (Newtown-Yardley Road). It can also be reached from Route 413 north to 413 Bypass.

STUDENT SERVICES

On campus, the nursing student can take advantage of the University's Counseling Center; Campus Ministry; the Cabaret, which offers one night a week of music and student entertainment; the Rainbow Connection, a support group for anyone who might feel different because of age, race, or ethnic background; the bookstore; volleyball activities; and three racquetball courts, a new weight room, and an auxiliary gym for personal conditioning. Nursing students can join the Delta Tau Chapter of Sigma Theta Tau, the international nursing honor society, as well as the strong and active Student Nurses Association at Holy Family (SNAHF), which participates in campus activities to promote health. The University's volunteer services offer opportunities for individuals to help at a variety of charitable agencies within the community.

THE NURSING STUDENT GROUP

Culturally diverse traditional and nontraditional students, full-time and part-time students, transfer students, and registered nurses are enrolled in the B.S.N. program.

Upon completion of the program, graduates usually find employment in hospitals and community agencies in or near the city of Philadelphia. A number of graduates each year are offered employment in agencies affiliated with the School of Nursing. Graduate follow-up surveys indicate a high degree of satisfaction with the program, and a growing number of graduates are pursuing advanced nursing education.

COSTS

The University has one of the most competitive tuition structures in the Philadelphia area. For the 2004–05 academic year, tuition was $7995 per semester for full-time students. The general fee is $250 per semester. The clinical nursing fee is $50–$150 per semester for full-time nursing students. Tuition for part-time students was $335 per credit for non-nursing and nursing courses and $380 per credit for nursing clinical courses. The clinical nursing fee for part-time nursing students was $150 per course. For graduate courses, tuition was $415 per credit hour and $465 per credit hour for nursing clinical courses.

FINANCIAL AID

In addition to Federal Pell Grants and Pennsylvania Higher Education Assistance Agency (PHEAA) grants, the financial aid program includes scholarships, grants-in-aid, loans, and work programs. Of particular interest is the Nursing Student Loan Program, which provides federal and institutional funds to aid eligible students pursing a career in nursing through low-interest, long-term loans with repayment period beginning nine months after withdrawal or when a student ceases to study on at least a half-time basis. For details, students should call the Financial Aid Office at 215-637-5538.

APPLYING

Holy Family University has a rolling admissions policy but encourages early application. High school students must submit an application form, a nonrefundable $25 fee, a high school transcript, SAT I scores, and a letter of recommendation. Transfer students must submit an application form, a nonrefundable $25 fee, previous college transcripts, high school transcripts (or GED test scores), and a letter of recommendation. Application forms are available from the addresses given below.

CORRESPONDENCE AND INFORMATION

For the B.S.N. program:
Director of Undergraduate Admissions
Holy Family University
Grant and Frankford Avenues
Philadelphia, Pennsylvania 19114-2094
Telephone: 215-637-3050
E-mail: undergra@holyfamily.edu
World Wide Web: http://www.holyfamily.edu

For the accelerated RN-B.S.N. program:
Director of Admissions and Marketing
Division of Extended Learning
Newtown Location
Holy Family University
1 Campus Drive
Newtown, Pennsylvania 18940
Telephone: 215-504-2000
World Wide Web: http://www.holyfamily.edu

For the M.S.N. program:
Director of Graduate Admissions
Holy Family University
Grant and Frankford Avenues
Philadelphia, Pennsylvania 19114-2094
Telephone: 215-637-3555
World Wide Web: http://www.holyfamily.edu

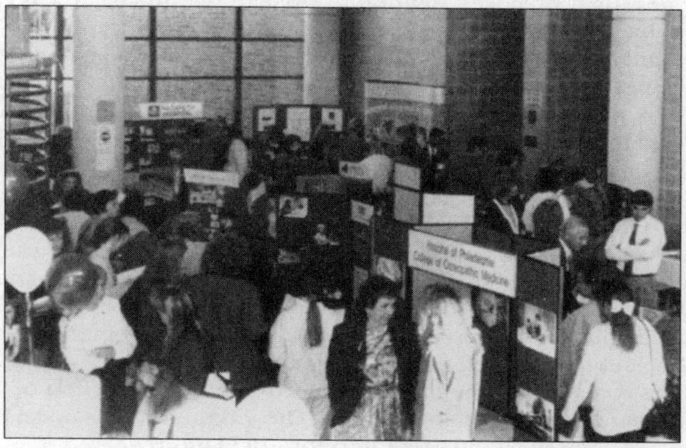

Nurse Recruiting Day at Holy Family University allows nursing students to explore job opportunities as recruiters from hospitals and health-care agencies visit the campus.

Illinois State University
Mennonite College of Nursing
Normal, Illinois

THE UNIVERSITY
Illinois State University was founded in 1857 and was the first public university in the state of Illinois. The mission of the University is to expand the horizons of knowledge and culture among students, colleagues, and the general public through teaching and research. As a multidimensional, residential university, it has one of the largest undergraduate programs in Illinois, with six colleges and thirty-seven academic departments that offer more than 160 major/minor options. The Graduate School coordinates forty master's, specialist, and doctoral programs. Illinois State University is highly committed to a student-centered focus as evidenced by approximately 91 percent of undergraduate credit hours being taught by faculty members and at least 73 percent of all classes having 30 or fewer students.

THE COLLEGE OF NURSING
Mennonite College of Nursing at Illinois State University began as a private, diploma program in 1918. Mennonite made the transition to an upper-division baccalaureate program in 1982 and began a graduate program in 1995. On July 1, 1999, the nursing college merged with Illinois State University and moved from the private to the public sector, making Mennonite the sixth college and first professional college at Illinois State University. The nursing program is located on the campus quad in a newly remodeled building with state-of-the-art facilities. The mission is to educate students to serve the citizens of Illinois and the global community, with a particular responsibility to address the nursing and health-care needs of urban and rural populations, especially the vulnerable and underserved. There is a dynamic community of learning in which reflective thinking and ethical decision making are valued. The College is committed to being purposeful, open, just, caring, disciplined, and celebratory. Students work closely with faculty members of Mennonite College of Nursing, who actively engage in research, write for publication, give professional presentations, and participate in clinical practice. Graduates possess outcome abilities of caring, critical thinking, communication, and professional practice. Mennonite College of Nursing is accredited by the Commission on Collegiate Nursing Education.

Current research activities of the faculty include decision making at end-of-life, nutritional adequacy in low-income pregnant women, HIV infection among women at high-risk, access to health care for the working poor, quality outcomes in long-term care, and use of touch therapy.

PROGRAMS OF STUDY
In the Prelicensure/Bachelor of Science in Nursing Program, students complete the University's General Education program or the Illinois Transferable General Education Core Curriculum, including required courses and additional requirements. To be admitted to the nursing major, completion of 59 semester hours is required. The nursing major requires completion of 65 semester hours in nursing courses. These requirements make up the 124 semester hours required for graduation.

The faculty of the nursing college provides a curriculum that responds to both the nursing needs of society and the learning needs of students. Students have frequent contact with faculty members on an individual and group basis. The nursing curriculum is four semesters of full-time study. Each semester provides for the practice of skills and application of knowledge through a variety of classroom and laboratory experiences.

The Registered Nurse/Bachelor of Science in Nursing (RN/B.S.N.) Completion Program at Mennonite College of Nursing offers full-time, accelerated three-semester plans and part-time plans. All RN/B.S.N. courses are offered online. Proficiency examinations and portfolio processes are available in select courses.

Thirty-three nursing hours are granted for prior lower-division courses upon successful completion of all general education requirements. Sixty-four nursing hours are required, of which 33 may be earned as escrow credit for prior learning. Requirements for the B.S.N. include a minimum of 123 hours, a 30-hour residency, a cumulative grade point average (GPA) of at least 2.0 on a 4.0 scale, and a grade of C or better in all required courses. Fifty-nine General Education hours are required for graduation. Additional University graduation requirements include a 3-hour global studies course and a University writing examination.

The Master of Science in Nursing (M.S.N.) Program offers two sequences, Family Nurse Practitioner (FNP) and Nursing Systems Administration (NSA), and two certificates, Nurse Educator Certificate (NEC) and Post-Master's Family Nurse Practitioner Certificate. The FNP sequence offers a 44-hour option or a 48-hour option with a thesis. The NSA sequence offers a 30-hour option or a 34-hour option with a thesis. The NSA specialty courses are offered online. NEC course work prepares graduates to function in the areas of nursing education and nursing service/clinical practice. Candidates for the certificate must complete a total of 15 credits. The Post-Master's FNP Certificate requires a minimum of 26 credits at Mennonite College of Nursing.

AFFILIATIONS WITH HEALTH-CARE FACILITIES
Mennonite College of Nursing has a clinical network of approximately fifty off-campus agencies, such as hospitals, nursing homes, public health departments, and community centers. Student experiences are extended to include surrounding communities in which specialty health services are provided to various clients. This type of clinical rotation allows students to have a complex, diverse orientation to multiple health-care approaches.

ACADEMIC FACILITIES
Milner Library at Illinois State University has more than 1.3 million cataloged books, 390,000 government publications, 1.8 million microforms, 460,000 maps, and 26,000 audio recordings. In addition, there is state-of-the-art technology in classrooms, including computer, video, and Internet resources. A distance education classroom/computer lab and futuristic clinical laboratories are available in Edwards Hall, which houses Mennonite College of Nursing.

LOCATION
Illinois State University is located in the community of Bloomington–Normal with a population of approximately 100,000. Bloomington–Normal is located in central Illinois, 137 miles southwest of Chicago and 164 miles northeast of St. Louis, and is one of the fastest-growing communities in Illinois. The University is near three major interstate highways and the

railway between St. Louis and Chicago. The local airport offers a wide range of flights on a daily basis.

STUDENT LIFE

Nursing students actively participate in the University-wide Honors Program and the Transcultural Program, which allows students the opportunity to examine nursing care in a location culturally different from central Illinois. In the past, students have had experiences in Texas, Kentucky, Montana, England, and Japan.

Illinois State University has thirteen residence halls with lifestyle options. A floor of one of these residence halls is reserved for Mennonite College of Nursing students.

THE NURSING STUDENT GROUP

Xi Pi, a chapter of nursing's honor society, Sigma Theta Tau International, is located at Mennonite College of Nursing. Students are eligible for application to the honor society and the Student Nursing Association (SNA). An additional opportunity for involvement is the Peer Support Program, in which outstanding students are selected to support incoming students.

All graduate students belong to the campuswide Graduate Student Organization. In addition, students can become involved in the Mennonite Graduate Student Organization, which is one of 250 registered student organizations at Illinois State University.

COSTS

For students who enrolled starting in fall 2004, tuition per credit hour was assessed at $160. General fees per semester hour were $43.20.

Graduate study costs were $145 per credit hour, with a fee assessment of $43.20.

FINANCIAL AID

The Financial Aid Office at Illinois State University administers from federal, state, institutional, and private sources to ensure that eligible students have access to an education. Prospective students should visit the Web site at http://www.infosys.ilstu.edu/depts/Finaid/ for further financial aid information.

Mennonite College of Nursing awards scholarships in conjunction with the Financial Aid Office and the Illinois State University Foundation. Scholarship information and application forms may be found at http://www.mcn.ilstu.edu by selecting "Prospective Students."

Graduate students may apply for graduate assistantships that include tuition waivers. Traineeships may be available for full-time nurse practitioner students.

APPLYING

For the Prelicensure/Bachelor of Science in Nursing Sequence, a total of 59 semester college hours is required to be considered for admission. Students must receive a C or better in designated required courses and have a minimum cumulative GPA of 2.7 on a 4.0 scale. Students may be admitted to the program following completion of their sophomore year in college. Class cohorts begin in the fall semester only. Applications received prior to January 2 for admission consideration the following fall receive preferential admission review. Academic preferences and early admission criteria are available upon request.

For the Registered Nurse/Bachelor of Science in Nursing Program, an applicant must be a graduate of a state-approved diploma school of nursing or an associate-degree nursing program, be licensed as a registered nurse in the state of Illinois, have completed specific required courses with a C or better, and submit one recommendation form. Applicants are considered for admission for fall and spring semesters.

For the Master of Science in Nursing Program, an applicant must hold a B.S.N. from an accredited program, have a minimum GPA of 3.0 for the last 60 semester hours of undergraduate course work, satisfactorily complete a graduate-level statistics course (300 level or higher), submit Graduate Record Examinations (GRE) scores and the GRE Writing Assessment, be licensed as a registered nurse in the state of Illinois, and submit a resume, three letters of reference, and an essay discussing professional and educational goals. GRE scores are not required for those applicants with a GPA of 3.4 or higher for the last 60 hours of undergraduate course work.

All applicants to the Nurse Educator Certificate Program must show evidence of current enrollment in an accredited master's degree nursing program or evidence of graduation from an accredited master's degree nursing program, complete a Nurse Educator Certificate application form, submit one reference from a person qualified to assess the applicant's potential to succeed as a nurse educator, and must meet general admission requirements as designated for Mennonite College of Nursing's Master of Science in Nursing Program.

For the Family Nurse Practitioner Post-Master's Certificate Program, course work is determined for each student after an assessment of the applicant's prior graduate nursing education to determine equivalency to the master's degree core and support courses.

CORRESPONDENCE AND INFORMATION:

Illinois State University
Mennonite College of Nursing
Campus Box 5810
Normal, Illinois 61790-5810
Telephone: 309-438-7400
World Wide Web: http://www.mcn.ilstu.edu

PROGRAM HEADS

Sara L. Campbell, D.N.S., RN, CNAA, BC; Associate Dean. (e-mail: slcampb2@ilstu.edu)

Pamela Lindsey, M.S., RN; Undergraduate Program Director. (e-mail: pllinds@ilstu.edu)

Brenda Recchia Jeffers, Ph.D., RN; Graduate Program Director. (e-mail: brjeffe@ilstu.edu)

Indiana University
School of Nursing
Indianapolis, Bloomington, and Columbus, Indiana

THE UNIVERSITY
Founded in 1820, Indiana University (IU) has grown from its modest beginnings into one of the oldest and largest universities in the Midwest and one of the nation's finest educational institutions. Offering 838 degree programs at eight campuses around the state, IU attracts students from every state in the United States and around the world. IU's residential campus at Bloomington and its urban center in Indianapolis form the core of the University, bringing a high-quality education within the reach of any student. IU is accredited by the North Central Association of Colleges and Schools.

THE SCHOOL OF NURSING
Since its inception as The Indiana University Training School for Nurses in 1914, the Indiana University School of Nursing (IUSON) has become one of the largest multipurpose schools of nursing in the United States. Ranked twelfth nationally (*U.S. News & World Report,* 1998), IUSON offers the following academic degrees, ranging from the associate to the doctoral levels: the Bachelor of Science in Nursing (B.S.N.), the Master of Science in Nursing (M.S.N.), and the Ph.D. in Nursing Science.

The School's B.S.N. and M.S.N. programs are accredited by the National League for Nursing Accrediting Commission (NLNAC). The B.S.N. and M.S.N. programs are also accredited by the Commission on Collegiate Nursing Education (CCNE), the B.S.N. program is accredited by the Indiana State Board of Nursing, and the School's continuing education department is accredited by the American Nurses Credentialing Center's Commission on Accreditation. IUSON is an agency member of the NLN, AACN, and CIC.

PROGRAMS OF STUDY
The B.S.N. degree program provides a comprehensive academic foundation in the sciences and humanities essential for preparing students for a generalist practice role. The baccalaureate program appeals to students wishing to combine general education with professional course work and also serves as a foundation for graduate study. (It is recommended that those interested in graduate studies enter nursing education at the B.S.N. level.) The program takes a minimum of four years of full-time study to complete. The program emphasizes health promotion, maintenance, and preventions as well as managing individuals and families coping with acute and chronic illnesses. Indiana University–Purdue University offers the B.S.N. degree to both traditional and second degree students. Indiana University–Purdue University at Columbus offers courses toward the completion of the LPN to A.S.N. mobility option. Indiana University Bloomington offers all required courses for the B.S.N. degree.

The goal of the M.S.N. degree program is to prepare graduates for leadership roles in advanced nursing practice, clinical specialization, and nursing administration. Majors are offered in twelve areas: adult health clinical nurse specialist studies, adult psychiatric/mental health nursing, child/adolescent psychiatric/mental health nursing, community health nursing, nursing administration, pediatric nurse practitioner studies, pediatric clinical nurse specialist studies, adult nurse practitioner studies, neonatal nurse practitioner studies, family nurse practitioner studies, acute-care nurse practitioner studies, and women's health nurse practitioner studies. Post-master's options are available in all clinical areas and in nursing administration and teacher education. Students select a major area of study when they apply for admission. Students may elect to follow a full- or part-time course of study. All degree requirements must be met within six years of initial enrollment.

The Ph.D. in Nursing Science Degree program, which builds on baccalaureate nursing education, is based on the beliefs that professional nursing is a scientific discipline and that it has a unique role and body of knowledge that can be expanded, applied, and validated through recognized methods of scholarly inquiry. The primary goal of the program is the preparation of scholars in one of the following focus areas: environments for health, acute and chronic health problems, health promotion, and family health adaptation. The 90-credit curriculum includes concentrations in theory, research, and statistics; nursing science and research; an external cognate minor; and a dissertation. The Ph.D. program is post-B.S.N. Students who hold either a B.S.N. or M.S.N. may apply. Thirty credits may be met by course work completed for the M.S.N.

Nurses wishing to pursue additional academic education at IUSON can also take advantage of several "mobility options." The LPN to A.S.N. mobility program enables students to apply previous nursing education toward earning an Associate of Science in Nursing degree. Graduates are eligible to take the registered nurse licensure examination. The associate/diploma RN to B.S.N. mobility option facilitates the application of previous course work toward the Bachelor of Science in Nursing degree. Nursing knowledge is substantiated through "bridging courses" rather than through testing. The associate/diploma RN to M.S.N. mobility program offers a unique opportunity for those individuals who have accumulated advanced nursing knowledge and skill through additional experiences. The RN to M.S.N. educational mobility option is available to qualified registered nurses who do not hold a baccalaureate degree in nursing but who have earned academic credit in addition to their initial registered nurse program. Included are those whose highest academic credential is the diploma in nursing or the A.S.N. degree. Specific mobility courses are offered on the Indianapolis, Bloomington, and Columbus campuses and through distance education, including the Internet.

AFFILIATIONS WITH HEALTH-CARE FACILITIES
The Indiana University Medical Center (IUMC), located on the Indiana University–Purdue University at Indianapolis (IUPUI) campus, includes the Schools of Nursing, Medicine, Social Work, Allied Health, and Dentistry. IUMC's extensive diagnostic clinics and five teaching hospitals are Indiana's primary referral hospitals and its chief centers for clinical instruction in the health professions. The School's commitment to practice is also reflected in the number of its innovative programs and ongoing cutting-edge research. The Maternity Outreach Mobilization (MOM) project provides prenatal care to needy women in Indianapolis. The Institute of Action Research for Community Health, dedicated to working with cities across the state to improve community health, has been designated a World Health Organization (WHO) Collaborating Center in Healthy Cities. The Mary Margaret Walther Program for Cancer Care Research Center, located on the IUPUI campus, is a leader in oncology care research.

ACADEMIC FACILITIES

Library facilities for student use are extensive. IUPUI facilities include the University Library, the School of Law Library, the School of Dentistry Library, the Medical Science Library, Herron School of Art Library, and a School of Nursing reference library. The Medical Science Library houses the largest and most complete health science library in Indiana. The multimillion-dollar University Library employs state-of-the-art electronic information systems technology.

LOCATION

The B.S.N., M.S.N., and Ph.D. nursing programs are offered on the IUPUI campus; Columbus Center offers the LPN to A.S.N. mobility option and selected general education courses for the B.S.N.; and the B.S.N. degree may be obtained at IU Bloomington. Graduate programs are offered through the campus of IUPUI in Indianapolis. Selected baccalaureate- and core master's-level nursing courses are offered over the Internet.

STUDENT SERVICES

The mission of the student services area of the School of Nursing is to help students attain their academic and professional goals. Support services for disadvantaged students are available; however, services may vary from campus to campus.

THE NURSING STUDENT GROUP

The headquarters of Sigma Theta Tau International, nursing's honor society, is located on the Indianapolis campus, where it was founded in 1922. All prenursing and nursing undergraduates are eligible for membership in the National Student Nurses Association and the Indiana Association of Nursing Students. Chi Eta Phi Sorority is a service organization open to all qualified undergraduate nursing students. The Minority Nursing Student Organization is a peer support group for minority nursing students. Membership in the RN to B.S.N. Organization is open to all registered nurses in the baccalaureate program.

COSTS

Tuition and fees vary by campus. Indiana residents pay $145.05 per credit hour for undergraduate courses and $194.10 per credit hour for graduate courses. Nonresidents pay approximately $451.15 per credit hour for undergraduate courses and $560.15 per credit hour for graduate courses. Students may also be responsible for student technology fees, student activity fees, and laboratory and other fees.

FINANCIAL AID

Financial aid, including scholarships, grants, and loans, is provided by the federal government, the state of Indiana, Indiana University, IUSON, and individual donors. Undergraduate students should contact the Office of Scholarships and Financial Aid at the campus of undergraduate attendance for information.

APPLYING

Students interested in the B.S.N. degree program must be accepted to IU and begin studies with required general education course work. Students who meet all application requirements are eligible to apply for competitive admission to the nursing program.

Requirements for unconditional admission to the M.S.N. program are as follows: a B.S.N. from an accredited program or its equivalent, a minimum 3.0 GPA on a 4.0 scale, a score of 400 or better on two of the three sections of the GRE, a current Indiana registered nurse license (international applicants must submit evidence of passing the Council of Graduates of Foreign Nursing Schools qualifying examination and must receive licensure in Indiana prior to enrollment), a TOEFL score of 550 or above for those whose native language is not English, completion of a 3-credit statistics course within the last seven years with at least a grade of B–, verification of ability to use computer technologies, and verification of physical assessment skills. Requirements for admission into the RN to M.S.N. mobility option are the same, except the student does not need a B.S.N. Students who meet the above requirements but whose highest credential in nursing is an A.S.N. degree or diploma are eligible for admission.

The criteria for consideration for admission to the Ph.D. program are a baccalaureate degree with a major in nursing from an accredited program or its equivalent; a baccalaureate cumulative GPA of 3.0 or higher on a 4.0 scale (for those holding a master's degree, a graduate GPA of 3.5 or higher is required); completion of a 3-credit statistics course with a grade of B or higher within seven years before the date of proposed enrollment; ability to secure current registered nurse licensure in Indiana; scores of 600 or better on all sections of the GRE; scores of 600 or better on the TOEFL for students whose first language is not English (a written test of English is also required); a two- to three-page essay; evidence of the capacity for original scholarship and research in nursing; three references; have a research mentor who must be a nursing faculty member with full IU graduate school status; and an interview.

CORRESPONDENCE AND INFORMATION

Office of Educational Services
Indiana University School of Nursing
1111 Middle Drive, NU 122
Indianapolis, Indiana 46202
Telephone: 317-274-2806
Fax: 317-274-2996
E-mail: nursing@iupui.edu
World Wide Web: http://nursing.iupui.edu

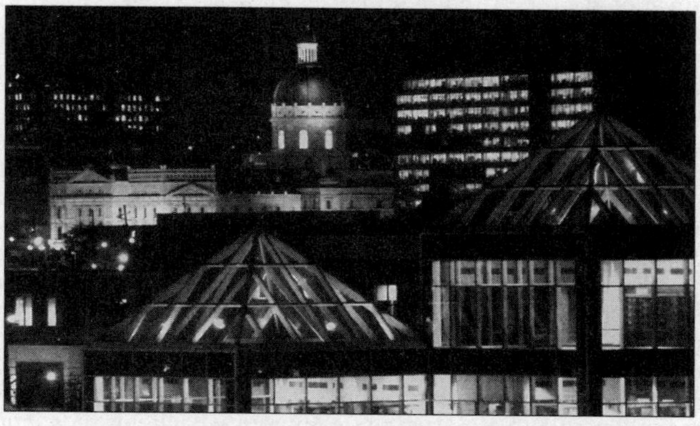

In the foreground is the IUPUI Medical Library. In the background is downtown Indianapolis.

The Johns Hopkins University
School of Nursing
Baltimore, Maryland

THE UNIVERSITY

Since its founding in 1876, Johns Hopkins University has been in the forefront of higher education. Originally established as an institution oriented toward graduate study and research, it is often called America's first true university. Today, the Johns Hopkins commitment to academic excellence continues in its eight academic divisions: Nursing, Medicine, Public Health, Arts and Science, Engineering, Continuing Studies, Advanced International Studies, and the Peabody Conservatory of Music. With a full-time enrollment of approximately 7,000 students, it is the smallest of the top-ranked universities in the United States and, by its own choice, remains small.

THE SCHOOL OF NURSING

The School of Nursing was established in 1983 by Johns Hopkins University. It is known worldwide for innovation and excellence in teaching, research, and patient care.

By choosing to attend Johns Hopkins University School of Nursing, students become leaders in the nursing profession. A Hopkins education provides a solid foundation on which to base a lifelong career in the ever-growing field of nursing. Hopkins students enjoy the advantages of an education at an institution with a worldwide reputation and an outstanding network of alumni who are willing to serve as guides and mentors. Students at the School of Nursing are given the opportunity to participate in designing an educational program tailored to their individual needs. A rigorous academic curriculum, which includes a strong scientific orientation, gives students the background to understand the health-care decisions they will make as professionals. Students learn in an atmosphere where excellence is expected, valued, and reinforced.

The School of Nursing emphasizes undergraduate research. Its graduates are prepared for professional practice through an educational process that emphasizes clinical excellence, critical thinking, and intellectual curiosity.

PROGRAMS OF STUDY

Johns Hopkins University School of Nursing prepares students for professional nursing practice through an educational process that combines a strong academic curriculum with intensive clinical experience. The program is built on the University's commitment to research, teaching, patient service, educational innovation, and excellence in clinical practice. The School's mission is to prepare its students academically and technologically for challenges of the future and to graduate professional nurses who can participate in all aspects of modern health care.

The School of Nursing offers an NLNAC-accredited upper-division baccalaureate program leading to a Bachelor of Science degree with a major in nursing. College graduates with a degree in any major other than nursing are eligible to apply to either the 13½-month accelerated program, which begins annually in June, or to the two-year traditional program, which begins in September.

The Johns Hopkins University School of Nursing has a collaborative program of study that integrates academic study at Johns Hopkins University and volunteer service in the Peace Corps. The program combines four semesters at the School of Nursing or the 13½-month accelerated program followed by Peace Corps training and two years of volunteer service. Returned Peace Corps Volunteers are eligible to participate in the Peace Corps Fellows program while enrolled in the school. This provides a unique opportunity for clinical education in community health nursing while meeting the human needs of low-income, underserved, and homeless families through preventive health services.

The School of Nursing also offers a Direct Entry to Combined B.S./M.S.N. Program. The School of Nursing offers an NLNAC-accredited master's program leading to the Master of Science in Nursing (M.S.N.) degree. The goal of the master's program is to prepare nurse experts in advanced practice and/or management for leadership in professional nursing practice and patient-centered health-care delivery. Master's study and research opportunities are available in selected clinical areas, health policy, and management of nursing and health-care services. The program broadens the perspective of students by requiring them to take innovative interdisciplinary approaches to the resolution of health-care problems. Graduates are prepared to work throughout the health-care system in both the public and private sectors, including community-based primary care, acute care, subacute care, specialty care, and integrated systems of managed care. Students planning a career path that focuses on nursing care for a specific population of patients may choose from several advanced practice nursing options. These include nurse practitioner in adult, family, or pediatric primary care; nurse practitioner in adult acute/critical care; health-systems management, clinical nurse specialist, or a combination of both management and clinical nurse specialist in a dual degree. Students may also choose a course of study leading to careers in public health nursing. Nurses with master's degrees in nursing are eligible to apply to the Post-Master's Nurse Practitioner Program, which also includes an adult, family, or pediatric focus, as well as adult acute/critical-care nurse practitioner. Other programs include a joint M.S.N./M.B.A. degree with the School of Professional Studies in Business and Education, a joint M.S.N./M.P.H. degree with the Bloomberg School of Public Health in public health nursing and public health, and a certificate program, Hopkins Business of Nursing, for mid-level career nurses, which is offered in conjunction with the School of Professional Studies in Business and Education.

The Ph.D. program prepares nurse scholars to conduct original research that advances the theoretical foundation of nursing practice and health-care delivery. The School offers Ph.D. students the combination of a strong nursing science base, a broad range of faculty expertise, and unmatched opportunities for creative interdisciplinary collaboration.

AFFILIATIONS WITH HEALTH-CARE FACILITIES

The Johns Hopkins Medical Institutions (JHMI) campus is part of a world-renowned academic health center that includes the Schools of Nursing, Medicine, and Public Health; the Johns Hopkins Hospital; and the William H. Welch Medical Library.

The Johns Hopkins Health System includes, in addition to Johns Hopkins Hospital, three other hospital campuses, one of which houses the National Institute on Aging Gerontology Center and the National Institute on Drug Abuse Addiction Research Center.

ACADEMIC FACILITIES

The William H. Welch Medical Library provides the Johns Hopkins Medical Institutions and its affiliates with information services that advance research, teaching, and patient care. The Welch Library Gateway menu leads library users to remote and local online databases, including the JHMI Online Catalog and complete MEDLINE; a dynamic array of other databases, including WelchWeb and JHMI InfoNet; and a growing number of databases and full-text journals offered by the Milton S. Eisenhower Library. The Nursing Information Resource Center is managed by the Welch Library and maintains a core collection of books to support student course work.

The Center for Nursing Research provides support services to the School of Nursing faculty members and students, such as consultation on research design and conduct, including data management and analysis; information on funding sources and grant application processes; advice on career development and continuing education and research; and other resources.

Three microcomputer, computer/interactive video laboratories are equipped with a computer network that contains seventy IBM-compatible microcomputers and laser printers.

The Nursing Research Laboratory is dedicated to research projects in nursing that incorporate basic biological science methods. The Research Laboratory consists of a dark room, microscopy facilities, tissue culture facilities, a core equipment area, an electrophysiologic lab, a vivarium, a cold room, a utility area, and bench space for research.

Three nursing practice labs are available to provide the student with an opportunity to gain experience and confidence in performing a wide variety of nursing technologies. Patient care stations in the laboratories, designed to closely approximate inpatient areas and stocked with necessary supplies, are available for students to practice both basic and advanced nursing technologies.

LOCATION

The School of Nursing is located on the campus of the Johns Hopkins Medical Institutions, including the School of Medicine, the Bloomberg School of Public Health, and the Johns Hopkins Hospital. Located 10 minutes away is the Homewood Campus of Johns Hopkins University, which is accessible to students via a free shuttle service.

STUDENT SERVICES

There are more than seventy student organizations within the University, including fraternities and sororities and social, religious, and cultural groups. Each class within the School of Nursing has a government board and a president. There is also the Student Government Association (SGA), which includes all divisions of the entire University. Each class has two representatives to the SGA, and anyone may attend the meetings.

THE NURSING STUDENT GROUP

The School of Nursing attracts a national and international student body of approximately 575 students, including undergraduate and graduate students.

COSTS

For the 2004–05 academic year, baccalaureate tuition was $22,224, and master's tuition was $24,216. For the M.S.N./M.P.H. and the Ph.D. programs, tuition was $34,884 and $29,616, respectively.

FINANCIAL AID

Johns Hopkins University School of Nursing attempts to provide financial assistance to all eligible accepted students. The School of Nursing assists those students who qualify for need-based aid. Such assistance is usually in the form of loans, grants, scholarships, and work-study programs. While most of the financial aid received by students is based on financial need, many students also benefit from awards based on academic merit and achievement.

APPLYING

The School seeks individuals who will bring to the student body the qualities of scholarship, motivation, and commitment.

A complete baccalaureate and master's application consists of an application form and a nonrefundable $75 application fee. Doctoral applicants pay an application fee of $100.

Applicants to the baccalaureate program are required to have three recommendations, official college transcripts, an official high school transcript (unless the applicant has already completed a college degree), and SAT I or ACT scores, if they are not more than five years old and the student does not already hold a bachelor's degree. A grade point average of at least 3.0 (on a 4.0 scale) is recommended. Personal interviews may be requested.

Applicants to the master's program are required to have graduated from a baccalaureate or master's degree program in nursing with a GPA of at least 3.0 (on a 4.0 scale), a current Maryland state nursing license, competitive scores on the Graduate Record Examinations (GRE), academic and professional references, and official transcripts from all previous schools attended. Personal interviews may be requested. Students interested in a Ph.D. program should contact the Office of Admissions and Student Services for individual counseling regarding entrance requirements.

International students whose native language is not English must submit official test score reports of the Test of English as a Foreign Language (TOEFL). In order to be considered for admission, nonpermanent residents must establish their ability to finance their education in the United States. International students must submit official records of all university-level course work. To be considered for transfer toward a degree, any courses listed on an international transcript must be submitted by the student to the World Education Service (WES). International RN students may have their transcripts evaluated by the Commission on Graduates of Foreign Nursing Schools (CGFNS). Students should contact the Office of Admissions and Student Services for additional information regarding WES and CGFNS.

CORRESPONDENCE AND INFORMATION

Office of Admissions and Student Services, Suite 113
School of Nursing
The Johns Hopkins University
525 North Wolfe Street
Baltimore, Maryland 21205-2110

THE DEAN

Martha N. Hill, Dean, Professor, and Director of Center for Nursing Research; Ph.D., RN, FAAN.

Anne E. Belcher, Senior Associate Dean for Academic Affairs; Ph.D., RN, FAAN.

Jerilyn Allen, Associate Dean for Research; Sc.D., RN, FAAN.

Sandra Angell, Associate Dean for Student Affairs; M.L.A., RN.

Claire Bogdanski, Associate Dean for Finance and Administration; M.B.A., CPA.

Jacquelyn Campbell, Associate Dean for Faculty Affairs; Ph.D., RN.

Deborah Wells, Associate Dean for Development and Alumni Relations; B.S.

Kennesaw State University
WellStar School of Nursing
Kennesaw, Georgia

THE UNIVERSITY

Kennesaw State University (KSU) is a public university in the University System of Georgia that is located in northwest greater metropolitan Atlanta. Chartered in 1963, KSU serves as a rich resource for the region's educational, economic, social, and cultural advancement, offering baccalaureate and professional master's degrees to its 17,000 students in the arts, humanities, sciences, and professional fields of business, social services, and nursing.

KSU offers a high-quality teaching/learning environment that sustains instructional excellence, serves a diverse student body, and promotes high levels of student achievement. It educates the whole person through a supportive campus climate, necessary services, and leadership development opportunities and promotes cultural, ethnic, racial, and gender diversity by practices and programs that embody the ideals of an open, democratic, and global society.

THE SCHOOL OF NURSING

Nursing at KSU began as an associate degree program in 1968. The Baccalaureate Degree Nursing Program was added in 1985 and included a generic baccalaureate degree option and an RN-B.S.N. completion program. In 1995, the associate degree program was discontinued and an M.S.N. program, to prepare primary-care nurse practitioners, accepted its first class. Both programs were merged into WellStar School of Nursing in 2001. All the baccalaureate nursing programs and the M.S.N. program are accredited by the Commission on Collegiate Nursing Education.

PROGRAMS OF STUDY

KSU offers baccalaureate and master's degree programs in nursing. The baccalaureate nursing program offers a generic B.S.N. program, an accelerated program for students with degrees in other fields, and an online B.S.N. completion option for registered nurses. The curriculum includes courses in the humanities and the biological and social sciences as well as the theoretical and clinical practice background necessary for the practice of professional nursing. Generic students are admitted twice annually to maintain smaller classes.

The B.S.N. accelerated track for degreed applicants is an intensive accelerated program for students who hold degrees in other disciplines from an accredited institution. The sixteen-month-program provides an excellent career migration for those with B.A.'s or B.S.'s from a variety of fields, particularly psychology, biology, the social sciences, and the humanities. The curriculum includes both theoretical and clinical nursing classes. Accelerated program students are admitted each year in August (fall semester) only and as full-time students. The B.S.N. accelerated track is offered at a satellite campus in Rome, Georgia, at the Floyd College campus.

The B.S.N. completion option for registered nurses is based on the statewide articulation plan formulated by nursing programs in the state of Georgia. Upon completion of a bridge course, registered nurse students receive credit for 24 semester hours of sophomore- and junior-level nursing courses and may enter the senior-level courses. This program admits students once a year and includes online, Web-based courses to provide flexible options for the working nurse. Emphasis at the senior level is on community and family nursing, career development, and professional growth. Clinicals are individually tailored to meet students' needs.

There are two M.S.N. programs. WellStar Primary-Care Nurse Practitioner Program prepares experienced registered nurses as primary-care nurse practitioners who are eligible for national certification as family or adult nurse practitioners. The M.S.N. in advanced care management and leadership is designed to provide experienced registered nurses with advanced preparation in clinical management and leadership with the option of preparing for certification as a CNS. Both programs are designed for working professional nurses, with all classes scheduled on alternate weekends. Students are admitted to the primary-care nurse practitioner program once a year in the fall.

AFFILIATIONS WITH HEALTH-CARE FACILITIES

WellStar School of Nursing has affiliations with more than sixty health and community agencies in the metropolitan Atlanta area and northwest Georgia. Two of the major reasons cited by students for choosing KSU are location and access to experience in both the major acute-care facilities in Atlanta and a tremendous diversity of other community-based health and social agencies.

The primary-care nurse practitioner program collaborates with more than 150 nurse practitioners, physicians, and physician assistants in a variety of primary-care settings. These professionals serve as clinical preceptors for the nurse practitioner students.

ACADEMIC FACILITIES

WellStar School of Nursing is located on the main campus of KSU. Modern classrooms, faculty offices, conference rooms, study areas, a learning resource center, a campus health center, and computer facilities are all located in the same building. The KSU library is housed in a 100,000-square-foot building and is networked with online computer databases and document retrieval facilities. Students have access to library resources, e-mail, and the Internet both on campus and from home computers. WellStar School of Nursing has a goal of increasing the use of technology in the classroom and has invested in many computer learning resources that are available to students.

LOCATION

Nestled in the hills just 20 miles north of metropolitan Atlanta, KSU is easily accessible to its 16,000 students. The 182-acre campus is memorable for its beautiful grounds, oak-lined streets, manicured lawns, and colorful flower beds. The University offers a diverse array of cultural enrichment opportunities for the community, including concerts, recitals, art exhibitions, plays, and lectures. It has NCAA national baseball, basketball, and softball championships. Its proximity to Atlanta offers a vast field of cultural and recreational opportunities, from theater productions and major art exhibits to professional football, basketball, baseball, and soccer.

STUDENT SERVICES

KSU encourages student involvement through more than forty campus activities, social fraternities and sororities, student government, student publications, and intramural and leisure programs. Support services include career planning and placement, personal counseling, financial aid, an Advisement

Center, a Wellness Center, and a special Lifelong Learning Center that caters to the nontraditional-age student. There are a limited child-care facility, a well-equipped gym, a campus health center, and a Student Development Center, which concentrates support services for minority, international, and special needs students.

THE NURSING STUDENT GROUP

KSU is a nontraditional, commuter university serving a diverse student body. There are more than 400 students enrolled in the undergraduate and graduate nursing programs. Generic students tend to be slightly older than traditional college-age students, with an average age of 27 years and a range of 20 to 54 years. RN-B.S.N. students average 35 years of age, with a range of 25 to 47 years. Approximately 10 percent of the students are male, and approximately 20 percent have a previous degree in another field. KSU has a growing population of international and historically underrepresented students.

Students in the master's program are professional nurses with a minimum of three years of experience. They work in a variety of settings scattered over the geographic region of northwest Georgia and the metropolitan Atlanta area.

COSTS

Tuition for full-time undergraduate students who are Georgia residents is approximately $1161 per semester (based on a two-semester year). Graduate student tuition is slightly higher. Nonresident fees for out-of-state students are an estimated $4645 per semester. On-campus housing is available. Additional university fees for student activities, parking, and technology cost $300 per semester. Special nursing expenses include an initial $150 to $200 required for the purchase of uniforms, a suitable watch, a stethoscope, and other supplies; a $305 testing fee is charged initially upon admission to the program; a $35 lab fee is charged for each required clinical nursing course per semester; and malpractice insurance coverage fees are charged every semester.

FINANCIAL AID

The University financial assistance program provides need-based, scholastic, and athletic scholarships. The Office of Student Financial Aid processes need-based scholarships and grants, government-guaranteed loans, and work-study programs. Co-op programs and Army and Air Force ROTC also help defray costs. In addition, KSU participates in the HOPE program for superior students. Nursing students are also eligible for Service Cancellable Loans and various targeted scholarships.

APPLYING

All B.S.N. applicants must have full admittance to the University, which requires an official transcript from high school and SAT I or ACT scores and/or official transcripts from each university attended, along with a $20 application fee.

Applications are taken during the fall and spring semester for acceptance into the following spring or fall generic B.S.N. class. Completion of seven of the twelve prerequisites with a grade point average of at least 2.7 is the minimum requirement for admission. Admission is competitive.

The B.S.N. accelerated track for degreed applicants is highly competitive. Since there are a limited number of spaces in the program, students must submit applications between June 1 and December 15 to be considered for fall semester admission to the classes beginning the next calendar year. Because of the program's accelerated pace, it is most advantageous for the student to discuss goals, timeline, and outside commitments with the nursing admissions coordinator to determine if the program is right for the student and to review specific admission requirements to the accelerated program, which include the completion of twelve prerequisites, a cumulative grade point average of 2.7 or better, and a professional letter of reference.

Registered nurses are admitted during the spring semester to begin the one-year completion program in summer. Students must complete fifteen prerequisite courses with a minimum grade point average of 2.7 and include a letter of reference for consideration.

Applications to the M.S.N. WellStar Primary-Care Nurse Practitioner Program must have a baccalaureate degree in nursing from an accredited institution, with a GPA of at least 3.0; a minimum of three years' full-time professional experience within the last five years involving direct patient care, documented in a professional resume; a current RN license in the state of Georgia; an acceptable score on the GRE; a statement of personal goals for the program; an undergraduate physical-assessment course; an undergraduate research course; and full admission into KSU.

CORRESPONDENCE AND INFORMATION

Fran Paul
Advising Coordinator
WellStar School of Nursing
Kennesaw State University
1000 Chastain Road, #1601
Kennesaw, Georgia 30144-5519
Telephone: 770-499-3211
770-423-6061
Fax: 770-423-6627
World Wide Web: http://www.kennesaw.edu/chhs/schoolofnursing/

Kent State University
College of Nursing
Kent, Ohio

THE UNIVERSITY

Founded in 1910, Kent State University is today ranked among the Doctoral/Research Universities–Extensive by the Carnegie Foundation and is the second-largest of Ohio's public universities. The eight-campus system throughout northeastern Ohio enrolls nearly 34,000 students. The Kent campus offers baccalaureate, master's, and doctoral study in the Colleges of Arts and Science, Business Administration, Communication and Information, Education, Fine and Professional Arts, and Nursing and the School of Technology. At the seven regional campuses, associate degrees in technical, business, and health fields are offered as well as lower-division baccalaureate study.

The University's primary concern is the student. There is a commitment to providing the academic atmosphere and curricular and extracurricular activities that stimulate curiosity, broaden perspective, enrich awareness, deepen understanding, establish disciplined habits of thought, prepare for a vocation, and help realize potential as an individual and as a responsible and informed citizen.

THE COLLEGE OF NURSING

The Kent State University College of Nursing, established in 1967, offers the most comprehensive program of study in nursing in Ohio, ranks in the 98th percentile in size in the nation, and enjoys a reputation for excellent academic performance, clinical knowledge, and leadership ability of its students and graduates. The associate degree in nursing (ADN) program is accredited by the National League for Nursing Accrediting Commission. The B.S.N. and M.S.N. programs are accredited by the Commission on Collegiate Nursing Education.

Since its founding, nursing at Kent State University has enjoyed continued growth, and today it is the largest college of nursing in Ohio. The mission of Kent State University College of Nursing reflects a commitment to furthering nursing knowledge, to excellence in instruction, and to preparing graduates who are able to address changing societal needs. There exists an academic atmosphere that fosters intellectual curiosity, develops professional and personal values, and facilitates the acquisition, interpretation, utilization, and expansion of nursing knowledge for the discipline and for professional practice.

Kent's faculty, skilled in the scholarship of teaching, discovery, application, and integration, fosters the intellectual life of the University. The College of Nursing's faculty members, who number more than 85, are active, creative contributors to the advancement of nursing knowledge and to the improvement of health-care delivery through teaching, research, and service activities at the local, regional, national, and international levels. The nursing faculty is composed of scholars, researchers, and those with strong clinical skills. Currently, 85 percent of the regular, full-time faculty members are doctorally prepared, and 4 are Fellows in the American Academy of Nursing. Teaching excellence and scholarly pursuits are hallmarks of the College of Nursing faculty.

PROGRAMS OF STUDY

The College of Nursing offers associate, baccalaureate, master's, and Ph.D. degree programs in nursing. The baccalaureate degree program accommodates generic as well as second-degree, licensed practical nurse, and registered nurse students. All nursing courses for RN students are offered in a Web-based format, distributed learning technologies are used for all senior-level courses in the B.S.N. program, and there is an accelerated option for second-degree students. The master's degree nursing program offers clinical concentrations in nursing of adults, including gerontology, psychiatric–mental health nursing, and parent-child nursing as well as functional concentrations in nurse practitioner clinical specialization and administration. Post-master's nurse practitioner certificate programs are also available in acute, family, and primary care as well as women's health, pediatrics, and psychiatric–mental health nursing. A Web-based certificate program in nursing education is also offered. In addition, dual-degree M.S.N./M.P.A. and M.S.N./M.B.A. options, as well as an interdisciplinary gerontology concentration, are available. There is also a Ph.D. in nursing program.

An associate degree in nursing program is offered on three regional campuses (Ashtabula, East Liverpool, and Tuscarawas). The associate degree program prepares practitioners to assume responsibility for the provision of technical nursing care.

The baccalaureate nursing program is an undergraduate program leading to the Bachelor of Science in Nursing degree. The curriculum includes courses in the humanities and biological and social sciences as well as theoretical knowledge and clinical practice in the discipline of nursing. Both generic students and nontraditional students (second-degree, RNs, and LPNs) are admitted to the program. There are currently more than 1,000 students enrolled in the baccalaureate program. The first two years of the baccalaureate program are available on several of the regional campuses; select upper-division courses and all course requirements for RN students to complete the B.S.N. are available at regional campuses. An accelerated program is available for students who hold a degree in another field.

The master's program is an accelerated graduate program leading to a Master of Science in Nursing degree. The purpose of this program is to prepare specialists for leadership and advanced practice roles in professional nursing. Enrollment in the master's program is more than 200, with approximately 65 percent of these students pursuing graduate study on a part-time basis.

The purpose of the Doctor of Philosophy (Ph.D.) degree program is to develop scholars in nursing who are informed about the many dimensions of scholarship, with balance, and synthesis among research, practice, and teaching. This program is conducted in collaboration with the University of Akron College of Nursing and rests on the belief that strength can be achieved through strong linkages among faculty members and students and among the diverse units of both universities. The program consists of five components: nursing knowledge; research methods, designs, and statistics; cognates; health-care and nursing policy; and the dissertation. Full- and part-time students are accommodated in this program.

A program of continuing nursing education is also offered. The College of Nursing is an Ohio Nurses Association–approved provider of continuing education and awards continuing education units (CEUs) for program offerings.

AFFILIATIONS WITH HEALTH-CARE FACILITIES

The College of Nursing has established affiliations with more than seventy-five health agencies throughout northeastern Ohio for clinical learning experiences. These range from large urban medical centers, including The Cleveland Clinic Foundation and University Hospitals of Cleveland, to small rural hospitals and clinics as well as a variety of long-term and community health-care agencies.

ACADEMIC FACILITIES

The College of Nursing is located in Henderson Hall, a building designed specifically to house the nursing programs. It contains classrooms, faculty offices, conference rooms, study areas, nursing multipurpose and computer laboratories, a learning resource center, a nursing research center, and a 250-seat auditorium. In addition, the excellent services and resources of the entire Kent State University are available. The twelve-story open-stack library is a member of the Association of Research Libraries and holds more than 1.5 million volumes, including an extensive collection of nursing and medical references. The basic science complex of Northeastern Ohio Universities College of Medicine is located 6 miles from the Kent campus and is an integral part of Kent State.

LOCATION

Located in Kent, Ohio (population approximately 30,000), the Kent campus is situated on a beautiful 2,264-acre tree-covered area. Close by are the metropolitan areas of Cleveland (35 miles), Akron (15 miles), Canton (35 miles), and Youngstown (35 miles). The seven regional campuses are located in communities 35–80 miles from the Kent campus. The most populous of Ohio's four quadrants, northeastern Ohio is an area rich with cultural and recreational activities. Among these are Kent's Porthouse Theatre and Blossom Music Center, summer home of the Cleveland Orchestra.

STUDENT SERVICES

A comprehensive array of student services are available through the College of Nursing Office of Student Affairs and the University's Michael Schwartz Student Service Center. In addition to academic services, health services, counseling and guidance, career planning and placement, financial aid, residential service, recreation, and student activities programming are provided. There are more than 200 undergraduate and graduate student organizations on campus that welcome members from throughout the University. Opportunities for participation in a variety of intercollegiate sports also exist.

THE NURSING STUDENT GROUP

Kent serves a talented, culturally rich student body from Ohio and around the world, including historically underrepresented and nontraditional students. Students in nursing reflect a microcosm of the University student body.

Students for Professional Nursing (SPN) is a very active student organization that provides opportunity for development of leadership skills, promoting health-care activities on campus, and facilitating socialization into the professional role. In addition, there is a chapter of the Ohio Nursing Students Association (ONSA) at Kent. Graduate students can take an active role in the University Graduate Student Senate and the Graduate Nurse Student Organization (GNSO).

COSTS

Kent State's tuition is set by the Board of Trustees. For current tuition information, students should visit the Bursar's Office's Web site (http://www.kent.edu/bursar).

FINANCIAL AID

Kent State University has developed a financial aid program to assist students who lack the necessary funds for a college education. This program consists of scholarships, loans, grants-in-aid, and part-time employment. In addition to the regular University financial aid, nursing students are eligible for financial assistance that is exclusively for nursing students and includes federal, armed services, and hospital tuition assistance. The College of Nursing also has a short-term emergency loan fund for nursing expenses. Registered nurses may find additional financial assistance through the clinical agencies with whom they are employed. Federal traineeships, graduate assistantships, scholarships, and special awards, such as the Ohio Board of Regents Scholars program, are additional sources of financial assistance for graduate students.

APPLYING

Applicants to the B.S.N. program need to submit a completed Kent State University application; a high school transcript; ACT or SAT scores (for students under 21 years of age); an official transcript from each college, university, or school attended; and a $30 application fee.

Students completing prenursing requirements with a GPA of 2.5 or higher and a 2.5 average or higher in the first-year science courses make application to the nursing sequence, which begins in the second year of the program. Registered nurses and persons holding a non-nursing degree are admitted directly to the College of Nursing.

Applicants to the master's program must have current Ohio licensure as a registered nurse, have a baccalaureate degree in upper-division nursing with supervised clinical practice from an accredited program, achieve a grade point average of at least 3.0 on a 4.0 scale from the undergraduate program, and have completed an elementary course in research methodology. In addition to an application form, $30 application fee, and official transcript, prospective students are asked to submit three letters of reference and an essay not exceeding 300 words describing previous education and experience, future professional goals, and reasons for seeking graduate nursing education. A satisfactory score on the Graduate Record Examinations is required for applicants with a GPA below 3.0. A preadmission interview is recommended.

Admission to the Joint Ph.D. in Nursing Program (JPDN) is determined by a review committee of JPDN faculty members. Each applicant must provide evidence of successful completion of a master's degree in nursing at an accredited program with a minimum grade point average of 3.0 on a 4.0 scale; evidence of current licensure or eligibility for licensure by the Ohio Board of Nursing; official reports of scores on the Graduate Record Examinations; a clear and succinct statement of the applicant's clearly defined career goals; a sample of written work that indicates logic and writing skills (an essay, term paper, thesis, published article, or professional report); and three letters of reference from professionals or professors who can adequately evaluate the applicant and the applicant's previous work and potential for success. Applicants must also complete a personal interview with a graduate faculty member to assess research interests and motivation for successful completion of doctoral study. Accepted applicants must register for courses within two years of acceptance into the JPDN.

CORRESPONDENCE AND INFORMATION

Student Affairs
College of Nursing
Henderson Hall
Kent State University
P.O. Box 5190
Kent, Ohio 44242-0001
Telephone: 330-672-7930
Fax: 330-672-2433
World Wide Web: http://www.kent.edu/nursing

Loma Linda University
School of Nursing
Loma Linda, California

THE UNIVERSITY

Loma Linda University is a Seventh-day Adventist educational health sciences institution located in southern California. More than 3,000 students are enrolled in Loma Linda University's eight schools. The Schools of Allied Health Professions, Dentistry, Medicine, Nursing, Pharmacy, Public Health, and Science and Technology and the Graduate School offer more than fifty-five programs.

The University is dedicated to promoting physical, intellectual, social, and spiritual growth in its faculty members and students and to transforming their daily activities into personal ministries. The University's mission, "To continue the healing and teaching ministry of Jesus Christ, to make man whole," describes the essence of what it stands for.

THE SCHOOL OF NURSING

The School of Nursing, established in 1905, has California Board of Registered Nursing approval and is accredited by the Commission on Collegiate Nursing Education until 2009.

The faculty members in the School of Nursing are known for their commitment to mentoring students and providing a rich learning environment. The School believes that one-on-one interaction between faculty members and students is the essence of study. Thus, its programs are orchestrated to consider individual needs and professional goals. Along with their focus on teaching, many of the faculty members maintain individual research programs with ongoing externally funded projects that provide opportunities for student involvement. They demonstrate both Christian values and competence in their scholarship and professions.

PROGRAMS OF STUDY

Loma Linda University School of Nursing offers students many choices in pursuing their nursing education. Three degree programs are offered through the School: the Bachelor of Science (B.S.), the Master of Science (M.S.), and the Doctor of Philosophy in nursing (Ph.D.).

The B.S. degree prepares students for professional nursing practice in acute and community settings. It may be completed in eight quarters after the initial year of prerequisites. Students may sit for boards after completing five to six quarters in this program and receive the A.S. degree. Advanced placement is available for LVNs, RNs, and students with baccalaureate degrees in other fields. Students with a baccalaureate degree in another field of study may complete the certificate in nursing in five quarters and enter Loma Linda University's M.S. program.

The A.S. to M.S. option is designed for the RN with current work experience (a minimum of three years) whose goal is the M.S. in nursing. The A.S. to M.S. option allows the student to enroll in up to 8 units of graduate-level core nursing courses that will apply towards the B.S. degree in nursing.

The M.S. degree program is designed to engage students in scientific inquiry and to apply their discoveries in a variety of clinical, teaching, and administrative settings. Graduate students may select a focus in advanced practice nursing as a nurse practitioner or clinical nurse specialist, in nursing administration, or in a combined-degree program. Post-master's certificate programs are also available through the graduate program in nursing. Upon completion of the M.S. degree, graduates are eligible for the appropriately related certification by the American Nurses Association and by the California Board of Registered Nursing.

The Ph.D. degree in nursing is designed to prepare nurse scholars for leadership in education, health-care administration, clinical practice, and research. It is expected that a doctorally prepared nurse scientist will be committed to the generation of knowledge critical to development of nursing science and practice.

ACADEMIC FACILITIES

The academic resources and the clinical facilities of the University constitute a rich environment for the nursing student, both in classroom instruction and in clinical experience. The University Medical Center and other hospitals and community agencies are used for student clinical experience.

LOCATION

Loma Linda University is centrally located in beautiful, sunny southern California. It is approximately 60 miles east of Los Angeles and is located in an enviable geographic location, offering the best of both urban and rural settings. Students can snow ski at Big Bear, enjoy outdoor recreation in the desert, go surfing at the beach, or experience the arts of Los Angeles.

STUDENT SERVICES

The University offers students a variety of services, including free access to Drayson Center, its 100,000-square-foot, state-of-the-art fitness/wellness facility. There is also a Student Association that represents the unified efforts of the student body to bring together, in purpose and activities, students from all programs and schools on the campus. Loma Linda University is also very involved in local as well as international outreach activities. International students receive guidance and assistance from the Office of International Student Services. Loma Linda University is committed to whole-person student development.

THE NURSING STUDENT GROUP

The School's primary responsibility is the education of students, who come from diverse ethnic and cultural backgrounds, enabling them to acquire the foundation of knowledge, skills, values, attitudes, and behaviors appropriate for their chosen academic or health-care ministry. A personal Christian faith that permeates the lives of the students is encouraged. Loma Linda University School of Nursing has a low student-faculty ratio, which ensures that nursing students receive personal attention from their professors. Graduates from the School are in high demand and are employed in large medical centers, community health centers, primary-care facilities, and small community hospitals.

COSTS

Tuition for the 2004–05 school year was $465 per credit unit. Tuition and fees vary according to degree level and program.

In addition to on-campus dormitories, there are a number of apartments within walking distance of the University. The Office of Student Affairs maintains information on local housing on their Web site at http://www.llu.edu/llu/housing. The surrounding cities of Redlands, Grand Terrace, and San Bernardino also have a number of apartments and condominiums.

FINANCIAL AID

Loma Linda University offers financial aid programs for eligible students with documented needs. A financial aid adviser is dedicated to assisting students with financial aid planning and debt-management counseling. In addition to tuition, a student should budget for room and board for a nine-month period if on-campus residence is desired. Books, uniforms, and other supplies must also be considered. Students who think they will be in need of financial assistance should apply early. Information is available from the LLU Student Financial Aid Office at 909-558-4509.

APPLYING

For the undergraduate program, new students are accepted for the fall, winter, and spring quarters. Applications can be found on the University's Web site (http://www.llu.edu). Students must have completed the nursing prerequisites with a GPA of 3.0 or better, schedule a personal interview with the admissions director, and take a nurse entrance exam.

For the M.S. program, students must have a B.S. degree and an undergraduate GPA of at least 3.0 and participate in an interview; the GRE is not required but recommended. A current California RN license is required for enrollment in clinical nursing courses. Nursing experience in the area of the desired clinical option is preferred before beginning graduate study.

For the Ph.D. program, students must possess a master's degree in nursing with a minimum 3.5 GPA at that level, have taken the GRE within the last five years and received satisfactory scores, participate in a personal interview, and show evidence of scholarly work.

CORRESPONDENCE AND INFORMATION

For the bachelor's degree:
Office of Admissions
School of Nursing
Loma Linda University
Loma Linda, California 92350
Telephone: 909-558-4923
800-422-4558 (toll-free)
E-mail: admissions_sn@sn.llu.edu
World Wide Web: http://www.llu.edu/llu/nursing

For the graduate degrees:
Office of Admissions
Graduate School
Loma Linda University
Loma Linda, California 92350
Telephone: 909-558-4529
800-422-4558 (toll-free)
E-mail: jbates@sn.llu.edu
World Wide Web: http://www.llu.edu/llu/grad/

Long Island University, Brooklyn Campus
School of Nursing
Brooklyn, New York

THE UNIVERSITY AND THE CAMPUS

Celebrating seventy-six years of access to the American dream through excellence in higher education, Long Island University is the nation's seventh-largest private university. The University offers 563 undergraduate, graduate, and doctoral-level degree programs and certificates. Nearly 700 full-time faculty members educate more than 31,000 students on six metropolitan-area campuses in Brooklyn, Brookville (C. W. Post), Southampton, Brentwood, Rockland, and Westchester, and at six overseas sites. The Arnold & Marie Schwartz College of Pharmacy and Health Sciences prepares students for successful careers in pharmacy and health care. The accomplishments of more than 116,000 living alumni testify to the success of the University's mission—to provide the highest level of education to people from all walks of life.

With more than 11,000 students and 250 certificate and undergraduate and graduate degree programs in the arts and media, the natural sciences, business, social policy, urban education, the health professions, and pharmacy, the Brooklyn Campus is distinguished by dynamic curricula reflecting the great urban community it serves. Students enjoy the benefits of living and learning in a multicultural environment that promotes growth and a progressive exchange of knowledge and ideas.

THE SCHOOL OF NURSING

The School of Nursing is exceptionally well positioned to fill the need for nursing professionals in the growing areas of health promotion; home care of the acutely, long-term, and chronically ill; and community health. The School offers the B.S. in nursing and an RN/B.S. Connection Program as well as the M.S. for adult nurse practitioners, family nurse practitioners, and geriatric nurse practitioners; the M.S. in Nursing: Executive Program for Nursing and Health Care Management, an advanced certificate for adult nurse practitioners, family nurse practitioners, and geriatric nurse practitioners; a B.S./M.S. Accelerated Program in Nursing/Executive Program for Nursing and Health Care Management; and a B.S./M.S. Accelerated Program for Nursing/Adult Nurse Practitioners. Graduates of the bachelor's program are eligible to take the examination for licensure of registered professional nurses in New York State. Registered professional nurses who have earned a diploma or associate degree at other institutions may apply credits toward completion of the Bachelor of Science degree through the RN/B.S. Connection Program.

PROGRAMS OF STUDY

The program leading to the B.S. in nursing is accredited by the Commission on Collegiate Nursing Education. It is designed to prepare students who are beginning nursing studies to develop the competencies essential for professional nursing practice, sit for the state licensure examination for registered nurses, and build a foundation for graduate study. The program's proximity to Manhattan creates the opportunity for clinical experiences in some of the world's most prestigious hospitals and health-care agencies. Candidates must successfully complete 128 credits, including 4 credits in non-core freshman courses; 36 credits in the humanities, social sciences, and sciences and mathematics; 62 credits in nursing requirements; 7 credits in distribution; and 19 credits in ancillary requirements. Graduates are able to incorporate knowledge synthesized from the nursing, humanities, psychosocial, and biophysical curriculum into all aspects of professional nursing practice; use critical thinking, communication, and therapeutic intervention skills; embody the characteristics of humanism and caring in the practice of nursing; facilitate adaptive responses of individuals and families within the community in the promotion, maintenance, and restoration of health; and assume leadership roles in structured and unstructured health-care settings. The program is also available to registered nurses seeking the baccalaureate degree through the RN/B.S. Connection Program. Registered nurses admitted into the program may receive up to 64 transfer credits, including required core curriculum, prerequisite, and distribution credits. Transferred credits may also include up to 31 credits in nursing courses for work previously completed. Flexible course schedules are available for the working professional.

The M.S. for adult nurse practitioners, M.S. for family nurse practitioners, and M.S. for geriatric nurse practitioners are designed to prepare advanced practice nurses in primary-care roles for adult and family populations. Clinical expertise is stressed, resulting in the graduate's ability to assess, diagnose, monitor, coordinate, and manage the health care of their clients in both primary- and acute-care settings; perform and interpret physical examinations and laboratory tests; select and prescribe appropriate drug therapy for common acute and chronic child and adult disorders; and articulate the role of the nurse practitioner as a collaborative member of the health team. Candidates for the degree must successfully complete 43 credits of theory, equivalent to 495 hours, and clinical laboratory work of 600 hours for the adult and geriatric programs and 49 credits and 900 clinical hours for the family nurse practitioner program.

An advanced certificate for adult nurse practitioners is also available to nurses who have earned a master's degree in nursing and are seeking clinical expertise in the advanced practice role for the care of adult clients. Candidates must successfully complete 35 credits of theory, equivalent to 360 hours, in addition to clinical laboratory work of 600 hours for the adult and geriatric programs and 41 credits and 900 clinical hours for the family nurse practitioner program.

The M.S. in Nursing: Executive Program for Nursing and Health Care Management provides a unique opportunity to educate the nurse executive with needed skills for today's complex health-care environment. The program combines both nursing and business courses, fulfilling the growing need for executive nurses who are responsible for multimillion-dollar budgets, cost-benefit analyses, reduction of overtime expenses, and staff. Graduates are prepared to assume leadership positions in hospitals, nursing homes, community health centers, HMOs, home-care agencies, consulting firms, and entrepreneurial ventures. Candidates must successfully complete 43 credits, including two semesters of internship experience in management of a nursing or health-care organization. The graduate programs are accredited by the Commission on Collegiate Nursing Education (CCNE).

AFFILIATIONS WITH HEALTH-CARE FACILITIES

Due to the campus's proximity to Manhattan, students often have the opportunity to learn through clinical experiences and after graduation obtain jobs in some of the top hospitals and health-care facilities in the world. The School's affiliates encompass a wide range of clinical health-care settings, including acute-care and community agencies and prestigious hospitals, such as Beth Israel Medical Center, Montefiore Medical Center, New York Methodist Hospital, Maimonides Medical Center, and St. Luke's–Roosevelt Hospital Center.

ACADEMIC FACILITIES

The campus has invested more than $40 million to construct and renovate buildings and academic facilities. The William Zeckendorf Health Sciences Center houses state-of-the-art classrooms and labs for students in nursing, pharmacy, and the health professions. Ten academic computing laboratories offer user-friendly environments to work on homework assignments, research, and class projects. Dorm rooms are wired for computers and Internet access. The Salena Library Learning Center provides access to more than 2.8 million library volumes University-wide as well as its own substantial collection of books, periodicals, microfilms, and recordings.

LOCATION

The 11-acre Brooklyn Campus is located in the heart of downtown Brooklyn, only minutes from Manhattan. Some of Brooklyn's richest cultural and historic attractions are within walking distance, including the Brooklyn Academy of Music, known for its innovative drama, music, and dance productions; the Brooklyn Heights Promenade, featuring world-famous panoramic views of the Manhattan skyline; the Brooklyn Bridge; and the Statue of Liberty. The campus is surrounded by neighborhoods the New York City Landmarks Preservation Commission recognizes as historic districts. Close to the campus are the Brooklyn Museum, Prospect Park, and the Brooklyn Botanic Garden.

STUDENT SERVICES

On any given day, students can participate in more than sixty on-campus clubs and organizations. Nursing students can also join the Nursing Association. The campus Frosh Center offers incoming students a support network that includes academic advising, financial aid service, counseling, tutoring, and computer-assisted instruction.

THE NURSING STUDENT GROUP

The undergraduate student body pursuing the B.S. in nursing is composed of students just beginning their nursing studies and practicing registered nurses who seek the baccalaureate degree. Upon completion of all requirements, these students are eligible to take the state licensure examination for registered professional nurses. The graduate student body pursuing the M.S. in nursing is composed of students preparing to become advanced practice nurses in primary-care roles. RN/B.S. students are normally registered nurses who already hold registered nurse licensure and are interested in earning the B.S. in nursing. Candidates for the M.S. in Nursing: Executive Program for Nursing and Health Care Management are nursing professionals interested in pursuing careers as nurse executives and administrators. The advanced certificate for adult nurse practitioners is available to nurses who have earned a master's degree and are seeking clinical expertise in the advanced practice role for the care of adult clients.

COSTS

Brooklyn Campus undergraduate tuition rates for 2004–05 were $651 per credit. Graduate tuition was $705 per credit. These rates do not include University fees of approximately $550 for student activities and specific programs or miscellaneous costs such as books, supplies, and personal expenses. On-campus room and board charges averaged $3140 per semester.

FINANCIAL AID

Ninety-three percent of undergraduate students attending the Brooklyn Campus receive financial aid to help meet college expenses. Parental contributions, government aid programs, Long Island University Scholarships, student earnings, loans, and scholarships from outside sources are all considered by the financial aid office when formulating a student's aid package. Full, partial, and transfer academic scholarships, Dean's Awards, and activity awards are available if the student qualifies. Complete details about all of these options are included in the Brooklyn Campus financial aid information publication, which is available through the admissions office. TAP and Pell grants are also available to those who qualify.

APPLYING

Before beginning the professional phase of the B.S. in nursing program, students must satisfy all proficiency requirements, complete all prerequisite courses, obtain a grade of 9.0 or above on the Nelson-Denny Reading Test, and have a minimum grade point average (GPA) of 2.5. In addition, a personal interview may be required. Prior to entry into the first nursing course, students are responsible for obtaining certification in cardiopulmonary resuscitation (CPR).

An application for admission; an official high school transcript, evidence of graduation from high school, or GED scores; SAT I or ACT test results; and a $30 application fee must be submitted to be considered for undergraduate admission. Transfer applicants must submit a completed transfer application form, an official transcript from all colleges previously attended, a $30 application fee, and financial aid records from all colleges previously attended.

To qualify for admission into the RN/B.S. Connection Program, registered nurses must possess a current RN license, be a graduate from an accredited nursing program, demonstrate evidence of clinical competency, and have at least a 2.5 cumulative grade point average from previous academic studies.

Acceptance requirements for the M.S. for nurse practitioners include a B.S. degree from a CCNE- or NLNAC-accredited school of nursing, with a minimum 3.0 GPA in the nursing major and at least a 2.5 overall GPA; a New York State RN license; two years of recent clinical experience or the equivalent; three professional references; and a personal interview. Research, statistics, and health-assessment courses or certificate are also a prerequisite but may be completed during the first year of graduate work. Registered nurses with non-nursing baccalaureate degrees may be able to qualify for entrance to the graduate program by validation of knowledge through required tests.

Acceptance requirements for the advanced certificate program include an M.S. from a CCNE- or NLNAC-accredited school of nursing with a minimum 3.0 GPA, a New York State RN license, two years of recent clinical experience or equivalent, three professional references, and a personal interview.

Acceptance requirements for the M.S. in Nursing: Executive Program for Nursing and Health Care Management include a B.S. degree from an NLNAC-accredited school of nursing, with a minimum 3.0 GPA in the nursing major and at least a 2.5 overall GPA; a New York State RN license; two years of recent clinical experience or the equivalent; three professional references; a personal interview; and research and statistics prerequisites, which may be completed during the first year of graduate work.

CORRESPONDENCE AND INFORMATION:

Kristin Cohen, Dean of Admissions
Office of Admissions
Long Island University, Brooklyn Campus
1 University Plaza
Brooklyn, New York 11201-5372
Telephone: 718-488-1011
Fax: 718-797-2399
E-mail: alan.chaves@liu.edu
World Wide Web: http://www.liu.edu

Dawn F. Kilts, Dean
School of Nursing, Room 401
Zeckendorf Health Sciences Center
Long Island University, Brooklyn Campus
1 University Plaza
Brooklyn, New York 11201-5372
Telephone: 718-488-1059
Fax: 718-780-4019
E-mail: dawn.kilts@liu.edu

Luther College
Department of Nursing
Decorah, Iowa

THE COLLEGE

Luther College, founded in 1861, is a four-year, residential liberal arts college of the Evangelical Lutheran Church in America. The College, which was founded by Norwegian immigrants, is an academic community of faith and learning where students of promise from all beliefs and backgrounds have the freedom to learn, to express themselves, to perform, to compete, and to grow. The College, located in Decorah, Iowa, is home to 2,575 students from thirty-four states and twenty-eight countries around the world. Thirty-five percent of the students are from the state of Iowa; 89 percent come from the four-state area of Iowa, Minnesota, Wisconsin, and Illinois. Each year, approximately 80 to 100 international students (3 percent of the student body) choose to study at Luther. The College offers more than sixty majors and preprofessional programs leading to the Bachelor of Arts degree.

THE DEPARTMENT OF NURSING

The goals of Luther's nursing program are to prepare nurses to function autonomously and interdependently with individuals, families, groups, and communities to promote, maintain, and restore optimal health in a variety of health-care settings. The nursing major, therefore, offers an integrated program of liberal arts and fourteen professional nursing courses. The program gives students a broad approach to nursing, providing a base for graduate study or immediate entry into the nursing profession. Following graduation with a Bachelor of Arts in nursing, Luther nursing students may write the National Council Licensure Examination for Registered Nurses (NCLEX-RN).

PROGRAMS OF STUDY

It is Luther's mission to produce well-rounded and capable students. In the context of a Christian, liberal arts institution, student nurses explore the sciences and the humanities in addition to their nursing courses. The first year provides a foundation in the liberal arts. An introductory course in nursing gives the student an overview of the nursing profession. Faculty members advise each student about career opportunities in nursing.

Students entering the nursing program should have a solid background in English, math, biology, and chemistry.

Clinical nursing courses begin in the fall of the sophomore year. Nursing courses at this level emphasize health assessment throughout the life span in a variety of settings. These learning experiences develop new communication and interpersonal skills.

Third-year students engage in a concentrated study of nursing concepts through caring for children and adults with physical and emotional problems. The sites for the clinical experiences include Rochester Methodist Hospital and St. Mary's Hospital, affiliates of the Mayo Medical Center, and the Federal Medical Center as well as a variety of community-based health-care agencies in Rochester, Minnesota.

The senior year provides final preparation for entry into the practice of professional nursing. Courses focus on promoting health and preventing illness in childbearing families and in community groups. One feature of the senior year is the assignment of an expectant mother to each nursing student. The student follows the mother through the pregnancy and is present at birth. Following graduation, an NCLEX review course is available to all nursing students.

AFFILIATIONS WITH HEALTH-CARE FACILITIES

Luther College conducts its clinical nursing experiences during the junior year at Mayo Medical Center facilities in Rochester, Minnesota, as well as a variety of community-based facilities. These affiliations afford students the opportunity for exposure to the most recent technical and personal strategies for effective nursing care. Additional clinical experiences occur with Winneshiek County Memorial Hospital, the Oneota Riverview Care Facility, the Winneshiek County Public Health Nursing Service, Minowa Cancer Detection, and a variety of community-based programs in Northeast Iowa.

ACADEMIC FACILITIES

The 800-acre campus includes the Preus Library, housing 350,000 volumes, 1,100 periodicals, and the College art collection. The library offers five online indexes and ten commercial online services and provides access to more than 480 other libraries. Modern, well-equipped laboratories in the Valders Hall of Science are supplemented by several other science-teaching facilities on campus, including a planetarium, a greenhouse, an herbarium, a live-animal center, a human anatomy laboratory, a natural history museum, and a psychology sleep laboratory. The science facilities also include an extensive field study area and two electron microscopes. Within easy walking distance of the campus, the field study area offers an ideal setting for studies in aquatic biology, ecology, and field biology. Five ponds, two reestablished prairies, marshes, wooded areas, and agricultural lands are available for classwork and independent study. The College has a fiber-based campus network connecting a variety of PC and Macintosh computers (in several environments) to shared computing resources and to the Internet. More than 400 microcomputers and terminals are available for student use throughout the campus.

LOCATION

The College is located in Decorah, a city of 8,500 people in the scenic bluff country of northeast Iowa. The Upper Iowa River, which runs through the campus, is one of twenty-seven rivers throughout the country designated as a National Scenic and Recreational River. Rich in Scandinavian heritage, Decorah is a popular recreation area, providing opportunities for canoeing, fishing, hunting, cross-country skiing, camping, hiking, cycling, and spelunking. Three airports are located within a 75-mile radius of Decorah: in Rochester, Minnesota; Waterloo, Iowa; and La Crosse, Wisconsin.

STUDENT SERVICES

Luther provides numerous student services in a setting that includes programming seven days a week. The Regents Center for recreation, the Centennial Union, and the Center for Faith and Life serve as hubs of student life activities. Students are involved in the governance of the College through involvement on college committees and student government organizations. Luther fields nineteen athletic teams and provides more than forty intramural activities. In addition, students from every academic department participate in the broad-based music program.

THE NURSING STUDENT GROUP

The Luther College nursing program enrolls approximately 100 students, with 20 to 25 students graduating annually. Since the program was established in 1978, the retention rate of nursing students from sophomore to senior year has typically been 90 percent. Nursing students generally have an average of more than 25 on the ACT and are challenged in a very rigorous program that prepares them well for the profession or for graduate study. Nursing students must achieve a Luther College grade point average of at least 2.3.

COSTS

For 2004–05, the comprehensive fee was $27,240, which included tuition, general fees, facilities fees, room, board, subscriptions to student publications, and admission to College-supported concerts, lectures, and other events. A room telephone, cable TV, computer access from residence hall rooms, and a health-service program are also included. Private music lessons are $200 per semester. It is estimated that an additional $3000 is adequate for books, clothing, entertainment, and other personal expenses.

FINANCIAL AID

More than 97 percent of all Luther students receive some financial aid in the form of grants, such as the Federal Pell Grant, scholarships from Luther and other sources, loans, and jobs on campus. Luther awards Regent and Presidential scholarships to applicants demonstrating superior academic achievement. The amount of aid given is determined by the College's analysis of the Free Application for Federal Student Aid. The priority deadline for a financial aid application is March 1 each year. Students receive notification of their aid awards after their acceptance for admission. All nursing students benefit from the Bernice Fischer Cross and Bert S. Cross Perpetual Endowment for the Luther College Mayo Nursing Program and Health Sciences Program. This endowment is used for equal-share assistance for the Luther College nursing students enrolled in the curriculum provided in the Mayo Medical Center in Rochester, Minnesota. This is not a need-based scholarship.

APPLYING

An application, SAT I or ACT scores, an educator's reference, a transcript of previous academic work, and a $25 application fee are required for admission. On-campus interviews are recommended but not required. Admission is selective. An applicant must be a graduate of an accredited high school and have completed at least 4 units of English, 3 units of mathematics, 3 units of social science, and 2 units of natural science. It is strongly recommended that the applicant have at least two years of a foreign language.

CORRESPONDENCE AND INFORMATION

Admissions Office
Luther College
Decorah, Iowa 52101
Telephone: 563-387-1287
800-458-8437 (toll-free)
Fax: 563-387-2159
E-mail: admissions@luther.edu
World Wide Web: http://www.luther.edu/~nursing

THE FULL-TIME FACULTY

Donna Kubesh, Department Head; Ph.D.; RN.
Corine Carlson, M.S.; RN.
Penny Leake, Ph.D.; RN.
Jayme Nelson, M.S.; RN.
Mary Overvold-Ronningen, M.S.; RN.

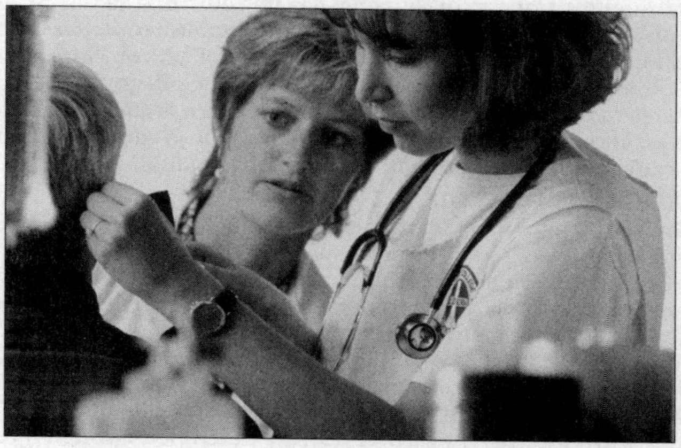

Luther College nursing students gain significant clinical experience in facilities associated with the Mayo Medical Center.

Marquette University
College of Nursing
Milwaukee, Wisconsin

MARQUETTE
UNIVERSITY

THE UNIVERSITY

Established in 1881, Marquette University is recognized for its rigorous core curriculum and professional preparation in the Jesuit tradition. An enrollment of 11,000 includes students from all fifty states and eighty countries. Colleges and Schools of the University include Arts and Sciences, Business Administration, Communication, Dental, Education, Engineering, Health Sciences, Law, and Nursing. The location in the heart of Milwaukee affords students opportunities to apply learning in partnership with the dynamic urban community. The Marquette experience is personally transformational as it prepares graduates to transform society for the better.

THE COLLEGE OF NURSING

Marquette's College of Nursing has its roots in 1898 as St. Joseph's Hospital School of Nursing and established its baccalaureate program as Marquette University College of Nursing in 1936 and master's program in 1938. The College focuses on excellence in clinical teaching and health care of the vulnerable, those at risk for adverse health outcomes. The graduate program is ranked among the top 20 percent in the nation.

PROGRAMS OF STUDY

The four-year Bachelor of Science in Nursing (B.S.N.) degree program provides a strong academic foundation in nursing, natural and social science, and humanities. Preparation for a professional nursing role is emphasized through the development of clinical, cognitive, and leadership skills and personal and professional values. Students are admitted as freshmen in the College of Nursing, which assures placement in clinical nursing courses. Nursing courses begin on the first day of enrollment. Clinical skills, introduced in the second year, are developed through seven clinical rotations in the junior and senior years. A low student-teacher ratio (8:1) affords personal attention in all clinical rotations, including adult care, maternity, mental health, pediatric, and community health and a synthesis course in a setting of the student's choice.

The 128-credit B.S.N. program includes courses in the humanities, physical-biological sciences, and social-behavioral sciences as well as electives and courses in the nursing major. A University Core of Common Studies is foundational for all majors at Marquette University. Lower-division nursing courses are Dimensions of Professional Nursing, Health Assessment, Foundations of Nursing Practice, Pathophysiology 1 and 2, and Pharmacotherapeutics. Upper-division courses include Nursing Research, Care of Adults*, Childbearing Family Nursing*, Mental Health Nursing*, Primary Health Care Concepts, Gerontological Nursing, Family Centered Nursing of Children*, Nursing of Communities*, Care of Acutely Ill Adults*, Nursing Synthesis*, and Nursing Leadership. The asterisk (*) denotes clinical practice courses.

There are additional options for students in the B.S.N. program. These include a nursing/psychology double major, B.S.N./premedicine studies, B.S.N./pre-DPT program, and Spanish for health professionals. There are ROTC programs with the Army, Air Force, and Navy. Study-abroad options are available in sixteen countries. Students may elect an internship at the Les Aspin Center for Government in Washington, D.C., working on health policy. The Advanced Nurse Scholar (ANS) program offers select freshmen entry to nurse practitioner or nurse midwifery M.S.N. programs.

The RN to B.S.N. program is available for ADN and diploma RNs. Prior course work is evaluated, and students may be awarded credits through credit transfer and a validation process. Typically, students take 50 to 70 additional credits to complete the 128-credit B.S.N.

Marquette University College of Nursing offers the Master of Science in Nursing (M.S.N.) degree and post-master's certificates that prepare graduates for advanced practice roles or leadership roles within health-care systems. Individuals may enter through four pathways: post-B.S.N., combined RN and M.S.N. for those with non-nursing bachelor's degrees (DE), RN to B.S.N. to M.S.N., and ADN-prepared nurses with bachelor's degrees in other disciplines. Graduates are academically eligible to seek formal professional certification as nurse practitioners, clinical nurse specialists, nurse midwives, or nurse administrators. Six specialty options are available: health-care systems leadership and advanced practice programs in nurse midwifery, children, adults, older adults, and acute care. Full-time students complete the 39–45 credit programs in four semesters.

A 51-credit post-M.S.N./Ph.D. program to prepare teachers/scholars focuses on knowledge generation related to vulnerable populations.

AFFILIATIONS WITH HEALTH-CARE FACILITIES

The College is affiliated with more than eighty health-care agencies in Wisconsin and the surrounding states. These agencies include the hospitals, clinics, and home care of public health departments, schools, parishes, long-term-care facilities, hospice, and clinics. Many of these agencies offer excellent student employment opportunities as well as financial aid and loan forgiveness programs.

ACADEMIC FACILITIES

Marquette is located on an 80-acre campus with excellent facilities. State-of-the-art libraries support student and faculty needs through their collections, services, and connections to worldwide resources. The Instructional Media Center provides a broad range of media support to faculty members and students. Information Technology Services offer voice and data communications and computer-based services to students all around campus, with Internet access from the residence hall rooms. The College of Nursing has five technology-enhanced classrooms and a well-equipped Learning Resource Center (LRC). The LRC provides computer access, media resources, and practice labs supplied with state-of-the-art models and equipment necessary to develop a solid foundation for clinical practice.

LOCATION

The College is located in a metropolitan area on the shore of Lake Michigan with a population of more than 1 million people. The city of Milwaukee is known as the city of festivals and for the friendliness of its residents (the Germans call it "gemütlichkeit"). Students can enrich their lives with theater, music, art, major-league sports, and world-class dining.

STUDENT SERVICES

Students take advantage of a wide range of student services including individual advising with a faculty member, student health services, a writing center, tutoring, counseling center, 160 student organizations, and the University ministry with a staff dedicated to students needs. Student development includes leadership and service opportunities. Marquette students and faculty members provide more than 100,000 hours of service per year. The University Task Force on Diversity attends to recruitment and the needs of a diverse group of students and faculty members and addresses multicultural appreciation.

THE NURSING STUDENT GROUP

Currently, there are more than 440 undergraduates enrolled from throughout the U.S. About 10 percent are students of color and about 9 percent are men. Nurses from Kenya, the Republic of Georgia, and other countries, attending Marquette for special programs, join them in some classes. In the past five years, nursing students have earned University student leadership awards and have competed in varsity soccer, basketball, tennis, and track and cross-country as well as club sports.

There are more than 190 graduate students enrolled. About 20 percent are full-time students and most are employed while attending classes. Graduates from the M.S.N. programs are employed in various leadership positions. These include hospital presidents, chief nursing officers of health-care systems, partners in group practices, nursing faculty members, clinical nurse specialists, nurse midwives, and nurse practitioners.

COSTS

The annual tuition for the undergraduate nursing program in 2004–05 was $21,550, and the cost for the graduate program was $660 per credit.

FINANCIAL AID

More than 90 percent of undergraduate students receive financial aid, including scholarships, grants, and low-interest loans. The rising demand for nurses has increased support for nursing education from federal and state sources as well as from health-care organizations. Applicants should complete the FAFSA (Free Application for Federal Student Aid) and work with the University's financial aid counselors to optimize support. Graduate student aid includes federal traineeships, teaching assistantships, research assistantships, Marquette University Tuition Scholarships, health-care agency tuition programs, and other option-specific dedicated scholarships.

APPLYING

Requirements for the prelicensure B.S.N. program include high school academic record; one year of algebra, geometry, biology, and chemistry; and ACT or SAT I scores. Interested students are encouraged to visit in person or on the Web. For detailed information, students should contact University Admissions toll-free at 800-222-6544.

Routes to admission to the M.S.N. program vary depending upon the student's background. Students who have a B.S.N., who are RNs who want to complete the accelerated B.S.N./M.S.N., or who have completed a degree in a discipline other than nursing may apply. Admission requirements include the completed Marquette University Graduate School application (available online at www.grad.mu.edu), three completed reference forms, an up-to-date resume, a brief goal statement, GRE scores, and an undergraduate GPA of 3.0 or better.

Direct Entry (DE) students are to have completed the following: bachelor's degree with a GPA of 3.0 or better; 5–6 credits in anatomy and physiology; 5–6 credits of another science, such as chemistry, biology, or microbiology; 3 credits of social science; and 3 credits of statistics.

Applications are accepted throughout the year for the fall or spring semesters. Financial aid applications are due by February 15 for the following fall semester. Direct Entry students begin as a cohort in the last week in May and complete the pre-M.S.N. course work and an initial 9 graduate credits in fifteen months. At the completion of the pre-M.S.N. phase, they are eligible to complete the professional licensing exam in the state of Wisconsin and proceed into their desired graduate option.

CORRESPONDENCE AND INFORMATION

College of Nursing
Marquette University
P.O. Box 1881
Milwaukee, Wisconsin 53201
Telephone: 414-288-3809
E-mail: judith.miller@marquette.edu (graduate)
janet.krejci@marquette.edu (undergraduate)
World Wide Web: http://www.marquette.edu/nursing

THE FACULTY

Lea Acord, Ph.D; RN. Dean and Educational Administration Professor.

Cheryl Anderson, M.S.N., M.A.; RN, CCRN. Health-care ethics.

Ruth Ann Belknap, Ph.D.; APRN, BC. Family violence in Hispanic women.

Kathleen Bobay Ph.D.; RN, CS, FNP. Health-care systems, measuring clinical nursing expertise.

Marilyn Bratt, Ph.D.; RN. Nurse residency programs.

Margaret Bull, Ph.D.; RN, FAAN. Continuity of care, community elder care.

Holli DeVon, Ph.D.; RN. Gender differences in symptoms of unstable angina.

Diane Dressler, M.S.N.; RN, CCRN, CCTC. Critical care, heart transplant, heart failure.

Richard J. Fehring, D.N.Sc.; RN, CNFPP, CNFPE. Natural family planning, adult health.

Marilyn Frenn, Ph.D.; RN. Health promotion, adolescent health.

Mary Beth Gosline, Ph.D.; RN, CS, CEN. Elder care, emergency care, education.

Kristin Haglund, M.S.N., Ph.D.; RN, FNP, PNP. Pediatric primary care, adolescent sexual behavior.

Lisa Hanson, D.N.Sc.; RN, CNM. Women's health, nurse midwifery care.

Kathryn Harrod, D.N.Sc.; RN, CNM. Caring behaviors in labor.

Karen Ivantic-Doucette, M.S.N.; RN-CS, ACRN, FNP. HIV/AIDS care, international health.

Kerry Kosmoski-Goepfert, Ph.D.; RN. Critical care, health-care systems.

Judith Kowatsch, M.S.N.; RN-C. Maternal-child care.

Janet Krejci, Ph.D.; RN, CNAA. Systems, health-care leadership development.

Mary Ann Lough, Ph.D.; RN. Community delivery systems, chronically ill elders.

Shelly Malin, Ph.D.; RN. Leadership development, children and families.

Ruth McShane, Ph.D.; RN. Family caregiving, chronic illness.

Judith F. Miller, Ph.D.; RN, FAAN. Hope, chronic illness, self-management.

Maureen O'Brien, Ph.D.; RN. Technology-dependent children.

Sandra Ramey, Ph.D.; RN. Cardiovascular risk factors, health promotion.

Polly Ryan, Ph.D.; RN. Behavior change, outcomes research.

Doris Schoneman, Ph.D.; RN, CS. Community health interventions and outcomes.

Christine Shaw, Ph.D.; RN, BC, FNP, ANP. Primary care of underserved.

Terry Tobin, M.S.N., M.P.H.; RN. Maternal-child care, women's health.

Leona VandeVusse, Ph.D.; RN, CNM. Primary care of women, birth stories.

Darlene Weis, Ph.D.; RN. Health policy, nursing values, international nursing.

Marianne Weiss, D.N.Sc.; RN. Pre-term labor, postpartum follow-up, outcomes.

Sarah A. Wilson, Ph.D.; RN. Community health and culture, dying and hospice.

Jill Winters, Ph.D.; RN. Critical care, music therapy, outcome measures, telehealth.

Medical College of Georgia
School of Nursing
Augusta, Georgia

THE COLLEGE
The Medical College of Georgia (MCG), Georgia's health sciences university, is located at Georgia's eastern border on the Savannah River and is the state's primary institution to educate health-care professionals. It is the third-largest of the thirty-four colleges and universities in the University System of Georgia, with approximately 2,500 students, interns, residents, and fellows. It is the largest single employer in the city of Augusta, with more than 5,000 faculty and staff members.

THE SCHOOL OF NURSING
In response to the wartime need for additional nurses, the University System of Georgia voted August 11, 1943, to offer courses in nursing education. This participation in the U.S. Cadet Nurse Corps paved the way for establishing a department of nursing at the University of Georgia the following fall. The program moved from Athens, Georgia, to Augusta in 1956 and became a part of the Medical College of Georgia. The School of Nursing, with a strong commitment to research, moved forward in its development as a university-based nursing program. In 1974, to meet Georgia's growing need for baccalaureate-prepared nurses, a free-standing, self-contained satellite campus was opened in Athens, Georgia. This campus, for more than twenty years, has consistently prepared one third of the graduates of the baccalaureate program each year. To assist faculty research, an essential component in graduate education, the Center for Nursing Research was established in 1987. In 1994, the Board of Regents approved more than $1.5 million to renovate the historic Stoney Building, where the School moved in January 1995. In 1996, a second satellite campus was created in cooperation with Gordon College to offer an RN to B.S.N. program using distance learning technology. In 1999, the family nurse practitioner program began to be offered by distance learning technology on the campus of Columbus State University, and in 2002, the RN/B.S.N. and RN to M.S.N. programs were offered on this campus.

The School of Nursing is accredited by the National League for Nursing Accrediting Commission and is a member agency of the Council of Baccalaureate and Higher Degree Programs. In addition, the School of Nursing has preliminary approval from the Commission on Collegiate Nursing Education.

The School of Nursing faculty has 36 full-time and 15 part-time members representing diverse areas of teaching and research.

PROGRAMS OF STUDY
Degrees offered are the Bachelor of Science in Nursing (B.S.N.), Master of Science in Nursing (M.S.N.) (clinical nurse specialist program), Master of Nursing (M.N.) (nurse practitioner programs and nursing anesthesia), and the Doctor of Philosophy (Ph.D.) in nursing. The baccalaureate program has a community-based curriculum that incorporates a wide variety of clinical experiences in inpatient, outpatient, and community settings. As part of the baccalaureate program, a B.S.N. completion program for registered nurses is offered online.

The Master of Science in Nursing program offers specialties in adult and community health nursing. The Master of Nursing program offers specialties in nursing anesthesia, family nurse practitioner studies, and pediatric nurse practitioner studies.

The doctoral program specialty is health care across the life span.

AFFILIATIONS WITH HEALTH-CARE FACILITIES
MCG's campus includes MCG Hospital, the Children's Medical Center, and more than eighty specialty clinics. Since 1956, MCG has operated the 540-bed teaching hospital and clinics, the Medical College of Georgia Health Care, Inc. The facility is a leading referral center for Georgia and the region. To meet the clinical learning needs of students and the baccalaureate program, more than 275 contracts exist between the School of Nursing and a variety of health-care agencies throughout Georgia and South Carolina.

ACADEMIC FACILITIES
The five-school campus of almost 90 acres includes forty-seven buildings, with construction of new buildings plus expansion and renovation of present buildings continuing the growth trend of the institution.

The University operates community outreach clinics in twenty-eight counties. Telemedicine sites are located throughout the state. The institution also has a satellite campus in Athens, Georgia, and delivers distance learning to students in Atlanta, Dalton, Barnesville, and Columbus. The University houses a large multimedia library that participates in the state library system, GALILEO, with MERLIN. GALILEO provides access to more than fifty databases and services pertinent to undergraduate studies. The library also offers an extensive public computing area with Macintosh and IBM-compatible microcomputers, terminals with access to MERLIN and GALILEO, and programs for word processing, spreadsheets, graphics, and other services. In addition, students have access to computers within their respective schools.

LOCATION
Augusta, the second-largest city in Georgia, is located on the south bank of the Savannah River, midway between the Great Smokey Mountains and the Atlantic Ocean. It is a growing and thriving city with a metropolitan-area population of around 400,000, and was recently ranked as the second most favorable place to live in Georgia. The area is known for its balmy climate, with an annual mean temperature of 64 degrees.

Founded in 1836 by General James Oglethorpe, Augusta is Georgia's second-oldest city. Augusta was Georgia's capital in 1778 and from 1785 to 1795. The city offers a wide array of cultural and recreational activities. Augusta has an impressive riverwalk, the site of many activities such as the Augusta Invitation Regatta, a national collegiate rowing event. The city also is a short drive from Lake Thurmond Reservoir, the site of such outdoor activities as waterskiing, swimming, boating, and camping. Augusta is world-renowned as the home of the Masters Golf Tournament.

Augusta has many associations dedicated to the performing and visual arts, including the Augusta Opera Association, the Augusta Ballet, the Augusta Players, the Augusta Children's Theatre, the Augusta Symphony, and the Augusta Art Association. The Medical College of Georgia, Augusta State University, and Paine College often bring prestigious films, speakers, and special events to the city.

Augusta offers exceptional shopping and features a downtown art and antiques district. The area's hundreds of restaurants range from fine to casual dining, featuring everything from ethnic specialties to burgers.

Augusta is within an easy 3-hour drive to Atlanta, the University of Georgia, the Atlantic Ocean, and the mountains.

Augusta is a leading health-care center of the Southeast and has a rapidly developing and diversified industrial base. The area's nine hospitals serve the Southeast and beyond.

STUDENT SERVICES

MCG's Student Health Services provides primary care for MCG students' medical, dental, and psychological needs. The Minority Academic Advisement Program ensures the recruitment and retention of minority students in schools through the University System of Georgia. The School of Nursing houses the Learning Resources Center, where students learn psychomotor skills needed to practice nursing. Students also have access to computers, audiovisual materials, nursing journals, and classroom materials.

THE NURSING STUDENT GROUP

Student life at the Medical College of Georgia offers many learning experiences in a variety of settings. The School of Nursing has approximately 200 undergraduate students and 100 graduate students in Augusta and approximately 130 undergraduate and 15 graduate students in Athens. The distance learning site in Barnesville serves approximately 20 RN students, and the distance site in Columbus accommodates approximately 10 students. Many student organizations are available to enhance the student's career, including the Georgia Association of Nursing Students (GANS); the IMHOTEP-Leadership Honor Society; MCG Student Government Association; Sigma Theta Tau, Beta Omicron Chapter; and Phi Chi Beta of Chi Eta Phi Sorority. The Augusta and Athens chapters of GANS are active on local, state, and national levels. Several students have held national offices. More than 90 percent of the graduating class of 2002 were offered employment opportunities at hospitals, outpatient clinics, nursing homes, day-care centers, and physicians' offices immediately upon graduating.

COSTS

Full-time tuition for 2003–04 was $1604 for in-state students and $6416 for out-of-state students per semester. Part-time tuition costs were $134 per credit hour for in-state students and $535 per credit hour for out-of-state students. On-campus housing costs range from $938 to $1750; off-campus room and board expenses range from $9000 to $13,000. Additional fees per term include a $38 activity fee, a $130 health fee (if taking 6 hours or more), a $50 Wellness Center fee, and a $75 technology fee. Books, uniforms, and equipment fees are approximately $400 to $800 per academic year.

FINANCIAL AID

For a copy of the *Student Financial Aid Bulletin,* students should contact the Financial Aid Office. A limited number of part-time employment opportunities are available through the MCG Personnel Office.

APPLYING

Admission to the Medical College of Georgia School of Nursing is based on high school graduation or its equivalent; scores on the SAT I or ACT; cumulative GPA, with some preference given for outstanding grades in courses supporting nursing; completion of all prerequisite course work; and references.

CORRESPONDENCE AND INFORMATION

Office of Academic Admissions
AA-170 Kelly Building
Medical College of Georgia
Augusta, Georgia 30912
Telephone: 706-721-2725
Fax: 706-721-0186
E-mail: underadm@mail.mcg.edu
gradadm@mail.mcg.edu
World Wide Web: http://www.mcg.edu/son

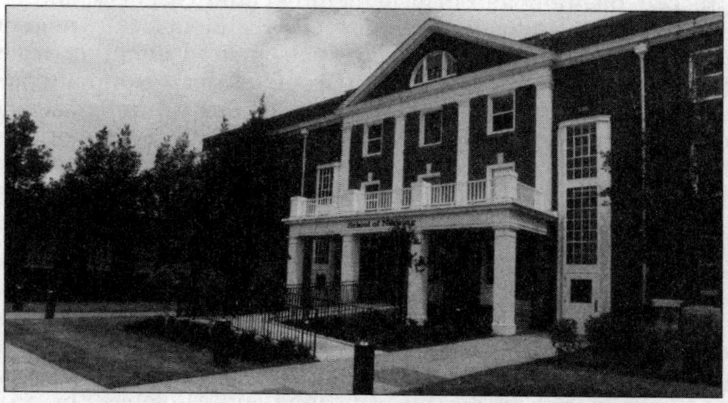

The School of Nursing was founded in 1943 and serves as the University System of Georgia's flagship nursing school, meeting the challenges of an evolving health-care system.

MGH Institute of Health Professions
Graduate Program in Nursing
Boston, Massachusetts

THE SCHOOL

The MGH Institute of Health Professions, founded in 1977, is an innovative graduate school affiliated with the internationally known Massachusetts General Hospital (MGH). The Institute offers programs in nursing, communication sciences and disorders, physical therapy, clinical investigation, and a new program in medical imaging. A faculty of more than 80 members, half of whom are practicing clinicians, teaches more than 600 students. The Institute is accredited by the New England Association of Schools and Colleges. The Graduate Program in Nursing is approved by the Board of Registration in Nursing of the Commonwealth of Massachusetts and is accredited by the National League for Nursing Accrediting Commission.

Located in Boston, the Institute was formed to meet the need for master clinicians—leaders in the health-care professions with an education formed by theory and simultaneous practice and based upon a thorough understanding of specialized clinical practice, planning and management of clinical services, and research. The Institute offers an impressive student-faculty ratio of 7:1, enabling students to receive personalized attention from faculty members. The setting also promotes small-group interactions that advance the health professions through interdisciplinary models of education, research, and practice. For more information, prospective students should consult the Institute's Web site, listed in this In-Depth Description.

THE NURSING PROGRAM

With internationally recognized faculty members who are researchers, clinicians, and mentors to students, the Graduate Program in Nursing is designed to prepare advanced practice nurses to assume leadership roles in the health-care system of the future. This includes engaging diverse individuals, families, groups, and communities in pursuit of healing and wholeness, by providing excellence and innovation in education, scholarship, and service.

The program is based on the philosophy that nursing is caring for the body, mind, and spirit of persons in relation to their environment at every level of human connection: individuals, families, groups, and communities. From this framework, nursing addresses promotion, maintenance, and restoration of health while underscoring the political, economic, and social forces that have impacted a person. These forces create a diverse environment within which nursing seeks to maximize health at every level of human existence.

The Graduate Program in Nursing is the largest program at the MGH Institute of Health Professions and has more than 200 students. The Master of Science in Nursing (M.S.N.) degree program accepts both college graduates and nurses with bachelor's degrees in nursing and other fields. A nondegree Certificate of Advanced Study (CAS) is available for RNs holding a master's degree in nursing. Registered nurses with an associate degree in nursing or diploma in nursing are also eligible for admission provided they have completed specific prerequisite general education requirements. Upon graduation, all students are eligible to take nurse practitioner certification examinations in their selected specialty or specialties.

PROGRAMS OF STUDY

The Graduate Program in Nursing offers the following programs of study, which are designed to be congruent with the individual student's prior preparation and professional goals: Master of Science in Nursing degree for college graduates (entry-level program); Master of Science in Nursing degree for registered nurses with an associate degree in nursing, a diploma in nursing, or a bachelor's degree in nursing or other discipline (RN-to-M.S. program); and Certificates of Advanced Study in primary care, psychiatric–mental health, and acute care for registered nurses holding a Master of Science degree in nursing (CAS program).

The entry-level program requires three years of full-time study (no summers) and consists of generalist and advanced practice courses. Upon successful completion of the generalist courses (at the end of the fall semester, year two), entry-level students are eligible to apply for and take the examination for registered nurse licensure (NCLEX-RN®). The Massachusetts Board of Registration in Nursing administers this examination. All entry-level students must achieve RN licensure prior to entering the final (third) year of their program. RN and CAS students may complete the program on a full- or part-time basis, with courses offered in the daytime, evenings, and during the summer. Total credits depend on the specialities selected.

All programs offer opportunities to develop specializations in a variety of areas. Current specialities include acute-care and primary-care specialities in family, pediatrics, and general adult. Dual primary-care specialties are available in adult/women's health, adult/gerontology, adult/HIV/AIDS, and adult/psychiatric–mental health. Upon graduation, all students are eligible to sit for one or more nurse practitioner certification examinations within selected clinical specialties. Prospective students should see the Institute's online catalog by visiting the Web site for additional information and curriculum plans.

The Graduate Program in Nursing has an outstanding faculty, with strong academic preparation and clinical expertise, reflecting diverse backgrounds and geographical origins. Faculty members practice in a variety of health-care settings and maintain active programs of clinical research in areas such as maternal-infant health, aging, women's health, HIV/AIDS, spirituality and health, and cultural diversity. Through their practice, research, and scholarship, faculty members provide excellent role models for student learning and professional practice.

Institute students have a high pass rate in both the RN licensure (NCLEX-RN) and Advanced Practice Certification exams. Over the past few years, 94–100 percent of first-time takers have passed the NCLEX-RN. All entry-level nursing students have successfully passed the exam prior to entering their third year of study. Advanced Practice Certification pass rates and scores are consistently above national averages.

AFFILIATIONS WITH HEALTH-CARE FACILITIES

The MGH Institute of Health Professions is affiliated with Massachusetts General Hospital and Partners HealthCare System. Established in 1994, Partners was created by the affiliation of Massachusetts General Hospital and Brigham and Women's Hospital. The Partners system also includes area community health centers and hospitals, the Institute, and many private primary-care practices throughout New England. Partners provides primary and specialty care and serves as a referral center for patients throughout the region and around the world. Its clinical facilities are an extraordinary resource for the education of health-care professionals. Affiliations also exist with a large number of clinical sites in the Boston area and nationwide. Students work with and are precepted by highly experienced clinicians in a wide variety of settings: community health centers, homeless shelters, outpatient clinics, elderly housing, private practices, health maintenance organizations, nurse-managed clinics, school-based clinics, and various acute-care settings, among others.

With more than 400 contractual agreements throughout the greater New England area, clinical learning offers the setting whereby theory is joined with practice to increase students' confidence in their skills, clinical judgment, and ability to make a valuable contribution to improving health care within society. In addition, many students find part-time work in these institutions during their course of study. Entry-level students often work full-time during the summer, first as patient care assistants and then as RNs during the second summer. This provides an opportunity to gain additional nursing experience prior to graduation.

ACADEMIC FACILITIES

Clinical and research opportunities are provided at MGH and in more than 500 other major health-care centers and community settings in the greater Boston area. Through MGH's Treadwell Library, which contains major basic science, medical, and nursing collections, students may access online computer databases and an extensive reference and periodical collection. The Institute's Ruth Sleeper Learning Center provides computers and modern technology for interactive learning.

LOCATION

Located in the historic Charlestown Navy Yard, overlooking Boston's famed waterfront, the Institute offers students a stimulating environment. There are numerous opportunities for extracurricular activities, including theaters, museums, concerts, and professional sports events. Boston has an excellent public transportation system and is located in proximity to rivers, lakes, mountains, and parks.

STUDENT SERVICES

The Office of Student Affairs offers a wide variety of student services, including student activities and programming. The office also advises student government, provides financial support for the National Student Nurses Association and student conferences, and oversees accommodations for students with disabilities.

THE NURSING STUDENT GROUP

Institute students come from a wide variety of disciplines and educational backgrounds. Entry-level students vary from new liberal arts or basic science graduates to students with a master's or Ph.D. degree and strong experience in another field. RN students also have diverse backgrounds and bring their unique nursing experience to share. The wide age range and diverse backgrounds enhance learning opportunities for all. Exposure to different ideas is provided, and the development of the skills and ability for critical thinking and collaboration are strengthened.

COSTS

Tuition for the 2004–05 academic year was $707 per credit hour, with the number of credits dependent on individual program requirements. A general student fee is assessed each semester for lab and clinical expenses, technical support, and student services. Books and supplies cost about $1500 per year.

FINANCIAL AID

Financial assistance is supplemental to the student's financial resources. Whenever possible, financial need is met through a combination of sources that may include federal loans, scholarships, graduate assistantships, and federal traineeships.

APPLYING

Entry-level students are graduates of baccalaureate programs in fields other than nursing and must complete prerequisite course work in anatomy, physiology, chemistry, microbiology, nutrition, and statistics before matriculation. Applicants may complete those prerequisites at the Institute in "Science Summer," the summer preceding matriculation. RN program students must hold a bachelor's degree in nursing, an associate degree in nursing, or a diploma in nursing. Prerequisites include a statistics course and a current RN license. Associate degree and diploma students are required to successfully complete additional general education prerequisites. All applicants must take the Graduate Record Examinations (GRE) unless they qualify for a waiver as explained in the Institute's application instructions. Advanced Practice Certificate applicants are not required to take the GRE. Prospective students should see the Institute's online catalog by visiting the Web site for admission application requirements and available nurse practitioner specialty areas.

CORRESPONDENCE AND INFORMATION

Office of Student Affairs
MGH Institute of Health Professions
P.O. Box 6357
Boston, Massachusetts 02114-0016
Telephone: 617-726-3140
Fax: 617-726-8010
E-mail: admissions@mghihp.edu
World Wide Web: http://www.mghihp.edu

THE FACULTY

Linda Andrist, Associate Professor; Ph.D., Brandeis; RNC, WHNP. Women's health research.

Deborah Bradford, Clinical Instructor; M.S.N., Boston College; RN, ANP.

Cheryl Cahill, Amelia Peabody Professor in Nursing Research; Ph.D., Michigan; RN.

Inge Corless, FAAN Professor; Ph.D., Brown; RN. HIV/AIDS and palliative-care research.

Deborah D'Avolio, Assistant Professor; Ph.D., Boston College; RN, ANP. Domestic violence research.

Patricia Fitzgerald, Clinical Instructor; M.S.N., Salem State; RN.

Elizabeth Friedlander, Clinical Assistant Professor; M.S.N., Simmons; RNC, ANP.

Alex Hoyt, Instructor; M.S.N., MGH Institute of Health Professions; RNC, FNP.

Veronica Kane, Assistant Professor; M.S.N., Yale; RNC, PNP.

Ursula Kelly, Clinical Assistant Professor; M.S.N., Massachusetts Worcester; APRN. Domestic violence in Latina women.

Ellen Long-Middleton, Assistant Professor; Ph.D., Boston College; RNC, FNP.

Patricia Lussier-Duynstee, Assistant Professor; Ph.D., Massachusetts; RN. Community health.

Talli McCormick, Clinical Assistant Professor; M.S.N., MGH Institute of Health Professions; RNC, GNP. Gerontology research.

Janice Bell Meisenhelder, Associate Professor; D.N.Sc., Boston University; RN. Spirituality research.

Jacqueline Sue Myers, Assistant Professor; Ph.D., George Mason; RN, PNP.

Patrice Nicholas, Professor; D.N.Sc., Boston University; M.P.H., Harvard; RNC, ANP.

Joanne O'Sullivan; Ph.D., M.S.N., Boston College; RN, FNP. Adolescent research.

Alexandra Paul-Simon, Assistant Professor; Ph.D., Boston College; RN.

Katherine Simmonds, Clinical Instructor; M.S.N., MGH Institute of Health Professions; RNC, WHNP.

Kathleen Solomon, Clinical Assistant Professor; M.S.N., Massachusetts Lowell; RNC, FNP.

Sharon Sullivan, Clinical Instructor; M.S., Boston University; RN.

Nancy Terres, Assistant Professor; Ph.D., Tufts; RN. Pediatric research.

John Twomey, Associate Professor; Ph.D., Virginia; RNC, PNP. Pediatric research.

Maria Winne, Clinical Instructor; M.S., Massachusetts Boston; RN.

Karen Wolf, Clinical Associate Professor; Ph.D., Brandeis; RNC, ANP. Historical research.

Michigan State University
College of Nursing
East Lansing, Michigan

THE UNIVERSITY

Founded in 1855 as an autonomous public institution of higher learning by and for the citizens of Michigan, Michigan State University (MSU) was designated the beneficiary of the Morrill Act endowment in 1863, making MSU one of the earliest land-grant institutions in the United States. Since then, MSU has evolved into an internationally esteemed university, offering a comprehensive spectrum of programs and attracting gifted professors, staff members, and students. The University seeks excellence in all programs and activities, and this challenge for high achievement creates a dynamic atmosphere. MSU fulfills the fundamental purposes of all major institutions of higher education: to seek, to teach, and to preserve knowledge. As a land-grant institution, the University meets these objectives in all its formal and informal education programs, in basic and applied research, and in public service. MSU remains an innovative, responsive public resource.

THE COLLEGE OF NURSING

The nursing program at Michigan State University began in 1950 as a generic baccalaureate program and has grown to include an RN to B.S.N. program; an accelerated second degree program; a master's degree with concentrations in advanced nursing practice, nursing education, and clinical nurse leader; and a doctoral (Ph.D.) program. Post-master's and postdoctoral opportunities also exist within the College. The College of Nursing (CON) was one of the MSU campus pioneers, through the Virtual University, in the use of the Internet for education delivery. Currently, the College offers two programs (RN to B.S.N. and M.S.N. in nursing education) completely online, and core courses in the nurse practitioner concentrations are also available online. Outreach programs are offered in collaboration with local community colleges and health-care agencies. Community-based clinical experience is an essential component of nursing education at MSU. More than 300 clinical preceptors and adjunct faculty members provide clinical instruction in more than 150 health-care agencies throughout Michigan.

PROGRAMS OF STUDY

The College of Nursing offers an undergraduate program leading to the Bachelor of Science degree with a major in nursing and graduate programs leading to the Master of Science in Nursing (M.S.N.) degree and the Doctor of Philosophy (Ph.D.) degree with a major in nursing. The focus of the undergraduate program is basic professional education; that of the master's program is the education of advanced practice nurses and nurse educators, while the Ph.D. program prepares nurse researchers.

The undergraduate nursing program provides a foundation for professional practice based on the biological, physical, and behavioral sciences and the humanities. The program is designed to prepare the student for nursing practice with individuals, families, and aggregates of persons in a variety of health states and health-care settings, including hospitals and community health agencies. With professional experience, the graduate may progress to beginning-level leadership positions. The program, which has been approved by the Michigan Board of Nursing and accredited by the Commission on Collegiate Nursing Education (CCNE), also provides a foundation for graduate study in nursing.

The Master of Science degree program utilizes an innovative curriculum that reflects the dynamic challenges facing the health-care system. The M.S.N. program currently prepares students for the role of nurse provider, specifically, as advanced nurse practitioners in family and adult nursing, clinical nurse leaders, and the role of nurse educator. Additional concentrations that reflect current and expanding roles are under development. Completion of a thesis is an optional component of the degrees.

The Doctor of Philosophy degree program with a major in nursing is designed with a major emphasis in health status and health outcomes research related to individuals and families within the context of community. The focus of the Ph.D. program is to prepare clinical researchers. Graduates conduct and facilitate research in a variety of academic, clinical, and community-based settings.

ACADEMIC FACILITIES

The MSU Libraries have an extensive research collection of more than 4 million volumes housed in the main library and fourteen branch libraries serving classroom buildings across the campus. The collection includes more than 28,000 periodicals, 200,000 maps, 40,000 sound recordings, Michigan and U.S. government documents, and publications of the United Nations and other international organizations. MSU is the nation's only university with three on-campus medical schools, graduating medical doctors, veterinarians, and osteopathic physicians. The College of Nursing is housed in the Life Sciences Building and includes a media laboratory, a demonstration laboratory for clinical skills, and a recently established technology classroom.

LOCATION

The property holdings of MSU at East Lansing total 5,192 acres. Of this, more than 2,000 acres are in existing or planned campus development; the remaining acres are devoted to experimental farms, outlying research facilities, and more than 700 acres of protected natural areas. Campus plantings serve as a vast collection for teaching and research. The collections include some 7,000 varieties of trees, shrubs, and vines. The W. J. Beal Botanical Garden is an outstanding campus resource with more than 3,000 plant species. Major buildings number about 200 on the contiguous campus; there are 46 lane-miles of roadways and 3.7 million square feet of walks.

STUDENT SERVICES

The MSU CON is committed to providing a high-quality nursing program for capable and motivated students from all backgrounds. Student supportive services provide opportunities to strengthen student achievement through academic counseling, free tutorial support, career and financial planning, and peer/professional counseling. College of Nursing faculty and staff members also work with University offices such as the Office of Supportive Services, the Learning Resource Center, and the Writing Center to provide comprehensive support for nursing students. The LEAP (Learning, Excelling, and Attaining Professionalism) Initiative provides targeted support and programs to students who are underrepresented in the nursing profession, including first-generation college students and students of color.

THE NURSING STUDENT GROUP

Nursing student organizations enhance the College's sense of community. The Nursing Student Advisory Council, an elected body representing all student levels, acts as the liaison between the faculty/administration and students. The MSU Chapter of the Nursing Student Association is active at the local and state levels. The Pre-Nursing Student Organization assists the College in matricular issues relevant to students prior to admission to the major. The College also has chapters of Sigma Theta Tau International, the Christian Nurses Fellowship, and Chi Eta Phi Sorority, Inc.

COSTS

Applicants are encouraged to refer to http://www.ctlr.msu.edu/studrec/ or http://www.ctlr.msu.edu/studrec/On-line_prog-_Fees.htm for the current tuition and fees information.

FINANCIAL AID

Financial aid is available for direct educational costs and for personal living expenses. Undergraduates are eligible for scholarships and grants from numerous sources, loans, and jobs. Graduate assistantships, private scholarships, Professional Nurse Traineeships, and MSU Fellowships are available through the College of Nursing. Graduate and research assistantships, which offer tuition waivers and pay monthly stipends, are also available. College scholarships from private donors of the College are available to students at all levels.

APPLYING

Applicants must submit their applications to the College of Nursing by March 1 of the year during which admission is sought for the undergraduate program and by February 1 for all graduate programs. Undergraduate applicants must complete the required prerequisite courses and have a minimum cumulative grade point average (GPA) of 2.5 and 2.2 in the sciences. Complete application criteria and packets are available at the Web site listed in the Correspondence and Information section.

Applicants to the Master of Science in Nursing program must have a minimum grade point average of 3.0 in the last two years of the baccalaureate degree and an approved statistics course within five years of the planned date of enrollment. RNs with a bachelor's degree in other fields are eligible to apply.

Applicants to the Ph.D. program must have a minimum GPA of 3.0 for all previous academic work, submit GRE scores (verbal, quantitative, and analytic) from within the last five years, hold an M.S.N. degree, and submit three references. Admission to both the M.S.N. and Ph.D. programs also includes an interview with the faculty.

CORRESPONDENCE AND INFORMATION

College of Nursing
A117 Life Sciences Building
East Lansing, Michigan 48824
Telephone: 517-353-4827
800-605-6424 (toll-free)
Fax: 517-432-8251
E-mail: nurse@msu.edu
World Wide Web: http://www.nursing.msu.edu/

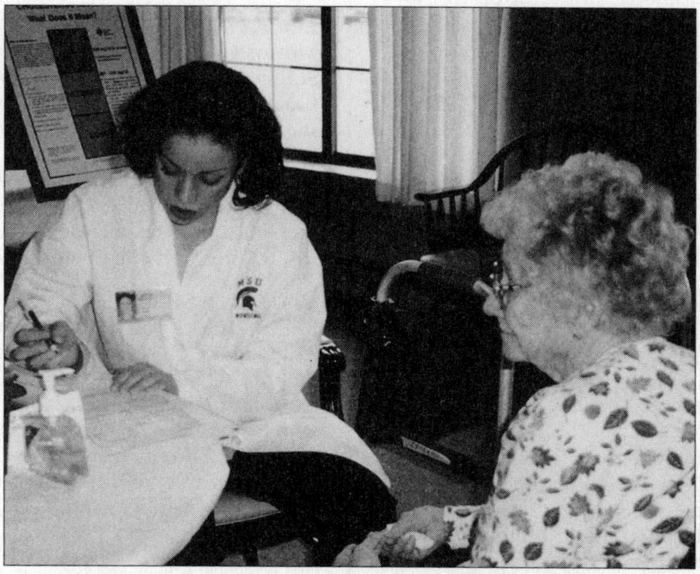

A B.S.N. student participates in College-sponsored community health screening.

Mount Carmel College of Nursing

MOUNT CARMEL
COLLEGE OF
NURSING

Columbus, Ohio

THE COLLEGE

Mount Carmel College of Nursing (MCCN) is a private, specialized institution of higher education offering a Bachelor of Science Degree in nursing, a Master of Science program in adult health, an RN to BSN Program, a Dietetic Internship Program, a nine-month Surgical Technology Program, and a Division of Continuing Education. The College's baccalaureate degree in nursing includes both the prelicensure program as well as a curriculum option called the RN to BSN Completion Program for registered nurses seeking a baccalaureate degree.

The College is accredited by the North Central Association of Colleges and Schools, and the nursing program is accredited by the National League for Nursing Accrediting Commission.

Mount Carmel College of Nursing is a subsidiary of Mount Carmel Health and boasts one of the largest undergraduate nursing programs among all Ohio private colleges with nursing programs. The learning is enhanced by experiences and opportunities made possible by the College's inclusion in Mount Carmel Health System, an integrated delivery system. Mount Carmel includes three acute-care hospitals, community outreach programs, hospice, home health, and ambulatory care centers.

Founded in 1903 by the Congregation of the Sisters of the Holy Cross, Mount Carmel offered a diploma program until 1993. In 1990, Mount Carmel College of Nursing was established. MCCN offers small classes, one-on-one instruction, and the opportunity to form lifelong friendships. A variety of cocurricular activities exists to enrich the college experience.

Mount Carmel College of Nursing is committed to respect for all persons, holistic development of individuals, and encouragement of social responsibility.

PROGRAMS OF STUDY

MCCN offers a comprehensive approach to health-care education. The Prelicensure Program leads to a Bachelor of Science degree in nursing. This traditional four-year program is designed for students without previous nursing experience. The first two years of study focus on completing general education requirements, which provide the foundation for the nursing program. Nursing studies begin in the sophomore year, when the curriculum combines hands-on clinical experiences with classroom theory. Nursing course work emphasizes clinical practice in a variety of acute-care hospitals and community-based centers. In addition to regular classes, the nursing and humanity seminars encourage students to explore personal health-related interests and provides them with rich cultural experiences.

The Advanced Placement Program allows students to transfer in all non-nursing courses from their first two years of study at other institutions of higher learning. When degree requirements (prerequisite courses completed) are met, a nursing degree can be obtained in five semesters. All transfer students must complete a twelve-week summer advanced-placement tract at the College prior to the fall semester start.

The RN to BSN Completion Program is designed for registered nurses who want to earn a Bachelor of Science degree in nursing. The registered nurse can complete degree requirements in four semesters of full-time study. Classes are scheduled one full day per week, so that RNs may work full-time if necessary. Class sizes are small and designed to meet the individual needs of the student. The program offers flexibility for the nurse seeking his or her level of expertise within the confines of course objectives.

A Master of Science program, which includes specialty tracks in palliative care and nursing education, began in 2003.

AFFILIATIONS WITH HEALTH-CARE FACILITIES

Clinical learning experiences are offered at several hospitals, including those within the Mount Carmel network and at Children's' Hospital in Columbus. Other clinical opportunities are conducted in conjunction with numerous community health agencies within central Ohio. Clinical sites may include Mount Carmel West Hospital, Mount Carmel East Hospital, Mount Carmel St. Ann's Hospital, Children's Hospital, neighboring elementary schools, Maryhaven Drug and Substance Abuse Center, and community-based agencies. The clinical areas of study offer students an excellent and well-rounded opportunity to experience all elements of nursing care in a variety of environments.

ACADEMIC FACILITIES

As part of a large health-care delivery system, students at MCCN have access to a full professional library. The library provides a full range of reference, bibliographic, and interlibrary loan services.

Students also have access to an on-site Learning Resource Center, which is designed specifically to support studies. The center includes a fully equipped computer lab for student use and a multimedia area that houses state-of-the-art instructional technology.

LOCATION

Mount Carmel College of Nursing is located on the near West Side of Columbus, Ohio, on the hospital campus of Mount Carmel West. With well over a million residents in its metropolitan area, Columbus is a diverse city. Mount Carmel is located just minutes from the exciting downtown area, which is conveniently located near shopping theaters, sporting events, and parks.

Columbus has all the benefits of a large city without losing the feeling of small-town warmth and spontaneity.

STUDENT SERVICES

MCCN has a full range of services to meet students' needs. There is a Student Union complete with kitchen, vending machines, and numerous sitting and reading areas; a gymnasium and exercise room; and Mount Carmel intramural sports, which include organized basketball, volleyball, and softball teams. A student nursing organization, SNAM, is an excellent resource for students to establish friendships while providing community service and enhancing their skills in the field of nursing.

For students wishing to live on campus, MCCN maintains full-service dormitories within the College for easy access to classes and the faculty. In addition, students, both commuter and resident, have access to three on-campus dining options: the hospital cafeteria, Wendy's, and Tim Hortons.

For those interested in spectator sports, the Ohio State University and other nearby colleges and universities have regularly scheduled sporting events. Sports fans can enjoy games hosted by the Columbus Clippers, a Triple-A farm baseball team of the New York Yankees; the Columbus Blue Jackets, a professional ice hockey team; and the Columbus Crew, a professional soccer team.

In addition, Columbus boasts an outstanding symphony orchestra, a jazz orchestra, numerous music clubs of all genres, both opera and ballet companies, and world-class shopping and entertainment facilities including Easton Town Center, Tuttle Mall, and the Columbus City Center.

THE NURSING STUDENT GROUP

More than 40 faculty members teach 600 students in the College's nursing programs. Faculty and staff members are committed to fostering personal and academic growth–an approach that transcends into such areas as graduation and retention rates, which are among the highest in the state and far surpass national averages. For those who need help academically, "Success in College" courses are available to promote academic improvement and development.

Mount Carmel's cultural environment is one that embraces diversity. The highly successful "Learning Trail Program" assists students of various cultural backgrounds by nurturing academic, personal, and professional growth through one-on-one consultation. Minority student retention and graduation rates far exceed national averages.

Diversity extends beyond the richness that people of different backgrounds bring to the campus. Outreach programs have enabled students to visit many places including a Native American Reservation, an Appalachian mining town, and Europe.

Job placement services are available both during college and upon graduation. As an undergraduate, many opportunities exist within Mount Carmel, including those in hospitals, hospice, and home care. While there are no guarantees, these positions often lead to the first employment opportunity after graduation. In addition, senior students find assistance with referrals, job placement, resume writing, and job-seeking skills.

COSTS

Fees range from approximately $5812 for the first year to $16,694 during the fourth year. Housing costs associated with living in the dormitory are $935 per semester for double occupancy.

FINANCIAL AID

Numerous financial aid options are available to students. Financial aid is awarded based on demonstrated financial need, scholastic achievement, and other considerations in the form of loans, employment opportunities, scholarships, and grants. Students may find assistance through the College's own financial aid programs and through federal programs. Representatives from the MCCN financial aid department can assist students in exploring various options.

APPLYING

Applicants with college credit must meet MCCN general admission requirements and must have earned a college GPA of 2.25 or higher. ACT or SAT scores need not be submitted if 30 hours of college credit have been successfully completed. Applicants should submit official transcripts from all colleges and universities attended. Transfer students must also submit an official high school transcript.

The following criteria are used for admission: A high school diploma (or GED) with a minimum cumulative GPA of 2.5 is required; a GPA of 3.0 is preferred. The applicant may submit evidence of a college GPA of 2.25 or higher in lieu of the high school GPA. High school course requirements are English, four courses; college preparatory math, two courses (three recommended); laboratory science, two courses (biology and chemistry); social science, two courses; foreign language, two courses (sign language is an option); and visual or performing arts, one course (two recommended). If any of the above courses are not passed in high school, the applicant is required to take these classes at the college level and earn a minimum grade of C (+/-). The courses must be completed prior to the applicant attending Mount Carmel College of Nursing. (All applicants must submit a transcript from high school.) All applicants must provide ACT or SAT scores, except applicants who have been out of high school more than five years or have at least 30 college/university credits. An essay is also required. To schedule a visit and tour, students should call either number listed below. For information about all programs within MCCN, students can contact the school via any of the methods listed below.

CORRESPONDENCE AND INFORMATION

Office of Admission
Mount Carmel College of Nursing
127 South Davis Avenue
Columbus, Ohio 43222
Telephone: 614-234-4CON
800-556-6942 (toll-free)
World Wide Web: http://www.mccn.edu

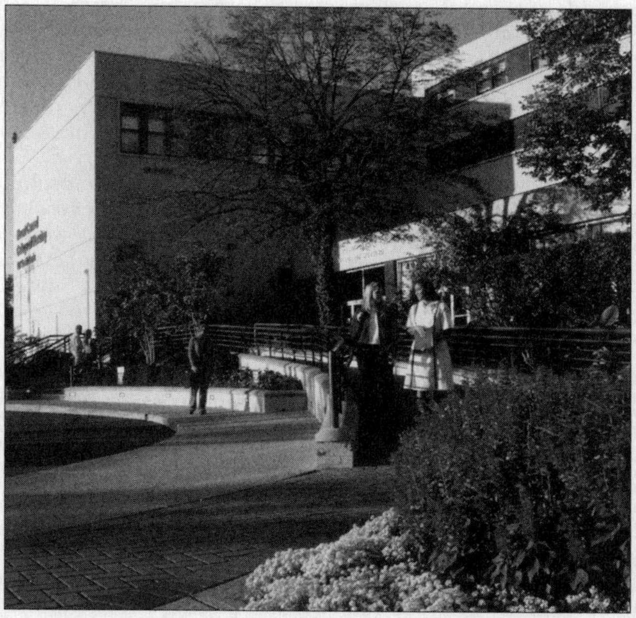

Individualized attention, small classes, and highly experienced and caring faculty members foster excellence in education at Mount Carmel College of Nursing.

Mount Saint Mary College
Division of Nursing
Newburgh, New York

THE COLLEGE

Mount Saint Mary College is a private, four-year liberal arts college for men and women with an enrollment of 2,600 students. With a favorable student-faculty ratio of 16:1, the Mount provides a warm and personal atmosphere. Mount Saint Mary College is a young, vibrant, growing school where group commitment is made to the individual student.

Since opening its doors in 1960, the College's basic goals have been the pursuit and dissemination of knowledge and the development of the capacity to discern and use it. The Mount maintains a firm belief in the value of a liberal arts education and a commitment to the Judeo-Christian traditions upon which is was founded. It retains the spirit of the intellectual, cultural, ethical, spiritual, and social philosophies of its founders.

The College's mission is to form a vital academic community characterized by the attitude that learning is a lifelong process. This process involves the ongoing acquisition of knowledge, skills, and experience and a continuing selection of values and a commitment to a value system.

THE DIVISION OF NURSING

Mount Saint Mary College's nursing program prepares students to practice as highly skilled professionals capable of meeting the demands of a rapidly evolving health-care system. Students who graduate from the Mount have a strong theoretical basis enhanced by development of clinical skills. This is achieved through nursing course work, clinical experiences, and a liberal arts background. Students apply what they learn in class directly to real-life experiences in their clinical experiences and cooperative education placements.

Intimate with today's ever-racing, ever-changing atmosphere, the faculty emphasizes a critical-thinking, problem-solving approach to nursing care. Students are prepared to work in multicultural health-care settings, where they utilize creative solutions to make independent patient care decisions. Students collaborate with other members of a health-care team to provide the best possible care.

PROGRAMS OF STUDY

The Bachelor of Science degree program in nursing prepares graduates for diverse careers in nursing and for graduate study. The program integrates professional nursing courses with a liberal arts education that emphasizes evidence-based practice, professional values, development of a strong knowledge base, skill competence, an appreciation of human and cultural diversity, and the development of leadership skills.

There are 120 credits required for the degree. In addition to the liberal arts core requirements and nursing courses, nursing students take multiple courses in biology and chemistry. The nursing program is accredited by the Commission on Collegiate Nursing Education.

The baccalaureate program offers several options for undergraduate study, including the traditional track (fall and spring semesters), evening accelerated track, and the RN Fast Track. Upon completion of all program requirements, graduates take the NCLEX for licensure as registered nurses.

Graduates are employed worldwide in hospitals, long-term-care facilities, community agencies, management, research, academia, government, private corporations, and professional organizations. Alumni have earned master's and doctoral degrees as well as certifications in many nursing specialty areas.

AFFILIATIONS WITH HEALTH-CARE FACILITIES

Mount Saint Mary College's nursing students begin working in health-care settings the second semester of the sophomore year and continue throughout their senior year. Students are assigned to a variety of hospitals and community agencies for clinical experiences. Assignments vary from semester to semester but typically include St. Luke's hospital in Newburgh, New York; St. Francis and Vassar Brothers hospitals in Poughkeepsie, New York; Cornwall Hospital in Cornwall, New York; Orange Medical Center in Goshen and Middletown, New York; Westchester Medical Center in Valhalla, New York; Danbury Hospital in Danbury, Connecticut; and VA Medical Centers as well as area health departments, community health centers, schools, homes, nursing homes, and senior citizens centers.

ACADEMIC FACILITIES

The fully computerized Curtin Memorial Library provides a state-of-the-art Integrated Online Library System that provides access to the library's holdings and an automated check-out system. Students are able to use the system from the library, the Academic Computer Center, and their dorm rooms. Students have access to online search services. These search services provide access to periodical databases with journal article citations and some full-text articles. The library has online access to First Search and the Expanded Academic Index. The library has several periodical databases on CD-ROM.

The library collection has more than 120,000 volumes, more than 1,100 periodical subscriptions, and an extensive video collection. The College coordinates an interlibrary loan program with public and private libraries throughout the Hudson Valley region.

The newly renovated Nursing Learning Resource Center (LRC) is open to nursing students to gain practical experience in nursing techniques. Hospital equipment and patient simulators are available to aid in the acquisition of nursing skills. The LRC also includes ten computer workstations with state-of-the-art interactive software to enhance learning.

Students have access to the campus network, online library resources, e-mail, and the Internet from residence halls and many other campus facilities via the Wireless Academic Network. The Academic Computer Center contains six separate computer facilities using the latest PC technology, including multimedia capabilities. Teaching facilities include modern classrooms equipped with television monitors, two 20-station PC classrooms, a state-of-the-art multimedia production center, faculty technology center, and the availability of laptops with LCD projection screens for computer presentations outside the laboratories.

LOCATION

Mount Saint Mary College's campus sits on the banks of the scenic Hudson River in a residential section of Newburgh, New York, approximately halfway between Albany and New York City. The campus is served by Stewart International Airport. The nearby Catskill Mountains offer recreational opportunities all year long, including ski trips and hikes.

STUDENT SERVICES

The Mount offers students more than classes, tests, and term papers. Students are encouraged to take advantage of the 30 clubs and organizations on campus. The Student Government Association is the legislative body for student life.

All undergraduate nursing majors belong to the Nursing Student Union (NSU) from the time they enter the College. NSU is an integral part of nursing students' experiences since its inception in the 1960s. This group offers students the opportunity to develop leadership skills by participating in college governance, networking, and community service activities. The organization is governed by students with the assistance of a nursing faculty adviser who is selected by the students. Students elect their own officers, administer their own budget, and determine their own agenda. All activities required for NSU events are planned and carried out by the students, including the invitation of speakers, printing invitations, and other program activities. Students also participate in health fairs and organize study groups for freshmen nursing students. Students may also get involved with the National Student Nurses Association and the international chapter of Sigma Theta Tau, the honor society for nursing. The experience of working together as a team and coordinating important events offers the students invaluable experience as they prepare for careers as professional nurses. Ninety percent of all nursing graduates are employed in the nursing field or enrolled in graduate school within six months of graduation.

THE NURSING STUDENT GROUP

The nursing program provides an opportunity for close interaction between faculty and students. All undergraduate nursing students belong to the Nursing Student Union from the time they enter as nursing majors until they graduate. The feasibility of establishing a chapter of the National Student Nurses Association is being explored, and it would provide numerous membership benefits beyond the College. Selected senior nursing students are invited to join the College's chapter of Sigma Theta Tau International, the honor society for nursing. A nursing student listserv keeps students and faculty members connected in a meaningful way.

COSTS

For the 2004–05 academic year, undergraduate tuition was $15,180. Graduate program tuition for the academic year was $554 per credit.

FINANCIAL AID

Mount Saint Mary College's financial aid program provides assistance in the form of federal, state, and campus-based scholarships, and grants, loans, and part-time employment for students who demonstrate academic potential but whose resources are insufficient to meet the costs of higher education. High-achieving students may also benefit from awards based solely on previous academic performance. Using March 15 as a priority date, students apply for financial aid by completing the admissions process and filing the Free Application for Federal Student Aid (FAFSA).

APPLYING

Students who wish to apply to the Mount's undergraduate nursing program should submit a completed application form and a $35 application fee to the Admissions Office. Students should also make arrangements for their high school transcript and SAT scores to be forwarded to the same office. Letters of recommendation, while not required, are strongly advised. Mount Saint Mary College operates on a rolling admissions policy. Once a student's file is complete, he or she is usually notified of the admissions decision within two to four weeks.

The graduate nursing division requires applicants to submit an application at least six weeks before the desired entry date. Applicants must submit a completed application form and fee; official transcripts from all institutions attended, undergraduate and graduate; a photocopy of New York State RN license/registration and malpractice insurance identification; official GRE or MAT scores; three letters of recommendation; a personal statement of interest; qualifications; career goals; official TOEFL score (if applicable); and a completed health form. Upon receipt of all documents the applicant will be notified and instructed to arrange an interview with the Program Coordinator.

CORRESPONDENCE AND INFORMATION

Director of Admissions
Mount Saint Mary College
330 Powell Avenue
Newburgh, New York 12550
Telephone: 845-569-3248
888-YES-MSMC (toll-free)
E-mail: mtstmary@msmc.edu
World Wide Web: http://www.msmc.edu

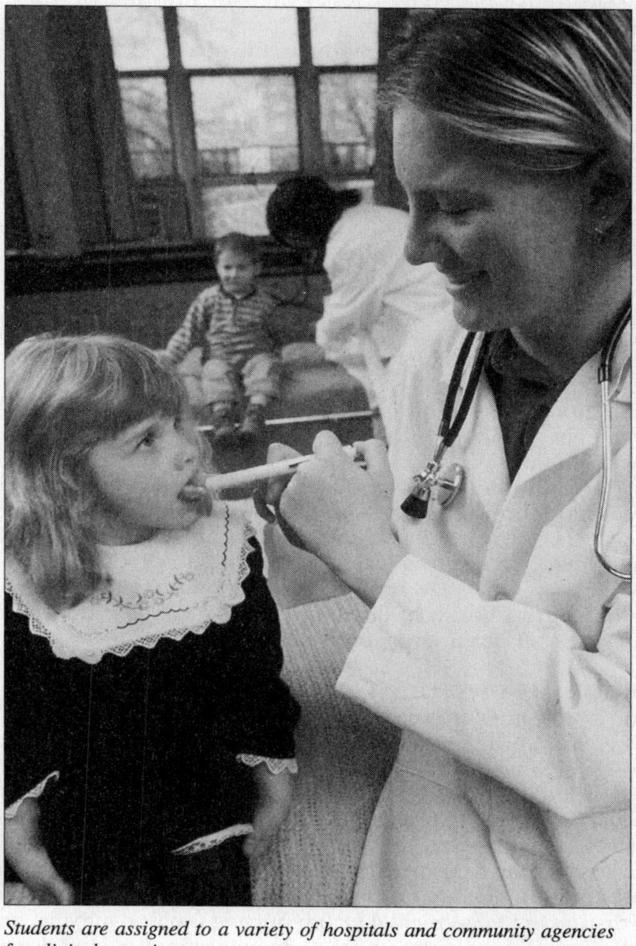

Students are assigned to a variety of hospitals and community agencies for clinical experiences.

New York University
Division of Nursing
New York, New York

THE UNIVERSITY

New York University (NYU), the largest private university in the country, was founded in 1831. NYU draws top students from every state and from 140 other countries. The University attracts a world-famous faculty and distinguished student body.

The University includes fourteen schools and colleges. In NYU's Division of Nursing, students have all the advantages and resources found only at a major research university, yet they are also part of a small college community that shares a commitment to the health and welfare of humanity. Exchanging ideas with scholars in health, education, and the arts assists nursing students' growth as professionals and people.

THE DIVISION OF NURSING

Excellence has placed New York University's Division of Nursing among the nation's top nursing programs. The intellectual energies of the faculty and students, the quality of the academic resources, and the rich interaction with a vibrant city provide a learning experience that is unique in its rigor and diversity. All programs—baccalaureate, master's, and doctorate—provide a dynamic balance between nursing theory and practice. These programs prepare graduates for leadership roles in direct care, administration, research, or teaching. They reflect the latest advances in knowledge and technology as well as today's modern health-care environment.

All of the Division of Nursing's full-time, tenure-track faculty members are doctorally prepared. Full-time clinical faculty members are all master's or doctorally prepared expert practitioners. Part-time faculty members hold at least a master's degree in their clinical specialty area. When students graduate, in addition to a wealth of knowledge and skills, they take with them the ability to think analytically—the hallmark of a successful nursing career.

NYU Division of Nursing alumni are in positions of leadership throughout the world, where they practice in diverse clinical, academic, and administrative settings. Many are making their mark through nursing science research. Others have forged new roles as entrepreneurs in private practice or as consultants to health insurers, pharmaceutical companies, and international health organizations.

PROGRAMS OF STUDY

The NYU Division of Nursing offers a four-year, generic B.S. program, which includes a special sequence of courses for registered nurses; a B.S. for college graduates, which may be completed in a regular track or fifteen-month accelerated track; a dual-degree B.S./M.A. program; an M.A. in nursing education; an M.A. in nursing administration; an M.A. in nursing informatics; an M.A. in advanced practice nursing adult acute care, adult primary care, geriatrics, adult/geriatrics, and pediatrics as well as mental health nursing, holistic nursing, and palliative care nursing; an M.A. in midwifery; a joint-degree program with the Wagner Graduate School of Public Service (M.A. in nursing administration/M.S. in management); and a Ph.D. in research and theory development in nursing science. The Division of Nursing also offers post-master's certificate programs in advanced nursing practice: administration, adult acute care, adult primary care, geriatrics, adult/geriatrics, pediatrics, mental health nursing, palliative care, holistic nursing, nursing informatics, and midwifery. The Division also offers M.A. subspecialty concentrations and post-master's certificates in children with special needs, substance abuse disorders, and home-health nursing and a master's completion sequence for certificate-prepared nurse practitioners and certified nurse midwives.

The B.S. program in nursing prepares students to manage the full scope of nursing care responsibilities in today's complex health-care environment. The nursing science curricula emphasize a humanistic approach that examines the social, emotional, and environmental context in which wellness and illness occur. Students examine the growth and development of the family structure, patterns that characterize different age groups, human behavior in health and illness, and the effects of chronic illness. In the classroom, students learn nursing theories, nursing process, and relevant knowledge. Students apply these theories in practice through laboratory and clinical study. Students gain experience in all clinical areas, including maternal-child health, adult medical-surgical nursing, community/psychiatric nursing, geriatric nursing, and nursing leadership. Students work with all ages and cultures in a range of settings.

The M.A. programs in advanced education in nursing science prepare students for leadership roles in management, nursing education, informatics, and advanced nursing practice. They are unique programs that subscribe to a philosophy and vision of nursing reflecting a commitment to human values and the advancement of nursing as a profession. The programs emphasize critical thinking, the development and use of a theoretical base for advanced practice, the application of evidence-based practice to further nursing practice knowledge, and the promotion of a professional identity. The 45- to 48-point curricula include a core in nursing theory, clinical advanced practice core, an area of concentration, and related cognates and electives. Graduates of the clinical programs are eligible to sit for ANCC and other certification examinations as Nurse Practitioners and/or Clinical Nurse Specialists or are eligible for American College of Nurse-Midwives certification and licensure as a professional midwife in New York State. All advanced practice nursing programs are registered by the state of New York as nurse practitioner programs. The Post-M.A. Advanced Certificate Programs require 12 to 30 points.

The Ph.D. program in research and theory development in nursing science educates scholars in the critical and creative study of human beings and their environment and prepares leaders to examine issues in nursing and health care. The required course work of approximately 54 points is taken in the Division of Nursing and other University departments on a full- or part-time basis. The curriculum is designed to provide a solid research foundation in quantitative and qualitative methods, which generates nursing knowledge and furthers theory development and substantive practice within the discipline.

AFFILIATIONS WITH HEALTH-CARE FACILITIES

The Division of Nursing offers clinical and practicum experience at many of the nation's foremost hospitals, including NYU Medical Center, Bellevue Hospital Center, Mt. Sinai Medical Center, St. Vincent's Hospital, Beth Israel Medical Center, and more than fifty other acute-care hospitals. Students also gain significant experience in community settings, including Visiting

Nurse Service, the Brooklyn Mobile Health Van, and other ambulatory and home-care settings.

ACADEMIC FACILITIES

NYU's Bobst Library is one of the largest open-stack research libraries in the world. Bobst is one of eight NYU libraries, including the Medical Center Library, to which nursing students have access. The Division of Nursing provides Nursing Arts Laboratories, which enable students to practice their nursing skills in a simulated hospital setting.

LOCATION

NYU is located in historic Greenwich Village, traditionally a community of artists and intellectuals. NYU's campus is within minutes of off-Broadway drama, Little Italy, Chinatown, and renowned museums. As an international center of finance, culture, and communications, New York City offers unmatched educational, internship, and social opportunities.

STUDENT SERVICES

The University offers students a variety of services and resources, including the Office of Counseling and Student Services; the Office for African American, Latino, and Asian American Services; the University Health Center; the Office of Career Services; the Coles Sports and Recreation Center; Information Technology Services; and the Henry and Lucy Moses Center for Students with Disabilities.

THE NURSING STUDENT GROUP

The student body represents most of the fifty states and many other countries. This diversification affords opportunities for rich and lasting relationships. The average student is a mature, self-directed individual who assumes both professional and academic responsibilities, often in addition to family commitments.

COSTS

Tuition and fees for 2004–05 were $30,094 (including nonrefundable registration and services fees) for full-time undergraduates. Graduate students paid $951 per point (plus nonrefundable registration and services fees).

FINANCIAL AID

Financial aid at NYU comes from many sources. In order to meet an applicant's financial need, the University may offer a package of aid that includes scholarships or grants, loans, or work-study programs. NYU requires the submission of the Free Application for Federal Student Aid (FAFSA).

The Division of Nursing offers a competitive financial aid program. Scholarships for full-time and part-time study are available. For master's and doctoral candidates, a number of fellowships and assistantships are available. Information on financial aid may be obtained from the Office of Financial Aid by calling 212-998-4444.

APPLYING

As baccalaureate program requirements differ for the generic, RN, college graduate, and dual B.S.-M.A. programs, interested students should contact the Division of Nursing Office of Enrollment Services at 212-998-5317 for specific requirements. For admission to the M.A. program, a candidate must have a baccalaureate nursing degree from an accredited nursing program. A minimum overall GPA of 3.0, RN licensure, two professional letters of reference, a goal statement, and an interview are also required. TOEFL scores are required for students whose native language is not English. Students who have not met the prerequisites of basic statistics and nursing research may take them while in the program. Applicants with an associate degree in nursing and a bachelor's degree in another field may apply to the M.A. program.

Admission requirements for the post-master's advanced certificate programs are a master's degree in nursing with a minimum 3.0 GPA. For admission to the Ph.D. program, the applicant must be a nurse with baccalaureate and master's degrees acceptable to NYU, with at least one degree in nursing. A minimum grade point average of 3.0 on a scale of 4.0 and GRE scores of at least 1000 are required. In addition, the applicant must submit a resume, demonstration of professional performance/contribution to the nursing profession, two professional reference letters, a three- to five-page goal statement, copies of GRE scores, and transcripts of college-level work.

CORRESPONDENCE AND INFORMATION

Office of Enrollment Services
Division of Nursing
New York University
246 Greene Street
New York, New York 10003-6677
Telephone: 212-998-5317
E-mail: nursing.programs@nyu.edu
World Wide Web: http://www.education.nyu.edu/nursing

THE FACULTY

Carolyn Auerhahn, Clinical Assistant Professor; Ed.D., Columbia.
Mary Brennan, Clinical Assistant Professor; M.S., Boston College.
Patricia Burkhardt, Clinical Associate Professor; M.P.H., Dr.P.H., Johns Hopkins.
Elizabeth Capezuti, Professor; Ph.D., Pennsylvania.
Barbara Carty, Clinical Associate Professor; Ed.D., Columbia.
Donna (Danuta) Clemmens, Assistant Professor; Ph.D., Connecticut.
Mei Fu, Assistant Professor; Ph.D., Missouri.
Terry Fulmer, Professor and Head, Division of Nursing; Ph.D., Boston College.
Judith Haber, Professor and Director, Master's and Post-Master's Programs; Ph.D., NYU.
Laura Hayman, Professor; Ph.D., Pennsylvania.
Nancy Jackson, Clinical Associate Professor; Ed.D., Columbia.
Kathleen Kenney, Clinical Associate Professor; M.S.N., SUNY at Stony Brook.
Christine Tassone Kovner, Professor; M.S.N., Pennsylvania; Ph.D., NYU.
Carla H. Mariano, Associate Professor; M.Ed., Ed.D., Columbia.
Linda Mayberry, Associate Professor; Ph.D., California, San Francisco.
Sandee McClowry, Associate Professor; Ph.D., California, San Francisco.
Diane O. McGivern, Professor; Ph.D., NYU.
Mathy Mezey, Independence Foundation Professor of Nursing Education; M.Ed., Ed.D., Columbia.
Madeline A. Naegle, Associate Professor; Ph.D., NYU.
Elizabeth Norman, Professor and Director, Doctoral Program, Division of Nursing; Ph.D., NYU.
Melanie Percy, Assistant Professor; Ph.D., South Carolina.
Hila Richardson, Clinical Professor; Dr.P.H., Columbia.
Deborah Sherman, Associate Professor; M.S.N., Pace; Ph.D., NYU.

Northeastern University
School of Nursing
Bouvé College of Health Sciences
Boston, Massachusetts

THE UNIVERSITY
Northeastern University is a private, urban university in Boston and a world leader in cooperative education (Co-op). The University is committed to achieving excellence through high-quality instruction in liberal and professional curricula and providing individuals with opportunities for access to an excellent education. The University has a distinguished, nationally and internationally known faculty of dedicated teachers, researchers, and scholars. The Bouvé College of Health Sciences at Northeastern University comprises the School of Nursing, the School of Pharmacy, and the School of Health Professions.

THE SCHOOL OF NURSING
The primary mission of the School of Nursing is to prepare nursing leaders for basic and advanced nursing practice that contributes to the health of the nation. Faculty members are actively engaged in nursing practice in a variety of health-care settings and conduct research in their specialty areas. Nursing students spend a substantial portion of their clinical time in the neighborhoods of Boston, working and learning with students from other health disciplines to address the needs of an urban population. Students receive clinical instruction in many of Boston's world-renowned hospitals.

PROGRAMS OF STUDY
The School offers a five-year cooperative education Bachelor of Science in Nursing (B.S.N.) degree program and an upper-division transfer-track into the B.S.N. program for students who meet the requirements for transferable college credit applicable to Northeastern's curriculum. An RN-to-B.S.N. track is also available.

The baccalaureate program is designed to prepare students to become professional nurses for practice in a variety of health-care settings, such as communities, hospitals, neighborhood health centers, schools, and homes. Faculty members focus educational efforts on preparing students to learn management of acute and episodic illnesses and complex chronic diseases of clients. Leadership development, case management, discharge planning, and economics of health care are essential components of the curriculum. The School aims to provide all students—including those with diverse backgrounds and changing career goals—with a broad-based education and the stimulus for ongoing personal and professional growth. The curriculum offers instruction in nursing theory and research, the humanities, and the biological, psychological, physical, and social sciences. More than 50 percent of the course work is in sciences and humanities.

The baccalaureate program alternates academic semesters with paid work experience in health-care settings. This combination of academic study and co-op experience produces an overall learning experience that gives greater meaning to the nursing academic program and direction to a student's career choice and development. Students work with a Co-op Coordinator to plan paid work experiences that meet their individual needs.

The program is accredited by the Commission on Collegiate Nursing Education and the National League for Nursing Accrediting Commission and approved by the Board of Registration in Nursing of the Commonwealth of Massachusetts. Successful completion of the baccalaureate program allows graduates to take the National Council Licensing Examination (NCLEX-RN) to become registered nurses.

The School offers two options for individuals who already have a baccalaureate degree in another field who seek a career change into nursing. They can enter the three-year, upper-division transfer-track program and receive a B.S.N. degree or they can enter the Direct Entry Program to earn a Master of Science degree with a major in nursing. This is a full-time program that combines 64 semester credit hours of RN-preparation course work, one 6- to 8-month cooperative education experience, and completion of one specialization in the Master of Science program (explained below), to prepare graduates as advanced practice nurses.

The School of Nursing offers a Master of Science degree program to prepare graduates as nurse practitioners, clinical specialists, nurse anesthetists, and managers. The master's program offers clinical specializations in administration; anesthesia; critical care; neonatal care; pediatric, adult, or family primary care; and psychiatric–mental health nursing. Within the framework of nursing science, the concepts of community-based care, emergent leadership, professional competence, and intra/interdisciplinary collaboration provide the foundation for advanced professional practice. The curriculum varies depending upon the specialization but generally requires 43 semester hours. It is designed so that students can pursue either full-time or part-time study. Full-time students can expect to complete the degree requirements in four semesters over two calendar years. Part-time students may take up to five years to complete the program. Classes are offered in the late afternoon and evening. Modifications in the curriculum exist to qualify for certification for various specialties. The B.S.N./M.S. program offers an innovative pathway for nurses holding a diploma or an associate degree in nursing to earn a joint B.S.N./M.S. degree; the program requires 67 semester hours for graduation. The M.S./M.B.A. degree program is a 70-semester-hour program that prepares nurses for executive-level management in health care. The nurse anesthesia program is a full-time, twenty-seven-month, 53-semester-hour program.

Certificates of Advanced Graduate Study are offered in all of the above specialization areas. These postgraduate programs are designed for nurses with a master's degree in nursing who seek further academic preparation to learn advanced practice skills in another specialization or to qualify for national certification.

AFFILIATIONS WITH HEALTH-CARE FACILITIES
The University's location in Boston enables the School to collaborate with some of the world's premier health-care organizations. Students have supervised clinical experiences in renowned teaching hospitals and co-op opportunities in a range of acute-care, rehabilitation, and community-health facilities. Noted health-care institutions with which the School affiliates include Beth Israel Deaconess Medical Center, Boston Medical Center, Brigham and Women's Hospital, Caritas St. Elizabeth's Medical Center, Dana-Farber Cancer Institute, Children's Hospital, Massachusetts General Hospital, and McLean Hospital as well as Healthcare for the Homeless, Spaulding Rehabilitation Hospital, regional Visiting Nurse associations, and many other highly regarded health-care systems. The School has a partnership with the city of Boston's Commission on Public Health, which allows unique opportunities to participate in the city's public health initiatives and neighborhood health centers.

ACADEMIC FACILITIES
In 2002, Bouvé College of Health Sciences opened the George D. Behrakis Health Sciences Center, a seven-story, 117,000-square-foot state-of-the-art building, housing classrooms, laboratories, and clinical facilities that simulate real health-care settings. The nursing laboratory has twelve student-centered practice areas, including fully equipped hospital stations and patient treatment areas. Nursing students practice assessment and procedural skills using simulators and mannequins across the life span.

Northeastern has several interdisciplinary centers and institutes that engage in research in collaboration with academic departments. The Division of Academic Computing provides students with access to computing resources. A high-speed data network links users and facilities on the central campus and three satellite campuses. In addition, the campus network is connected via the Internet to computing resources around the world. University libraries contain more than 893,000 bound volumes, 2.1 million microfilms, 150,000 documents, 8,585 periodical subscriptions, and 18,861 audio, video, and software titles. A central library contains technologically sophisticated services, including online catalog and circulation systems, a gateway to external networked information resources, and a network of CD-ROM optical disk databases.

LOCATION

Northeastern's 67-acre Boston campus is in the heart of the Back Bay section of the city, between the Museum of Fine Arts and Symphony Hall and a short walk from Fenway Park. At Northeastern, students discover that part of the adventure of going to college in Boston is exploring the cultural, educational, historical, and recreational offerings of the city. In addition, Cape Cod and the North Shore of Massachusetts are easily reached by car or public transportation for swimming, surfing, and boating. The scenic areas of northern New England are accessible for skiing, hiking, and mountain climbing.

STUDENT SERVICES

The University has many resources and service offices to meet student needs. These include the University Health and Counseling Services, the Cabot Physical Education Center, the Marino Recreational Center (open 24 hours a day, seven days a week), the campus bookstore, Academic Computing Services, Campus Ministry, housing, dining services, the International Student Office, the English Language Center, the John D. O'Bryant African-American Institute, the Latino/a Student Cultural Center, and the Center for Counseling and Student Development. The Bouvé College of Health Sciences Office of Student Services offers academic advising and schedules tutorial sessions and other activities.

THE NURSING STUDENT GROUP

There are approximately 700 students enrolled in the School of Nursing: just under 600 undergraduates and 115 graduate students. They represent a wide variety of academic, professional, and cultural backgrounds. Nursing students come all across the United States as well as from Asia, Europe, and Africa. Approximately 5 percent of the nursing students are men.

COSTS

For 2004–05, freshman tuition was $26,750, room and board cost $9810, and other mandatory student fees were approximately $300. Graduate tuition per semester hour was $825 for full- and part-time students. Full-time mandatory fees ranged from $224 to $2000, depending on the specialty. Books and supplies averaged $800 for the academic year.

FINANCIAL AID

The University operates a substantial aid program designed to make attendance at Northeastern feasible for all qualified students. By coordinating the resources of the University and various public and private scholarship programs, the Office of Student Financial Services was able to provide more than $100 million to more than 10,000 students in 2004–05. Approximately 81 percent of the freshman class received some form of financial aid. Financial aid is based on need and academic merit and may consist of grants, loans, work-study employment, or any combination of these three items. To apply, incoming undergraduate students must file a Free Application for Federal Student Aid (FAFSA) and a CSS PROFILE form with the College Scholarship Service by the priority filing date of February 15. Graduate students must file the FAFSA and an Institutional Aid Application.

Northeastern awards need-based financial aid to graduate students through the Federal Perkins Loan, Federal Work-Study, and Federal Stafford Student Loan programs. The University also offers a limited number of minority fellowships and Martin Luther King, Jr. Scholarships. In addition, the graduate school offers financial assistance through teaching, research, and administrative assistantship awards. Assistantship awards vary and can include tuition remission and stipends. Nurse traineeship funds are also available for graduate students in their clinical year.

APPLYING

Admission to Northeastern is selective and competitive. For the 2004–05 academic year, the University received 24,400 applications for 2,800 places in the freshman class. In building a diverse and talented class, the University seeks to enroll students who have been successful academically and who have shown a strong commitment to school and community through extracurricular activities. Students who have earned strong grades in a rigorous college-preparatory program, are innovative and creative, and who possess leadership abilities are most successful in the University's admission process. December 15 is the deadline for priority consideration for freshmen for September admission, merit scholarships, and admission to the Honors Program. February 1 is the general deadline for September admission. Freshmen who apply for the fall entrance date by February 1 are mailed a decision between March 1 and April 1. If accepted for fall admission, freshmen are required to send a tuition deposit by May 1 to secure a place in the class. For transfer students, the priority deadline for the fall is May 1. Campus tours and group information sessions are held daily and are available without an appointment.

Applicants to the graduate program should have earned a baccalaureate degree in nursing from a program accredited by the Commission on Collegiate Nursing Education or by the National League for Nursing Accrediting Commission. The B.S.N./M.S. program, however, allows nurses who have graduated from accredited diploma and associate degree programs to pursue graduate study. The Direct Entry Program allows applicants with a bachelor's degree in a field other than nursing to be admitted as a graduate student in nursing. An elementary statistics course is a prerequisite for all applicants.

Admission requirements include a satisfactory scholastic record, an official copy of all college transcripts, satisfactory scores on the General Test of the Graduate Record Examinations (GRE), the Miller Analogies Test (MAT), or the Graduate Management Admission Test (GMAT) for M.S./M.B.A. applicants. Three letters of recommendation, a personal goal statement, one to two years of current professional nursing practice, and current registration to practice nursing in the United States are also required. There are some modifications in the requirements for the Direct Entry program, the B.S.N./M.S. program, and for international students, including the submission of TOEFL scores by international students whose native language is not English. The application fee is $50 for the graduate programs. Students may be admitted in the fall, spring, or summer semesters, depending on the program of study; however, students interested in full-time study should submit their application by March 1 for the fall semester. Applications for the nurse anesthesia specialization are due December 1 and applications for the Direct Entry program are due February 1 for admission in the fall semester. Special needs students are welcome.

CORRESPONDENCE AND INFORMATION

Office of Undergraduate Admissions
150 Richards Hall
Northeastern University
360 Huntington Avenue
Boston, Massachusetts 02115
Telephone: 617-373-2200
617-373-3100 (TTY)
Fax: 617-373-8780
E-mail: admissions@neu.edu
World Wide Web: http://www.admissions.neu.edu

Graduate Application Inquiries and Application Requests
Bouvé College of Health Sciences
120 Behrakis Health Science Center
Northeastern University
Boston, Massachusetts 02115-5096
Telephone: 617-373-3125
Fax: 617-373-4701
E-mail: bouvegrad@neu.edu
World Wide Web: http://www.bouve.neu.edu

THE DEAN

Nancy Hoffart, Dean and Professor, School of Nursing; Ph.D., RN.

Quinnipiac University
Department of Nursing
Hamden, Connecticut

THE UNIVERSITY

Quinnipiac University, founded in 1929, is an independent, coeducational, nonsectarian institution. It is primarily a residential university on an attractive New England campus. Quinnipiac employs a large undergraduate faculty (265 full-time members) relative to the size of its undergraduate student body (5,089), keeping the University-wide student-faculty ratio at 16:1. The full graduate and undergraduate enrollment is 7,121. The University maintains an extensive network of professional associations with the health, business, and education communities through prominent clinical programs and internship placements.

THE DEPARTMENT OF NURSING

The baccalaureate nursing program at Quinnipiac University was instituted in 1991, with the first class graduating in 1995. The National Council Licensure Examination for Registered Nurses (NCLEX-RN) pass rate is greater than 90 percent. There are currently 12 full-time faculty members and about 25 adjunct faculty members.

The undergraduate curriculum is an upper-division major. Students admitted to the professional component in the junior year must have attained a cumulative grade point average of 2.67. Continued good standing requires that the cumulative as well as the semester grade point average of 2.67 be maintained for the remainder of the program.

The nursing curriculum at Quinnipiac fosters professional socialization for future roles and responsibilities within the profession. Graduates of the program are prepared as generalists to begin the practice of professional nursing with sound theoretical foundations and more than 800 hours of diverse clinical practice experiences. Graduates are also prepared for graduate study. In addition to the generalist perspective, the curriculum provides an introductory specialty focus in which senior students may select a precepted experience.

PROGRAMS OF STUDY

All programs within the School of Health Sciences are based on a comprehensive foundation in the liberal arts and sciences. Students may attend on a part-time or full-time basis. A state-of-the-art advanced skills laboratory, utilizing resources from other health-related disciplines, is used for teaching advanced skills.

Accredited by the National League for Nursing Accrediting Commission (NLNAC), Quinnipiac's bachelor's degree program in nursing offers the theoretical and clinical education students need to enter professional nursing practice. Graduates of the program are eligible to take the NCLEX-RN exam and are well prepared for graduate study in nursing. In addition to the traditional four-year program, an innovative accelerated option is available to non-nurse college graduates.

Students admitted to the accelerated B.S.N. option earn a second baccalaureate degree in nursing in one calendar year of full-time study that commences in May. A third B.S.N. option exists for registered nurses with a diploma or an associate degree who wish to earn a B.S.N.

Because nursing involves a wide range of responsibilities, the program takes a holistic approach to the sciences, health-care theory, and the techniques of nursing. Quinnipiac's nursing faculty members also introduce their students to the cultural, social, and economic implications of health-care management.

Beginning with the first nursing course, students benefit from well-equipped labs, detailed simulations of health-care facilities, patient-oriented education, and highly effective field experiences.

The graduate nursing program, also accredited by the NLNAC, seeks to prepare professional nurses at an advanced theoretical and clinical practice level in order to address present and potential societal health need. Three available tracks are adult nurse practitioner, family nurse practitioner, and forensic nurse clinical specialist. Post-master's certificate tracks in adult and family nurse practice are also available. Quinnipiac's M.S.N. includes core courses that cover advanced concepts and theoretical foundations of nursing, research methods, and health-care policy and economics.

AFFILIATIONS WITH HEALTH-CARE FACILITIES

The school's strong affiliates with health-care providers in the area allow students to complete clinical work at such institutions as Yale–New Haven Hospital, New Britain General Hospital, the Hospital of St. Raphael, and Veterans Administration Medical Center, Mid-State Medical Center, as well as in private practices, clinics, and other health-care centers.

ACADEMIC FACILITIES

Modern buildings surround 500 acres of rolling fields and streams, adjacent to Sleeping Giant State Park. Library holdings total 304,857, with 4,291 periodicals. Quinnipiac is one of the most wired campuses in the country, and this is reflected in its academic facilities and programs. All incoming students must purchase a University recommended laptop computer for use in the classroom. Students also use their computers for e-mail and for access to online library resources and the Internet. Students can reach all of these online services from the data network in their dorm rooms or from the wireless network that covers the library and classrooms.

The technologically advanced portion of the nursing curriculum is supported by grants that afford students an opportunity to practice with sophisticated equipment in the clinical skills practice lab prior to actual clinical practice. Innovative software provides computer-assisted learning with a variety of simulated patient-care situations that challenge the student to use critical-thinking skills.

LOCATION

Quinnipiac's campus is located in suburban Hamden, Connecticut, a southern New England town 8 miles from metropolitan New Haven and 25 miles from Hartford. It is easily reached via the New England Turnpike (Interstate 95), Interstate 91, the Wilbur Cross Parkway (Merritt Parkway), and Interstate 84. There are two major airports within 45 minutes of the campus. Area attractions include the Yale Repertory Theater; the Schubert, Long Wharf, and Oakdale Theaters; the Peabody Museum; dance clubs; museums; and cinemas.

STUDENT SERVICES

Quinnipiac University has a variety of resources and services to meet the needs of students, including a 28,000-square-foot state-of-the-art recreation and fitness center, the Learning Center, the International Student Club, and the Counseling and Career Services Center.

THE NURSING STUDENT GROUP

Students in the nursing program come from a wide variety of backgrounds and geographic locations. The majority are resident full-time students. Quinnipiac's low student-faculty ratio of 16:1 ensures that nursing students receive personal attention from their professors. Graduates are employed in large medical centers, community health centers, primary-care facilities, and small community hospitals.

COSTS

Tuition costs for the 2004–05 academic year were $21,540 for full-time enrollment (16 credit hours per semester). Room and board costs were $9900, and student fees were $960. Additional expenses include books, lab fees, immunizations, uniforms, malpractice insurance, CPR certification, and travel to and parking at clinical sites.

FINANCIAL AID

Approximately 68 percent of freshmen receive financial aid, with freshman awards averaging $13,091 through a combination of grants (not to be repaid), student loans, and on-campus jobs. The University offers merit-based scholarships; the admissions application deadline for these is February 1. Students should complete and submit the Free Application for Federal Student Aid (FAFSA) to the federal processor by March 1.

APPLYING

Students may file an application early in their senior year of high school. The results of the SAT I or ACT should be forwarded to Quinnipiac University. The University has a rolling admissions policy. In November, students are notified about four weeks after the application and required documents are received. Early application is recommended to assure consideration for the program of choice. Freshman students generally have a 3.4 GPA or better average in college-preparatory courses (transfer students have a 3.0 GPA or better), rank in the top 30 percent of their high school class, and have an average combined score of 1100 on the SAT I.

CORRESPONDENCE AND INFORMATION

Joan Isaac Mohr, Vice President and Dean
Carla M. Knowlton, Director
Undergraduate Admissions
Quinnipiac University
275 Mount Carmel Avenue
Hamden, Connecticut 06518
Telephone: 203-582-8600
800-462-1944 (toll-free)
Fax: 203-582-8906
E-mail: admissions@quinnipiac.edu
World Wide Web: http://www.quinnipiac.edu

THE FACULTY

Cynthia Barrere, Associate Professor of Nursing; Ph.D., Connecticut.
E. Jane Bower, Associate Professor of Nursing; Ph.D., Adelphi.
Janet Dombroski, Assistant Professor of Nursing; M.S.N., Pace.
Anne Durkin, Associate Professor of Nursing; Ph.D., Connecticut.
Mary Helming, Assistant Professor of Nursing.
Laima Karosas, Assistant Professor of Nursing; M.S.N., Yale.
Jeanne LeVasseur, Associate Professor of Nursing; Ph.D., Connecticut.
Elizabeth McGann, Professor of Nursing and Department Chair; D.N.Sc., Yale.
Barbara Moynihan, Associate Professor of Nursing; Ph.D., Connecticut.
Lisa O'Connor, Assistant Professor of Nursing; M.S.N., Hartford.
Lynn Price, Associate Professor of Nursing; J.D., George Washington.
Janice Thompson, Associate Professor of Nursing; Ph.D., Adelphi.

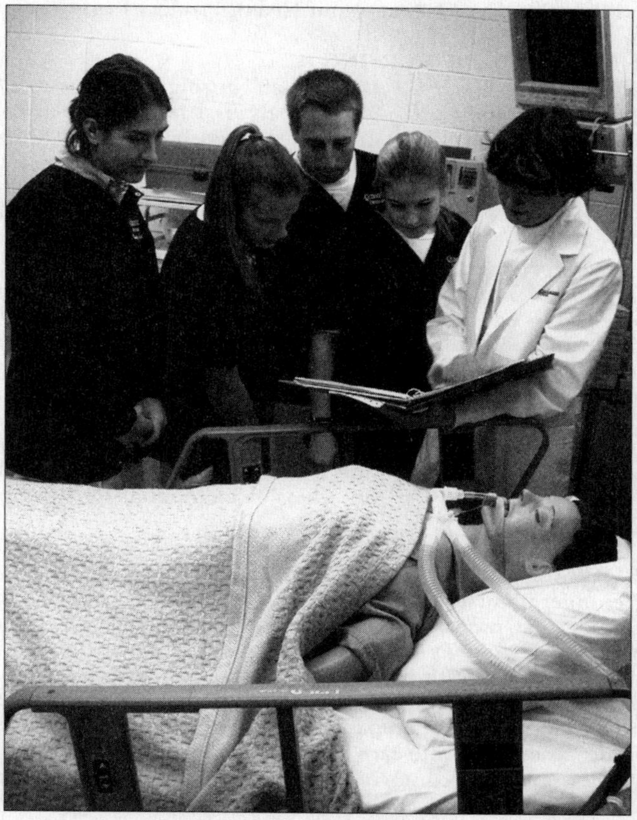

Nursing students utilize the critical-care laboratory.

Regis College
Center for Health Sciences, Nursing Program
Weston, Massachusetts

THE COLLEGE

Regis College is a small, Catholic, liberal arts and sciences college for undergraduate women and graduate-level men and women. Founded in 1927 by the Congregation of the Sisters of Saint Joseph of Boston, their members desired to put their resources to use for the good of society through education. The College is consistently rated among the top small liberal arts colleges in the North in "America's Best Colleges" by *U.S. News & World Report.* Regis College offers bachelor's degrees in a wide variety of majors and master's degrees in Nursing, Teaching, Organizational and Professional Communication, Leadership and Organizational Change, and Health Product Regulation.

THE DIVISION OF NURSING

Established in 1983, the Division of Nursing began as a B.S. degree completion program for registered nurses. A weekend track was started in 1989 and was selected by the Army Nurse Corps as an educational pathway that would fulfill reserve nurse's military obligations while he or she earned a baccalaureate degree. The first military weekend group graduated in 1992. The programs now include a B.S.N. program and a graduate program with a variety of traditional and accelerated tracks. The nursing programs reflect the mission of Regis College—to educate individuals to attain personal and career goals, while also addressing the changing needs of society. The faculty is dedicated to excellence in teaching and is committed to the integration of theory and practice in professional nursing. Students can expect a challenging educational experience in a supportive environment. The nursing programs are fully accredited by the National League for Nursing Accrediting Commission and offer flexible options for study on a full- or part-time basis.

PROGRAMS OF STUDY

The undergraduate program offers a B.S.N., a four-year course of study that prepares individuals for professional practice as registered nurses. This program integrates study in the liberal arts and sciences with professional nursing education. Students gain diverse clinical experiences within the greater Boston area and develop skills that prepare them to provide care to clients in a wide variety of health-care settings.

The graduate program offers a Master of Science with a focus in nursing leadership for diverse health-care systems or nurse practitioner. The nurse practitioner track offers three primary-care options: pediatric, family, and psychiatric mental health nurse practitioner. An accelerated curriculum track is designed for non-nurses who hold a baccalaureate degree in a field other than nursing. This track requires the completion of certain prerequisite courses and requires three years, including two summers of study. Students take the NCLEX-RN exam after sixteen months, and a B.S.N. is awarded at the end of the second year. Students have the option of exiting the program with the B.S.N. At the completion of the third year, the M.S. is awarded, and students are eligible to take nurse practitioner certification examinations.

The RN to B.S. to M.S. Upward Mobility track allows students with an associate degree or diploma in nursing to earn both the B.S. and M.S. within one curriculum. Students have the option of exiting the program with the B.S.N. Registered nurses who have a baccalaureate degree in a discipline other than nursing may enter this accelerated pathway as well. Classes are offered during the day, in the evening, on weekends, and during the summer. For RNs, post-master's certificates and certificates in nursing leadership and in nursing education are also offered.

AFFILIATIONS WITH HEALTH-CARE FACILITIES

The Nursing programs at Regis College offer a wide variety of health-care settings in which students may obtain enriching clinical experiences appropriate for their educational and professional goals. Students are placed in ambulatory, acute-, subacute-, and long-term-care facilities; nurse-managed clinics in homeless shelters; elementary and secondary schools; and elderly and low-income housing in both urban and suburban settings. Qualified nurse practitioner students have the opportunity to complete a portion of the clinical requirement in approved national or international settings. The Nursing Program also offers on-site work place courses for the master's degree programs for registered nurses employed in the Boston area, including the Lahey Clinic, St. Elizabeth's Hospital, and Hallmark Health Systems.

ACADEMIC FACILITIES

The Regis College Library provides resources and services to meet the research and study needs of undergraduate and graduate students and faculty members. The library contains 140,000 volumes and 787 current periodical subscriptions in print. Regis College Library has approximately 115 nursing periodicals in paper format plus more than 600 nursing journal titles containing full-text articles that are available through the library's subscriptions to online nursing databases. The library also has thousands of nursing books, including a large reference collection and an extensive collection located in the library stacks.

LOCATION

Regis College is located on a beautiful 168-acre residential campus 12 miles west of Boston, home to some of the world's leading educational, cultural, and health-care facilities. The College is easily accessible by major highways and is linked to metropolitan public transportation by a free campus shuttle bus.

STUDENT SERVICES

Regis College offers a wide range of student services, including the Fine Arts Center, which includes a 650-seat Eleanor Welch Casey Theatre and the Carney Art Gallery. The Athletic Facility features a regulation 75-foot pool with outdoor patio and sun deck plus a fitness center. The Student Union Building houses the main dining room and College café, the campus bookstore, and the post office. On-campus housing is available for undergraduates. Qualified nursing students are invited to join Sigma Theta Tau, the international nursing honor society.

THE NURSING STUDENT GROUP

There are approximately 450 graduate nursing students. Master's-prepared nurses have gone on to hold distinguished positions in every area of the health-care industry, including administration, clinical practice, academia, and government.

COSTS

Tuition for 2004–05 is $395 per credit for undergraduate nursing courses, $1050 per course for non-nursing undergraduate courses, and $515 per credit for graduate courses. Full-time tuition for undergraduate and graduate students is $10,250 per semester. Summer tuition depends on the number of credits carried. VISA, MasterCard, or Discover may be used for tuition payment. A tuition payment plan is also available. For further information, students should contact the Controller's Office at 781-768-7200. The total cost of the program varies depending upon the number of credits transferred or granted by examination or articulation.

FINANCIAL AID

The Regis College Office of Financial Aid is located in College Hall, Room 121. Students interested in applying for financial aid may request information by calling 781-768-7180. Prospective students should investigate sources of financial assistance, including loans, employer tuition remission, and scholarships. The Higher Education Information Center (telephone: 617-536-0200; Web site: http://www.heic.org), located in the Boston Public Library at Copley Square, houses a national financial aid database.

APPLYING

All nursing applicants are processed through the Regis College Office of Admission and are considered on a rolling basis. Applicants must submit a completed application, including a resume, a signed personal statement, three confidential letters of recommendation, and official transcripts from the nursing program and/or colleges attended. Scores from the Graduate Record Examinations (GRE) or Miller Analogies Test (taken within the past five years) are required for admission to the graduate program. Prospective students should inquire about opportunities to waive this requirement. There is a $30 application fee. Information about the GRE is available from the Educational Testing Service, P.O. Box 6000, Princeton, New Jersey 08541-6000, or by calling 609-771-7670. Information about the Miller Analogies Test may be obtained by calling the Psychological Corporation toll-free at 800-622-3231. A minimum GPA of 3.0 in all course work, including undergraduate, a diploma program or an associate degree, and prerequisite courses, is advised. A interview is required of all applicants.

RN applicants must be graduates of accredited diploma, associate degree, or baccalaureate programs in nursing. Documentation of individual malpractice insurance and a current Massachusetts license to practice as a registered nurse must be provided four weeks prior to clinical courses. Regis College offers registered nurses the opportunity for advanced placement through CLEP and other Advanced Placement examinations. For further information, prospective students should contact the Center for Health Sciences, Nursing Program.

CORRESPONDENCE AND INFORMATION

Ms. Claudia Pouravelis, Graduate Admission Counselor
Regis College
235 Wellesley Street
Weston, Massachusetts 02493-1571
Telephone: 781-768-7058
866-GET-REGIS (toll-free)
Fax: 781-768-7071
E-mail: nursing@regiscollege.edu
World Wide Web: http://www.regiscollege.edu

THE FACULTY

Antoinette Hays, Associate Professor and Center Director for Nursing; Ph.D., Brandeis.
Maureen Beirne-Streff, Visiting Associate Professor of Nursing; Ed.D., Boston University.
Michael Bilozur, Assistant Professor of Biology; Ph.D., Boston College.
Nancy Bittner, Assistant Professor of Nursing; Ph.D., Rhode Island.
Fran Borger-Klempner, Lecturer in of Nursing; M.S., Catholic University.
Patricia Ciarleglio, Lecturer in Nursing and Placement Coordinator; M.S., Regis College.
Karen Crowley, Lecturer in Nursing; M.S., Simmons; FNP.
Mary Crowley, Nursing Laboratory Coordinator; M.S., Boston University.
Patricia Dardano, Associate Professor of Nursing; D.N.Sc., Boston University.
Rosemarie Fuller, Lecturer in Nursing; M.S.N., Illinois.
Eda George, Assistant Professor of Nursing; Ph.D., Brandeis.
Joanne Hyde, Lecturer in Nursing; M.S., Boston University.
Sheila Juliani, Lecturer in Nursing; M.S.N., Northeastern.
Philip Jutras, Associate Professor of Management; Ed.M., Massachusetts Boston; Ph.D., Boston College.
Marylou Kelleher, Lecturer in Nursing; M.S., Regis College.
Margaret Knight, Assistant Professor of Nursing; Ph.D., Rhode Island.
Mary Lombard, Professor of Biology; Ph.D., Boston College.
Naser Mahmoud, Lecturer in Pharmacology; Pharm.D., Massachusetts College of Pharmacy.
Barbara Marcel, Lecturer in Psychology; Ph.D., Northeastern.
Luanne Nugent, Lecturer in Nursing; M.S., Boston University.
Kenneth Peterson, Lecturer in Nursing; M.S., Massachusetts Amherst.
Susan Sawyer, Assistant Professor of Nursing; Ph.D., Massachusetts Amherst.
Elizabeth Selover, Lecturer in Nursing; M.S., Simmons.
Colleen Simonelli, Lecturer in Nursing; M.S., Boston College.
Mary Smalarz, Associate Professor in Nursing; Ed.D., Boston University.
Rosmin Suleman, Lecturer in Pharmacology; M.S., Massachusetts College of Pharmacy.
Donna Williams, Lecturer in Nursing; M.S., Massachusetts Medical Center.

Sacred Heart University
Department of Nursing
Fairfield, Connecticut

THE UNIVERSITY

Sacred Heart University, established in 1963, is a coeducational independent institution of higher learning in the Catholic intellectual tradition whose primary objective is to prepare men and women to live in and make contributions to the human community. From its founding, the University has been recognized for its caring approach to students. This expresses the University's belief that each student is born with a unique set of qualities and skills. Sacred Heart University is committed to combining education for life with preparation for professional excellence. The current undergraduate enrollment is approximately 3,000 full-time students. Extracurricular activities include fraternities, sororities, student government, the student newspaper, the yearbook, a student radio station, academic clubs in almost every area of study, the debate club, the International Club, La Hispanidad, and intramural sports programs. Sacred Heart University offers men's and women's competition in NCAA Division I baseball, basketball, bowling, crew, cross-country, equestrian, fencing, field hockey, football, golf, ice hockey, lacrosse, soccer, softball, swimming, tennis, track and field (indoor and outdoor), volleyball, and wrestling. The University's football team was the Division IA national champion in 2001.

THE DEPARTMENT OF NURSING

Nursing at Sacred Heart University is an integral part of the overall University, whose aim is to assist in the development of people who are knowledgeable of self, rooted in faith, educated in mind, compassionate in heart, responsive to social and civic obligations, and prepared to contribute to an ever-changing world. The nursing faculty believes that nursing is an evolving professional discipline, grounded in the liberal arts, sciences, and humanities. These disciplines support the science and art of nursing, providing the framework for practice, development of new knowledge, and nursing education.

With dramatic change occurring within the health-care environment, nurses play an increasingly important role in improving the delivery of care through their critical-thinking skills and holistic perspective, while ensuring that patients receive the care and services required. Thus, professional nurses are prepared to assess and analyze the health of individuals and communities, make diagnoses regarding human responses to health needs, create plans for providing care, and perform those activities calling for professional nurse skills, while continuously evaluating and modifying care to obtain the best patient outcomes. Working collaboratively with other members of the health-care team, nurses serve as advocates for patients and families within health-care facilities and in communities.

The nursing curriculum at Sacred Heart University incorporates both traditional hospital and community practice settings to ensure that students have access to state-of-the-art care and the opportunity to develop the essential skills of clinical practice. Nursing graduates of Sacred Heart University are prepared as generalists, ready to assume the practice of professional nursing with a solid foundation in nursing and health-care theory and demonstrated clinical competency. In addition, the development of interdisciplinary collaboration and leadership skills along with the use of advanced educational technology (including a skills lab and Web-based assignments and courses) prepare graduates for a variety of challenging positions and future graduate study. Hallmarks of the Sacred Heart University nursing programs include strong emphasis on the spiritual and ethical implications of health care, the impact of diversity on patients and caregivers, the health of individuals within communities, and special consideration of the needs of the growing population of older people (gerontology). The Sacred Heart nursing program was recently recognized by the American Association of Colleges of Nursing and the Hartford Institute for Geriatric Nursing for implementation of an innovative curriculum in geriatric nursing.

The nursing faculty comprises highly experienced professionals recognized as experts among their peers, representing the major clinical specialties within nursing. The full-time faculty works closely with selectively recruited adjunct faculty members who provide special skills and focus areas. The nursing faculty has developed a strong network of committed adjunct faculty members and educational preceptors who share generously of their time and expertise with students and the programs. Graduates are highly sought after by prospective employers for their high NCLEX pass rates and outstanding skills.

PROGRAMS OF STUDY

Programs of undergraduate study offered are a B.S.N. program for beginning and transfer students and an RN–B.S.N. program with the option of Web-based courses for all didactic course work for RNs with an associate degree or diploma in nursing. Graduate study concentrations lead to an M.S.N. and include family nurse practitioner studies or patient-care services administration, with the option of a dual M.S.N.–M.B.A. degree. Starting in January 2003, administration courses in nursing were added on the World Wide Web, enabling students to select a distance learning option at the graduate level. An RN–M.S.N. program and a post-master's certificate option in family nurse practitioner studies are also offered.

The B.S.N. program introduces core nursing courses in the sophomore year, including foundations of practice and health assessment. Medical-surgical nursing and obstetrics and pediatric content are the focus of the junior year. The junior and senior years build upon earlier knowledge, increasing the complexity and number of patients cared for while developing the expected leadership, communication, evaluation, and critical-thinking skills. A significant amount of actual clinical practice experience is optimized through clinical laboratory practice and preparation that includes one-to-one interaction and feedback. Students may elect an opportunity for focused study in a variety of areas, including gerontology, community health, and critical care. Service learning activities are planned in several courses, coupling real-world experience with learning objectives. Each undergraduate student has a laptop computer equipped with wireless campus technology to promote more online access to information and a host of related resources.

The RN–B.S.N. program is a highly flexible course of study that is influenced by the individuals' professional goals and experiences. Students may elect traditional classroom experiences, a Web-based curriculum, or a combination of both to fulfill the requirements of the B.S.N.

The family nurse practitioner major prepares graduates for advanced practice across the life span. This rigorous curriculum incorporates traditional and interactive classroom activities, case-study analysis, demonstration and clinical laboratory and supervised clinical practice with an expert preceptor. Completion results in an M.S.N. or, for nurses already prepared at the master's level, a certificate, qualifying graduates to take a national certification examination.

The patient-care services program prepares RNs for positions of administrative responsibility within health-care organizations. Contemporary leadership theory and practice are examined within the context of the dramatically changing health-care environment to ensure that graduates are prepared to lead the next generation of health-care providers. Students have the option to enroll for a dual M.S.N.-M.B.A. degree if they meet entry requirements.

AFFILIATIONS WITH HEALTH-CARE FACILITIES

More than eight acute-care hospitals and a large variety of health-care facilities and organizations are within 30 minutes of the campus, providing a rich resource of learning experiences in virtually every major clinical practice area. Opportunities for internships and other experiential programs are in place and are increasing due to employer demand and the growing nursing shortage.

ACADEMIC FACILITIES

The University's library contains more than 164,000 volumes, 2,157 periodical titles, and 110,000 nonprint items such as videotapes, audiocassettes, phonodiscs, microforms, filmstrips, and slide sets. It also provides online database searching services. There are 4,823 volumes for the health sciences, as well as 106 periodicals in nursing.

Sacred Heart University is in the sixth year of its Student Mobile Computing Program. Full-time students receive a Dell laptop computer. The campus has been transformed into a wireless networked environment.

The Nursing Laboratory is divided into inpatient (hospital bed stations with full body models) and clinic (examination tables and related materials for an office) settings, and it is equipped to support practice of core nursing skills at the undergraduate level and advanced clinical skills for graduate students. The classroom portion of the lab allows for demonstration during class periods, using a variety of supplemental learning techniques. The inventory of audiovisual equipment and supplies, including videos, computers, and anatomical models, is expanded each year. Software includes programs on nutrition, NCLEX practice tests, and comprehensive NCLEX review. Students have full access to the University library and the Internet.

LOCATION

Ideally located in beautiful Fairfield County in southwestern Connecticut, Sacred Heart University is 1 hour northeast of New York City, 2½ hours southwest of Boston, and 1 hour southwest of the capital city of Hartford. More than half of the 56-acre campus is surrounded by a thirty-six-hole golf course. The campus location promotes easy accessibility to shopping, dining, and cultural and leisure activities.

STUDENT SERVICES

A five-year Strategic Plan provides a road map for the University as it strives to meet the needs of today's students. The plan calls for the construction of new facilities as well as the implementation of new academic, athletic, and social programs. Seven new residence halls have opened in the last five years. A $17-million health and recreation complex opened in 1997. Sacred Heart University is committed to providing students with extensive services to complement their education. The University Learning Center offers tutoring and assistance in basic study skills.

THE NURSING STUDENT GROUP

Students in the nursing program represent diverse cultural groups, economic levels, and geographical regions, although most live within 2 hours of campus. Full- and part-time study are possible for both undergraduate and graduate study; however, most students in the generic B.S.N. program study full-time, with about two thirds living in local campus housing. RN–B.S.N. and graduate students study mostly part-time and live at home. Full-time graduate students and designated part-time students may be eligible for financial support through federal traineeship grants and other sources of financial aid.

There is an active Student Nurses Association, a significant number of loyal alumni involved in numerous program efforts, and a strong chapter of Sigma Theta Tau, the honor society for nursing. Faculty members are committed to individualized advisement, and a low faculty-student ratio is designed to provide meaningful educational experiences. More than 96 percent of recent graduates are employed or pursue graduate study within six months of graduation.

COSTS

Tuition for academic year 2003–04 was $20,268 for full-time undergraduate students and $355 per credit for part-time students. Room and board totaled $8900. Graduate nursing students paid $420 per credit.

FINANCIAL AID

Sacred Heart University maintains a strong commitment to provide higher education to as many students as possible by making available scholarships, grants, loans, and part-time employment. Financial aid packages are developed by combining Sacred Heart University's own resources with a variety of federal and state financial aid programs. Eighty-five percent of all students receive some form of financial aid.

APPLYING

Applications to the nursing program are processed through the Admissions Office for freshman, transfer, and graduate students. Freshman students apply for matriculation into the nursing major during their second semester. Transfer and RN–B.S.N. students may request admission interviews with the Nursing Program Director to ascertain compliance with eligibility requirements and proposed plan of study. Prospective students should refer to the Sacred Heart University admission section for detailed information regarding admission deadlines and notifications.

CORRESPONDENCE AND INFORMATION

Office of Admissions
Sacred Heart University
5151 Park Avenue
Fairfield, Connecticut 06825-1000
Telephone: 203-371-7880
E-mail: halucha@sacredheart.edu
World Wide Web: http://www.sacredheart.edu/

Dori Taylor Sullivan, Director
Nursing Programs
Sacred Heart University
5151 Park Avenue
Fairfield, Connecticut 06825-1000
Telephone: 203-371-7715

THE FACULTY

Dori Taylor Sullivan, Associate Professor and Director; Ph.D., Connecticut; RNC. Administration/adult medical-surgical.

Anne M. Barker, Associate Professor; Ed.D., Columbia; RN. Administration.

Susan DeNisco, Clinical Assistant Professor; M.S., Pace; APRN. Family nurse practitioner.

Kathleen S. Fries, Instructor; M.S.N., Sacred Heart; RN. Maternal–child health.

Michael R. Hargrave, Instructor; M.B.A., Rensselaer; M.S.N., Rochester. Medical-surgical, leadership.

Carol Kravitz, Clinical Assistant Professor; M.S.N., SUNY at Binghamton; APRN. Pediatric nurse practitioner.

Cynthia K. O'Sullivan, Instructor; M.S.N., Pennsylvania; RN. Critical care/medical-surgical.

Linda L. Strong, Assistant Professor; Ed.D., Columbia; RN. Community health.

Constance E. Young, Associate Professor; Ed.D., Columbia; RN. Medical-surgical, ethics.

Saint Anthony College of Nursing

Rockford, Illinois

THE COLLEGE

Saint Anthony College of Nursing is an upper-division college, offering the last two years of a four-year program for a Bachelor of Science in Nursing. The College of Nursing educates nurses in the science of nursing and the art of life. Students are encouraged to think freely and creatively and become excellent decision makers. The Bachelor of Science in Nursing degree program balances the study of science and liberal arts so graduates are prepared to face challenges in and out of the workplace.

The Sisters of the Third Order opened the Saint Anthony School of Nursing in 1915. During the early 1990s, the institution became a baccalaureate degree–granting institution and changed its name to Saint Anthony College of Nursing. During the school's history, more than 2,600 of its graduates have joined the nursing profession.

The mission of Saint Anthony College of Nursing is to provide an upper-division baccalaureate nursing education. The College is a private, Catholic institution serving students from local, state, and national areas. Implementing the philosophy of the Saint Anthony College of Nursing, which reflects that of the Sisters of the Third Order of Saint Francis, the College prepares individuals to function as caring, competent professional nurses in beginning leadership roles and as knowledgeable consumers of nursing research. These professional nurses are prepared to participate in the emerging health needs of a changing society.

PROGRAMS OF STUDY

The College offers the final two years of a four-year Bachelor of Science in Nursing (B.S.N.) degree. These two years consist of nursing theory courses and extensive clinical practice experience. The College provides more than 700 hours of direct clinical experience in a variety of acute-care settings, including a Level 1 trauma center. Students also gain experience working in ambulatory care settings, such as home health care, mental health clinics, community agencies, and clinics. Student gain clinical experience with children, adults, and geriatric patients.

There is also a program with which actively licensed Illinois-registered professional nurses can earn a B.S.N. degree (RN to B.S.N.). RNs should contact the Student Affairs Office for information about earning credits for licensure and certifications. A Student at Large program is available for those who wish to enroll without pursuing a degree or who wish to start nursing courses prior to full acceptance.

ACADEMIC FACILITIES

In addition to the facilities of the OSF Saint Anthony Medical Center, students take advantage of the Sister Mary Linus Learning Resource Center, which provides access to a wide variety of both physical and online research material, as well as the recently built skills lab, where equipment, procedures, and safety are learned prior to patient contact.

LOCATION

Saint Anthony College of Nursing is located in Rockford, Illinois, which is 75 miles northwest of Chicago. Rockford is well-known for its industrial corporations and agriculture. Many recreational and cultural opportunities are available in this community of 160,000. In addition to Saint Anthony College of Nursing, there are three other institutions of higher education, three hospitals, a State of Illinois mental health and developmental center, and numerous health-care agencies located in the greater Rockford area.

COSTS

Tuition for the fall 2005 semester is $7700 per semester for full-time students and $482 per credit hour for part-time students. Also required are a $50 application fee, $200 tuition deposit, $50 computer fee, and other miscellaneous fees. Book prices vary. Each student is also required to pay a $13 annual Professional Liability Insurance Fee. There are several payment options, including cash, check, or credit card. The College reserves the right to revise fees at any time.

FINANCIAL AID

The primary purpose of the financial aid program is to assure that students who want to attend but who need monetary assistance have the ability to do so. Students must be enrolled in at least 6 credits during a semester and make satisfactory progress. In addition to federal and state programs, several College, community, and health-agency grants are available. To apply for financial aid, a student must complete the Free Application for Federal Student Aid (FAFSA). For additional information, students should contact the College Financial Aid Officer.

APPLYING

A total of 32 prerequisite credits and one of the prenursing sciences (anatomy and physiology, microbiology, or organic chemistry) must have been completed with an overall grade point average of 2.5 on a 4.0 scale in order to be considered for provisional acceptance. Courses must have been taken at a regionally accredited college or university for a grade of C or above to be considered for transfer credits. Credit may also be awarded for acceptable scores on AP or CLEP tests (as recommended by the American Council on Education) in appropriate subject areas. A total of 64 prerequisite credits must be completed before starting the nursing program. A written statement of personal, professional, educational, and career goals must be completed on campus at the time of the personal interview. This statement is reviewed for both content and ability to communicate effectively.

Three acceptable professional references must be submitted, including one from a current or recent instructor. The other two references should be from a current or recent employer, another instructor, or a school counselor. For those applicants whose primary language is not English, a minimum TOEFL score of 550 is required.

Admitted students must be in good physical and mental health and be able to carry out the functions of a nursing student as determined by the College. A physical exam within six months of entrance into the B.S.N. degree program is required. Specific health requirements are determined by the College and/or government and clinical agency mandates, including verification of immunizations (tetanus/diphtheria, polio, measles, and mumps), a statement regarding history of chicken pox, rubella titer (students must prove immunity to rubella and rubeola), and a two-step TB skin test no earlier than three weeks before classes begin (an annual TB skin test thereafter and/or annual TB assessment by the College nurse). Affiliated agencies where students have clinical experience may require additional tests. Students are notified by the College when testing is requested by these agencies. Obtaining necessary examinations and tests is the responsibility of the student.

A completed application for admission to the B.S.N. degree program must be submitted to the Office of Student Services with the appropriate application fee. Evidence of successful completion of cardiopulmonary resuscitation training (to be updated annually) must be submitted in accordance with the College's CPR policy. Verification of health/accident and auto insurance (if operating a motor vehicle) must be on file in the Student Services Office. Professional liability insurance is required. A Transfer/Withdrawal/Dismissal Form must be completed if an applicant has attended another nursing or professional health-care program but did not satisfactorily complete it.

CORRESPONDENCE AND INFORMATION

Cheryl Delgado
Admissions Representative
Saint Anthony College of Nursing
5658 East State Street
Rockford, Illinois 61008-2468
Telephone: 815-227-2141
Fax: 815-395-2275
E-mail: cheryldelgado@sacn.edu
World Wide Web: http://www.sacn.edu

San Diego State University
School of Nursing
San Diego, California

THE UNIVERSITY

San Diego State University (SDSU) was founded in 1897 and in 1971 became part of the California State University and College systems. Today San Diego State University is the largest campus in the CSU system and one of the largest in the western United States. SDSU is a major urban university with strong research programs. More than 30,000 students attend classes in sixty-nine different disciplines on a 271-acre campus. Repeatedly named by college presidents in *U.S. News & World Report* surveys as one of the outstanding comprehensive universities in the western United States, SDSU provides education in a wide variety of humanities, sciences, fine and performing arts, and professional disciplines. The mission-style architecture and broad, flowered walkways give the campus its unique southern California quality and charm.

THE SCHOOL OF NURSING

The School of Nursing is part of the College of Health and Human Services and was established as a baccalaureate program with the University in 1953. Since then, the nursing program has maintained continuous national accreditation. The School is accredited by the Commission on Collegiate Nursing Education, the American College of Nurse-Midwives, the Commission on Teacher Credentialing, and the California State Board of Nursing. In 1982, the School of Nursing opened the Master of Science degree program in community health and nursing systems administration. The critical-care concentration began admitting students in 1985, the pediatric specialization began in 1989, and the school nursing program began in 1993. The family nurse practitioner program began in 1994 and the nurse midwifery program in 1995. The advanced practice program for care of adults and the elderly opened in 1996, preparing nurse practitioners and critical-care specialists. The School admits RNs to the baccalaureate nursing program and offers a health services credential for school nurses. All baccalaureate graduates qualify for the California Public Health Certificate of Nursing.

The tenured faculty members and several lecturers in the School of Nursing are doctorally prepared and conduct research in a wide variety of clinical areas. Some of the research interests of the faculty include stress and coping in children, psychosocial issues of critically ill children, parent-infant relationships, infertility, physiological alterations in the neonate, evoked-potential responses, tissue oxygenation, administrative issues, cross-cultural nursing, and genetics. The faculty members are also experts in a variety of research methodologies, including the historical, qualitative, and quantitative methodologies.

PROGRAMS OF STUDY

The baccalaureate program prepares nurses who can function at a beginning level of practice in a wide variety of settings. It also prepares students with the basis for graduate study at the master's and doctoral levels. Undergraduate students are given opportunities to acquire knowledge from the natural and social sciences, to develop critical thinking and professional decision-making abilities, to utilize current research in the application of the nursing process, to develop leadership potential and accountability in professional practice, to become aware of the emerging roles of the professional nurse and of the social forces and trends affecting health and health-care systems, and to balance professional and personal growth and values. Satisfactory completion of 128 credits is required for graduation. Students may sit for the California licensing exam after completing seven semesters of the prescribed program of full-time study. Part-time study is also permitted.

The Master of Science degree in nursing is offered in one of three major concentrations: nursing systems administration, community health nursing, and advanced practice nursing of adults and the elderly (including specialization in primary care and acute care). Students in community health may specialize in public health, midwifery, or school nursing. Graduates of the program are prepared to function as midlevel and executive-level nursing administrators, nurse practitioners, or clinical nurse specialists. In addition to the clinical or administrative focus, all graduates of the program are prepared for beginning roles as nurse researchers. These roles may involve critical analysis of research, application of research findings to clinical practice, data collection for larger collaborative nursing and medical studies, and acting as principal investigators.

The graduate program requires a minimum of 39 semester units; however some specialties, such as NP and midwifery, require more. All specialties may be completed in two years of full-time study. Part-time study is also permitted. Students take between 12 and 15 units of core courses that investigate nursing research, theory, professional issues, and organizational systems. The remaining units are devoted to courses supporting the clinical specialty. All students may complete a master's thesis, project, or comprehensive exam. Students receive guided supervision throughout their thesis research.

AFFILIATIONS WITH HEALTH-CARE FACILITIES

The School of Nursing is affiliated with more than 120 different health-care agencies. All the major community hospitals, the Department of Health, schools, HMOs, jails, hospices, community clinics, home health agencies, and doctors' offices provide learning experiences for the SDSU nursing students. Patients are also seen in their homes.

ACADEMIC FACILITIES

The School of Nursing has its own media, computer, and skills labs. Students also have access to the College Computer Lab and the University's mainframe and microcomputer facilities. The University Computer Center provides equipment, software, and technical personnel to support student research.

The University library has more than 1 million volumes and subscribes to more than 175 periodicals related to nursing and health care. The library provides general reference services and a specific librarian and related services for nursing. The School also has easy access to the Bio-Medical Library of the University of California, San Diego, as well as surrounding hospital libraries.

The SDSU Institute for Nursing was founded in 1988 and includes eight San Diego health-care institutions. The institute promotes collaborative research between service and academia through multisite studies. Its purpose is to promote collaboration in the conduct, dissemination, and utilization of nursing research that contributes to the quality of patient care.

LOCATION

San Diego is the seventh-largest city in the United States. San Diego County is the southernmost county of California, covering 4,255 square miles and ending at the United States–Mexico border. The climate is semi-arid with a mean temperature of 70 degrees year-round. The Pacific Ocean and the beaches are approximately a 20-minute drive west from the campus. The mountains are 30 miles east, and the desert is 80 miles northeast. San Diego offers diverse cultural, athletic, and recreational activities.

STUDENT SERVICES

Services are many and varied. Some examples are Campus Tours, Career Services, Counseling and Psychological Services, Disabled Student Services, Educational Opportunity/Ethnic Affairs, Health Services, On-Campus Housing for Singles, International Student Center, Ombudsmen, Student Athlete Academic Support Services, the Student Resource Center, Leisure Connection, Recreational Sports Office, and Mission Bay Aquatic Center.

THE NURSING STUDENT GROUP

There are currently more than 500 undergraduate and more than 100 graduate full- and part-time students enrolled in the School of Nursing. The SDSU School of Nursing is the largest supplier of nurses to San Diego and Imperial counties of southern California. The student body is diverse in ethnic background and geographic origin. The University provides many opportunities for students to participate on School and University committees and in activities. Graduates of the SDSU nursing programs have been actively recruited for both beginning and advanced practice positions in agencies throughout the United States.

COSTS

Registration fees for California residents in 2004–05 were $1468 for undergraduates and $1711 for graduate students. Tuition for nonresidents (U.S. and international) was $339 per unit in addition to the registration fees cited above. Additional academic fees include application fees, thesis binding fees, and graduation charges. Students are also required to have professional liability insurance ($1.3 million minimum) and transportation.

Although most students choose to live in off-campus housing, University housing is available. The cost of living in San Diego is comparable to that in other large metropolitan areas.

FINANCIAL AID

Financial aid is available in a variety of forms. Information on student loans, grants, and fellowships is available from the Financial Aid Office. Professional nurse traineeships and graduate assistantships are offered to graduate students through the School of Nursing. In addition to the direct student aid offered through the University, employment opportunities with a variety of educational benefits are available in nearby health-care agencies.

APPLYING

The application process has two steps. First, an application is made online to the University through Admissions and Records; a second application is made to the School of Nursing. For deadlines and criteria, students should contact the School of Nursing office.

CORRESPONDENCE AND INFORMATION

School of Nursing
San Diego State University
San Diego, California 92182-0254
Telephone: 619-594-5357
Fax: 619-594-2765
World Wide Web: http://nursing.sdsu.edu

THE FACULTY

Gwen Anderson, Associate Professor and Associate Director of Research; Ph.D., Boston College; RN.
Janet L. Blenner, Professor; Ph.D., NYU; FAAN.
Betty Broom, Associate Professor; Ph.D., Texas at Austin.
Nancy Coffin-Romig, Lecturer and RN-B.S. Advisor; D.N.Sc., San Diego.
Lorraine Fitzsimmons, Associate Professor; D.N.S., Indiana; FNP.
Joan M. Flagg, Associate Professor; Ph.D., Texas at Austin.
Rosemary Gaines, Lecturer; M.N., UCLA.
Kay Gilbert, Lecturer; Ph.D., Texas at Austin.
Sue A. Hadley, Associate Professor and Graduate Advisor; D.N.S., Indiana; NP.
Jan Hall, Lecturer; M.S.N., San Diego State.
Gail Hanscom, Lecturer; M.S.N., Boston University; M.A., San Diego State; FNP.
Janet R. Heineken, Professor; Ph.D., Denver.
Lauren Hunter, Assistant Professor; Ph.D., San Diego; RN, CNM.
Major King, Assistant Professor; Ph.D., UCLA.
Nancy Lischke, Lecturer; M.N., UCLA.
Linda Long, Lecturer; M.S.N., California State, Los Angeles.
Doris McCarthy, Lecturer; M.S.N., M.A., San Diego State.
Mary Ellin Miller, Lecturer; M.S.N., San Diego.
Rita I. Morris, Associate Professor; Ph.D., American.
Lien Ngo-Nguyen, Lecturer; M.N., Phoenix.
Becky C. Palmer, Assistant Professor; Ph.D., British Columbia.
Mary Beth Parr, Lecturer; M.S.N., Virginia.
Jane Rapps, Lecturer; D.N.Sc., San Diego.
Richard C. Reed, Associate Professor and College of Health and Human Services Associate Dean for Student Affairs; Ed.D., Tulsa.
Lembi Saarmann, Associate Professor and Associate Director of the Graduate Program; Ed.D., Columbia.
Julia Smith, Assistant Professor; Ph.D., San Diego.
Eunyoung Eunice Suh, Lecturer; Ph.D., Pennsylvania.
Toni Sullivan, Distinguished Visiting Professor; Ed.D., Utah.
Nancy Sweeney, Assistant Professor; D.N.Sc., Widener.
Patricia Wahl, Professor and Director; Ph.D., Cincinnati; FAAN.
Carolyn L. Walker and Undergraduate Advisor, Professor; Ph.D., Utah.

Thomas Edison State College
Program in Nursing
Trenton, New Jersey

THE COLLEGE

Thomas Edison State College provides flexible, high-quality collegiate learning opportunities for self-directed adults. Cited as "one of the brighter stars of higher learning" by the *New York Times* and identified by *Forbes* magazine as one of the top twenty colleges and universities in the nation in the use of technology to create learning opportunities for adults, Thomas Edison State College provides high-quality higher education to adults wherever they live and work. Founded in 1972, Thomas Edison State College enables adult students to complete associate, baccalaureate, and master's degrees through distance learning and the assessment of prior learning.

THE NURSING PROGRAM

The Thomas Edison State College Bachelor of Science in Nursing (B.S.N.) degree program for registered nurses (RNs) currently licensed in the United States admitted its first students in October 1983. Initiated in response to a need for additional opportunities for RNs in New Jersey to earn a B.S.N. degree, the program was initially offered as an examination-based program. The program was reorganized as an online distance learning program in 2001 and made available to RNs throughout the United States. Consistent with the mission of the College, the program continues to offer open and rolling admissions with multiple credit-earning options and no residency requirement. Enrollment continues to increase, with more than 350 students currently enrolled.

The nursing program uses off-site nurse educators from a variety of nursing education and service settings to develop, implement, and evaluate the program. All nursing educators have a minimum of a master's degree in nursing, with approximately 80 percent prepared at the doctoral level and many tenured at their home institution. As a distance learning program, the B.S.N. degree program has the opportunity to draw these nurse educators from throughout the United States, resulting in a diverse and experienced group of nurse educators. The B.S.N. degree program is accredited by the National League for Nursing Accrediting Commission and the New Jersey Board of Nursing.

PROGRAMS OF STUDY

The B.S.N. degree program is flexible and self-paced and allows for different methods of learning and degree completion. The program requires a minimum of 120 semester hours of credit; 60 in general education, 48 in nursing, and 12 in free electives. RNs who have completed an associate degree in nursing program or an RN diploma program may have 20 credits applied from previous nursing course work toward the 48-credit nursing component. A total of 80 credits may be accepted from a community college, and up to 60 credits may be awarded to diploma graduates based on current licensure. There is no age restriction on credits transferred to meet general-education requirements or lower-division nursing requirements. All upper-division nursing credits must be from an accredited baccalaureate, higher-degree nursing program, or other Thomas Edison State College–approved credit-earning methods, and these credits must be newer than ten years if completed prior to application to Thomas Edison State College. All credits applied to the nursing component must have a grade equivalent of C or better.

There are eight requirements in the 28-credit upper-division nursing requirement, all of which may be satisfied by twelve-week online courses offered quarterly by the College. All nursing courses are 3 credits each, with the exception of the final nursing course, Community Health Nursing, which is 7 credits. Nonenrolled RNs may take two online nursing courses prior to enrollment in the program, with the exception of the final two courses, Independent Study and Community Health Nursing, which are restricted to RNs enrolled in the Thomas Edison State College B.S.N. program and require evidence of current licensure and malpractice insurance. The online nursing courses are independent, highly interactive courses that require student participation in online group discussions at least three times weekly in addition to readings and the online submission of written assignments. There are no proctored examinations for the online courses; assessment of learning by the online course mentors occurs via the online group discussion participation and written assignments. Graduations occur quarterly, but there is no time limit for degree completion.

ACADEMIC FACILITIES

Thomas Edison State College students use the rich library research facilities of the New Jersey State Library, which is an affiliate of Thomas Edison State College. Students also have access to the Virtual Academic Libraries Environment (VALE), a consortium of fifty-two New Jersey colleges and universities, which provides access to a network of research libraries.

LOCATION

Thomas Edison State College is located in the capital city of Trenton, New Jersey, but its reach is global. Students live and study in all fifty states and more than seventy other countries. The College's campus comprises the Kelsey Building at 101 West State Street and the adjacent Townhouse Complex, the Academic Center at 167 West Hanover Street, and the Kuser Mansion at 315 West State Street. The College's state-of-the-art facilities, from electronic classrooms and computer labs to a corporate-style education conference room and other amenities, allow Thomas Edison State College to link students and mentors at dozens of colleges throughout the country and around the world.

STUDENT SERVICES

The Thomas Edison State College Bachelor of Science in Nursing degree program is distinctive in that it is completed entirely at a distance, therefore, students in the program do not require traditional campus-based services. The College offers all core student services via the Internet through iTESC®, a suite of online services. Also through the Internet, students have access to such services as course and test registration and payment; displaying of registration schedules, course and mentor availability, and grades; displaying and updating of student information; online course and mentor evaluations; and other services.

In addition to technical support provided by the College's Office of Management Information Systems (MIS), a technical support mentor is embedded in the online nursing program. This mentor answers questions and provides support for students and other mentors when any technological issue may arise.

B.S.N. degree students have access to all academic advisement services provided by the College, including the availability of an academic adviser for nursing. Enrolled students may access advisement services by the U.S. Postal Service, fax, e-mail, telephone, or in-person appointments. All College and program publications provided to students may also be accessed on the College Web site.

THE NURSING STUDENT GROUP

Students in the Thomas Edison State College B.S.N. degree program are typically midcareer professionals with a wide variety of nursing practice and management experiences. The average student is 42 years old. Of the more than 350 students enrolled in the B.S.N. degree program during the 2004–05 academic year, nearly all were actively employed in nursing. Approximately 9 percent of the enrolled students were men, and the program enjoyed a 24 percent diversity rate.

COSTS

The tuition for the 2004–05 academic year was $260 per credit for New Jersey residents and $374 per credit for out-of-state residents. There was a $75 nonrefundable application fee and a one-time $300 B.S.N. Credential Review Fee. The estimated cost for books and supplies for the online nursing courses is $100 per course.

FINANCIAL AID

Nursing students support their study primarily with employer tuition aid and loans. Unsubsidized loans are available to all accepted applicants. The Thomas Edison State College Office of Financial Aid & Veterans' Affairs is available to assist students.

APPLYING

Applicants to the B.S.N. degree program must be RNs who are currently licensed in the United States; have proficiency in using a computer; browsing the Web, sending and receiving Internet mail; and have access to PowerPoint software. Minimum system requirements are access to the Internet, an Internet browser such as Netscape 4.4 or newer or Internet Explorer 4.4 or newer, and the ability to send and receive e-mail. Applicants must submit the completed College application with nonrefundable fee to the College's Office of Admissions; have all official college transcripts and college-level examination score reports and notarized copy of current RN license sent to the College's Office of the Registrar. The completed B.S.N. Credential Review Form and fee must be submitted to the Office of the Bursar to enroll in the program.

CORRESPONDENCE AND INFORMATION

Renee San Giacomo
Director of Admissions
Thomas Edison State College
101 West State Street
Trenton, New Jersey 08608-1176
Telephone: 888-442-8372 (toll-free)
Fax: 609-984-8447
E-mail: info@tesc.edu
World Wide Web: http://www.tesc.edu

Thomas Jefferson University
Department of Nursing
Philadelphia, Pennsylvania

THE UNIVERSITY

Thomas Jefferson University, one of the oldest and largest academic health centers in the United States, is made up of Jefferson Medical College, one of the largest private medical schools in the country; Jefferson College of Graduate Studies, for advanced study in the basic medical sciences; and Jefferson College of Health Professions (JCHP). The University shares its campus with Thomas Jefferson University Hospital, one of the nation's premier health-care facilities, and is a member of Jefferson Health System, a regional, integrated health-care delivery system. JCHP provides innovative academic programs for a highly qualified, culturally diverse student population. The College focuses on generating new health-care knowledge through scholarship and applied, collaborative, and interdisciplinary research.

THE DEPARTMENT OF NURSING

Thomas Jefferson University has a long and distinguished history of providing men and women with the kind of nursing education that can be found at few educational institutions in the nation. Nursing education has been an integral part of Jefferson since its inception in 1891 as The Jefferson Medical College Hospital School of Nursing. The Department of Nursing was established in 1970 in the College of Health Professions.

Graduates of the undergraduate program are awarded the Associate of Science in Nursing (A.S.N.) degree or Bachelor of Science in Nursing (B.S.N.) degree, and graduates of the graduate program are awarded the Master of Science in Nursing (M.S.N.) degree. The programs are fully accredited by the American Association of Colleges of Nursing Commission on Collegiate Nursing Education (CCNE) through 2011.

Jefferson nursing faculty members, the majority of whom are doctorally prepared, have a deep commitment to their roles as teachers and to the professional development of students. Undergraduate and graduate students have the opportunity to participate in faculty research, scholarly activities, and practice, as well as to collaborate in interdisciplinary University projects. The Department currently enrolls approximately 300 undergraduates, the majority of whom are full-time, and more than 150 graduate students, the majority of whom enroll on a part-time basis.

PROGRAMS OF STUDY

The A.S.N. curriculum offered by the Department of Nursing prepares students to serve as generalists in the role of caregiver in a hospital or in-patient setting. Students complete 68 credits of general education and nursing course work, completing the A.S.N. program in two academic years. This program is offered at the Methodist Hospital campus in south Philadelphia and the Geisinger Medical Center campus in Danville, Pennsylvania.

The B.S.N. curriculum offered by the Department of Nursing is an upper-division program that emphasizes interdisciplinary education among students in the health professions. Students enter the nursing major at Jefferson after completing 59 lower-division credits in the sciences and humanities. The B.S.N. program at Jefferson balances the liberal arts, sciences, humanities, and professional nursing preparation and emphasizes health promotion, maintenance, and disease prevention as well as managing individuals and families coping with acute and chronic illness. Students complete 62 to 64 nursing credits at Jefferson. Full-time and part-time options are available. Graduates are prepared to practice professional nursing as generalists in a variety of health-care settings. The undergraduate program is among the most progressive in the United States.

The RN-B.S.N. program is designed to educate registered nurses who graduated from diploma or associate degree nursing programs for an increased leadership role in nursing. Students complete 60 credits of sciences and humanities in lower-division courses prior to entering the nursing major at Jefferson. Thirty-five upper-division credits are awarded for previous nursing knowledge. The Department offers the unique opportunity for RN students to earn 10.5 of the remaining upper-division credits through Portfolio Assessment of previous nursing knowledge. This enables RN students to begin the program in their senior year and complete the program in two semesters of full-time study or two years of part-time study. RNs can earn the B.S.N. totally online.

The RN-B.S.N./M.S.N. option allows RN students who have obtained their basic nursing education through either a diploma or associate degree program to qualify for admission to graduate nursing education through a combined B.S.N./M.S.N. program. The goal of the option is to provide a mechanism for RN students to earn the B.S.N. and M.S.N. degrees in a seamless integrated curriculum. An Accelerated Pathway option is available to RN students with a baccalaureate degree in a field other than nursing. Twenty-seven of the 36 credits required to earn the M.S.N. can be completed online.

Two programs leading to the B.S.N. and M.S.N. degrees are available to highly motivated, academically talented students who hold a bachelor's degree in a field other than nursing. The Accelerated Pathway to the M.S.N. for Second-Degree Students enables prelicensure students to earn both degrees in three academic years of full-time study. (A similar program is available for RNs.) The Facilitated Academic Coursework Tract (FACT) is a more intense program that enables prelicensure students to complete both degrees in two calendar years of full-time study.

The Master of Science in Nursing program prepares nurses for advanced and sophisticated clinical practice. The graduate program offers nurse practitioner, clinical nurse specialist, and post-master's certificate programs in acute care, adult health, community systems administration, oncology, and pediatrics, as well as a family nurse practitioner option. In addition, a family nurse practitioner/community systems administration integrated program is available, as are programs in neonatal nurse practitioner studies and informatics.

The curriculum is predicated on the Department of Nursing's belief that professional nursing is an art and a science that incorporates theory, research, and clinical practice. The curriculum is organized using a core curriculum concept. All core and many support courses are available both in the classroom and via the Internet. All specialty areas require 36 credits.

AFFILIATIONS WITH HEALTH-CARE FACILITIES

The University shares its campus with Thomas Jefferson University Hospital, one of the nation's premier health-care facilities. The multi-institutional Jefferson Health System and other leading hospitals and agencies throughout the region offer outstanding learning opportunities in a broad array of health-care settings.

ACADEMIC FACILITIES

Scott Library provides resources and facilities for study and research by graduate and undergraduate students and faculty and staff members. In addition to the extensive holding of books and periodicals, direct online access to full-text periodicals is available.

The computing services available to the University community are extensive. JeffLine provides access to the Internet. In addition to computing stations located throughout Scott Library, the Department Learning Resource Center houses computers and computer classrooms that are available to students and faculty members. The Learning Resource Center also maintains extensive holdings of a wide variety of audiovisual materials, training models, computer software programs, and simulations as well as a clinical learning laboratory.

LOCATION

Thomas Jefferson University is located in historic Center City, Philadelphia, the fifth-largest city in the United States. It is within walking distance of many places of historic and cultural interest. Theaters, museums, art galleries, and historic areas are just a few blocks away. Convenient bus, rail, and subway lines offer transportation to Jefferson as well as to a variety of interesting attractions.

STUDENT SERVICES

The University has many resources and services available to meet the needs of students. These include academic advising, counseling, housing, student health, tutoring, day care, fitness facilities, computing services, student organizations, and career services.

THE NURSING STUDENT GROUP

Students enrolled in the undergraduate and graduate programs represent a diverse group in terms of age, gender, ethnicity, cultural background, socioeconomic status, and religious orientation. Approximately 28 percent of the students indicate that they are members of minority ethnic groups. About 25 percent of the undergraduate students are registered nurses pursuing the B.S.N. Nursing students are active in University-wide student organizations and activities as well as nursing-specific organizations and activities. Last year's pass rate on the RN licensing examination was 97.8 percent, the highest among baccalaureate and associate degree programs in the region. By comparison, the national pass rate was 86.7 percent, and Pennsylvania's pass rate was 79.94 percent. Jefferson's graduates are highly respected and recruited. Its job placement rate is 100 percent, and graduates receive multiple offers.

COSTS

Tuition for full-time B.S.N. students for the 2004–05 academic year was $20,194. Part-time tuition was $726 per credit. Tuition for full-time M.S.N. students was $23,069. Part-time tuition was $800 per credit. The twelve-month FACT fee was $25,324.

FINANCIAL AID

Jefferson is committed to meeting the financial needs of its students. More than 75 percent of the current students receive financial assistance. Aid can include Federal Pell Grants, National Direct Student Loans, the College Work-Study Program, Air Force ROTC scholarships, nursing scholarships, nursing loans, state grants, work scholarships, state-guaranteed loans, and academic scholarships. Completed applications must be received by the Financial Aid Office no later than May 1 to ensure the maximum award.

APPLYING

Prospective students should apply as soon as possible after September 1 for the following year. Applications to the B.S.N. program are accepted and evaluated on an ongoing basis, but priority consideration is given to applications received by March 1. Along with a completed application, applicants must submit transcripts for all college work, a personal statement of academic and professional intent, and two letters of recommendation. A high school transcript is required for PACE applicants. Qualified applicants should have completed 59 prerequisite credits prior to entry into the program. Science courses that are more than ten years old require additional validation. The Test of English as a Foreign Language and the Test of Written English are required of all applicants for whom English is not the native language. Admission takes place in the fall.

Applicants to the Accelerated Pathway to the M.S.N. program must submit a completed application, transcripts of all college work, a personal statement of academic and professional intent, three letters of recommendation, and GRE or MAT scores. Admission takes place in the fall.

Applicants to the RN-B.S.N. program are required to submit a completed application, official transcripts from previous schools, a personal statement of academic and professional intent, and two letters of recommendation. Qualified applicants should have completed the 60 prerequisite credits prior to entry into the program. The Test of English as a Foreign Language and the Test of Written English are required of all applicants for whom English is not the native language. Admission takes place in fall or spring.

Applications to the M.S.N. program are accepted on an ongoing basis. Full-time students begin the program in the summer semester. Part-time students may begin in the fall, spring, or summer semester. Admission requirements include a bachelor's degree in nursing; competitive scores on the GRE or MAT; RN licensure; a minimum of one year of clinical experience; undergraduate courses in statistics, nursing research, and physical assessment; computer literacy; three letters of reference; a resume; and a personal statement addressing professional goals.

CORRESPONDENCE AND INFORMATION

Office of Admissions
Thomas Jefferson University
130 South 9th Street
Edison Building, Suite 1610
Philadelphia, Pennsylvania 19107-5233
Telephone: 215-503-8890
877-JEFF-CHP (toll-free)
Fax: 215-503-7241
World Wide Web: http://www.jefferson.edu/jchp

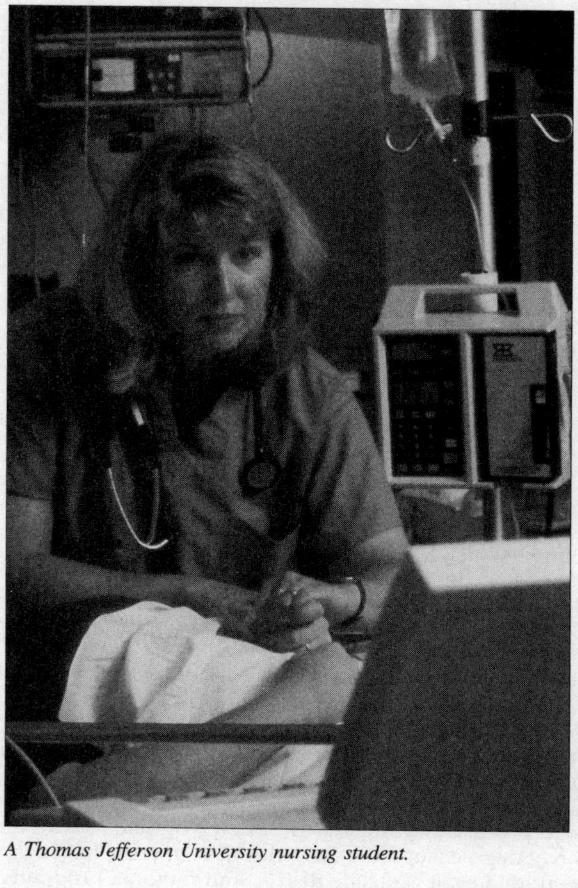

A Thomas Jefferson University nursing student.

The University of Akron
College of Nursing
Akron, Ohio

THE UNIVERSITY
The University of Akron (UA) is the public research university for northern Ohio. Founded in 1870, it is the only public university in Ohio with a science/engineering program ranked among the nation's top five by *U.S. News & World Report.* The University of Akron excels in such areas as polymer science, gerontological nursing, global business, and marketing.

The University of Akron is also a world leader in creating new materials for the new economy; a national leader in the development, protection, management, and commercialization of intellectual property; and a regional leader in information technology initiatives.

UA's polymer science and engineering program is ranked second in the nation, serves Ohio's $22-billion polymer industry, and includes NASA-supported nanotechnology initiatives. The University also has strong ties with business leaders, including IT partnerships with IBM, Cisco Systems, and TimeWarner.

Serving more than 22,300 students, the University offers more than 400 associate, bachelor's, master's, doctoral, and law degree programs and approximately 100 certificate programs through ten degree-granting colleges at its main campus in Akron and its Wayne College branch campus in Orrville and at sites throughout Medina and Summit counties.

Professionals who want to improve their careers can select from a wide range of workshops and courses, including weekend programs offering degrees at an accelerated pace, through the University of Akron's Workforce Development and Continuing Education Division.

The University of Akron offers its students the "Akron Advantage," a series of initiatives that provide exceptional benefits for UA students. The Akron Advantage includes the New Landscape for Learning program, a $200-million, multiyear campus improvement program that will add six new buildings and 30 acres of green space to the campus; the Career Advantage network, which guarantees every student, regardless of major, the opportunity to obtain practical experience in their chosen fields before graduation; and Technology Without Boundaries℠, an initiative to provide students with the latest learning technologies, from online and Web-enhanced courses, to distance-learning classrooms and wireless laptop computers. For more information about the Akron Advantage, students should visit the University's Web site (listed below) or call 800-655-4884 (toll-free).

THE COLLEGE OF NURSING
Founded in 1967, the College has a long tradition of excellence. The College offers multiple educational programs designed to meet the needs of both students aspiring to become professional nurses and practicing professional nurses seeking career advancement.

Located on the campus in Mary Gladwin Hall, the College offers the basic baccalaureate program (B.S.N.), an accelerated B.S.N. for students who hold a bachelor's degree in an area other than nursing, an RN/B.S.N. sequence for registered nurse graduates of associate degree and diploma programs, an LPN/B.S.N. sequence for licensed practical nurses aspiring to become professional nurses, the Master of Science in Nursing (M.S.N.) degree, and the RN/M.S.N. sequence for registered nurse graduates of associate degree and diploma programs who meet graduate standards. The University of Akron and Kent State University offer a Joint Ph.D. in Nursing (JPDN) program, a single doctoral program with a single, unified doctoral nursing faculty and student body. The program prepares scholars in nursing with balanced preparation to be researchers, educators, administrators, consultants, or entrepreneurs.

There are 42 full-time and 16 part-time faculty members. Twenty-five full-time faculty members (59 percent) hold doctoral degrees. The remainder have master's degrees in nursing, with many having earned certification in advanced practice specialty areas.

The College offers clinical experiences for students in a wide variety of traditional and nontraditional settings and with diverse patient populations, including care of adults in hospitals, community agencies, and homes; care of well and ill elderly; care of newborns and children; care of persons with mental health problems in hospitals and community agencies; critical care; and extended care and rehabilitation.

The College is approved by the Ohio Board of Nursing, accredited by the National League for Nursing Accrediting Commission (NLNAC), and holds preliminary approval from the Commission on Collegiate Nursing Education (CCNE).

International study in nursing through a summer elective course is often available.

PROGRAMS OF STUDY
The basic baccalaureate program leading to the B.S.N. degree and RN licensure is a four-year program that is balanced between nursing courses and University courses. Students enter the program after completing one year of prerequisite University courses. The nursing courses span three years, with clinical experiences in each semester of the program. The senior year features a senior practicum that is designed to give the student greater depth in an area of the student's choosing. A Cooperative Education Program is available to combine work and study.

A fifteen-month accelerated B.S.N. program is open to students who already hold a bachelor's degree and have completed prerequisite courses. All science courses must have been taken within the last five years.

The RN/B.S.N. sequence has been serving the educational needs of registered nurses since 1980. The sequence features learning contracts to allow flexible hours for clinical requirements and classroom time scheduled one day per week. Once students are admitted to the College, they can complete the sequence in one calendar year of full-time study; a part-time option is available. There is no testing required for admission. An outreach RN/B.S.N. sequence is offered at the Lorain County Community College campus and Wayne College.

The LPN/B.S.N. sequence was begun in 1990. The College was one of the first baccalaureate programs in the country to offer a sequence for LPNs. This sequence features testing for advanced placement and credit for prior learning. The LPN can finish the baccalaureate program in four semesters if advanced placement is earned.

The Master of Science in Nursing (M.S.N.) degree program prepares graduates for roles in advanced practice or advanced role preparation in administration. Within the advanced practice options, students may choose adult/gerontological health nursing, behavioral health nursing, child and adolescent health nursing, or nurse anesthesia tracks. Advanced practice options include preparation as a nurse practitioner or clinical nurse specialist. All M.S.N. graduate students take a common core and advanced practice or role options that include advanced clinical experiences.

The RN/M.S.N. sequence is designed for RN graduates of associate degree and diploma programs who meet graduate admission criteria. Students take three years to complete the sequence, which includes baccalaureate and master's course work. Through this program, the student receives both the B.S.N. and M.S.N. degrees.

An M.P.H. consortium program exists with the Northeast Ohio University College of Medicine (NEOUCOM).

ACADEMIC FACILITIES

The College has a state-of-the-art learning resources center that includes simulated patient care areas and a computer laboratory. The College also has a Center for Nursing, which links the College to the community and is used by clients for health-care services and by the faculty and students as a practice and research site. The nursing library holdings are contained in the Science and Technology Library of the University. Nursing students have full access to all the facilities and services of the entire University.

LOCATION

Located in the northeast region of Ohio, Akron offers a wide variety of recreational, business, and cultural activities. The area is perfect for recreational activities that encompass all seasons. The University's presence in northeast Ohio provides numerous opportunities in major collegiate, amateur, and professional sports, concerts, cultural events, and commerce, all within easy driving distance and many accessible via public transportation. On campus, the Ohio Ballet, Emily Davis Art Gallery, University Orchestra, Opera/Musical Theatre, concerts, recitals, choral programs, Touring Arts Program, University Theatre, Repertory Dance Company, and professional artists performing at Edwin J. Thomas Performing Arts Hall contribute to the University's rich cultural environment.

Blossom Music Center, summer home of the Cleveland Orchestra, is located 20 minutes north of the campus. The city of Cleveland with all its fine recreational, sports, and cultural offerings is just 40 minutes from the University.

STUDENT SERVICES

The University has many resource and service offices to meet student needs. Campus resources include the Academic Advisement Center, Adult Resource Center, Sixty Plus Program, Placement Services, Student Employment, Career Placement Services, Student Volunteer Program, Counseling and Testing Center, Financial Aid Office, Student Health Services, Pan-African Culture and Research Center, Office of International Programs, Office of Multicultural Development, Peer Counseling Program, Office of Accessibility, and writing, reading, and math developmental laboratories.

Undergraduate and graduate student organizations exist to involve students in the governance of the College. The Delta Omega chapter of Sigma Theta Tau, the international honor society of nursing, is housed within the College. The Collegiate Nursing Club, which is open to all undergraduate students, is affiliated with the National Student Nurses Association.

A campus natatorium, indoor track, and fitness rooms are all open to nursing students.

THE NURSING STUDENT GROUP

Enrollment in the undergraduate program is 407; it is 207 in the graduate program. Full-time and part-time students are represented in both programs. Postbaccalaureate students, RNs, LPNs, transfer students, and new high school graduates are represented in the College. About 10 percent of each entering B.S.N. class in the undergraduate program are men.

COSTS

Undergraduate tuition and fees for the 2004–05 academic year for Ohio residents were $313 per credit up to 11.5 credits or a $3755 flat fee per semester for 12 to 15 credits. Nonresidents paid a $274.36 per-credit surcharge.

Graduate tuition costs for the 2004–05 academic year were $328 per credit for Ohio residents. There was a $218 per-credit surcharge for nonresidents.

Additional costs include housing, transportation, books, course laboratory fees, immunizations, CPR certification, uniforms, and liability insurance.

FINANCIAL AID

Financial aid is available through the University as well as the College of Nursing. The University offers a variety of scholarships, grants, loans, student assistantships, work-study opportunities, and graduate assistantships. The College offers a variety of scholarships, graduate assistantships, and Federal Graduate Nurse Traineeships.

APPLYING

Students applying for the baccalaureate program must have completed one year of prerequisite college/university courses and have earned at least a 2.75 grade point average in those prerequisite courses. Applicants must be enrolled at the University of Akron for the spring semester prior to admission and are ranked according to grade point average in science courses after completion of the spring semester. Each year, 140 students are admitted into the undergraduate program. Course work begins in the fall.

Students entering the LPN/B.S.N. sequence must have completed two years of prerequisite college/university courses with a minimum overall college grade point average of 2.75. Course work begins in the spring semester.

Requirements for the RN/B.S.N. sequence include completion of prerequisite courses and current Ohio RN licensure. Course work begins in the summer.

Students applying to the M.S.N. program must hold a baccalaureate degree in nursing from an NLNAC-accredited nursing program; complete prerequisite courses; submit scores from the GRE taken within the last five years, an essay, and three letters of reference; and hold a current Ohio RN license.

CORRESPONDENCE AND INFORMATION

Office of Student Affairs
College of Nursing
The University of Akron
Akron, Ohio 44325-3701
Telephone: 888-477-7887 (toll-free)

Office of Undergraduate Admissions
The University of Akron
Akron, Ohio 44325-2001
Telephone: 330-972-7100

Office of Graduate Admissions
The University of Akron
Akron, Ohio 44325-2101
Telephone: 330-972-7663

Office of Financial Aid
The University of Akron
Akron, Ohio 44325-6211
Telephone: 330-972-7032
World Wide Web: http://www.uakron.edu

University of Alabama in Huntsville
College of Nursing
Huntsville, Alabama

THE UNIVERSITY

The University of Alabama in Huntsville (UAH), one of the three campuses comprising the University of Alabama System, is accredited by the Commission on Colleges of the Southern Association of Colleges and Schools to award bachelor's, master's, and doctoral degrees. Nestled in the rolling foothills of north central Alabama, Huntsville is internationally renowned for its high technology industry and its ties to the U.S. space program. UAH was one of the original group of colleges and universities to be designated a Space Grant College. UAH is the only institution offering both undergraduate and graduate nursing programs in north Alabama and is the area's center for research activities in nursing.

The modern 350-acre UAH campus has thirty-one major buildings, including the College of Nursing. UAH has more than 6,900 students and more than 300 full-time faculty members, 89 percent with terminal degrees.

THE COLLEGE OF NURSING

The College of Nursing offers the Bachelor of Science in Nursing (B.S.N.) degree and the Master of Science in Nursing (M.S.N.) degree as well as a Post-master's Family Nurse Practitioner Certificate. The undergraduate and graduate programs are designed to give the student the theoretical and experiential bases for current and future practice. The College of Nursing is accredited by the National League for Nursing Accrediting Commission and the Collegiate Commission on Nursing Education and is approved by the Alabama Board of Nursing.

Although nursing is becoming highly specialized, it remains, fundamentally, a caring profession. UAH took both of these aspects into consideration when designing its curriculum in nursing. In addition to focusing on essentials of nursing in hospitals, the curriculum also emphasizes community-based practice and primary care. When the revised curriculum for the College of Nursing was submitted for approval, the Alabama Board of Nursing applauded the efforts of the UAH College of Nursing in developing an innovative and forward-looking program for preparing students to function in the rapidly changing nursing field.

The 40 faculty members in the College of Nursing place a high priority on teaching and individual attention to students. The undergraduate student-faculty ratio in clinical areas is less than 10:1. The professors have an ongoing concern with some of the most significant issues in nursing today, including breast cancer research, nursing ethics, health care to underserved rural populations, space research, and health policy.

PROGRAMS OF STUDY

The Bachelor of Science in Nursing (B.S.N.) degree provides the nursing theory, science, humanities, and behavioral science preparation necessary for the full scope of professional nursing responsibilities and provides the knowledge base necessary for advanced education in specialized clinical practice. Building on the foundation provided by 60 semester hours of general education requirements, the baccalaureate curriculum provides extensive clinical opportunities in the context of a holistic, family-centered, community-based approach. Computer technology is integrated throughout the curriculum. A minimum of 129 semester hours are required for the B.S.N.; 69 semester hours must be in nursing.

The UAH College of Nursing also offers a specialized B.S.N. curriculum designed for registered nurses. This program recognizes the unique abilities and needs of registered nurse students and builds on students' existing knowledge and experience. Classes for registered nurses meet only one day a week to accommodate work schedules as much as possible. This twelve-month program offers both full- and part-time attendance options. The students in the RN/B.S.N. program must also earn 128 semester hours of credit. Registered nurse students receive 32 semester hours of validated nursing credit for previous nursing knowledge and take an additional 37 semester hours of nursing at UAH. The RN-M.S.N. Early Decision Option is available to associate degree–prepared RNs. Nurses who decide early in their course of study that they wish to receive both a B.S.N. and an M.S.N. can complete both in a seven-semester sequence.

The graduate program in nursing leads to the Master of Science in Nursing degree. This program focuses on preparation for advanced nursing practice. It prepares graduates to assume leadership roles in the direct delivery of care as nurse practitioners in primary care (family nurse practitioners) and in acute care (acute-care nurse practitioners and adult health clinicians) or in the administration of health-care delivery systems (nursing administration). The M.S.N. program can be completed in four semesters, although other options are also available for students who prefer a slower pace. Graduate courses are taught one day a week to accommodate the majority of students who continue to practice while pursuing the M.S.N. The length of the program varies by specialty and ranges from 39 to 42 semester hours. Both thesis and nonthesis options are available. Nurse practitioner students complete 588 clinical hours, adult health clinicians complete 546 clinical hours, and nursing administration students complete 336 clinical hours.

The Graduate Certificate in Nursing Education is a five-course, 15-semester-hour program offered to graduate and postgraduate nursing students. The post-M.S.N. family nurse practitioner certificate program is designed for individuals who have already earned a master's degree in nursing and who desire additional preparation for family nurse practitioner certification. The program is three semesters in length.

ACADEMIC FACILITIES

Located in the center of the UAH main campus, the Nursing Building is a spacious, four-story structure that houses state-of-the-art equipment, lecture rooms, and laboratories for teaching nursing. The building also contains faculty and administrative offices. A Learning Resource Center, equipped with a comprehensive selection of audiovisual materials, is available to students for independent study and group learning activities. A well-equipped computer lab in the Learning Resource Center is available for use by all nursing students.

Located adjacent to the Nursing Building, the UAH library has a collection of 412,571 volumes and receives some 2,766 periodicals. The library houses both monographs and journals useful to nursing students. Students are also able to use the Medical Library at the University of Alabama School of Medicine–Huntsville Program, which is located in the heart of the city's medical district.

Clinical experiences are arranged in a variety of appropriate settings within the Huntsville area, which serves as a regional center for state-of-the-art health care. With three major hospitals in Huntsville and a wide variety of health-care facilities located close by, adequate resources are available to offer students a broad array of clinical nursing experiences.

LOCATION

The University is located in Huntsville, Alabama, adjacent to Cummings Research Park and close to Redstone Arsenal and NASA's Marshall Space Flight Center. A wonderful mix of modern amenities and old Southern charm, Huntsville is a regional center for arts, entertainment, industry, and medicine. Located in the foothills of the Appalachian Mountain chain, Huntsville is 4 hours from Memphis and Atlanta and approximately 2 hours from Birmingham and Nashville.

STUDENT SERVICES

UAH provides a full-range of student services for all members of the student body. These services include the student counseling center, wellness center, tutorial services, academic advisement center, and office of multicultural affairs.

The College of Nursing funds and supports its own Office of Student Affairs to meet the needs of all students enrolled in the College. Located in the Nursing Building and staffed by student services professionals, the Office of Student Affairs provides assistance with admissions, academic advisement and registration services, information on financial aid, and referral services.

The University also provides a rich and varied extracurricular program. There are more than 100 student clubs and organizations on campus, including dozens of honor societies, preprofessional clubs, and sororities and fraternities. Cabarets, films, dances, concerts, and lectures are offered throughout the year. In addition to a full slate of intramural activities, UAH fields varsity teams in eight sports.

THE NURSING STUDENT GROUP

Approximately 400 undergraduate and 200 graduate students, representing a wide variety of ages, ethnic backgrounds, and experiences, make up the diverse students body in the College of Nursing.

COSTS

Tuition and fees for the 2004–05 academic year were approximately $2650 per semester for baccalaureate students. Graduate tuition and fees were approximately $3100 per semester. Uniforms, liability insurance, physical examinations, CPR certification, and Hepatitis B immunizations are required upon admission. For RN/B.S.N. students, additional expenses may include fees for "Credit by Validation."

FINANCIAL AID

Various types of financial aid are available based on scholastic performance and financial need. While some institutional scholarships are awarded solely on a student's academic record, many require demonstration of financial need. Interested students should contact the Office of Financial Aid and complete both a UAH scholarship application and the Free Application for Federal Student Aid.

Federal Professional Nurse Traineeships are available to eligible graduate students. Applications are provided to students after they accept their offer of admission. Some graduate assistantships are also available each academic year.

APPLYING

All applicants for admission to the B.S.N. degree program of the College of Nursing must complete UAH admission requirements, be admitted as regular degree-seeking students, and declare nursing as their major. Students are admitted to the upper division once a year for fall semester. Admission to the upper-division nursing major is competitive. A separate application for the upper-division nursing major must be completed on forms provided by the College of Nursing and received by March 1 preceding the fall semester for which admission is sought. Each lower-division course requirement for the nursing major must be completed with a minimum grade of C prior to admission to the upper division.

RN/B.S.N. students are admitted once a year. Registered nurse students must submit proof of current licensure in the state of Alabama. Recent graduates of associate degree or diploma nursing programs who are not yet licensed may be admitted to complete lower-division course work, but they will not be admitted to the upper-division clinical component of the program until they are licensed. Each lower-division course requirement must be completed with at least a grade of C prior to admission to the RN/B.S.N. program. The deadline for applications is March 1 preceding the fall semester for which admission is sought.

An RN-M.S.N. early decision option is available to associate degree–prepared RNs so they may complete the B.S.N. and the M.S.N. in a seven-semester sequence.

M.S.N. students are admitted once a year for fall semester. The application deadline for priority consideration is April 15 preceding the fall semester for which admission is sought. Applicants must have a B.S.N. from an accredited program, a minimum GPA of 3.0, current GRE or MAT scores, three references, satisfactory completion of a basic statistics course, and an Alabama nursing license. Admission is competitive.

Post-masters students are admitted once a year for summer semester. The application deadline is April 1. Applicants must have an M.S.N., credit for graduate-level health assessment and pathophysiology, two references, and completed an applicant's statement.

Prior to admission to any program, students are advised through the College of Nursing Office of Student Affairs. All interested students should contact the Office of Student Affairs for detailed program information, admission requirements, and application deadlines.

CORRESPONDENCE AND INFORMATION

Office of Student Affairs
NB 207
UAH College of Nursing
Huntsville, Alabama 35899

Telephone: 256-824-6742
Fax: 256-824-6026
E-mail: nursing@email.uah.edu
World Wide Web: http://onlinenurse.nb.uah.edu
http://www.uah.edu

The University of Arizona
College of Nursing
Tucson, Arizona

THE UNIVERSITY OF ARIZONA® COLLEGE OF NURSING

THE UNIVERSITY

The University of Arizona was organized as a land-grant college by action of the Legislative Assembly of the Territory of Arizona in 1885. The University is organized into twelve schools and eighteen colleges with an enrollment of 36,932 students, of whom 7,387 are graduate students. Students come from all fifty states and more than 100 countries. The University of Arizona (Carnegie Doctoral/Research University–Extensive) offers a broad spectrum of undergraduate and graduate programs in more than 150 departments and fields. Doctoral degrees are offered in ninety fields, including nursing. The University is one of sixty-three research universities in the United States and Canada elected to the Association of American Universities. The University is internationally known for its excellent faculty, groundbreaking research, and top-ranked programs. The University is accredited by the North Central Association of Colleges and Schools.

The College of Nursing is one of five academic units within the Arizona Health Sciences Center (AHSC), known nationally for its contributions to health care and research. Each year, $85 million in research grants and gifts expands the ability of the AHSC to conduct basic and applied research to improve the health of the residents of the state. The AHSC has strong interdisciplinary programs, including gerontology, neuroscience, public health, and rural health.

THE COLLEGE OF NURSING

The College of Nursing, founded in 1956, currently serves 447 students: 303 undergraduate and 144 graduate, 83 of whom are doctoral students. The College of Nursing is a learning community that provides undergraduate and graduate education, generates and expands nursing knowledge, and provides service to the community. The College offers extraordinary educational and research opportunities through the Center of Injury Mechanisms and Related Responses, the Research Resource Center, and the Center on Aging, one of many Centers of Excellence. These centers provide consultation on research design and data analysis, on research and educational grant proposals, and on conduct proposal reviews. Centers also offer educational opportunities directed toward improving the health of the Arizona citizenry. The Center on Aging is an interdisciplinary program in gerontology and geriatric care. Numerous rural and border health interdisciplinary programs offer exceptional educational experiences. The College has international partnership programs with Mahidol University in Bangkok, Thailand, and the Autonomous University of Nuevo Leon in Monterrey, N.L., Mexico. Both partnerships provide opportunities for graduate student and faculty exchange, collaborative research projects, and international colleagueship. Since 1997, the faculty has engaged in the Faculty Praxis Plan to strive toward linking educational, research, and service activities to local, state, national, and international health needs. The College of Nursing is accredited by the Commission on Collegiate Nursing Education (2002–12).

PROGRAMS OF STUDY

The College offers a Bachelor of Science in Nursing (B.S.N.) for traditional students and a fourteen-month accelerated B.S.N. program for college graduates. The B.S.N. program prepares the professional nurse through extensive study in the concepts and skills of patient assessment, patient-care management, and evaluation of patient-care outcomes and the impact of ethical, legal, and technological strategies. Traditional program students begin the nursing major in the third semester of the eight-semester program.

The College offers a Master of Science (M.S.) and a doctoral degree (Ph.D.) with a major in nursing that maximizes the use of online technology. The M.S. program has three options: nurse practitioner (NP), health-care systems (HCS), and nursing informatics (NI). The NP option provides nurses with advanced preparation as adult nurse practitioners (ANP), family nurse practitioners (FNP), or psychiatric–mental health nurse practitioners (PMHNP). The NP focus is on the nurse as a primary-care provider knowledgeable about health assessment, primary prevention, health maintenance, and illness management. The HCS focus is on conducting evaluations that assist leaders in making decisions about health-care delivery and improving client, provider, and organizational outcomes. The NI focus is on using technology more effectively and on designing, implementing, and evaluating health-care information systems. Graduate certificate programs are available online in rural health, informatics, health-care systems, and nurse practitioner options.

The state-of-the-art Ph.D. program is delivered online and is designed to prepare scientists to conduct theory-based research in nursing, to engage in scholarly dialogue, and to contribute to the development of nursing knowledge. The doctoral program curriculum is designed as a full-time, three-year, 64-credit post-master's program, or a full-time, four-year, 79-credit postbaccalaureate program. The program provides a learning matrix of course work, collegial relationships, community networks, mentored research, and collaboration in scholarship.

World-renowned researchers and scholars mentor students in one of three research focal areas: health-care systems, injury mechanisms and biobehavioral responses, and vulnerable populations. In addition to the doctoral program, the College has predoctoral and postdoctoral research training fellowships in injury mechanisms and related responses. Research assistantships and scholarships are also available. Graduates of the doctoral program provide national and international leadership that advances the discipline and profession of nursing. *U.S. News & World Report* (2001) ranked the College of Nursing's graduate programs among the top twenty in the United States (top 4 percent, according to the dean).

ACADEMIC FACILITIES

The University library system, which consists of three large but separate facilities, contains approximately 7 million items, including books, periodicals, microforms, maps, government publications, manuscripts, and nonbook media. College facilities for student learning and research include a Patient Care Learning Center, Office of Research, Computer Laboratory, Behavioral Studies Laboratory, and Biological Studies Laboratory.

LOCATION

The University of Arizona College of Nursing is located in Tucson, Arizona, in the southern section of the Sonoran Desert 45 miles north of the Mexican border. Tucson is a city of 750,000 people, with a rich Western history and culture influenced by Native Americans, Mexicans, and American pioneers. The wealth of educational, cultural, and recreational opportunities attracts students and visitors from around the world. The environment of southern Arizona is pristine, with wondrous sunrises and sunsets highlighting the mountain ranges that surround the city. The city shares common borders with the Tohono O'Odam and the Pasqua Yaqui Indian Nations and is surrounded by rugged mountains rising to more than 9,000 feet. Southern Arizona has more than 300 days of sunshine per year, more than any other region in the U.S.

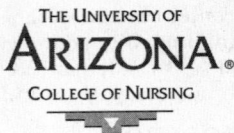

STUDENT SERVICES

The University provides various services and opportunities to promote students' intellectual and social growth and physical health. These include recreation facilities, student organizations, and honor societies. There is an active student governing organization as well as specialized academic support and clinical services.

THE NURSING STUDENT GROUP

The College of Nursing is committed to recruiting a diverse population of national and international students to study at the University. Of the 447 students, 303 are undergraduate and 144 are graduate students. The student body includes those of African-American, Native American, Asian, European-American, and Hispanic heritage.

COSTS

Tuition for full-time B.S.N., M.S., and Ph.D. students for the 2004–05 academic year ranged from $2049 to $4174. Tuition costs are among the lowest in the nation. Tuition for the accelerated B.S.N. program for college graduates is paid by sponsoring health-care organizations of Tucson.

FINANCIAL AID

The University of Arizona provides access to a wide range of federal, state, and private financial aid to students through the University's Office of Student Financial Aid. Assistance is available to students based on financial need, academic merit, and program of study. The College oversees the distribution of an abundance of merit- and need-based financial awards in the form of scholarships, fellowships, and the Federal Advanced Education Nursing Traineeships for graduate students.

APPLYING

Application materials and instructions for each educational program are available online at the College's Web site, which is listed in the Correspondence and Information section. Deadline dates for application vary according to program level. The College holds information meetings on the various programs throughout the year.

CORRESPONDENCE AND INFORMATION

Office of Student Affairs
College of Nursing
The University of Arizona
P.O. Box 210203
Tucson, Arizona 85721-0203
Telephone: 520-626-3808
800-288-6158 (toll-free)
Fax: 520-626-6424
E-mail: info@nursing.arizona.edu
YourOnlinePhD@nursing.arizona.edu
World Wide Web: http://www.nursing.arizona.edu

THE FACULTY

Terry Badger, Professor; Ph.D., Texas at Austin, 1986; FAAN. Behavioral interventions/chronic illness.

Judith Berg, Associate Professor; Ph.D., California, San Francisco, 1997. Menopause symptom management in breast cancer survivors.

Joyceen Boyle, Professor and Associate Dean, Academic Affairs; Ph.D., Utah, 1982; FAAN. Cultural aspects of health.

Linda Chapman, Clinical Associate Professor; D.N.Sc., California, San Francisco, 1990. Expectant fathers during labor and birth.

Janice Crist, Assistant Professor; Ph.D., Oregon Health Sciences, 1999. Mexican elders, family decision making, in-home care.

Neva Crogan, Assistant Professor; Ph.D., Washington State, 1998. Improving the nutritional status and QOL of older adults in nursing homes.

Sandra Cromwell, Associate Professor; Ph.D., Arizona, 1992. Behavioral change in Mexican-American sedentary older women.

Judith Effken, Associate Professor; Ph.D., Connecticut, 1993. Clinical information displays to improve trauma outcomes.

Carmen Eribes, Clinical Associate Professor; Ph.D., California, San Francisco, 1997. Community health and occupational health; health promotion and risk reduction.

Melissa Goldsmith, Clinical Assistant Professor; Ph.D., Arizona. Health behavior among women, cervical cancer screening behavior, postpartum smoking relapse.

Kathleen Insel, Assistant Professor; Ph.D., Arizona, 1993. Aging and medication adherence.

Marjorie Isenberg, Professor and Dean; D.N.Sc., Boston University, 1978; FAAN. Testing Orem's Self-Care Deficit Theory, international collaboration for testing self-care nursing science.

Elaine Jones, Associate Professor; Ph.D., Arizona, 1986. Family functioning: deaf parents with nondeaf children.

Jacqueline Kelley, Clinical Professor; N.D., M.P.H., Case Western Reserve, 1996. Adolescent pregnancy, fetal alcohol syndrome.

Gerri Lamb, Associate Professor; Ph.D., Arizona, 1987; FAAN. Health policy and economics.

Lois Loescher, Assistant Professor; Ph.D., Arizona, 2001. Cancer prevention and control, cancer genetic risk.

Marylyn Morris McEwen, Associate Professor; Ph.D., Arizona, 2003. Mexican immigrants' understanding and experience with latent tuberculosis infection and factors that influence preventive treatment.

Cheryl McNiece, Clinical Assistant Professor; Ph.D., Arizona, 2002. Oncology and pain management.

Carrie Merkle, Associate Professor; Ph.D., Arizona State, 1990; FAAN. Prolactin and endothelial wound repair in vitro.

Cathleen Michaels, Assistant Professor; Ph.D., Texas Woman's, 1985; FAAN. Women's mammography.

Petra Miketova, Research Assistant Professor; Ph.D., Arizona, 1997. Cellular membrane damage with chemotherapeutic agents.

Ki Moore, Professor and Director; D.N.Sc., California, San Francisco, 1985; FAAN. Biobehavioral interventions to improve CNS outcomes in children with leukemia.

Carolyn Murdaugh, Associate Dean for Research; Ph.D., Arizona, 1982. Cardiovascular, quality of life.

Linda Phillips, Professor; Ph.D., Arizona, 1986; FAAN. Traumatic brain injury.

Pamela Reed, Professor; Ph.D., Wayne State, 1982; FAAN. Nursing philosophy and spirituality.

Sally Reel, Clinical Professor and Associate Dean, Academic Practice; Ph.D., Virginia, 1994; FAAN. Rural health care and school violence.

Leslie Ritter, Assistant Professor; Ph.D., Arizona, 1996. Mechanism of injury after stroke or cerebral ischemia.

Rita Snyder, Associate Professor; Ph.D., Arizona, 1983. Information technology.

Amy Tsang, Assistant Professor; Ph.D., California, San Francisco, 1995. Disease severity, symptoms, self-efficacy, and physical activity.

Joyce Verran, Professor and Director; Ph.D., Arizona, 1982; FAAN. Nurse-sensitive patient outcomes.

Deborah Vincent, Associate Professor; Ph.D., Michigan, 1998. Cost-effectiveness, type 2 diabetes in Latinos, alternative health-care delivery models.

Shu-Fen Wung, Associate Professor; Ph.D., California, San Francisco, 1999. ECG criteria for posterior myocardial infarction.

University of Cincinnati
College of Nursing
Cincinnati, Ohio

THE UNIVERSITY

The University of Cincinnati (UC), founded in 1819, is a multifaceted learning and research center. As a large, urban, state university it represents a diverse community with many opportunities. The University's mission is to function as a model for freedom of intellectual exchange and to provide the highest quality learning environment, world-renowned scholarship, and innovation. Its commitment to building a community of students and faculty and staff members where individuals appreciate and respect diversity is demonstrated through the Just Community program. Alumni and faculty members of the University are proven leaders, inventors, artists, and scholars in many disciplines. The University is one of 150 universities in the 2000 Carnegie Classification that were classified as Doctoral/ Research Universities–Extensive.

The University's campus features the best of both worlds—it is large enough to offer vast educational opportunities, yet small enough to feel cozy. With seventeen colleges and an annual enrollment of approximately 34,000 students, UC offers more than 445 programs of study. However, from one end of the campus to the other is only a 20-minute walk. To learn more about UC, students should visit the University's Web site at http://www.uc.edu.

THE COLLEGE OF NURSING

In 2003, *U.S. News & World Report* ranked the UC College of Nursing in the top 6 percent of baccalaureate and higher degree programs. The College has a long history of excellence in nursing education. In 1916 it became the first baccalaureate program in nursing in the United States. In addition to the Bachelor of Science in Nursing (B.S.N.), the College offers Master of Science in Nursing (M.S.N.) and Doctor of Philosophy (Ph.D.) in nursing programs. The College prepares beginning and advanced practitioners of professional nursing to function in a variety of settings with diverse populations. Opportunities abound for practicing nurses to maintain, improve, and expand their competencies.

The College is fully accredited by the Commission of Collegiate Nursing Education (CCNE). The appropriate graduate programs are fully accredited by the Council on Accreditation of Nurse Anesthesia Educational Programs and the Division of Accreditation of the American College of Nurse Midwives. The Pediatric Nurse Practitioner Program is recognized by the National Certification Board of Pediatric Nurse Practitioners and Nurses.

The College is an integral part of the University and its Medical Center. Cooperative relations among the units of the University, myriad health-care settings, and the diversity of the greater Cincinnati community facilitate creative approaches for leadership and excellence in nursing. The College is a World Health Organization Collaborating Center affiliate.

The faculty members of the College are well prepared to provide excellent classroom and clinical instruction. The College employs 60 full-time faculty members. Many faculty members are nationally certified in a clinical area of specialization. They contribute to the improvement of the profession and health care through their outstanding teaching, research, and service.

The Institute for Nursing Research, which is a collaborative effort with Patient Care Services at University Hospital, fosters health-related research. Major research foci are injury and violence, substance abuse, symptom management, and oncology. Multiple NIH grants have been received to promote research in these areas.

PROGRAMS OF STUDY

The College's B.S.N. program options include a traditional track and an RN/B.S.N. track. The prenursing year for traditional students exposes them to nursing through the course Success in College and Nursing. The B.S.N. curriculum provides a foundation for community-focused professional practice with individuals and families having a variety of health-care needs. Community-focused professional practice includes acute care in hospitals as well as other health-care environments. Emphasis is placed on clinical competence, critical thinking, professional roles, participation in multidisciplinary teams, and a commitment to continued learning. Full- or part-time study is possible.

The master's program prepares nurses for advanced practice nursing and for leadership and management in diverse health-care environments. It offers an accelerated pathway for individuals holding baccalaureate degrees in fields other than nursing who wish to become advanced practice nurses. The master's curriculum consists of core courses plus courses in the student's selected area of clinical focus. A scholarly project is required for degree completion. Upon completion of the program, graduates meet current national specialty certification requirements for advanced practice in their chosen field. Nurse practitioner preparation in acute care and adult, family, pediatric, neonatal, and women's health is offered. Clinical nurse specialist options include acute and ambulatory care, community health, occupational health, and psychiatric nursing. Other options are nurse anesthesia, nurse midwifery, and nursing service administration (including an M.S.N./M.B.A. option). Post-master's certificate programs for practitioners, psychiatric nursing, and genetics are available.

The doctoral program focuses on the preparation of nurses for positions of leadership in academic and health services institutions and health policy agencies. The curriculum is designed with a core of required courses and a cognate area of the student's choosing to support preparation for research in a defined area. Students may enter the doctoral program upon completion of a B.S.N. or M.S.N. degree. Doctoral students are required to be in residence for full-time study during three of five consecutive quarters, excluding those for a dissertation.

AFFILIATIONS WITH HEALTH-CARE FACILITIES

The Medical Center and main University campuses are contiguous. Units in the Medical Center in addition to the College of Nursing include the Colleges of Allied Health Sciences, Pharmacy, and Medicine. Some affiliated institutions adjacent to the Medical Center are the University Hospital, the Veterans Affairs Medical Center, the Cincinnati Children's Hospital Medical Center, the Shriners Burns Institute, the Cincinnati Center for Developmental Disorders, and the Cincinnati Health Department. The College is affiliated with multiple hospitals, home care services, community agencies, and health service providers. Cooperative relationships provide rich educational, clinical, and research resources.

ACADEMIC FACILITIES

The College has numerous academic resources. The resources include multiple libraries and on-site research and technology support.

The College's Solomon P. Levi Library is one of the best nursing libraries and houses more than 300 journals relevant to nursing. In addition, the library connects to all the University libraries and OhioLINK, the statewide online catalog. These connections provide students, wherever they are, with access to the second-largest library system in the country.

The College's Research Institute provides grant development and project management assistance, statistical consultation, and data management support.

Among the technology resources are an equipped classroom for live interactive distance learning, a learning center incorporating clinical practice laboratories, a twenty-three-station student computer lab, online teaching materials, and faculty support for development of electronic resources and use of the University's online delivery system. All classrooms are equipped with projection and computer systems to assist faculty members in facilitating learning.

LOCATION

The University is only 10 minutes from downtown Cincinnati, so students can easily benefit from city activities. The city is big enough to have nationally renowned arts organizations and major-league sports, yet small enough to take pride in its neighborhood cafés and scenic parks. Cincinnati is known for its restaurants, riverfront recreation areas, and festivals such as Oktoberfest and the Appalachian Fair. Cincinnati is accessible by various modes of transportation and is the hub of a network of interstate highways.

STUDENT SERVICES

Education does not stop at the academic doors. The University is a place where students are continually learning, sharing, and growing. Students may choose to live in residence halls or take part in a variety of clubs. Diversity is an important part of the University community, with a number of ethnic organizations, services, and events. Students take part in intramural sports, attend College Conservatory of Music concerts and plays, or sometimes just hang out.

The College's Office of Student Affairs provides academic counseling and support services for students in every program of the College. The office offers a variety of orientation and career development programs to help students attain their professional goals. Coordinators for each program assist students and make the students' use of general University services easier.

There are many opportunities for student growth outside of the College's classroom and clinical settings. Some students have taken advantage of opportunities for international experiences. Undergraduate and graduate students participate in a variety of student government, philanthropic, and social organizations. Undergraduate students are active in the National Student Nurse Association. Students in all programs who excel in scholarship, research, or clinical practice are recognized through induction into the College's Beta Iota chapter of Sigma Theta Tau, the international honor society for nursing, and through College, University, and national awards.

THE NURSING STUDENT GROUP

The students in all programs in the College of Nursing represent diverse backgrounds in age, gender, ethnicity, nationality, and experience. The undergraduate program enrollment comprises approximately 375 students, about 20 percent of whom are registered nurses returning for baccalaureate degrees. The master's program enrollment averages 200 students, about 60 percent of whom are enrolled full-time. The doctoral program has 50 students, most of whom are enrolled full-time. Graduates of the College are sought by local, state, and national employers.

COSTS

Tuition and fees for the entire three-quarter academic year in 2004–05 were approximately $6936 for undergraduates and $8094 for graduate students who are full-time Ohio residents. Full-time nonresident student tuition was $17,319 for undergraduates and $13,080 for graduate students per year. Tuition per credit hour was $193 (undergraduate, Ohio resident), $482 (undergraduate, nonresident), $270 (graduate, Ohio resident), and $498 (graduate, nonresident). Health insurance and parking, if needed, are additional costs.

University housing costs are approximately $7474 per year for residence hall room and board and $488 to $695 per month for apartments. For those who wish to live off campus, Cincinnati offers reasonable, suitable housing for rent.

FINANCIAL AID

Financial assistance for students derives from a variety of sources such as College and University scholarships, low-interest loans, University Graduate Assistantships, and Professional Nurse Traineeship funds. Scholarships, assistantships, and traineeships are awarded on a competitive basis. The majority of full-time graduate students receive some type of financial assistance.

APPLYING

B.S.N. program applicants should obtain program information and application materials from the University's Office of Admissions. All traditional freshman are admitted to prenursing. Applicants who qualify as Academic Scholars at the time of admission to prenursing are guaranteed admission to the nursing major if they maintain grades of C or better in all required prenursing courses, with a minimum GPA of 2.5 in these courses. For all other applicants and transfer students, admission into the nursing major is on a competitive basis.

The application process for the M.S.N. and Ph.D. programs is handled through the College's Office of Student Affairs. Program and financial aid information as well as application materials are available on the Web at http://www.uc.edu. Graduate Record Examinations (GRE) scores are required as part of the admission process. TOEFL scores are required of all applicants whose native language is not English. Applicants who have completed the application process by January 1 are given priority consideration for fall admission and financial assistance. For individuals seeking admission to the nurse anesthesia major, the application deadline is October 1 for each class that starts the following September.

CORRESPONDENCE AND INFORMATION

Office of Student Affairs
College of Nursing
University of Cincinnati
P.O. Box 210038
Cincinnati, Ohio 45221-0038
Telephone: 513-558-3600
Fax: 513-558-7523
E-mail: nursing@uc.edu
World Wide Web: http://www.uc.edu
http://www.nursing.uc.edu

University of Connecticut
School of Nursing
Storrs, Connecticut

THE UNIVERSITY

The University of Connecticut is a modern, multifaceted institution with more than 24,000 students, 95,000 alumni, and 120 major buildings on 3,100 acres at the main campus in Storrs, three professional schools, and five regional campuses in other parts of the state. The library houses more than 2 million volumes. The University Health Center, which houses the Schools of Medicine and Dental Medicine and the University Hospital, is located in Farmington, about 40 miles from the main campus in Storrs. Since its founding in 1881, the University has grown steadily and dramatically to fulfill its mandated objectives as a provider of high-quality public education, research, and public service. The University is the state's land-grant, sea-grant, and space-grant institution. It is one of only two Carnegie Foundation Research I universities in New England. In 1995, the state of Connecticut enacted UCONN 2000, a $1-billion infrastructure program that has created an unprecedented transformation in the University.

THE SCHOOL OF NURSING

The School of Nursing was founded in 1942 and graduated its first baccalaureate class in 1947. During its history, the School has grown in size and stature. In addition to the baccalaureate program, which now has an enrollment of more than 400, the School offers a master's program with six subspecialty areas of study. The master's program has an enrollment of 150. An RN-to-M.S. program and a Ph.D. program are offered, and there is a new accelerated RN program, the Master's Entry Into Nursing (MEIN) Program. Relevant programs are approved by the Connecticut State Board of Examiners for Nursing and accredited by the National League for Nursing Accrediting Commission. In addition, they have received preliminary approval from the Commission on Collegiate Nursing Education.

The School's 21 full-time faculty members are prepared at the doctoral level, and 20 part-time clinical faculty members have at least a master's degree in a clinical specialty. The School also has access to more than 100 adjunct clinical faculty members from a wide variety of agencies in the state to serve as preceptors for graduate students.

PROGRAMS OF STUDY

The undergraduate program provides an opportunity to combine general education with professional preparation in nursing. The curriculum requires four academic years. Courses in the social, behavioral, and biological sciences and in the humanities serve as a foundation for the nursing major. The nursing major is concentrated in the junior and senior years with introductory courses presented in the first and second years. Upon successful completion of the undergraduate program, students receive the Bachelor of Science degree and are eligible for examination for licensure as registered nurses. Graduates of a baccalaureate program with a major in nursing may prepare for professional careers in any specialty track.

The University offers master's preparation in the following areas: nurse practitioner, with emphases in acute care, neonatal, and primary care, and clinical nurse specialist, with emphases in community health, neonatal, and critical care. There is also a master's degree program in patient care system administration. Dual-degree options are available in public health in combination with the community health nursing program (M.S./M.P.H.) and in business administration in combination with any of the other specialty tracks (M.S./M.B.A.). Upon successful completion of the three- or four-semester master's program, students receive the Master of Science degree.

Registered nurses without baccalaureate degrees may enroll in a modified sequence of courses leading to the master's degree in nursing (RN-M.S.). Those who meet the eligibility criteria may earn 30 transfer credits in nursing under the Connecticut Articulation Model for Nurse Educational Mobility or through portfolio review.

The Master's Entry Into Nursing program allows individuals with a baccalaureate degree in a non-nursing field to sit for the nursing board exams after one year of intensive study. The student can then enter the master's program in nursing.

The Ph.D. program in nursing prepares nurse leaders who will advance the scientific body of knowledge that is unique to professional nursing practice. Educational experiences are offered in nursing theory development, in philosophy of nursing science, in qualitative and quantitative research methods, and in advanced statistics. Study in specialty areas further supports the individual's area of clinical interest. Doctoral students entering the program are mentored by a faculty member with expertise and ongoing research activities in the clinical specialty of interest to the student.

AFFILIATIONS WITH HEALTH-CARE FACILITIES

Students receive their clinical experiences in a wide variety of settings, in both rural and urban areas. The School is affiliated with about seventy-five health-care agencies within a 35-mile radius of the campus. These include not only hospitals but schools, day-care centers, extended-care facilities, community health agencies, ambulatory centers, physicians' offices, industry, mental health clinics, inpatient facilities, well-child and obstetrical clinics, and other related settings, such as Alcoholics Anonymous, Lamaze, and La Leche meetings.

ACADEMIC FACILITIES

The University's Homer Babbidge Library is a rich storehouse of valuable information. Ranked among the country's top thirty for research resources, it has a strong book collection in nursing and the physical and social sciences. The journal collection includes more than 500 titles devoted to nursing. With seating for 3,000, the library provides access to data with a 24-hour online catalog computer system.

The University Computer Center provides access to the mainframe system nearly 24 hours a day from any of the 1,700 terminals throughout the campus, from PCs attached to the campus network, or via modem. The center's personal computing facilities include in-house IBM and Macintosh labs as well as several labs in dorms and academic buildings.

Well-equipped nursing laboratories provide a practice site for undergraduate students to facilitate the transfer of knowledge from theory to actual practice. Students practice newly acquired skills in the new, state-of-the-art simulation laboratory before performing them on actual patients in clinical settings. The School's Center for Nursing Research facilitates student and faculty research by providing statistical consultation, editorial assistance, mentoring, and research support.

The Josephine A. Dolan Collection is a premier collection of nursing artifacts in the nation and is located on campus in

Storrs Hall. The papers of Josephine Dolan as well as records of other leaders and organizations and records that document major activities and events in nursing history are located in the Archives of Nursing Leadership at the Thomas J. Dodd Research Center on the Storrs campus.

LOCATION

The School of Nursing is located on the main campus of the University in Storrs, Connecticut, which is 30 miles east of Hartford, 2½ hours from New York City, and 90 minutes from Boston. Storrs is a small community with the clean air and quiet rural atmosphere of eastern Connecticut. Cultural and sports activities abound in the area. The University sponsors numerous theater and musical activities throughout the year, and the cultural activities available in Hartford, New Haven, Boston, and New York City are all close enough to attend on a regular basis. The University has numerous facilities for the active sports enthusiast. For the sports fan, the very competitive Big East basketball season highlights the full slate of intercollegiate sports events.

STUDENT SERVICES

The University offers many services to meet student needs. These include services for students with physical and/or learning disabilities, career counseling and placement, student health and personal counseling, and tutoring and other academic support services. There are a number of centers offering students opportunities to meet and socialize with other students from similar backgrounds. The Rainbow Center joins the Centers for African-American, Asian-American, Puerto Rican, Latino, Slavic, Jewish, and Women Students in enhancing campus diversity. Each has an active schedule of social and educational events usually highlighting events and studies important in its culture.

THE NURSING STUDENT GROUP

The population is diverse with respect to age, gender, and ethnicity. The majority of undergraduate students attend full-time. Approximately half of the undergraduates choose to live on campus. However, an increasing number of students are older, working adults who attend part-time while maintaining either full-time or part-time employment. The majority of graduate students attend part-time.

COSTS

Tuition and fees and room and board costs for those who live on campus for each academic year are listed in the online catalogs (undergraduate and graduate) at the University's home page.

FINANCIAL AID

All students who estimate that they may be unable to pay the cost of their education through their own resources are encouraged to apply for financial assistance. This assistance, in the form of scholarships, grants, loans, and part-time employment, is administered by the Student Financial Aid Office. The application deadline is February 15. In addition to this need-based assistance, graduate students may be awarded graduate assistantships, fellowships, and traineeships. There are merit-based scholarships for undergraduate students.

APPLYING

Undergraduate students apply to the Undergraduate Admissions Office. They must submit an application, a secondary school record, SAT scores, official transcripts of all postsecondary work completed, and a completed residence affidavit. Upon receipt of all information necessary to complete the application, the admissions office notifies the applicant of the decision by mail.

Graduate students submit two applications, one to the Graduate School and one to the School of Nursing. Students must submit an application, letters of reference, a personal statement, a completed residence affidavit, and transcripts of all postsecondary work to the Graduate School Admissions Office. Students must have an undergraduate total GPA of 3.0 or better from a nursing program accredited by the NLNAC or the AACN to be considered for regular admission. In addition to those of the Graduate School, requirements for admission to the School of Nursing include a baccalaureate degree in nursing from an accredited nursing program or, for nurses without baccalaureate degrees, completion of the specially designed course sequence for upper-division nursing content; current nurse licensure in Connecticut; skills in health assessment; and a personal interview. In addition, admission to the doctoral program requires a minimum total master's degree GPA of 3.25, submission of GRE scores, completion of a graduate-level course in multivariate statistics, and submission of any published works or scholarly papers. The School of Nursing admissions committees make admission recommendations to the Graduate School. Notification of decisions is made by mail from the Graduate School.

CORRESPONDENCE AND INFORMATION

Office of Academic Advising Center
School of Nursing
University of Connecticut
231 Glenbrook Road, Unit 2026
Storrs, Connecticut 06269-2026
Telephone: 860-486-1968
E-mail: nuradm11@uconnvm.uconn.edu
World Wide Web: http://www.nursing.uconn.edu

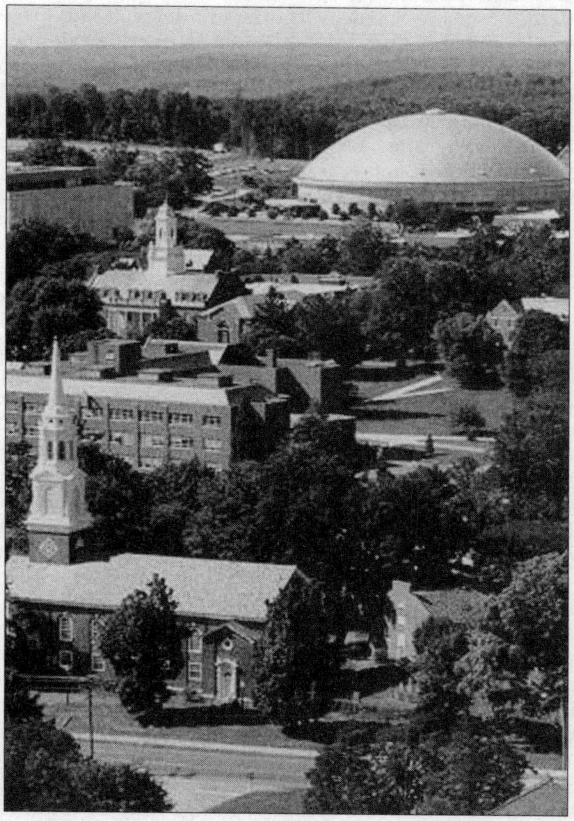

A view of the campus.

University of Delaware
Department of Nursing
Newark, Delaware

THE UNIVERSITY

The University of Delaware has grown from its founding as a small private academy in 1743 to a major university. As one of the oldest land-grant institutions, as well as a sea-grant, space-grant, and urban-grant institution, Delaware offers an impressive collection of educational resources. Undergraduates may choose to major in one or more of over 100 academic majors. The University's distinguished faculty includes internationally known scientists, authors, and teachers who are committed to continuing the University of Delaware's tradition in providing one of the highest-quality undergraduate educations available.

The University comprises seven colleges: Agricultural and Natural Resources; Arts and Sciences; Business and Economics; Engineering; Health and Nursing Sciences; Human Services, Education, and Public Policy; and Marine Sciences. Together, the colleges offer more than 100 majors. Enrollment in the fall 2004 semester was 20,713 students, including 16,023 undergraduates, 3,395 graduate students and doctoral students, and 1,295 continuing education students.

THE DEPARTMENT OF NURSING

The Department of Nursing is housed within the College of Health and Nursing Sciences. It offers undergraduate programs for traditional nursing students, accelerated students, and registered nurses, all leading to the Bachelor of Science in Nursing (B.S.N.) degree. The Department also offers a graduate program leading to the Master of Science in Nursing (M.S.N.) degree. All programs are fully accredited by the National League for Nursing Accrediting Commission and hold preliminary approval from the Commission on Collegiate Nursing Education.

PROGRAMS OF STUDY

The traditional undergraduate program is available to beginning students of nursing, including new high school graduates, transfer students, and change-of-major students. This program requires 122 semester credits for completion. In the freshman year, nursing majors are introduced to the profession through course work and lab experiences while developing a firm foundation in the essential science and liberal arts courses. In the sophomore year, students complete all of the essential science courses and most of the liberal arts courses while further developing clinical and decision-making skills in nursing through simulation and laboratory experiences. In the junior year, there is an expansion of nursing knowledge in both essential and specialty clinical nursing domains while completing associated field experiences. Finally, senior-level nursing students enter a residency period in which they are immersed in clinical experiences for the entire year in order to enhance their nursing knowledge and to prepare them for entry into practice. Students may elect to take selected courses during winter or summer sessions. Honors courses and a nursing honors program are available to qualified undergraduate students. In addition, the Department of Nursing is actively involved in the University Study Abroad Program.

An accelerated program of study is available for adults who have previously earned a baccalaureate degree. This option allows students to pursue a course of study whereby they complete all of their nursing requirements (60 credits) in fifteen months. To pursue this option, the student must have completed all prerequisite courses and have earned a 3.0 GPA or higher prior to beginning any nursing courses.

The Baccalaureate for the Registered Nurse (BRN) is an innovative program for RNs who are graduates of associate degree or diploma programs. The BRN major requires 120 credits for program completion. The program is offered in an online format and is available to RNs nationwide. All students must, however, attend two 1-credit weekend experiences. This format provides the needed flexibility for busy adult students who pursue degree completion while continuing to work full- or part-time. The program can be completed in fifteen months but must be completed within five years of the first nursing course. The BRN program utilizes a work site model for exam proctoring. Any health-care facility, industry wellness center, or community college can become a participating work site. There are currently 181 work sites spanning multiple states and one other country. Graduates of accredited associate degree and diploma programs who are licensed may directly transfer up to 30 credits in nursing as evidence of their basic nursing knowledge. State-of-the-art technologies are used to facilitate communication, advisement, and course work among and between students and faculty members. Full library access is provided via the Internet. A Special Programs Information Line (toll-free number) augments course-related communication.

An online RN-M.S.N. option is also offered to RNs who are graduates of associate degree or diploma programs. Qualified applicants can complete the B.S.N. and M.S.N. requirements concurrently in the RN to M.S.N. program, which requires 134 credits for graduation. Health services administration and clinical nurse specialties will be offered through this program.

The graduate program includes core concepts in advanced nursing practice as well as concepts that are specific to the areas of specialization. The curriculum is built on the theories and professional practice students have obtained at the baccalaureate level of nursing education and provides a foundation for future doctoral study. Research is an area of emphasis in graduate study. Students may elect to complete a thesis, a nonthesis scholarly project, or a 3-credit research utilization course.

The graduate program prepares clinical nurse specialists (CNS) in children's health, adult health, and adult or child psychiatric specialties, adult and family nurse practitioners, and health services administrators. Students in the CNS concentrations complete 34 credit hours, with emphasis on the three spheres of influence: clients (patients/families/communities), nursing personnel, and health organizations and networks.

The adult nurse practitioner concentration requires 40 credit hours, while the family nurse practitioner concentration requires 43 credit hours, with the clinical emphasis in primary care. Health services administration students must complete 37 credit hours and are prepared to assume leadership positions as health-care managers. Students may elect to enroll full-time or part-time.

Post-master's certificate programs are available in all areas for students who already hold a Master of Science degree in nursing. Clinical nurse specialists and nurse practitioners are eligible to sit for the national certification examinations and have exceptionally high pass rates. The health services administration concentration and CNS concentrations utilize

Web-based or Web-enhanced delivery systems. Other core and selected specialty courses may also be offered in a Web-based format.

ACADEMIC FACILITIES

The University libraries contain more than 2.6 million volumes of books and bound periodicals, 3.3 million items in microtext, and subscriptions to more than 12,000 periodicals. The libraries provide access to more than 6,800 online full-text journals and to more than 230 networked databases. DELCAT is the library's online catalog, giving information for materials located in the libraries and on the libraries' Web site (http://www.lib.udel.edu/). The libraries offer an online reference service, online interlibrary loan forms, and electronic reserves for selected courses. Special library services are available for distance learning students.

The information technology resources available at the University of Delaware are unparalleled. The University's commitment to providing a superior technology environment enables students and faculty members to pursue academic studies and to conduct the business of campus life with ease and efficiency.

Students use a wide range of technology in their academic work. In all disciplines, students use electronic mail, word processing, and tools to search the Internet for information. All University classrooms are connected to the campus network, enabling faculty members to use a wide variety of multimedia services and devices in their teaching. Many classrooms have Internet connections at student seats to facilitate the use of laptop computers. Instructional video is broadcast over the University television network, and many classes include special viewings as part of course requirements.

Students on campus can connect their own computers directly to the campus network from their residence hall rooms. Off-campus students can dial in to the network from surrounding regions. General-access computing sites are available for student use on campus, and these have network ports to connect laptop computers. The Morris Library carrels also have network ports. Wireless access areas are also available in common areas across the campus, including Morris Library, student centers, and residence hall lounges.

The Department of Nursing has two general practice labs, a critical-care lab, and an examination suite for nurse practitioner students. A clinical simulation laboratory and resource center provide students with a safe clinical practice site prior to direct patient care. Students may access a computer laboratory housed in the building. The college also houses a large state-of-the-art instructional TV studio where nursing courses and support courses are taught and prepared for use in the distance delivery system. Faculty members are committed to the development and integration of technologies in the teaching/learning process.

LOCATION

Situated in the small, picturesque town of Newark, Delaware, the University's main campus is less than 2½ hours from the metropolitan bustle of New York City, Baltimore, Philadelphia, and Washington, D.C. The campus is convenient to an impressive array of major clinical facilities as well as cultural and recreational resources.

STUDENT SERVICES

The University has many resources and services to meet individual student needs. These include the Student Support Services Program, the University Writing Center, the Center for Counseling and Student Development, the Mathematical Sciences Teaching and Learning Center, the English Language Institute, and the Career Planning and Placement Office.

The Division of Special Programs works collaboratively with all departments within the college to coordinate technology-related learning activities. Continuing professional education programs and credit courses delivered locally and in a distance format are another focus of the division. Two 16-hour certificate programs, Cognitive Therapy: Interventions for Healthcare Providers and Cognitive Therapy: Advanced Applications for Healthcare Providers, are currently available. Educational partnerships with health-care institutions and community agencies provide interdisciplinary educational and research opportunities.

Undergraduate nursing students are encouraged to participate in the local chapter of the National Student Nurses Organization and/or the Black Student Nursing Organization. Registered nurse students have their own electronic support group.

THE NURSING STUDENT GROUP

Approximately 580 students are enrolled in the traditional undergraduate program, including 70 adult students pursuing the accelerated degree option. In addition, 130 matriculated RN students are enrolled in the BRN program. Enrollment in the graduate program is approximately 55.

COSTS

For the 2004–05 academic year, tuition was $6304 for undergraduate Delaware residents and $15,990 for nonresidents. Tuition covers registration for 12 to 17 credits per semester. Students taking fewer than 12 credits were charged $263 per credit hour for Delaware residents and $667 per credit hour for nonresidents. Room and board costs were $3640.

FINANCIAL AID

In most cases, the University awards aid on the basis of need. Financial aid may include grants, loans, and employment opportunities. The University also offers a number of scholarships based on academic proficiency alone. Students have been able to successfully obtain nurse traineeships, National Student Nurses Association scholarships, and other specialty scholarships.

APPLYING

Applicants to the undergraduate degree programs can apply online (http://www.udel.edu/viewbook) or can request an application by contacting the Admission's Office (302-831-8125). Applicants to the graduate program can request an application online (http://www.udel.edu/gradoffice) or by contacting the Office of Graduate Studies (302-831-2129). The application deadlines are February 15 for fall admission and November 15 for spring admission. For information regarding specific requirements, students should contact the appropriate unit in the college.

CORRESPONDENCE AND INFORMATION

For information about the traditional and accelerated nursing programs and graduate program:

Department of Nursing
College of Health and Nursing Sciences
University of Delaware
Newark, Delaware 19716

Telephone: 302-831-1253
E-mail: ud-nursing@udel.edu
World Wide Web: http://www.udel.edu/nursing

For information about the RN-B.S.N. and RN-M.S.N. distance learning program, the online RN Refresher course, and certificate programs:

Division of Special Programs
College of Health and Nursing Sciences
University of Delaware
Newark, Delaware 19716

Telephone: 800-UOD-NURS (toll-free)
E-mail: dsp-email@udel.edu
World Wide Web: http://www.udel.edu/DSP

University of Illinois at Chicago
College of Nursing
Chicago, Illinois

THE UNIVERSITY

The University of Illinois at Chicago (UIC) serves approximately 25,000 students, who reflect the ethnic and racial diversity of Chicago itself. Seventy-five percent of these students come from Cook County and 48 percent are residents of Chicago. The Colleges of Nursing, Medicine, Pharmacy, Dentistry, and Health and Human Development Sciences and the School of Public Health are located within the 305-acre west side Medical Center District about 2 miles west of downtown Chicago. The district has the world's largest concentration of public and private health-care facilities and includes the University of Illinois at Chicago Medical Center, Cook County Hospital, Rush-Presbyterian-St. Luke's Medical Center, West Side Veterans Administration Medical Center, Institute for Juvenile Research, Illinois State Psychiatric Institute, and Illinois State Pediatric Institute.

THE COLLEGE OF NURSING

The UIC College of Nursing is consistently recognized as one of the top ten nursing programs in the United States. The mission of the College includes the triad of university functions—teaching, research, and service—providing university education in nursing to meet the present and future needs of society. In 2003, the College was third in total NIH research and research training dollars, and in 2003, it was ranked seventh out of 142 schools of nursing by *U.S. News & World Report.* The nurse midwifery program was ranked third among its competitors. Fully accredited by the Commission on Collegiate Nursing Education (CCNE), the College offers programs leading to the degrees of Bachelor of Science in Nursing (B.S.N.), Master of Science (M.S.) in nursing sciences, and Doctor of Philosophy (Ph.D.) in nursing sciences. The College, which has provided high-quality education since 1951, is currently designated as a WHO Collaborating Centre for Nursing and Midwifery. The faculty includes 16 members of the American Academy of Nursing. Worldwide, alumni are a source of leadership in academic, health-system, corporate, and political arenas.

PROGRAMS OF STUDY

Transfer students are admitted to the generic baccalaureate program in Chicago and Urbana-Champaign. The program, which prepares beginning nurses to function in a variety of settings, requires 57 liberal arts and sciences semester hours and 63 nursing semester hours for graduation. Students may complete the program in two years. RN-B.S.N. students applying to the program offered in Chicago, Quad Cities, and Urbana-Champaign must meet the transfer admission requirements, which include 57 semester hours of liberal arts and sciences course work and a cumulative GPA of at least 2.5 (A=4.0). Completion of three NLN Mobility Profile II examinations and three transition courses determine credit by exemption for up to 33 semester hours of nursing course work, leaving 30 semester hours of nursing course work, which may be completed in four semesters.

The master's program prepares nurses for advanced practice roles, with emphasis on basic, clinical, and nursing sciences; knowledge of health systems and environment; and understanding of professional issues of advanced practice roles, while a research focus is maintained. The roles are clinical nurse specialist, which utilizes advanced information within a specialty to manage complex health problems, and nurse practitioner, which emphasizes the comprehensive care of patients as well as the ability to manage the complex problems addressed by the specialty.

Within each specialty and option, there are several concentrations of study. These include administrative studies in nursing (alone or combined as a dual-degree option with an M.B.A. or health informatics), medical-surgical nursing (acute care, geriatric, adult), maternal-child nursing (nurse midwifery; women's health; pediatric, including PNP; perinatal), public health nursing (dual-degree option with an M.P.H., school health, community nurse specialist, family nurse practitioner, occupational health nursing), and psychiatric–mental health nursing.

Master's courses are offered at at all locations and may use teleconference or videoconferencing. The 36 required semester hours include statistics, nursing inquiry I & II, health environment and systems, and issues of advanced practice in nursing (10 semester hours); advanced nursing courses (23–36 semester hours); electives (2–3 semester hours); a thesis (5 semester hours) or a research project (3 semester hours); and a final examination. More than 36 semester hours are required to complete most of the specialty concentrations.

Post-master's programs are available in most of the study options. This prepares individuals to sit for examinations for certification in these fields.

The Ph.D. program develops leaders in nursing who influence the provision of health care through systematic investigation, education, policy development and implementation, and expert professional practice. Major areas of research include administration, physiological and psychological studies related to the care of the acutely and chronically ill, health promotion and maintenance, stress and coping, narcolepsy, quality of life, community health nursing, women's health, family, and gerontological nursing. The Ph.D. degree requires 96 semester hours, including nursing theory (6 semester hours), statistics (6 semester hours), research methods (6 semester hours), advanced nursing and non-nursing courses (15 semester hours), independent research (31 semester hours), and a previously completed M.S. program (32 semester hours). A preliminary oral examination, dissertation, and final oral examination are required to earn the Ph.D. in nursing sciences.

The B.S.N. to Ph.D. program allows the exceptional student to proceed directly from the B.S.N. to the Ph.D. in nursing science degrees.

Through the CIC, a consortium of the Midwest's "Big Ten" universities and the University of Chicago, doctoral students may register for course work or independent study in the other universities of the CIC and work with experts in their research areas. The Graduate Entry Program is designed for students who hold baccalaureate degrees in other fields and wish to pursue a master's degree in nursing.

ACADEMIC FACILITIES

UIC libraries hold more than 5.7 million items, including more than 6,000 current periodicals and more than 500,000 bound periodical volumes, books, government documents, and audiovisual items housed in the Library of the Health Sciences, which is the regional medical library for 2,700 medical libraries in ten states from Ohio to the Dakotas. The Interlibrary Loan Service is offered to students and faculty and staff members, and the libraries of two other Chicago institutions, the University of Chicago and Northwestern University, are available for use by graduate students. The Academic Computer Center provides computing and network support for instructional and research needs of the University's students and faculty and staff members.

LOCATION

Situated 2 miles west of Chicago's downtown, UIC is surrounded by world-renowned architecture, theater, art, music, and sports activities. Easily accessible from both airports by public transportation and the Eisenhower Expressway, the College is located in a historic neighborhood, currently the center of a new, rapidly growing residential and professional community.

STUDENT SERVICES

The Center for Excellence provides an array of services from career counseling and academic skills courses to personal counseling and assistance for disabled students. Other services include two fitness/recreation centers, a child-care center, the Office of International Studies, and support organizations such as African American Academic Network, Latin American Recruitment and Education Services, and the Native American Support Program for members of minority groups.

THE NURSING STUDENT GROUP

Students reflect the ethnic and racial diversity of Chicago itself. UIC has long provided solid academic training for first-generation college students from the city's numerous ethnic groups and currently provides opportunities to students returning to school following a significant absence due to other career or family responsibilities. About 10 percent of those enrolled in the undergraduate program are men. Even though University housing is available, 85 percent of Chicago students commute or live in apartments near the campus.

COSTS

For 2004–05, full-time tuition and fees per semester for undergraduates were $4042 for Illinois residents and $9666 for nonresidents. For full-time graduate students, tuition and fees were $6195 for Illinois residents and $11,802 for nonresidents. Part-time undergraduate tuition ranged from $1902 to $3023 for Illinois residents and from $3777 to $6772 for nonresidents; part-time graduate study ranged from $2620 to $4458 for Illinois residents and from $4489 to $8196 for nonresidents. On-campus housing was available in Chicago for approximately $7000 for two semesters; costs may vary depending on location.

FINANCIAL AID

Several financial assistance programs are available through the Office of Student Financial Aid. Applications for financial aid in the form of research or training assistantships, fellowships, traineeships, and tuition waivers are submitted to the College of Nursing. These financial aid awards are made from the College's resources. The College of Nursing makes recommendations to the Graduate College for such awards as University Fellowships and the Abraham Lincoln Graduate Fellowship.

APPLYING

Applicants for the B.S. degree must have completed the following liberal arts and sciences requirements: English composition I and II; microbiology; general and organic chemistry; anatomy; physiology; 6 semester hours of social science; 6 semester hours of humanities, nutrition, and life span, human growth, and development; and a cultural diversity course. A minimum cumulative GPA of 2.5 (A=4.0) and a minimum GPA of 2.0 in natural science courses are required. Applicants must submit two letters of recommendation, a personal statement, a College information form, and a prerequisite evaluation form. The applicant to the RN-B.S.N. program must have a current RN license or be scheduled to take the NCLEX at the first opportunity after graduation from a diploma or associate degree nursing program accredited by the NLNAC.

M.S. applicants must have a current RN license (several specialty concentrations require an Illinois license) and either a B.S.N. degree from a CCNE- or NLNAC-accredited program or a B.S. degree from an accredited institution in a field other than nursing; a minimum GPA of 3.0 (A=4.0); introductory courses in statistics and research methods or their equivalent; GRE General Test scores (or GMAT scores for the M.S. dual-degree M.B.A. or health informatics option); TOEFL scores (for international students); a statement of career goals; a curriculum vitae; three letters of reference; and a faculty interview. The GRE requirement may be waived for students holding a 3.25 GPA (A=4.0) in the final 60 hours of their bachelor's degree program.

Ph.D. applicants must meet the requirements for entry into the M.S. program, possess an M.S. degree from a CCNE- or NLNAC-accredited program, and present evidence of potential for advanced scholarship. The applicant who has a B.S. degree from an accredited nursing program and an M.S. degree in a field other than nursing is eligible for consideration for admission. The GRE requirement is not waived for Ph.D. applicants. Applicants for the Graduate Entry Program must meet all requirements for entry into the M.S. program and must take the GRE (no waiver available).

Prospective applicants should contact the College of Nursing Office of Academic Programs for specific application deadlines and priority application dates. Applications for the B.S.N., selected M.S., and the Ph.D. programs are accepted for fall only. Admission to several of the M.S. options is for any term.

CORRESPONDENCE AND INFORMATION

Office of Academic Programs
College of Nursing (M/C 802)
University of Illinois at Chicago
845 South Damen Avenue
Chicago, Illinois 60612-7350
Telephone: 312-996-7800
Fax: 312-996-8066
E-mail: con@uic.edu
World Wide Web: http://www.uic.edu/nursing

University of Maryland
School of Nursing
Baltimore, Maryland

THE UNIVERSITY

The University of Maryland's Baltimore campus includes six professional schools: Nursing, Medicine, Dentistry, Pharmacy, Social Work, and Law; the Graduate School; the Maryland Institute for Emergency Medical Systems; the University of Maryland Medical Center; and the Veterans Affairs Medical Center. It was established in 1807 and currently enrolls nearly 6,000 students and has 1,600 faculty members.

The University of Maryland's Baltimore campus is one of the fastest-growing biomedical research centers in the United States and maintains more than $300 million in sponsored-program support. Its unique composition enables it to address health care, public policy, and social issues through multidisciplinary research, scholarship, and community action. The School's location in the Baltimore-Washington-Annapolis triangle maximizes opportunities for student placements and collaboration with government agencies, health-care institutions, and life science industries.

THE SCHOOL OF NURSING

The School of Nursing, established in 1889 by Louisa Parsons, has been instrumental in strengthening nursing education and shaping the profession. Its mission is to provide leadership through undergraduate, graduate, and continuing education programs as well as research and service of the highest quality.

Maryland consistently ranks among the top ten schools of nursing in the United States. The School awarded its first M.S. degree in 1954 and its first Ph.D. degree in 1984. Alumni include more than 20,000 nurses, and current enrollment is 1,400. The faculty members are internationally renowned for their research and clinical expertise, their innovative instructional programs, and their state-of-the-art models for nurse-managed delivery of health-care services. (Senior faculty members and administrators are listed in the faculty section.)

The School is organized into two departments: Family and Community Health and Organizational Systems and Adult Health. Graduate specialties in nursing informatics and anesthesia remain among only a few in the nation. Flexible and combined programs of study that accelerate degree completion are in place. The School uses and operates a variety of nurse-managed clinics that serve as practicum sites for students. These include Open Gates, a community health center serving the medically underserved; the Governor's Wellmobiles, mobile health clinics that provide screening, treatment, and referral for children and their families and the homeless; fifteen school-based wellness centers that provide primary care for students; the Senior Care Center that provides geriatric assessment and primary care to low-income seniors; the South West Family, a center that provides health services and helps teenage parents stay in school; and a pediatric ambulatory clinic that provides primary-care services for the surrounding community.

PROGRAMS OF STUDY

The B.S.N. program is an upper-division, professional program accredited by the National League for Nursing Accrediting Commission (NLNAC). It is based on prerequisite courses that provide a liberal education and support the study of nursing. A flexible undergraduate track that may be completed on a full- or part-time basis is available—traditional baccalaureate and registered nurse. The traditional baccalaureate track requires students to complete 59 prerequisite credits before matriculation. The registered nurse track includes RN to B.S.N., RN to B.S.N. online, and RN to M.S. options. Students must complete 59 prerequisite credits and are awarded 30 additional credits for prior nursing course work. They then transfer and matriculate with 89 credits as seniors.The accelerated RN to M.S. option is designed for nurses with baccalaureate degrees in other disciplines or for RNs who do not have baccalaureate degrees but have the interest and ability to pursue leadership and specialty preparation at the master's level.

The NLNAC-accredited M.S. program focuses on specialization and a commitment to and involvement in the development and refinement of nursing knowledge. The program prepares graduates in nineteen specialty areas as acute-care nurse practitioners, primary-care nurse practitioners, nurse midwives, advanced practice nurses, nurse anesthetists, clinical research managers, and administrators. An M.S./M.B.A. joint degree and an accelerated M.S. program are also offered.

The Ph.D. program is designed for nurses who are committed to leadership in the discovery and refinement of nursing knowledge through research. The program allows students to focus on study, which examines the theoretical and empirical bases for nursing actions in a variety of clinical settings, or on research, which focuses on the study of nursing systems or the theoretical and empirical bases for educational, administrative, and/or policy-related nursing actions. Individual research interests and career goals determine the specialty area chosen. A Ph.D./M.B.A. joint-degree program is also offered. Most students enter the doctoral program after earning a master's degree; however, a postbaccalaureate entry option is available.

AFFILIATIONS WITH HEALTH-CARE FACILITIES

The School is affiliated with the University of Maryland Medical System, which includes University Hospital, Maryland Cancer Center, and R Adams Cowley Shock Trauma Center. Affiliations also are established with the Veterans Affairs Medical Center and more than 400 additional hospitals, community health centers, health maintenance organizations, health departments, private practices, community clinics, and schools throughout the region and the state.

ACADEMIC FACILITIES

The University's Health Sciences Library is the regional medical library for the Southeastern states and is part of the National Library of Medicine's biomedical information network. It houses more than 340,000 volumes and 2,300 current journal subscriptions. Campus computer resources include mainframe and microcomputer support for faculty and staff members and students; electronic access enables them to exchange information on and off campus.

The School's computer laboratories include 105 workstations, a computerized teaching theater, and an interactive video laboratory that utilizes advanced computerized clinical simulations and decision-making models that enable students to practice clinical skills and critical decision making at their own pace. Clinical simulation laboratories allow students to practice nursing skills using equipment designed to replicate patient-care situations. "Standardized patients" allow students to practice their clinical skills in a controlled environment prior to demonstrating them in actual clinical settings. Distance learning technology provides interactive classes involving students from across the state.

LOCATION

Baltimore combines the attractions of contemporary urban living with the advantages of a location within an educational hub composed of thirty colleges and universities. The School of Nursing is part of a district called UniversityCenter. Several blocks from campus are Oriole Park at Camden Yards and the Inner Harbor, which includes the National Aquarium and the Maryland Science Center. UniversityCenter is easily accessible; Baltimore-Washington International Airport is nearby, the Baltimore Metro and Light Rail System connects the campus to neighboring counties, the University operates a shuttle service, and student parking is available.

STUDENT SERVICES

The School provides programs that support the academic experience. It conducts seminars to improve writing skills, test taking, study habits, and time management and maintains a peer tutoring program. The School also conducts career placement and development seminars and advises student government and professional organizations. The University's student resources include student health, counseling, athletic facilities, residence life, student development, the student union, and financial aid.

THE NURSING STUDENT GROUP

Approximately 800 students are enrolled in the B.S.N. program, 500 in the M.S. program, and 96 in the Ph.D. program. Of the undergraduates, 40 percent are enrolled in the RN to B.S.N. option. Nearly 25 percent of the traditional students are enrolled in the accelerated second degree option. Approximately 90 percent enrolled in the traditional baccalaureate option attend full-time.

COSTS

Tuition in 2004–05 for the B.S.N. program was $6506 for full-time in-state students, $285 per credit for part-time in-state students, $16,745 for full-time out-of-state students, and $427 per credit for part-time out-of-state students. Graduate tuition is on a per-credit basis. In-state graduate tuition was $380 per credit, and out-of-state graduate tuition was $681 per credit. Additional educational expenses, including books, insurance, immunizations, and fees, for full-time students average $2600 per year.

FINANCIAL AID

The School's scholarship program is based on academic achievement. Students may receive assistance in meeting educational expenses through grants, scholarships, loans, and part-time employment. Federal Graduate Nurse Traineeships and graduate assistantships are also available for qualified full-time students in the master's and doctoral programs.

APPLYING

B.S.N. applicants are expected to have a minimum 3.0 GPA. Accelerated second degree B.S.N. applicants must have a minimum 3.0 GPA and submit letters of recommendation. Admission to the baccalaureate program is competitive; the mean GPA of accepted students is above 3.0. Applications for fall admission to all B.S.N. options must be submitted by April 1. Applications for spring admission to all B.S.N. options must be submitted by September 1.

M.S. applicants must have a minimum 3.0 GPA and a B.S.N. from an NLNAC-accredited program.

All Ph.D. applicants, except those in the accelerated B.S.N. to Ph.D. option, must have a minimum 3.0 GPA and a master's degree in nursing from an NLNAC-accredited program. The GRE is required for all graduate applicants. Students should contact the Office of Student Affairs and Admissions for complete information on admission requirements.

CORRESPONDENCE AND INFORMATION

Office of Admissions and Student Affairs
University of Maryland School of Nursing
655 West Lombard Street, Suite 102
Baltimore, Maryland 21201
Telephone: 410-706-0501
866-687-7386 (toll-free)
E-mail: admission@son.umaryland.edu
Internet: http://nursing.umaryland.edu

THE ADMINISTRATION

Janet D. Allan, Professor and Dean; Ph.D., Berkeley; RN, CS, FAAN.

Barbara Covington, Associate Dean, Information and Learning Technologies; Ph.D., Texas A&M: RN.

Ruth Harris, Professor and Chair of Adult Health and Education, Administration, Informatics, and Health Policy; Ph.D., Maryland; RN, FAAN.

Louise S. Jenkins, Associate Professor of Adult Health and Director of Graduate Programs; Ph.D., Maryland; RN.

Mary Etta E. Mills, Associate Professor, Organizational Systems and Adult Health, and Assistant Dean for Baccalaureate Studies; Sc.D., Johns Hopkins; RN, CNAA.

Kathryn Montgomery, Assistant Professor and Associate Dean for Organizational Partnership and Outreach; ?????.

Patricia G. Morton, Professor of Organizational Systems and Adult Health Nursing and Assistant Dean for Master's Studies; Ph.D., Maryland; RN, CRNP, FAAN.

Maria Oros, Associate Dean, Clinical Practice and External Affairs; M.S., Towson; RN.

Barbara Smith, Associate Dean for Research; Ph.D., RN, FACSM, FAAN.

Sue Ann Thomas, Assistant Dean for Doctoral Studies, Organizational Systems, and Adult Health Nursing; Ph.D., Maryland; RN, FAAN.

University of Massachusetts Worcester
Graduate School of Nursing
Worcester, Massachusetts

UMASS

THE UNIVERSITY

The University of Massachusetts Worcester (UMW) was founded by proclamation of the governor and an act of the legislature to meet the health-care needs of the residents of the commonwealth of Massachusetts. Its basic mission is to serve the people of the commonwealth through national distinction in health sciences education, research, public service, and clinical care.

Today, the 67-acre campus located in Worcester comprises the School of Medicine, the Graduate School of Biomedical Sciences, and the Graduate School of Nursing. The campus's hospital and clinics are part of UMass Memorial Health Care, a nonprofit, integrated clinical system created in April 1998 by the merger of the UMass clinical system and Memorial Health Care. The UMW campus is one of a small number of freestanding, university-based academic health sciences campuses in the United States and, as the sponsor of educational and service programs in health-care throughout the commonwealth, UMW is a local, regional, and statewide health resource.

THE GRADUATE SCHOOL OF NURSING

In its relatively brief history, the Graduate School of Nursing (GSN) at the University of Massachusetts Worcester has developed exceptional clinical leaders, faculty members, and scientists for nursing and health workforce development. The GSN is renowned for its focus on facilitating high-quality, cost-effective graduate nursing education for the citizens of the commonwealth and the region as it prepares professional and advanced practice nurses to become leaders, practitioners, scientists, and educators at the master's, post-master's, and doctoral levels. One of the few nursing schools in New England based at an academic health sciences center, the GSN offers interdisciplinary research, clinical service, and education within a collaborative health professions environment.

PROGRAMS OF STUDY

Within the GSN master's program, several pathway options lead to the preparation of advanced practice nurses and nurse educators. Advanced nursing specialties include: adult ambulatory/community-care nurse practitioner, adult acute/critical-care nurse practitioner, dual track with gerontological nurse practitioner, and nurse educator. The pathways are the traditional master's pathway for registered nurses with a baccalaureate degree in nursing, the pre-master's pathway for registered nurses who posses an associate degree in nursing and a baccalaureate degree in a field other than nursing, and the Graduate Entry Pathway (GEP) for individuals with a baccalaureate degree in a field other than nursing, which leads first to registered nurse licensure and then to advanced nursing specialties.

The Ph.D. in nursing program began in 1994 at UMW through a collaborative arrangement with the University of Massachusetts Amherst campus. This innovative doctoral program utilizes the resources of the University's Worcester health sciences campus and the Amherst comprehensive campus. Faculty members are shared between the two nursing schools, blending and enhancing resources for doctoral students. The doctoral program promotes mentorship in research and scholarship among its faculty members and students for the advancement of nursing science and practice.

ACADEMIC FACILITIES

The GSN is distinctive as the only nursing school in the commonwealth with its sole focus on graduate nursing education. It shares its campus resources and facilities with the commonwealth's only public medical school, the University of Massachusetts Medical School, and its clinical partner, UMass Memorial Health Care, making the GSN one of the only three nursing schools in New England based at an academic health sciences center. The GSN's focus and location generate rich, interdisciplinary health professions education that offers real-world opportunities to create cutting-edge models of collaborative education, research, and practice.

The Lamar Soutter Library serves as the National Library of Medicine's New England Regional Medical Library, one of eight such regional libraries nationwide, exhibiting medical information products offered by the National Library of Medicine and providing training seminars and presentations that teach health professionals and consumers how to gain access to useful information.

LOCATION

Located in central Massachusetts, 40 miles west of Boston, Worcester is the third-largest city in New England and the hub of economic activity in the area. Complementing its health-care, insurance, education, biotechnology, and finance industries, Worcester and surrounding towns host fourteen colleges and universities. Worcester's central location also makes it ideal for visits to favorite New England attractions, including Cape Cod, a 90-minute drive southeast; Newport, Rhode Island, a 60-minute drive southeast; and Boston, a 45-minute drive east.

STUDENT SERVICES

Major areas of responsibility of School Services are Matriculation Services and Pre-Matriculation Programs. Matriculation Services include financial aid, registrar/student record, student ADA support, and Weather Watch. Pre-Matriculation Programs include Outreach Programs for Minority and Disadvantaged Students (High School Health Careers Program and the Summer Enrichment Program), the Office of Science Education (the Worcester Pipeline Collaborative and the Regional Science Resource Center), and the Undergraduate Summer Research Fellowship Program.

The Graduate Student Nursing Organization's (GSNO) purpose is to foster communication, coordination, and continuity among graduate students and the administration and faculty members of the University of Massachusetts Worcester, the Graduate School of Nursing, and the University community. Membership includes all full-time and part-time students enrolled in the graduate school of the UMass Worcester, GSN. Monthly meetings are conducted by elected GSNO officers, with open GSNO meetings held quarterly.

THE NURSING STUDENT GROUP

There are approximately 120 students enrolled at the Graduate School or Nursing: 17 collaborative Ph.D. students, 57 traditional master's students, and 46 Graduate Entry Pathway students. Students are primarily from Massachusetts, but many come from other parts of New England and across the United States. Students range in age from 21 to 64.

COSTS

In 2004, tuition for the pre-master's pathway, traditional master's pathway, post-master's certificate programs, and Ph.D. program was $110 per credit for in-state students and $410 per credit for out-of-state students. For the Graduate Entry Pathway, tuition was $21,000 for the first year, $13,511 for the second year, and $9044 for the third year for in-state students and $30,992 for the first year, $20,698 for the second year, and $16,260 for the third year for out-of-state students. Fees cost approximately $2591. Tuition and fees are subject to change.

FINANCIAL AID

Students who believe their resources are insufficient to fund their graduate education may apply for financial aid. To be eligible for financial assistance, students must be accepted for admission or enrolled in good standing and making satisfactory academic progress. In addition, they must neither owe a repayment on a Federal Pell Grant, Federal Supplemental Educational Grant, or State Student Incentive Grant nor be in default on a Federal Perkins Loan (formerly National Direct Student Loan), Federal Stafford Loan (formally Guaranteed Student Loan), Federally Insured Student Loan, Federal SLS, or Federal PLUS or Federal ALAS Loan received for study at any postsecondary institution. Furthermore, students must demonstrate financial need to be eligible for most, although not all, financial aid programs. Because financial aid is awarded annually, all financial aid recipients must reapply each year.

APPLYING

Admission to the Graduate School of Nursing is granted by the faculty. Students who wish to be considered for the degree of Master of Science must submit their applications and supporting materials to the University of Massachusetts Worcester, Graduate School of Nursing. The GSN has posted deadlines for admission for each pathway in the master's program. Applicants are encouraged to submit materials in advance of posted deadlines. Applicants are reviewed individually on the basis of previous academic achievement, Graduate Record Examination (GRE) scores, professional experience, and personal attributes. Each application also is reviewed to determine whether prerequisites have been met for acceptance into the Master of Science degree program. Admission criteria vary slightly for the Graduate Entry Pathway and the traditional or pre-master's pathway.

CORRESPONDENCE AND INFORMATION:

Graduate School of Nursing
University of Massachusetts Worcester
55 Lake Avenue North
Worcester, Massachusetts 01655-0002
Telephone: 508-856-5801
E-mail: GSNAdmissions@umassmed.edu
World Wide Web: http://www.umassmed.edu/gsn

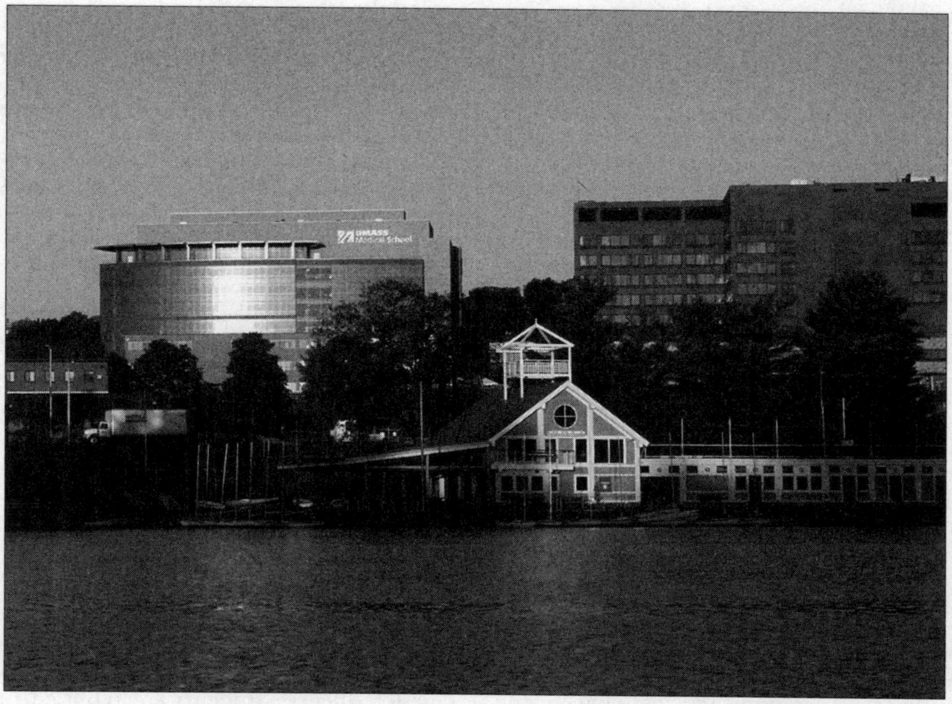

UMass Worcester Medical School.

University of Michigan
School of Nursing
Ann Arbor, Michigan

THE UNIVERSITY
The University of Michigan, located in Ann Arbor, Michigan, has more than 445,000 alumni worldwide. Graduates of the University have made substantial contributions to intellectual, scientific, and cultural growth. Its internationally ranked faculty, supported by the most advanced research programs, prepares students to teach, lead, heal, and innovate in the global society of the twenty-first century. The University of Michigan is consistently ranked among the nation's top ten universities.

THE SCHOOL OF NURSING
The University of Michigan School of Nursing has held an unsurpassed reputation of excellence for more than 100 years, because it has kept pace with advances in knowledge and technology and trends in health care. The School of Nursing is also unparalleled in terms of its distinguished faculty, with more than 90 percent of all tenure-track faculty members doctorally prepared. This caliber of faculty preparation enhances the balance between clinical and theoretical experiences for students.

Matching faculty strength with current societal needs has led to the formation of three School-supported, interdisciplinary Centers of Excellence where educational, clinical, and research initiatives are fostered. Results influence nursing science, practice, and public health policy. The centers are focused on three areas: enhancement and restoration of cognitive function, advancing the science of health promotion and risk reduction across the life span, and concepts of frailty and vulnerability as applied to life's later stages. Each center offers periodic forums where members present results of their research. Students in undergraduate and graduate programs can apply to become a Center Scholar in one of the centers. In addition to the Centers of Excellence, the Grants and Research Office works with the program areas to maintain an exciting and productive research environment in the School of Nursing. The center stimulates, coordinates, and facilitates research through a variety of functions such as consulting on research design and data analysis, assisting in the preparation of grant proposals, and identifying reviewers for proposals before submission for external funding.

PROGRAMS OF STUDY
Nursing education is an investment in the future of health care in terms of both the individual nurse and the overall health-care delivery system. The School of Nursing is strongly committed to the concept that nurses must continue to be challenged educationally in order to meet the rigors of a highly complex, diverse profession.

The Bachelor of Science in Nursing (B.S.N.) degree is the basis for a career in nursing. The School of Nursing's four-year B.S.N. program offers applicants direct admission as freshmen. Transfer students may be admitted to the second-year level of the program, depending upon the course work they have already completed and the availability of openings in the second year. As of fall 2004, the School offers an accelerated B.S.N. program for students with bachelor's degrees in other fields. Students in the accelerated Second Career program will be able to complete a B.S.N. degree and prepare for the registered nurse NCLEX exam and licensing in twelve months. If a student would like to pursue an advanced degree in nursing, a University of Michigan School of Nursing Master of Science or post-baccalaureate Ph.D. degree may be completed.

In addition to the four-year B.S.N. program, the School offers a B.S.N. completion program in Ann Arbor, Traverse City, and Kalamazoo for the A.D.N. or diploma nurse. The School's RN to M.S. program combines undergraduate and graduate studies for highly motivated RNs. This program may be completed in three to four part-time years, depending on the master's specialty.

At the Master of Science level, the School of Nursing, through the University's Horace H. Rackham School of Graduate Studies, offers advanced practice certification and clinical nurse specialist programs. Program offerings include nursing business and health systems with a focus in nursing informatics, nursing management/administration, nursing and health-care policy, or entrepreneurial nursing (Web-based format); dual degrees in nursing and business administration, nursing and information, and nursing and health services administration; medical-surgical nursing; adult or pediatric acute-care nurse practitioner; psychiatric–mental health nursing; psychiatric–mental health nurse practitioner; gerontological nursing; gerontological nurse practitioner; adult primary-care adult nurse practitioner (a women's health/childbearing families post-master's certificate option); family nurse practitioner; occupational health nursing; community care/home health nursing; infant, child, and adolescent health primary-care pediatric nurse practitioner; and nurse midwifery (with a concentration in women's health). Some programs offer post-master's options; some programs are available through On Job/On Campus.

The On Job/On Campus Program is flexible, offering students an opportunity to learn while maintaining work and family responsibilities. Classes are scheduled for one long weekend a month for twenty to twenty-two months. The emphasis of the program is on home health-care nursing, occupational health nursing, and community care nursing.

The curriculum plan of the master's programs is implemented through four major components: core courses, specialization courses, cognates, and a master's project. Core courses, which are required in all master's-level programs, fall into three subject categories: theory development, leadership, and research. Nursing specialization courses are designed to prepare students for advanced nursing practice in their respective areas of study. Cognate courses related to a student's program are selected from other University of Michigan graduate areas. All master's degree students are required to complete a master's project that involves participation in research or that is practice or policy oriented.

The School's Ph.D. program prepares an exclusive community of nurse-scientists capable of developing new knowledge necessary to support and advance nursing practice. This postbaccalaureate program is predicated on a strong foundation of clinical expertise and framed within a nursing perspective. Graduates of this prestigious and rigorous program have assumed leadership positions in every area of nursing, including health-care policy, academe, professional organizations, and health-care settings.

The School of Nursing has offered postdoctoral study opportunities since 1987. Currently, this training is offered in health promotion and risk reduction, women's health disparities, and neurobehavior, with support from the National Institutes of Health. The goal of the health promotion and risk reduction training program is to develop scientists capable of sustaining independent research careers focused on generating knowledge about health promotion and risk reduction within the theoretical perspective of nursing science. The goal of the women's health disparities training program is to prepare scientists in an interdisciplinary environment to address women's health needs across the lifespan. The goal of the neurobehavior training program is to develop scientists capable of sustaining independent research careers focused on generating knowledge about human responses and behaviors associated with altered brain functioning.

ACADEMIC FACILITIES
There are more than 7 million volumes in the nineteen libraries on the University's campus. Also on campus are nine museums, several hospitals, hundreds of laboratories and institutes, and more than 12,000 microcomputers.

LOCATION
The University of Michigan is located in Ann Arbor, a city well-known for its parks, rivers, and historical heritage. Ann Arbor's designation as an "All-America City" complements its well-earned title, "Research Center of the Midwest."

STUDENT SERVICES
The University of Michigan has many services available to students, including the Affirmative Action Office, Career Planning and Placement, Center for the Education of Women, Services for Students with Disabilities, the International Center, Minority Student Services, Office of Multicultural Affairs, Office of the Ombudsman, Sexual Assault Prevention and Awareness Center, Student Legal Services, Student Organization Development Center, University Health Center, and a multitude of academic and personal counseling services.

THE NURSING STUDENT GROUP
Of the 887 students registered at the School, 653 are undergraduates. The total student body includes students of color (African Americans, Native Americans, Asians, and Hispanics). The University of Michigan School of Nursing is proud of its continued commitment to a diverse student body.

COSTS
For 2004–05, full-time tuition costs per term for resident undergraduate lower-division courses were $3966; for nonresidents, $12,877. For resident graduate students, full-time tuition costs were $4486; for nonresidents, $13,792.

FINANCIAL AID
Financial assistance based on need is available through the Office of Financial Aid. It may consist of a combination of grants, scholarships, and loans, including Nursing Student Loans and work-study opportunities. A limited number of need-based grants and loans are available after enrollment directly through the School of Nursing. Graduate assistance can be obtained from various sources. Some Graduate Student Teaching and Graduate Student Research Assistantships are available within the School of Nursing. Fellowships and scholarships are available through the Horace H. Rackham School of Graduate Studies.

APPLYING
The deadline for applications to the projected Second Career program is September 15 for the following fall term. The deadline for applications to B.S.N. and RN/B.S.N. programs is February 1. Application to the Master of Science nursing programs is based on a rolling admissions plan. The master's degree programs admit fall and winter. The deadline for applications to the Ph.D. program is December 1 for the following fall term. To request additional information about University of Michigan School of Nursing programs or to inquire about the application deadline, students should call 734-763-5985 or 800-458-8689 (toll-free).

CORRESPONDENCE AND INFORMATION

All University of Michigan Nursing Programs:
Office of Academic Affairs
School of Nursing
University of Michigan
400 North Ingalls, #1160
Ann Arbor, Michigan 48109-0482
Telephone: 734-647-0109
Fax: 734-647-1419
E-mail: umnursing@umich.edu
World Wide Web: http://www.nursing.umich.edu/

Undergraduate Admissions:
Office of Undergraduate Admissions
1220 Student Activities Building
University of Michigan
Ann Arbor, Michigan 48109-1316

Graduate Admissions:
Horace H. Rackham School of Graduate Studies
University of Michigan
915 East Washington
Ann Arbor, Michigan 48109-1070

Postdoctoral Program:
Dr. Richard W. Redman, Director
Doctoral and Postdoctoral Studies
School of Nursing
University of Michigan
400 North Ingalls Building, Room 1154
Ann Arbor, Michigan 48109-0482
Telephone: 734-764-9454
Fax: 734-763-6668
E-mail: rwr@umich.edu

University of Minnesota, Twin Cities Campus
School of Nursing
Minneapolis, Minnesota

THE UNIVERSITY
The University of Minnesota, with its four campuses, ranks among the top twenty universities in the United States. It is both a state land-grant university, with a strong tradition of education and public service, and a major research institution with scholars of national and international reputation. The Academic Health Center on the Minneapolis campus comprises the Medical School, School of Dentistry, School of Nursing, School of Public Health, and College of Pharmacy.

THE SCHOOL OF NURSING
Established in 1909, the School of Nursing holds the distinction of being the first continuing nursing program on a university campus. The School of Nursing assumes responsibility for improving nursing care through its programs in nursing education, research, and community service.

PROGRAMS OF STUDY
The School of Nursing offers three degrees: the Bachelor of Science in Nursing, the Master of Science with a major in nursing, and the Doctor of Philosophy with a major in nursing. A Post-Baccalaureate Certificate program is also offered. The baccalaureate, postbaccalaureate, and master's programs are accredited by the Commission on Collegiate Nursing Education (the CCNE does not accredit doctoral programs).

The baccalaureate program is a three-year major admitting approximately 130 students each fall to two campuses: Minneapolis and Rochester, Minnesota.

The Post-Baccalaureate Certificate program is a graduate-level program that spans sixteen months. The courses overlap those of the M.S. program, and prerequisites must be completed prior to entry. Entry to this program is competitive and is limited to 30 students. Students should contact the School of Nursing for information about the prerequisites.

The Graduate School offers the Master of Science degree with a major in nursing under two plans: Plan A (thesis option) and Plan B (nonthesis option). The M.S. program offers seventeen areas of study through Plan B, some of which are offered as Web-based programs. Areas of study include clinical nurse specialist (adult health, gerontological, pediatric, psych–mental health), nurse practitioner (family, pediatric, gerontological, women's health), nursing administration, children with special health-care needs nursing, public health nursing (adolescent health), nursing education, nurse midwifery, and nurse anesthesia. An M.P.H./M.S. dual degree is also available. The M.S. program can be completed in approximately two years of full-time study.

The Ph.D. program is research oriented and is designed to prepare creative and productive scholars in nursing.

ACADEMIC FACILITIES
The University library system is the seventeenth largest in North America, lending more books and journal articles to other libraries than any other in the nation. Students have access to more than 20,000 computer workstations as well as the clinics and laboratories of the Fairview University Medical Center.

LOCATION
The Twin Cities area, with more than 2 million people, is the metropolitan and cultural center of the upper Midwest. The Minnesota Orchestra, the Tyrone Guthrie Theater, and a rich array of art galleries, museums, and small theaters provide extensive cultural opportunities. Outdoor recreation is exceptional. Numerous lakes within the metropolitan area offer various sports activities throughout the year.

STUDENT SERVICES
The University provides a host of support services for students, including Boynton Health Service, disability services, International Study and Travel Center, student unions, Minnesota Women's Center, Sexual Violence Program, Student Diversity Institute, University Counseling & Consulting Service, student cultural centers, and more.

THE NURSING STUDENT GROUP
The School of Nursing enrolls about 800 students. The B.S.N. program has approximately 390 students; the master's program, 330 students; and the Ph.D. program, 40 students. There are 60 students in the Post-Baccalaureate Certificate Program.

COSTS
Tuition in 2004–05 for the B.S.N. program was $3339 for 13 or more credits per semester for residents and $9154 for 13 or more credits per semester for nonresidents. For full-time graduate students, tuition (6 to 14 credits) was $4087 per semester for residents and $7637 for nonresidents. Per-semester fees include a University fee, $400; Student Services Fee, $276; and Technology Fee, $110, for a total of $786.

FINANCIAL AID
Financial aid resources include graduate fellowships, graduate teaching and research assistantships, scholarships from the School of Nursing Foundation, traineeship grants, and loans from the Office of Student Financial Services.

APPLYING
Requirements for B.S.N. program applicants include applicable prerequisite course work prior to application, a preferred minimum grade point average of 2.8 on a 4.0 scale in the prerequisites and a preferred minimum 2.5 cumulative GPA, and a profile statement. The application deadline is February 1 for the following fall semester.

Applicants to the Post-Baccalaureate Certificate program must have completed a baccalaureate degree in a non-nursing area and have completed applicable prerequisite course work. Successful applicants typically have a cumulative GPA of at least 3.0 from their degree-granting institution. Application requirements include two letters of reference and essay question completion. The application deadline is December 15 for the following fall.

M.S. program applicants must have an RN license and a bachelor's degree with a major in nursing or, if the degree is not in nursing, evidence of ability in health promotion, community health nursing, leadership, and teaching. Application requirements include two letters of reference and the completion of profile essays. Application deadlines are August 1, November 1, and January 1. For the nurse practitioner, clinical nurse specialist, and nurse midwifery areas of study, priority is given to applicants who submit their applications by the November 1 deadline.

Applicants to the Ph.D. program must have a master's degree or a bachelor's degree with an exceptionally strong record in the physical or behavioral sciences. Applicants must submit GRE scores, two letters of reference, and a profile statement. Admission and fellowship applications must be received by October 1 for the fall semester.

CORRESPONDENCE AND INFORMATION

UMTC School of Nursing
5-160 Weaver-Densford Hall
308 Harvard Street Southeast
Minneapolis, Minnesota 55455
Telephone: 612-624-4454
World Wide Web: http://www.nursing.umn.edu

THE FACULTY

Melissa D. Avery, Associate Professor; Ph.D., Minnesota. Exercise as a therapeutic intervention for women with gestational diabetes, maternal nutrition and other antenatal factors influencing infant birth weight, outcomes of nurse midwifery care.

Linda H. Bearinger, Professor; Ph.D., Minnesota. Public health issues and interventions among adolescents, health decision-making among at-risk populations.

Donna Z. Bliss, Associate Professor; Ph.D., Pennsylvania. Effects of dietary fiber on the colon.

Linda Chlan, Assistant Professor; Ph.D., Minnesota. Effects of music on anxiety and discomfort in mechanically ventilated patients.

Laura J. Duckett, Associate Professor; Ph.D., Minnesota. Maternal employment and breast-feeding.

Sandra R. Edwardson, Professor; Ph.D., Minnesota. Cost-quality trade-offs in nursing services, elderly self-care behavior.

Ann Garwick, Associate Professor; Ph.D., Minnesota. Children with chronic disabilities and their families.

Linda Gerdner, Assistant Professor; Ph.D., Iowa. Management of agitation in persons with Alzheimer's disease and related disorders (ADRD), culturally sensitive care in persons with ADRD and their family caregivers.

Cynthia Gross, Professor; Ph.D., Yale. Quality of life outcomes of persons after transplantation and during drug therapy; quality of life and health status in patients with lung disorders, diabetes, or renal failure; reliability and validity of quality of life instruments and clinical assessments for research.

Laila Gulzar, Assistant Professor; Ph.D. International and interorganizational collaboration, cross-cultural health and cultural competence, nursing curing Islamic civilization (sixth through twelfth centuries), women's access to primary health care, health-care experiences of immigrants.

Linda Halcón, Assistant Professor; Ph.D., Minnesota. Public health nursing, epidemiology.

Helen E. Hansen, Associate Professor; Ph.D., Kansas. Nursing administration, health-care delivery systems, health team collaboration, leadership.

Susan Henly, Associate Professor; Ph.D., Minnesota. Psychometric methods for nursing research; covariance structures analysis, bonding, and maternal role development; social context for breast-feeding.

Felicia Schanche Hodge, Professor; Dr.P.H., Berkeley. Native American health with focuses on community intervention in areas of diabetes, cancer control, substance abuse, health promotion, and smoking cessation and control.

Catherine Juve, Associate Education Specialist; Ph.D., Minnesota. Substance abuse in pregnancy.

Merrie J. Kaas, Associate Professor; D.N.Sc., California, San Francisco. Older women's mental health, mental health/illness in long-term care.

Madeleine Kerr, Associate Professor; Ph.D., Michigan. Health promotion interventions with workers, research with Mexican-American and other ethnic/racial groups, occupational health: health protective behaviors.

Kathleen E. Krichbaum, Associate Professor; Ph.D., Minnesota. Factors contributing to quality of care for the elderly in nursing homes, clinical teaching effectiveness, evaluating clinical learning.

Barbara J. Leonard, Professor; Ph.D., Minnesota. Child health care, care of children with special health-care needs.

Marsha L. Lewis, Associate Professor; Ph.D., Minnesota. Clinical and client decision making, quality of life for the chronically mentally ill.

Joan Liaschenko, Associate Professor; Ph.D., California, San Francisco. Ethics, nursing practice, nursing humanities, philosophy of nursing, psychiatric nursing, home-care nursing.

Linda L. Lindeke, Associate Professor; Ph.D., Minnesota. Advanced nursing practice, high-risk infants.

Ruth D. Lindquist, Associate Professor; Ph.D., Minnesota. Risks of and response to cardiovascular disease, personal control and quality of life in health care, alterations in homeostatic function in elderly, critical care.

Margaret Moss, Assistant Professor; D.S.N., Texas–Houston Health Science Center. Gerontology, minority aging, American Indians and aging.

Christine Mueller, Associate Professor; Ph.D., Maryland. Clinical and cost outcomes for nursing home residents using research-based clinical protocols and organizational interventions via advanced practice nurses; staffing in long-term-care facilities.

Carol O'Boyle, Assistant Professor; Ph.D., Minnesota. International health, infectious disease and control, nursing theory and learning.

Cynthia Peden-McAlpine, Assistant Professor; Ph.D., Adelphi. Expert thinking in nursing practice, critical care and public health nursing, nurse executive practice, moral aspects of thinking in nursing practice, phenomenological and hermeneutic methodology.

Margaret Plumbo, Instructor; M.S., Minnesota. Women's health, depression and the family, adolescent IDDM and the family.

Cheryl Robertson, Assistant Professor; Ph.D., Minnesota. Effects of war, repression, and torture on the health of families and communities, focusing on models that promote resilience and health systems capacity development.

Roxanne Struthers, Assistant Professor; Ph.D., Minnesota. Home health care and community health nursing for individuals, families, and communities on Native American reservations; alternative healing practices.

Jean Wyman, Professor; Ph.D., Washington (Seattle). Gerontological nursing, urinary incontinence, fall prevention and exercise in the elderly.

University of Pennsylvania
School of Nursing
Philadelphia, Pennsylvania

THE UNIVERSITY

The University of Pennsylvania (Penn) is an independent, nonsectarian institution. As one of the finest universities in the country, it offers an outstanding array of resources for both undergraduate and graduate students. The excellence of its many schools offers students the opportunity to take elective courses across the campus in a wide range of subjects, making it one of the major centers for learning and research in the nation. Penn will be graduating the student of the twenty-first century from a seamless academic community. This concept provides a framework that fosters student and faculty collaboration across the University, enhancing opportunities for a diversified approach to education and research.

THE SCHOOL OF NURSING

Penn is the only Ivy League institution offering a baccalaureate nursing program that begins day one, master's programs in nursing, and doctoral nursing study. The University of Pennsylvania Medical Center began training professional nurses in 1886. Today the School of Nursing at Penn offers one of the most progressive and highly regarded programs in the country.

The University of Pennsylvania School of Nursing is consistently ranked among the nation's top graduate schools of nursing in a major survey conducted by *U.S. News & World Report.* In determining its rankings, the criteria considered were the School's reputation for scholarship, curriculum, research, and the quality of the faculty and students. The undergraduate nursing program is listed in *Ruggs Book of Colleges* as high school guidance counselors' first choice for nursing.

The University has virtually all of its undergraduate and graduate facilities—including its hospitals, libraries, and laboratories—on one campus, giving nursing students access to people, ideas, and information on a multitude of subjects. Nursing students have matchless opportunities for clinical experience at the world-renowned University of Pennsylvania Health System, the Children's Hospital of Philadelphia, the Penn Nursing Network (nurse-managed clinical practices), and the Philadelphia VA Medical Center in addition to many other clinical agencies and health-care institutions in the Philadelphia region.

At Penn, nursing students are taught and advised by a faculty that is nationally and internationally recognized for its leadership in education, practice, and research. Undergraduate and graduate students often take advantage of the opportunity to participate in faculty research and scholarly publications. The Penn faculty members have a deep commitment to their role as teachers as well as to the development of professional and personal alliances between students and faculty.

PROGRAMS OF STUDY

The School of Nursing offers a Bachelor of Science in Nursing (B.S.N.) degree with a program that balances the liberal arts, science, and professional nursing preparation. Courses in the nursing major emphasize interpersonal communication, critical-thinking skills, clinical competence, and research. Special opportunities include nursing-specific study-abroad programs; a joint-degree program, dual-degree options, and minors in Penn's College of Arts and Sciences, Annenberg School for Communication, Wharton School, and School of Engineering and Applied Science; and submatriculation (initiating pursuit of a graduate degree while working toward the completion of the B.S.N.) into Penn's School of Law or one of the School of Nursing's sixteen M.S.N. specialties.

In 1997, the University initiated an undergraduate joint degree program offered by the School of Nursing and the Wharton School. Graduates will be awarded a B.S.N. from the School of Nursing and Bachelor of Science in Economics from the Wharton School with a concentration in health-care management and policy. Additional programs include a health communication minor with the Annenberg School for Communication, and a B.S.N./Ph.D. option.

Penn offers an accelerated program allowing students already holding a baccalaureate degree to complete a B.S.N. or B.S.N./M.S.N. degree. These second-degree accelerated programs build on an individual's present level of education so that students need only complete required nursing-specific courses.

The RN Return Program is designed to educate hospital diploma and associate degree RNs for an increased leadership role in nursing through the earning of a B.S.N. degree. Previous college and university courses are evaluated for transfer credit, and many clinical nursing courses may be challenged by taking specified Excelsior College examinations.

The School of Nursing offers the Master of Science in Nursing (M.S.N.) degree, including nurse practitioner programs in adult acute care, adult health, adult oncology, family health, gerontology, neonatal, pediatrics, pediatric acute/chronic, pediatric critical-care, pediatric oncology, and women's health. Advanced practice specialist programs include the nurse anesthesia, nurse midwifery, and the psychiatric–mental health advanced practice programs. Administration programs are also available in health leadership and nursing and health-care administration. There are also many special options at Penn Nursing, including unique opportunities and minors. There are four unique opportunities: adult home care, clinical nurse specialist, occupational/environmental health, and perinatal. Students enrolled in graduate programs may apply for one of ten minors, which include adult acute care, adult oncology, behavioral health, forensic science, gerontology, health informatics, health leadership, nursing and health-care administration, palliative care, and women's health studies. An M.S.N. in nursing administration/M.B.A. is offered in conjunction with the Wharton School, and an M.S.N./M.P.H. is offered in conjunction with the School of Medicine. A post-master's teacher education program is also available.

The School of Nursing recognizes the evolving nature of health care and the desire on the part of many nurses to expand or alter current roles and responsibilities. It is possible to pursue post-master's work, which is designed for those who already possess a master's degree in nursing and are interested in either extending their knowledge and skill in their current area of practice or changing to a new area of nursing practice. Students also have the option of designing their own curriculum to include two or more programs.

The mission of the doctoral program of the University of Pennsylvania School of Nursing is to prepare nurse scientists for successful careers, particularly in research-intensive environments. Graduates of this program will be leaders who will move the science of nursing forward through the conduct and dissemination of research for the advancement of nursing practice. These nurse scientists will take responsibility to shape and advance health care, with the ultimate goal of improving the public's health through the integration of theory, research, and practice.

The educational experience focuses on the processes of knowing and an examination of substantive bodies of knowledge. Development as a researcher is fostered through exposure to the philosophic and methodological aspects of nursing and related basic and applied disciplines.

For students with a special interest, there are also joint programs, such as a Ph.D. in nursing and a master's in bioethics or a Ph.D. in nursing and an M.B.A. from the Wharton School. M.S.N./Ph.D. and M.S./Ph.D. options are also available.

ACADEMIC FACILITIES

The Penn Library holds more than 5 million printed volumes and 3.8 million items in microform and subscribes to more than 40,000 current serial subscriptions. The library also houses 196,474 bound volumes in health and 9,552 electronic journals. The University library system processes 362,000 reference and information transactions per year.

The Mathias J. Brunner Instructional Technology Center, located within the School, is a state-of-the-art facility featuring virtual learning and patient-care simulation.

Specialized centers at the School of Nursing include the Center for Nursing Research; Center for Urban Health Research; International Center of Research for Women, Children and Families; the Center for Health Outcomes and Policy Research; the Center for the Study of the History of Nursing; the Center for Gerontologic Nursing Science; and the Hartford Center of Geriatric Nursing Excellence.

LOCATION

Philadelphia is the fifth-largest metropolitan area in the United States. The four undergraduate schools and twelve graduate schools of the University are located on a 260-acre tract on the west side of the Schuylkill River. Unified by a network of pedestrian walkways and almost entirely closed off to cars, the campus contributes to the sense of community that is characteristic of Penn. Although situated in a major urban setting just across the river and less than 2 miles from the center of Philadelphia, the University is surrounded by a largely residential community known as University City.

STUDENT SERVICES

The University campus, and the School of Nursing specifically, have many resources and services available to meet the needs a diverse student body. These include cultural centers, religious organizations, academic advising, counseling, housing, dining, student health, tutoring, day care, athletic facilities, and computing services.

THE NURSING STUDENT GROUP

The School of Nursing population is a diverse group of students. The School is an intimate niche within the University enabling students to receive personalized attention from the faculty and staff. School of Nursing faculty members advise nursing students, further enhancing student-faculty interaction.

COSTS

Tuition for full-time B.S.N. students for the 2004–05 academic year was $27,544. Part-time tuition was $3518 per course. Tuition for full-time M.S.N. students was $26,973; it was $3392 per course part-time. Full-time Ph.D. students are fully funded with a stipend and tuition support for the first four years. Part-time Ph.D. tuition was $3720 per course in 2004–05.

FINANCIAL AID

Penn is committed to meeting the financial need of all of its students. Many different sources of aid are available. Scholarships, grants, low-interest student loans, and teaching and research assistantships are awarded appropriately, based on a student's need and level of study. Financial aid counseling is available for individual consultation and support. Students are encouraged to work directly with the School to help them develop the means to support their education.

APPLYING

Freshman applicants to the B.S.N. program should be completing a general college-preparatory program in high school. They must also take the new SAT with writing, administered by the College Board beginning March 2005. Students should verify testing with the admission counselor in the School of Nursing. If taking the ACT, applicants are required to take the new ACT with writing, administered by the ACT beginning February 2005.

Prospective freshman students can apply under one of two admissions plans. The Early Decision Plan is for those applicants who have decided that the University of Pennsylvania School of Nursing is their first-choice college and agree to attend if accepted. Applications are due by November 1, with decisions mailed in mid-December. Regular decision applications to the School of Nursing are due by January 1, and students are notified by the end of February.

Transfer students are admitted for the fall semester only. The application deadline is March 15, with notification beginning early May.

B.S.N./M.S.N. and B.S.N. second degree applicants must apply by October 15 for June or September admission and will hear by late February. The Graduate Record Examinations (GRE) are required for B.S.N./M.S.N. applicants.

It is important that applicants to all of the baccalaureate options arrange a personal interview with an admissions counselor in the School of Nursing. This interview will afford students an opportunity to learn more about the specific program they are considering and to better understand the course work required to complete the B.S.N. degree. Online applications are available.

All master's and doctoral applicants must have completed an accredited baccalaureate nursing program, have taken a course in basic statistics, and have nursing licensure. Applicants should interview with the appropriate program director and must submit, along with the completed application forms, GRE General Test scores, transcripts, references, and essays. Applicants who have earned a GPA of 3.2 or higher in their baccalaureate nursing program may be eligible for the GRE waiver program. International students must submit results from the TOEFL and GRE and may be asked to have their foreign transcripts evaluated in a Full Educational Course-by-Course Report by the Commission on Graduates of Foreign Nursing Schools or World Education Services. Applications are accepted on a rolling basis for most M.S.N. programs; however, applicants are encouraged to submit applications early to secure clinical placement and maximum financial aid. Applications to the M.S.N./Ph.D. program are due on November 1. Applications for the doctoral program must be submitted by December 15.

For more information, to request written materials, or for access to the online application, prospective students should access the School's World Wide Web site.

CORRESPONDENCE AND INFORMATION

Office of Enrollment Management
School of Nursing
University of Pennsylvania
420 Guardian Drive
Philadelphia, Pennsylvania 19104-6096
Telephone: 215-898-4271
866-867-6877 (toll-free)
Fax: 215-573-8439
E-mail: admissions@nursing.upenn.edu
World Wide Web: http://www.nursing.upenn.edu

University of Phoenix Online
School of Nursing
Phoenix, Arizona

THE UNIVERSITY

Founded in 1976, University of Phoenix is the nation's largest private accredited university. The University provides a relevant, real-world education to working adults at more than 139 campuses and learning centers in the U.S., Puerto Rico, Canada, and via the Internet. University of Phoenix is dedicated to the educational needs of working professionals and their employers. The commitment to the adult learner is unequivocal: the University has awarded bachelor's and master's degrees to more than 171,600 graduates, using an innovative learning format that makes higher education more accessible, efficient, and relevant. The University is accredited by the Higher Learning Commission and is a member of the North Central Association of Colleges and Schools (NCA). In addition, the nursing programs are accredited by the National League for Nursing Accrediting Commission (NLNAC).

The University of Phoenix Online is part of the University of Phoenix. Founded in 1989, University of Phoenix Online was among the first accredited universities to provide college degree programs via the Internet. In addition to nursing, complete degree programs in business, management, e-business, technology, criminal justice, and education are also offered. University of Phoenix Online provides students with the same quality education, curriculum, faculty, and resources offered at more than 139 University of Phoenix campuses and learning centers. A commitment to educational excellence and unsurpassed student service has made the University a leading accredited online university in the United States.

THE SCHOOL OF NURSING

University of Phoenix Online offers a comprehensive online nursing program that provides unparalleled convenience and flexibility for the RN who seeks advanced education. High academic standards, commitment to quality, and intensely focused programs have earned the University a reputation for leadership in both the academic and nursing communities. A distinguished blend of proven academic practices and innovative instructional delivery systems has helped to build the university, with a growing network of campuses and learning centers throughout the United States. The goal is to provide all nursing students with the means to be more effective at their jobs so that they may reap the rewards that follow.

The Online Campus has approximately 8,000 faculty members. The degree programs are taught by proven professionals who bring a unique blend of academic and experiential insight to every course they teach. Faculty members are carefully chosen both for their success in their own careers and for their ability and desire to effectively facilitate a challenging and rewarding learning environment. All NUR courses in the M.S.N. program are taught by doctoral-prepared faculty members. Faculty members hold master's or doctoral degrees and possess an average of fifteen years of current practical experience in the fields relating to the subjects they teach. Each instructor is skilled in the unique craft of providing course instruction, direction, and feedback to students physically distant from the classroom. This integration of advanced academic preparation, communications expertise, and current professional experience ensures that students learn real-world application. All of the nursing courses are taught by practitioner faculty members who are as familiar with client care and current health-care/nursing issues as they are with academics.

PROGRAMS OF STUDY

The Bachelor of Science in Nursing (B.S.N.) program is a two-year program designed to develop the professional knowledge and skills of working registered nurses. The curriculum is built upon a foundation of biological, physical, and social sciences that contribute to the science of nursing. The liberal arts components enhance the development of the intellectual, social, and cultural aspects of the professional nurse. The degree program uses an instructional program with behavioral objectives that concentrate on the development of the nurse's role as caregiver, teacher, and manager of care. Utilizing a self-care framework, working registered nurses are prepared as generalists who are able to apply professional skills and knowledge to nursing, clients, and health-care systems. Nursing students can complete their degrees 100 percent online, and clinical course work is done locally with no need for travel.

The Bachelor of Science in health-care services is an applied degree, about two years in length, intended to equip students with the knowledge and basic skills for employment in the health-care environment. Graduates blend the human side of health care with business management practices and navigate effectively as managers in the growing industry of health care. Graduates exhibit flexibility, sensitivity, and effective communication, whether working with individuals, with a team, or within health-care systems. Total credits required for the degree program are 120.

The Master of Science in Nursing (M.S.N.) program is also a two-year program designed to develop and enhance the knowledge and skills of registered nurses. It is designed for nurses who want to pursue more advanced positions in today's challenging health-care environment. The program blends nursing theory with advanced practice concepts necessary to successfully work within the structure, culture, and mission of any size health-care organization or educational setting. The M.S.N. program consists of three major areas: the core, the major, and the cognate. The core incorporates the major foci of a Master of Science in Nursing degree: the theory of nursing, ethical nursing issues, and the influence of nursing research on the advanced practice of nursing. The major includes advanced course work in nursing: management of families and aggregates, administration, and education. The cognate includes course work concerning today's health-care environment: health-care infrastructure, health-care finance, and data-based decision making. The program requires the completion of 39 credits. Graduate students are permitted to waive up to 9 credits by transferring comparable graduate-level course work taken at other accredited colleges or universities.

A B.S.N. to M.S.N. pathway program is also available for those University of Phoenix Online B.S.N. graduates who would like to continue in the Master of Science in Nursing program. In addition, a bridge program is available for registered nurses who hold a non-B.S.N. bachelor's degree. The bridge program consists of taking three courses from the B.S.N. program prior to admission to the M.S.N. program.

The Master of Business Administration/Health Care Management (M.B.A./HCM) degree program is a two-year, 46-credit program that is designed for professionals seeking management positions in the health-care field. The program is structured with two primary goals in mind. The first is to provide students with a broad-based understanding of current management tools and techniques with practical application in the health-care industry. The second goal is to prepare students to manage human and material resources effectively and efficiently within the health-care environment. The program emphasizes fundamental curriculum, critical thinking, and decision making that has been positioned for the changing requirements and dynamics of the health-care industry. Students are required to give due consideration to the broader implications of decisions, such as the potential effect on governmental relations, marketing, human resources, and finances and operations. Students develop additional expertise with regard to solutions for persistant management problems through the completion of an applied management science project, which relates the student's professional interests or responsibilities to the goal of improved managerial functioning.

The Master of Health Administration program prepares leaders who can effectively respond to the dynamic and ever-changing health-care industry. These individuals have a capacity to critically examine and evaluate issues and trends and are empowered to influence the destiny of the global health-care system. The curriculum is tailored to the needs of the health-care leader/manager by providing content in finance, policy, research, technology, quality improvement, economics, marketing, and strategic planning. In addition, students are also asked to complete course work related to their area of concentration, such as public health, long-term care, and health informatics. The Master of Health Administration is a two-year, 40-credit-hour program.

The dual M.S.N./M.B.A./HCM degree program is designed to provide nurses with a unique blend of advanced nursing and business management skills to manage today's innovative health-care delivery systems. The program combines essentials from both degree programs to provide students with the knowledge and skills necessary to enhance and support patient services. The M.B.A./HCM program emphasizes the identification, analysis, and solution of complex management problems that require technical understanding and balanced decision making. Although a functional knowledge of accounting, finance, and management underlies the program, equal attention is given to the development of report writing, oral reporting, and group process skills. This program is three years in length and requires 61 credits.

ACADEMIC FACILITIES

The Online program relies on computer communications to link faculty members and students from around the world into interactive learning groups. Class size is limited to 15 students for maximum interaction. Degrees are completed entirely online for the convenience of working adults who find it difficult or impossible to attend classes at fixed times and places.

LOCATION

Once enrolled in an online degree program, students log on to the computer conferencing system five days each week to participate in class discussions. Students work online, sending and receiving material to and from class groups, while conducting most of their communication and course work offline.

STUDENT SERVICES

University of Phoenix Online offers its students exceptional customer service. An experienced Nursing Admissions Counselor is available to help answer all questions regarding programs, start dates, financing, and the application process. A free "pre-evaluation" of potential credits for prior education or work experience can also be requested. Once the application and fees have been received, an adviser processes the application, ships the software, helps order textbooks and course materials, and gets the student into class. During class, students have access to a full range of online research libraries and services. Every instructor provides guidance and feedback on student progress.

THE NURSING STUDENT GROUP

University courses are designed for working adults who have busy work schedules and full personal lives. The average age of entering University of Phoenix students is approximately 36 years, with a household income of $70,000 to $79,000. Nearly 60 percent of entering students have at least eleven years of work experience, and about 60 percent of students receive some tuition assistance from their employers—double the national average for adult students at other institutions.

COSTS

Undergraduate nursing tuition is $385 per credit, and graduate nursing tuition is $430 per credit. There is an application fee of $100 and a graduation fee of $55. Textbook costs vary by course.

FINANCIAL AID

Several low-interest financial aid options are available, even to individuals with a high income. University of Phoenix participates in many financial aid programs, including the Federal Stafford Student Loan, the Federal PLUS Loan, and the Federal Pell Grant. The University does not charge students for processing financial aid applications. For further details about eligibility and to receive application forms, students should speak with a financial adviser.

APPLYING

Applicants must be employed in a nursing role or have access to an appropriate health-care organization environment. Nursing students must have a diploma or associate degree in nursing, with a cumulative GPA of at least 2.0 and a current RN license. One hallmark of the B.S.N. program is that there is no testing of prior nursing knowledge if the RN is in good standing within the state of practice. Graduate students must have an undergraduate nursing degree or other related health-care degree from a regionally accredited college or university, with a cumulative GPA of 2.5 or better (3.0 for prior graduate work). Students must also be currently employed, with a minimum of three years' work experience as an RN (or two years' work experience as an RN plus one year in a health-care–related field). RNs who have a non-nursing bachelor's degree take three bridge courses from the B.S.N. program prior to being eligible for graduate M.S.N. course work. Unless students rely on international transcripts for admission, all that is needed to begin the first course are a completed application, enrollment agreement, and disclosure form. While students are in their first three classes, academic counselors work with them to complete transcript requests, the Comprehensive Cognitive Assessment, and any other items necessary for formal registration. To apply for admission, students should visit http://myapply.phoenix.edu/apply/formslogin.asp.

CORRESPONDENCE AND INFORMATION:

Admissions Department
University of Phoenix Online
3157 East Elwood Street
Phoenix, Arizona 85034
Telephone: 877-611-3390 (toll-free in U.S.)
Fax: 602-387-6440
World Wide Web: http://www.uopx.com/petersons

University of Pittsburgh
School of Nursing
Pittsburgh, Pennsylvania

THE UNIVERSITY

Founded in 1787, the University of Pittsburgh is the oldest institution of higher education west of the Allegheny Mountains. It is an independent, state-related, nonsectarian coeducational institution offering a variety of undergraduate and graduate programs. Total enrollment at the Pittsburgh campus is approximately 27,000, including nearly 9,000 graduate and professional students. In recognition of the strength of its graduate programs, the University was elected in 1974 to the Association of American Universities, an organization of the fifty-eight most respected graduate and research institutions in North America.

THE SCHOOL OF NURSING

Founded in 1939 as an independent school of the University, the School of Nursing strives to have a positive impact on the quality of health care for all segments of the population through its teaching, research, and service. It offers educational programs that anticipate and reflect the health-care needs of the region, state, and nation, resulting in the awarding of 7,305 baccalaureate degrees, 2,923 master's degrees, and 159 doctoral degrees to nursing students. There are approximately 800 nursing students, so students benefit from the low student-faculty ratio and small class sizes of the School of Nursing as well as from the extensive resources and enrichment opportunities of a major research university and medical center.

The School is known nationally for the strengths of its clinical and research programs. Students benefit from the variety and excellence of available clinical sites, including nurse-managed nurse practitioner clinics. Faculty members who teach clinical courses have their own clinical practice in order to share their knowledge and enhance their skills. Current faculty and student research programs reflect the breadth of patient populations and health-care problems that are under investigation.

PROGRAMS OF STUDY

Study options available at the undergraduate level include the baccalaureate program, the accelerated second-degree B.S.N., and programs designed especially for registered nurses (RNs). Baccalaureate students typically enter as freshmen unless they have completed all required freshman courses and are accepted into the sophomore class. The 124-credit curriculum emphasizes the basic liberal arts and sciences the first year and initiates the clinical phase the second year. The last two years include a variety of clinical experiences culminating in a leadership/transition course where seniors work closely with nurse preceptors. Many undergraduates choose to complete an independent study with faculty mentors. Graduates are eligible to take the National Council Licensure Examination (NCLEX) to become RNs. Registered nurse options are the RN-B.S.N. or RN-M.S.N. programs, where the B.S.N. can be earned in less than one year of full-time study or longer for part-time study.

The accelerated second-degree B.S.N. program is designed to enable students with a previous baccalaureate degree to earn a baccalaureate degree in nursing. This is an intensive, fast-paced program that builds upon a student's previous education while providing science and nursing content to enable students to earn a B.S.N. degree within three terms of full-time study. Admission to this option is highly competitive and is based upon proven academic achievement and grades earned in prerequisite courses. Two of the accelerated courses and one of the prerequisite courses are master's-level courses. Successful completion of this program earns the student 11 credits toward the M.S.N. degree, should the student decide to pursue a master's degree in nursing at the University of Pittsburgh School of Nursing.

Postbaccalaureate certificates include health-care genetics, health-care management, and school nurse certification.

Graduate programs of study lead to the M.S.N. and Ph.D. degrees. Professional nurses who want to pursue a graduate degree have several choices at the School. In the advanced practice arena, the School of Nursing prepares students for the role of a nurse anesthetist, nurse practitioner, or clinical nurse specialist. Nurse practitioner options include acute-care nurse practitioner, with a concentration in adult health, cardiopulmonary, critical care, oncology, or a directed option, and primary-care nurse practitioner, with options in family, pediatrics, psychiatric, or adult. There is also an opportunity to obtain a clinical nurse specialist degree in medical/surgical or psychiatric nursing. A second option is the specialized role. This role could include a focus in administration, education, informatics, or research.

The advanced practice option varies from 41 to 52 credits. The curriculum consists of core courses, advanced nursing practice specialty courses, role development courses, and electives. Core courses include health promotion, pathophysiology, physical diagnosis, pharmacology, nursing theory and research, and the research practicum. The specialized role option is 40 credits in length. The curriculum consists of core courses, specialty cognates, and focused electives. Core courses include research theory and practicum, health-care outcomes, informatics, and a specialized practicum. Minors are also available in nursing education, nursing research, nursing informatics, or nursing administration as well as the school nurse certificate and management certificate for health professionals. For those who have a current master's degree, a second master's option is also available, and a thesis is optional. There are post-M.S.N. certificate options in administration, education, informatics, and health-care genetics as well as five nurse practitioner options.

The Ph.D. program prepares scholars to extend scientific knowledge that advances the science and practice of nursing and to contribute to the scientific base of other disciplines. The curriculum includes courses in the history and philosophy of science, nursing theory development, the structure of nursing knowledge, issues influencing leadership and public policy in nursing and health, advanced statistics, quantitative research methods, research methodologies, instrumentation, and a research practicum with an experienced researcher. An area of research emphasis, which matches a faculty member's research emphasis, is selected by the student early in the program. Current faculty research initiatives include adolescent health, health-care outcomes, chronic disorders, critical care, health promotion, and mental health. The culminating requirement is a dissertation.

Two options exist for completing the doctoral program. The traditional M.S.N.–Ph.D. option is for students with a traditional master's degree with a clinical specialty focus. This option requires the completion of 64 credits. A one-term, full-time residency is required; however, the remainder of the degree requirements may be completed through either full- or part-time study. The B.S.N.-Ph.D. option is for individuals who wish to focus on research and prepare for a research career and does not require a master's degree or lead to a master's degree with a clinical specialty focus. This option requires full-time study to complete 95–97 credits.

ACADEMIC FACILITIES

Nursing students have access to the Maurice and Laura Falk Library of the Health Sciences, with 2,697 journals and 429,581 volumes, and to the University Library System, with 2,919,302 items. The School of Nursing Learning Resources Center (LRC) provides reference services, a nursing skills practice laboratory, computer laboratory, small television studio, and a graphics laboratory. The LRC computer laboratory is open 60 hours per week and provides microcomputer capability and access to the University mainframe computer system and to the Internet. Students also use the University's computer labs, which are located around the campus.

LOCATION

The University's 136-acre campus is situated in Oakland, the heart of Pittsburgh's educational, medical, and cultural center. Within walking distance of the campus are theaters, art galleries, museums, libraries, and concert halls.

Pittsburgh has consistently been named one of the nation's most livable cities in various national surveys. Most students and many faculty members live within walking distance of the University, in either Oakland, Squirrel Hill, or Shadyside. These areas abound in ethnic restaurants and in shops of all varieties, reflecting the cosmopolitan background of the residents. Most people find that Pittsburgh is a friendly, warm, active, exciting, and comfortable city in which to live.

STUDENT SERVICES

The University offers students a wide variety of services, including outpatient health care at the Student Health Service; career development, learning skills, and psychological services; veterans and disabled student services; numerous student activities; and child care.

THE NURSING STUDENT GROUP

In 2003–04, the School of Nursing enrolled 614 undergraduate students and 388 graduate students. Many were already registered nurses who were working toward B.S.N., M.S.N., or Ph.D. degrees in order to improve their career mobility, assume a new role, or increase their personal satisfaction.

COSTS

Undergraduate tuition per term in 2004–05 for full-time study was $6374 for in-state and $12,392 for out-of-state students. Tuition per credit for part-time study was $455 for in-state and $885 for out-of-state students. Full-time student fees were $664. On-campus housing costs ranged from $1407 to $2785 per term. Available meal plan options varied from $285 to $1805 per term.

Graduate tuition per term in 2004–05 for full-time study was $7299 for in-state and $10,031 for out-of-state students. Tuition per credit for part-time study was $599 for in-state and $823 for out-of-state students. Full-time student fees were $584.

FINANCIAL AID

The University awards financial assistance to both undergraduate and graduate students through scholarships, loans, part-time employment, work-study, and School of Nursing awards. Freshman applicants apply by March 1 and continuing students by April 1.

Master's students receive a variety of financial aid through the School of Nursing, including Professional Nurse Traineeships for full-time study, University tuition aid for part-time study, specified scholarships, loans, graduate student assistant positions, and out-of-state student tuition awards.

Doctoral students also receive aid from the School. Out-of-state full-time students who meet specific criteria pay in-state tuition rates due to school-based scholarships. Many full-time doctoral students have graduate assistant, researcher, or teaching fellow positions, which are primarily merit-based, pay a stipend, and include a tuition scholarship and individual health insurance. These students work 10–20 hours per week, and many have excellent experiences on faculty research projects or teaching. Workshops on applying for predoctoral and postdoctoral training grant fellowships are provided. In addition, other scholarships and part-time tuition aid are available. Students should apply for all School-based aid by June 1 and should contact the Student Services Office for further information.

APPLYING

Applicants to all programs should present appropriate transcripts, admission test scores, and other required material by the deadline date. For the latest and most complete admission information, applicants should contact the Student Services Office. High school applicants and those applying for transfer from another college or university should contact the University Office of Admissions and Financial Aid at 412-624-PITT to receive information and an application. Admission decisions are made on a rolling basis, but applicants should apply as early as possible. Registered nurse applicants are admitted on a rolling basis for all terms.

Undergraduate prelicensure applicants are evaluated primarily on the basis of their high school or previous college-level academic work, with an emphasis on performance in science courses. For high school applicants or transfer applicants with fewer than 24 credits, SAT I scores as well as the student's high school record are considered.

Master's applicants must have a baccalaureate degree in nursing, a current license to practice, and one to two years of experience (for full-time study). Admission decisions are based upon a faculty interview, professional goals, previous academic performance, and GRE or MAT scores, if required by the program. Applications are due January 1 for the anesthesia program, for full-time and part-time study. Applications for full-time study for all other programs must be made by August 1 for fall term, December 1 for spring term, and April 1 for summer term. Applicants for part-time study may be admitted to any term on a rolling admissions basis as long as spaces are available.

Doctoral applicants must have a baccalaureate degree in nursing, documentation of academic success in an appropriate master's program, evidence of competence in scholarly research and the ability to communicate in writing, and satisfactory GRE scores. Admission decisions are based upon previous academic performance, faculty interviews, professional and research goals, a match between the applicant's research interest and those of available faculty members, and GRE scores. Applications are accepted on a rolling basis.

CORRESPONDENCE AND INFORMATION

Student Services
School of Nursing
University of Pittsburgh
3500 Victoria Street
Pittsburgh, Pennsylvania 15261
Telephone: 412-624-4586
888-747-0794 (toll-free)
Fax: 412-624-2409
E-mail: rgartley@pitt.edu
World Wide Web: http://www.nursing.pitt.edu

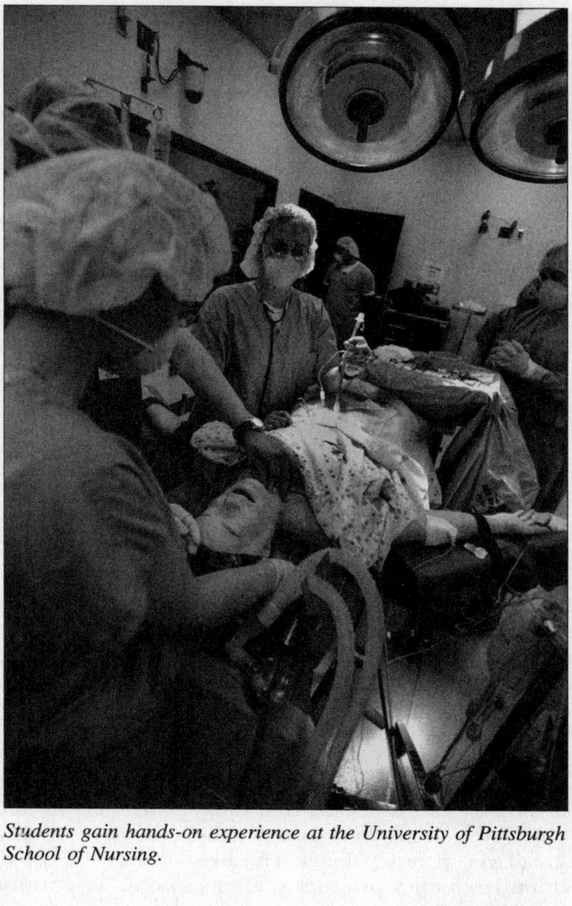

Students gain hands-on experience at the University of Pittsburgh School of Nursing.

University of St. Francis
College of Nursing and Allied Health
Joliet, Illinois

THE UNIVERSITY

The University of St. Francis (USF) is a national leader in offering educational opportunities to health-care professionals. Founded in 1920 by the Sisters of St. Francis of Mary Immaculate, the University's mission includes utilizing high-quality programming to address unmet educational needs.

More than 4,125 students are served in various graduate and undergraduate programs at locations throughout the nation, including nearly 1,500 students at the University's main campus in Joliet, Illinois.

The University of St. Francis faculty is committed to teaching. The University has 83 full-time faculty members, more than half of whom have terminal degrees. Sixty adjunct faculty members bring a variety of academic and professional experience to the classroom. Faculty advisers are an integral part of the USF experience.

USF faculty members are invested in the success of their students, both academically and personally. Nursing faculty members are strong clinicians. Their intense commitment to health care and to patients ensures that students are challenged academically while still offered a personal, caring support system.

About 85 percent of USF students find employment or enter graduate school within six months of graduation.

The University of St. Francis is fully accredited by the Higher Learning Commission and is a member of the North Central Association of Colleges and Schools (Web site: http://www.higherlearningcommission.org; telephone: 312-263-0456). The University also is accredited by the National League for Nursing Accrediting Commission (NLNAC).

THE COLLEGE OF NURSING AND ALLIED HEALTH

Founded in 1920, the University of St. Francis' College of Nursing and Allied Health has educated three generations of nurses, who are recognized throughout the regional health-care arena as exceptional clinicians and dedicated professionals.

The University promotes hands-on learning and partners with 133 health-care organizations to provide meaningful clinical experiences for its students. Supervisors at these organizations say that USF students are among the best prepared, most enthusiastic, and most inquiring of the nursing students with whom they work. The many areas of health care—hospitals, home health, managed care, primary-care clinics, public health, hospice care, long-term care, and mental health—are addressed in the curriculum and made available to students through clinical experiences. The nursing program focuses on the development of critical-thinking skills, cultural awareness, and patient advocacy as areas that help students excel in the dynamic health-care field.

USF is one of the few schools in the nation to provide its prenursing and premed students with the opportunity to regularly use state-of-the-art learning tools. These include A.D.A.M., revolutionary software that allows students to dissect a virtual cadaver in more detail. The new start of the art virtual simulation laboratory provides students with an opportunity to practice skills on mannequins in a safe environment.

The College of Nursing, in keeping with the University's Franciscan tradition, also subscribes to the values of respect, compassion, service, and integrity, believed to be essential to becoming a caring, effective health-care professional.

The passing rates of USF nursing graduates on the state licensure examination are above the national average pass rate. The NCLEX passing rate for the past academic year of nursing graduates was 91 percent.

PROGRAMS OF STUDY

The College of Nursing and Allied Health offers the Bachelor of Science in Nursing (B.S.N.) program in the traditional format for incoming freshmen and for transfer students and as a Fast Track option for registered nurses with an ADN or diploma. Course work may be available through traditional classroom study and online.

The four-year and transfer programs are based in a strong liberal arts component of general education that enhances the critical-thinking skills necessary for the scientific inquiry of nursing studies. Once in the nursing program, course work is intensive and focused. Students learn not only science and nursing proficiencies but also about themselves as people and caregivers.

The RN-B.S.N. Fast Track is an online program designed to provide an educational opportunity for registered nurses to obtain a baccalaureate degree in nursing. Students may attend full- or part-time. Advanced-placement credit is awarded upon submission of transcripts from an associate or diploma nursing program.

The Master of Science in Nursing (M.S.N.) program has two tracks of study: nurse practitioner and clinical nurse specialist, with concentrations in gerontology and/or nursing education. The nurse practitioner track at the Joliet campus prepares the student to provide primary health care in the community setting and in inpatient facilities. The Albuquerque, New Mexico, campus offers the family nurse practitioner program. Both campuses offer on-site and online courses. After completion of their studies, graduate students are eligible to take the adult, family, or gerontology nurse practitioner or the clinical nurse specialist national certification exam and apply for advanced practice licensure.

The Master of Science in physician assistant studies at the University of St. Francis is a nationally focused, graduate-level program in primary-care medicine. The program educates students to provide high-quality diagnostic and therapeutic medical services with physician supervision. Consistent with the mission of the University of St. Francis, physician assistant students are educated to provide health care to a variety of patient populations, with a special emphasis on the underserved. This program, located in Albuquerque, is a full-time, twenty-seven-month professional education program. The program consists of fifteen months of classroom and laboratory instruction followed by twelve months of supervised clinical rotations. Students must complete the entire twenty-seven-month program at the University of St. Francis. Upon successful completion of the program, students are awarded a Master of Science degree in physician assistant studies and are eligible to take the national certifying examination. This program has received probationary accreditation by ARC-PA.

The College of Nursing and Allied Health at USF also offers Bachelor of Science degrees in medical technology, nuclear medicine technology, radiography, and radiation therapy. USF is one of only two universities in Illinois that offers a B.S. degree in radiation therapy.

AFFILIATIONS WITH HEALTH-CARE FACILITIES
Key to students becoming exceptional, caring nurses are the hands-on learning experiences gained only through clinical settings. USF students may have clinical experiences with any of 208 health-care organizations. The University maintains working relationships with high-quality health-care organizations such as Hope Children's Hospital, Silver Cross Hospital, the Will County Health Department, Provena Saint Joseph Medical Center, and Saint James Hospital. The University's relationship with the nearby Provena Saint Joseph Medical Center offers educational opportunities rich in practical application.

Working relationships extend to the areas of hospitals, home health, managed care, primary clinics, public health, hospice care, long-term care (nursing homes), and public health. Students may even choose to learn about health care in other countries. One student recently studied the health-care system of Norway and spent a summer at the University of Oslo.

ACADEMIC FACILITIES
The College of Nursing and Allied Health is housed at the Provena Saint Joseph Medical Center complex, about 5 minutes from the Wilcox Street campus. The College of Nursing has classrooms, learning laboratories, a computer center, a library, a student lounge, and an auditorium.

In fall 2005, the College of Nursing and Allied Health is scheduled to be in state-of-the-art facilities in the newly renovated Motherhouse, built in 1881 by the University's founders.

The University of St. Francis also has a center in Albuquerque, where the physician assistant studies program and the Master of Science in Nursing family nurse practitioner program are offered.

LOCATION
The University of St. Francis campus is in a historic residential district known as Joliet's Cathedral area. The University is 35 miles southwest (about 45 minutes) of Chicago and is easily accessible by major roadways and trains. The University also offers classes at a variety of health-care facilities throughout the nation.

STUDENT SERVICES
The University of St. Francis is committed to educating students both in the classroom and through activities outside the classroom. A variety of student clubs and organizations are available as well as volunteer activities. Student Affairs sponsors many entertainment events as well as the Student Government Association. Cultural musical events, which bring internationally and nationally acclaimed performers to the University, are sponsored through the Featured Performances series. Exhibits that bring the works of regionally recognized artists to campus also are planned.

THE NURSING STUDENT GROUP
The University of St. Francis has 406 students in its nursing programs. Of the total, 68 are in the RN-B.S.N. Fast Track program, 371 are women, and 107 are members of minority groups. About 175 are part-time students. University of St. Francis nursing program graduates enjoy a 100 percent placement rate.

COSTS
Tuition and fees for full-time students are $17,670; room and board are $6180. Fast Track tuition is $380 per credit hour.

FINANCIAL AID
The University of St. Francis is committed to assisting students in obtaining a high-quality, private education. The University spent nearly $4 million in institutional aid and scholarships in addition to nearly $6 million in federal and state assistance to enable students to attend USF. In order to apply for all forms of federal, state, and USF assistance, students must complete a financial aid application form. USF prefers that students complete the Free Application for Federal Student Aid (FAFSA). M.S.N. students can apply for Advanced Nursing Education Traineeship funds awarded to the University. Several students have received scholarships from Johnson & Johnson's The Promise of Nursing Campaign.

APPLYING
Freshmen are admitted in the fall and spring. Students should take the ACT or SAT and visit the campus for an interview by April 1. Entrance exams should be taken in the spring of the junior year or the fall of the senior year in high school. Applications should be filed by August 15 for fall entry and December 1 for spring entry, along with high school transcripts and an application fee of $25. Notification is on a rolling basis.

Transfer students anticipating enrollment as nursing majors should submit applications for admission and have transcripts forwarded to the Admissions one year to one semester in advance of their projected entry semester.

RN-B.S.N. Fast Track and Master of Science in Nursing students should submit transcripts from previously attended schools. Physician assistant studies students should complete the admissions process through Central Application Service for Physician Assistants (CASPA) at http://www.caspaonline.org.

Informational packet requests may be obtained from the Admissions Office via e-mail.

CORRESPONDENCE AND INFORMATION
University of St. Francis
500 Wilcox Street
Joliet, Illinois 60435
Telephone: 815-740-5037
800-735-7500 (toll-free)
E-mail: admissions@stfrancis.edu
World Wide Web: http://www.stfrancis.edu

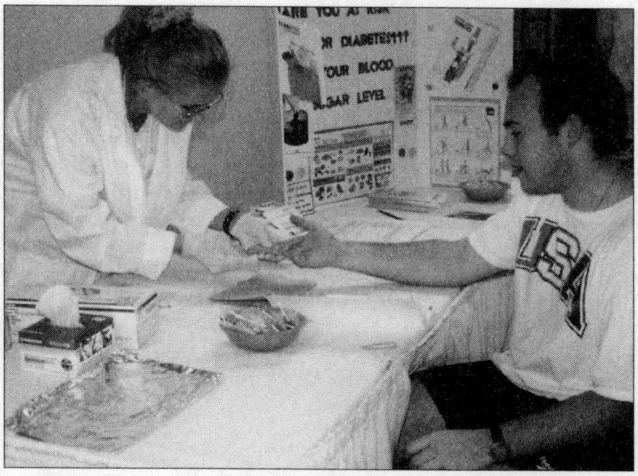

To gain practical experience and as part of their community health outreach, nursing students conduct two health fairs each year.

University of San Diego
Hahn School of Nursing and Health Science
San Diego, California

THE UNIVERSITY

The University of San Diego (USD) is an independent, Roman Catholic university founded in 1949. With a holistic philosophy, USD seeks to foster competence, international and cultural sensitivity, professional responsibility, and a spirit of volunteerism in each student. The University places a special emphasis on the exploration of human values and welcomes non-Catholics as well as Catholic students and faculty members.

The 180-acre hilltop campus, known for its Spanish Renaissance architecture, overlooks Mission Bay with breathtaking views of the Pacific Ocean and San Diego Bay. USD's central location offers students easy access to the San Diego area.

The University comprises five academic units: the College of Arts and Sciences and the Schools of Business Administration, Education, Law, and Nursing. Total enrollment in the fall 2004 semester was 7,486 (4,908 undergraduates, 1,114 law students, and 1,548 graduate students).

THE SCHOOL OF NURSING AND HEALTH SCIENCE

Founded in 1974 through an endowment by the late Philip Y. Hahn, the School of Nursing and Health Science was established to offer the Bachelor of Science in Nursing (B.S.N.) for registered nurses. Following the graduation of the first class in 1976, the Master of Science in Nursing (M.S.N.) program was established. The B.S.N. and M.S.N. programs are accredited by the Commission on Collegiate Nursing Education. The Doctor of Nursing Science (D.N.Sc.) program was approved in 1985, and the first D.N.Sc. degree was awarded in May 1989. In December 1998, the Board of Trustees approved the change of the doctoral program from D.N.Sc. to Ph.D.

The mission of the Hahn School of Nursing and Health Science is to be at the forefront of the discipline of nursing by providing excellence in the quality of the School's baccalaureate and graduate programs through its teaching, by strengthening the knowledge base for nursing practice through research, and by providing leadership for the discipline through its faculty members and graduates.

All of the School's full-time, tenure-track faculty members are doctorally prepared. Part-time faculty members hold at least a master's degree in their clinical specialty area. The School also has the services of a rich cadre of clinical, administrative, and educational preceptors.

The School is centrally located and occupies a beautifully appointed building constructed in 1978 through federal funds and matching funds from Murial Hahn, the widow of Philip Y. Hahn. The youngest and smallest of the five academic units of the University, the School of Nursing and Health Science offers educational programs at the undergraduate, master's, and doctoral levels.

PROGRAMS OF STUDY

The Hahn School of Nursing and Health Science offers the B.S.N. for RNs, the Accelerated RN to M.S.N., the Master's Entry Program in Nursing (for non-RNs), the M.S.N., a joint M.B.A./ M.S.N. with the School of Business Administration, and the Ph.D. Post-M.S.N. Adult, Family, and Pediatric Nurse Practitioner Certificates; an Adult Clinical Nurse Specialist Certificate; and a Health Care Systems Certificate are also offered.

The B.S.N. program, with an upper-division major in nursing, is structured for graduates of hospital diploma and associate degree programs who have met the specified prerequisite admission requirements.

The M.S.N. program is built upon the baccalaureate degree in nursing and emphasizes research, theory, and practice. The M.S.N. program prepares adult nurse practitioners with an option in gerontology, family nurse practitioners, pediatric nurse practitioners, adult clinical nurse specialists, and nurse administrators for leadership and managerial roles in client-care services administration in health-care organizations. A Latino health-care option and an integrative health-care option are available within the adult, family, and pediatric nurse practitioner tracks. Each of the tracks shares a common core of knowledge and is designed to prepare an advanced practice nurse in the respective area.

The Accelerated RN to M.S.N. program is designed for nurses holding a diploma or an associate degree who want to pursue the M.S.N. degree. The program of study leads to the awarding of the B.S.N. degree and eligibility for certification as a public health nurse in the state of California, as well as the M.S.N. degree. The program offers the same specialty options as the M.S.N.

The Master's Entry Program in Nursing (MEPN) is intended for individuals with a baccalaureate in another discipline. The program is designed for the person seeking a new career in nursing. The first year of the three-year MEPN program provides the student with the general foundation in nursing. The remaining two years of the program are spent preparing the graduate student for a master's degree in a specialty area. The program of study leads to the awarding of the M.S.N. degree and offers the same specialty options as the M.S.N. program.

The Ph.D. program is designed to prepare nurse scholars who will advance knowledge in the discipline through the extension of the theoretical base of nursing and the application of knowledge to professional practice. The program provides learning opportunities that emphasize theory development, research, and leadership ability in response to social, political, and ethical issues in global health care.

AFFILIATIONS WITH HEALTH-CARE FACILITIES

The School is affiliated with a wide variety of clinical resources, including UCSD Medical Center, Sharp Health Care (Hospitals and Clinics), Scripps Health (Hospitals and Clinics), Children's Hospital, Veterans Administration Hospital, Kaiser Permanente, and Balboa Naval Hospital. Because of its focus on health promotion, a large number of community agencies are utilized, including schools, home health agencies, the San Diego Department of Health Services, HMOs, and community clinics.

ACADEMIC FACILITIES

The University provides students access to state-of-the-art computer laboratories and the Helen K. and James C. Copley Library, which houses 450,000 volumes, 351,000 titles, and 2,200 print periodicals subscriptions and access to about 18,000 current periodicals in electronic form, including a well-serviced health sciences collection. Students and faculty members have access to the School of Law Legal Research Center as well as additional resources in area medical and health sciences libraries. The San Diego Library Circuit, a collaborative effort among San Diego State University; the University of California,

San Diego; California State University, San Marcos; and the University of San Diego, allows access to an additional 2 million titles. The Media Center, a division of Copley Library, supports the instructional function of the University by providing nonprint information services such as videotapes and audiotapes.

The Hahn School of Nursing and Health Science houses its own Computer Lab and Learning Resource Center. The Computer Lab provides students with an up-to-date lab that is equipped with fifteen computer stations. The Learning Resource Center is provided for the student to listen to and view selected instructional media such as videotapes, audiotapes, and sound/slide presentations. The center also produces audiovisual software and overhead transparencies for faculty and student use.

LOCATION

Located on the southern tip of California, San Diego offers a wide variety of recreational, business, science, art, and cultural activities. With an average temperature of 64 degrees in February and 76 degrees in August, the area is perfect for biking, jogging, tennis, softball, and all aquatic sports. San Diego is also noted for a world-famous zoo, museums, Spanish missions, Sea World, and major sports programs. The proximity to Mexico provides an excellent opportunity for gaining firsthand insights into Mexican culture. The International Airport, downtown, Mission Bay, and the Aquatic Center are just a few minutes from the campus.

STUDENT SERVICES

The University has many resources and services designed to meet student needs. These include the Manchester Family Child Development Center (child care and development), Health Center, Sports and Recreation Center, bookstore, post office, Academic Computing Services, Campus Ministry, housing, dining services, and the Hahn University Center and its facilities, including the Multicultural Center. The International Resource Center and International Student Association offer personal and academic advising and activities.

THE NURSING STUDENT GROUP

All students in the Hahn School of Nursing and Health Science, except the students in the first year of the MEPN program, are registered nurses and most are practicing, at least part-time. Depending on their experience and the level of program being pursued, students are employed in positions as varied as beginning-level practitioner to nurse educator to middle- or top-level health-care administrator.

COSTS

Tuition costs for the 2004–05 academic year were $920 per unit for the B.S.N., $905 per unit for the M.S.N., and $920 per unit for the doctoral program. Since all students are registered nurses, they seldom live in campus housing. However, living expenses, including room and board, transportation, and personal expenses, are estimated at approximately $10,500. Other educational expenses, including books, immunizations, instruments, insurance, travel to clinical sites, and student fees, total approximately $5000.

FINANCIAL AID

The primary purpose of the financial aid program at USD is to provide financial assistance to students who, without such aid, would be unable to attend the University. Financial need is met by a combination of scholarships, grants, graduate fellowships, loans, and graduate assistantships. Federal Graduate Nurse Traineeships are offered through the School.

APPLYING

Applicants to all nursing degree programs, except the Master's Entry Program, must have California nursing licensure as an RN and professional liability and malpractice insurance. The B.S.N., Accelerated RN to M.S.N., and MEPN programs require completion of all nursing program prerequisites prior to admission and a GPA of 3.0 on a 4.0 scale. The master's and post-master's programs further require a B.S.N. or an M.S.N., respectively, from an approved, accredited institution; a minimum GPA of 3.0 on a 4.0 scale; a 3-unit course in statistics; and one to two years of professional nursing practice is preferred. Additional requirements for the doctoral program include a minimum of one year's experience in clinical nursing beyond the B.S.N. and a minimum graduate school GPA of 3.5 on a 4.0 scale. Applicants with non-nursing baccalaureate or master's degrees may be considered for admission to the M.S.N. and Ph.D. programs, respectively. All applicants must show proof of required immunizations and screening tests, including a recent physical examination. Students should contact the appropriate office at the University for complete information about admission requirements and application deadlines.

CORRESPONDENCE AND INFORMATION

Office of Undergraduate Admissions
University of San Diego
5998 Alcala Park
San Diego, California 92110-2492
Telephone: 619-260-4506
Fax: 619-260-6836

Office of Graduate Admissions
University of San Diego
5998 Alcala Park
San Diego, California 92110-2492
Telephone: 619-260-4524
Fax: 619-260-4158
World Wide Web: http://www.sandiego.edu/academics/nursing

THE FACULTY

Cheryl Ahern-Lehmann, Associate Clinical Professor; Ph.D., Claremont and San Diego State; RN.
Mary Jo Clark, Professor; M.S.N., Texas Woman's; Ph.D., Texas at Austin; RN.
Cynthia A. Connelly, Associate Professor; M.S.N., San Diego; Ph.D., Rhode Island; RN.
Jane M. Georges, Associate Professor; M.S.N., California, San Francisco; Ph.D., Washington (Seattle); RN.
Sally B. Hardin, Professor and Dean; M.S.N., Illinois at Chicago; Ph.D., Illinois at Urbana-Champaign; RN.
Diane C. Hatton, Professor; D.N.Sc., California, San Francisco; RN.
Anita J. Hunter, Associate Professor; Ph.D., Connecticut; RN.
Susan Instone, Associate Professor; D.N.Sc., San Diego; RN.
Kathleen S. James, Associate Professor; D.N.Sc., San Diego; RN.
Young-Shin Lee, Assistant Professor; M.S.N., Seoul National; Ph.D., Texas at Austin; RN.
Sharon McGuire, Assistant Professor; M.S.N., Miami; Ph.D., San Diego; O.P., RN.
Mary-Rose Mueller, Associate Professor; M.S.N., San Diego; Ph.D., California, San Diego; RN.
Allen J. Orsi, Associate Professor; M.S.N., Columbia; Ph.D., Pennsylvania; RN.
Patricia Quinn, Instructor; M.S., California, San Francisco; RN.
Linda Robinson, Associate Professor; Ph.D., Pennsylvania; RN.
Patricia Roth, Professor; M.S.N., Arizona; Ed.D., USC; RN.
Nancy Jex Sabin, Instructor; M.S., California, San Francisco; RN.
Vince Salyers, Assistant Professor; M.S.N., San Francisco State; Ed.D., San Francisco; RN.

University of Southern Indiana
School of Nursing and Health Professions
Evansville, Indiana

THE UNIVERSITY
The University of Southern Indiana (USI), established in 1965, is a comprehensive public university offering undergraduate and graduate degrees. The University is composed of five schools—the Schools of Nursing and Health Professions, Science and Engineering, Business, Education and Human Services, and Liberal Arts.

The University of Southern Indiana has a strong tradition of commitment to education excellence. In 1996, the University and the School of Nursing began offering Internet-based courses and programs for students. Undergraduate programs in nursing, health services, and imaging sciences and graduate programs in nursing, health administration, and occupational therapy are available online from the School of Nursing and Health Professions.

On-campus facilities include a student health center, a bookstore, athletic facilities, a computer center, and a comprehensive library that provides online reference materials.

THE SCHOOL OF NURSING AND HEALTH PROFESSIONS
The School of Nursing and Health Professions was founded in 1988 as the first state-supported baccalaureate nursing program in southern Indiana. In 1996, the School initiated a master's degree program in nursing. The School also offers a post-master's nurse practitioner certificate program as well as other programs designed to meet the needs of practicing nurses in today's health-care environment.

Recognizing the complexity of health care, the School has developed an undergraduate and graduate nursing curriculum designed to prepare students efficiently and expertly. This curriculum emphasizes clinical nursing competence and uses a wide array of learning resources. Faculty members have expertise and strong clinical practice backgrounds in their areas of teaching.

The School of Nursing and Health Professions has taken a lead role in the development of distance education courses and programs. The RN-B.S.N., RN-M.S.N., and M.S.N. nursing programs may be completed through the Internet. In addition to these nursing programs, the School of Nursing and Health Professions offers online programs in health services, health administration, and radiologic and imaging sciences. Additional information may be obtained through the School's Web site at http://health.usi.edu.

PROGRAMS OF STUDY
The baccalaureate nursing program is designed to prepare the professional nurse to plan, implement, and evaluate health care for individuals, families, and groups in institutional and community settings. The undergraduate nursing program is based on a planned progression of courses arranged to build upon previous knowledge and to develop skills and performance at an increasing level of competence. Students are required to complete 128 credits to receive the degree, including the University core curriculum courses supportive to the nursing major and 70 hours of nursing courses. Students enrolled in the baccalaureate program may elect to sit for the registered nurse licensure exam at the end of the third year of the program. The student is then awarded an associate degree and may complete the fourth year of nursing courses on a part-time or full-time basis.

The second degree accelerated B.S.N. program is designed for students who already hold a baccalaureate degree in another discipline. Once the prerequisite courses—Chemistry, Anatomy and Physiology, Microbiology, Nutrition, and Statistics—are completed, the student enrolls in nursing courses and completes the baccalaureate degree in nursing in sixteen months.

Registered nurses with an associate degree or diploma are provided the opportunity to obtain a baccalaureate degree in nursing through the RN-B.S.N. completion option. The nursing courses required for this option are provided online. The flexibility of the RN-B.S.N. option provides nurses with the opportunity to complete the course requirements in their own home and on their own schedule with reasonable costs. The RN-B.S.N. curriculum is built upon a foundation of biological, physical, and social sciences and acknowledgment of previously learned nursing content. No further testing of prior knowledge is required for nurses who hold a valid RN license and are in good standing in their current employment position.

The RN-M.S.N. program is designed for registered nurses with an associate degree or diploma who are interested in graduate nursing education and preparation for an advanced practice nursing role. The program builds on a student's prior learning and requires three years of practice experience as a registered nurse. Students, in consultation with a faculty adviser, develop a plan of study that is based on prior learning and the student's selected graduate study major. After successful completion of University core courses, 13–14 hours of undergraduate nursing courses, and successful completion of 12 hours of graduate course credits, a Bachelor of Science in Nursing degree is awarded. At this point in their program of study, students are granted full admission into the graduate program. After successful completion of the remaining required graduate nursing courses, students are awarded an M.S.N.degree.

The Master of Science in Nursing is offered for nurses seeking advanced education in professional nursing. The graduate program prepares nurses for advanced practice as acute care nurse practitioners, clinical nurse specialists, family nurse practitioners, nurse educators, and nurse managers/leaders. The graduate degree is awarded upon the completion of 39 to 42 credits, dependent upon the focus of graduate nursing education. Post-master's certificate programs are available for clinical nurse specialist, nurse practitioner, nursing managers/leaders, and nursing education.

The baccalaureate and graduate nursing programs are accredited by the Commission on Collegiate Nursing Education. The 24 members of the nursing faculty represent diverse areas of teaching and research.

AFFILIATIONS WITH HEALTH-CARE FACILITIES
The School of Nursing and Health Professions is affiliated with a variety of clinical resources, including hospitals, community agencies, physician practice groups, HMOs, schools, clinics, home health agencies, senior centers, and day-care centers that are used throughout the program of study. Written agreements are established with health-care facilities located conveniently from a student's home community.

ACADEMIC FACILITIES

The David L. Rice Library houses about 341,000 volumes, 7,800 listening and viewing materials, and 600,000 items in microformat and subscribes to 41 electronic online databases with more than 12,000 full-text online journals. The library is fully automated for literature searches and online full-text journal searches. More than 1,100 online nursing and health-care journals are available for enrolled students.

The Computer Center has campus labs throughout the University. A variety of color graphics, database management systems, simulations, and models software is available for students.

The Charles E. Day Learning Resource Center, located in the School of Nursing and Health Professions, includes a learning laboratory with the latest technology. The learning laboratory simulates the hospital and home settings with appropriate and supportive models and supplies.

LOCATION

Evansville, Indiana, with a population of approximately 135,000, is a unique city. It is big enough to provide metropolitan amenities but small enough to have small-town charm and hospitality. Located at a horseshoe bend on the Ohio River, Evansville has a long and colorful history. The campus is conveniently located 7 miles from downtown Evansville.

STUDENT LIFE

A wide variety of organizations and activities contribute to the total education of the on-campus student. More than eighty student organizations provide activities that include student government, leadership academy, career organizations, multicultural center, athletics, student publications, and a student-operated radio station.

Two nursing organizations include the USI Association of Nursing Students and the Omicron Psi chapter of Sigma Theta Tau, International Nursing Honor Society. Both organizations provide students with the opportunity to develop leadership skills; to participate in local, regional, and national nursing forums; and to work collaboratively with nursing school faculty members.

THE NURSING STUDENT GROUP

In fall 2004, the School of Nursing enrolled more than 400 undergraduate and 200 graduate nursing students. The diversity of the nursing student population is representative of the general population of its geographic area.

COSTS

In 2004–05, undergraduate tuition for in-state students was $135 per credit hour or $2050 per semester for full-time study (15 hours). For graduate students, in-state tuition was $195 per credit or $1750 per semester for full-time study (9 hours). University fees were $90 per semester. Other fees and housing costs are determined on an individual basis.

FINANCIAL AID

USI offers a wide variety of financial assistance programs through various federal and state programs. Several scholarships are also offered through contributions made to the School by alumni and patrons. The amounts and types of financial assistance that a student receives are determined by the eligibility of the applicant for each program.

APPLYING

Applicants for the B.S.N. program must first be admitted to the University. A second application is then submitted to the nursing program. Students must have a high school GPA of at least 3.0 (on a 4.0 scale) and must have a minimum SAT (or comparable standardized exam) score of 1000. High school chemistry and biology are recommended. Transfer applicants must have a minimum GPA of 2.7. The acceptable grade in science courses is a C or better. Applicants for the second degree accelerated B.S.N. program must have a minimum 3.0 GPA on a 4.0 scale in their previous degree, a 2.7 or better GPA in the prerequisite courses, and complete an on-site interview and writing requirement.

RN-B.S.N. applicants must hold a current registered nurse license in one of the fifty states or territories, meet general University requirements for admission, and have graduated from an accredited nursing program with a minimum GPA of 2.5.

RN-M.S.N. applicants must have three years experience as a registered nurse, hold a current, unencumbered RN license, and must have a minimum GPA of 3.0.

Applicants to the master's and post-master's degree programs are required to have a current license as a registered nurse in one of the fifty states or territories, hold an earned B.S. or M.S. degree in nursing from an accredited school, have a minimum GPA of 3.0, have practiced as an RN for 2,000 hours within the last five years, and provide letters of reference.

Admission and enrollment services are available online at the Web site listed.

CORRESPONDENCE AND INFORMATION

Deborah Bookout
Student Advising Coordinator
University of Southern Indiana
School of Nursing and Health Professions
8600 University Boulevard
Evansville, Indiana 47712
Telephone: 812-465-1150
E-mail: dbookout@usi.edu
World Wide Web: http://health.usi.edu

The University of Tampa
Department of Nursing
Tampa, Florida

THE UNIVERSITY

The University of Tampa (UT), founded in 1931, is a medium-sized, residential, private university that integrates the richness of the liberal arts tradition with twenty-first-century technology and innovative teaching strategies. The College of Liberal Arts and Sciences and the College of Business offer more than sixty-five fields of undergraduate study and preprofessional programs. Graduate programs in business and nursing and an Evening College complement the curriculum.

The 190 full-time faculty members include distinguished scholars, authors, artists, and educators who promote student- and community-responsive learning opportunities. The 5,000 currently enrolled students experience classes in small, personalized settings that balance "learning by thinking" with "learning by doing."

In an innovative first-year program, students explore global issues and cultures, examine career possibilities, and refine their critical-thinking and communication skills. Students, representing fifty states and territories and nearly 100 countries, find their academic experience at UT to be an enriching one that encourages a global perspective, provides opportunities to apply their skills and knowledge throughout the curriculum, and prepares them for future career challenges. For qualifying students, the Honors Program offers expanded opportunities for instruction, internships, and study abroad.

Eighty percent of UT's eight residence halls are new within the past six years, and 70 percent of all full-time students live on campus. The new Vaughn Center and residence hall complex serves as the new hub of campus life.

UT has one of the nation's best NCAA Division II sports programs. Spartan athletes compete on fourteen men's and women's varsity teams. The swimming pool, tennis courts, jogging track, outdoor volleyball and basketball courts, crew training facility, and modern fitness center are enjoyed by all, making sunshine, sports, and fitness hallmarks of the UT experience.

The University of Tampa is accredited by the Southern Association of Colleges and Schools to award associate, baccalaureate, and master's degrees. In addition, the University is accredited for teacher education by the Florida State Board of Education. The Florida State Approving Agency for Veterans' Training recognizes the University with approval for veterans' educational benefits. The University is an associate member of the European Council of International Schools (ECIS), a European accrediting association. All nursing programs are accredited by the National League for Nursing Accrediting Commission (NLNAC), and the University is a member of the American Association of Colleges of Nursing and the National Organization of Nurse Practitioner Faculties.

THE DEPARTMENT OF NURSING

The Department of Nursing admitted its first class in 1981 and graduated its charter class in 1984. The B.S.N. completion program gained accreditation from the National League for Nursing Accrediting Commission (NLNAC) in 1986. The Master of Science in Nursing (M.S.N.) degree program was awarded NLNAC accreditation in 1998. Master's degree options include family and adult nurse practitioner studies and nursing education. Post-master's certificates may be earned in each of these concentrations.

PROGRAMS OF STUDY

In 2002, UT began a traditional four-year Bachelor of Science in Nursing (B.S.N.) program (accredited by the NLNAC in 2003), helping to round out a slate of offerings that already included RN to B.S.N. completion and RN/B.S.N./M.S.N. tracks. The RN to B.S.N. program allows RN graduates of diploma and associate degree programs to complete the B.S.N. degree, and it provides a foundation for graduate education. RNs with associate degrees who seek a Master of Science in Nursing (M.S.N.) degree enroll in the RN to B.S.N./M.S.N. option, enabling the qualified RN to complete both the B.S.N. and M.S.N. degrees more rapidly than in traditional programs. In this option, when required undergraduate courses are completed, students are awarded the B.S.N. Certain undergraduate courses are then replaced by graduate-level courses.

The master's degree program offers family nurse practitioner and adult nurse practitioner concentrations. UT's newest graduate nursing concentration, nursing education, responds to the critical shortage of nurse educators throughout the nation. It is the only nursing education program in west central Florida.

Many nurses seeking graduate degrees choose one of the nurse practitioner concentrations because of the opportunity to impact patient care decisions and health-care policy with greater autonomy. UT's nursing education concentration is poised to add significantly to the number of nurse educators who will have positive effects on the nursing shortage.

All of these programs recognize that nursing is a very different career than it was prior to the explosion of new information, new technology, new pharmacology, and the demands of a burgeoning health-care consumer population. Along with judgment and critical thinking, UT's nursing programs prepare graduates who are superbly educated, empowered, ethical, and politically articulate. Nurses are educated to have authority—not only when they occupy high-level positions, but at the bedside.

AFFILIATIONS WITH HEALTH-CARE FACILITIES

In keeping with the University's commitment to hands-on, real-world learning, UT's nursing programs enjoy affiliations with more than 120 Tampa Bay–area clinical facilities. There are twenty-five hospitals and nearly 1,000 doctor's offices in Hillsborough County alone. Tampa General Hospital, an 877-bed acute-care facility and level one trauma center, has established a partnership with UT that has enabled the implementation of the new four-year B.S.N. program. A $700,000 state-of-the-art clinical laboratory utilizing computer-generated simulations as well as simulated human models is available for UT nursing students at Tampa General Hospital. This laboratory provides students with opportunities to learn and practice their nursing skills with the latest technology available.

The Tampa Bay area is rich in clinical experience opportunities. Specialty facilities and expert health-care professionals enrich the education of UT nursing students through their willingness to precept, mentor, and teach in the University's programs. Myriad opportunities for challenging positions in all aspects of health await those graduates who choose to remain in Florida following graduation.

ACADEMIC FACILITIES

For nursing and all students, the Macdonald-Kelce Library is well-equipped to meet the diversified needs of college students. It has more than 250,000 bound volumes and some 1,600 periodicals. In addition, the library is a member of the Tampa Bay Library Consortium, which provides delivery of books and research materials from a variety of member libraries. UTOPIA, an electronic online catalog, allows patrons to search other libraries and databases, check the status of their accounts, and even read government documents. Students can access UTOPIA from home, residence hall, or office or anywhere an online computer can be found.

Many of UT's classrooms are tech supported, but the Computer Resources Center is the technological center of the University. It offers hands-on experience in a laboratory environment, combining practical application with theoretical instruction. The entire campus is linked by a high-speed campus computer network, and all members of the UT community have free Internet access and e-mail. All students in every residence hall have their own computer jacks, and they may use one of the many computer labs located in convenient areas on campus.

LOCATION

Surrounding the UT campus is Tampa, a vibrant, ethnically and culturally diverse, modern city located on the west central coast of Florida. Once a sleepy southern town, Tampa's boom began in the 1950s and continues unabated in the 2000s. An imposing skyline continues to burst into bloom over a cityscape that was almost entirely flat just two decades ago. Tampa is just an hour west of Orlando's Disney attractions and 30 minutes from beautiful gulf beaches.

A million residents now inhabit the city and surrounding Hillsborough County, with more than 2 million in the four-county Tampa–St. Petersburg–Clearwater metroplex (commonly referred to simply as "Tampa Bay") and 4 million in the eleven-county region. Tampa is the educational, medical, cultural, economic, business, shipping, entertainment, and legal center of it all, and the community is involved with its premier private university. More than 700 Tampa Bay community leaders serve on University boards and advisory groups.

STUDENT SERVICES

Leadership opportunities abound in an atmosphere of individual discovery and development fostered by the University's active campus life, including Greek life, more than 110 student clubs and organizations, and service learning opportunities. A cocurricular transcript option gives UT graduates a resume-enhancing edge with prospective employers and graduate schools. Professionals in the Academic Center for Excellence (ACE), the Saunders Writing Center, and the Academic Advising and Career Services offices help students stay on track academically.

THE NURSING STUDENT GROUP

There are 195 students currently enrolled in UT nursing programs: 50 in the B.S.N. completion program, 100 in the M.S.N. and postgraduate certificate programs, and 45 in the Department's four-year B.S.N program. The B.S.N. completion and graduate programs are designed for adult learners who attend part-time, primarily in the evenings, the majority already working in various health-care settings in the Tampa Bay community. Applying from many parts of the country, most four-year students are residential and attend full-time during the day. Because of the critical shortage of nurses to serve a growing population of acutely ill and elderly patients, many graduates select employment in Florida, where they receive excellent salaries and benefits.

COSTS

Undergraduate tuition and fee costs for the 2004–05 academic year are $18,172 for full-time study. Room and board charges average $6670 for a double room for the academic year. Graduate tuition (for graduate-level courses only) is $390 per credit hour. Additional fees for books, supplies, lab fees, etc., also apply, and vary by semester.

FINANCIAL AID

Special Florida and federal financial aid incentives are in place to encourage students to pursue nursing degrees. UT awards institutional financial aid based on merit and need to full-time undergraduate students. Some graduate assistantships and federal traineeships are awarded to M.S.N. students each year. Students are encouraged to explore outside funding sources such as employers and health-related agencies. All students pursuing at least half-time study are eligible for loans. Information on financial assistance is available online at http://www.ut.edu or by calling the Financial Aid Office at 813-253-6219.

APPLYING

Admission application forms are available on the University's Web site for downloading or completion online. Applications for admission to the RN to B.S.N. and M.S.N. programs are evaluated on a rolling basis, and students may enter in the fall, spring, or summer terms.

Undergraduate students apply to the four-year baccalaureate nursing program by first applying to the University, completing the regular UT undergraduate admissions application. Official transcripts from all schools attended, SAT or ACT scores, an essay, and a recommendation from a guidance counselor or teacher are required. Acceptance to the University does not constitute admission to the nursing program. Separate application is made to the nursing program once pre-nursing requirements (28 credits) have been met. Meeting minimal requirements does not guarantee admission to this high-demand, limited-enrollment program. Four-year B.S.N. students are admitted to the nursing program each spring for the fall term only.

Admission to the RN to B.S.N. program requires the applicant to be currently licensed in Florida as a registered nurse. Applicants who provide proof of eligibility for licensure may attend the first semester, but they must have obtained a Florida RN license by the end of that semester to continue in the program. Applicants to this program must also provide official transcripts from each college attended. Special admission applications are required for the M.S.N. program. Admission to the M.S.N. program requires current Florida licensure as an RN, a GPA of 3.0 or higher in the last 60 credit hours of college/university courses, a computer course, and successful completion of the GRE. Two professional letters of reference, a resume, and a personal statement about the decision to pursue graduate work and career goals are also required. Applicants with baccalaureate degrees in a discipline other than nursing may enroll in the pre-M.S.N. program to complete additional course work prior to full admission to the M.S.N. degree program.

CORRESPONDENCE AND INFORMATION:

Admissions Office
University of Tampa
401 West Kennedy Boulevard
Tampa, Florida 33606
Telephone: 813-253-6273
Fax: 813-258-7398
E-mail: nursing@ut.edu
World Wide Web: http://www.ut.edu

University of Wisconsin–Madison
School of Nursing
Madison, Wisconsin

SCHOOL OF NURSING
University of Wisconsin-Madison

THE UNIVERSITY

In achievement and prestige, the University of Wisconsin–Madison (UW–Madison) has long been recognized as one of America's great universities. Founded in 1849, it is today one of the nation's largest public land-grant institutions, with an international reputation as a leading teaching and research university. As stated in the *Vision for the Future,* the University's mission is "to create, integrate, transfer and apply knowledge." The University offers a complete spectrum of liberal arts studies, professional programs, and student activities. With more than 40,000 students, the student body is diverse and cosmopolitan.

THE SCHOOL OF NURSING

The School of Nursing has had a strong commitment to enhancing health care since its beginning in 1924. Consistently ranked among top nursing schools for graduate education and research, the School is an integral part of the UW–Madison health sciences complex. Members of the faculty are academically well prepared and recognized as scholars, researchers, expert clinicians and teachers, and leaders in the profession.

The School offers a Bachelor of Science degree in nursing, a Master of Science degree and a Doctor of Philosophy degree with a major in nursing, and opportunities for postdoctoral research. In fall 2004, the School enrolled 271 students in the baccalaureate nursing major, 53 returning RN students, 129 students in the M.S. program, 3 students in post-master's nurse practitioner options, and 40 students in the Ph.D. and postdoctoral programs.

PROGRAMS OF STUDY

The Bachelor of Science program prepares individuals for entry-level professional practice and provides a basis for leadership roles and graduate study. The 124-credit curriculum comprises course work in general education, nursing practice, and electives. Students are admitted to the nursing major in the junior year. An Honors Program is offered, providing opportunities for high-ability students who seek greater depth and challenge in their educational experience. Students have the opportunity to complete the nursing component of the program either at the UW–Madison campus or the Western Campus for Nursing located at Gundersen Lutheran Medical Center in LaCrosse, Wisconsin. An Early Entry Ph.D. option is designed for undergraduaute students who are interested in research careers in nursing.

The Collaborative Nursing Program (CNP), of which the UW–Madison School of Nursing is a partner, is offered for registered nurse students seeking a baccalaureate degree. The program is offered to Wisconsin residents via the Internet and the combined resources of five University of Wisconsin System nursing schools.

An RN/B.S./M.S. accelerated track is offered for registered nurses who are highly motivated, who have a high level of academic achievement, and whose educational goal is a master's or a doctoral education. The faculty recognizes that RN students have acquired considerable knowledge and clinical competency through previous education and professional employment and is committed to assisting them in meeting their career goals.

The purpose of the Master of Science degree program is to prepare nurses for leadership roles in advanced clinical practice and education or to provide a basis for further research preparation. A minimum of 36 graduate credits is required, although many of the program options require additional credits in order to meet national credentialing requirements. The master's curriculum is reflective of faculty expertise and scholarship, as well as the standards and guidelines of the profession, and is designed to maintain a high standard of scholarship and prepare individuals with in-depth knowledge and experience in their selected areas of practice. Students select both a clinical and a functional role focus. Clinical population options are adult health and illness, geriatric, medical-surgical, pediatric, psychiatric–mental health, and women's health nursing. The nurse practitioner options include acute care, adult, geriatric, pediatric, psychiatric mental health, and women's health. New program initiatives include the NET option (an online sequence that prepares nurse educators for tomorrow) and a dual-degree M.S./M.P.H. program. Program graduates are eligible for national certification and reimbursable professional practice. In Wisconsin, graduates can apply to become Advanced Practice Nurse Prescribers. Students and alumni consistently evaluate the master's program as strong, and graduates have been highly successful in attaining professional certification and finding positions.

Established in 1984, the Ph.D. program in nursing is characterized by an early and continuous training in research, a strong scientific base in nursing, and a minor in a related discipline. The purpose of the program is to prepare nurses to assume major roles in the development, evaluation, and dissemination of knowledge about phenomena of interest in nursing. Graduates become the scholars and teachers who move the nursing profession forward through systematic inquiry into nursing issues. The curriculum leading to the doctorate includes seven components: existing and evolving knowledge in nursing, methods of nursing inquiry, research ethics, nursing doctoral seminars, course work in a minor field, teaching and learning, and research/dissertation credits. Graduates of the program have assumed faculty positions at major universities in the United States, Canada, and many other countries and have been awarded postdoctoral fellowships to further their research. Doctoral and postdoctoral funding is available as part of an NINR-funded training program in patient-centered interventions. The Bolliger Post Doctoral Fellowship provides funding for nurse researchers to work on their individual research under the direction of a senior faculty member in the School of Nursing.

AFFILIATIONS WITH HEALTH-CARE FACILITIES

Faculty and staff members maintain affiliations with many health, education, and social service agencies throughout urban and rural Wisconsin, including the Wisconsin Department of Health and Family Services and many public health deparments, schools, and hospitals. The School is especially committed to performing research and providing student clinical experiences in health professional shortage areas, as exemplified by participation in the Area Health Education Centers (AHEC) of Wisconsin.

ACADEMIC FACILITIES

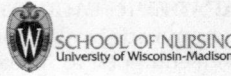

A new Health Sciences Learning Center provides the Schools of Medicine, Nursing, and Pharmacy with state-of-the-art classrooms, computer resources, and distance education facilities as well as a comprehensive health sciences library. Educational resources for both on-campus and distance students include online access to library journals, Web-based course materials, and videoconferencing technologies. Collaborative arrangements with a number of campus departments expand the practice, education, and research experiences open to students.

LOCATION

Madison, situated on an isthmus between Lakes Mendota and Monona, is a midsize city with a population of about 225,000, known for its natural beauty. With its good economy, low crime rate, and abundance of cultural and recreational activities, Madison ranks consistently among the top cities in the country. Its central location, 90 miles from Milwaukee, 120 miles from Chicago, and 250 miles from Minneapolis, places it within easy driving distance of these major metropolitan areas.

STUDENT SERVICES

Advisers are available in the B.S. program to help students interpret curriculum and academic requirements and plan a balanced program. They also assist with academic problems and acquaint students with campus resources. At the graduate level, students may select, or are assigned, a faculty adviser with whom they plan their program of study. A writing course is taught in the School for graduate students. The School's multicultural affairs coordinator provides specialized assistance as needed and refers students to campus and community resources. The campus offers a wide variety of support services for students, including the International Student Services Office, the McBurney Disability Resource Center, the Multicultural Student Center, and many others.

THE NURSING STUDENT GROUP

The student body comprises students from throughout the U.S. and abroad. The School is committed to recruitment, admission, retention, and graduation of students who are members of minority groups. The student view is welcomed and important. Students serve as voting members on School of Nursing committees.

COSTS

For 2004–05, full-time tuition and fees for resident undergraduate students were $5866; they were $19,866 for nonresidents. Full-time tuition and fees for resident graduate students were $8320; they were $23,590 for nonresidents.

FINANCIAL AID

The campus Office of Student Financial Services awards financial aid based on need. Financial aid packages consist of loans, grants, and work-study assistance. The School of Nursing administers a number of scholarships to qualified nursing students. Scholarships in varying amounts are awarded annually, and some are renewable as long as the recipient is in good academic standing. Several forms of financial aid are available for graduate students. These include traineeships, fellowships, scholarships, research and teaching assistantships, and loans. Advanced Opportunity Fellowships are available for qualified minority or economically disadvantaged nonminority students. The School is committed to funding full-time students in the Ph.D. program.

APPLYING

Admission to the nursing major is available in the fall semester only. The deadline for applying is February 1. Individuals may be considered for admission as prenursing students in the fall, spring, and summer sessions, provided they are entering as beginning freshmen or transfer students with more than 24 college credits. The deadline for freshmen and prenursing transfer students is February 1 for summer and fall and October 1 for spring. Admission to the prenursing classification is no guarantee of admission to the nursing major.

Graduate application deadlines depend on the program of interest. Master's and post-master's applications are due March 1 for fall enrollment and October 1 for spring semester enrollment. For the Ph.D. program, applications are due January 15 for fall enrollment and September 15 for spring enrollment.

Prospective students are encouraged to visit the School of Nursing's Web site for more detailed information about admission requirements.

CORRESPONDENCE AND INFORMATION

School of Nursing
University of Wisconsin–Madison
600 Highland Avenue
Madison, Wisconsin 53792-2455
Fax: 608-263-5296
World Wide Web: http://www.son.wisc.edu

Undergraduate Admissions, Office K6/146
Telephone: 608-263-5166
E-mail: ugadmin@mailplus.wisc.edu

Graduate Admissions, Office K6/145B
Telephone: 608-263-5180
E-mail: admit@mhub.son.wisc.edu

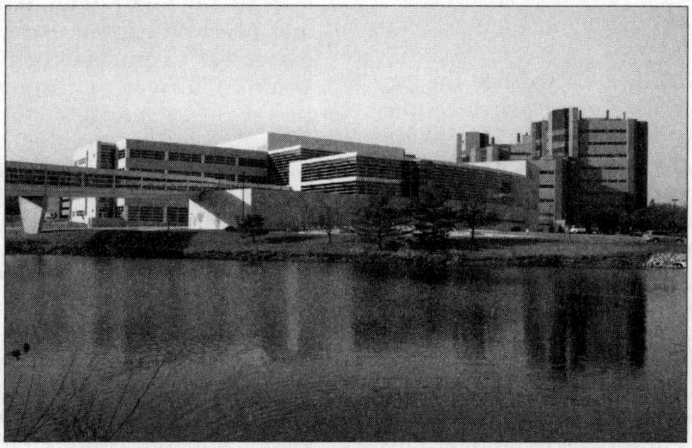

The Health Sciences Learning Center on the UW–Madison campus.

University of Wisconsin–Milwaukee
College of Nursing
Milwaukee, Wisconsin

THE UNIVERSITY
The University of Wisconsin–Milwaukee (UWM) was established in 1956 with the merger of the University of Wisconsin Extension Center in Milwaukee and Wisconsin State College. Since then, UWM has flourished into a major part of the intellectual, cultural, and economic life of southeastern Wisconsin. Ranked by the Carnegie Foundation as a research institution, UWM supports a dynamic academic community of nearly 26,000 students, 1,350 faculty and instructional staff members, and 1,900 staff members. As Wisconsin's premier urban research university, UWM offers more than 100 undergraduate majors and sub-majors, forty-eight master's programs, and eighteen doctoral programs in thirteen schools and colleges. A recent renaissance exemplified by the Milwaukee Idea, UWM's embodiment of community-university engagement, has resulted in a high level of excitement and productivity campuswide.

THE COLLEGE OF NURSING
Since its inception in 1965, the College of Nursing has been dedicated to providing academic programs of the highest quality that are at the forefront of nursing. The programs are nationally ranked, and the faculty is widely recognized for achievements and innovations.

Reflective of its commitment to the urban community, the College operates the Institute for Urban Health Partnerships, which oversees four Community Nursing Centers that offer the unique ability to integrate the multiple missions of an urban university through outstanding opportunities for student learning, faculty practice, research, and community service.

Bachelor of Science in Nursing and Master of Science and Doctor of Philosophy degrees in nursing are available through programs that provide a solid academic foundation for nursing in a variety of settings. In addition to the pursuit of knowledge, the UWM College of Nursing creates an environment that values and supports personal growth. In fall 2004, the College enrolled 1,349 students in the baccalaureate nursing major, 72 returning RN students, 116 students in master's programs, and 77 students in the doctoral program.

PROGRAMS OF STUDY
The 124-credit baccalaureate curriculum is based on an integrated, nursing-centered model intended to provide optimum preparation for practice as a professional nurse. There are two baccalaureate options available. The traditional option, also offered through a consortial program at the UW-Parkside campus, is for students who do not have a prior college degree. The accelerated option is for nonnurse college graduates. Both programs include course work relevant to professional practice, delivery of nursing care, systems for care delivery, and leadership skill development appropriate to current dynamic and diverse health-care settings.

The College also participates in a unique cooperative arrangement to bring nursing education to students in remote areas, using the latest in distance education technology. This Collaborative Nursing Program (CNP), a cooperative effort of five UW System Colleges of Nursing, enables registered nurse students to complete a baccalaureate degree.

Study in the master's program prepares students to participate in planning and implementing advanced practice nursing to meet the special needs of clients, particularly in urban communities. Within this program, the student may elect a family nurse practitioner option or a clinical nurse specialist option specializing in community health, adult health, maternal-child health, psychiatric–mental health, or systems management. Both options require 46 credits, providing eligibility for graduates to sit for a variety of certification exams.

In addition to these traditional programs, two distinctive options are also in place. A Post-Master's Family Nurse Practitioner Certificate option is available for registered nurses who have completed a master's degree in nursing but who desire preparation as family nurse practitioners. This option requires 21 credits. The second option is a Post–Nurse Practitioner option for baccalaureate-prepared certified nurse practitioners seeking a master's degree. This program requires 25 credits and can be completed in three consecutive semesters of weekend course work and distance learning.

Also offered at the graduate level is the Health Professional Educational Certificate, designed to provide health professionals, such as nurses, respiratory therapists, and occupational therapists, with additional preparation in educational principles and theory to support them in their roles as educators of students, staff members, and clients.

The College of Nursing, in collaboration with the UWM School of Business Administration, also offers an M.S. in nursing/M.B.A. degree program. Graduates of this dual program are prepared to assume leadership roles in nursing administration, health-care administration, and management.

Established in 1984, the Ph.D. curriculum includes a required research core that facilitates the development of skills to analyze and generate knowledge in the field of nursing. The historical evolution of nursing science is studied in regard to its philosophical and empirical antecedents, and current nursing science is studied through explorations of the interrelationships among the theory, research, and practice of nursing. Preparation for a role as nurse scientist, responding to and shaping public policy for the health and social needs of the public, also is addressed. Specialty courses enable students to focus on a specific nursing phenomenon and develop a sound theoretical and research base of expertise in this area of interest. Students may elect to pursue their programs of study in a traditional (on-site) format or through online study (Web-based instruction).

A B.S. to Ph.D. option is also offered to nurses who want to pursue research and scholarship goals consistent with doctoral-level education. This track does not include the clinical advanced practice preparation provided through the master's program.

ACADEMIC FACILITIES
The College maintains state-of-the-art resources to support a rich academic environment. The Nursing Learning Resource Center, serving students, faculty members, and the community, is an integral component of both the undergraduate and graduate curriculums. This college laboratory is a mediated and simulated learning environment in which students perform skills foundational to safe nursing practice. Used as a resource in the development and evaluation of media, the center also houses a modern, well-equipped computer laboratory.

In the Harriet H. Werely Center for Nursing Research and Evaluation, staff members work to develop the research potential of faculty members, students, and the greater nursing community. Personnel offer consultation in design, methodology, data analysis, computer programming, grant proposal writing, and writing for publication.

The Center for Cultural Diversity and Health houses a collection of comprehensive health behavior information for culturally diverse groups in the Milwaukee community. The center provides students, faculty members, and health professionals stimulating learning opportunities in health care for culturally diverse groups through continuing education seminars, clinical practice models, and research, to meet the health needs of culturally diverse groups.

The College's Center for Nursing History includes the Inez G. Hinsvark Historical Gallery, a unique learning resource located on the ground floor of Frances Cunningham Hall. The significant role of nurses in history is brought to life by artifacts, mementos, and photographs as well as borrowed collections.

LOCATION

UWM's 93-acre campus is located on Milwaukee's Upper East Side, one of the city's most attractive residential areas, and is a short walk from historic Lake Park and the beautiful Lake Michigan shoreline. Milwaukee possesses a wealth of cultural and recreational resources. These include the Milwaukee Art Museum, Milwaukee Public Museum, Milwaukee County Zoo, Summerfest, theaters, concert halls, restaurants, parks, professional sports events, and ethnic festivals.

STUDENT SERVICES

Advisers are available to undergraduate students to assist in interpreting curriculum and academic requirements and planning a balanced course of study. A separate adviser is assigned to continuing RN students as well as to the UW-Parkside consortial students. Students may make appointments with their advisers or simply drop in, as time allows, or utilize telephone or e-mail communications. Regular group advising sessions are also offered. Tutorial support in the basic sciences and study groups are among the services offered through the College's Academic Enrichment Center, in addition to the academic support services available to all students on the greater UWM campus.

Graduate students, in addition to their general student services adviser, also may select or are assigned a faculty member with whom they collaborate closely to establish and complete their advanced course of study.

THE NURSING STUDENT GROUP

The student body is a diverse group of individuals pursuing their academic goals in both traditional and nontraditional ways. Students come to UWM from throughout the country and the world, as well as the state of Wisconsin. The College of Nursing maintains a close relationship with two sister schools in South Korea, with exchanges of students and faculty members occurring often.

Graduates of the various programs have found exciting and rewarding positions as nursing professionals, advanced practitioners, researchers, and educators throughout the Metro-Milwaukee area, the Midwest, and beyond.

COSTS

For 2004–05, full-time tuition and fees for resident undergraduate students were $5835, and they were $18,587 for nonresidents. Full-time tuition and fees for resident graduate students were $8131, and they were $22,497 for nonresidents.

FINANCIAL AID

The campus Financial Aid Office awards financial aid based on need. Financial aid packages consist of loans, grants, and work-study assistance. The College of Nursing administers a number of scholarships to qualified students. Scholarships in varying amounts are awarded annually. Financial aid available to graduate students includes traineeships, fellowships, scholarships, research and teaching assistantships, and loans.

APPLYING

Students who seek to enter the nursing major in September must submit applications by the preceding January 15; for January entrance, the deadline is the preceding July 15. Students who have completed 15 credits or required courses with a cumulative GPA of 3.5 or higher may be eligible for earlier admission. Individuals may be considered for admission as prenursing students in the fall and spring as beginning freshmen or transfer students. Admission to the prenursing classification is no guarantee of admission to the nursing professional program.

Graduate application deadlines depend on the program of interest. Master's applications are due to the UWM Graduate School by January 1 and to the College of Nursing by February 1 for fall enrollment and to the UWM Graduate School by September 1 and to the College of Nursing by October 1 for spring semester enrollment. For the Ph.D. program, applications are due to the UWM Graduate School and to the College of Nursing by February 1 for fall enrollment. Applications received after these dates are reviewed on a rolling basis.

Prospective students are encouraged to visit the College of Nursing Web site for more detailed information about admission requirements.

CORRESPONDENCE AND INFORMATION

College of Nursing
University of Wisconsin–Milwaukee
1921 East Hartford Avenue
P.O. Box 413
Milwaukee, Wisconsin 53211-3060
Fax: 414-229-6474
E-mail: www.asknursing@uwm.edu
World Wide Web: http://www.nursing.uwm.edu

Donna Wier, Senior Adviser
Undergraduate Admissions
Student Affairs Office
Room 129-Cunningham Hall
Telephone: 414-229-5481
E-mail: ddw@uwm.edu

Jacqueline Davit, RN Advisor
RN Completion Program Admissions
Student Affairs Office
Room 129, Cunningham Hall
Telephone: 414-229-4662
E-mail: jdavit@uwm.edu

Ahnalee Brincks, Academic Advisor
Graduate Admissions
Student Affairs Office
Room 129, Cunningham Hall
Telephone: 414-229-5474
E-mail: brincks@uwm.edu

Ursuline College
The Breen School of Nursing
Pepper Pike, Ohio

THE COLLEGE

Ursuline College is a Catholic liberal arts college offering baccalaureate and graduate programs. Founded as a women's college in 1871, Ursuline's students remain predominantly women. The College is committed to helping both women and men achieve their goals.

Ursuline's nationally recognized core curriculum encourages students to explore their identities and life goals. Ursuline takes a holistic approach to learning, encouraging students to rely on their studies, not only as a means for launching a successful career but also for enjoying a happy and meaningful life. This integrated approach is truly reflective of a new generation of students who, along with the faculty, serve as catalysts for the dynamic learning environment at Ursuline. That culture and small classes provide more than 1,400 students with individual attention and special care.

THE SCHOOL OF NURSING

Nursing has been a vital program at Ursuline College since 1975. Today, The Breen School of Nursing has the largest academic program on campus. The School offers B.S.N. and M.S.N. degree programs and post-master's certificates. B.S.N. graduates score exceptionally well on the NCLEX exam, with a 100 percent pass rate in 1998, 2001, and 2003. At the M.S.N. level, the palliative care program is the first of its kind in the country; the case management program is the only one of its kind in the area.

The Breen School of Nursing offers its professional programs within Ursuline's values-based learning environment. An individualized approach enables students to enjoy personal instruction, learn material in greater depth, and gain experience in a wide variety of health-care environments. The Breen School's graduates are sought by employers, who find them to be well prepared and flexible in adapting to new settings. The School has more than 2,000 graduates, many of whom hold leadership positions. In addition to a highly qualified full-time faculty, the M.S.N. program has visiting professors who are nationally recognized leaders in nursing.

PROGRAMS OF STUDY

The Breen School offers programs that prepare nurses for the health-care marketplace of the future, at both the basic (B.S.N.) and advanced practice (M.S.N.) levels.

The B.S.N. program provides a broad foundation by combining Ursuline's liberal studies core with an intensive three-year sequence in the nursing major. Qualified students are admitted directly into nursing. The B.S.N. program (129 credits, 58 of which are in nursing) can be completed in four years. Unique classroom and clinical assignments enable students to develop critical-thinking, communication, technical, and leadership skills. Students complete clinical rotations in renowned health-care institutions in the greater Cleveland area. The School's holistic and values-based nursing program provides a framework for students to learn about the caring and ethical side of health care, pass the NCLEX licensing exam, and adapt to practice in the twenty-first century. There are accelerated tracks for RNs, LPNs, and for those who have earned a bachelor's degree in another discipline. Students may combine traditional, accelerated, and Web courses.

The M.S.N. program prepares advanced practice nurses as clinical nurse specialists (CNS) and nurse practitioners (NP). The faculty believes that the different roles of advanced practice nursing are more similar than different so CNS and NP students have several classes together. The emphasis at the graduate level is on refining analytical skills, developing a clearer ability to connect theory to practice, and enhancing professional skills. All programs have a strong clinical component where caring, communication, and critical thinking are emphasized. There are four tracks: care management, palliative care, adult nurse practitioner, and family nurse practitioner. The number of credit hours required for the M.S.N. degree is 39, with the exception of the family nurse practitioner track, which requires 42 credit hours. Courses are offered in the evenings and on Saturdays in an accelerated model. Students may choose to complete the clinical practicum in the greater Cleveland area or at an alternate location. The palliative care post-M.S.N. track is available via distance learning. Graduates are eligible to take advanced practice certification exams.

The care management track is a cutting-edge program that prepares students as leaders in outcomes-based practice, quality improvement, and fiscally sound resource management. Students develop a subspecialty area of expertise throughout the program. The palliative care track focuses on care when a cure is no longer possible. Emphasis is on comprehensive care of the mind, body, and spirit through collaborative practice with other health-care providers. The adult nurse practitioner track focuses on health promotion and disease prevention of adults with acute and chronic diseases. The family nurse practitioner track focuses on primary health care across the life cycle with an emphasis on health maintenance, disease prevention, counseling, and education.

AFFILIATIONS WITH HEALTH-CARE FACILITIES

The Breen School of Nursing is affiliated with numerous internationally renowned and community-based health-care agencies throughout the greater Cleveland area. M.S.N. students may elect to do their practicum in another state or country.

ACADEMIC FACILITIES

Ursuline's library, well-known to health professionals in the area, houses more than 125,400 volumes, 369 periodical subscriptions, and 3,641 electronic subscriptions. Membership in OhioLINK and a comprehensive media collection provide access to thousands of additional resources. One of the reference librarians is a liaison with the School of Nursing. Other campus resources include media and computer centers. The College has five dedicated rooms for computers, plus individual computers in numerous locations, including the residence halls. Students enjoy classes in the new Bishop Anthony M. Pilla Student Learning Center, which houses a state-of-the-art nursing skills lab.

LOCATION

Ursuline College is located on a beautiful campus in Pepper Pike, a residential suburb approximately 12 miles from downtown Cleveland. The surrounding area has many restaurants and stores, including a large mall just 10 minutes from campus. The Cleveland area offers a multitude of activities such as music, art, science, parks, and sports. Ursuline is easily accessible from Route 271 or via the RTA. For students looking to combine a quiet but serious academic life with the cultural excitement of a major city, Ursuline College provides these unique advantages.

STUDENT SERVICES

In addition to sports, the College provides a fitness center, personal and career counseling, mentoring and cooperative education programs, campus ministry, and an Office for Multicultural Affairs. The Academic Support and Learning Disabilities Center provides academic support services for all students, including assistance with study, testing, and writing skills. Tutoring is available in reading, writing, math, and science. The Program for Academic Success (PAS) was designed to help students who are not prepared for college-level work, especially in math and science.

THE NURSING STUDENT GROUP

Although Ursuline remains a women's college, men are welcome and represent approximately 7 percent of the students who are enrolled in nursing. Most students come from Ohio and surrounding states and represent different ethnic, racial, cultural, religious, and economic backgrounds. Currently, the School of Nursing has approximately 325 undergraduate and 70 graduate students.

COSTS

In 2004–05, undergraduate tuition was $599 per credit hour. Full-time students usually carry 12 to 16 credits. Graduate tuition was $639 per credit hour.

FINANCIAL AID

The Office of Financial Aid administers a number of institutional, state, and federal programs. Financial assistance may include a combination of scholarships, loans, grants, and work-study opportunities. To apply for financial aid, students must complete the Free Application for Federal Student Aid (FAFSA) and the Ursuline College Financial Aid Application. Approximately 85 percent of undergraduates in nursing receive financial aid.

APPLYING

Undergraduate and graduate applications are accepted on a rolling basis. Admission to the B.S.N. program is through the Office of Admission. In addition to criteria for clear admission to the College, applicants seeking admission to the B.S.N. program directly from high school need to have successfully completed algebra, biology (with lab), and chemistry (with lab), each with a grade of 2.5 the first time the courses were taken for credit. Students may transfer college courses in which they have earned a grade of 2.0.

Admission to the M.S.N. program is through The Breen School of Nursing. Admission criteria include an official transcript verifying completion of an accredited baccalaureate program with a GPA of 3.0. The MAT or GRE may be required of applicants whose GPA is less than 3.0.

CORRESPONDENCE AND INFORMATION

For the Undergraduate Program:
Sarah Carr
Director of Admission
Ursuline College
2550 Lander Road
Pepper Pike, Ohio 44124-4398
Telephone: 440-449-4203
888-URSULINE (toll-free)
Fax: 440-684-6138
World Wide Web: http://www.ursuline.edu

For the Graduate Program:
Carol H. Waggoner, Ph.D., RN
Director, Graduate Program
The Breen School of Nursing
Ursuline College
2550 Lander Road
Pepper Pike, Ohio 44124-4398
Telephone: 440-449-3425
Fax: 440-449-4267
E-mail: cwaggoner@ursuline.edu
World Wide Web: http://www.ursuline.edu

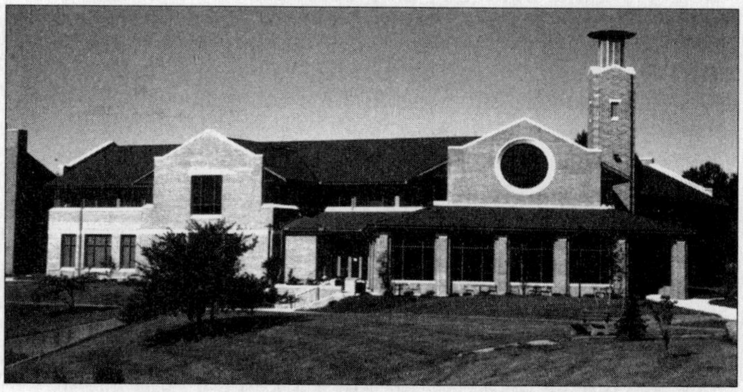

Located on 112 scenic acres in Pepper Pike, Ohio—just 12 miles east of Cleveland—the Breen School of Nursing is a student's pathway to success.

Vanderbilt University
School of Nursing
Nashville, Tennessee

THE UNIVERSITY
Vanderbilt University was established in 1873 through a $1-million donation by Commodore Cornelius Vanderbilt. Vanderbilt University offers a full range of undergraduate programs as well as forty-one master's degree programs and forty Ph.D. programs. There are more than 1,600 full-time faculty members and a diverse student population of almost 10,000.

THE SCHOOL OF NURSING
For more than ninety years, Vanderbilt University School of Nursing (VUSN) has been providing innovative educational opportunities for its students. The School's proudest tradition is educating nurses who are impassioned professionals capable of meeting—and exceeding—the demands of a constantly evolving profession. By 1926, the School had grown from its initiation as the Vanderbilt Hospital Training School (1909) to a school of nursing, offering a diploma in nursing combined with studies in arts and sciences, leading to a B.S. degree. In 1933, VUSN offered the first B.S.N. in Tennessee and became a charter member of the Association of Collegiate Schools of Nursing (ACSN), which later became the National League for Nursing Accrediting Commission (NLNAC), under which the program is currently accredited. The nurse-midwifery program is accredited by the American College of Nurse-Midwives. In 1985, VUSN introduced the Prespecialty "Bridge" Pathway to the master's program, replacing the B.S.N. degree program. The Prespecialty "Bridge" Pathway offers multiple entry options for students seeking to become advanced practice nurses, including those with 78 hours of college credit, an associate degree or diploma in nursing and 78 hours of college credit, or a B.S.N. Recognizing that some nurses who may have earned master's degrees in nursing would like additional or different specialties, VUSN offers a post-master's option. In 1993, the Ph.D. in Nursing Science program was established.

PROGRAMS OF STUDY
Vanderbilt University School of Nursing offers a Master of Science in Nursing (M.S.N.) with multiple entry options. Applicants with a Bachelor of Science in Nursing, an associate degree in nursing and 78 semester hours of college credit, a diploma in nursing and 78 semester hours of college credit, a bachelor's degree in another field, or at least 78 semester hours of college credit are eligible to apply to the program.

The M.S.N. degree is offered with the following specialties: clinical management, health systems management, nurse midwifery, nursing informatics, primary-care nurse practitioner (adult, adult/gerontology dual certification, family, pediatric, or women's health), specialty-care nurse practitioner (acute care, neonatal, pediatric acute care, or psychiatric–mental health), and a joint management and Master of Business Administration (M.S.N./M.B.A. dual degree). The School offers numerous focus areas, including cardiovascular disease management, clinical research management, emergency response management, forensic nursing, oncology, palliative care, transplant services, and trauma. Many of the programs are delivered in a modified distance format to accommodate individuals who work full-time and/or maintain residence outside middle Tennessee. International exchange opportunities are available.

Applicants with a Bachelor of Science in Nursing (B.S.N.) from an NLNAC-accredited program are admitted directly to the specialty year for a 39-semester-hour program of studies in all specialties except nurse midwifery, which is 52 semester hours. Admission to the School of Nursing without a B.S.N. degree is possible through the generalist nursing Prespecialty/M.S.N. program. Students with an associate degree in nursing and 78 semester hours of college credit or a diploma in nursing and 78 semester hours of college credit may enter the program and earn the Master of Science in Nursing degree in five semesters of full-time study. Students with a baccalaureate degree in another field or at least 78 semester hours of college credit may enter the program and earn an M.S.N. degree in six semesters of full-time study.

The Ph.D. in Nursing Science program is designed for highly qualified individuals who hold graduate degrees in nursing and are interested in careers in nursing science. Areas of concentration include the study of individual, family, and community responses to health and illness and the outcomes of care-delivery practices. Students are exposed to theory generating and theory testing methods responsive to health-care needs across the life span.

The Ph.D. in Nursing Science curriculum is organized into three broad areas: phenomena of concern in nursing science; scientific inquiry, including application, testing, and generation of theory; and a minor in an area of the student's interest that supports the student's focus of study. Students work with faculty mentors who guide and oversee their educational experiences from the time of admission through the completion of the degree requirements. They participate in intensive research experiences connected with faculty research projects and are exposed to a variety of research designs and analysis techniques.

The faculty members of the School of Nursing are committed to the educational preparation of a group of nurse scholars who can lead the nation in demonstrating how well-conceived, theory-based nursing research verifies and extends the body of nursing knowledge. Faculty members are experienced scholars whose research is funded by national and private foundations and who serve as leaders in several specialty areas in nursing and health care.

AFFILIATIONS WITH HEALTH-CARE FACILITIES
Vanderbilt University School of Nursing offers its students opportunities to complete clinical courses, conduct inquiry, and learn in diverse settings. The School maintains more than 1,000 contracts with clinical practices in hospitals, communities, health departments, private practices, clinics, outpatient facilities, home-health agencies, skilled-care facilities, nursing homes, schools, and industries. Many of these sites are in urban settings in Nashville, rural areas of Tennessee, and several other states. The Vanderbilt University Medical Center maintains a reputation for excellence in teaching, practice, and research and provides students with a tertiary academic setting, where patients receive exemplary care from creative health-care teachers and scholars.

ACADEMIC FACILITIES
The Jean and Alexander Heard Library is the collective name for all of the libraries at Vanderbilt, which have a combined collection of more than 2 million volumes. In addition to the Central library, the Biomedical, Divinity, Education, Law, Management, and Science libraries serve their respective schools and disciplines. The state-of-the-art Annette and Irwin Eskind Biomedical Library provides students with access to worldwide information through the very best in informatic retrieval and management technology. Traditional library services, book stacks, and comfortable reading areas are also provided along with technology training assistance.

The focal point of scholarship at the School of Nursing is the Joint Center for Nursing Research (JCNR), which is housed on the fifth floor of Godchaux Hall. Although research and scholarship activities occur throughout the School and are interwoven into all aspects of academic life at Vanderbilt, the center serves as the central resource, repository, and facilitator of faculty member, student, and nursing staff member scholarship. Its mission is to facilitate scholarly activity and thereby promote new knowledge and improved care delivery to the community and the nation. It achieves this mission through the established relationships between the School of Nursing, the University, and affiliated health-care agencies.

A complete collection of software programs for word processing, statistical analysis, slide and graphics preparation, spreadsheet applications, power analysis calculations, and qualitative data analysis are available for use by faculty members and students. Reference materials pertaining to research design, methods, instruments, and analysis are also available. Weekly research and scholarship-related luncheon seminars are held and are open to faculty members, students, and staff members of member hospitals.

Vanderbilt's computing resources include a campuswide integrated network with full Internet connectivity that is supported by several departmental-level units: Academic Computing & Information Services (ACIS), Network Computing Services, the Biomedical Informatics Center, and the Helene Fuld Instructional Media Center (HFIMC). Combined, these units provide a full range of services, including Web development and server administration, consultation, training, 24/7 help-desk troubleshooting, and learning resource research, procurement, and management.

The HFIMC is the primary provider of instructional technology support at VUSN. Its inventory includes computer labs with twenty-five new-model, business-class computers; nine multimedia presentation computers; digital AV/data recording and distribution equipment; and Web servers—all linked by a 100-Mb Ethernet network. There is also network capability at every seat of the main lecture hall and in the student lounge. Direct access to the Internet and to the Vanderbilt computer network gives users ready access to many online services, such as the research databases of the VU Medical Center and the Vanderbilt University Jean and Alexander Heard Library, and shared productivity tools. Other HFIMC resources include an AV viewing room with VCRs and 35mm slide viewers, group meeting rooms, and a software library with videotapes, audiotapes, CD-ROMs, and interactive videodiscs. Using methods such as threaded conferences and streaming video, VUSN continues to expand its initiatives that are aimed at distributing as many learning resources as possible to the home desktops of students.

LOCATION

Vanderbilt is located on a 333-acre parklike campus approximately 1½ miles from downtown Nashville, providing a peaceful setting within an urban environment. Long known as a center of banking, finance, and publishing, this capital city of Tennessee is a unique blend of Southern hospitality and cosmopolitan diversity that ranks high in the "quality of life" surveys. Nashville has an international airport and is easily accessible from interstate highways.

STUDENT SERVICES

Vanderbilt provides its students with a comprehensive list of services, including the Career Center, Psychological and Counseling Services, Student Health Center, the Office of International Services, the Child Care Center, the Bishop Joseph Johnson Black Cultural Center, and the Margaret Cuninggim Women's Center, as well as security escort services, shuttle bus services, and graduate student and family housing.

THE NURSING STUDENT GROUP

Vanderbilt University School of Nursing has been successful in attracting students from diverse educational backgrounds and work experiences. Approximately 60 percent of the class began the program in the 2004 academic year without a background in nursing. These individuals will enter the nursing profession prepared as advanced practice nurses after two full calendar years (six semesters) of study. Ages of class members range from 20 to 56, and 9 percent of the students are men. The School's diverse student body includes Asian Americans, African Americans, American Indians, and Hispanic students, in addition to international students.

COSTS

Tuition for the M.S.N. program for the 2004–05 academic year was $810 per semester hour for all students. Tuition for the Ph.D. in Nursing Science program is $1213 per semester hour. Tuition for both programs is subject to change.

Expenses for books and supplies vary according to specialty. Equipment such as tape recorders and diagnostic tools is required for certain specialties. Other charges include laboratory fees, student activities and recreation fees, liability insurance coverage, and hospitalization insurance.

FINANCIAL AID

Financial aid is available from several sources for full-time M.S.N. students. All students who wish to apply for financial aid and scholarships must apply to the School of Nursing no later than May 1 for the next academic year. Information about financial aid for M.S.N. students can be obtained from the School of Nursing Admissions Office.

Information about financial aid for Ph.D. students can be obtained from the University's Office of Financial Aid, located at 2309 West End Avenue, Nashville, Tennessee 37203-1725 (telephone: 615-322-3591). Tuition reimbursement is given to all full-time Ph.D. students; all tuition is covered, except for dissertation credit hours.

APPLYING

Admission requirements for applicants to the M.S.N. program include a minimum 3.0 GPA, three letters of recommendation, a statement of career goals, an interview survey, and a minimum GRE score of 1000 on the verbal and quantitative components and 3.5 on the analytical component or a GMAT score of 550 or better.

Admission to the Ph.D. in Nursing Science program is through the University's Graduate School, which has oversight responsibility for all doctoral programs in the University. Application materials are returned to the School of Nursing.

Successful applicants to the Ph.D. in Nursing Science program are those whose previous academic performance, letters of reference, Graduate Record Examinations (GRE) scores, and personal statement meet admission standards for the School of Nursing and the University Graduate School. In addition, because of the importance of research oversight in doctoral education, only students whose research and career goals fit with the School's areas of concentration are considered for admission. All applicants are interviewed by the Director of the Doctoral Program and 2 doctoral faculty members.

CORRESPONDENCE AND INFORMATION:

For information on the M.S.N. and Ph.D. in Nursing Science programs:

Admissions Office
Vanderbilt University School of Nursing
226 Godchaux Hall
21st Avenue South
Nashville, Tennessee 37240

Telephone: 615-322-3800
Fax: 615-343-0333
E-mail: vusn-admissions@vanderbilt.edu
World Wide Web: http://www.mc.vanderbilt.edu/nursing/

Villanova University
College of Nursing
Villanova, Pennsylvania

College of Nursing
VILLANOVA
UNIVERSITY

THE UNIVERSITY

Villanova University is an independent coeducational institution of higher learning founded by the Augustinians, one of the oldest teaching orders in the Catholic Church. Since its beginning in 1842, the University's Augustinian character has been evident in its devotion to the principles of scholarship, community, and the relationship between mind and heart as well as in its commitment to producing graduates with strong moral values and proficient skills.

Villanova is a comprehensive university with undergraduate academic colleges in the areas of commerce and finance, engineering, liberal arts and sciences, and nursing. The University offers selected master's and doctoral degrees, including the Master of Science in Nursing (M.S.N.) and Ph.D. in nursing, and maintains a highly regarded School of Law. Villanova's student body of more than 10,000 represents almost every state in the nation as well as forty-four countries. Approximately 50 percent of its undergraduates are men.

THE COLLEGE OF NURSING

The College of Nursing, founded in 1953, has the distinction of being the first collegiate nursing program under Catholic auspices in Pennsylvania, the largest nursing college in the commonwealth within a private university, and the only nursing program in the country under Augustinian sponsorship. All of the programs offered by the College—baccalaureate, master's, doctoral, and continuing education—are fully accredited. There are approximately 5,500 alumni of the degree-granting programs, and the College currently enrolls approximately 470 undergraduates, the majority of whom are full-time, and 180 graduate students, most of whom enroll on a part-time basis.

The faculty believes that education provides students with opportunities to develop habits of critical, constructive thought so that they may make discriminating judgments in their search for the truth. This type of intellectual development can best be attained in a teaching-learning environment that fosters sharing of knowledge, skills, and attitudes as well as inquiry toward the development of new knowledge. The faculty members and students comprise a community of learners and teacher-scholars. Approximately 80 percent of the full-time faculty members in the College hold an earned doctorate, and many are actively engaged in research. The faculty, however, has teaching as its primary commitment, and most of the teaching is carried out by full-time faculty members.

The College, in conjunction with the University's Office of International Studies, offers a sophomore year abroad in the baccalaureate program at the University of Manchester in Manchester, England. There are a growing number of students sponsored by international organizations who are attending the master's program, and the College is exploring opportunities to expand international experiences for its students. The continuing education program offers a variety of workshops, seminars, conferences, self-study activities, and short courses and a post-master's certificate in nursing administration. All of these options are designed to assist practicing nurses to advance, maintain, and provide high-quality health care.

PROGRAMS OF STUDY

Villanova awards the Bachelor of Science in Nursing (B.S.N.) degree after completion of 136 credits, 75 of which are in nursing; the remaining 61 are in arts and science. The program integrates a liberal education with the ideals, knowledge, and skills of professional nursing practice under the direction of a qualified faculty. Baccalaureate education prepares individuals for professional nursing practice in a variety of health-care settings and for continuous personal and educational growth, including entrance into graduate education in nursing. The College welcomes applications from adults who wish to begin preparation for a career in nursing. These include individuals who possess undergraduate and/or graduate degrees in other fields as well as adults entering college for the first time. Part-time study is possible during the introductory level of the program. Full-time study is required during the clinical portion of the program. Graduates from diploma and associate degree nursing programs are eligible for admission to the baccalaureate program. Through a series of nursing examinations and clinical validation, a registered nurse student may demonstrate current nursing knowledge, earning 45 credits in nursing. A maximum of 50 percent of the credits from the total curriculum may be transferred by either adult learners or registered nurse students.

The M.S.N. program at Villanova University requires the completion of 45 credits and prepares nurses for roles as nurse practitioners; nurse anesthetists; case management administrators; educators; and health-care administrators. The curriculum includes core courses (including research, theory, and leadership), clinical courses (including a practicum in adult, community, gerontology, parent-child, or psychiatric–mental health nursing), free electives, an independent study course, and role-related courses (including a practicum). No thesis is required; however, students who wish to work with faculty members who are conducting research or who wish to engage in a research-oriented independent study project are encouraged to do so and are assisted in the endeavor.

The Villanova nursing doctoral program leads to the Ph.D. degree and prepares nurses as forward-thinking teacher scholars for academic careers in higher education. Graduates are well-prepared to teach diverse populations of students in a variety of educational and clinical settings using state-of-the-art technology. They provide leadership as the architects of curricula and members of evaluative bodies, are active contributors to the advancement and development of theory and research, and assume the varied roles of faculty members within academic institutions. The doctoral program combines innovative and traditional modalities, offering distance learning opportunities in the fall and spring semesters and on-site experience during summer sessions. The program was designed with a maximum of 51 credits; the length of the program varies depending on previous education, currency of graduate education, and individual needs.

AFFILIATIONS WITH HEALTH-CARE FACILITIES

The College of Nursing is affiliated with more than seventy health-care agencies in the Greater Philadelphia area that provide settings for undergraduate and graduate student clinical experiences. These facilities include hospitals in large medical centers, community hospitals, extended-care facilities, home-health agencies, schools, industrial health settings, senior citizen and community health centers, HMOs, insurance companies, and managed-care agencies.

ACADEMIC FACILITIES

The Falvey Memorial Library provides resources and facilities for study and research by graduate and undergraduate students, faculty members, and visiting scholars. It houses more than 650,000 volumes, of which more than 22,000 are nursing or nursing-related. The library has an extensive periodicals section with 251 nursing and nursing-related holdings. Library services include computerized literature searches with direct access to the National Library of Medicine databases and extensive instructional media services, including a professionally staffed video studio for the production of sophisticated video materials. In addition to the general University library and extensive interlibrary loan access, students in the College of Nursing have access to the Law Library and that of the College of Commerce and Finance. The computing services available to the University community are extensive, with computer stations located throughout the campus. In addition to those available in the primary computing center, the College of Nursing Learning Resource Center houses computers and interactive video systems that are available for the exclusive use of its students and faculty. The Learning Resource Center also maintains extensive holdings of a wide variety of audiovisual materials, training models, computer software programs, and simulations to support the teaching enterprise. Students and faculty members have access to the fully staffed Center during extended weekday and selected weekend hours.

LOCATION

With its more than 220 landscaped acres in one of the most beautiful residential areas in America, the Villanova campus is among the showplaces in the suburban Philadelphia area. Located on the prestigious Main Line, with a station on its campus, Villanova is easily accessible by train from Philadelphia. It also lies in proximity to several major highways that make the Philadelphia airport as well as the New York and Washington, D.C., areas easily accessible. Such a location provides students with safe and easy access to the cultural and recreational opportunities available in Philadelphia and makes those of New York and Washington, D.C., readily available as well.

STUDENT SERVICES

Villanova University offers a wide variety of student services. Campus Ministry promotes a sense of community through the coordination of a variety of programs that are of a religious and human service character with a view to aiding students with their spiritual and personal growth. A full array of student activities, including a theater, Greek system, music activities, intramural and intercollegiate sports, and a fitness center, are available. Such opportunities facilitate the total development of students, promote a spirit of community, provide opportunities for students to interact with other individuals who have varied interests, and provide the supports necessary to succeed academically. In addition, student health services, a counseling center, career planning and placement services, a writing center, and study skills resources are available to all students.

THE NURSING STUDENT GROUP

Most of the individuals enrolled in the undergraduate program are full-time students who began their nursing studies directly after completing high school. Approximately 20 percent of the B.S.N. population are registered nurses or adult learners. Graduates are employed in major health-care facilities, universities, or other settings throughout the country, and approximately 30 percent have completed or are enrolled in graduate programs. Approximately 90 percent of the individuals enrolled in the M.S.N. program are part-time students with several years experience as nurses. Students in the program received their undergraduate education in a wide variety of institutions, and the number of international students enrolled in the master's program is increasing steadily. Graduates of this program hold positions of leadership, such as nurse practitioner, nurse anesthetist, administrator, educator, and case manager, in some of the most prestigious health-care institutions in the country. Approximately 20 percent of the M.S.N. graduates have completed or are enrolled in doctoral programs.

COSTS

Full-time tuition for the undergraduate program in the 2004–05 academic year is $27,350. The per-credit rate for part-time undergraduate courses is $580, and general fees are $300. For the 2004–05 academic year, tuition for the master's program is $560 per credit, with a general University fee of $60 per semester. For the 2004–05 academic year, tuition for the doctoral program is $700 per credit.

FINANCIAL AID

Undergraduate financial aid is granted on the basis of need and scholastic ability and includes Villanova University scholastic grants, student loans, federal grants, state grants, and scholarships from outside sources such as corporations, unions, charitable trusts, and service clubs. The University financial aid office assists applicants in this process. Financial assistance is available to graduate students in the form of graduate assistantships, professional nurse traineeships, scholarships, and loans.

APPLYING

Admission to the undergraduate program is based on evaluation of high school grade point average, SAT I scores, rank in class, participation in extracurricular activities, and recommendations of teachers and counselors. Applications must be submitted by January 7, and applicants are notified of their admission decision on an ongoing basis.

For transfer students, adult learners, and registered nurses, applications must be received no later than November 15 (for January entrance) or April 15 (for September entrance). Criteria used to evaluate these applicants include complete transcripts from previous schools, quality point average at a previously attended institution, and evidence of honorable withdrawal from previously attended institution(s). Transcripts from a secondary school are required if the applicant has never attended an institution of higher learning.

Applications to the M.S.N. program are accepted on an ongoing basis, and students may begin the program in the fall, spring, or summer terms. Admission requirements include the B.S.N., a minimum of one year recent clinical practice in nursing, acceptable scores on the MAT or GRE, undergraduate statistics, physical assessment, three letters of reference from professional nurses, and a personal statement of career goals.

Applicants to the doctoral program should submit all materials by February 15 in the year prior to enrollment. Materials include the application form, curriculum vitae, application fee, three references, evidence of scholarly writing, essay, official transcripts, GRE scores from the last five years, and TOEFL scores (international students only). Applicants are notified of acceptance early in the spring semester so that they can plan to attend the on-campus orientation and summer session.

CORRESPONDENCE AND INFORMATION

Office of Undergraduate Admission
Villanova University
800 East Lancaster Avenue
Villanova, Pennsylvania 19085
Telephone: 610-519-4453
Fax: 610-519-6450

Graduate Nursing Program
Office of University Admission
Villanova University
800 East Lancaster Avenue
Villanova, Pennsylvania 19085-1690
Telephone: 610-519-4934
Fax: 610-519-7650

Virginia Commonwealth University
School of Nursing
Richmond, Virginia

THE UNIVERSITY

A public, urban university located in the state capital, Virginia Commonwealth University (VCU) was founded in 1838. VCU is ranked by the Carnegie Foundation as one of the nation's top research universities and is one of only three such universities in the state. VCU is composed of two campuses, the Monroe Park Campus and the Medical College of Virginia Campus. More than 24,000 students attend VCU, with 28 percent of the students representing minority groups.

VCU's Medical College of Virginia Campus is home to the Schools of Nursing, Allied Health, Pharmacy, Dentistry, and Medicine. The VCU Medical Center is one of the most comprehensive teaching hospitals in the country.

THE SCHOOL OF NURSING

The School of Nursing originated in 1893 and has evolved from a basic diploma program to a school of more than 600 students, with multiple programs at the baccalaureate, master's, and doctoral degree levels. In addition, the School of Nursing offers post-master's certificate programs. The School of Nursing takes pride in its long history of service to the profession of nursing and continues to be a leader in nursing education in Virginia and the country.

PROGRAMS OF STUDY

Beginning in 2003, the School of Nursing offers several new programs, including an accelerated track in the undergraduate program for non-nursing college graduates and an RN-M.S. program for registered nurses who graduated from a diploma or associate degree program in nursing.

The School of Nursing offers programs leading to B.S., M.S., and Ph.D. degrees in nursing. The School offers post-master's certificate practitioner programs in adult, acute care, child, family, and women's health and post-master's certificate programs in psychiatric–mental health, nursing administration and leadership, and nursing in faith communities.

The undergraduate program encompasses the traditional, accelerated B.S., and RN-B.S. weekend programs. Students can enter the traditional undergraduate program as freshmen or may transfer into the nursing program as sophomores after finishing their first year of study in VCU's College of Humanities and Science or at another college or university. Non-nursing college graduates may complete their bachelor's degree in nursing in a year-round, five-semester program. Registered nurses can obtain their bachelor's degree by attending class once a month in the RN-B.S. weekend program. This flexible program can be completed in three semesters of study and is offered in multiple sites across the state of Virginia. Academically talented registered nurses may apply to the RN-M.S. program.

The master's program is designed to prepare graduates for advanced nursing practice as nurse practitioners, clinical nurse specialists, and nurse leaders.

The School offers an entry-level master's program for individuals with bachelor's degrees in disciplines other than nursing. The accelerated second-degree program is a year-round, full-time program that begins in the summer and offers study in adult health–acute (clinical nurse specialist studies (CNS) and nurse practitioner studies (NP) tracks), adult health—primary (NP track), child health (NP track), family health (NP track), nursing administration and leadership, psychiatric–mental health nursing (CNS and NP tracks), and women's health (NP track). Upon graduation, students are eligible for certification as nurse practitioners or clinical nurse specialists in their chosen specialty area.

The traditional master's program offers full-time and part-time study in adult health–acute (CNS and NP tracks), adult health—primary (NP track), child health (NP track), family health (NP track), nursing administration and leadership, integrative psychiatric mental health (CNS, NP, and HN tracks), and women's health (NP track). Registered nurses with a bachelor's degree in another discipline may enter the traditional master's program but are also required to complete selected undergraduate upper-division nursing courses.

The goal of the doctoral program in nursing is the preparation of scholars to develop knowledge in the discipline of nursing. The Ph.D. program has four areas of inquiry from which students choose. They then study with faculty members who have programs of research related to some aspect of the focus area. The four areas are healing, biobehavioral clinical research, immunocompetence, and risk and resilience.

AFFILIATIONS WITH HEALTH-CARE FACILITIES

The School of Nursing is affiliated with a wide variety of health-care agencies within and outside the metropolitan Richmond area. These include major health-care agencies such as the VCU Medical Center and Hunter Holmes McGuire VA Medical Center as well as other acute- and primary-care settings, ambulatory practice sites, schools, and community health centers.

ACADEMIC FACILITIES

The University library facilities include Cabell and Tompkins-McCaw Libraries. The combined collections in these libraries total more than 1.23 million volumes. The comprehensive collections of Tompkins-McCaw Library are a designated resource library for the Southeastern states in the National Network of Libraries in Medicine. The University Library Services are extensively automated, with almost 900 databases available for searching and more than 100 public-access workstations.

LOCATION

The city of Richmond, located on the James River, provides a backdrop for an energetic academic and social life on the Virginia Commonwealth campuses. The University is located 2 hours from the nation's capital, the Blue Ridge Mountains, the

Appalachian Trail, and the Atlantic Ocean. The School of Nursing is housed on the Medical Campus, which is located near the state capitol and the government and financial centers of downtown Richmond.

STUDENT SERVICES

The University and School offer a comprehensive array of student services at both the undergraduate and graduate levels. These include academic advising by professional faculty and staff members, academic support services within the School and University, a career and placement center, services for students with disabilities, counseling, and student activities.

THE NURSING STUDENT GROUP

The School of Nursing enrolls approximately 295 traditional undergraduate students and 285 RN-B.S. weekend students. In the graduate program, there are approximately 103 accelerated second-degree students, 118 traditional master's students, and 33 doctoral students.

COSTS

The 2004–05 in-state resident full-time undergraduate tuition and fees were $5084, and out-of-state tuition and fees were $17,248. In-state graduate tuition and fees were $7370, and out-of-state tuition and fees were $17,248.

FINANCIAL AID

Financial aid is available through the University's Financial Aid Office. The School of Nursing offers scholarships for full-time study. Full-time doctoral students receive a stipend and scholarships covering tuition and fees and serve as teaching or research assistants.

APPLYING

All programs use a self-managed application process and require standardized test scores of all applicants. Suggested application deadlines are as follows: entry-level master's and accelerated B.S. programs and doctoral program, December 1; traditional undergraduate program, January 15; traditional master's program, February 1; RN-B.S. weekend program, March 15; and doctoral program, February 1. Monthly information sessions are offered at the School of Nursing.

CORRESPONDENCE AND INFORMATION

Office of Enrollment & Student Services
School of Nursing
Virginia Commonwealth University
P.O. Box 980567
Richmond, Virginia 23298-0567
Telephone: 804-828-5171
800-828-9451 (toll-free)
Fax: 804-828-7743
World Wide Web: http://www.nursing.vcu.edu

THE FACULTY

Sadeeka Al-Majid, Assistant Professor; Ph.D., Wisconsin–Madison.

Anne Boyle, Collateral Assistant Professor; Ph.D., Virginia.

Marie Chapin, Clinical Instructor; M.S.N., Virginia Commonwealth.

Richard Cowling, Associate Professor; Ph.D., NYU.

Ann Cox, Collateral Assistant Professor; Ph.D.; Virginia Commonwealth.

Carol Cutler, Collateral Assistant Professor; D.N.Sc., Catholic University.

Anthony DeLellis, Associate Professor and Assistant Dean; Ph.D., Virginia.

Lauren Goodloe, Director of Nursing and Vice President, Patient Care Services; Ph.D., Virginia Commonwealth.

Mary Jo Grap, Associate Professor; Ph.D., Georgia State.

Patricia Gray, Associate Professor and Chair; Ph.D., Utah.

Debra Hearington, Collateral Assistant Professor; M.S., Virginia Commonwealth.

JoAnne Henry, Associate Professor; Ph.D., Virginia.

Sharon Humenick, Professor; Ph.D., Texas at Austin.

Rita Jablonski, Collateral Associate Professor; M.S.N., Pennsylvania.

Edward Kardos, Collateral Instructor and Director of Development; B.S., James Madison.

Phyllis Kritek, Professor; Ph.D., Illinois.

Nancy Langston, Professor and Dean; Ph.D., Georgia State.

Judith Lewis, Associate Professor; Ph.D., Brandeis.

Susan Lipp, Collateral Instructor and Director of Enrollment and Student Services; M.S.N., North Carolina at Chapel Hill.

Nancy McCain, Professor; Ph.D., Alabama at Birmingham.

Martha Moon, Associate Professor; Ph.D., California, San Francisco.

Cindy Munro, Associate Professor; Ph.D., Virginia Commonwealth.

Rita Pickler, Associate Professor and Chair; Ph.D., Virginia.

Gayle Roux, Assistant Professor; Ph.D., Georgia State.

Jeanne Salyer, Associate Professor; Ph.D., Virginia Commonwealth.

Eileen Scaringi, Clinical Assistant Professor; M.S.N., MGH Institute of Health Professions.

Donna Taliaferro, Associate Professor; Ph.D., Texas Woman's.

Inez Tuck, Professor and Chair Dean; Ph.D., North Carolina at Greensboro.

Janet Younger, Professor and Associate Dean; Ph.D., Virginia.

Washburn University
School of Nursing
Topeka, Kansas

THE UNIVERSITY

Washburn University was founded in 1865 as a small private school, but today it has evolved into a comprehensive public university with an enrollment of approximately 6,500 students. The University is governed by its own 9-member Board of Regents. It receives its funding from the city of Topeka, the state of Kansas, student tuition, and private endowments. The University comprises five major academic units: the College of Arts and Sciences and the Schools of Law, Business, Nursing, and Applied Studies. The University offers associate, bachelor's, and master's degrees and the Juris Doctor as well as certificate programs in a number of areas. Diverse educational, cultural, and aesthetic experiences are provided through the University for the citizens of Topeka and northeast Kansas, but the University actually enrolls students from all 105 counties in the state and from across the nation and serves a growing number of international students.

THE SCHOOL OF NURSING

The baccalaureate nursing program was established in 1974 in response to a local and statewide need for more nurses and strong community-based support for baccalaureate nursing education. The nursing program maintains both state and national accreditation. It is designed to prepare women and men for careers in professional nursing. The focus of the program is the study of the individual and family life process from conception through aging in varying stages of health within the context of community and in a variety of settings. The baccalaureate nursing program is based on the belief that each human being is a unitary, living, open system and is continuously engaged in a mutual dynamic process with the environment. The Science of Unitary Human Beings is the conceptual framework upon which the nursing program is based and is derived from the work of nursing theorist Martha E. Rogers. The principles of helicy, resonancy, and integrality provide the basis for understanding the mutual process between human beings and the environment and provide for the organization of knowledge essential to the science and practice of nursing. A nursing curriculum is implemented to assist the learner in viewing the person as a unified whole.

PROGRAMS OF STUDY

The School of Nursing has an enrollment of approximately 200 generic and RN undergraduate students majoring in nursing. This population includes beginning college students, college transfer students, second career students, and adult learners. The upper-division nursing curriculum builds upon the lower-division courses in the humanities and the natural and social sciences. Students enter the nursing major with a foundation of liberal arts and general education. Nursing courses are designed to facilitate the professional development of students and the integration of knowledge. The general education component and supporting courses for the major comprise a total of 65 credit hours and the major in nursing is 59 credit hours, with a total of 124 hours required for the B.S.N. degree. The curriculum is designed to be completed in four academic years. During the final semester of study, the School also offers its students the opportunity to participate in international education in community health nursing. Current affiliating institutions include Queen's University in Belfast, Northern Ireland, and Mikkeli Polytechnic in Savonlinna, Finland. Students from these institutions, in turn, affiliate with Washburn in the areas of community health and acute-care nursing.

Two articulation programs for obtaining the B.S.N. degree are also offered; one for registered nurses from associate degree and hospital diploma programs, and one for practical or vocational nurse graduates. Articulating RN and LPN students meet the same general education requirements as generic students; however, advanced standing and transfer credit allowances are offered for both lower-division and upper-division courses upon evaluation of their prior education and determination of course content equivalence. All nursing courses in the RN to B.S.N. articulation plan are offered via the Internet and Interactive Television (ITV).

In addition to the baccalaureate program, the School of Nursing provides opportunities for continuing education for registered nurses, practical nurses, and mental health technicians. A certificate in school nursing is offered for RN students.

AFFILIATIONS WITH HEALTH-CARE FACILITIES

An advantage of the School is its urban focus and access to Topeka's extensive medical-care complex, which provides excellent facilities for clinical learning experiences. Clinical laboratory takes place in a variety of community clinics, hospitals, public health agencies, nursery schools, Head Start programs, physicians' offices, youth centers, mental health centers, senior centers, and private homes. The normal developmental processes and health needs of individuals, families, and groups form the basis for the selection of student learning experiences throughout Topeka and in surrounding communities. Students have opportunities to work with persons of all ages and diverse cultural backgrounds.

ACADEMIC FACILITIES

The School of Nursing is located in the Kelsey H. and Edna B. Petro Allied Health Center, a 126,000-square-foot modern facility that also houses the Department of Health, Physical Education and Exercise Science and the Department of Athletics. The School of Nursing provides a state-of-the-art science learning center, a health assessment clinic, and a computer laboratory within the Petro building.

Students in the School of Nursing have easy access to Mabee Library, Bennett Computer Center, the Henderson Learning Resources and Instructional Media Center, classroom buildings, and the Memorial Union, Bookstore, and Administration Building. Students are provided open parking spaces on campus.

The University owns and operates an educational television station, KTWU, in a new facility on campus. Semester course offerings are available over the KTWU network, reaching several areas of the state. KTWU-ETV provides both local and PBS programming and frequent national satellite teleconferences. The University's libraries provide automated online catalog and circulation services.

LOCATION

Located in the center of the United States and the heart of the Midwest, Washburn University is also in the geographical center of Topeka, the capital city of Kansas. The city of Topeka radiates a Midwestern friendliness and provides regional shopping, cultural events, and entertainment. The University cooperates with local businesses, health-care organizations, social agencies, educational institutions, and labor and government entities to bring the highest quality educational and recreational opportunities to Washburn students and the citizens of northeast Kansas. Topeka is known for its zoo, civic symphony, civic theater, and art museums as well as for its proximity to Kansas City and major sports programs.

STUDENT SERVICES

A wide variety of student services are offered to complement the academic programs and provide for the students' well-rounded education. Some of the services available to students include the University Child Development Center and Day Care Program; the Center for Learning and Student Success (CLASS), which includes academic enrichment, advising, counseling, placement, and study skills programs; International Student Center; Disabled Student Services; Veteran Affairs; Minority Affairs; Health Services; Campus Ministry; Office of Student Life and Campus Activities; and Computer Services. Student organizations, including Student Nurses of Washburn (SNOW), Sigma Theta Tau honor society for nursing, Phi Kappa Phi, and other honor societies are available to Washburn students. Student publications, intercollegiate athletics, and fraternities and sororities offer extracurricular activities for students. Freshman students can experience living in the state-of-the-art Living Learning Center, a 400-bed dormitory located in the center of campus. Apartment-style housing is available on campus for students beyond their freshman year.

THE NURSING STUDENT GROUP

Students in the School of Nursing are primarily from Kansas. Students range in age from 21 to 51 years old, and the average age is 26. Approximately one third of the students are married and have dependents. Many students commute to campus from areas within the city, some come from as far as 130 miles, and others live on campus. The School of Nursing has an 11 percent minority and 1 percent international student enrollment.

COSTS

Tuition for the 2004–05 academic year was $150 per credit hour with an activity fee of $31 per credit hour for 6 credit hours or more for undergraduate Kansas resident students. For nonresidents, tuition was $305 per credit with an activity fee of $31 per credit hour for 6 credit hours or more. The tuition and fee structure includes parking, the student newspaper and yearbook, admission to all athletic events, and Washburn Student Health Service. Other costs include books, immunizations and laboratory tests required for the health physical, personal health insurance, liability insurance (currently paid by Washburn University for all nursing students), CPR certification, uniforms, laboratory supplies, health assessment equipment, travel to clinical sites, graduation costs (invitations, caps, gowns), photo for School composite, and NCLEX examination and RN licensure application fees. These additional costs are estimated at $2000 per year.

FINANCIAL AID

Nursing students with above-average academic records and/or a demonstrated financial need may apply for scholarships, grants-in-aid, or loans through the University Financial Aid Office. The School of Nursing has a number of nursing scholarship endowments that are awarded annually to nursing students through the School of Nursing.

APPLYING

Students may apply for admission to the nursing major following completion of at least 30 semester hours of specified prerequisite School of Nursing requirements with a minimum cumulative grade point average of 2.7 on a 4.0 scale. Students must be admitted to Washburn University before applying to the School of Nursing. Both the University application form and the School of Nursing application form are available online. The School of Nursing application form is available for downloading. The School of Nursing application must be submitted along with college transcripts to the nursing office by November 1 for consideration for fall admission and by May 15 for spring admission.

The number of students admitted to the major each year is determined by an enrollment management plan and is based on adequacy of clinical placements, availability of teaching faculty, and University resources. Students are selected for admission without discrimination on the basis of sex, race, color, national origin, religion, ancestry, age, disability, or sexual preference.

CORRESPONDENCE AND INFORMATION

Washburn University School of Nursing
1700 College Avenue
Topeka, Kansas 66621
Telephone: 785-231-1010 Ext. 1525
Fax: 785-231-1032
E-mail: nursing@washburn.edu
World Wide Web: http://www.washburn.edu/sonu/

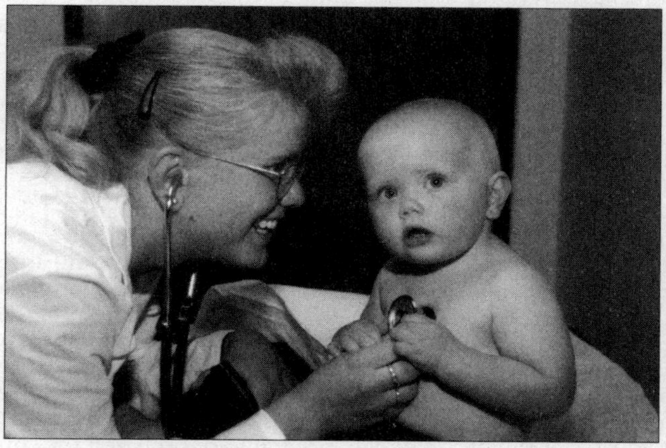

WU nursing student checks baby's heart rate.

Wayne State University
College of Nursing
Detroit, Michigan

THE UNIVERSITY

Wayne State University (WSU) is among the nation's eighty-eight distinguished public and private universities with the Carnegie Research University I classification. The University is accredited by the North Central Association of Colleges and Schools. High-quality educational programs are offered in more than 600 fields of study leading to more than 300 different degrees at the bachelor's, master's, and doctoral levels. WSU's main campus encompasses 184 acres of landscaped, tree-lined pedestrian malls and ninety-eight research and educational buildings of classic and contemporary design. The multicultural urban context of the University provides a rich environment for student learning.

THE COLLEGE OF NURSING

The College of Nursing is regionally, nationally, and internationally recognized for educating graduate and undergraduate students as practitioners and scholars who provide leadership for the profession and discipline of nursing. The College is committed to research and scholarly activity that contributes to the body of knowledge of care and the human health experience in diverse environmental contexts. Moreover, the College excels in the development, application, and dissemination of knowledge to promote the health and well-being of society through teaching, research, and public service. Wayne State University College of Nursing is consistently ranked among the top graduate schools of nursing in the nation (*U.S. News & World Report*). The College of Nursing, established in 1945 as an autonomous academic unit within the University, is accredited by the National League for Nursing Accrediting Commission and the Commission for Collegiate Nursing Education. Innovative program options at the undergraduate, master's, and doctoral levels are available for learners from diverse backgrounds. The focal areas of research excellence at the College are self-care and caregiving and urban health. The College's undergraduate program is ranked seventh in the nation in Gourman's ratings of leading schools of nursing.

PROGRAMS OF STUDY

The College of Nursing offers programs leading to B.S.N., M.S.N., and Ph.D. in nursing degrees. The College offers graduate certificates in transcultural nursing and nursing education. Interdisciplinary graduate certificates in gerontology and infant mental health are also available. Within the baccalaureate program, options are available for applicants with diverse academic experience, including a traditional option for high school graduates, an accelerated option for college graduates with degrees in disciplines other than nursing, and an option for registered nurses. Graduates of the baccalaureate program are prepared for entry into professional practice. For academically talented registered nurses, an accelerated RN-M.S.N. program is available. The M.S.N. program is designed to prepare nurses for advanced nursing practice in the care of culturally diverse individuals, families, groups, and communities in a variety of health-care settings. The program educates nurses to assume leadership roles as nurse practitioners and clinical nurse specialists. The course experiences are designed to enhance the ability of students to think critically and creatively, engage in scientific inquiry, and use knowledge to direct nursing practice. Within the M.S.N. program, students may study within the following areas of specialization: adult primary-care nursing; gerontological nurse practitioner studies; adult acute-care nursing; adult critical-care nursing; advanced practice nursing with women, neonates, children, and midwifery; community health nursing; and psychiatric–mental health nurse practitioner studies.

The Ph.D. in nursing program is designed to prepare researchers and scholars who will provide leadership to the profession and discipline of nursing, the program emphasizes the development of the student's capacity to make significant, original contributions to nursing knowledge. The curriculum focuses on scientific inquiry and consists of a series of nursing seminars that address research methods, knowledge development, and the substantive domains of the discipline. The courses are designed to enhance the ability of students to develop and test new or extant nursing theories and acquire skill in the use of both qualitative and quantitative research methods. Three optional paths toward the Ph.D. degree in nursing are offered: two paths for students entering the program with a bachelor's degree in nursing and one path for those entering with a master's degree in nursing.

AFFILIATIONS WITH HEALTH-CARE FACILITIES

The College of Nursing is affiliated with a wide variety of health-care agencies (approximately 100) within and outside metropolitan Detroit. These include major health-care agencies such as the Detroit Medical Center, Henry Ford Health System, St. John's Health System, and the Oakland County Health Department as well as primary-care settings, ambulatory practice sites, schools, and community health centers.

ACADEMIC FACILITIES

The University library facilities include Purdy/Kresge, Science and Engineering, Shiffman Medical, and David Adamany Undergraduate Libraries. Together these campus libraries provide approximately 2.2 million books, with 400,000 covering health topics. Periodical subscriptions number 12,500, of which 2,500 are health-care related. CINAHL and MEDLINE are available.

Through the Learning Resource Center (LRC), the College of Nursing provides computer-assisted instruction programs, interactive video programs, videotapes, and audiotapes for group or individualized student instruction. Auxiliary to the LRC is the Physical Assessment Learning Laboratory, which provides the facilities for students to acquire and master knowledge and skills in assessment and nursing technology. The Center for Health Research provides services to the faculty and graduate students in the form of consultation services and technical assistance.

LOCATION

Wayne State University is located in the cultural center of Detroit, within walking distance of the Detroit Institute of Arts, the Detroit Historical Museum, Science Museum, International Institute, Museum of African American History, Detroit Medical Center, and the main branch of the Detroit Public Library. With easy access to numerous facilities by car or bus, students can enjoy the Detroit Symphony Orchestra, Broadway shows, and performances by well-known entertainers at the Fisher theater, the Fox theater, and the Masonic Temple. Historic Bricktown, lively Greektown, and the renowned Renaissance Center are also nearby.

STUDENT SERVICES

The College of Nursing has a full array of student services at both the undergraduate and graduate levels. These include academic advising by professional staff and faculty members, academic support services within the College and within the University, placement services, services for students with disabilities, housing, personal counseling, and student activities.

THE NURSING STUDENT GROUP

The College of Nursing enrolls approximately 350 undergraduates, 150 master's students, and 60 doctoral students. The College's undergraduate student population is predominantly from the greater metropolitan area. The graduate programs represent a culturally diverse student population with representation from throughout North America, South America, Europe, and Africa. Graduates of master's and doctoral programs in nursing are in great demand, and employment opportunities are excellent throughout the nation.

COSTS

Undergraduate tuition during the 2004–05 academic year was $187.50 per credit hour for state residents and $431.60 per credit hour for nonresidents. These rates reflect junior/senior, upper-division status. Graduate tuition was $339.15 per credit hour for state residents and $683.35 per credit hour for nonresidents. A $98.50 registration fee and a per-credit-hour omnibus fee of $14.30 for undergraduates or $21.50 for graduate students (for no more than 12 credit hours for undergraduates) were also required.

FINANCIAL AID

Opportunities for assistance with educational expenses are available to students through the University's Office of Scholarship and Financial Aid and the College of Nursing. Federal, state, and institutional funds are available based on financial need and academic merit. Assistance for both full- and part-time study is available through scholarships and fellowships, teaching and research assistantships, professional nurse traineeships, and nursing loans. Early application is essential.

APPLYING

All students must apply to both the University and the College of Nursing. To be considered for admission, undergraduate applicants must complete a minimum of 30 credits with a minimum honor point average of 2.5 in prerequisite courses. Students must file a B.S.N. application for admission, including transcripts, by March 31 for fall term admission. Selection is based on scholarship in prerequisite course work. To qualify for admission, applicants for graduate study must have completed a baccalaureate program in nursing (or the equivalent) accredited by the NLNAC and must have current RN licensure. Selection is based on GRE scores, an autobiographical and goals statement, scholastic achievement, and professional references. Application deadlines for admission to the Master of Science in Nursing program are two months prior to the term of admission. The Ph.D. priority application deadline is four months prior to the start of the term of admission. Applications received after the priority deadline are considered if space is available.

CORRESPONDENCE AND INFORMATION

Office for Student Affairs
College of Nursing
Wayne State University
Detroit, Michigan 48202

Telephone: 313-577-4082
888-837-0847 (toll-free)
Fax: 313-577-6949
World Wide Web: http://www.nursing.wayne.edu

THE FACULTY

Adult Health

Nancy Artinian, Professor; Ph.D., Wayne State, 1988. Stress in spouses and families of coronary bypass surgery patients.

Ramona Benkert, Assistant Professor; Ph.D., Michigan, 2002. Cross-racial health care: Racial identity and cultural mistrust in primary care.

Stephen Cavanagh, Professor and Associate Dean; Ph.D., Texas at Austin, 1987. Stroke, arthritis, and hypertension in the elderly.

Jean E. Davis, Associate Professor; Ph.D., Arizona, 1987. Sleep and sleep disorders in vulnerable populations.

Patricia A. Jarosz, Assistant Professor; Ph.D., Michigan, 2001. Obesity and binge eating.

Helene J. Krouse, Professor and Assistant Dean; Ph.D., Boston College, 1984. Quality of life and sleep problems in allergy and asthma patients.

Marilyn Oermann, Professor; Ph.D., Pittsburgh, 1980. Clinical teaching and evaluation in nursing education.

Rosalind M. Peters, Assistant Professor; Ph.D., Wayne State, 2001. Self-care for hypertension and prevention of kidney disease.

Barbara Pieper, Professor; Ph.D., Wayne State, 1980. Management of pressure ulcers.

Barbara K. Redman, Professor and Dean; Ph.D., Washington (Seattle), 1966. Ethics, patient education, and health policy.

Virginia Rice, Professor; Ph.D., Michigan, 1982. Health promotion and smoking cessation.

April Vallerand, Assistant Professor; Ph.D., Pennsylvania, 1995. Pain management and functional status in patients with chronic pain.

Linda Weglicki, Assistant Professor; Ph.D., Michigan, 1999. Adolescent health: Risk behaviors such as adolescent pregnancy; tobacco prevention and cessation.

Family, Community, and Mental Health

Karen Aroian, Professor; Ph.D., Washington (Seattle), 1988. Immigrant and minority health, cross-cultural research methods.

Cynthia A. Danford, Assistant Professor; Ph.D., California, San Francisco, 2002. Child behavior and health outcomes, parent-child interaction cross-culturally.

Mary J. Denyes, Associate Professor; Ph.D., Michigan, 1980. Self-care nursing research in children's pain.

Naomi E. Ervin, Associate Professor and Assistant Dean; Ph.D., Michigan, 1980. Quality of community health nursing care, access to nursing services.

Judith Floyd, Professor; Ph.D., Wayne State, 1982. Management of sleep problems across the life span.

Linda Ann Lewandowski, Associate Professor; Ph.D., Massachusetts Amherst, 1988. Children and families coping with violence, abuse, and/or trauma.

Judith Fry McComish, Assistant Professor; Ph.D., Wayne State, 1984. Infant mental health, high risk mothers and their infants.

Christine W. Saltzberg, Assistant Professor (clinical); Ph.D., Cornell, 2002. Epistemological reflection and development, ethics and health policy, uncertainty, wisdom and nursing expertise.

Stephanie Myers Schim, Assistant Professor; Ph.D., Wayne State, 1997. Community health, leadership, end-of-life care.

Patricia Thornburg, Clinical Assistant Professor; Ph.D., Cincinnati, 1993. Child health promotion, lived experiences of caregivers.

Deborah S. Walker, Associate Professor; D.N.Sc., UCLA, 1994. Models of prenatal care delivery and perinatal outcomes, especially psychosocial outcomes; evidence-based care and innovative uses of information technology in midwifery clinical care and education.

Feleta Wilson, Associate Professor; Ph.D., Wayne State, 1991. Patients' literacy levels and patient education.

Westminster College
School of Nursing and Health Sciences
Salt Lake City, Utah

THE COLLEGE
Founded in 1875, Westminster College is the only private, comprehensive, liberal arts college in Utah and one of the few in the Intermountain West. The College prepares its 2,500 students for success through a strong foundation of liberal education combined with cutting-edge professional programs at both the undergraduate and graduate levels. Students are exposed to cultural diversity and learn to value differences among people. Westminster College has been ranked as a top-tier institution for value in *U.S. News & World Report* for the tenth consecutive year and is the only institution in Utah to be included in the *Colleges of Distinction* guidebook.

THE SCHOOL OF NURSING AND HEALTH SCIENCES
The School of Nursing and Health Sciences began in 1894 when the Board of Directors established the first training school for nurses in Utah. The School operated as a diploma program out of St. Marks' Hospital, then moved to Westminster College and began offering a Bachelor of Science (B.S.) degree in nursing; the first class graduated in 1972. In 1995, the School added a master's program and began preparing family nurse practitioners (FNP). In 2006, the School (now the School of Nursing and Health Sciences) is scheduled to relocate to the new Health, Wellness, and Athletic Center. Both the bachelor's and master's programs are accredited by the Commission of Collegiate Nursing Education (CCNE).

The curriculum contains core courses in literature, science, psychology, and sociology followed by study in specialty areas such as pediatrics, critical care, obstetrics, and medical-surgical nursing. Students learn critical-thinking and communication skills so they can make important decisions about patient care and promote their well-being.

PROGRAMS OF STUDY
The Bachelor of Science in nursing program prepares professional nurse generalists to meet the health-care needs of society and continue lifelong personal and professional development. Graduates of the program are eligible to take the National Licensing Examination for Registered Nurses (NCLEX-RN) and are prepared to provide professional nursing care based on knowledge derived from theory and research. Students synthesize a broad range of knowledge into the practice of professional nursing and influence the quality of nursing and health care within a variety of practice settings.

This undergraduate program may be completed in four years. Students must complete 128 credits to earn the B.S. degree, including 4 credits in a foreign language, 24 credits in liberal arts courses, 57 in prerequisite science courses, and the rest in nursing courses. Students who qualify for admission to Westminster College may declare a nursing major at that time and be admitted to the nursing program but do not progress into clinical nursing courses until after completing the prerequisite courses, in fall of the sophomore year, with a grade of C or better.

The Master of Science in Nursing (M.S.N.) program prepares nursing professionals for the advanced practice role of family nurse practitioner (FNP). The program enhances students' understanding of theoretical, empirical, and practical knowledge related to advanced practice nursing. Graduates are prepared to establish therapeutic nurse/client relationships, use a holistic approach in health care, and promote the advanced nurse practitioner role in health care.

A full-time student may complete the program within five semesters, including one summer semester. A minimum of 42 semester hours plus 504 hours of clinical practice are required for graduation. Upon graduation, M.S.N. students are eligible to sit for the American Nurse Credential Center (ANCC) or the American Academy of Nurse Practitioners (AANP) certification exams and apply for Utah licensure as advanced practice registered nurses (APRN) with prescriptive authority.

A Family Nurse Practitioner Certificate option is also available for the nationally certified adult nurse practitioner (ANP), gerontological nurse practitioner (GNP), or pediatric nurse practitioner (PNP) who wishes to become a family nurse practitioner (FNP). Students complete a minimum of 19 credits—9 in theory and 10 are clinical practice (420 clinical clock hours). Those students who do not hold a current Utah Advanced Practice License with prescriptive privileges must work with their faculty adviser to prepare an individualized plan of study.

AFFILIATIONS WITH HEALTH-CARE FACILITIES
For clinical experience, students are assigned to leading health-care delivery systems, hospitals, clinics, and community settings to be exposed to high-technology equipment, hands-on procedures, and state-of-the-art information technology. These clinical assignments are located throughout the Salt Lake Valley. Most valuable of all is the experience students gain by giving direct care to patients and their families.

ACADEMIC FACILITIES
The Giovale Library holds an expansive collection of up-to-date books and journals. The library also has the latest in technology, including approximately 95 online databases, e-books, and e-journals; a wireless network; a General Computing Lab with forty-seven workstations, a Writing Center, and an Assistive Technology Lab. The library also has links to an extensive number of education journals and databases as well as other libraries located in Utah. In 2006, the third floor of the Health, Wellness, and Athletic Center is scheduled to become home to the nursing program, providing classrooms, offices, and a simulation laboratory with state-of-the-art mannequins to support experiential learning sessions for students at all levels of nursing education.

LOCATION
The School of Nursing and Health Sciences is only 10 minutes from downtown Salt Lake City and 20 minutes from world-class bouldering. Salt Lake offers ten major ski and snowboard resorts as well as sixteen national parks, monuments, and recreational areas. Backpacking, mountain biking, kayaking, mountain climbing, canyoneering, spelunking, and rafting are all within easy reach of the campus. Salt Lake also has several cultural events, including jazz and alternative music venues, theater, and multiple dance companies. Other arts organizations include the Utah Symphony and Opera and the Sundance Film Festival.

STUDENT SERVICES
Student Nurses of Westminster (SNOW) is the undergraduate student nursing club at Westminster College. Meetings are held

monthly in Malouf Hall. The Health, Wellness, and Athletic Center, the future home of the nursing program, also holds a multiuse fitness complex featuring a gymnasium, a climbing wall, a racquetball court, and a swimming pool. The Shaw Student Center includes the cafeteria, bookstore, Career Resource Center, Campus Ministry, and Campus Counseling offices.

THE NURSING STUDENT GROUP

Graduates are qualified to work in a variety of health-care settings developing health-care plans and providing treatment. They work as independent primary-care providers in underserved areas, as members of multidisciplinary health-care teams in urban settings, in collaboration with physicians in medical practices, clinics, schools, and a variety of community settings. More than 70 percent of students expect to work as family nurse practitioners after graduation. Recent alumni have found positions in nursing education, management, ambulatory care, acute care, advanced practice, research, and flight nursing. In 2004, graduates of the M.S.N. program posted a 100 percent pass rate on the certification exam administered by the ANCC.

COSTS

Undergraduate tuition is $18,192 plus an additional $290 in fees. Room and board, including meals, is $5636 for a double room and $6306 for a single. Graduate tuition is $732 per credit hour, or $11,712 for full-time tuition (16 credit hours). Students also pay a student activity fee of $22 to $42, a student publication fee of $3, and a technology fee of $50 to $100, depending on the number of credits taken in a given semester. Graduate students living on the campus pay $3050 to $3720 per year for a single or double room and $2586 for meals. There is no married housing available on campus.

FINANCIAL AID

Approximately 98 percent of applicants to the undergraduate program receive some form of financial assistance; the average package is more than $12,000. Types of assistance offered to nursing students at the graduate level include loans, tuition reimbursement, and payment plans.

APPLYING

Westminster applicants to the B.S. in nursing program submit an application in the fall of their sophomore year, which should include transcripts from all schools attended, three letters of recommendation, the number of hours completed at Westminster, and a typed letter of intent. Transfer students (not RN or LPN students) must also include a letter of recommendation from their school's dean of nursing. RN and LPN students from another school must be a graduate of an accredited practical nursing program and submit proof of a valid current Utah practical nurse license in good standing.

CORRESPONDENCE AND INFORMATION

Westminster College
School of Nursing and Health Sciences
1840 South 1300 East
Salt Lake City, Utah 84105
Telephone: 801-832-2150
Fax: 801-832-3110
E-mail: admissions@westminster.edu
World Wide Web: http://www.westminstercollege.edu/nursing

THE FACULTY

Marilyn Chan, Associate Professor; Ed.D. candidate, Utah; M.S.N., Utah, 1987; RN, CPNP. Well-child issues, SIDS, child moral development, family kinetic drawings, ADHD-LD, medical ethics, health care and health promotion from infancy through adolescence.

Yeou-Lan Chen, Professor; Ph.D., Utah, 1991; RN. Theoretical foundation of nursing, traditional Chinese medicine, Chinese philosophy and culture, community nursing, complementary medicine/healing.

Carol Cheney, Assistant Professor; M.S.N., Westminster, 1977; APRN. Family practice, emergency medicine, humanitarian services.

Jean A. Dyer, Dean; Ph.D., Maine, 2004; M.S.N., Salem State, 1994. Program development, nursing management, international nursing education, curriculum design, research, theory, learning styles assessment.

Diane Forster-Burke, Professor; M.S., Utah, 1987; RN. Wellness, community health, school nursing, health-related legislation, political activism, complementary health-care practices, high-quality health care, nursing regulation, parish nursing.

Rhonda Lucey, Assistant Professor; M.S.N., Utah, 1997; APRN, ANCC. Health assessment, young adult and women's health, OB/GYN, medical-surgical nursing.

Marsha Morton, Professor; M.A., Iowa, 1981; RN. Gerontological nursing, adult health nursing, transcultural nursing, ethics, HIV/AIDS.

Sheryl Steadman, Assistant Professor; Ph.D., Utah, 2003; APRN. Nursing leadership, community mental health, student teaching/learning, standards of professional nursing practice.

Tao Tan, Instructor; B.S.; AP. Chinese medicine.

Sheri Tesseyman, Assistant Professor; Ph.D. candidate, Utah; M.S.N., Brigham Young, 1989; RN. Community nursing, intensive care, management.

Diane Van Os, Professor; M.S., Utah, 1980. Work with homeless; children's health issues, including abuse and poverty; chronic health problems.

Bonnie Walkingshaw, Professor; M.S., Utah, 1969; RN. Positioning of the acute stroke patient for the prevention of contractures, delineation between technical and professional nursing education, information technology literacy in nursing and nursing education, diabetes, holistic health and wellness.

Stephanie Zimmer, Assistant Professor; M.S.N., Utah, 1988; FNP. Women's health issues across the lifespan; complementary medicine applications; aromatherapy; wellness, prevention, and health education; hospice, grief and loss, and support groups.

Widener University
School of Nursing
Chester, Pennsylvania

THE UNIVERSITY
Founded in 1821, Widener University is a leading metropolitan university that offers a learning environment in which curricula are connected to societal issues through civic engagement. The University provides a unique combination of liberal arts and professional education. It has a distinct student focus in which dynamic teaching, active scholarship, personal attention, and experiential learning are key components. Located in Pennsylvania and Delaware, Widener is composed of eight schools and colleges offering degree programs at the associate, baccalaureate, master's, and doctoral levels. Total enrollment in fall 2004 was 6,694 students, including 2,375 full-time undergraduates, 1,775 graduate students, and 1,878 School of Law students.

THE SCHOOL OF NURSING
Widener's School of Nursing has a long and rich tradition with its origins in the Crozer Foundation of Chester, Pennsylvania. The College of Nursing of the Crozer Foundation was already well established when it became part of Widener in 1970. The School has been continuously accredited by the National League for Nursing Accrediting Commission (NLNAC) since 1972 and continually approved by the Pennsylvania State Board of Nursing. The School maintains two educational sites, one on the Main Campus in Chester and another, for graduate students only, on the Harrisburg Campus. Widener's School of Nursing offers programs for students at the bachelor's, master's, and doctoral level. In addition to the full-time day program, there is an accelerated program for second-degree students, a part-time evening/weekend program, a part-time evening/weekend RN/B.S.N. program, an RN/B.S.N./M.S.N. program, and an RN/M.S.N. accelerated program for RNs with a baccalaureate degree in another discipline. The School's first master's program—in burn, emergency, and trauma—was introduced at Widener in 1980 as the third program of its type and the first in the Northeastern United States. At present, the School offers the Master of Science in Nursing (M.S.N.) and post-master's certificates in the advanced practice specialties of emergency/critical care nursing, adult health nursing, community-based nursing, psychiatric/mental health nursing, nurse educator, and family nurse practitioner. The Doctor of Nursing Science program originated in 1983 and graduated its first student in 1987. An accelerated M.S.N. to Doctor of Nursing Science program, supported by a Department of Health and Human Services Grant, was introduced in fall 2004.

PROGRAMS OF STUDY
The baccalaureate program, leading to licensing as a registered nurse, prepares graduates with a broad education in liberal arts and sciences as well as depth in professional knowledge and skills. In the first two years of the program, undergraduates concentrate on courses in biological and behavioral sciences, humanities, and electives. Upper-level nursing courses build on initial nursing courses as well the integration of knowledge and theories gained from the humanities, social sciences, and natural sciences. Undergraduate students with a cumulative GPA of 3.0 or higher may take up to 6 graduate nursing credits as part of their undergraduate program.

The RN/B.S.N. option, which builds on previous education and experience, is designed for registered nurses employed in the work arena and is scheduled in a part-time weekend format. Registered nurses are granted 31 credits upon matriculation to the School. Nursing courses prepare registered nurses for an expanded professional role to meet the challenges of changing health-care needs. The RN/B.S.N./M.S.N. option is for students who choose to begin graduate course work as undergraduates.

Options for the Master of Science in Nursing are as follows: Adult health nursing (38 credits) focuses on the advanced practice role by providing a broad foundation in health promotion/disease prevention, concepts of illness care and case management, community and environmental issues, and rehabilitation. Community-based nursing (38 credits) explores the advanced practice role and the health-care needs of individuals, the community, and medically underserved populations. Emergency/critical care nursing (38 credits) provides advanced education to enable professional nurses to plan and implement expert nursing care for critically ill clients or those experiencing a health emergency. Clinical competence, a system perspective, and the role of the advanced practice nurse as a change agent are emphasized. Psychiatric/mental health nursing (39 credits) prepares advanced practice nurses for a variety of mental health settings. The nurse educator option (38–41 credits) prepares graduates for faculty roles within a specific clinical specialty. Students can choose the nurse educator option in adult health, community-based, and emergency/critical care nursing specialties. The family nurse practitioner option (46 credits) prepares the professional nurse to be a provider of primary care to individuals and families across their life spans. A holistic approach to management of family health through interdisciplinary collaboration is a primary emphasis of this advanced practice role.

Post-master's certificates in all M.S.N. disciplines are available for students who wish to continue advancing themselves after obtaining the master's degree.

The RN/M.S.N. accelerated program is designed for RNs with a baccalaureate degree in another discipline. These students take, or transfer from another accredited school of nursing, three undergraduate foundation courses before being admitted to the graduate program.

The primary goal of Widener's doctoral program in nursing is the preparation of nurse scholars for educational leadership roles. Graduates are ready to create and disseminate to the public new knowledge gained from disciplined inquiry related to nursing and nursing education. Students in the program have clinical expertise in nursing at the master's level. Requirements for graduation include completion of at least 48 credits of doctoral course work in nursing beyond the master's degree as well as a minimum of 15 credits of dissertation advisement.

AFFILIATIONS WITH HEALTH-CARE FACILITIES
Widener undergraduate students begin their clinical education in the junior year and complete a total of 680 hours of actual clinical experience in a variety of agencies. Clinical experiences for graduate students take place in various acute and primary practice sites in rural and urban settings. Multiple hospitals, schools, and community health-care agencies in Pennsylvania, New Jersey, and Delaware are used for clinical experiences for both graduate and undergraduate students. Examples include Crozer-Chester Medical Center, Mercy Catholic Medical System, the University of Pennsylvania Health System, Children's Hospital of Philadelphia, and A. I. DuPont Institute.

ACADEMIC FACILITIES
Widener's Wolfgram Memorial Library houses close to 250,000 volumes of books, 175,000 microforms, and 2,000 periodicals as well as audiovisual and other nonprint media. Of these, 12,162 are nursing related and 18,135 are health related. Examples of Web-based resources available to students are CINAHL, MEDLINE, PsychInfo, PsycARTICLES, ERIC, Registry of Nursing Research, and the Online Journal of Knowledge Synthesis for Nursing. Widener's Nursing Learning Resource Center, located in the School

of Nursing, gives students practice in simulated clinical settings to prepare them for actual hands-on patient experiences. The Nursing Learning Resource Center houses videotapes, computer-assisted instruction, models, and films. The University also provides state-of-the-art computer labs, and dormitories are wired for Internet use.

LOCATION

Rolling green lawns and an eclectic mixture of architecture characterize Widener's spacious campus in Chester, Pennsylvania. The University is ideally located at the intersection of Route 320 and I-95, near the Philadelphia International Airport, with direct access from I-476. It is just 12 miles southwest of Philadelphia in historic Delaware County. New York City and Washington, D.C., are roughly within a 2-hour drive. The New Jersey beaches and the famous Brandywine River Valley are also nearby. The Harrisburg Campus is located in a suburban setting on 21 acres, 7 miles from downtown Harrisburg.

STUDENT SERVICES

Academic support services include freshman academic advising, tutoring by faculty members and peers, and an early-warning program for incoming freshmen. Individualized writing and reading assistance is provided through the Writing Center and the Reading and Academic Skills Center. A Math Center is also available. The Career Advising and Placement Services (CAPS) Office houses an extensive career library and assists students with career development. Widener has more than sixty student organizations, including the Black Student Union, Commuter Student Organization, Student Government, International Club, and Rotaract Club. In addition, Widener offers NCAA Division III varsity sports and intramural and recreational opportunities for all students.

THE NURSING STUDENT GROUP

Of the more than 535 students in the School of Nursing, 377 are enrolled in the undergraduate program. Undergraduates are expected to be active members of the Widener University Student Nurses' Association (WUSNA), the State Nurses' Association of Pennsylvania (SNAP), and the National Student Nurses' Association (NSNA). These associations provide opportunities for the exchange of ideas and the pursuit of common educational and professional interests. WUSNA officers are elected from the ranks of all classes. Representatives frequently attend the national convention.

All students are eligible for membership in the Eta Beta chapter of the Honor Society of nursing, Sigma Theta Tau International. Candidates for membership are chosen each fall from students enrolled in the baccalaureate and graduate programs.

The School of Nursing Alumni Association (SONAA) actively supports the school with participation in student events and recruitment activities as well as with service and monetary contributions.

COSTS

Tuition costs for the 2004–05 academic year were $23,000 for full-time undergraduate students and $565 per credit for part-time undergraduate nursing students. Graduate nursing tuition was $600 per credit for master's programs and $620 per credit for doctoral study. The cost of room and board ranged from $8100 to $10,700, depending on the accommodations selected. On-campus housing is guaranteed to undergraduates for all four years.

FINANCIAL AID

In 2004, approximately 90 percent of Widener nursing undergraduates received financial aid in the form of grants, loans, scholarships (some specifically for nursing majors), and employment. Eligibility for aid is based on need as well as academic merit.

APPLYING

Admission is competitive. All applicants are evaluated individually to determine their potential for academic success. Widener bases admission decisions on the strength of academic preparation, recommendations, extracurricular activities, personal qualifications, and the pattern of testing on various standardized tests. Since the University has a rolling admissions policy, students are notified of the admission decision soon after their application is completed. Admission into the master's program requires an undergraduate degree, a minimum GPA of 3.0 in the bachelor's program, and a current license as a registered nurse. Admission into the doctoral program requires a minimum GPA of 3.5 from an accredited master's program in nursing, a current license as a registered nurse, a graduate statistics course with a grade of at least C, and graduate courses in nursing theories and conceptional models.

CORRESPONDENCE AND INFORMATION:

Marguerite M. Barbiere, Dean
School of Nursing
Widener University
One University Place
Chester, Pennsylvania 19013-5792
Telephone: 610-499-4214
Fax: 610-499-4216
E-mail: Marguerite.M.Barbiere@widener.edu

Jane Brennan, Assistant Dean
Undergraduate Program
Telephone: 610-499-4210
E-mail: Jane.M.Brennan@widener.edu

Mary Walker, Assistant Dean
Graduate Programs
Telephone: 610-499-4208
E-mail: Mary.B.Walker@widener.edu

Ann M. Herring, Director of Special Programs
RN/B.S.N./M.S.N. Programs
Telephone: 610-499-4209
E-mail: amherring@mail.widener.edu

THE FACULTY

Marguerite M. Barbiere, Ed.D., Dean of Nursing and Professor.
Jane M. Brennan, D.N.Sc., Assistant Dean for Undergraduate Programs and Associate Professor.
Mary B. Walker, Ed.D., Assistant Dean for Graduate Programs and Associate Professor.

Lois R. Allen, Ph.D., Professor.
Mary Baumberger-Henry, D.N.Sc., Assistant Professor.
Elizabeth W. Bayley, Ph.D., Professor.
Lynne C. Borucki, Ph.D., Assistant Professor.
Tammie Calabrese, M.S.N., Lecturer.
Norma Jean Colby, M.S.N., Lecturer.
Shirlee Drayton-Brooks, Ph.D., CRNP, Director of the Family Nurse Practitioner Program.
Mary Francis, M.S.N., Lecturer.
Lynn E. Kelly, Ph.D., Associate Professor.
Judith Ann Kilpatrick, D.N.Sc., Assistant Professor.
Anne M. Krouse, Ph.D., Assistant Professor.
Margaret A. Miller, Ph.D., Associate Professor.
Marye O'Reilly-Knapp, D.N.Sc., Assistant Professor.
Barbara J. Patterson, Ph.D., Associate Professor.
Joyce Rasin, Ph.D., Associate Professor
Janice L. Reilly, Ed.D., Assistant Professor.
Mary Ellen Santucci, D.N.Sc., Assistant Professor
Rose Schwartz, M.S.N., Visiting Lecturer.
Doris C. Vallone, Ph.D., Assistant Professor.
Juanita Watson, Ph.D., Assistant Professor.
Joan Webb, M.S.N., Lecturer.
Andrea M. Wolf, M.S.N., CRNP, Lecturer.

Wright State University
College of Nursing and Health
Dayton, Ohio

WRIGHT STATE UNIVERSITY™

THE UNIVERSITY

Wright State University is a comprehensive, state-assisted institution that was founded in 1964 and was granted full university status in 1967. It serves nearly 16,000 students in 100 undergraduate programs and nearly fifty master's, Ph.D., and professional degree programs. The University is composed of eight academic units: Business, Education and Human Services, Engineering and Computer Science, Liberal Arts, Medicine, Nursing and Health, Professional Psychology, and Science and Mathematics.

Wright State is a metropolitan university. It is committed to providing leadership in addressing the educational, social, and cultural needs of the Greater Miami Valley and to promoting the economic and technological development of the region through a strong program of basic and applied research and professional service. Wright State is dedicated to excellence in teaching, research, and service.

Wright State seeks to enroll achievement-oriented traditional and nontraditional students and maintains an open admissions policy for undergraduates.

THE COLLEGE OF NURSING AND HEALTH

The College of Nursing and Health's baccalaureate program began in 1973, and the first students were admitted to the master's program in 1978. The College currently enrolls approximately 600 undergraduate and 200 graduate students.

In 1984, the College entered into a collaborative agreement with the Division of Nursing at Miami Valley Hospital to form a Center for Excellence in Nursing. Through collaboration with nursing staff members, this agreement affords unique opportunities for research, clinical practice, and education for students and the faculty.

The College of Nursing and Health reflects the broader mission of the University by providing excellent educational programs that prepare nurses for a dynamic health-care environment. As part of a metropolitan university, the College accepts the obligation to extend its resources to the surrounding region. It provides leadership to address regional health needs and forms partnerships with other disciplines, institutions, and organizations to cooperatively address health-related community problems. The clinical education programs are structured to provide students with a solid foundation in health assessment, health promotion, community-based practice, and primary health-care concepts.

All of the College's full-time tenure-track faculty members are doctorally prepared. Faculty members teaching in the B.S.N. and M.S. programs have a wealth of clinical expertise. In addition, students gain a breadth and depth of knowledge from nurses serving as preceptors for clinical practicum courses.

PROGRAMS OF STUDY

The College of Nursing and Health offers the B.S.N. degree, the M.S. degree, a joint M.S./M.B.A. degree in conjunction with the Raj Soin College of Business, and a school nurse certificate program in collaboration with the College of Education and Human Services. For RNs with a baccalaureate degree in a traditional discipline area other than nursing, there is a bridge program that allows students to earn the master's degree after completion of a limited number of undergraduate nursing courses. The B.S.N. and M.S. programs are accredited by the National League for Nursing Accrediting Commission (NLNAC), and the M.B.A. program is accredited by AACSB International–The Association to Advance Collegiate Schools of Business.

The baccalaureate program emphasizes health and well-being across the life span and prepares graduates for entry into professional practice as generalists. The program provides entry options for both prelicensure students and RN students who have completed an associate degree or diploma program in nursing. RNs are offered a program that includes transition courses that integrate their previous learning with the new knowledge provided in a baccalaureate program. Courses for RNs are offered on campus and broadcast to the outreach off-campus sites one day a week or online via the Internet. The program may be completed in two calendar years of full-time study by RNs with an associate degree. The baccalaureate program accommodates both full-time and part-time students.

The master's program educates nurses for advanced leadership roles in practice and administration as well as for doctoral study in nursing. The curriculum offers students the opportunity to prepare for roles as clinical nurse specialists in adult health or community health; nurse practitioners in the family nurse practitioner, acute-care nurse practitioner, or pediatric nurse practitioner majors, some of which have an option for post-master's study; school nurses; or nurse administrators in the nurse administrator major or the dual-degree (M.S./M.B.A.) program.

The master's program accommodates both full-time and part-time students, with most classes offered in the late afternoon and evening. The sequence of course offerings is flexible. Students must complete all requirements for the degree within five years.

ACADEMIC FACILITIES

The College of Nursing and Health is housed in University Hall. Clinical instructional facilities are abundant and varied. The College has contracts with more than 200 agencies in the area, including hospitals, rehabilitation centers, county health departments, nursing homes, school systems, senior citizen centers, day-care centers, and other community-based settings, which can be used for clinical experiences and research.

For research, both the Dunbar Library and the Fordham Health Sciences Library provide abundant resources. The Dunbar Library also provides media production services and facilities. The University's Statistical Consulting Center and the College's Center for Nursing and Health Research provide support for research design and data analysis. The College also has a computer laboratory that includes interactive video programs for classroom and independent learning.

LOCATION

The campus is located in a rural-suburban setting 10 miles east of Dayton, a business and manufacturing center with a metropolitan population approaching 1 million. The University is adjacent to Wright Patterson Air Force Base, which is a center for Air Force research and procurement. A variety of recreational, cultural, art, science, and business activities are available in the metropolitan area. Transportation to the campus via RTA is available from throughout the Miami Valley. The Dayton International Airport and downtown are less than 25 miles from the campus.

STUDENT SERVICES

The University has many resources and a variety of services for both undergraduate and graduate students. Since Wright State is a leader in providing support and accessibility to students with disabilities, a broad range of physical and academic services are available. In addition, Wright State has an International Student Program, a Child Development Center, an on-campus bookstore, Campus Ministry, six housing communities, dining services, Bolinga Cultural Resources Center, Student Health Services, Counseling Services, and the Nutter Center for sports and recreation.

THE NURSING STUDENT GROUP

There are approximately 600 undergraduate students and 200 graduate students in the College of Nursing and Health. Many of the undergraduate students are employed at least part-time and attend school full-time. Most graduate students are employed full-time in area health-care agencies in a variety of clinical and administrative positions and pursue the part-time plan.

COSTS

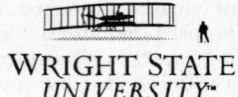

Tuition for undergraduate students in 2004–05 was $197 per credit hour (in-state) and $381 per credit hour (out-of-state); full-time tuition for 11 to 18 credit hours was $2159 per quarter (in-state) and $4164 per quarter (out-of-state). Tuition for graduate students was $271 per credit hour (in-state) and $458 per credit hour (out-of-state); full-time tuition for 11 to 18 credit hours was $2884 per quarter (in-state) and $4889 per quarter (out-of-state). Other expenses include books, immunizations, uniforms, insurance, and travel to clinical sites.

FINANCIAL AID

A number of scholarships based on academic excellence, as well as grants based on financial need, are available for undergraduate students. Graduate assistantships and Professional Nurse Traineeships are available for students who meet the criteria. Graduate academic fellowships, awarded on the basis of academic merit, are also available. Need-based Federal Perkins and Federal Stafford Student Loans are available to students who qualify.

APPLYING

To be eligible for admission, undergraduate students must be matriculated at the University, complete all designated prerequisite courses with a grade of C or better, and have a cumulative GPA of at least 2.5.

Graduate applicants must have an overall undergraduate GPA of at least 3.0 or an overall GPA of at least 2.7 with a 3.0 or better in the last 90 quarter hours (60 semester hours); have a B.S.N. degree from a college or university that is accredited by a nationally recognized body for nursing education accreditation or a bachelor's degree in a field other than nursing and be a registered nurse with selected support and professional nursing bridge courses; and have an Ohio RN license. All application materials for fall quarter should be submitted by April 15. Applications received after that date are considered on a space-available basis.

CORRESPONDENCE AND INFORMATION

Office of Admissions
E148 Student Union
Wright State University
3640 Colonel Glenn Highway
Dayton, Ohio 45435
Telephone: 937-775-5700

School of Graduate Studies
E344 Student Union
Wright State University
3640 Colonel Glenn Highway
Dayton, Ohio 45435
Telephone: 937-775-2976

THE FACULTY

Janice Belcher, Associate Professor; M.S., Ohio State (mental health); Ph.D., Virginia Commonwealth (nursing administration).

Barbara Bogan, Assistant Professor; M.S., Ohio State (nursing).

Ann Bowling, Clinical Instructor; M.S.N., Cincinnati (pediatric nurse practitioner).

S. Jean Budding, Clinical Assistant Professor; M.S., Wright State (nursing administration).

Annette Canfield, Clinical Instructor; M.S., Wright State (education).

Candace Cherrington, Assistant Professor; M.N., Kansas (adult health); Ph.D., Ohio State (nursing).

Donna Miles Curry, Associate Professor; M.S.N., Saint Louis (nursing of children); Ph.D., Ohio State (family relations and human development).

Latanya Davis, Clinical Instructor; M.S., Wright State (family nurse practitioner).

Jane Doorley, Clinical Assistant Professor; M.S., Wright State (rehabilitation/community health nursing).

Kathi Flanders, Clinical Instructor; M.S.N., Cincinnati (family nurse practitioner).

Barbara Fowler, Professor and Director of Research; M.S.N., Cincinnati (parent/child nursing); Ed.D., Cincinnati (curriculum and instruction, nursing education); D.N.Sc., Rush (community nurse practitioner).

Cynthia Gibbons, Assistant Professor; M.S.N., Kentucky (parent/child nursing); Ph.D., Pittsburgh (nursing).

Margaret Clark Graham, Professor; M.S.N., Vanderbilt (family nurse practitioner); Ph.D., Ohio State (community health education).

Bobbe Gray, Assistant Professor; M.S.N., (maternal nursing), Ph.D., (nursing), Case Western Reserve.

Laura Herbert, Clinical Instructor; M.S., Wright State (community health nursing).

Carol Holdcraft, Assistant Professor and Assistant Dean; M.S.N., Cincinnati (adult psychiatric nursing); D.N.S., Indiana (nursing).

Cindra Holland, Clinical Instructor; M.S., Wright State (adult health).

Jane Hutcheson, Clinical Instructor; M.S., Wright State (rehabilitation/community health).

Catherine Johnson, Clinical Assistant Professor; M.S., Ohio State (nursing); M.S., Wright State (family nurse practitioner).

Lynne Kelley, Clinical Assistant Professor; M.P.H., Emory (health policy); M.S.N., Cincinnati (maternal-child health).

Judie Lincks, Clinical Instructor; M.S., Wright State (nursing administration).

Yueh-Feng Lu, Assistant Professor; M.S., Wright State (adult health); Ph.D., Case Western Reserve (nursing).

Mary Lynd, Assistant Professor; Ph.D., Texas Woman's (nursing).

Gina Maiocco, Assistant Professor; Ph.D., Utah (nursing).

Patricia Martin, Professor and Dean; M.S., Wright State (rehabilitation/community health nursing); Ph.D., Case Western Reserve (nursing).

Gail Moddeman, Assistant Professor; M.S., Wright State (nursing administration); Ph.D., Kentucky (nursing).

Virginia Nehring, Associate Professor; M.S.N., Yale (community health); Ph.D., Walden (nursing research, education).

Robin Osterman, Clinical Instructor; M.S.N., Cincinnati (psychiatric nursing).

Susan Praeger, Professor; M.S., New York Medical College (nursing); Ed.D., Northern Colorado (humanistic nursing education).

Cynthia Price, Clinical Instructor; M.S., Ball State (nursing leadership).

Leatha Ross, Clinical Instructor; M.S., Wright State (family nurse practitioner).

Kristine A. Scordo, Associate Professor; M.S., Ohio State (cardiovascular nursing); Ph.D., Ohio State (cardiac physiology).

Elizabeth Sorensen, Assistant Professor; M.S., New Hampshire (nursing administration); Ph.D., Ohio State (nursing research).

Ann Stalter, Clinical Instructor; M.S., Wright State (nursing administration).

Kim Stewart, Clinical Instructor; M.S., Wright State (adult health nursing).

Alice Teall, Clinical Assistant Professor; M.S., Wright State (family nurse practitioner).

Martha Teter, Clinical Assistant Professor; M.S., Wright State (nursing, family nurse practitioner); M.S., Dayton (education/counseling).

June Tierney, Clinical Assistant Professor; M.S.N., Cincinnati (psychiatric nursing).

Rose Tobin, Clinical Instructor; M.S., Adelphi (parent-child nursing).

Patricia Vermeersch, Assistant Professor; M.S., Case Western Reserve (gerontological nursing); Ph.D., Case Western Reserve (clinical nursing research).

Tara Withrow, Clinical Instructor; M.S.N., Xavier (nursing administration).

Joyce Zurmehly, Assistant Professor; M.S.N., Bellarmine (nursing education); Ph.D., Walden (health services).

INDEXES

Baccalaureate Programs

Accelerated Baccalaureate

Alabama
University of South Alabama, College of Nursing, *Mobile* (BSN)

Arizona
Arizona State University, College of Nursing, *Tempe* (BSN)
Grand Canyon University, Samaritan College of Nursing, *Phoenix* (BSN)
Northern Arizona University, Department of Nursing, *Flagstaff* (BSN)
University of Phoenix–Phoenix Campus, College of Health and Human Services, *Phoenix* (BSN)
University of Phoenix–Southern Arizona Campus, College of Health and Human Services, *Tucson* (BSN)

California
Azusa Pacific University, School of Nursing, *Azusa* (BSN)
California State University, Long Beach, Department of Nursing, *Long Beach* (BSN)
Mount St. Mary's College, Department of Nursing, *Los Angeles* (BSN)
University of Phoenix–Northern California Campus, College of Health and Human Services, *Pleasanton* (BSN)
University of Phoenix–Sacramento Campus, College of Health and Human Services, *Sacramento* (BSN)
University of Phoenix–San Diego Campus, College of Health and Human Services, *San Diego* (BSN)

Colorado
Regis University, Department of Nursing, *Denver* (BSN)
University of Northern Colorado, School of Nursing, *Greeley* (BS)
University of Phoenix–Southern Colorado Campus, College of Health and Human Services, *Colorado Springs* (BSN)

District of Columbia
The Catholic University of America, School of Nursing, *Washington* (BSN)
Howard University, Division of Nursing, *Washington* (BSN)

Florida
Barry University, School of Nursing, *Miami Shores* (BSN)
University of Miami, School of Nursing, *Coral Gables* (BSN)
University of Phoenix–Orlando Campus, College of Health and Human Services, *Maitland* (BSN)
University of Phoenix–Tampa Campus, College of Health and Human Services, *Tampa* (BSN)
University of South Florida, College of Nursing, *Tampa* (BS)

Georgia
Georgia State University, School of Nursing, *Atlanta* (BS)
Kennesaw State University, School of Nursing, *Kennesaw* (BSN)

Hawaii
Hawai'i Pacific University, School of Nursing, *Honolulu* (BSN)

Idaho
Boise State University, Department of Nursing, *Boise* (BS)

Illinois
Loyola University Chicago, Marcella Niehoff School of Nursing, *Chicago* (BSN)
Southern Illinois University Edwardsville, School of Nursing, *Edwardsville* (BS)

Indiana
Saint Mary's College, Department of Nursing, *Notre Dame* (BS)
Valparaiso University, College of Nursing, *Valparaiso* (BSN)

Iowa
Allen College, Program in Nursing, *Waterloo* (BSN)
Mercy College of Health Sciences, Division of Nursing, *Des Moines* (BSN)

Kansas
MidAmerica Nazarene University, Division of Nursing, *Olathe* (BSN)

Louisiana
University of Louisiana at Monroe, Nursing, *Monroe* (BS)

Maine
University of Maine, School of Nursing, *Orono* (BSN)
University of Maine at Fort Kent, Department of Nursing, *Fort Kent* (BSN)

Massachusetts
Regis College, Department of Nursing, *Weston* (BSN)
Simmons College, Department of Nursing, *Boston* (BS)

Michigan
Northern Michigan University, College of Nursing and Allied Health Science, *Marquette* (BSN)
University of Phoenix–West Michigan Campus, College of Health and Human Services, *Grand Rapids* (BSN)

Missouri
Graceland University, School of Nursing, *Independence* (BSN)
Research College of Nursing, College of Nursing, *Kansas City* (BSN)
Saint Louis University, School of Nursing, *St. Louis* (BSN)
University of Missouri–St. Louis, College of Nursing, *St. Louis* (BSN)
William Jewell College, Department of Nursing, *Liberty* (BS)

Nebraska
Clarkson College, Department of Nursing, *Omaha* (BSN)
University of Nebraska Medical Center, College of Nursing, *Omaha* (BSN)

Nevada
University of Nevada, Reno, Orvis School of Nursing, *Reno* (BSN)

New Jersey
Fairleigh Dickinson University, Metropolitan Campus, Henry P. Becton School of Nursing and Allied Health, *Teaneck* (BSN)

New Mexico
University of Phoenix–New Mexico Campus, College of Health and Human Services, *Albuquerque* (BSN)

New York
Adelphi University, School of Nursing, *Garden City* (BS)
Hartwick College, Department of Nursing, *Oneonta* (BS)
Mount Saint Mary College, Division of Nursing, *Newburgh* (BSN)
New York University, Division of Nursing, *New York* (BS)

Ohio
Cleveland State University, Department of Nursing, *Cleveland* (BSN)
Kent State University, College of Nursing, *Kent* (BSN)

Oklahoma
Southern Nazarene University, School of Nursing, *Bethany* (BS)
University of Phoenix–Oklahoma City Campus, College of Health and Human Services, *Oklahoma City* (BSN)
University of Phoenix–Tulsa Campus, College of Health and Human Services, *Tulsa* (BSN)

Oregon
Oregon Health & Science University, School of Nursing, *Portland* (BS)

Pennsylvania
College Misericordia, Department of Nursing, *Dallas* (BSN)
Holy Family University, School of Nursing and Allied Health Professions, *Philadelphia* (BSN)
Thomas Jefferson University, Department of Nursing, *Philadelphia* (BSN)
University of Pennsylvania, School of Nursing, *Philadelphia* (BSN)

Puerto Rico
Inter American University of Puerto Rico, Metropolitan Campus, Carmen Torres de Tiburcio School of Nursing, *San Juan* (BSN)

South Carolina
Lander University, School of Nursing, *Greenwood* (BSN)
Medical University of South Carolina, College of Nursing, *Charleston* (BSN)

South Dakota
South Dakota State University, College of Nursing, *Brookings* (BS)

Tennessee
Belmont University, School of Nursing, *Nashville* (BSN)
Carson-Newman College, Department of Nursing, *Jefferson City* (BSN)
The University of Memphis, Loewenberg School of Nursing, *Memphis* (BSN)
The University of Tennessee Health Science Center, College of Nursing, *Memphis* (BSN)

Texas
Texas Christian University, Harris School of Nursing, *Fort Worth* (BSN)

Virginia
Hampton University, Department of Nursing, *Hampton* (BS)
Marymount University, School of Health Professions, *Arlington* (BSN)
Old Dominion University, Department of Nursing, *Norfolk* (BSN)

Wisconsin
Bellin College of Nursing, Nursing Program, *Green Bay* (BSN)
University of Wisconsin-Oshkosh, College of Nursing, *Oshkosh* (BSN)

Alberta
University of Calgary, Faculty of Nursing, *Calgary* (BN)

Newfoundland and Labrador
Memorial University of Newfoundland, School of Nursing, *St. John's* (BN)

Nova Scotia

Dalhousie University, School of Nursing, *Halifax* (BScN)

St. Francis Xavier University, Department of Nursing, *Antigonish* (BScN)

Saskatchewan

University of Saskatchewan, College of Nursing, *Saskatoon* (BSN)

Accelerated Baccalaureate for Second Degree

Alabama

Auburn University, School of Nursing, *Auburn University* (BSN)

Arizona

Arizona State University, College of Nursing, *Tempe* (BSN)

Northern Arizona University, Department of Nursing, *Flagstaff* (BSN)

The University of Arizona, College of Nursing, *Tucson* (BSN)

Arkansas

University of Arkansas for Medical Sciences, College of Nursing, *Little Rock* (BSN)

California

California State University, Long Beach, Department of Nursing, *Long Beach* (BSN)

Loma Linda University, School of Nursing, *Loma Linda* (BS)

Colorado

University of Colorado at Colorado Springs, Beth-El College of Nursing and Health Sciences, *Colorado Springs* (BSN)

Connecticut

Fairfield University, School of Nursing, *Fairfield* (BS)

Quinnipiac University, Department of Nursing, *Hamden* (BSN)

Saint Joseph College, Department of Nursing, *West Hartford* (BS)

Delaware

University of Delaware, Department of Nursing, *Newark* (BSN)

District of Columbia

Georgetown University, School of Nursing and Health Studies, *Washington* (BSN)

Howard University, Division of Nursing, *Washington* (BSN)

Florida

Barry University, School of Nursing, *Miami Shores* (BSN)

Florida Atlantic University, College of Nursing, *Boca Raton* (BSN)

Florida International University, School of Nursing, *Miami* (BSN)

Jacksonville University, School of Nursing, *Jacksonville* (BSN)

University of Central Florida, School of Nursing, *Orlando* (BSN)

University of Miami, School of Nursing, *Coral Gables* (BSN)

University of North Florida, School of Nursing, *Jacksonville* (BSN)

Georgia

Emory University, Nell Hodgson Woodruff School of Nursing, *Atlanta* (BSN)

Kennesaw State University, School of Nursing, *Kennesaw* (BSN)

Idaho

Idaho State University, Department of Nursing, *Pocatello* (BSN)

Illinois

Blessing-Rieman College of Nursing, *Quincy* (BSN)

Lewis University, Program in Nursing, *Romeoville* (BSN)

Rush University, College of Nursing, *Chicago* (BSN)

West Suburban College of Nursing, *Oak Park* (BSN)

Indiana

Ball State University, School of Nursing, *Muncie* (BS)

Indiana University-Purdue University Indianapolis, School of Nursing, *Indianapolis* (BSN)

Indiana University South Bend, Division of Nursing and Health Professions, *South Bend* (BSN)

Marian College, Department of Nursing and Nutritional Science, *Indianapolis* (BSN)

Purdue University, School of Nursing, *West Lafayette* (BS)

University of Southern Indiana, School of Nursing and Health Professions, *Evansville* (BSN)

Iowa

Allen College, Program in Nursing, *Waterloo* (BSN)

Mercy College of Health Sciences, Division of Nursing, *Des Moines* (BSN)

Kansas

MidAmerica Nazarene University, Division of Nursing, *Olathe* (BSN)

Kentucky

Bellarmine University, Donna and Allan Lansing School of Nursing and Health Sciences, *Louisville* (BSN)

Northern Kentucky University, Department of Nursing, *Highland Heights* (BSN)

Spalding University, School of Nursing, *Louisville* (BSN)

University of Louisville, School of Nursing, *Louisville* (BSN)

Louisiana

University of Louisiana at Lafayette, College of Nursing, *Lafayette* (BSN)

Maine

University of Southern Maine, College of Nursing and Health Professions, *Portland* (BS)

Maryland

The Johns Hopkins University, School of Nursing, *Baltimore* (BS)

Salisbury University, Program in Nursing, *Salisbury* (BS)

University of Maryland, School of Nursing, *Baltimore* (BSN)

Villa Julie College, Nursing Division, *Stevenson* (BS)

Massachusetts

Curry College, Division of Nursing, *Milton* (BS)

Regis College, Department of Nursing, *Weston* (BSN)

Simmons College, Department of Nursing, *Boston* (BS)

University of Massachusetts Amherst, School of Nursing, *Amherst* (BS)

Michigan

Michigan State University, College of Nursing, *East Lansing* (BSN)

Saginaw Valley State University, Crystal M. Lange College of Nursing and Health Sciences, *University Center* (BSN)

University of Michigan, School of Nursing, *Ann Arbor* (BSN)

Wayne State University, College of Nursing, *Detroit* (BSN)

Minnesota

Concordia College, Department of Nursing, *Moorhead* (BA)

Minnesota State University Mankato, School of Nursing, *Mankato* (BS)

Missouri

Graceland University, School of Nursing, *Independence* (BSN)

Lester L. Cox College of Nursing and Health Sciences, Department of Nursing, *Springfield* (BSN)

Research College of Nursing, College of Nursing, *Kansas City* (BSN)

Saint Louis University, School of Nursing, *St. Louis* (BSN)

University of Missouri-Columbia, Sinclair School of Nursing, *Columbia* (BSN)

Nebraska

Creighton University, School of Nursing, *Omaha* (BSN)

Nebraska Methodist College, Department of Nursing, *Omaha* (BSN)

University of Nebraska Medical Center, College of Nursing, *Omaha* (BSN)

New Jersey

Fairleigh Dickinson University, Metropolitan Campus, Henry P. Becton School of Nursing and Allied Health, *Teaneck* (BSN)

Seton Hall University, College of Nursing, *South Orange* (BSN)

University of Medicine and Dentistry of New Jersey, School of Nursing, *Newark* (BSN)

William Paterson University of New Jersey, Department of Nursing, *Wayne* (BSN)

New Mexico

New Mexico State University, Department of Nursing, *Las Cruces* (BSN)

University of New Mexico, College of Nursing, *Albuquerque* (BSN)

New York

Adelphi University, School of Nursing, *Garden City* (BS)

The College of New Rochelle, School of Nursing, *New Rochelle* (BSN)

Columbia University, School of Nursing, *New York* (BS)

Dominican College, Division of Nursing, *Orangeburg* (BSN)

Hartwick College, Department of Nursing, *Oneonta* (BS)

New York University, Division of Nursing, *New York* (BS)

Pace University, Lienhard School of Nursing, *New York* (BS)

State University of New York Downstate Medical Center, College of Nursing, *Brooklyn* (BS)

University at Buffalo, The State University of New York, School of Nursing, *Buffalo* (BS)

University of Rochester, School of Nursing, *Rochester* (BS)

North Carolina

Duke University, School of Nursing, *Durham* (BSN)

The University of North Carolina at Chapel Hill, School of Nursing, *Chapel Hill* (BSN)

Ohio

Capital University, School of Nursing, *Columbus* (BSN)

Cleveland State University, Department of Nursing, *Cleveland* (BSN)

Kent State University, College of Nursing, *Kent* (BSN)

The University of Akron, College of Nursing, *Akron* (BSN)

Ursuline College, The Breen School of Nursing, *Pepper Pike* (BSN)

Wright State University, College of Nursing and Health, *Dayton* (BSN)

Oklahoma

Oklahoma City University, Kramer School of Nursing, *Oklahoma City* (BSN)

Oregon
Linfield College, School of Nursing, *McMinnville* (BSN)

Pennsylvania
College Misericordia, Department of Nursing, *Dallas* (BSN)
Drexel University, College of Nursing and Health Professions, *Philadelphia* (BSN)
Duquesne University, School of Nursing, *Pittsburgh* (BSN)
Edinboro University of Pennsylvania, Department of Nursing, *Edinboro* (BS)
Temple University, Department of Nursing, *Philadelphia* (BSN)
Thomas Jefferson University, Department of Nursing, *Philadelphia* (BSN)
University of Pennsylvania, School of Nursing, *Philadelphia* (BSN)
University of Pittsburgh, School of Nursing, *Pittsburgh* (BSN)
Villanova University, College of Nursing, *Villanova* (BSN)
Waynesburg College, Department of Nursing, *Waynesburg* (BSN)
Wilkes University, Department of Nursing, *Wilkes-Barre* (BS)

South Carolina
Lander University, School of Nursing, *Greenwood* (BSN)

Tennessee
Belmont University, School of Nursing, *Nashville* (BSN)
East Tennessee State University, College of Nursing, *Johnson City* (BSN)
Union University, School of Nursing, *Jackson* (BSN)
The University of Memphis, Loewenberg School of Nursing, *Memphis* (BSN)
The University of Tennessee Health Science Center, College of Nursing, *Memphis* (BSN)

Texas
Texas A&M University–Corpus Christi, School of Nursing and Health Sciences, *Corpus Christi* (BSN)
Texas Christian University, Harris School of Nursing, *Fort Worth* (BSN)
The University of Texas Health Science Center at Houston, School of Nursing, *Houston* (BSN)
The University of Texas Medical Branch, School of Nursing, *Galveston* (BSN)

Virginia
George Mason University, College of Nursing and Health Science, *Fairfax* (BSN)
Marymount University, School of Health Professions, *Arlington* (BSN)
Norfolk State University, Department of Nursing, *Norfolk* (BSN)
Shenandoah University, Division of Nursing, *Winchester* (BSN)
Virginia Commonwealth University, School of Nursing, *Richmond* (BS)

West Virginia
West Virginia University, School of Nursing, *Morgantown* (BSN)

Wisconsin
University of Wisconsin–Milwaukee, College of Nursing, *Milwaukee* (BSN)
University of Wisconsin–Oshkosh, College of Nursing, *Oshkosh* (BSN)

Alberta
University of Calgary, Faculty of Nursing, *Calgary* (BN)

Nova Scotia
Dalhousie University, School of Nursing, *Halifax* (BScN)
St. Francis Xavier University, Department of Nursing, *Antigonish* (BScN)

Accelerated LPN to Baccalaureate

California
San Francisco State University, School of Nursing, *San Francisco* (BSN)

District of Columbia
Howard University, Division of Nursing, *Washington* (BSN)

Illinois
Bradley University, Department of Nursing, *Peoria* (BSN)
MacMurray College, Department of Nursing, *Jacksonville* (BSN)

Kansas
MidAmerica Nazarene University, Division of Nursing, *Olathe* (BSN)

Michigan
Northern Michigan University, College of Nursing and Allied Health Science, *Marquette* (BSN)

New York
Dominican College, Division of Nursing, *Orangeburg* (BSN)

Ohio
Ursuline College, The Breen School of Nursing, *Pepper Pike* (BSN)

Pennsylvania
Edinboro University of Pennsylvania, Department of Nursing, *Edinboro* (BS)
The University of Scranton, Department of Nursing, *Scranton* (BS)
Wilkes University, Department of Nursing, *Wilkes-Barre* (BS)

Virginia
George Mason University, College of Nursing and Health Science, *Fairfax* (BSN)
Marymount University, School of Health Professions, *Arlington* (BSN)
Norfolk State University, Department of Nursing, *Norfolk* (BSN)

West Virginia
Alderson-Broaddus College, Department of Nursing, *Philippi* (BSN)

Nova Scotia
St. Francis Xavier University, Department of Nursing, *Antigonish* (BScN)

Accelerated RN Baccalaureate

Alabama
The University of Alabama at Birmingham, School of Nursing, *Birmingham* (BSN)

Arizona
Arizona State University, College of Nursing, *Tempe* (BSN)
Grand Canyon University, Samaritan College of Nursing, *Phoenix* (BSN)
University of Phoenix Online Campus, College of Health and Human Services, *Phoenix* (BSN)

Arkansas
University of Arkansas for Medical Sciences, College of Nursing, *Little Rock* (BSN)

California
Azusa Pacific University, School of Nursing, *Azusa* (BSN)
Loma Linda University, School of Nursing, *Loma Linda* (BS)
University of Phoenix–Southern California Campus, College of Health and Human Services, *Costa Mesa* (BSN)

Colorado
University of Phoenix–Colorado Campus, College of Health and Human Services, *Lone Tree* (BSN)

Connecticut
Saint Joseph College, Department of Nursing, *West Hartford* (BS)

Delaware
Wilmington College, Division of Nursing, *New Castle* (BSN)

District of Columbia
Howard University, Division of Nursing, *Washington* (BSN)

Florida
Florida Gulf Coast University, School of Nursing, *Fort Myers* (BSN)
University of Phoenix–Fort Lauderdale Campus, College of Health and Human Services, *Fort Lauderdale* (BSN)
University of Phoenix–Jacksonville Campus, College of Health and Human Services, *Jacksonville* (BSN)

Georgia
Albany State University, College of Health Professions, *Albany* (BSN)
Columbus State University, Nursing Program, *Columbus* (BSN)
Georgia Southern University, School of Nursing, *Statesboro* (BSN)
Georgia State University, School of Nursing, *Atlanta* (BS)
Piedmont College, School of Nursing, *Demorest* (BSN)

Hawaii
University of Phoenix–Hawaii Campus, College of Health and Human Services, *Honolulu* (BSN)

Illinois
Benedictine University, Department of Nursing, *Lisle* (BSN)
Bradley University, Department of Nursing, *Peoria* (BSN)
DePaul University, Department of Nursing, *Chicago* (BS)
Lakeview College of Nursing, *Danville* (BSN)
Lewis University, Program in Nursing, *Romeoville* (BSN)
Millikin University, School of Nursing, *Decatur* (BSN)
Olivet Nazarene University, Division of Nursing, *Bourbonnais* (BSN)
University of St. Francis, College of Nursing and Allied Health, *Joliet* (BSN)

Indiana
Indiana University Kokomo, Indiana University School Of Nursing, *Kokomo* (BSN)
University of Indianapolis, School of Nursing, *Indianapolis* (BSN)

Iowa
Allen College, Program in Nursing, *Waterloo* (BSN)
Mount Mercy College, Department of Nursing, *Cedar Rapids* (BSN)

Kansas
MidAmerica Nazarene University, Division of Nursing, *Olathe* (BSN)
Tabor College, Department of Nursing, *Hillsboro* (BSN)

Kentucky
Midway College, Program in Nursing (Baccalaureate), *Midway* (BSN)
Spalding University, School of Nursing, *Louisville* (BSN)
University of Louisville, School of Nursing, *Louisville* (BSN)

Louisiana
University of Phoenix–Louisiana Campus, College of Health and Human Services, *Metairie* (BSN)

Maryland
College of Notre Dame of Maryland, Department of Nursing, *Baltimore* (BS)
Columbia Union College, Nursing Department, *Takoma Park* (BS)
Salisbury University, Program in Nursing, *Salisbury* (BS)
Villa Julie College, Nursing Division, *Stevenson* (BS)

Massachusetts
Regis College, Department of Nursing, *Weston* (BSN)
University of Massachusetts Amherst, School of Nursing, *Amherst* (BS)
Worcester State College, Department of Nursing, *Worcester* (BS)

Michigan
Madonna University, College of Nursing and Health, *Livonia* (BSN)
University of Phoenix–Metro Detroit Campus, College of Health and Human Services, *Southfield* (BSN)

Minnesota
The College of St. Scholastica, Department of Nursing, *Duluth* (BA)

Missouri
Graceland University, School of Nursing, *Independence* (BSN)

Nebraska
University of Nebraska Medical Center, College of Nursing, *Omaha* (BSN)

Nevada
University of Nevada, Las Vegas, Department of Nursing, *Las Vegas* (BSN)

New Jersey
College of Saint Elizabeth, Department of Nursing, *Morristown* (BSN)
Felician College, Department of Professional Nursing–BSN, *Lodi* (BSN)
Rutgers, The State University of New Jersey, Camden College of Arts and Sciences, Department of Nursing, *Camden* (BS)

New Mexico
New Mexico State University, Department of Nursing, *Las Cruces* (BSN)

New York
Daemen College, Department of Nursing, *Amherst* (BS)
Dominican College, Division of Nursing, *Orangeburg* (BSN)
Medgar Evers College of the City University of New York, Department of Nursing, *Brooklyn* (BSN)
Molloy College, Department of Nursing, *Rockville Centre* (BS)
Mount Saint Mary College, Division of Nursing, *Newburgh* (BSN)
Pace University, Lienhard School of Nursing, *New York* (BS)
Roberts Wesleyan College, Division of Nursing, *Rochester* (BS)
State University of New York at Binghamton, Decker School of Nursing, *Binghamton* (BS)
State University of New York Institute of Technology, School of Nursing and Health Systems, *Utica* (BS)
University of Rochester, School of Nursing, *Rochester* (BS)

North Carolina
East Carolina University, School of Nursing, *Greenville* (BSN)

Ohio
College of Mount St. Joseph, Department of Nursing, *Cincinnati* (BSN)
Kent State University, College of Nursing, *Kent* (BSN)
Miami University, Department of Nursing, *Hamilton* (BSN)
The Ohio State University, College of Nursing, *Columbus* (BSN)
Otterbein College, Program in Nursing, *Westerville* (BSN)
Ursuline College, The Breen School of Nursing, *Pepper Pike* (BSN)
Walsh University, Department of Nursing, *North Canton* (BSN)

Oklahoma
Bacone College, Department of Nursing, *Muskogee* (BSN)
Northeastern State University, Department of Nursing, *Tahlequah* (BSN)
Oklahoma Wesleyan University, Division of Nursing, *Bartlesville* (BSN)

Pennsylvania
Carlow University, Division of Nursing, *Pittsburgh* (BSN)
College Misericordia, Department of Nursing, *Dallas* (BSN)
DeSales University, Department of Nursing and Health, *Center Valley* (BSN)
Duquesne University, School of Nursing, *Pittsburgh* (BSN)
Eastern University, Program in Nursing, *St. Davids* (BSN)
Edinboro University of Pennsylvania, Department of Nursing, *Edinboro* (BS)
Gwynedd-Mercy College, School of Nursing, *Gwynedd Valley* (BSN)
Immaculata University, Department of Nursing, *Immaculata* (BSN)
La Roche College, Department of Nursing and Nursing Management, *Pittsburgh* (BSN)
Mount Aloysius College, Department of Nursing, *Cresson* (BSN)
Thomas Jefferson University, Department of Nursing, *Philadelphia* (BSN)
University of Pennsylvania, School of Nursing, *Philadelphia* (BSN)
Waynesburg College, Department of Nursing, *Waynesburg* (BSN)
West Chester University of Pennsylvania, Department of Nursing, *West Chester* (BSN)
Wilkes University, Department of Nursing, *Wilkes-Barre* (BS)

South Carolina
Lander University, School of Nursing, *Greenwood* (BSN)
University of South Carolina Upstate, Mary Black School of Nursing, *Spartanburg* (BSN)

Tennessee
East Tennessee State University, College of Nursing, *Johnson City* (BSN)
King College, School of Nursing, *Bristol* (BSN)
The University of Memphis, Loewenberg School of Nursing, *Memphis* (BSN)
The University of Tennessee, College of Nursing, *Knoxville* (BSN)
The University of Tennessee at Martin, Department of Nursing, *Martin* (BSN)
The University of Tennessee Health Science Center, College of Nursing, *Memphis* (BSN)

Texas
The University of Texas at Tyler, Program in Nursing, *Tyler* (BSN)
The University of Texas Health Science Center at Houston, School of Nursing, *Houston* (BSN)

Utah
University of Phoenix–Utah Campus, College of Health and Human Services, *Salt Lake City* (BSN)

Vermont
University of Vermont, Department of Nursing, *Burlington* (BS)

Virginia
George Mason University, College of Nursing and Health Science, *Fairfax* (BSN)
Hampton University, Department of Nursing, *Hampton* (BS)
Marymount University, School of Health Professions, *Arlington* (BSN)

West Virginia
Alderson-Broaddus College, Department of Nursing, *Philippi* (BSN)
Marshall University, College of Nursing and Health Professions, *Huntington* (BSN)
West Liberty State College, Department of Health Sciences, *West Liberty* (BSN)

Wisconsin
Cardinal Stritch University, Ruth S. Coleman College of Nursing, *Milwaukee* (BSN)

Ontario
Ryerson University, Program in Nursing, *Toronto* (BScN)

Quebec
Université du Québec à Chicoutimi, Program in Nursing, *Chicoutimi* (BNSc)

Saskatchewan
University of Saskatchewan, College of Nursing, *Saskatoon* (BSN)

ADN to Baccalaureate

Alabama
Troy University, School of Nursing, *Troy* (BSN)
Tuskegee University, Program in Nursing, *Tuskegee* (BSN)
University of South Alabama, College of Nursing, *Mobile* (BSN)

Arizona
Northern Arizona University, Department of Nursing, *Flagstaff* (BSN)
University of Phoenix Online Campus, College of Health and Human Services, *Phoenix* (BSN)
University of Phoenix–Phoenix Campus, College of Health and Human Services, *Phoenix* (BSN)
University of Phoenix–Southern Arizona Campus, College of Health and Human Services, *Tucson* (BSN)

Arkansas
Arkansas Tech University, Program in Nursing, *Russellville* (BSN)
Harding University, College of Nursing, *Searcy* (BSN)
University of Arkansas at Monticello, Division of Nursing, *Monticello* (BSN)
University of Arkansas for Medical Sciences, College of Nursing, *Little Rock* (BSN)

California
Azusa Pacific University, School of Nursing, *Azusa* (BSN)
Biola University, Department of Nursing, *La Mirada* (BS)
California State University, Chico, School of Nursing, *Chico* (BSN)
California State University, Fresno, Department of Nursing, *Fresno* (BSN)
California State University, Fullerton, Department of Nursing, *Fullerton* (BSN)
California State University, Sacramento, Division of Nursing, *Sacramento* (BSN)
California State University, San Bernardino, Department of Nursing, *San Bernardino* (BSN)
California State University, Stanislaus, Department of Nursing, *Turlock* (BSN)
Dominican University of California, Program in Occupational Therapy, *San Rafael* (BSN)
Humboldt State University, Department of Nursing, *Arcata* (BSN)
Mount St. Mary's College, Department of Nursing, *Los Angeles* (BSN)

Point Loma Nazarene University, School of Nursing, *San Diego* (BSN)
San Francisco State University, School of Nursing, *San Francisco* (BSN)
Sonoma State University, Department of Nursing, *Rohnert Park* (BSN)
University of California, Los Angeles, School of Nursing, *Los Angeles* (BS)
University of Phoenix–Northern California Campus, College of Health and Human Services, *Pleasanton* (BSN)
University of Phoenix–Sacramento Campus, College of Health and Human Services, *Sacramento* (BSN)
University of Phoenix–San Diego Campus, College of Health and Human Services, *San Diego* (BSN)
University of Phoenix–Southern California Campus, College of Health and Human Services, *Costa Mesa* (BSN)
University of San Diego, Hahn School of Nursing and Health Sciences, *San Diego* (BSN)

Colorado
Colorado State University-Pueblo, Department of Nursing, *Pueblo* (BSN)
Mesa State College, Department of Nursing and Radiologic Sciences, *Grand Junction* (BSN)
Metropolitan State College of Denver, Department of Health Professions, *Denver* (BS)
University of Phoenix–Colorado Campus, College of Health and Human Services, *Lone Tree* (BSN)
University of Phoenix–Southern Colorado Campus, College of Health and Human Services, *Colorado Springs* (BSN)

Connecticut
Sacred Heart University, Program in Nursing, *Fairfield* (BS)
Southern Connecticut State University, Department of Nursing, *New Haven* (BSN)
University of Hartford, College of Education, Nursing, and Health Professions, *West Hartford* (BSN)

District of Columbia
Georgetown University, School of Nursing and Health Studies, *Washington* (BSN)
Howard University, Division of Nursing, *Washington* (BSN)
University of the District of Columbia, Nursing Education Program, *Washington* (BSN)

Florida
Barry University, School of Nursing, *Miami Shores* (BSN)
Florida Southern College, Department of Nursing, *Lakeland* (BSN)
Jacksonville University, School of Nursing, *Jacksonville* (BSN)
St. Petersburg College, Department of Nursing, *St. Petersburg* (BSN)
University of Phoenix–Fort Lauderdale Campus, College of Health and Human Services, *Fort Lauderdale* (BSN)
University of Phoenix–Jacksonville Campus, College of Health and Human Services, *Jacksonville* (BSN)
University of Phoenix–Orlando Campus, College of Health and Human Services, *Maitland* (BSN)
University of Phoenix–Tampa Campus, College of Health and Human Services, *Tampa* (BSN)
University of South Florida, College of Nursing, *Tampa* (BS)
The University of Tampa, Department of Nursing, *Tampa* (BSN)
University of West Florida, Department of Nursing, *Pensacola* (BSN)

Georgia
Albany State University, College of Health Professions, *Albany* (BSN)
Armstrong Atlantic State University, Program in Nursing, *Savannah* (BSN)
Brenau University, School of Health and Science, *Gainesville* (BSN)
Georgia Southern University, School of Nursing, *Statesboro* (BSN)
Kennesaw State University, School of Nursing, *Kennesaw* (BSN)
Medical College of Georgia, School of Nursing, *Augusta* (BSN)
University of Phoenix–Atlanta Campus, College of Health and Human Services, *Atlanta* (BSN)

Guam
University of Guam, College of Nursing and Health Sciences, *Mangilao* (BSN)

Hawaii
University of Hawaii at Hilo, Department in Nursing, *Hilo* (BSN)
University of Hawaii at Manoa, School of Nursing and Dental Hygiene, *Honolulu* (BS)
University of Phoenix–Hawaii Campus, College of Health and Human Services, *Honolulu* (BSN)

Idaho
Idaho State University, Department of Nursing, *Pocatello* (BSN)
Lewis-Clark State College, Division of Nursing and Health Sciences, *Lewiston* (BSN)

Illinois
Illinois State University, Mennonite College of Nursing, *Normal* (BSN)
MacMurray College, Department of Nursing, *Jacksonville* (BSN)
McKendree College, Department of Nursing, *Lebanon* (BSN)
Rockford College, Department of Nursing, *Rockford* (BSN)
Rush University, College of Nursing, *Chicago* (BSN)
Saint Francis Medical Center College of Nursing, Baccalaureate Nursing Program, *Peoria* (BSN)
Saint Xavier University, School of Nursing, *Chicago* (BSN)
West Suburban College of Nursing, *Oak Park* (BSN)

Indiana
Bethel College, Department of Nursing, *Mishawaka* (BSN)
Indiana University East, Division of Nursing, *Richmond* (BSN)
Indiana University–Purdue University Indianapolis, School of Nursing, *Indianapolis* (BSN)
Indiana Wesleyan University, Division of Nursing, *Marion* (BS)

Iowa
Allen College, Program in Nursing, *Waterloo* (BSN)
Briar Cliff University, Department of Nursing, *Sioux City* (BSc PN)
Iowa Wesleyan College, Division of Health and Natural Sciences, *Mount Pleasant* (BSN)
Mercy College of Health Sciences, Division of Nursing, *Des Moines* (BSN)

Kansas
Emporia State University, Newman Division of Nursing, *Emporia* (BSN)
Kansas Wesleyan University, Department of Nursing Education, *Salina* (BSN)
MidAmerica Nazarene University, Division of Nursing, *Olathe* (BSN)
University of Kansas, School of Nursing, *Kansas City* (BSN)
Washburn University, School of Nursing, *Topeka* (BSN)

Kentucky
Bellarmine University, Donna and Allan Lansing School of Nursing and Health Sciences, *Louisville* (BSN)
Midway College, Program in Nursing (Baccalaureate), *Midway* (BSN)

Louisiana
McNeese State University, College of Nursing, *Lake Charles* (BSN)
Northwestern State University of Louisiana, College of Nursing, *Shreveport* (BSN)
University of Louisiana at Lafayette, College of Nursing, *Lafayette* (BSN)
University of Louisiana at Monroe, Nursing, *Monroe* (BS)
University of Phoenix–Louisiana Campus, College of Health and Human Services, *Metairie* (BSN)

Maine
University of Southern Maine, College of Nursing and Health Professions, *Portland* (BS)

Maryland
Coppin State University, Helene Fuld School of Nursing, *Baltimore* (BSN)
Salisbury University, Program in Nursing, *Salisbury* (BS)
Villa Julie College, Nursing Division, *Stevenson* (BS)

Massachusetts
Anna Maria College, Department of Nursing, *Paxton* (BSN)
Atlantic Union College, Department of Nursing, *South Lancaster* (BSN)
Fitchburg State College, Department of Nursing, *Fitchburg* (BSN)
Framingham State College, Department of Nursing, *Framingham* (BS)
Regis College, Department of Nursing, *Weston* (BSN)
Salem State College, Nursing Department, *Salem* (BSN)
Simmons College, Department of Nursing, *Boston* (BS)

Michigan
Andrews University, Department of Nursing, *Berrien Springs* (BS)
Madonna University, College of Nursing and Health, *Livonia* (BSN)
Northern Michigan University, College of Nursing and Allied Health Science, *Marquette* (BSN)
Spring Arbor University, Program in Nursing, *Spring Arbor* (BSN)
University of Phoenix–Metro Detroit Campus, College of Health and Human Services, *Southfield* (BSN)
University of Phoenix–West Michigan Campus, College of Health and Human Services, *Grand Rapids* (BSN)
Western Michigan University, College of Health and Human Services, *Kalamazoo* (BS)

Mississippi
Delta State University, School of Nursing, *Cleveland* (BSN)
Mississippi University for Women, Division of Nursing, *Columbus* (BSN)
University of Mississippi Medical Center, Program in Nursing, *Jackson* (BSN)
University of Southern Mississippi, School of Nursing, *Hattiesburg* (BSN)
William Carey College, School of Nursing, *Hattiesburg* (BSN)

Missouri
Deaconess College of Nursing, *St. Louis* (BSN)
Graceland University, School of Nursing, *Independence* (BSN)
Lester L. Cox College of Nursing and Health Sciences, Department of Nursing, *Springfield* (BSN)
Maryville University of Saint Louis, Nursing Program, School of Health Professions, *St. Louis* (BSN)
Missouri Southern State University, Department of Nursing, *Joplin* (BSN)
Southwest Missouri State University, Department of Nursing, *Springfield* (BSN)

Webster University, Department of Nursing, *St. Louis* (BSN)

Montana

Montana State University–Northern, College of Nursing, *Havre* (BSN)

Nebraska

Clarkson College, Department of Nursing, *Omaha* (BSN)
College of Saint Mary, Division of Health Care Professions, *Omaha* (BSN)
Nebraska Methodist College, Department of Nursing, *Omaha* (BSN)
Nebraska Wesleyan University, Department of Nursing, *Lincoln* (BSN)
Union College, Division of Health Sciences, *Lincoln* (BSN)
University of Nebraska Medical Center, College of Nursing, *Omaha* (BSN)

Nevada

University of Nevada, Las Vegas, Department of Nursing, *Las Vegas* (BSN)
University of Nevada, Reno, Orvis School of Nursing, *Reno* (BSN)

New Hampshire

Rivier College, Department of Nursing and Health Sciences, *Nashua* (BS)

New Jersey

College of Saint Elizabeth, Department of Nursing, *Morristown* (BSN)
Kean University, Department of Nursing, *Union* (BSN)
Monmouth University, Marjorie K. Unterberg School of Nursing, *West Long Branch* (BSN)
Saint Peter's College, Nursing Program, *Jersey City* (BSN)
William Paterson University of New Jersey, Department of Nursing, *Wayne* (BSN)

New Mexico

University of Phoenix–New Mexico Campus, College of Health and Human Services, *Albuquerque* (BSN)

New York

College of Mount Saint Vincent, Division of Nursing, *Riverdale* (BS)
College of Staten Island of the City University of New York, Department of Nursing, *Staten Island* (BS)
Daemen College, Department of Nursing, *Amherst* (BS)
D'Youville College, Department of Nursing, *Buffalo* (BSN)
Elmira College, Program in Nursing Education, *Elmira* (BS)
Medgar Evers College of the City University of New York, Department of Nursing, *Brooklyn* (BSN)
State University of New York at New Paltz, Department of Nursing, *New Paltz* (BSN)
State University of New York at Plattsburgh, Department of Nursing, *Plattsburgh* (BS)
State University of New York College at Brockport, Department of Nursing, *Brockport* (BSN)
State University of New York Institute of Technology, School of Nursing and Health Systems, *Utica* (BS)
State University of New York Upstate Medical University, College of Nursing, *Syracuse* (BS)
University at Buffalo, The State University of New York, School of Nursing, *Buffalo* (BS)
University of Rochester, School of Nursing, *Rochester* (BS)
York College of the City University of New York, Program in Nursing, *Jamaica* (BS)

North Carolina

East Carolina University, School of Nursing, *Greenville* (BSN)
Lees-McRae College, Nursing Program, *Banner Elk* (BSN)
Lenoir-Rhyne College, Program in Nursing, *Hickory* (BS)
Queens University of Charlotte, Division of Nursing, *Charlotte* (BSN)
The University of North Carolina at Chapel Hill, School of Nursing, *Chapel Hill* (BSN)
The University of North Carolina at Charlotte, School of Nursing, *Charlotte* (BSN)
The University of North Carolina at Greensboro, School of Nursing, *Greensboro* (BSN)
Winston-Salem State University, Department of Nursing, *Winston-Salem* (BSN)

North Dakota

Dickinson State University, Department of Nursing, *Dickinson* (BSN)
Medcenter One College of Nursing, Medcenter One College of Nursing, *Bismarck* (BSN)
University of North Dakota, College of Nursing, *Grand Forks* (BSN)

Ohio

Case Western Reserve University, Frances Payne Bolton School of Nursing, *Cleveland* (BSN)
Cleveland State University, Department of Nursing, *Cleveland* (BSN)
Kent State University, College of Nursing, *Kent* (BSN)
Medical College of Ohio, School of Nursing, *Toledo* (BSN)
Shawnee State University, Department of Nursing, *Portsmouth* (BSN)
The University of Akron, College of Nursing, *Akron* (BSN)

Oklahoma

East Central University, Department of Nursing, *Ada* (BS)
Oklahoma City University, Kramer School of Nursing, *Oklahoma City* (BSN)
Oklahoma Panhandle State University, Bachelor of Science in Nursing Program, *Goodwell* (BSN)
Oklahoma Wesleyan University, Division of Nursing, *Bartlesville* (BSN)
Oral Roberts University, Anna Vaughn School of Nursing, *Tulsa* (BSN)
University of Phoenix–Oklahoma City Campus, College of Health and Human Services, *Oklahoma City* (BSN)
University of Phoenix–Tulsa Campus, College of Health and Human Services, *Tulsa* (BSN)

Pennsylvania

Bloomsburg University of Pennsylvania, Department of Nursing, *Bloomsburg* (BSN)
Clarion University of Pennsylvania, School of Nursing, *Oil City* (BSN)
DeSales University, Department of Nursing and Health, *Center Valley* (BSN)
Drexel University, College of Nursing and Health Professions, *Philadelphia* (BSN)
Edinboro University of Pennsylvania, Department of Nursing, *Edinboro* (BS)
Gwynedd-Mercy College, School of Nursing, *Gwynedd Valley* (BSN)
Holy Family University, School of Nursing and Allied Health Professions, *Philadelphia* (BSN)
Marywood University, Department of Nursing, *Scranton* (BSN)
Mount Aloysius College, Department of Nursing, *Cresson* (BSN)
University of Pennsylvania, School of Nursing, *Philadelphia* (BSN)
University of Pittsburgh, School of Nursing, *Pittsburgh* (BSN)
University of Pittsburgh at Bradford, Department of Nursing, *Bradford* (BSN)
The University of Scranton, Department of Nursing, *Scranton* (BS)
Villanova University, College of Nursing, *Villanova* (BSN)
Widener University, School of Nursing, *Chester* (BSN)
Wilkes University, Department of Nursing, *Wilkes-Barre* (BS)

Puerto Rico

Inter American University of Puerto Rico, Metropolitan Campus, Carmen Torres de Tiburcio School of Nursing, *San Juan* (BSN)
University of Puerto Rico, Medical Sciences Campus, School of Nursing, *San Juan* (BSN)

Rhode Island

University of Rhode Island, College of Nursing, *Kingston* (BS)

South Carolina

Charleston Southern University, Wingo School of Nursing, *Charleston* (BSN)
Medical University of South Carolina, College of Nursing, *Charleston* (BSN)

South Dakota

Mount Marty College, Nursing Program, *Yankton* (BSc PN)
Presentation College, Department of Nursing, *Aberdeen* (BSN)

Tennessee

Belmont University, School of Nursing, *Nashville* (BSN)
East Tennessee State University, College of Nursing, *Johnson City* (BSN)
Southern Adventist University, School of Nursing, *Collegedale* (BS)
Tennessee Wesleyan College, Fort Sanders Nursing Department, *Knoxville* (BSN)
The University of Memphis, Loewenberg School of Nursing, *Memphis* (BSN)
The University of Tennessee at Chattanooga, School of Nursing, *Chattanooga* (BSN)
The University of Tennessee at Martin, Department of Nursing, *Martin* (BSN)
The University of Tennessee Health Science Center, College of Nursing, *Memphis* (BSN)

Texas

Lamar University, Department of Nursing, *Beaumont* (BSN)
Southwestern Adventist University, Department of Nursing, *Keene* (BS)
Tarleton State University, Department of Nursing, *Stephenville* (BSN)
Texas A&M University–Corpus Christi, School of Nursing and Health Sciences, *Corpus Christi* (BSN)
The University of Texas at Brownsville, Department of Nursing, *Brownsville* (BSN)
The University of Texas at El Paso, School of Nursing, *El Paso* (BSN)
The University of Texas at Tyler, Program in Nursing, *Tyler* (BSN)
The University of Texas Health Science Center at Houston, School of Nursing, *Houston* (BSN)
The University of Texas Health Science Center at San Antonio, School of Nursing, *San Antonio* (BSN)
University of the Incarnate Word, Program in Nursing, *San Antonio* (BSN)
West Texas A&M University, Division of Nursing, *Canyon* (BSN)

Utah

University of Phoenix–Utah Campus, College of Health and Human Services, *Salt Lake City* (BSN)
Weber State University, Program in Nursing, *Ogden* (BSN)

Vermont

Norwich University, Division of Nursing, *Northfield* (BSN)
Southern Vermont College, Department of Nursing, *Bennington* (BSN)

BACCALAUREATE PROGRAMS
ADN to Baccalaureate

Virginia
Eastern Mennonite University, Department of Nursing, *Harrisonburg* (BSN)
Hampton University, Department of Nursing, *Hampton* (BS)
Jefferson College of Health Sciences, Nursing Education Program, *Roanoke* (BSN)
Marymount University, School of Health Professions, *Arlington* (BSN)
Shenandoah University, Division of Nursing, *Winchester* (BSN)
University of Virginia, School of Nursing, *Charlottesville* (BSN)
Virginia Commonwealth University, School of Nursing, *Richmond* (BS)

Washington
Gonzaga University, Department of Nursing, *Spokane* (BSN)
Pacific Lutheran University, School of Nursing, *Tacoma* (BSN)
Walla Walla College, School of Nursing, *College Place* (BS)

West Virginia
Fairmont State University, School of Nursing/Allied Health Adm., *Fairmont* (BSN)
Mountain State University, Program in Nursing, *Beckley* (BSN)
Shepherd University, Department of Nursing Education, *Shepherdstown* (BSN)

Wisconsin
Alverno College, Division of Nursing, *Milwaukee* (BSN)
Concordia University Wisconsin, Division of Nursing, *Mequon* (BSN)
Marian College of Fond du Lac, Nursing Studies Division, *Fond du Lac* (BSN)
University of Wisconsin–Madison, School of Nursing, *Madison* (BS)

Quebec
Université du Québec en Outaouais, Département des Sciences Infirmières, *Gatineau* (BScN)

Baccalaureate for Second Degree

Alabama
Samford University, Ida V. Moffett School of Nursing, *Birmingham* (BSN)
The University of Alabama at Birmingham, School of Nursing, *Birmingham* (BSN)
The University of Alabama in Huntsville, College of Nursing, *Huntsville* (BSN)

Arizona
Arizona State University, College of Nursing, *Tempe* (BSN)

Arkansas
University of Arkansas, Eleanor Mann School of Nursing, *Fayetteville* (BSN)

California
Biola University, Department of Nursing, *La Mirada* (BS)
California State University, Chico, School of Nursing, *Chico* (BSN)
California State University, Fresno, Department of Nursing, *Fresno* (BSN)
California State University, Fullerton, Department of Nursing, *Fullerton* (BSN)
Dominican University of California, Program in Occupational Therapy, *San Rafael* (BSN)
Humboldt State University, Department of Nursing, *Arcata* (BSN)
Point Loma Nazarene University, School of Nursing, *San Diego* (BSN)
Sonoma State University, Department of Nursing, *Rohnert Park* (BSN)
University of San Francisco, School of Nursing, *San Francisco* (BSN)

Colorado
Colorado State University-Pueblo, Department of Nursing, *Pueblo* (BSN)

Connecticut
Fairfield University, School of Nursing, *Fairfield* (BS)
Saint Joseph College, Department of Nursing, *West Hartford* (BS)

District of Columbia
The Catholic University of America, School of Nursing, *Washington* (BSN)
Howard University, Division of Nursing, *Washington* (BSN)

Florida
Barry University, School of Nursing, *Miami Shores* (BSN)
Jacksonville University, School of Nursing, *Jacksonville* (BSN)
University of Miami, School of Nursing, *Coral Gables* (BSN)
University of South Florida, College of Nursing, *Tampa* (BS)

Georgia
Armstrong Atlantic State University, Program in Nursing, *Savannah* (BSN)
Georgia Southwestern State University, School of Nursing, *Americus* (BSN)

Illinois
Saint Anthony College of Nursing, Saint Anthony College of Nursing, *Rockford* (BSN)
West Suburban College of Nursing, *Oak Park* (BSN)

Indiana
Purdue University Calumet, School of Nursing, *Hammond* (BS)

Iowa
Allen College, Program in Nursing, *Waterloo* (BSN)
Clarke College, Department of Nursing and Health, *Dubuque* (BS)
Morningside College, Department of Nursing Education, *Sioux City* (BSN)

Kansas
Washburn University, School of Nursing, *Topeka* (BSN)

Maryland
Coppin State University, Helene Fuld School of Nursing, *Baltimore* (BSN)
The Johns Hopkins University, School of Nursing, *Baltimore* (BS)

Massachusetts
Anna Maria College, Department of Nursing, *Paxton* (BSN)
Regis College, Department of Nursing, *Weston* (BSN)
Salem State College, Nursing Department, *Salem* (BSN)
Simmons College, Department of Nursing, *Boston* (BS)

Michigan
Eastern Michigan University, Department of Nursing, *Ypsilanti* (BSN)
Grand Valley State University, Russell B. Kirkhof School of Nursing, *Allendale* (BSN)
Madonna University, College of Nursing and Health, *Livonia* (BSN)
Saginaw Valley State University, Crystal M. Lange College of Nursing and Health Sciences, *University Center* (BSN)
Western Michigan University, College of Health and Human Services, *Kalamazoo* (BS)

Minnesota
College of St. Catherine, Department of Nursing, *St. Paul* (BS)

Missouri
Missouri Southern State University, Department of Nursing, *Joplin* (BSN)
Research College of Nursing, College of Nursing, *Kansas City* (BSN)
Southwest Missouri State University, Department of Nursing, *Springfield* (BSN)

Nebraska
Clarkson College, Department of Nursing, *Omaha* (BSN)
University of Nebraska Medical Center, College of Nursing, *Omaha* (BSN)

New Jersey
Fairleigh Dickinson University, Metropolitan Campus, Henry P. Becton School of Nursing and Allied Health, *Teaneck* (BSN)
Rutgers, The State University of New Jersey, Camden College of Arts and Sciences, Department of Nursing, *Camden* (BS)
Rutgers, The State University of New Jersey, College of Nursing, *Newark* (BS)
Seton Hall University, College of Nursing, *South Orange* (BSN)

New York
Adelphi University, School of Nursing, *Garden City* (BS)
College of Mount Saint Vincent, Division of Nursing, *Riverdale* (BS)
The College of New Rochelle, School of Nursing, *New Rochelle* (BSN)
D'Youville College, Department of Nursing, *Buffalo* (BSN)
New York University, Division of Nursing, *New York* (BS)
St. John Fisher College, Nursing Program, *Rochester* (BS)
State University of New York College at Brockport, Department of Nursing, *Brockport* (BSN)
University of Rochester, School of Nursing, *Rochester* (BS)
Wagner College, Department of Nursing, *Staten Island* (BS)

North Carolina
East Carolina University, School of Nursing, *Greenville* (BSN)
Queens University of Charlotte, Division of Nursing, *Charlotte* (BSN)
The University of North Carolina at Greensboro, School of Nursing, *Greensboro* (BSN)
Winston-Salem State University, Department of Nursing, *Winston-Salem* (BSN)

Ohio
Kent State University, College of Nursing, *Kent* (BSN)
Wright State University, College of Nursing and Health, *Dayton* (BSN)

Oklahoma
Oklahoma Wesleyan University, Division of Nursing, *Bartlesville* (BSN)

Pennsylvania
Bloomsburg University of Pennsylvania, Department of Nursing, *Bloomsburg* (BSN)
Carlow University, Division of Nursing, *Pittsburgh* (BSN)
Cedar Crest College, Department of Nursing, *Allentown* (BS)
College Misericordia, Department of Nursing, *Dallas* (BSN)
Eastern University, Program in Nursing, *St. Davids* (BSN)
Edinboro University of Pennsylvania, Department of Nursing, *Edinboro* (BS)
Indiana University of Pennsylvania, Department of Nursing and Allied Health, *Indiana* (BSN)
La Salle University, School of Nursing, *Philadelphia* (BSN)

Neumann College, Program in Nursing and Health Sciences, *Aston* (BS)
Thomas Jefferson University, Department of Nursing, *Philadelphia* (BSN)
University of Pennsylvania, School of Nursing, *Philadelphia* (BSN)
The University of Scranton, Department of Nursing, *Scranton* (BS)
Villanova University, College of Nursing, *Villanova* (BSN)
Widener University, School of Nursing, *Chester* (BSN)

Rhode Island
Rhode Island College, Department of Nursing, *Providence* (BS)

South Carolina
Lander University, School of Nursing, *Greenwood* (BSN)

South Dakota
Presentation College, Department of Nursing, *Aberdeen* (BSN)

Tennessee
Belmont University, School of Nursing, *Nashville* (BSN)
Cumberland University, Rudy School of Nursing and Health Professions, *Lebanon* (BSN)
The University of Memphis, Loewenberg School of Nursing, *Memphis* (BSN)
The University of Tennessee at Chattanooga, School of Nursing, *Chattanooga* (BSN)
The University of Tennessee Health Science Center, College of Nursing, *Memphis* (BSN)

Texas
Texas A&M University–Corpus Christi, School of Nursing and Health Sciences, *Corpus Christi* (BSN)
Texas Woman's University, College of Nursing, *Denton* (BS)
University of Mary Hardin-Baylor, College of Nursing, *Belton* (BSN)
The University of Texas Health Science Center at Houston, School of Nursing, *Houston* (BSN)

Utah
Westminster College, St. Mark's-Westminster School of Nursing and Health Sciences, *Salt Lake City* (BSN)

Virginia
Eastern Mennonite University, Department of Nursing, *Harrisonburg* (BSN)
Hampton University, Department of Nursing, *Hampton* (BS)
Marymount University, School of Health Professions, *Arlington* (BSN)
Norfolk State University, Department of Nursing, *Norfolk* (BSN)

Washington
Seattle University, College of Nursing, *Seattle* (BSN)

West Virginia
Mountain State University, Program in Nursing, *Beckley* (BSN)
West Virginia University, School of Nursing, *Morgantown* (BSN)

Wisconsin
Alverno College, Division of Nursing, *Milwaukee* (BSN)
Edgewood College, Program in Nursing, *Madison* (BS)
University of Wisconsin–Oshkosh, College of Nursing, *Oshkosh* (BSN)

Alberta
University of Alberta, Faculty of Nursing, *Edmonton* (BScN)
University of Calgary, Faculty of Nursing, *Calgary* (BN)

British Columbia
The University of British Columbia, School of Nursing, *Vancouver* (BSN)

Manitoba
Brandon University, School of Health Studies, *Brandon* (BN)

Nova Scotia
Dalhousie University, School of Nursing, *Halifax* (BScN)

Ontario
McMaster University, School of Nursing, *Hamilton* (BScN)

Generic Baccalaureate

Alabama
Auburn University, School of Nursing, *Auburn University* (BSN)
Auburn University Montgomery, School of Nursing, *Montgomery* (BSN)
Jacksonville State University, College of Nursing and Health Sciences, *Jacksonville* (BSN)
Samford University, Ida V. Moffett School of Nursing, *Birmingham* (BSN)
Spring Hill College, Division of Nursing, *Mobile* (BSN)
Troy University, School of Nursing, *Troy* (BSN)
Tuskegee University, Program in Nursing, *Tuskegee* (BSN)
The University of Alabama, Capstone College of Nursing, *Tuscaloosa* (BSN)
The University of Alabama at Birmingham, School of Nursing, *Birmingham* (BSN)
The University of Alabama in Huntsville, College of Nursing, *Huntsville* (BSN)
University of Mobile, School of Nursing, *Mobile* (BSN)
University of North Alabama, College of Nursing and Allied Health, *Florence* (BSN)
University of South Alabama, College of Nursing, *Mobile* (BSN)

Alaska
University of Alaska Anchorage, School of Nursing, *Anchorage* (BS)

Arizona
Arizona State University, College of Nursing, *Tempe* (BSN)
Grand Canyon University, Samaritan College of Nursing, *Phoenix* (BSN)
Northern Arizona University, Department of Nursing, *Flagstaff* (BSN)
The University of Arizona, College of Nursing, *Tucson* (BSN)

Arkansas
Arkansas State University, Department of Nursing, *Jonesboro, State University* (BSN)
Arkansas Tech University, Program in Nursing, *Russellville* (BSN)
Harding University, College of Nursing, *Searcy* (BSN)
Henderson State University, Department of Nursing, *Arkadelphia* (BSN)
University of Arkansas, Eleanor Mann School of Nursing, *Fayetteville* (BSN)
University of Arkansas at Pine Bluff, Department of Nursing, *Pine Bluff* (BSN)
University of Arkansas for Medical Sciences, College of Nursing, *Little Rock* (BSN)
University of Central Arkansas, Department of Nursing, *Conway* (BSN)

California
Azusa Pacific University, School of Nursing, *Azusa* (BSN)
Biola University, Department of Nursing, *La Mirada* (BS)
California State University, Bakersfield, Program in Nursing, *Bakersfield* (BSN)
California State University, Chico, School of Nursing, *Chico* (BSN)
California State University, Fresno, Department of Nursing, *Fresno* (BSN)
California State University, Hayward, Department of Nursing and Health Sciences, *Hayward* (BS)
California State University, Long Beach, Department of Nursing, *Long Beach* (BSN)
California State University, Los Angeles, School of Nursing, *Los Angeles* (BS)
California State University, Sacramento, Division of Nursing, *Sacramento* (BSN)
California State University, Stanislaus, Department of Nursing, *Turlock* (BSN)
Dominican University of California, Program in Occupational Therapy, *San Rafael* (BSN)
Humboldt State University, Department of Nursing, *Arcata* (BSN)
Loma Linda University, School of Nursing, *Loma Linda* (BS)
Mount St. Mary's College, Department of Nursing, *Los Angeles* (BSN)
Point Loma Nazarene University, School of Nursing, *San Diego* (BSN)
Samuel Merritt College, School of Nursing, *Oakland* (BSN)
San Diego State University, School of Nursing, *San Diego* (BSN)
San Francisco State University, School of Nursing, *San Francisco* (BSN)
San Jose State University, School of Nursing, *San Jose* (BS)
Sonoma State University, Department of Nursing, *Rohnert Park* (BSN)
University of San Francisco, School of Nursing, *San Francisco* (BSN)

Colorado
Colorado State University-Pueblo, Department of Nursing, *Pueblo* (BSN)
Mesa State College, Department of Nursing and Radiologic Sciences, *Grand Junction* (BSN)
Regis University, Department of Nursing, *Denver* (BSN)
University of Colorado at Colorado Springs, Beth-El College of Nursing and Health Sciences, *Colorado Springs* (BSN)
University of Colorado at Denver and Health Sciences Center—Health Sciences Program, School of Nursing, *Denver* (BS)
University of Northern Colorado, School of Nursing, *Greeley* (BS)

Connecticut
Fairfield University, School of Nursing, *Fairfield* (BS)
Quinnipiac University, Department of Nursing, *Hamden* (BSN)
Sacred Heart University, Program in Nursing, *Fairfield* (BS)
Saint Joseph College, Department of Nursing, *West Hartford* (BS)
Southern Connecticut State University, Department of Nursing, *New Haven* (BSN)
Western Connecticut State University, Department of Nursing, *Danbury* (BS)

Delaware
Delaware State University, Department of Nursing, *Dover* (BSN)
University of Delaware, Department of Nursing, *Newark* (BSN)
Wesley College, Graduate Nursing Program, *Dover* (BSN)

District of Columbia
The Catholic University of America, School of Nursing, *Washington* (BSN)
Georgetown University, School of Nursing and Health Studies, *Washington* (BSN)
Howard University, Division of Nursing, *Washington* (BSN)

Florida
Barry University, School of Nursing, *Miami Shores* (BSN)

BACCALAUREATE PROGRAMS

Generic Baccalaureate

Bethune-Cookman College, School of Nursing, *Daytona Beach* (BSN)
Florida Agricultural and Mechanical University, School of Nursing, *Tallahassee* (BSN)
Florida Atlantic University, College of Nursing, *Boca Raton* (BSN)
Florida Gulf Coast University, School of Nursing, *Fort Myers* (BSN)
Florida Hospital College of Health Sciences, Department of Nursing, *Orlando* (BS)
Florida International University, School of Nursing, *Miami* (BSN)
Florida State University, School of Nursing, *Tallahassee* (BSN)
Jacksonville University, School of Nursing, *Jacksonville* (BSN)
Nova Southeastern University, College of Allied Health and Nursing, *Fort Lauderdale* (BSN)
University of Central Florida, School of Nursing, *Orlando* (BSN)
University of Florida, College of Nursing, *Gainesville* (BSN)
University of Miami, School of Nursing, *Coral Gables* (BSN)
University of North Florida, School of Nursing, *Jacksonville* (BSN)
University of South Florida, College of Nursing, *Tampa* (BS)
The University of Tampa, Department of Nursing, *Tampa* (BSN)
University of West Florida, Department of Nursing, *Pensacola* (BSN)

Georgia

Albany State University, College of Health Professions, *Albany* (BSN)
Armstrong Atlantic State University, Program in Nursing, *Savannah* (BSN)
Brenau University, School of Health and Science, *Gainesville* (BSN)
Clayton College & State University, Department of Nursing, *Morrow* (BSN)
Columbus State University, Nursing Program, *Columbus* (BSN)
Emory University, Nell Hodgson Woodruff School of Nursing, *Atlanta* (BSN)
Georgia Baptist College of Nursing of Mercer University, Department of Nursing, *Atlanta* (BSN)
Georgia College & State University, School of Health Sciences, *Milledgeville* (BSN)
Georgia Southern University, School of Nursing, *Statesboro* (BSN)
Georgia Southwestern State University, School of Nursing, *Americus* (BSN)
Georgia State University, School of Nursing, *Atlanta* (BS)
Kennesaw State University, School of Nursing, *Kennesaw* (BSN)
Medical College of Georgia, School of Nursing, *Augusta* (BSN)
University of West Georgia, Department of Nursing, *Carrollton* (BSN)
Valdosta State University, College of Nursing, *Valdosta* (BSN)

Guam

University of Guam, College of Nursing and Health Sciences, *Mangilao* (BSN)

Hawaii

Hawai'i Pacific University, School of Nursing, *Honolulu* (BSN)
University of Hawaii at Hilo, Department in Nursing, *Hilo* (BSN)
University of Hawaii at Manoa, School of Nursing and Dental Hygiene, *Honolulu* (BS)

Idaho

Boise State University, Department of Nursing, *Boise* (BS)
Idaho State University, Department of Nursing, *Pocatello* (BSN)
Lewis-Clark State College, Division of Nursing and Health Sciences, *Lewiston* (BSN)
Northwest Nazarene University, School of Health and Science, *Nampa* (BSN)

Illinois

Aurora University, School of Nursing, *Aurora* (BSN)
Blessing–Rieman College of Nursing, *Quincy* (BSN)
Bradley University, Department of Nursing, *Peoria* (BSN)
Chicago State University, College of Nursing and Allied Health Professions, *Chicago* (BSN)
Elmhurst College, Deicke Center for Nursing Education, *Elmhurst* (BSN)
Illinois State University, Mennonite College of Nursing, *Normal* (BSN)
Illinois Wesleyan University, School of Nursing, *Bloomington* (BSN)
Lakeview College of Nursing, *Danville* (BSN)
Lewis University, Program in Nursing, *Romeoville* (BSN)
Loyola University Chicago, Marcella Niehoff School of Nursing, *Chicago* (BSN)
MacMurray College, Department of Nursing, *Jacksonville* (BSN)
Millikin University, School of Nursing, *Decatur* (BSN)
Northern Illinois University, School of Nursing, *De Kalb* (BS)
North Park University, School of Nursing, *Chicago* (BS)
Olivet Nazarene University, Division of Nursing, *Bourbonnais* (BSN)
Rockford College, Department of Nursing, *Rockford* (BSN)
Rush University, College of Nursing, *Chicago* (BSN)
Saint Anthony College of Nursing, Saint Anthony College of Nursing, *Rockford* (BSN)
Saint Francis Medical Center College of Nursing, Baccalaureate Nursing Program, *Peoria* (BSN)
St. John's College, Department of Nursing, *Springfield* (BSN)
Saint Xavier University, School of Nursing, *Chicago* (BSN)
Southern Illinois University Edwardsville, School of Nursing, *Edwardsville* (BS)
Trinity Christian College, Department of Nursing, *Palos Heights* (BSN)
University of Illinois at Chicago, College of Nursing, *Chicago* (BSN)
University of St. Francis, College of Nursing and Allied Health, *Joliet* (BSN)
West Suburban College of Nursing, *Oak Park* (BSN)

Indiana

Anderson University, Department of Nursing, *Anderson* (BSN)
Ball State University, School of Nursing, *Muncie* (BS)
Bethel College, Department of Nursing, *Mishawaka* (BSN)
Goshen College, Department of Nursing, *Goshen* (BSN)
Indiana State University, School of Nursing, *Terre Haute* (BS)
Indiana University Bloomington, Department of Nursing–Bloomington Division, *Bloomington* (BSN)
Indiana University East, Division of Nursing, *Richmond* (BSN)
Indiana University Kokomo, Indiana University School Of Nursing, *Kokomo* (BSN)
Indiana University Northwest, School of Nursing and Health Professions, *Gary* (BSN)
Indiana University–Purdue University Indianapolis, School of Nursing, *Indianapolis* (BSN)
Indiana University South Bend, Division of Nursing and Health Professions, *South Bend* (BSN)
Indiana University Southeast, Division of Nursing, *New Albany* (BSN)
Indiana Wesleyan University, Division of Nursing, *Marion* (BS)
Marian College, Department of Nursing and Nutritional Science, *Indianapolis* (BSN)
Purdue University, School of Nursing, *West Lafayette* (BS)
Purdue University Calumet, School of Nursing, *Hammond* (BS)
Saint Mary's College, Department of Nursing, *Notre Dame* (BS)
University of Evansville, Department of Nursing, *Evansville* (BSN)
University of Indianapolis, School of Nursing, *Indianapolis* (BSN)
University of Saint Francis, Department of Nursing, *Fort Wayne* (BSN)
University of Southern Indiana, School of Nursing and Health Professions, *Evansville* (BSN)
Valparaiso University, College of Nursing, *Valparaiso* (BSN)

Iowa

Allen College, Program in Nursing, *Waterloo* (BSN)
Briar Cliff University, Department of Nursing, *Sioux City* (BSc PN)
Clarke College, Department of Nursing and Health, *Dubuque* (BS)
Coe College, Department of Nursing, *Cedar Rapids* (BSN)
Grand View College, Division of Nursing, *Des Moines* (BSN)
Iowa Wesleyan College, Division of Health and Natural Sciences, *Mount Pleasant* (BSN)
Morningside College, Department of Nursing Education, *Sioux City* (BSN)
Mount Mercy College, Department of Nursing, *Cedar Rapids* (BSN)
St. Ambrose University, Program in Nursing (BSN), *Davenport* (BSN)
The University of Iowa, College of Nursing, *Iowa City* (BSN)

Kansas

Baker University, School of Nursing, *Topeka* (BSN)
Bethel College, Department of Nursing, *North Newton* (BSN)
Emporia State University, Newman Division of Nursing, *Emporia* (BSN)
Fort Hays State University, Department of Nursing, *Hays* (BSN)
Kansas Wesleyan University, Department of Nursing Education, *Salina* (BSN)
MidAmerica Nazarene University, Division of Nursing, *Olathe* (BSN)
Newman University, Division of Nursing, *Wichita* (BSN)
Pittsburg State University, Department of Nursing, *Pittsburg* (BSN)
Southwestern College, Nursing Program, *Winfield* (BSN)
University of Kansas, School of Nursing, *Kansas City* (BSN)
Washburn University, School of Nursing, *Topeka* (BSN)
Wichita State University, School of Nursing, *Wichita* (BSN)

Kentucky

Bellarmine University, Donna and Allan Lansing School of Nursing and Health Sciences, *Louisville* (BSN)
Berea College, Department of Nursing, *Berea* (BS)
Eastern Kentucky University, Department of Baccalaureate and Graduate Nursing, *Richmond* (BSN)
Midway College, Program in Nursing (Baccalaureate), *Midway* (BSN)
Morehead State University, Department of Nursing and Allied Health Sciences, *Morehead* (BSN)
Murray State University, Department of Nursing, *Murray* (BSN)
Northern Kentucky University, Department of Nursing, *Highland Heights* (BSN)

Spalding University, School of Nursing, *Louisville* (BSN)
Thomas More College, Program in Nursing, *Crestview Hills* (BSN)
University of Kentucky, Graduate School Programs in the College of Nursing, *Lexington* (BSN)
University of Louisville, School of Nursing, *Louisville* (BSN)

Louisiana
Dillard University, Division of Nursing, *New Orleans* (BSN)
Grambling State University, School of Nursing, *Grambling* (BSN)
Louisiana College, Department of Nursing, *Pineville* (BSN)
Louisiana State University Health Sciences Center, School of Nursing, *New Orleans* (BSN)
McNeese State University, College of Nursing, *Lake Charles* (BSN)
Nicholls State University, Department of Nursing, *Thibodaux* (BSN)
Northwestern State University of Louisiana, College of Nursing, *Shreveport* (BSN)
Our Lady of Holy Cross College, Division of Nursing, *New Orleans* (BSN)
Southeastern Louisiana University, College of Nursing and Health Sciences, *Hammond* (BS)
Southern University and Agricultural and Mechanical College, School of Nursing, *Baton Rouge* (BSN)

Maine
Husson College, School of Nursing, *Bangor* (BSN)
University of Maine, School of Nursing, *Orono* (BSN)
University of Maine at Fort Kent, Department of Nursing, *Fort Kent* (BSN)
University of Southern Maine, College of Nursing and Health Professions, *Portland* (BS)

Maryland
Columbia Union College, Nursing Department, *Takoma Park* (BS)
Coppin State University, Helene Fuld School of Nursing, *Baltimore* (BSN)
The Johns Hopkins University, School of Nursing, *Baltimore* (BS)
Salisbury University, Program in Nursing, *Salisbury* (BS)
Towson University, Department of Nursing, *Towson* (BS)
University of Maryland, School of Nursing, *Baltimore* (BSN)
Villa Julie College, Nursing Division, *Stevenson* (BS)

Massachusetts
American International College, Division of Nursing, *Springfield* (BSN)
Boston College, William F. Connell School of Nursing, *Chestnut Hill* (BS)
Curry College, Division of Nursing, *Milton* (BS)
Elms College, Division of Nursing, *Chicopee* (BS)
Endicott College, Major in Nursing, *Beverly* (BS)
Northeastern University, School of Nursing, *Boston* (BSN)
Regis College, Department of Nursing, *Weston* (BSN)
Salem State College, Nursing Department, *Salem* (BSN)
Simmons College, Department of Nursing, *Boston* (BS)
University of Massachusetts Amherst, School of Nursing, *Amherst* (BS)
University of Massachusetts Boston, College of Nursing and Health Sciences, *Boston* (BS)
University of Massachusetts Dartmouth, College of Nursing, *North Dartmouth* (BSN)
University of Massachusetts Lowell, Department of Nursing, *Lowell* (BS)
Worcester State College, Department of Nursing, *Worcester* (BS)

Michigan
Andrews University, Department of Nursing, *Berrien Springs* (BS)
Calvin College, Department of Nursing, *Grand Rapids* (BSN)
Eastern Michigan University, Department of Nursing, *Ypsilanti* (BSN)
Grand Valley State University, Russell B. Kirkhof School of Nursing, *Allendale* (BSN)
Hope College, Department of Nursing, *Holland* (BSN)
Lake Superior State University, Department of Nursing, *Sault Sainte Marie* (BSN)
Madonna University, College of Nursing and Health, *Livonia* (BSN)
Michigan State University, College of Nursing, *East Lansing* (BSN)
Northern Michigan University, College of Nursing and Allied Health Science, *Marquette* (BSN)
Oakland University, School of Nursing, *Rochester* (BSN)
Saginaw Valley State University, Crystal M. Lange College of Nursing and Health Sciences, *University Center* (BSN)
University of Detroit Mercy, McAuley School of Nursing, *Detroit* (BSN)
University of Michigan, School of Nursing, *Ann Arbor* (BSN)
University of Michigan–Flint, Department of Nursing, *Flint* (BSN)
Wayne State University, College of Nursing, *Detroit* (BSN)
Western Michigan University, College of Health and Human Services, *Kalamazoo* (BS)

Minnesota
Bethel University, Department of Nursing, *St. Paul* (BSN)
College of Saint Benedict, Department of Nursing, *Saint Joseph* (BS)
College of St. Catherine, Department of Nursing, *St. Paul* (BS)
The College of St. Scholastica, Department of Nursing, *Duluth* (BA)
Concordia College, Department of Nursing, *Moorhead* (BA)
Gustavus Adolphus College, Department of Nursing, *St. Peter* (BA)
Minnesota Intercollegiate Nursing Consortium, *Northfield* (BA)
Minnesota State University Mankato, School of Nursing, *Mankato* (BS)
St. Cloud State University, Department of Nursing Science, *St. Cloud* (BS)
St. Olaf College, Department of Nursing, *Northfield* (BA)
University of Minnesota, Twin Cities Campus, School of Nursing, *Minneapolis* (BSN)
Winona State University, College of Nursing, *Winona* (BSN)

Mississippi
Alcorn State University, School of Nursing, *Natchez* (BSN)
Delta State University, School of Nursing, *Cleveland* (BSN)
Mississippi College, School of Nursing, *Clinton* (BSN)
Mississippi University for Women, Division of Nursing, *Columbus* (BSN)
University of Mississippi Medical Center, Program in Nursing, *Jackson* (BSN)
University of Southern Mississippi, School of Nursing, *Hattiesburg* (BSN)
William Carey College, School of Nursing, *Hattiesburg* (BSN)

Missouri
Avila University, Department of Nursing, *Kansas City* (BSN)
Central Missouri State University, Department of Nursing, *Warrensburg* (BS)
Graceland University, School of Nursing, *Independence* (BSN)
Lester L. Cox College of Nursing and Health Sciences, Department of Nursing, *Springfield* (BSN)
Maryville University of Saint Louis, Nursing Program, School of Health Professions, *St. Louis* (BSN)
Missouri Southern State University, Department of Nursing, *Joplin* (BSN)
Missouri Western State College, Department of Nursing, *St. Joseph* (BSN)
Research College of Nursing, College of Nursing, *Kansas City* (BSN)
Saint Louis University, School of Nursing, *St. Louis* (BSN)
Saint Luke's College, Nursing College, *Kansas City* (BSN)
Southeast Missouri State University, Department of Nursing, *Cape Girardeau* (BSN)
Southwest Missouri State University, Department of Nursing, *Springfield* (BSN)
Truman State University, Program in Nursing, *Kirksville* (BSN)
University of Missouri–Columbia, Sinclair School of Nursing, *Columbia* (BSN)
University of Missouri–Kansas City, School of Nursing, *Kansas City* (BSN)
University of Missouri–St. Louis, College of Nursing, *St. Louis* (BSN)
William Jewell College, Department of Nursing, *Liberty* (BS)

Montana
Carroll College, Department of Nursing, *Helena* (BA)

Nebraska
Clarkson College, Department of Nursing, *Omaha* (BSN)
College of Saint Mary, Division of Health Care Professions, *Omaha* (BSN)
Creighton University, School of Nursing, *Omaha* (BSN)
Midland Lutheran College, Department of Nursing, *Fremont* (BSN)
Nebraska Methodist College, Department of Nursing, *Omaha* (BSN)
Union College, Division of Health Sciences, *Lincoln* (BSN)
University of Nebraska Medical Center, College of Nursing, *Omaha* (BSN)

Nevada
University of Nevada, Las Vegas, Department of Nursing, *Las Vegas* (BSN)
University of Nevada, Reno, Orvis School of Nursing, *Reno* (BSN)

New Hampshire
Colby-Sawyer College, Department of Nursing, *New London* (BS)
University of New Hampshire, Department of Nursing, *Durham* (BS)

New Jersey
Bloomfield College, Division of Nursing, *Bloomfield* (BSN)
The College of New Jersey, School of Nursing, *Ewing* (BSN)
Fairleigh Dickinson University, Metropolitan Campus, Henry P. Becton School of Nursing and Allied Health, *Teaneck* (BSN)
Felician College, Department of Professional Nursing–BSN, *Lodi* (BSN)
Rutgers, The State University of New Jersey, Camden College of Arts and Sciences, Department of Nursing, *Camden* (BS)
Rutgers, The State University of New Jersey, College of Nursing, *Newark* (BS)
Seton Hall University, College of Nursing, *South Orange* (BSN)
University of Medicine and Dentistry of New Jersey, School of Nursing, *Newark* (BSN)
William Paterson University of New Jersey, Department of Nursing, *Wayne* (BSN)

New Mexico

New Mexico State University, Department of Nursing, *Las Cruces* (BSN)
University of New Mexico, College of Nursing, *Albuquerque* (BSN)

New York

Adelphi University, School of Nursing, *Garden City* (BS)
College of Mount Saint Vincent, Division of Nursing, *Riverdale* (BS)
The College of New Rochelle, School of Nursing, *New Rochelle* (BSN)
Dominican College, Division of Nursing, *Orangeburg* (BSN)
D'Youville College, Department of Nursing, *Buffalo* (BSN)
Elmira College, Program in Nursing Education, *Elmira* (BS)
Hartwick College, Department of Nursing, *Oneonta* (BS)
Hunter College of the City University of New York, Hunter-Bellevue School of Nursing, *New York* (BS)
Lehman College of the City University of New York, Department of Nursing, *Bronx* (BS)
Long Island University, Brooklyn Campus, School of Nursing, *Brooklyn* (BS)
Molloy College, Department of Nursing, *Rockville Centre* (BS)
Mount Saint Mary College, Division of Nursing, *Newburgh* (BSN)
Nazareth College of Rochester, Department of Nursing, *Rochester* (BS)
New York University, Division of Nursing, *New York* (BS)
Pace University, Lienhard School of Nursing, *New York* (BS)
Roberts Wesleyan College, Division of Nursing, *Rochester* (BS)
The Sage Colleges, Division of Nursing, *Troy* (BS)
St. John Fisher College, Nursing Program, *Rochester* (BS)
State University of New York at Binghamton, Decker School of Nursing, *Binghamton* (BS)
State University of New York at New Paltz, Department of Nursing, *New Paltz* (BSN)
State University of New York at Plattsburgh, Department of Nursing, *Plattsburgh* (BS)
State University of New York College at Brockport, Department of Nursing, *Brockport* (BSN)
University at Buffalo, The State University of New York, School of Nursing, *Buffalo* (BS)
Utica College, Department of Nursing, *Utica* (BS)
Wagner College, Department of Nursing, *Staten Island* (BS)

North Carolina

Barton College, School of Nursing, *Wilson* (BSN)
East Carolina University, School of Nursing, *Greenville* (BSN)
Lenoir-Rhyne College, Program in Nursing, *Hickory* (BS)
North Carolina Agricultural and Technical State University, School of Nursing, *Greensboro* (BSN)
North Carolina Central University, Department of Nursing, *Durham* (BSN)
Queens University of Charlotte, Division of Nursing, *Charlotte* (BSN)
The University of North Carolina at Chapel Hill, School of Nursing, *Chapel Hill* (BSN)
The University of North Carolina at Charlotte, School of Nursing, *Charlotte* (BSN)
The University of North Carolina at Greensboro, School of Nursing, *Greensboro* (BSN)
The University of North Carolina at Wilmington, School of Nursing, *Wilmington* (BS)
Western Carolina University, Department of Nursing, *Cullowhee* (BSN)
Winston-Salem State University, Department of Nursing, *Winston-Salem* (BSN)

North Dakota

Minot State University, Department of Nursing, *Minot* (BSN)
North Dakota State University, Tri-College University Nursing Consortium, *Fargo* (BSN)
University of Mary, Division of Nursing, *Bismarck* (BSN)
University of North Dakota, College of Nursing, *Grand Forks* (BSN)

Ohio

Capital University, School of Nursing, *Columbus* (BSN)
Case Western Reserve University, Frances Payne Bolton School of Nursing, *Cleveland* (BSN)
Cleveland State University, Department of Nursing, *Cleveland* (BSN)
College of Mount St. Joseph, Department of Nursing, *Cincinnati* (BSN)
Franciscan University of Steubenville, Department of Nursing, *Steubenville* (BSN)
Kent State University, College of Nursing, *Kent* (BSN)
Lourdes College, Nursing Department, *Sylvania* (BSN)
Malone College, School of Nursing, *Canton* (BSN)
Medical College of Ohio, School of Nursing, *Toledo* (BSN)
Mercy College of Northwest Ohio, Division of Nursing, *Toledo* (BSN)
Mount Carmel College of Nursing, Baccalaureate Nursing Program, *Columbus* (BSN)
The Ohio State University, College of Nursing, *Columbus* (BSN)
Otterbein College, Program in Nursing, *Westerville* (BSN)
The University of Akron, College of Nursing, *Akron* (BSN)
University of Cincinnati, College of Nursing, *Cincinnati* (BSN)
Ursuline College, The Breen School of Nursing, *Pepper Pike* (BSN)
Walsh University, Department of Nursing, *North Canton* (BSN)
Wright State University, College of Nursing and Health, *Dayton* (BSN)
Xavier University, Department of Nursing, *Cincinnati* (BSN)

Oklahoma

East Central University, Department of Nursing, *Ada* (BS)
Langston University, School of Nursing and Health Professions, *Langston* (BSN)
Oklahoma Baptist University, School of Nursing, *Shawnee* (BSN)
Oklahoma City University, Kramer School of Nursing, *Oklahoma City* (BSN)
Oklahoma Wesleyan University, Division of Nursing, *Bartlesville* (BSN)
Oral Roberts University, Anna Vaughn School of Nursing, *Tulsa* (BSN)
Southern Nazarene University, School of Nursing, *Bethany* (BS)
University of Central Oklahoma, Department of Nursing, *Edmond* (BSN)
University of Oklahoma Health Sciences Center, College of Nursing, *Oklahoma City* (BSN)
University of Tulsa, School of Nursing, *Tulsa* (BSN)

Oregon

Linfield College, School of Nursing, *McMinnville* (BSN)
Oregon Health & Science University, School of Nursing, *Portland* (BS)
University of Portland, School of Nursing, *Portland* (BSN)

Pennsylvania

Alvernia College, Nursing, *Reading* (BSN)
Bloomsburg University of Pennsylvania, Department of Nursing, *Bloomsburg* (BSN)
Carlow University, Division of Nursing, *Pittsburgh* (BSN)
Cedar Crest College, Department of Nursing, *Allentown* (BS)
College Misericordia, Department of Nursing, *Dallas* (BSN)
DeSales University, Department of Nursing and Health, *Center Valley* (BSN)
Duquesne University, School of Nursing, *Pittsburgh* (BSN)
East Stroudsburg University of Pennsylvania, Department of Nursing, *East Stroudsburg* (BS)
Edinboro University of Pennsylvania, Department of Nursing, *Edinboro* (BS)
Gannon University, Villa Maria School of Nursing, *Erie* (BSN)
Holy Family University, School of Nursing and Allied Health Professions, *Philadelphia* (BSN)
Indiana University of Pennsylvania, Department of Nursing and Allied Health, *Indiana* (BSN)
La Salle University, School of Nursing, *Philadelphia* (BSN)
Mansfield University of Pennsylvania, Robert Packer Department of Health Sciences, *Mansfield* (BSN)
Marywood University, Department of Nursing, *Scranton* (BSN)
Messiah College, Department of Nursing, *Grantham* (BSN)
Moravian College, St. Luke's School of Nursing, *Bethlehem* (BS)
Neumann College, Program in Nursing and Health Sciences, *Aston* (BSN)
The Pennsylvania State University University Park Campus, School of Nursing, *State College, University Park* (BS)
Saint Francis University, Department of Nursing, *Loretto* (BSN)
Temple University, Department of Nursing, *Philadelphia* (BSN)
Thomas Jefferson University, Department of Nursing, *Philadelphia* (BSN)
University of Pennsylvania, School of Nursing, *Philadelphia* (BSN)
University of Pittsburgh, School of Nursing, *Pittsburgh* (BSN)
The University of Scranton, Department of Nursing, *Scranton* (BS)
Villanova University, College of Nursing, *Villanova* (BSN)
Waynesburg College, Department of Nursing, *Waynesburg* (BSN)
West Chester University of Pennsylvania, Department of Nursing, *West Chester* (BSN)
Widener University, School of Nursing, *Chester* (BSN)
Wilkes University, Department of Nursing, *Wilkes-Barre* (BS)
York College of Pennsylvania, Department of Nursing, *York* (BS)

Puerto Rico

Inter American University of Puerto Rico, Metropolitan Campus, Carmen Torres de Tiburcio School of Nursing, *San Juan* (BSN)
Pontifical Catholic University of Puerto Rico, Department of Nursing, *Ponce* (BSN)
Universidad Adventista de las Antillas, Department of Nursing, *Mayagüez* (BSN)
University of Puerto Rico at Arecibo, Department of Nursing, *Arecibo* (BSN)
University of Puerto Rico at Humacao, Department of Nursing, *Humacao* (BS)
University of Puerto Rico, Mayagüez Campus, Department of Nursing, *Mayagüez* (BSN)
University of Puerto Rico, Medical Sciences Campus, School of Nursing, *San Juan* (BSN)
University of the Sacred Heart, Program in Nursing, *San Juan* (BSN)

Rhode Island

Rhode Island College, Department of Nursing, *Providence* (BS)

Salve Regina University, Department of Nursing, *Newport* (BS)
University of Rhode Island, College of Nursing, *Kingston* (BS)

South Carolina
Charleston Southern University, Wingo School of Nursing, *Charleston* (BSN)
Clemson University, School of Nursing, *Clemson* (BS)
Lander University, School of Nursing, *Greenwood* (BSN)
South Carolina State University, Department of Nursing, *Orangeburg* (BSN)
University of South Carolina, College of Nursing, *Columbia* (BSN)
University of South Carolina Upstate, Mary Black School of Nursing, *Spartanburg* (BSN)

South Dakota
Augustana College, Department of Nursing, *Sioux Falls* (BA)
Mount Marty College, Nursing Program, *Yankton* (BSc PN)
Presentation College, Department of Nursing, *Aberdeen* (BSN)
South Dakota State University, College of Nursing, *Brookings* (BS)

Tennessee
Austin Peay State University, School of Nursing, *Clarksville* (BSN)
Baptist College of Health Sciences, Nursing Division, *Memphis* (BSN)
Belmont University, School of Nursing, *Nashville* (BSN)
Carson-Newman College, Department of Nursing, *Jefferson City* (BSN)
Cumberland University, Rudy School of Nursing and Health Professions, *Lebanon* (BSN)
East Tennessee State University, College of Nursing, *Johnson City* (BSN)
King College, School of Nursing, *Bristol* (BSN)
Middle Tennessee State University, School of Nursing, *Murfreesboro* (BSN)
Tennessee State University, School of Nursing, *Nashville* (BSN)
Tennessee Technological University, School of Nursing, *Cookeville* (BSN)
Tennessee Wesleyan College, Fort Sanders Nursing Department, *Knoxville* (BSN)
Union University, School of Nursing, *Jackson* (BSN)
The University of Memphis, Loewenberg School of Nursing, *Memphis* (BSN)
The University of Tennessee, College of Nursing, *Knoxville* (BSN)
The University of Tennessee at Chattanooga, School of Nursing, *Chattanooga* (BSN)
The University of Tennessee at Martin, Department of Nursing, *Martin* (BSN)
The University of Tennessee Health Science Center, College of Nursing, *Memphis* (BSN)

Texas
Abilene Intercollegiate School of Nursing, *Abilene* (BSN)
Baylor University, Louise Herrington School of Nursing of Baylor University, *Dallas* (BSN)
East Texas Baptist University, Department of Nursing, *Marshall* (BSN)
Lamar University, Department of Nursing, *Beaumont* (BSN)
Midwestern State University, Nursing Program, *Wichita Falls* (BSN)
Prairie View A&M University, College of Nursing, *Houston* (BSN)
Tarleton State University, Department of Nursing, *Stephenville* (BSN)
Texas A&M International University, Canseco School of Nursing, *Laredo* (BSN)
Texas A&M University–Corpus Christi, School of Nursing and Health Sciences, *Corpus Christi* (BSN)
Texas Christian University, Harris School of Nursing, *Fort Worth* (BSN)
Texas Tech University Health Sciences Center, School of Nursing, *Lubbock* (BSN)
Texas Woman's University, College of Nursing, *Denton* (BS)
University of Mary Hardin-Baylor, College of Nursing, *Belton* (BSN)
The University of Texas at Arlington, School of Nursing, *Arlington* (BSN)
The University of Texas at Austin, School of Nursing, *Austin* (BSN)
The University of Texas at El Paso, School of Nursing, *El Paso* (BSN)
The University of Texas at Tyler, Program in Nursing, *Tyler* (BSN)
The University of Texas Health Science Center at Houston, School of Nursing, *Houston* (BSN)
The University of Texas Health Science Center at San Antonio, School of Nursing, *San Antonio* (BSN)
The University of Texas Medical Branch, School of Nursing, *Galveston* (BSN)
The University of Texas–Pan American, Department of Nursing, *Edinburg* (BSN)
University of the Incarnate Word, Program in Nursing, *San Antonio* (BSN)
West Texas A&M University, Division of Nursing, *Canyon* (BSN)

Utah
Brigham Young University, College of Nursing, *Provo* (BS)
University of Utah, College of Nursing, *Salt Lake City* (BS)
Westminster College, St. Mark's-Westminster School of Nursing and Health Sciences, *Salt Lake City* (BSN)

Vermont
Norwich University, Division of Nursing, *Northfield* (BSN)
University of Vermont, Department of Nursing, *Burlington* (BS)

Virgin Islands
University of the Virgin Islands, Division of Nursing, *Saint Thomas* (BS)

Virginia
Eastern Mennonite University, Department of Nursing, *Harrisonburg* (BSN)
George Mason University, College of Nursing and Health Science, *Fairfax* (BSN)
Hampton University, Department of Nursing, *Hampton* (BS)
James Madison University, Department of Nursing, *Harrisonburg* (BSN)
Liberty University, Department of Nursing, *Lynchburg* (BSN)
Lynchburg College, School of Health Sciences and Human Performance, *Lynchburg* (BS)
Marymount University, School of Health Professions, *Arlington* (BSN)
Old Dominion University, Department of Nursing, *Norfolk* (BSN)
Radford University, School of Nursing, *Radford* (BSN)
Shenandoah University, Division of Nursing, *Winchester* (BSN)
University of Virginia, School of Nursing, *Charlottesville* (BSN)
The University of Virginia's College at Wise, Department of Nursing, *Wise* (BSN)
Virginia Commonwealth University, School of Nursing, *Richmond* (BS)

Washington
Intercollegiate College of Nursing/Washington State University, *Spokane* (BSN)
Northwest University, The Mark and Huldah Buntain School of Nursing, *Kirkland* (BS)
Pacific Lutheran University, School of Nursing, *Tacoma* (BSN)
Seattle Pacific University, School of Health Sciences, *Seattle* (BSN)
Seattle University, College of Nursing, *Seattle* (BSN)
University of Washington, School of Nursing, *Seattle* (BSN)
Walla Walla College, School of Nursing, *College Place* (BS)

West Virginia
Alderson-Broaddus College, Department of Nursing, *Philippi* (BSN)
Marshall University, College of Nursing and Health Professions, *Huntington* (BSN)
Mountain State University, Program in Nursing, *Beckley* (BSN)
Shepherd University, Department of Nursing Education, *Shepherdstown* (BSN)
University of Charleston, Department of Nursing, *Charleston* (BSN)
West Liberty State College, Department of Health Sciences, *West Liberty* (BSN)
West Virginia University, School of Nursing, *Morgantown* (BSN)
West Virginia Wesleyan College, Department of Nursing, *Buckhannon* (BSN)

Wisconsin
Alverno College, Division of Nursing, *Milwaukee* (BSN)
Bellin College of Nursing, Nursing Program, *Green Bay* (BSN)
Columbia College of Nursing/Mount Mary College Nursing Program, *Milwaukee* (BSN)
Concordia University Wisconsin, Division of Nursing, *Mequon* (BSN)
Edgewood College, Program in Nursing, *Madison* (BS)
Marian College of Fond du Lac, Nursing Studies Division, *Fond du Lac* (BSN)
Marquette University, College of Nursing, *Milwaukee* (BSN)
Milwaukee School of Engineering, School of Nursing, *Milwaukee* (BSN)
University of Wisconsin–Eau Claire, College of Nursing and Health Sciences, *Eau Claire* (BSN)
University of Wisconsin–Madison, School of Nursing, *Madison* (BS)
University of Wisconsin–Milwaukee, College of Nursing, *Milwaukee* (BSN)
University of Wisconsin–Oshkosh, College of Nursing, *Oshkosh* (BSN)
Viterbo University, School of Nursing, *La Crosse* (BSN)

Wyoming
University of Wyoming, Fay W. Whitney School of Nursing, *Laramie* (BSN)

Alberta
University of Calgary, Faculty of Nursing, *Calgary* (BN)
The University of Lethbridge, School of Health Sciences, *Lethbridge* (BN)

British Columbia
British Columbia Institute of Technology, School of Health Sciences, *Burnaby* (BScN)
Kwantlen University College, Faculty of Community and Health Sciences, *Surrey* (BSN)
Malaspina University-College, Department of Nursing, *Nanaimo* (BScN)
Okanagan University College, Nursing Department, *Kelowna* (BSN)
Trinity Western University, Department of Nursing, *Langley* (BScN)
The University of British Columbia, School of Nursing, *Vancouver* (BSN)
University of Northern British Columbia, Nursing Programme, *Prince George* (BSN)

Manitoba
Brandon University, School of Health Studies, *Brandon* (BN)

BACCALAUREATE PROGRAMS
Generic Baccalaureate

University of Manitoba, Faculty of Nursing, *Winnipeg* (BN)

New Brunswick
University of New Brunswick Fredericton, Faculty of Nursing, *Fredericton* (BN)

Newfoundland and Labrador
Memorial University of Newfoundland, School of Nursing, *St. John's* (BN)

Nova Scotia
Dalhousie University, School of Nursing, *Halifax* (BScN)
St. Francis Xavier University, Department of Nursing, *Antigonish* (BScN)

Ontario
Brock University, Department of Nursing, *St. Catharines* (BScN)
Lakehead University, School of Nursing, *Thunder Bay* (BSN)
McMaster University, School of Nursing, *Hamilton* (BScN)
Nipissing University, Nursing Department, *North Bay* (BScN)
Queen's University at Kingston, School of Nursing, *Kingston* (BNSc)
Ryerson University, Program in Nursing, *Toronto* (BScN)
University of Ottawa, School of Nursing, *Ottawa* (BScN)
University of Toronto, Faculty of Nursing, *Toronto* (BScN)
The University of Western Ontario, School of Nursing, *London* (BScN)
University of Windsor, School of Nursing, *Windsor* (BScN)
York University, School of Nursing, Atkinson Faculty of Liberal and Profesional Studies, *Toronto* (BScN)

Prince Edward Island
University of Prince Edward Island, School of Nursing, *Charlottetown* (BScN)

Quebec
McGill University, School of Nursing, *Montréal* (BScN)
Université du Québec en Outaouais, Département des Sciences Infirmières, *Gatineau* (BScN)

Saskatchewan
University of Saskatchewan, College of Nursing, *Saskatoon* (BSN)

International Nurse to Baccalaureate

California
Humboldt State University, Department of Nursing, *Arcata* (BSN)

Hawaii
Hawai'i Pacific University, School of Nursing, *Honolulu* (BSN)

Iowa
Morningside College, Department of Nursing Education, *Sioux City* (BSN)

Massachusetts
Salem State College, Nursing Department, *Salem* (BSN)

Nebraska
Nebraska Wesleyan University, Department of Nursing, *Lincoln* (BSN)
University of Nebraska Medical Center, College of Nursing, *Omaha* (BSN)

New Jersey
College of Saint Elizabeth, Department of Nursing, *Morristown* (BSN)

New York
Long Island University, Brooklyn Campus, School of Nursing, *Brooklyn* (BS)
University at Buffalo, The State University of New York, School of Nursing, *Buffalo* (BS)

Oklahoma
Oklahoma Wesleyan University, Division of Nursing, *Bartlesville* (BSN)

Pennsylvania
Duquesne University, School of Nursing, *Pittsburgh* (BSN)
Holy Family University, School of Nursing and Allied Health Professions, *Philadelphia* (BSN)
Neumann College, Program in Nursing and Health Sciences, *Aston* (BS)
Villanova University, College of Nursing, *Villanova* (BSN)

South Dakota
Mount Marty College, Nursing Program, *Yankton* (BSc PN)

Texas
The University of Texas at Tyler, Program in Nursing, *Tyler* (BSN)

LPN to Baccalaureate

Arkansas
Arkansas State University, Department of Nursing, *Jonesboro, State University* (BSN)
Arkansas Tech University, Program in Nursing, *Russellville* (BSN)
Harding University, College of Nursing, *Searcy* (BSN)
University of Arkansas, Eleanor Mann School of Nursing, *Fayetteville* (BSN)
University of Arkansas at Monticello, Division of Nursing, *Monticello* (BSN)
University of Central Arkansas, Department of Nursing, *Conway* (BSN)

California
Biola University, Department of Nursing, *La Mirada* (BS)
California State University, Chico, School of Nursing, *Chico* (BSN)
California State University, Stanislaus, Department of Nursing, *Turlock* (BSN)
Dominican University of California, Program in Occupational Therapy, *San Rafael* (BSN)
Humboldt State University, Department of Nursing, *Arcata* (BSN)
Sonoma State University, Department of Nursing, *Rohnert Park* (BSN)

Colorado
Colorado State University-Pueblo, Department of Nursing, *Pueblo* (BSN)
Mesa State College, Department of Nursing and Radiologic Sciences, *Grand Junction* (BSN)

Delaware
Delaware State University, Department of Nursing, *Dover* (BSN)
Wesley College, Graduate Nursing Program, *Dover* (BSN)

District of Columbia
Howard University, Division of Nursing, *Washington* (BSN)

Florida
Barry University, School of Nursing, *Miami Shores* (BSN)

Georgia
Armstrong Atlantic State University, Program in Nursing, *Savannah* (BSN)
Georgia Southern University, School of Nursing, *Statesboro* (BSN)

Hawaii
Hawai'i Pacific University, School of Nursing, *Honolulu* (BSN)

Idaho
Boise State University, Department of Nursing, *Boise* (BS)
Idaho State University, Department of Nursing, *Pocatello* (BSN)
Lewis-Clark State College, Division of Nursing and Health Sciences, *Lewiston* (BSN)

Illinois
Blessing–Rieman College of Nursing, *Quincy* (BSN)
Chicago State University, College of Nursing and Allied Health Professions, *Chicago* (BSN)
MacMurray College, Department of Nursing, *Jacksonville* (BSN)
Saint Xavier University, School of Nursing, *Chicago* (BSN)

Indiana
Ball State University, School of Nursing, *Muncie* (BS)
Bethel College, Department of Nursing, *Mishawaka* (BSN)
Indiana State University, School of Nursing, *Terre Haute* (BS)
Marian College, Department of Nursing and Nutritional Science, *Indianapolis* (BSN)

Iowa
Briar Cliff University, Department of Nursing, *Sioux City* (BSc PN)
Morningside College, Department of Nursing Education, *Sioux City* (BSN)

Kansas
Bethel College, Department of Nursing, *North Newton* (BSN)
Emporia State University, Newman Division of Nursing, *Emporia* (BSN)
Newman University, Division of Nursing, *Wichita* (BSN)
Washburn University, School of Nursing, *Topeka* (BSN)

Louisiana
Grambling State University, School of Nursing, *Grambling* (BSN)
Nicholls State University, Department of Nursing, *Thibodaux* (BSN)
Northwestern State University of Louisiana, College of Nursing, *Shreveport* (BSN)
University of Louisiana at Monroe, Nursing, *Monroe* (BS)

Massachusetts
Salem State College, Nursing Department, *Salem* (BSN)
Simmons College, Department of Nursing, *Boston* (BS)

Missouri
Maryville University of Saint Louis, Nursing Program, School of Health Professions, *St. Louis* (BSN)
Missouri Western State College, Department of Nursing, *St. Joseph* (BSN)
Southwest Missouri State University, Department of Nursing, *Springfield* (BSN)

Montana
Montana State University–Bozeman, College of Nursing, *Bozeman* (BSN)

Nebraska
Clarkson College, Department of Nursing, *Omaha* (BSN)
Nebraska Methodist College, Department of Nursing, *Omaha* (BSN)
Union College, Division of Health Sciences, *Lincoln* (BSN)
University of Nebraska Medical Center, College of Nursing, *Omaha* (BSN)

New York
Dominican College, Division of Nursing, *Orangeburg* (BSN)
Molloy College, Department of Nursing, *Rockville Centre* (BS)
Nazareth College of Rochester, Department of Nursing, *Rochester* (BS)
State University of New York College at Brockport, Department of Nursing, *Brockport* (BSN)

North Carolina
North Carolina Agricultural and Technical State University, School of Nursing, *Greensboro* (BSN)
Queens University of Charlotte, Division of Nursing, *Charlotte* (BSN)
The University of North Carolina at Greensboro, School of Nursing, *Greensboro* (BSN)

North Dakota
Dickinson State University, Department of Nursing, *Dickinson* (BSN)
Minot State University, Department of Nursing, *Minot* (BSN)
North Dakota State University, Tri-College University Nursing Consortium, *Fargo* (BSN)
University of Mary, Division of Nursing, *Bismarck* (BSN)
University of North Dakota, College of Nursing, *Grand Forks* (BSN)

Ohio
Kent State University, College of Nursing, *Kent* (BSN)
Lourdes College, Nursing Department, *Sylvania* (BSN)
Otterbein College, Program in Nursing, *Westerville* (BSN)
The University of Akron, College of Nursing, *Akron* (BSN)

Oklahoma
Langston University, School of Nursing and Health Professions, *Langston* (BSN)
Oklahoma Baptist University, School of Nursing, *Shawnee* (BSN)
Oklahoma Wesleyan University, Division of Nursing, *Bartlesville* (BSN)
University of Central Oklahoma, Department of Nursing, *Edmond* (BSN)

Pennsylvania
East Stroudsburg University of Pennsylvania, Department of Nursing, *East Stroudsburg* (BS)
Edinboro University of Pennsylvania, Department of Nursing, *Edinboro* (BS)
Holy Family University, School of Nursing and Allied Health Professions, *Philadelphia* (BSN)
La Salle University, School of Nursing, *Philadelphia* (BSN)
Marywood University, Department of Nursing, *Scranton* (BSN)
Waynesburg College, Department of Nursing, *Waynesburg* (BSN)

South Dakota
Mount Marty College, Nursing Program, *Yankton* (BSc PN)
Presentation College, Department of Nursing, *Aberdeen* (BSN)

Tennessee
Baptist College of Health Sciences, Nursing Division, *Memphis* (BSN)
Cumberland University, Rudy School of Nursing and Health Professions, *Lebanon* (BSN)
East Tennessee State University, College of Nursing, *Johnson City* (BSN)
Union University, School of Nursing, *Jackson* (BSN)
The University of Memphis, Loewenberg School of Nursing, *Memphis* (BSN)

Texas
Tarleton State University, Department of Nursing, *Stephenville* (BSN)
The University of Texas at Tyler, Program in Nursing, *Tyler* (BSN)
The University of Texas Health Science Center at San Antonio, School of Nursing, *San Antonio* (BSN)
West Texas A&M University, Division of Nursing, *Canyon* (BSN)

Virginia
Eastern Mennonite University, Department of Nursing, *Harrisonburg* (BSN)
Hampton University, Department of Nursing, *Hampton* (BS)
Marymount University, School of Health Professions, *Arlington* (BSN)
Shenandoah University, Division of Nursing, *Winchester* (BSN)

Washington
Pacific Lutheran University, School of Nursing, *Tacoma* (BSN)
Walla Walla College, School of Nursing, *College Place* (BS)

West Virginia
Alderson-Broaddus College, Department of Nursing, *Philippi* (BSN)
Mountain State University, Program in Nursing, *Beckley* (BSN)

Wisconsin
Alverno College, Division of Nursing, *Milwaukee* (BSN)
Concordia University Wisconsin, Division of Nursing, *Mequon* (BSN)

Alberta
Athabasca University, Centre for Nursing and Health Studies, *Athabasca* (BN)

British Columbia
Malaspina University-College, Department of Nursing, *Nanaimo* (BScN)

Manitoba
Brandon University, School of Health Studies, *Brandon* (BN)

LPN to RN Baccalaureate

Alabama
University of Mobile, School of Nursing, *Mobile* (BSN)

Arkansas
Harding University, College of Nursing, *Searcy* (BSN)
University of Arkansas, Eleanor Mann School of Nursing, *Fayetteville* (BSN)

California
California State University, Sacramento, Division of Nursing, *Sacramento* (BSN)
Dominican University of California, Program in Occupational Therapy, *San Rafael* (BSN)
Point Loma Nazarene University, School of Nursing, *San Diego* (BSN)
Sonoma State University, Department of Nursing, *Rohnert Park* (BSN)

Colorado
Colorado State University-Pueblo, Department of Nursing, *Pueblo* (BSN)
Mesa State College, Department of Nursing and Radiologic Sciences, *Grand Junction* (BSN)

District of Columbia
Howard University, Division of Nursing, *Washington* (BSN)

Florida
Barry University, School of Nursing, *Miami Shores* (BSN)

Illinois
MacMurray College, Department of Nursing, *Jacksonville* (BSN)

Iowa
Iowa Wesleyan College, Division of Health and Natural Sciences, *Mount Pleasant* (BSN)

Kansas
Wichita State University, School of Nursing, *Wichita* (BSN)

Louisiana
University of Louisiana at Lafayette, College of Nursing, *Lafayette* (BSN)

Massachusetts
Salem State College, Nursing Department, *Salem* (BSN)

Michigan
Madonna University, College of Nursing and Health, *Livonia* (BSN)
Northern Michigan University, College of Nursing and Allied Health Science, *Marquette* (BSN)

Missouri
Missouri Southern State University, Department of Nursing, *Joplin* (BSN)

Nebraska
Midland Lutheran College, Department of Nursing, *Fremont* (BSN)

North Carolina
The University of North Carolina at Greensboro, School of Nursing, *Greensboro* (BSN)

North Dakota
Medcenter One College of Nursing, Medcenter One College of Nursing, *Bismarck* (BSN)
University of North Dakota, College of Nursing, *Grand Forks* (BSN)

Ohio
Malone College, School of Nursing, *Canton* (BSN)

Oklahoma
University of Tulsa, School of Nursing, *Tulsa* (BSN)

Pennsylvania
Bloomsburg University of Pennsylvania, Department of Nursing, *Bloomsburg* (BSN)
Carlow University, Division of Nursing, *Pittsburgh* (BSN)
Holy Family University, School of Nursing and Allied Health Professions, *Philadelphia* (BSN)
The University of Scranton, Department of Nursing, *Scranton* (BS)
Wilkes University, Department of Nursing, *Wilkes-Barre* (BS)
York College of Pennsylvania, Department of Nursing, *York* (BS)

South Dakota
Mount Marty College, Nursing Program, *Yankton* (BSc PN)

Tennessee
Belmont University, School of Nursing, *Nashville* (BSN)
The University of Tennessee at Martin, Department of Nursing, *Martin* (BSN)

Texas
The University of Texas at Tyler, Program in Nursing, *Tyler* (BSN)
The University of Texas Health Science Center at San Antonio, School of Nursing, *San Antonio* (BSN)

Virginia
Hampton University, Department of Nursing, *Hampton* (BS)
Marymount University, School of Health Professions, *Arlington* (BSN)
Shenandoah University, Division of Nursing, *Winchester* (BSN)

West Virginia
Alderson-Broaddus College, Department of Nursing, *Philippi* (BSN)

BACCALAUREATE PROGRAMS
LPN to RN Baccalaureate

Fairmont State University, School of Nursing/Allied Health Adm., *Fairmont* (BSN)

British Columbia
Okanagan University College, Nursing Department, *Kelowna* (BSN)

RN Baccalaureate

Alabama
Auburn University Montgomery, School of Nursing, *Montgomery* (BSN)
Jacksonville State University, College of Nursing and Health Sciences, *Jacksonville* (BSN)
Samford University, Ida V. Moffett School of Nursing, *Birmingham* (BSN)
Tuskegee University, Program in Nursing, *Tuskegee* (BSN)
The University of Alabama, Capstone College of Nursing, *Tuscaloosa* (BSN)
The University of Alabama at Birmingham, School of Nursing, *Birmingham* (BSN)
The University of Alabama in Huntsville, College of Nursing, *Huntsville* (BSN)
University of Mobile, School of Nursing, *Mobile* (BSN)
University of North Alabama, College of Nursing and Allied Health, *Florence* (BSN)
University of South Alabama, College of Nursing, *Mobile* (BSN)

Alaska
University of Alaska Anchorage, School of Nursing, *Anchorage* (BS)

Arizona
Northern Arizona University, Department of Nursing, *Flagstaff* (BSN)

Arkansas
Arkansas State University, Department of Nursing, *Jonesboro, State University* (BSN)
Arkansas Tech University, Program in Nursing, *Russellville* (BSN)
Harding University, College of Nursing, *Searcy* (BSN)
University of Arkansas, Eleanor Mann School of Nursing, *Fayetteville* (BSN)
University of Arkansas at Monticello, Division of Nursing, *Monticello* (BSN)
University of Arkansas for Medical Sciences, College of Nursing, *Little Rock* (BSN)
University of Central Arkansas, Department of Nursing, *Conway* (BSN)

California
Biola University, Department of Nursing, *La Mirada* (BS)
California State University, Bakersfield, Program in Nursing, *Bakersfield* (BSN)
California State University, Chico, School of Nursing, *Chico* (BSN)
California State University, Dominguez Hills, Program in Nursing, *Carson* (BSN)
California State University, Fresno, Department of Nursing, *Fresno* (BSN)
California State University, Fullerton, Department of Nursing, *Fullerton* (BSN)
California State University, Hayward, Department of Nursing and Health Sciences, *Hayward* (BS)
California State University, Long Beach, Department of Nursing, *Long Beach* (BSN)
California State University, Los Angeles, School of Nursing, *Los Angeles* (BS)
California State University, Northridge, Nursing Program, *Northridge* (BSN)
California State University, Sacramento, Division of Nursing, *Sacramento* (BSN)
California State University, San Bernardino, Department of Nursing, *San Bernardino* (BSN)
Dominican University of California, Program in Occupational Therapy, *San Rafael* (BSN)
Holy Names University, Department of Nursing, *Oakland* (BSN)
Humboldt State University, Department of Nursing, *Arcata* (BSN)
Loma Linda University, School of Nursing, *Loma Linda* (BS)
National University, Department of Nursing, *La Jolla* (BSN)
Point Loma Nazarene University, School of Nursing, *San Diego* (BSN)
San Diego State University, School of Nursing, *San Diego* (BSN)
San Francisco State University, School of Nursing, *San Francisco* (BSN)
Sonoma State University, Department of Nursing, *Rohnert Park* (BSN)
University of San Diego, Hahn School of Nursing and Health Sciences, *San Diego* (BSN)

Colorado
Colorado State University-Pueblo, Department of Nursing, *Pueblo* (BSN)
Mesa State College, Department of Nursing and Radiologic Sciences, *Grand Junction* (BSN)
Metropolitan State College of Denver, Department of Health Professions, *Denver* (BS)
Regis University, Department of Nursing, *Denver* (BSN)
University of Colorado at Colorado Springs, Beth-El College of Nursing and Health Sciences, *Colorado Springs* (BSN)
University of Colorado at Denver and Health Sciences Center—Health Sciences Program, School of Nursing, *Denver* (BS)
University of Northern Colorado, School of Nursing, *Greeley* (BS)

Connecticut
Central Connecticut State University, Department of Counseling and Family Therapy, *New Britain* (BSN)
Fairfield University, School of Nursing, *Fairfield* (BS)
Quinnipiac University, Department of Nursing, *Hamden* (BSN)
Sacred Heart University, Program in Nursing, *Fairfield* (BS)
Saint Joseph College, Department of Nursing, *West Hartford* (BS)
Southern Connecticut State University, Department of Nursing, *New Haven* (BSN)
University of Connecticut, School of Nursing, *Storrs* (BS)
University of Hartford, College of Education, Nursing, and Health Professions, *West Hartford* (BSN)
Western Connecticut State University, Department of Nursing, *Danbury* (BS)

Delaware
University of Delaware, Department of Nursing, *Newark* (BSN)
Wilmington College, Division of Nursing, *New Castle* (BSN)

District of Columbia
Georgetown University, School of Nursing and Health Studies, *Washington* (BSN)
Howard University, Division of Nursing, *Washington* (BSN)

Florida
Barry University, School of Nursing, *Miami Shores* (BSN)
Bethune-Cookman College, School of Nursing, *Daytona Beach* (BSN)
Florida Atlantic University, College of Nursing, *Boca Raton* (BSN)
Florida Hospital College of Health Sciences, Department of Nursing, *Orlando* (BS)
Florida International University, School of Nursing, *Miami* (BSN)
Florida State University, School of Nursing, *Tallahassee* (BSN)
Jacksonville University, School of Nursing, *Jacksonville* (BSN)
Nova Southeastern University, College of Allied Health and Nursing, *Fort Lauderdale* (BSN)
St. Petersburg College, Department of Nursing, *St. Petersburg* (BSN)
University of Central Florida, School of Nursing, *Orlando* (BSN)
University of Florida, College of Nursing, *Gainesville* (BSN)
University of Miami, School of Nursing, *Coral Gables* (BSN)
University of North Florida, School of Nursing, *Jacksonville* (BSN)
University of South Florida, College of Nursing, *Tampa* (BS)
The University of Tampa, Department of Nursing, *Tampa* (BSN)
University of West Florida, Department of Nursing, *Pensacola* (BSN)

Georgia
Albany State University, College of Health Professions, *Albany* (BSN)
Armstrong Atlantic State University, Program in Nursing, *Savannah* (BSN)
Clayton College & State University, Department of Nursing, *Morrow* (BSN)
Emory University, Nell Hodgson Woodruff School of Nursing, *Atlanta* (BSN)
Georgia Baptist College of Nursing of Mercer University, Department of Nursing, *Atlanta* (BSN)
Georgia College & State University, School of Health Sciences, *Milledgeville* (BSN)
Georgia Southwestern State University, School of Nursing, *Americus* (BSN)
Georgia State University, School of Nursing, *Atlanta* (BS)
Kennesaw State University, School of Nursing, *Kennesaw* (BSN)
LaGrange College, Department of Nursing, *LaGrange* (BSN)
Medical College of Georgia, School of Nursing, *Augusta* (BSN)
North Georgia College & State University, Department of Nursing, *Dahlonega* (BSN)
Piedmont College, School of Nursing, *Demorest* (BSN)
Thomas University, Division of Nursing, *Thomasville* (BSN)
University of Phoenix–Atlanta Campus, College of Health and Human Services, *Atlanta* (BSN)
University of West Georgia, Department of Nursing, *Carrollton* (BSN)
Valdosta State University, College of Nursing, *Valdosta* (BSN)

Guam
University of Guam, College of Nursing and Health Sciences, *Mangilao* (BSN)

Hawaii
Hawai'i Pacific University, School of Nursing, *Honolulu* (BSN)
University of Hawaii at Hilo, Department in Nursing, *Hilo* (BSN)
University of Hawaii at Manoa, School of Nursing and Dental Hygiene, *Honolulu* (BS)

Idaho
Boise State University, Department of Nursing, *Boise* (BS)
Lewis-Clark State College, Division of Nursing and Health Sciences, *Lewiston* (BSN)

Illinois
Aurora University, School of Nursing, *Aurora* (BSN)
Blessing–Rieman College of Nursing, *Quincy* (BSN)
Chicago State University, College of Nursing and Allied Health Professions, *Chicago* (BSN)

Elmhurst College, Deicke Center for Nursing Education, *Elmhurst* (BSN)
Governors State University, Division of Nursing, Communication Disorders, Occupational Therapy, and Physical Therapy, *University Park* (BS)
Illinois State University, Mennonite College of Nursing, *Normal* (BSN)
Illinois Wesleyan University, School of Nursing, *Bloomington* (BSN)
Lakeview College of Nursing, *Danville* (BSN)
Loyola University Chicago, Marcella Niehoff School of Nursing, *Chicago* (BSN)
MacMurray College, Department of Nursing, *Jacksonville* (BSN)
Northern Illinois University, School of Nursing, *De Kalb* (BS)
Rockford College, Department of Nursing, *Rockford* (BSN)
Rush University, College of Nursing, *Chicago* (BSN)
Saint Anthony College of Nursing, Saint Anthony College of Nursing, *Rockford* (BSN)
Southern Illinois University Edwardsville, School of Nursing, *Edwardsville* (BS)
Trinity Christian College, Department of Nursing, *Palos Heights* (BSN)
West Suburban College of Nursing, *Oak Park* (BSN)

Indiana

Ball State University, School of Nursing, *Muncie* (BS)
Bethel College, Department of Nursing, *Mishawaka* (BSN)
Goshen College, Department of Nursing, *Goshen* (BSN)
Indiana State University, School of Nursing, *Terre Haute* (BS)
Indiana University East, Division of Nursing, *Richmond* (BSN)
Indiana University Northwest, School of Nursing and Health Professions, *Gary* (BSN)
Indiana University–Purdue University Fort Wayne, Department of Nursing, *Fort Wayne* (BS)
Indiana University–Purdue University Indianapolis, School of Nursing, *Indianapolis* (BSN)
Indiana University South Bend, Division of Nursing and Health Professions, *South Bend* (BSN)
Indiana University Southeast, Division of Nursing, *New Albany* (BSN)
Marian College, Department of Nursing and Nutritional Science, *Indianapolis* (BSN)
Purdue University, School of Nursing, *West Lafayette* (BS)
Purdue University Calumet, School of Nursing, *Hammond* (BS)
University of Saint Francis, Department of Nursing, *Fort Wayne* (BSN)
University of Southern Indiana, School of Nursing and Health Professions, *Evansville* (BSN)
Valparaiso University, College of Nursing, *Valparaiso* (BSN)

Iowa

Allen College, Program in Nursing, *Waterloo* (BSN)
Briar Cliff University, Department of Nursing, *Sioux City* (BSc PN)
Clarke College, Department of Nursing and Health, *Dubuque* (BS)
Coe College, Department of Nursing, *Cedar Rapids* (BSN)
Grand View College, Division of Nursing, *Des Moines* (BSN)
Iowa Wesleyan College, Division of Health and Natural Sciences, *Mount Pleasant* (BSN)
Mercy College of Health Sciences, Division of Nursing, *Des Moines* (BSN)
Morningside College, Department of Nursing Education, *Sioux City* (BSN)
St. Ambrose University, Program in Nursing (BSN), *Davenport* (BSN)
The University of Iowa, College of Nursing, *Iowa City* (BSN)

Kansas

Baker University, School of Nursing, *Topeka* (BSN)
Bethel College, Department of Nursing, *North Newton* (BSN)
Emporia State University, Newman Division of Nursing, *Emporia* (BSN)
Fort Hays State University, Department of Nursing, *Hays* (BSN)
Kansas Wesleyan University, Department of Nursing Education, *Salina* (BSN)
MidAmerica Nazarene University, Division of Nursing, *Olathe* (BSN)
Newman University, Division of Nursing, *Wichita* (BSN)
Pittsburg State University, Department of Nursing, *Pittsburg* (BSN)
Southwestern College, Nursing Program, *Winfield* (BSN)
University of Kansas, School of Nursing, *Kansas City* (BSN)
Washburn University, School of Nursing, *Topeka* (BSN)
Wichita State University, School of Nursing, *Wichita* (BSN)

Kentucky

Bellarmine University, Donna and Allan Lansing School of Nursing and Health Sciences, *Louisville* (BSN)
Eastern Kentucky University, Department of Baccalaureate and Graduate Nursing, *Richmond* (BSN)
Midway College, Program in Nursing (Baccalaureate), *Midway* (BSN)
Morehead State University, Department of Nursing and Allied Health Sciences, *Morehead* (BSN)
Murray State University, Department of Nursing, *Murray* (BSN)
Northern Kentucky University, Department of Nursing, *Highland Heights* (BSN)
University of Kentucky, Graduate School Programs in the College of Nursing, *Lexington* (BSN)

Louisiana

Dillard University, Division of Nursing, *New Orleans* (BSN)
Grambling State University, School of Nursing, *Grambling* (BSN)
Louisiana State University Health Sciences Center, School of Nursing, *New Orleans* (BSN)
Loyola University New Orleans, Program in Nursing, *New Orleans* (BSN)
Nicholls State University, Department of Nursing, *Thibodaux* (BSN)
Northwestern State University of Louisiana, College of Nursing, *Shreveport* (BSN)
Southeastern Louisiana University, College of Nursing and Health Sciences, *Hammond* (BS)
University of Louisiana at Lafayette, College of Nursing, *Lafayette* (BSN)
University of Louisiana at Monroe, Nursing, *Monroe* (BS)

Maine

Husson College, School of Nursing, *Bangor* (BSN)
Saint Joseph's College of Maine, Department of Nursing, *Standish* (BSN)
University of Maine, School of Nursing, *Orono* (BSN)
University of Maine at Fort Kent, Department of Nursing, *Fort Kent* (BSN)
University of New England, Department of Nursing, *Biddeford* (BSN)

Maryland

Bowie State University, Department of Nursing, *Bowie* (BSN)
College of Notre Dame of Maryland, Department of Nursing, *Baltimore* (BS)
Coppin State University, Helene Fuld School of Nursing, *Baltimore* (BSN)
The Johns Hopkins University, School of Nursing, *Baltimore* (BS)
Towson University, Department of Nursing, *Towson* (BS)
University of Maryland, School of Nursing, *Baltimore* (BSN)
Villa Julie College, Nursing Division, *Stevenson* (BS)

Massachusetts

American International College, Division of Nursing, *Springfield* (BSN)
Atlantic Union College, Department of Nursing, *South Lancaster* (BSN)
Curry College, Division of Nursing, *Milton* (BS)
Elms College, Division of Nursing, *Chicopee* (BS)
Emmanuel College, Department of Nursing, *Boston* (BSN)
Endicott College, Major in Nursing, *Beverly* (BS)
Fitchburg State College, Department of Nursing, *Fitchburg* (BSN)
Northeastern University, School of Nursing, *Boston* (BSN)
Regis College, Department of Nursing, *Weston* (BSN)
Simmons College, Department of Nursing, *Boston* (BS)
University of Massachusetts Amherst, School of Nursing, *Amherst* (BS)
University of Massachusetts Boston, College of Nursing and Health Sciences, *Boston* (BS)
University of Massachusetts Dartmouth, College of Nursing, *North Dartmouth* (BSN)
University of Massachusetts Lowell, Department of Nursing, *Lowell* (BS)

Michigan

Eastern Michigan University, Department of Nursing, *Ypsilanti* (BSN)
Ferris State University, Department of Nursing and Dental Hygiene, *Big Rapids* (BSN)
Grand Valley State University, Russell B. Kirkhof School of Nursing, *Allendale* (BSN)
Lake Superior State University, Department of Nursing, *Sault Sainte Marie* (BSN)
Madonna University, College of Nursing and Health, *Livonia* (BSN)
Michigan State University, College of Nursing, *East Lansing* (BSN)
Oakland University, School of Nursing, *Rochester* (BSN)
Saginaw Valley State University, Crystal M. Lange College of Nursing and Health Sciences, *University Center* (BSN)
University of Detroit Mercy, McAuley School of Nursing, *Detroit* (BSN)
University of Michigan, School of Nursing, *Ann Arbor* (BSN)
University of Michigan–Flint, Department of Nursing, *Flint* (BSN)
Wayne State University, College of Nursing, *Detroit* (BSN)
Western Michigan University, College of Health and Human Services, *Kalamazoo* (BS)

Minnesota

Bemidji State University, Department of Nursing, *Bemidji* (BS)
Bethel University, Department of Nursing, *St. Paul* (BSN)
College of St. Catherine, Department of Nursing, *St. Paul* (BS)
Minnesota State University Mankato, School of Nursing, *Mankato* (BS)
Minnesota State University Moorhead, Tri-College University Nursing Consortium, *Moorhead* (BSN)
Winona State University, College of Nursing, *Winona* (BSN)

Mississippi

Alcorn State University, School of Nursing, *Natchez* (BSN)
Mississippi College, School of Nursing, *Clinton* (BSN)

University of Mississippi Medical Center, Program in Nursing, *Jackson* (BSN)
University of Southern Mississippi, School of Nursing, *Hattiesburg* (BSN)

Missouri

Central Missouri State University, Department of Nursing, *Warrensburg* (BS)
Deaconess College of Nursing, *St. Louis* (BSN)
Graceland University, School of Nursing, *Independence* (BSN)
Jewish Hospital College of Nursing and Allied Health, Division of Nursing, *St. Louis* (BSN)
Lester L. Cox College of Nursing and Health Sciences, Department of Nursing, *Springfield* (BSN)
Maryville University of Saint Louis, Nursing Program, School of Health Professions, *St. Louis* (BSN)
Missouri Southern State University, Department of Nursing, *Joplin* (BSN)
Missouri Western State College, Department of Nursing, *St. Joseph* (BSN)
Saint Louis University, School of Nursing, *St. Louis* (BSN)
Southeast Missouri State University, Department of Nursing, *Cape Girardeau* (BSN)
Southwest Baptist University, College of Nursing, *Bolivar* (BSN)
Truman State University, Program in Nursing, *Kirksville* (BSN)
University of Missouri–Columbia, Sinclair School of Nursing, *Columbia* (BSN)
University of Missouri–Kansas City, School of Nursing, *Kansas City* (BSN)
University of Missouri–St. Louis, College of Nursing, *St. Louis* (BSN)
Webster University, Department of Nursing, *St. Louis* (BSN)

Montana

Montana State University–Bozeman, College of Nursing, *Bozeman* (BSN)
Montana State University–Northern, College of Nursing, *Havre* (BSN)

Nebraska

Creighton University, School of Nursing, *Omaha* (BSN)
Midland Lutheran College, Department of Nursing, *Fremont* (BSN)
Nebraska Wesleyan University, Department of Nursing, *Lincoln* (BSN)
University of Nebraska Medical Center, College of Nursing, *Omaha* (BSN)

Nevada

University of Nevada, Reno, Orvis School of Nursing, *Reno* (BSN)

New Hampshire

Rivier College, Department of Nursing and Health Sciences, *Nashua* (BS)
Saint Anselm College, Department of Nursing, *Manchester* (BS)
University of New Hampshire, Department of Nursing, *Durham* (BS)

New Jersey

Bloomfield College, Division of Nursing, *Bloomfield* (BSN)
College of Saint Elizabeth, Department of Nursing, *Morristown* (BSN)
Fairleigh Dickinson University, Metropolitan Campus, Henry P. Becton School of Nursing and Allied Health, *Teaneck* (BSN)
Felician College, Department of Professional Nursing-BSN, *Lodi* (BSN)
Kean University, Department of Nursing, *Union* (BSN)
Monmouth University, Marjorie K. Unterberg School of Nursing, *West Long Branch* (BSN)
New Jersey City University, Department of Nursing, *Jersey City* (BSN)
The Richard Stockton College of New Jersey, Program in Nursing, *Pomona* (BSN)
Rutgers, The State University of New Jersey, College of Nursing, *Newark* (BS)
Saint Peter's College, Nursing Program, *Jersey City* (BSN)
Seton Hall University, College of Nursing, *South Orange* (BSN)
Thomas Edison State College, Program in Nursing, *Trenton* (BSN)
University of Medicine and Dentistry of New Jersey, School of Nursing, *Newark* (BSN)
William Paterson University of New Jersey, Department of Nursing, *Wayne* (BSN)

New Mexico

Eastern New Mexico University, Department of Allied Health—Nursing, *Portales* (BSN)
University of New Mexico, College of Nursing, *Albuquerque* (BSN)

New York

Adelphi University, School of Nursing, *Garden City* (BS)
The College of New Rochelle, School of Nursing, *New Rochelle* (BSN)
College of Staten Island of the City University of New York, Department of Nursing, *Staten Island* (BS)
Daemen College, Department of Nursing, *Amherst* (BS)
Dominican College, Division of Nursing, *Orangeburg* (BSN)
D'Youville College, Department of Nursing, *Buffalo* (BSN)
Elmira College, Program in Nursing Education, *Elmira* (BS)
Excelsior College, School of Nursing, *Albany* (BSN)
Hartwick College, Department of Nursing, *Oneonta* (BS)
Hunter College of the City University of New York, Hunter-Bellevue School of Nursing, *New York* (BS)
Keuka College, Division of Nursing, *Keuka Park* (BS)
Lehman College of the City University of New York, Department of Nursing, *Bronx* (BS)
Long Island University, Brooklyn Campus, School of Nursing, *Brooklyn* (BS)
Long Island University, C.W. Post Campus, Program in Nursing, *Brookville* (BS)
Mercy College, Program in Nursing, *Dobbs Ferry* (BScN)
Molloy College, Department of Nursing, *Rockville Centre* (BS)
Mount Saint Mary College, Division of Nursing, *Newburgh* (BSN)
Nazareth College of Rochester, Department of Nursing, *Rochester* (BS)
New York University, Division of Nursing, *New York* (BS)
Roberts Wesleyan College, Division of Nursing, *Rochester* (BS)
The Sage Colleges, Division of Nursing, *Troy* (BS)
St. John Fisher College, Nursing Program, *Rochester* (BS)
St. Joseph's College, New York, Department of Nursing, *Brooklyn* (BSN)
State University of New York at New Paltz, Department of Nursing, *New Paltz* (BSN)
State University of New York at Plattsburgh, Department of Nursing, *Plattsburgh* (BS)
State University of New York College at Brockport, Department of Nursing, *Brockport* (BSN)
State University of New York Downstate Medical Center, College of Nursing, *Brooklyn* (BS)
State University of New York Institute of Technology, School of Nursing and Health Systems, *Utica* (BS)
University of Rochester, School of Nursing, *Rochester* (BS)
Utica College, Department of Nursing, *Utica* (BS)
York College of the City University of New York, Program in Nursing, *Jamaica* (BS)

North Carolina

Cabarrus College of Health Sciences, Louise Harkey School of Nursing, *Concord* (BSN)
East Carolina University, School of Nursing, *Greenville* (BSN)
Gardner-Webb University, School of Nursing, *Boiling Springs* (BSN)
North Carolina Agricultural and Technical State University, School of Nursing, *Greensboro* (BSN)
Southeastern North Carolina Nursing Consortium, *Pembroke* (BSN)
The University of North Carolina at Chapel Hill, School of Nursing, *Chapel Hill* (BSN)
The University of North Carolina at Charlotte, School of Nursing, *Charlotte* (BSN)
The University of North Carolina at Greensboro, School of Nursing, *Greensboro* (BSN)
The University of North Carolina at Wilmington, School of Nursing, *Wilmington* (BS)
Western Carolina University, Department of Nursing, *Cullowhee* (BSN)
Winston-Salem State University, Department of Nursing, *Winston-Salem* (BSN)

North Dakota

Dickinson State University, Department of Nursing, *Dickinson* (BSN)
Medcenter One College of Nursing, Medcenter One College of Nursing, *Bismarck* (BSN)
Minot State University, Department of Nursing, *Minot* (BSN)
University of Mary, Division of Nursing, *Bismarck* (BSN)
University of North Dakota, College of Nursing, *Grand Forks* (BSN)

Ohio

Ashland University, Department of Nursing, *Ashland* (BSN)
Capital University, School of Nursing, *Columbus* (BSN)
Case Western Reserve University, Frances Payne Bolton School of Nursing, *Cleveland* (BSN)
Cedarville University, Department of Nursing, *Cedarville* (BSN)
Cleveland State University, Department of Nursing, *Cleveland* (BSN)
Franciscan University of Steubenville, Department of Nursing, *Steubenville* (BSN)
Kent State University, College of Nursing, *Kent* (BSN)
Kettering College of Medical Arts, Division of Nursing, *Kettering* (BSN)
Lourdes College, Nursing Department, *Sylvania* (BSN)
Malone College, School of Nursing, *Canton* (BSN)
Mercy College of Northwest Ohio, Division of Nursing, *Toledo* (BSN)
Miami University, Department of Nursing, *Hamilton* (BSN)
Mount Carmel College of Nursing, Baccalaureate Nursing Program, *Columbus* (BSN)
Ohio University, School of Nursing, *Athens* (BSN)
Otterbein College, Program in Nursing, *Westerville* (BSN)
Shawnee State University, Department of Nursing, *Portsmouth* (BSN)
The University of Akron, College of Nursing, *Akron* (BSN)
University of Cincinnati, College of Nursing, *Cincinnati* (BSN)
University of Phoenix–Cleveland Campus, College of Health and Human Services, *Independence* (BSN)
Wright State University, College of Nursing and Health, *Dayton* (BSN)

Oklahoma

Langston University, School of Nursing and Health Professions, *Langston* (BSN)

Northeastern State University, Department of Nursing, *Tahlequah* (BSN)
Oklahoma Baptist University, School of Nursing, *Shawnee* (BSN)
Oklahoma Wesleyan University, Division of Nursing, *Bartlesville* (BSN)
University of Central Oklahoma, Department of Nursing, *Edmond* (BSN)
University of Tulsa, School of Nursing, *Tulsa* (BSN)

Oregon
Linfield College, School of Nursing, *McMinnville* (BSN)
Oregon Health & Science University, School of Nursing, *Portland* (BS)

Pennsylvania
Alvernia College, Nursing, *Reading* (BSN)
Bloomsburg University of Pennsylvania, Department of Nursing, *Bloomsburg* (BSN)
California University of Pennsylvania, Department of Nursing, *California* (BSN)
Cedar Crest College, Department of Nursing, *Allentown* (BS)
Clarion University of Pennsylvania, School of Nursing, *Oil City* (BSN)
College Misericordia, Department of Nursing, *Dallas* (BSN)
DeSales University, Department of Nursing and Health, *Center Valley* (BSN)
Drexel University, College of Nursing and Health Professions, *Philadelphia* (BSN)
East Stroudsburg University of Pennsylvania, Department of Nursing, *East Stroudsburg* (BS)
Edinboro University of Pennsylvania, Department of Nursing, *Edinboro* (BS)
Gannon University, Villa Maria School of Nursing, *Erie* (BSN)
Gwynedd-Mercy College, School of Nursing, *Gwynedd Valley* (BSN)
Holy Family University, School of Nursing and Allied Health Professions, *Philadelphia* (BSN)
Immaculata University, Department of Nursing, *Immaculata* (BSN)
Indiana University of Pennsylvania, Department of Nursing and Allied Health, *Indiana* (BSN)
Kutztown University of Pennsylvania, Department of Nursing, *Kutztown* (BSN)
La Roche College, Department of Nursing and Nursing Management, *Pittsburgh* (BSN)
La Salle University, School of Nursing, *Philadelphia* (BSN)
Mansfield University of Pennsylvania, Robert Packer Department of Health Sciences, *Mansfield* (BSN)
Marywood University, Department of Nursing, *Scranton* (BSN)
Millersville University of Pennsylvania, Department of Nursing, *Millersville* (BSN)
Moravian College, St. Luke's School of Nursing, *Bethlehem* (BS)
Neumann College, Program in Nursing and Health Sciences, *Aston* (BS)
Pennsylvania College of Technology, School of Health Sciences, *Williamsport* (BSN)
The Pennsylvania State University University Park Campus, School of Nursing, *State College, University Park* (BS)
Saint Francis University, Department of Nursing, *Loretto* (BSN)
Temple University, Department of Nursing, *Philadelphia* (BSN)
Thomas Jefferson University, Department of Nursing, *Philadelphia* (BSN)
University of Pennsylvania, School of Nursing, *Philadelphia* (BSN)
University of Pittsburgh, School of Nursing, *Pittsburgh* (BSN)
University of Pittsburgh at Bradford, Department of Nursing, *Bradford* (BSN)
The University of Scranton, Department of Nursing, *Scranton* (BS)
Villanova University, College of Nursing, *Villanova* (BSN)
Widener University, School of Nursing, *Chester* (BSN)
Wilkes University, Department of Nursing, *Wilkes-Barre* (BS)
York College of Pennsylvania, Department of Nursing, *York* (BS)

Puerto Rico
Universidad Adventista de las Antillas, Department of Nursing, *Mayagüez* (BSN)

Rhode Island
Rhode Island College, Department of Nursing, *Providence* (BS)
Salve Regina University, Department of Nursing, *Newport* (BS)
University of Rhode Island, College of Nursing, *Kingston* (BS)

South Carolina
Charleston Southern University, Wingo School of Nursing, *Charleston* (BSN)
Clemson University, School of Nursing, *Clemson* (BS)
Lander University, School of Nursing, *Greenwood* (BSN)
Medical University of South Carolina, College of Nursing, *Charleston* (BSN)
South Carolina State University, Department of Nursing, *Orangeburg* (BSN)
University of South Carolina, College of Nursing, *Columbia* (BSN)

South Dakota
Augustana College, Department of Nursing, *Sioux Falls* (BA)
Mount Marty College, Nursing Program, *Yankton* (BSc PN)
Presentation College, Department of Nursing, *Aberdeen* (BSN)
South Dakota State University, College of Nursing, *Brookings* (BS)

Tennessee
Aquinas College, Department of Nursing, *Nashville* (BSN)
Austin Peay State University, School of Nursing, *Clarksville* (BSN)
Baptist College of Health Sciences, Nursing Division, *Memphis* (BSN)
Belmont University, School of Nursing, *Nashville* (BSN)
Carson-Newman College, Department of Nursing, *Jefferson City* (BSN)
Cumberland University, Rudy School of Nursing and Health Professions, *Lebanon* (BSN)
Lincoln Memorial University, Department of Nursing, *Harrogate* (BSN)
Middle Tennessee State University, School of Nursing, *Murfreesboro* (BSN)
Tennessee State University, School of Nursing, *Nashville* (BSN)
Tennessee Technological University, School of Nursing, *Cookeville* (BSN)
Tennessee Wesleyan College, Fort Sanders Nursing Department, *Knoxville* (BSN)
Union University, School of Nursing, *Jackson* (BSN)
The University of Memphis, Loewenberg School of Nursing, *Memphis* (BSN)
The University of Tennessee Health Science Center, College of Nursing, *Memphis* (BSN)

Texas
Abilene Intercollegiate School of Nursing, *Abilene* (BSN)
Angelo State University, Department of Nursing, *San Angelo* (BSN)
East Texas Baptist University, Department of Nursing, *Marshall* (BSN)
Lamar University, Department of Nursing, *Beaumont* (BSN)
Lubbock Christian University, Department of Nursing, *Lubbock* (BSN)
Midwestern State University, Nursing Program, *Wichita Falls* (BSN)
Prairie View A&M University, College of Nursing, *Houston* (BSN)
Southwestern Adventist University, Department of Nursing, *Keene* (BS)
Stephen F. Austin State University, Division of Nursing, *Nacogdoches* (BSN)
Texas A&M International University, Canseco School of Nursing, *Laredo* (BSN)
Texas A&M University–Corpus Christi, School of Nursing and Health Sciences, *Corpus Christi* (BSN)
Texas A&M University–Texarkana, Nursing Department, *Texarkana* (BSN)
Texas Woman's University, College of Nursing, *Denton* (BS)
University of Mary Hardin-Baylor, College of Nursing, *Belton* (BSN)
The University of Texas at Arlington, School of Nursing, *Arlington* (BSN)
The University of Texas at Austin, School of Nursing, *Austin* (BSN)
The University of Texas at Tyler, Program in Nursing, *Tyler* (BSN)
The University of Texas Health Science Center at San Antonio, School of Nursing, *San Antonio* (BSN)
The University of Texas Medical Branch, School of Nursing, *Galveston* (BSN)
The University of Texas–Pan American, Department of Nursing, *Edinburg* (BSN)

Utah
University of Utah, College of Nursing, *Salt Lake City* (BS)
Utah Valley State College, Department of Nursing, *Orem* (BSN)
Westminster College, St. Mark's-Westminster School of Nursing and Health Sciences, *Salt Lake City* (BSN)

Vermont
Norwich University, Division of Nursing, *Northfield* (BSN)
Southern Vermont College, Department of Nursing, *Bennington* (BSN)
University of Vermont, Department of Nursing, *Burlington* (BS)

Virgin Islands
University of the Virgin Islands, Division of Nursing, *Saint Thomas* (BS)

Virginia
Hampton University, Department of Nursing, *Hampton* (BS)
Liberty University, Department of Nursing, *Lynchburg* (BSN)
Marymount University, School of Health Professions, *Arlington* (BSN)
Norfolk State University, Department of Nursing, *Norfolk* (BSN)
Old Dominion University, Department of Nursing, *Norfolk* (BSN)
Radford University, School of Nursing, *Radford* (BSN)
Shenandoah University, Division of Nursing, *Winchester* (BSN)
University of Virginia, School of Nursing, *Charlottesville* (BSN)
The University of Virginia's College at Wise, Department of Nursing, *Wise* (BSN)

Washington
Gonzaga University, Department of Nursing, *Spokane* (BSN)
Intercollegiate College of Nursing/Washington State University, *Spokane* (BSN)
Seattle Pacific University, School of Health Sciences, *Seattle* (BSN)

BACCALAUREATE PROGRAMS

RN Baccalaureate

University of Washington, School of Nursing, *Seattle* (BSN)

West Virginia

Alderson-Broaddus College, Department of Nursing, *Philippi* (BSN)
Bluefield State College, Program in Nursing, *Bluefield* (BSN)
Fairmont State University, School of Nursing/Allied Health Adm., *Fairmont* (BSN)
Mountain State University, Program in Nursing, *Beckley* (BSN)
Shepherd University, Department of Nursing Education, *Shepherdstown* (BSN)
West Virginia University, School of Nursing, *Morgantown* (BSN)
West Virginia Wesleyan College, Department of Nursing, *Buckhannon* (BSN)

Wisconsin

Alverno College, Division of Nursing, *Milwaukee* (BSN)
Concordia University Wisconsin, Division of Nursing, *Mequon* (BSN)
Marquette University, College of Nursing, *Milwaukee* (BSN)
Milwaukee School of Engineering, School of Nursing, *Milwaukee* (BSN)
University of Wisconsin–Eau Claire, College of Nursing and Health Sciences, *Eau Claire* (BSN)
University of Wisconsin–Green Bay, BSN–LINC Online RN–BSN Program, *Green Bay* (BSN)
University of Wisconsin–Madison, School of Nursing, *Madison* (BS)
University of Wisconsin–Milwaukee, College of Nursing, *Milwaukee* (BSN)
University of Wisconsin–Oshkosh, College of Nursing, *Oshkosh* (BSN)
Viterbo University, School of Nursing, *La Crosse* (BSN)

Wyoming

University of Wyoming, Fay W. Whitney School of Nursing, *Laramie* (BSN)

Alberta

Athabasca University, Centre for Nursing and Health Studies, *Athabasca* (BN)
University of Alberta, Faculty of Nursing, *Edmonton* (BScN)
University of Calgary, Faculty of Nursing, *Calgary* (BN)
The University of Lethbridge, School of Health Sciences, *Lethbridge* (BN)

British Columbia

Kwantlen University College, Faculty of Community and Health Sciences, *Surrey* (BSN)
Malaspina University-College, Department of Nursing, *Nanaimo* (BScN)
Okanagan University College, Nursing Department, *Kelowna* (BSN)
The University of British Columbia, School of Nursing, *Vancouver* (BSN)

Manitoba

Brandon University, School of Health Studies, *Brandon* (BN)
University of Manitoba, Faculty of Nursing, *Winnipeg* (BN)

New Brunswick

Université de Moncton, School of Nursing, *Moncton* (BScN)

Newfoundland and Labrador

Memorial University of Newfoundland, School of Nursing, *St. John's* (BN)

Nova Scotia

Dalhousie University, School of Nursing, *Halifax* (BScN)
St. Francis Xavier University, Department of Nursing, *Antigonish* (BScN)

Ontario

Brock University, Department of Nursing, *St. Catharines* (BScN)
Lakehead University, School of Nursing, *Thunder Bay* (BSN)
McMaster University, School of Nursing, *Hamilton* (BScN)
Ryerson University, Program in Nursing, *Toronto* (BScN)
Trent University, Nursing Program, *Peterborough* (BScN)
University of Ottawa, School of Nursing, *Ottawa* (BScN)
The University of Western Ontario, School of Nursing, *London* (BScN)
University of Windsor, School of Nursing, *Windsor* (BScN)
York University, School of Nursing, Atkinson Faculty of Liberal and Profesional Studies, *Toronto* (BScN)

Quebec

McGill University, School of Nursing, *Montréal* (BScN)
Université de Sherbrooke, Department of Nursing, *Sherbrooke* (BScN)
Université du Québec à Chicoutimi, Program in Nursing, *Chicoutimi* (BNSc)
Université du Québec à Rimouski, Program in Nursing, *Rimouski* (BScN)
Université du Québec en Outaouais, Département des Sciences Infirmières, *Gatineau* (BScN)

Saskatchewan

University of Saskatchewan, College of Nursing, *Saskatoon* (BSN)

RPN to Baccalaureate

California

San Jose State University, School of Nursing, *San Jose* (BS)

Illinois

University of Illinois at Chicago, College of Nursing, *Chicago* (BSN)

Maine

Saint Joseph's College of Maine, Department of Nursing, *Standish* (BSN)

Missouri

Deaconess College of Nursing, *St. Louis* (BSN)

Nebraska

University of Nebraska Medical Center, College of Nursing, *Omaha* (BSN)

Ohio

Franciscan University of Steubenville, Department of Nursing, *Steubenville* (BSN)

Alberta

University of Alberta, Faculty of Nursing, *Edmonton* (BScN)

British Columbia

British Columbia Institute of Technology, School of Health Sciences, *Burnaby* (BScN)

Saskatchewan

University of Saskatchewan, College of Nursing, *Saskatoon* (BSN)

MASTER'S DEGREE PROGRAMS

Accelerated AD/RN to Master's

California
California State University, Fullerton, Department of Nursing, *Fullerton* (MSN)
University of San Diego, Hahn School of Nursing and Health Sciences, *San Diego* (MSN, MSN/MBA)

Connecticut
Sacred Heart University, Program in Nursing, *Fairfield* (MSN, MSN/MBA)
Saint Joseph College, Department of Nursing, *West Hartford* (MS)

Delaware
Wesley College, Graduate Nursing Program, *Dover* (MSN)

Massachusetts
Simmons College, Department of Nursing, *Boston* (MS, MSN/MS)

Michigan
Madonna University, College of Nursing and Health, *Livonia* (MSN, MSN/MSBA)
University of Detroit Mercy, McAuley School of Nursing, *Detroit* (MSN)
Wayne State University, College of Nursing, *Detroit* (MSN)

Missouri
Southwest Missouri State University, Department of Nursing, *Springfield* (MSN)

New York
Columbia University, School of Nursing, *New York* (MS, MS/MBA, MS/MPH)
Daemen College, Department of Nursing, *Amherst* (MSN)
D'Youville College, Department of Nursing, *Buffalo* (MS)
Pace University, Lienhard School of Nursing, *New York* (MS)
State University of New York Institute of Technology, School of Nursing and Health Systems, *Utica* (MS)
University at Buffalo, The State University of New York, School of Nursing, *Buffalo* (MS)
University of Rochester, School of Nursing, *Rochester* (MS, MSN/PhD)

Ohio
Case Western Reserve University, Frances Payne Bolton School of Nursing, *Cleveland* (MSN, MSN/MA, MSN/MBA, MSN/MPH, MSN/PhD)

Pennsylvania
DeSales University, Department of Nursing and Health, *Center Valley* (MSN, MSN/MBA)
Drexel University, College of Nursing and Health Professions, *Philadelphia* (MSN)
University of Pennsylvania, School of Nursing, *Philadelphia* (MSN, MSN/MBA, MSN/MPH, MSN/PhD)
The University of Scranton, Department of Nursing, *Scranton* (MS)
Wilkes University, Department of Nursing, *Wilkes-Barre* (MS)

Tennessee
Vanderbilt University, School of Nursing, *Nashville* (MSN, MSN/MBA)

Texas
Texas A&M University–Corpus Christi, School of Nursing and Health Sciences, *Corpus Christi* (MSN)
The University of Texas at Tyler, Program in Nursing, *Tyler* (MSN, MSN/MBA)
The University of Texas Health Science Center at Houston, School of Nursing, *Houston* (MSN, MSN/MPH)

Wisconsin
Marquette University, College of Nursing, *Milwaukee* (MSN, MSN/MBA)

Accelerated Master's

Alabama
University of South Alabama, College of Nursing, *Mobile* (MSN)

California
University of San Francisco, School of Nursing, *San Francisco* (MSN)

Colorado
Colorado State University-Pueblo, Department of Nursing, *Pueblo* (MS)

Florida
University of Miami, School of Nursing, *Coral Gables* (MSN)

Georgia
Albany State University, College of Health Professions, *Albany* (MSN)

Illinois
Lewis University, Program in Nursing, *Romeoville* (MSN, MSN/MBA)

Massachusetts
Simmons College, Department of Nursing, *Boston* (MS, MSN/MS)

Mississippi
University of Mississippi Medical Center, Program in Nursing, *Jackson* (MSN)

New York
Long Island University, C.W. Post Campus, Program in Nursing, *Brookville* (MS)

Ohio
College of Mount St. Joseph, Department of Nursing, *Cincinnati* (MN)
The Ohio State University, College of Nursing, *Columbus* (MS)
Ursuline College, The Breen School of Nursing, *Pepper Pike* (MSN)

Oklahoma
Southern Nazarene University, School of Nursing, *Bethany* (MS)

Pennsylvania
Carlow University, Division of Nursing, *Pittsburgh* (MSN)
Thomas Jefferson University, Department of Nursing, *Philadelphia* (MSN)
The University of Scranton, Department of Nursing, *Scranton* (MS)
Waynesburg College, Department of Nursing, *Waynesburg* (MSN, MSN/MBA)
Widener University, School of Nursing, *Chester* (MSN)

South Carolina
Medical University of South Carolina, College of Nursing, *Charleston* (MSN)

Tennessee
Vanderbilt University, School of Nursing, *Nashville* (MSN, MSN/MBA)

Washington
Pacific Lutheran University, School of Nursing, *Tacoma* (MSN)

Wisconsin
Cardinal Stritch University, Ruth S. Coleman College of Nursing, *Milwaukee* (MSN)

Accelerated Master's for Non-Nursing College Graduates

California
Azusa Pacific University, School of Nursing, *Azusa* (MSN)
San Francisco State University, School of Nursing, *San Francisco* (MSN)
University of San Francisco, School of Nursing, *San Francisco* (MSN)

Colorado
Colorado State University-Pueblo, Department of Nursing, *Pueblo* (MS)

Kentucky
Spalding University, School of Nursing, *Louisville* (MSN)

Massachusetts
Boston College, William F. Connell School of Nursing, *Chestnut Hill* (MS, MSN/MA, MSN/MBA)
Regis College, Department of Nursing, *Weston* (MSN)
Salem State College, Nursing Department, *Salem* (MSN, MSN/MBA)
Simmons College, Department of Nursing, *Boston* (MS, MSN/MS)

New York
Columbia University, School of Nursing, *New York* (MS, MS/MBA, MS/MPH)
University of Rochester, School of Nursing, *Rochester* (MS, MSN/PhD)

Ohio
Case Western Reserve University, Frances Payne Bolton School of Nursing, *Cleveland* (MSN, MSN/MA, MSN/MBA, MSN/MPH, MSN/PhD)
The Ohio State University, College of Nursing, *Columbus* (MS)
University of Cincinnati, College of Nursing, *Cincinnati* (MSN, MSN/MBA)

Pennsylvania
University of Pennsylvania, School of Nursing, *Philadelphia* (MSN, MSN/MBA, MSN/MPH, MSN/PhD)

Tennessee
Vanderbilt University, School of Nursing, *Nashville* (MSN, MSN/MBA)

Virginia
University of Virginia, School of Nursing, *Charlottesville* (MSN, MSN/MA, MSN/MBA, MSN/PhD, MSN/HSM)
Virginia Commonwealth University, School of Nursing, *Richmond* (MS, MS/MPH)

Wisconsin
Marquette University, College of Nursing, *Milwaukee* (MSN, MSN/MBA)

Accelerated Master's for Nurses with Non-Nursing Degrees

California
Azusa Pacific University, School of Nursing, *Azusa* (MSN)
California State University, Los Angeles, School of Nursing, *Los Angeles* (MS)

San Francisco State University, School of Nursing, *San Francisco* (MSN)
University of San Francisco, School of Nursing, *San Francisco* (MSN)

Connecticut
Sacred Heart University, Program in Nursing, *Fairfield* (MSN, MSN/MBA)

Illinois
Bradley University, Department of Nursing, *Peoria* (MSN)

Massachusetts
Simmons College, Department of Nursing, *Boston* (MS, MSN/MS)

New Jersey
Kean University, Department of Nursing, *Union* (MSN, MSN/MPA)

New York
Columbia University, School of Nursing, *New York* (MS, MS/MBA, MS/MPH)

Ohio
Case Western Reserve University, Frances Payne Bolton School of Nursing, *Cleveland* (MSN, MSN/MA, MSN/MBA, MSN/MPH, MSN/PhD)
College of Mount St. Joseph, Department of Nursing, *Cincinnati* (MN)

Pennsylvania
Waynesburg College, Department of Nursing, *Waynesburg* (MSN, MSN/MBA)

South Carolina
Medical University of South Carolina, College of Nursing, *Charleston* (MSN)

Tennessee
The University of Memphis, Loewenberg School of Nursing, *Memphis* (MSN)
The University of Tennessee, College of Nursing, *Knoxville* (MSN)
Vanderbilt University, School of Nursing, *Nashville* (MSN, MSN/MBA)

Texas
Texas A&M University–Corpus Christi, School of Nursing and Health Sciences, *Corpus Christi* (MSN)

Virginia
Virginia Commonwealth University, School of Nursing, *Richmond* (MS, MS/MPH)

Washington
Seattle University, College of Nursing, *Seattle* (MSN)

Accelerated RN to Master's

Alabama
The University of Alabama at Birmingham, School of Nursing, *Birmingham* (MSN, MSN/MPH)

California
California State University, Bakersfield, Program in Nursing, *Bakersfield* (MSN)
California State University, Los Angeles, School of Nursing, *Los Angeles* (MS)
University of San Diego, Hahn School of Nursing and Health Sciences, *San Diego* (MSN, MSN/MBA)

Connecticut
Sacred Heart University, Program in Nursing, *Fairfield* (MSN, MSN/MBA)
Saint Joseph College, Department of Nursing, *West Hartford* (MS)

Delaware
Wesley College, Graduate Nursing Program, *Dover* (MSN)

Florida
Jacksonville University, School of Nursing, *Jacksonville* (MSN, MSN/MBA)
The University of Tampa, Department of Nursing, *Tampa* (MSN)

Georgia
Georgia Southern University, School of Nursing, *Statesboro* (MSN)

Indiana
Purdue University Calumet, School of Nursing, *Hammond* (MS)
University of Saint Francis, Department of Nursing, *Fort Wayne* (MSN)

Kentucky
Spalding University, School of Nursing, *Louisville* (MSN)

Massachusetts
Northeastern University, School of Nursing, *Boston* (MS, MSN/MBA)
Simmons College, Department of Nursing, *Boston* (MS, MSN/MS)

Michigan
Madonna University, College of Nursing and Health, *Livonia* (MSN, MSN/MSBA)
University of Michigan, School of Nursing, *Ann Arbor* (MS, MS/MBA, MS/MPH)

Mississippi
University of Mississippi Medical Center, Program in Nursing, *Jackson* (MSN)

New York
Daemen College, Department of Nursing, *Amherst* (MSN)
Pace University, Lienhard School of Nursing, *New York* (MS)
State University of New York Institute of Technology, School of Nursing and Health Systems, *Utica* (MS)
University of Rochester, School of Nursing, *Rochester* (MS, MSN/PhD)

North Carolina
Queens University of Charlotte, Division of Nursing, *Charlotte* (MSN, MSN/MBA)

Ohio
Kent State University, College of Nursing, *Kent* (MSN, MSN/MBA, MSN/MPA)
University of Cincinnati, College of Nursing, *Cincinnati* (MSN, MSN/MBA)

Pennsylvania
Clarion University of Pennsylvania, School of Nursing, *Oil City* (MSN)
College Misericordia, Department of Nursing, *Dallas* (MSN)
DeSales University, Department of Nursing and Health, *Center Valley* (MSN, MSN/MBA)
Duquesne University, School of Nursing, *Pittsburgh* (MSN, MSN/MBA)
Thomas Jefferson University, Department of Nursing, *Philadelphia* (MSN)
University of Pennsylvania, School of Nursing, *Philadelphia* (MSN, MSN/MBA, MSN/MPH, MSN/PhD)
The University of Scranton, Department of Nursing, *Scranton* (MS)
Waynesburg College, Department of Nursing, *Waynesburg* (MSN, MSN/MBA)
Wilkes University, Department of Nursing, *Wilkes-Barre* (MS)

South Carolina
Medical University of South Carolina, College of Nursing, *Charleston* (MSN)

Tennessee
Southern Adventist University, School of Nursing, *Collegedale* (MSN, MSN/MBA)
The University of Tennessee, College of Nursing, *Knoxville* (MSN)
Vanderbilt University, School of Nursing, *Nashville* (MSN, MSN/MBA)

Virginia
Radford University, School of Nursing, *Radford* (MSN)

Washington
Gonzaga University, Department of Nursing, *Spokane* (MSN)
Intercollegiate College of Nursing/Washington State University, *Spokane* (MN)

Wisconsin
Marquette University, College of Nursing, *Milwaukee* (MSN, MSN/MBA)
University of Wisconsin–Madison, School of Nursing, *Madison* (MS)

Quebec
Université du Québec à Chicoutimi, Program in Nursing, *Chicoutimi* (MSN)

Master's

Alabama
Jacksonville State University, College of Nursing and Health Sciences, *Jacksonville* (MSN)
Samford University, Ida V. Moffett School of Nursing, *Birmingham* (MSN, MSN/MBA)
Troy University, School of Nursing, *Troy* (MSN)
The University of Alabama, Capstone College of Nursing, *Tuscaloosa* (MSN, MSN/MA, MSN/MBA)
The University of Alabama at Birmingham, School of Nursing, *Birmingham* (MSN, MSN/MPH)
The University of Alabama in Huntsville, College of Nursing, *Huntsville* (MSN)
University of Mobile, School of Nursing, *Mobile* (MSN)
University of South Alabama, College of Nursing, *Mobile* (MSN)

Alaska
University of Alaska Anchorage, School of Nursing, *Anchorage* (MS)

Arizona
Arizona State University, College of Nursing, *Tempe* (MS, MS/MPH)
Grand Canyon University, Samaritan College of Nursing, *Phoenix* (MS)
Northern Arizona University, Department of Nursing, *Flagstaff* (MS)
The University of Arizona, College of Nursing, *Tucson* (MS)
University of Phoenix Online Campus, College of Health and Human Services, *Phoenix* (MSN, MSN/MBA)
University of Phoenix–Phoenix Campus, College of Health and Human Services, *Phoenix* (MSN, MSN/MBA)
University of Phoenix–Southern Arizona Campus, College of Health and Human Services, *Tucson* (MSN, MSN/MBA)

Arkansas
Arkansas State University, Department of Nursing, *Jonesboro, State University* (MSN)
University of Arkansas, Eleanor Mann School of Nursing, *Fayetteville* (MSN)
University of Central Arkansas, Department of Nursing, *Conway* (MSN)

California
Azusa Pacific University, School of Nursing, *Azusa* (MSN)
California State University, Bakersfield, Program in Nursing, *Bakersfield* (MSN)
California State University, Chico, School of Nursing, *Chico* (MSN)
California State University, Dominguez Hills, Program in Nursing, *Carson* (MSN)
California State University, Fresno, Department of Nursing, *Fresno* (MSN)

California State University, Fullerton, Department of Nursing, *Fullerton* (MSN)
California State University, Long Beach, Department of Nursing, *Long Beach* (MSN, MS/MHSA)
California State University, Los Angeles, School of Nursing, *Los Angeles* (MS)
California State University, Sacramento, Division of Nursing, *Sacramento* (MS)
Dominican University of California, Program in Occupational Therapy, *San Rafael* (MSN)
Holy Names University, Department of Nursing, *Oakland* (MSN, MSN/MBA)
Loma Linda University, School of Nursing, *Loma Linda* (MS, MS/MA, MS/MPH)
Mount St. Mary's College, Department of Nursing, *Los Angeles* (MSN)
Point Loma Nazarene University, School of Nursing, *San Diego* (MSN)
Samuel Merritt College, School of Nursing, *Oakland* (MSN)
San Francisco State University, School of Nursing, *San Francisco* (MSN)
San Jose State University, School of Nursing, *San Jose* (MS)
Sonoma State University, Department of Nursing, *Rohnert Park* (MSN)
University of California, Los Angeles, School of Nursing, *Los Angeles* (MSN, MSN/MBA)
University of California, San Francisco, School of Nursing, *San Francisco* (MS)
University of Phoenix–Northern California Campus, College of Health and Human Services, *Pleasanton* (MSN, MSN/MBA)
University of Phoenix–Sacramento Campus, College of Health and Human Services, *Sacramento* (MSN, MSN/MBA)
University of Phoenix–San Diego Campus, College of Health and Human Services, *San Diego* (MSN, MSN/MBA)
University of Phoenix–Southern California Campus, College of Health and Human Services, *Costa Mesa* (MSN, MSN/MBA)
University of San Diego, Hahn School of Nursing and Health Sciences, *San Diego* (MSN, MSN/MBA)
University of San Francisco, School of Nursing, *San Francisco* (MSN)

Colorado
Colorado State University-Pueblo, Department of Nursing, *Pueblo* (MS)
Regis University, Department of Nursing, *Denver* (MS)
University of Colorado at Colorado Springs, Beth-El College of Nursing and Health Sciences, *Colorado Springs* (MSN, MSN/MBA)
University of Colorado at Denver and Health Sciences Center—Health Sciences Program, School of Nursing, *Denver* (MS, MSN/MBA)
University of Phoenix–Colorado Campus, College of Health and Human Services, *Lone Tree* (MSN, MSN/MBA)
University of Phoenix–Southern Colorado Campus, College of Health and Human Services, *Colorado Springs* (MSN, MSN/MBA)

Connecticut
Fairfield University, School of Nursing, *Fairfield* (MSN)
Quinnipiac University, Department of Nursing, *Hamden* (MSN)
Sacred Heart University, Program in Nursing, *Fairfield* (MSN, MSN/MBA)
Saint Joseph College, Department of Nursing, *West Hartford* (MS)
University of Connecticut, School of Nursing, *Storrs* (MS, MSN/MBA, MSN/MPH)
University of Hartford, College of Education, Nursing, and Health Professions, *West Hartford* (MSN, MSN/MSOB)
Western Connecticut State University, Department of Nursing, *Danbury* (MS)
Yale University, School of Nursing, *New Haven* (MSN, MSN/MBA, MSN/MPH)

Delaware
University of Delaware, Department of Nursing, *Newark* (MSN)
Wesley College, Graduate Nursing Program, *Dover* (MSN)
Wilmington College, Division of Nursing, *New Castle* (MSN, MSN/MBA, MSN/MS)

District of Columbia
The Catholic University of America, School of Nursing, *Washington* (MSN, MA/MSM)
Georgetown University, School of Nursing and Health Studies, *Washington* (MS)
Howard University, Division of Nursing, *Washington* (MSN)

Florida
Barry University, School of Nursing, *Miami Shores* (MSN, MSN/MBA)
Florida Agricultural and Mechanical University, School of Nursing, *Tallahassee* (MSN)
Florida Atlantic University, College of Nursing, *Boca Raton* (M Sc N)
Florida Gulf Coast University, School of Nursing, *Fort Myers* (MSN)
Florida International University, School of Nursing, *Miami* (MSN)
Florida State University, School of Nursing, *Tallahassee* (MSN, MSN/MS)
Jacksonville University, School of Nursing, *Jacksonville* (MSN, MSN/MBA)
University of Central Florida, School of Nursing, *Orlando* (MSN)
University of Miami, School of Nursing, *Coral Gables* (MSN)
University of North Florida, School of Nursing, *Jacksonville* (MSN)
University of Phoenix–Fort Lauderdale Campus, College of Health and Human Services, *Fort Lauderdale* (MSN, MSN/MBA)
University of Phoenix–Jacksonville Campus, College of Health and Human Services, *Jacksonville* (MSN, MSN/MBA)
University of Phoenix–Orlando Campus, College of Health and Human Services, *Maitland* (MSN, MSN/MBA)
University of Phoenix–Tampa Campus, College of Health and Human Services, *Tampa* (MSN, MSN/MBA)
University of South Florida, College of Nursing, *Tampa* (MS, MSN/MPH)
The University of Tampa, Department of Nursing, *Tampa* (MSN)

Georgia
Albany State University, College of Health Professions, *Albany* (MSN)
Armstrong Atlantic State University, Program in Nursing, *Savannah* (MSN, MN/MHSA)
Brenau University, School of Health and Science, *Gainesville* (MSN)
Emory University, Nell Hodgson Woodruff School of Nursing, *Atlanta* (MSN, MSN/MPH)
Georgia Baptist College of Nursing of Mercer University, Department of Nursing, *Atlanta* (MSN)
Georgia College & State University, School of Health Sciences, *Milledgeville* (MSN, MSN/MBA)
Georgia Southern University, School of Nursing, *Statesboro* (MSN)
Georgia State University, School of Nursing, *Atlanta* (MS)
Kennesaw State University, School of Nursing, *Kennesaw* (MSN)
Medical College of Georgia, School of Nursing, *Augusta* (MSN)
North Georgia College & State University, Department of Nursing, *Dahlonega* (MS)
University of West Georgia, Department of Nursing, *Carrollton* (MSN)
Valdosta State University, College of Nursing, *Valdosta* (MSN)

Hawaii
Hawai'i Pacific University, School of Nursing, *Honolulu* (MSN, MSN/MBA)
University of Hawaii at Manoa, School of Nursing and Dental Hygiene, *Honolulu* (MS)
University of Phoenix–Hawaii Campus, College of Health and Human Services, *Honolulu* (MSN, MSN/MBA)

Idaho
Idaho State University, Department of Nursing, *Pocatello* (MS)

Illinois
Bradley University, Department of Nursing, *Peoria* (MSN)
DePaul University, Department of Nursing, *Chicago* (MS)
Illinois State University, Mennonite College of Nursing, *Normal* (MSN)
Loyola University Chicago, Marcella Niehoff School of Nursing, *Chicago* (MSN, MSN/MBA, MSN/MDIV)
Northern Illinois University, School of Nursing, *De Kalb* (MS, MSN/MPH)
North Park University, School of Nursing, *Chicago* (MS, MSN/MA, MSN/MBA)
Olivet Nazarene University, Division of Nursing, *Bourbonnais* (MSN)
Rush University, College of Nursing, *Chicago* (MSN, MSN/MBA)
Saint Francis Medical Center College of Nursing, Baccalaureate Nursing Program, *Peoria* (MSN)
Saint Xavier University, School of Nursing, *Chicago* (MSN, MSN/MBA)
Southern Illinois University Edwardsville, School of Nursing, *Edwardsville* (MS)
University of Illinois at Chicago, College of Nursing, *Chicago* (MS, MS/MBA)

Indiana
Anderson University, Department of Nursing, *Anderson* (MSN, MSN/MBA)
Ball State University, School of Nursing, *Muncie* (MS)
Bethel College, Department of Nursing, *Mishawaka* (MSN)
Indiana State University, School of Nursing, *Terre Haute* (MS)
Indiana University–Purdue University Fort Wayne, Department of Nursing, *Fort Wayne* (MS)
Indiana University–Purdue University Indianapolis, School of Nursing, *Indianapolis* (MSN, MSN/MPH)
Indiana Wesleyan University, Division of Nursing, *Marion* (MS)
Purdue University, School of Nursing, *West Lafayette* (MS)
Purdue University Calumet, School of Nursing, *Hammond* (MS)
University of Indianapolis, School of Nursing, *Indianapolis* (MSN, MSN/MBA)
University of Saint Francis, Department of Nursing, *Fort Wayne* (MSN)
University of Southern Indiana, School of Nursing and Health Professions, *Evansville* (MSN)
Valparaiso University, College of Nursing, *Valparaiso* (MSN)

Iowa
Allen College, Program in Nursing, *Waterloo* (MSN)
Briar Cliff University, Department of Nursing, *Sioux City* (MSN)
Clarke College, Department of Nursing and Health, *Dubuque* (MSN)
The University of Iowa, College of Nursing, *Iowa City* (MSN, MSN/MBA, MSN/MPH)

Kansas
Fort Hays State University, Department of Nursing, *Hays* (MSN)

Washburn University, School of Nursing, *Topeka* (MSN)
Wichita State University, School of Nursing, *Wichita* (MSN, MSN/MBA)

Kentucky

Bellarmine University, Donna and Allan Lansing School of Nursing and Health Sciences, *Louisville* (MSN, MSN/MBA)
Eastern Kentucky University, Department of Baccalaureate and Graduate Nursing, *Richmond* (MSN)
Murray State University, Department of Nursing, *Murray* (M Sc N)
Spalding University, School of Nursing, *Louisville* (MSN)
University of Kentucky, Graduate School Programs in the College of Nursing, *Lexington* (MSN)
University of Louisville, School of Nursing, *Louisville* (MSN)

Louisiana

Grambling State University, School of Nursing, *Grambling* (MSN)
Louisiana State University Health Sciences Center, School of Nursing, *New Orleans* (MN)
Loyola University New Orleans, Program in Nursing, *New Orleans* (MSN)
McNeese State University, College of Nursing, *Lake Charles* (MSN)
Northwestern State University of Louisiana, College of Nursing, *Shreveport* (MSN)
Southeastern Louisiana University, College of Nursing and Health Sciences, *Hammond* (MSN)
Southern University and Agricultural and Mechanical College, School of Nursing, *Baton Rouge* (MSN)
University of Louisiana at Lafayette, College of Nursing, *Lafayette* (MSN)
University of Phoenix–Louisiana Campus, College of Health and Human Services, *Metairie* (MSN, MSN/MBA)

Maine

Husson College, School of Nursing, *Bangor* (MSN)
Saint Joseph's College of Maine, Department of Nursing, *Standish* (MSN, MSN/MA)
University of Maine, School of Nursing, *Orono* (MSN)
University of Southern Maine, College of Nursing and Health Professions, *Portland* (MS, MS/MBA)

Maryland

Bowie State University, Department of Nursing, *Bowie* (MSN)
Coppin State University, Helene Fuld School of Nursing, *Baltimore* (MSN)
The Johns Hopkins University, School of Nursing, *Baltimore* (MSN, MSN/MBA, MSN/MPH, MSN/PhD)
Salisbury University, Program in Nursing, *Salisbury* (MS)
Towson University, Department of Nursing, *Towson* (MS)
University of Maryland, School of Nursing, *Baltimore* (MS, MS/MBA)

Massachusetts

American International College, Division of Nursing, *Springfield* (MSN)
Boston College, William F. Connell School of Nursing, *Chestnut Hill* (MS, MSN/MA, MSN/MBA)
Fitchburg State College, Department of Nursing, *Fitchburg* (M Sc)
MGH Institute of Health Professions, Program in Nursing, *Boston* (MS)
Northeastern University, School of Nursing, *Boston* (MS, MSN/MBA)
Regis College, Department of Nursing, *Weston* (MSN)
Salem State College, Nursing Department, *Salem* (MSN, MSN/MBA)
Simmons College, Department of Nursing, *Boston* (MS, MSN/MS)
University of Massachusetts Amherst, School of Nursing, *Amherst* (MS, MS/MPH)
University of Massachusetts Boston, College of Nursing and Health Sciences, *Boston* (MS)
University of Massachusetts Lowell, Department of Nursing, *Lowell* (MS)
University of Massachusetts Worcester, Graduate School of Nursing, *Worcester* (MS)
Worcester State College, Department of Nursing, *Worcester* (MS)

Michigan

Andrews University, Department of Nursing, *Berrien Springs* (MS)
Eastern Michigan University, Department of Nursing, *Ypsilanti* (MSN)
Grand Valley State University, Russell B. Kirkhof School of Nursing, *Allendale* (MSN, MSN/MBA)
Madonna University, College of Nursing and Health, *Livonia* (MSN, MSN/MSBA)
Michigan State University, College of Nursing, *East Lansing* (MSN)
Northern Michigan University, College of Nursing and Allied Health Science, *Marquette* (MSN)
Oakland University, School of Nursing, *Rochester* (MSN)
Saginaw Valley State University, Crystal M. Lange College of Nursing and Health Sciences, *University Center* (MSN)
University of Detroit Mercy, McAuley School of Nursing, *Detroit* (MSN)
University of Michigan, School of Nursing, *Ann Arbor* (MS, MS/MBA, MS/MPH)
University of Michigan–Flint, Department of Nursing, *Flint* (MSN)
University of Phoenix–Metro Detroit Campus, College of Health and Human Services, *Southfield* (MSN, MSN/MBA)
University of Phoenix–West Michigan Campus, College of Health and Human Services, *Grand Rapids* (MSN, MSN/MBA)
Wayne State University, College of Nursing, *Detroit* (MSN)

Minnesota

Bethel University, Department of Nursing, *St. Paul* (MA)
College of St. Catherine, Department of Nursing, *St. Paul* (MA)
The College of St. Scholastica, Department of Nursing, *Duluth* (MA)
Concordia College, Department of Nursing, *Moorhead* (MS)
Minnesota State University Mankato, School of Nursing, *Mankato* (MSN)
Minnesota State University Moorhead, Tri-College University Nursing Consortium, *Moorhead* (MS)
University of Minnesota, Twin Cities Campus, School of Nursing, *Minneapolis* (MS, MS/MPH)
Winona State University, College of Nursing, *Winona* (MS)

Mississippi

Alcorn State University, School of Nursing, *Natchez* (MSN)
Delta State University, School of Nursing, *Cleveland* (MSN)
Mississippi University for Women, Division of Nursing, *Columbus* (MSN)
University of Mississippi Medical Center, Program in Nursing, *Jackson* (MSN)
University of Southern Mississippi, School of Nursing, *Hattiesburg* (MSN)
William Carey College, School of Nursing, *Hattiesburg* (MSN)

Missouri

Central Missouri State University, Department of Nursing, *Warrensburg* (MS)
Graceland University, School of Nursing, *Independence* (MSN)
Jewish Hospital College of Nursing and Allied Health, Division of Nursing, *St. Louis* (MSN)
Maryville University of Saint Louis, Nursing Program, School of Health Professions, *St. Louis* (MSN)
Research College of Nursing, College of Nursing, *Kansas City* (MSN)
Saint Louis University, School of Nursing, *St. Louis* (MSN, MSN/MPH)
Southeast Missouri State University, Department of Nursing, *Cape Girardeau* (MSN)
Southwest Missouri State University, Department of Nursing, *Springfield* (MSN)
University of Missouri–Columbia, Sinclair School of Nursing, *Columbia* (MS)
University of Missouri–Kansas City, School of Nursing, *Kansas City* (MSN)
Webster University, Department of Nursing, *St. Louis* (MSN)

Montana

Montana State University–Bozeman, College of Nursing, *Bozeman* (MN)

Nebraska

Clarkson College, Department of Nursing, *Omaha* (MSN)
Creighton University, School of Nursing, *Omaha* (MS)
Nebraska Methodist College, Department of Nursing, *Omaha* (MSN)
Nebraska Wesleyan University, Department of Nursing, *Lincoln* (MSN)
University of Nebraska Medical Center, College of Nursing, *Omaha* (MSN)

Nevada

University of Nevada, Las Vegas, Department of Nursing, *Las Vegas* (MSN)
University of Nevada, Reno, Orvis School of Nursing, *Reno* (MS, MSN/MPH)

New Hampshire

Rivier College, Department of Nursing and Health Sciences, *Nashua* (MS, MS/MBA)
University of New Hampshire, Department of Nursing, *Durham* (MS)

New Jersey

The College of New Jersey, School of Nursing, *Ewing* (MSN)
Fairleigh Dickinson University, Metropolitan Campus, Henry P. Becton School of Nursing and Allied Health, *Teaneck* (MSN)
Felician College, Department of Professional Nursing–BSN, *Lodi* (MSN)
Kean University, Department of Nursing, *Union* (MSN, MSN/MPA)
Monmouth University, Marjorie K. Unterberg School of Nursing, *West Long Branch* (MSN)
Rutgers, The State University of New Jersey, Camden College of Arts and Sciences, Department of Nursing, *Camden* (MS)
Rutgers, The State University of New Jersey, College of Nursing, *Newark* (MS, MS/MPH)
Saint Peter's College, Nursing Program, *Jersey City* (MSN)
Seton Hall University, College of Nursing, *South Orange* (MSN, MSN/MA, MSN/MBA)
University of Medicine and Dentistry of New Jersey, School of Nursing, *Newark* (MSN)
William Paterson University of New Jersey, Department of Nursing, *Wayne* (MSN)

New Mexico

New Mexico State University, Department of Nursing, *Las Cruces* (MSN)
University of New Mexico, College of Nursing, *Albuquerque* (MSN, MSN/MALAS, MSN/MPA, MSN/MPH)
University of Phoenix–New Mexico Campus, College of Health and Human Services, *Albuquerque* (MSN, MSN/MBA)

New York
Adelphi University, School of Nursing, *Garden City* (MS, MS/MBA)
College of Mount Saint Vincent, Division of Nursing, *Riverdale* (MSN)
The College of New Rochelle, School of Nursing, *New Rochelle* (MS)
College of Staten Island of the City University of New York, Department of Nursing, *Staten Island* (MS)
Columbia University, School of Nursing, *New York* (MS, MS/MBA, MS/MPH)
Daemen College, Department of Nursing, *Amherst* (MSN)
Dominican College, Division of Nursing, *Orangeburg* (MS)
D'Youville College, Department of Nursing, *Buffalo* (MS)
Excelsior College, School of Nursing, *Albany* (MS)
Hunter College of the City University of New York, Hunter-Bellevue School of Nursing, *New York* (MS, MS/MPH)
Lehman College of the City University of New York, Department of Nursing, *Bronx* (MS)
Long Island University, Brooklyn Campus, School of Nursing, *Brooklyn* (MS)
Long Island University, C.W. Post Campus, Program in Nursing, *Brookville* (MS)
Mercy College, Program in Nursing, *Dobbs Ferry* (MS)
Mount Saint Mary College, Division of Nursing, *Newburgh* (MS)
Nazareth College of Rochester, Department of Nursing, *Rochester* (MS)
New York University, Division of Nursing, *New York* (MA, MS/MA)
Pace University, Lienhard School of Nursing, *New York* (MS)
St. John Fisher College, Nursing Program, *Rochester* (MS)
State University of New York at Binghamton, Decker School of Nursing, *Binghamton* (MS)
State University of New York Institute of Technology, School of Nursing and Health Systems, *Utica* (MS)
State University of New York Upstate Medical University, College of Nursing, *Syracuse* (MS)
University at Buffalo, The State University of New York, School of Nursing, *Buffalo* (MS)
University of Rochester, School of Nursing, *Rochester* (MS, MSN/PhD)

North Carolina
Duke University, School of Nursing, *Durham* (MSN, MSN/MBA, MSN/MCM)
East Carolina University, School of Nursing, *Greenville* (MSN)
Gardner-Webb University, School of Nursing, *Boiling Springs* (MSN, MSN/MBA)
Queens University of Charlotte, Division of Nursing, *Charlotte* (MSN, MSN/MBA)
The University of North Carolina at Charlotte, School of Nursing, *Charlotte* (MSN, MSN/MHA)
The University of North Carolina at Greensboro, School of Nursing, *Greensboro* (MSN, MSN/MBA)
The University of North Carolina at Wilmington, School of Nursing, *Wilmington* (MSN)
Western Carolina University, Department of Nursing, *Cullowhee* (MSN)
Winston-Salem State University, Department of Nursing, *Winston-Salem* (MSN)

North Dakota
North Dakota State University, Tri-College University Nursing Consortium, *Fargo* (MS)
University of Mary, Division of Nursing, *Bismarck* (MSN)
University of North Dakota, College of Nursing, *Grand Forks* (MS)

Ohio
Capital University, School of Nursing, *Columbus* (MSN)
Case Western Reserve University, Frances Payne Bolton School of Nursing, *Cleveland* (MSN, MSN/MA, MSN/MBA, MSN/MPH, MSN/PhD)
Cleveland State University, Department of Nursing, *Cleveland* (MSN, MSN/MBA)
Franciscan University of Steubenville, Department of Nursing, *Steubenville* (MSN)
Kent State University, College of Nursing, *Kent* (MSN, MSN/MBA, MSN/MPA)
Malone College, School of Nursing, *Canton* (MSN)
Medical College of Ohio, School of Nursing, *Toledo* (MSN)
Mount Carmel College of Nursing, Baccalaureate Nursing Program, *Columbus* (MS)
The Ohio State University, College of Nursing, *Columbus* (MS)
Otterbein College, Program in Nursing, *Westerville* (MSN)
The University of Akron, College of Nursing, *Akron* (MSN)
University of Cincinnati, College of Nursing, *Cincinnati* (MSN, MSN/MBA)
University of Phoenix–Cleveland Campus, College of Health and Human Services, *Independence* (MSN)
Ursuline College, The Breen School of Nursing, *Pepper Pike* (MSN)
Wright State University, College of Nursing and Health, *Dayton* (MS, MS/MBA)
Xavier University, Department of Nursing, *Cincinnati* (MSN, MSN/MBA)

Oklahoma
Oklahoma City University, Kramer School of Nursing, *Oklahoma City* (MSN, MSN/MBA)
Southern Nazarene University, School of Nursing, *Bethany* (MS)
University of Oklahoma Health Sciences Center, College of Nursing, *Oklahoma City* (MS)
University of Phoenix–Oklahoma City Campus, College of Health and Human Services, *Oklahoma City* (MSN, MSN/MBA)
University of Phoenix–Tulsa Campus, College of Health and Human Services, *Tulsa* (MSN, MSN/MBA)

Oregon
University of Portland, School of Nursing, *Portland* (MS)

Pennsylvania
Bloomsburg University of Pennsylvania, Department of Nursing, *Bloomsburg* (MSN, MSN/MBA)
Carlow University, Division of Nursing, *Pittsburgh* (MSN)
Clarion University of Pennsylvania, School of Nursing, *Oil City* (MSN)
College Misericordia, Department of Nursing, *Dallas* (MSN)
DeSales University, Department of Nursing and Health, *Center Valley* (MSN, MSN/MBA)
Drexel University, College of Nursing and Health Professions, *Philadelphia* (MSN)
Duquesne University, School of Nursing, *Pittsburgh* (MSN, MSN/MBA)
Edinboro University of Pennsylvania, Department of Nursing, *Edinboro* (MSN)
Gannon University, Villa Maria School of Nursing, *Erie* (MSN)
Gwynedd-Mercy College, School of Nursing, *Gwynedd Valley* (MSN)
Holy Family University, School of Nursing and Allied Health Professions, *Philadelphia* (MSN)
Immaculata University, Department of Nursing, *Immaculata* (MSN)
Indiana University of Pennsylvania, Department of Nursing and Allied Health, *Indiana* (MSN)
La Roche College, Department of Nursing and Nursing Management, *Pittsburgh* (MSN)
La Salle University, School of Nursing, *Philadelphia* (MSN, MSN/MBA)
Mansfield University of Pennsylvania, Robert Packer Department of Health Sciences, *Mansfield* (MSN)
Marywood University, Department of Nursing, *Scranton* (MSN)
Millersville University of Pennsylvania, Department of Nursing, *Millersville* (MSN)
Neumann College, Program in Nursing and Health Sciences, *Aston* (MS)
The Pennsylvania State University University Park Campus, School of Nursing, *State College, University Park* (MS)
Temple University, Department of Nursing, *Philadelphia* (MSN)
Thomas Jefferson University, Department of Nursing, *Philadelphia* (MSN)
University of Pennsylvania, School of Nursing, *Philadelphia* (MSN, MSN/MBA, MSN/MPH, MSN/PhD)
University of Pittsburgh, School of Nursing, *Pittsburgh* (MSN)
The University of Scranton, Department of Nursing, *Scranton* (MS)
Villanova University, College of Nursing, *Villanova* (MSN)
West Chester University of Pennsylvania, Department of Nursing, *West Chester* (MSN)
Widener University, School of Nursing, *Chester* (MSN)
Wilkes University, Department of Nursing, *Wilkes-Barre* (MS)
York College of Pennsylvania, Department of Nursing, *York* (MS)

Puerto Rico
University of Puerto Rico, Medical Sciences Campus, School of Nursing, *San Juan* (MSN)
University of the Sacred Heart, Program in Nursing, *San Juan* (MSN)

Rhode Island
University of Rhode Island, College of Nursing, *Kingston* (MS)

South Carolina
Clemson University, School of Nursing, *Clemson* (MS)
Medical University of South Carolina, College of Nursing, *Charleston* (MSN)
University of South Carolina, College of Nursing, *Columbia* (MSN, MSN/MPH)

South Dakota
Augustana College, Department of Nursing, *Sioux Falls* (MA)
South Dakota State University, College of Nursing, *Brookings* (MS)

Tennessee
Belmont University, School of Nursing, *Nashville* (MSN)
Carson-Newman College, Department of Nursing, *Jefferson City* (MSN)
East Tennessee State University, College of Nursing, *Johnson City* (MSN)
Southern Adventist University, School of Nursing, *Collegedale* (MSN, MSN/MBA)
Tennessee Technological University, School of Nursing, *Cookeville* (MSN, M Sc N)
Union University, School of Nursing, *Jackson* (MSN)
The University of Memphis, Loewenberg School of Nursing, *Memphis* (MSN)
The University of Tennessee, College of Nursing, *Knoxville* (MSN)
The University of Tennessee at Chattanooga, School of Nursing, *Chattanooga* (MSN)
The University of Tennessee Health Science Center, College of Nursing, *Memphis* (MSN)

Texas
Abilene Intercollegiate School of Nursing, *Abilene* (MSN)
Angelo State University, Department of Nursing, *San Angelo* (MSN)
Baylor University, Louise Herrington School of Nursing of Baylor University, *Dallas* (MSN)

MASTER'S DEGREE PROGRAMS
Master's

Lamar University, Department of Nursing, *Beaumont* (MSN)
Prairie View A&M University, College of Nursing, *Houston* (MSN)
Texas A&M International University, Canseco School of Nursing, *Laredo* (MSN)
Texas A&M University–Corpus Christi, School of Nursing and Health Sciences, *Corpus Christi* (MSN)
Texas Christian University, Harris School of Nursing, *Fort Worth* (MSN)
Texas Tech University Health Sciences Center, School of Nursing, *Lubbock* (MSN, MSN/MBA)
Texas Woman's University, College of Nursing, *Denton* (MS, MSN/MHA)
The University of Texas at Arlington, School of Nursing, *Arlington* (MSN, MSN/MBA, MSN/MPH)
The University of Texas at Austin, School of Nursing, *Austin* (MSN, MSN/MBA)
The University of Texas at El Paso, School of Nursing, *El Paso* (MSN)
The University of Texas at Tyler, Program in Nursing, *Tyler* (MSN, MSN/MBA)
The University of Texas Health Science Center at Houston, School of Nursing, *Houston* (MSN, MSN/MPH)
The University of Texas Health Science Center at San Antonio, School of Nursing, *San Antonio* (MSN, MSN/MPH)
The University of Texas Medical Branch, School of Nursing, *Galveston* (MSN)
The University of Texas–Pan American, Department of Nursing, *Edinburg* (MSN)
University of the Incarnate Word, Program in Nursing, *San Antonio* (MSN, MSN/MBA)
West Texas A&M University, Division of Nursing, *Canyon* (MSN)

Utah
Brigham Young University, College of Nursing, *Provo* (MS)
University of Phoenix–Utah Campus, College of Health and Human Services, *Salt Lake City* (MSN, MSN/MBA)
Westminster College, St. Mark's-Westminster School of Nursing and Health Sciences, *Salt Lake City* (MSN)

Vermont
University of Vermont, Department of Nursing, *Burlington* (MS)

Virginia
George Mason University, College of Nursing and Health Science, *Fairfax* (MSN, MSN/MBA)
Hampton University, Department of Nursing, *Hampton* (MS)
James Madison University, Department of Nursing, *Harrisonburg* (MSN)
Jefferson College of Health Sciences, Nursing Education Program, *Roanoke* (MSN)
Liberty University, Department of Nursing, *Lynchburg* (MSN)
Marymount University, School of Health Professions, *Arlington* (MSN)
Old Dominion University, Department of Nursing, *Norfolk* (MSN)
Radford University, School of Nursing, *Radford* (MSN)
Shenandoah University, Division of Nursing, *Winchester* (MSN)
University of Virginia, School of Nursing, *Charlottesville* (MSN, MSN/MA, MSN/MBA, MSN/PhD, MSN/HSM)
Virginia Commonwealth University, School of Nursing, *Richmond* (MS, MS/MPH)

Washington
Intercollegiate College of Nursing/Washington State University, *Spokane* (MN)
Pacific Lutheran University, School of Nursing, *Tacoma* (MSN)
Seattle Pacific University, School of Health Sciences, *Seattle* (MSN, MN/MBA)
Seattle University, College of Nursing, *Seattle* (MSN)
University of Washington, School of Nursing, *Seattle* (MN, MN/MPH, MSN/MHA)

West Virginia
Marshall University, College of Nursing and Health Professions, *Huntington* (MSN)
Mountain State University, Program in Nursing, *Beckley* (MSN)
West Virginia University, School of Nursing, *Morgantown* (MSN)
Wheeling Jesuit University, Department of Nursing, *Wheeling* (MSN)

Wisconsin
Bellin College of Nursing, Nursing Program, *Green Bay* (MSN)
Concordia University Wisconsin, Division of Nursing, *Mequon* (MSN)
Edgewood College, Program in Nursing, *Madison* (MS)
Marian College of Fond du Lac, Nursing Studies Division, *Fond du Lac* (MSN)
Marquette University, College of Nursing, *Milwaukee* (MSN, MSN/MBA)
University of Wisconsin–Eau Claire, College of Nursing and Health Sciences, *Eau Claire* (MSN)
University of Wisconsin–Madison, School of Nursing, *Madison* (MS)
University of Wisconsin–Milwaukee, College of Nursing, *Milwaukee* (MS, MSN/MBA)
University of Wisconsin–Oshkosh, College of Nursing, *Oshkosh* (MSN)
Viterbo University, School of Nursing, *La Crosse* (MSN)

Wyoming
University of Wyoming, Fay W. Whitney School of Nursing, *Laramie* (MS)

Alberta
Athabasca University, Centre for Nursing and Health Studies, *Athabasca* (MN)
University of Alberta, Faculty of Nursing, *Edmonton* (MN)
University of Calgary, Faculty of Nursing, *Calgary* (MN)
The University of Lethbridge, School of Health Sciences, *Lethbridge* (M Sc)

British Columbia
The University of British Columbia, School of Nursing, *Vancouver* (MSN)
University of Victoria, School of Nursing, *Victoria* (MN)

New Brunswick
Université de Moncton, School of Nursing, *Moncton* (M Sc N)
University of New Brunswick Fredericton, Faculty of Nursing, *Fredericton* (MN)

Newfoundland and Labrador
Memorial University of Newfoundland, School of Nursing, *St. John's* (MN)

Nova Scotia
Dalhousie University, School of Nursing, *Halifax* (MN, MN/MHSA)

Ontario
McMaster University, School of Nursing, *Hamilton* (M Sc, MSN/PhD)
Queen's University at Kingston, School of Nursing, *Kingston* (M Sc)
University of Ottawa, School of Nursing, *Ottawa* (M Sc N)
University of Toronto, Faculty of Nursing, *Toronto* (MN, MN/MBA)
The University of Western Ontario, School of Nursing, *London* (M Sc N)
University of Windsor, School of Nursing, *Windsor* (M Sc)

Quebec
McGill University, School of Nursing, *Montréal* (M Sc)
Université de Sherbrooke, Department of Nursing, *Sherbrooke* (M Sc)
Université du Québec à Rimouski, Program in Nursing, *Rimouski* (M Sc N)
Université du Québec en Outaouais, Département des Sciences Infirmières, *Gatineau* (M Sc N)

Saskatchewan
University of Saskatchewan, College of Nursing, *Saskatoon* (MN)

Master's for Non-Nursing College Graduates

California
Samuel Merritt College, School of Nursing, *Oakland* (MSN)
San Francisco State University, School of Nursing, *San Francisco* (MSN)
University of California, San Francisco, School of Nursing, *San Francisco* (MS)
University of San Diego, Hahn School of Nursing and Health Sciences, *San Diego* (MSN, MSN/MBA)
University of San Francisco, School of Nursing, *San Francisco* (MSN)

Colorado
Colorado State University-Pueblo, Department of Nursing, *Pueblo* (MS)

Connecticut
Yale University, School of Nursing, *New Haven* (MSN, MSN/MBA, MSN/MPH)

District of Columbia
Georgetown University, School of Nursing and Health Studies, *Washington* (MS)

Illinois
DePaul University, Department of Nursing, *Chicago* (MS)
University of Illinois at Chicago, College of Nursing, *Chicago* (MS, MS/MBA)

Maine
University of Southern Maine, College of Nursing and Health Professions, *Portland* (MS, MS/MBA)

Massachusetts
MGH Institute of Health Professions, Program in Nursing, *Boston* (MS)
Northeastern University, School of Nursing, *Boston* (MS, MSN/MBA)
Regis College, Department of Nursing, *Weston* (MSN)
Simmons College, Department of Nursing, *Boston* (MS, MSN/MS)
University of Massachusetts Worcester, Graduate School of Nursing, *Worcester* (MS)

Nebraska
University of Nebraska Medical Center, College of Nursing, *Omaha* (MSN)

New York
Columbia University, School of Nursing, *New York* (MS, MS/MBA, MS/MPH)
University of Rochester, School of Nursing, *Rochester* (MS, MSN/PhD)

Ohio
Case Western Reserve University, Frances Payne Bolton School of Nursing, *Cleveland* (MSN, MSN/MA, MSN/MBA, MSN/MPH, MSN/PhD)
Medical College of Ohio, School of Nursing, *Toledo* (MSN)
The Ohio State University, College of Nursing, *Columbus* (MS)
University of Phoenix–Cleveland Campus, College of Health and Human Services, *Independence* (MSN)

Oklahoma
University of Oklahoma Health Sciences Center, College of Nursing, *Oklahoma City* (MS)

Oregon
University of Portland, School of Nursing, *Portland* (MS)

Pennsylvania
Thomas Jefferson University, Department of Nursing, *Philadelphia* (MSN)
Wilkes University, Department of Nursing, *Wilkes-Barre* (MS)

Tennessee
The University of Memphis, Loewenberg School of Nursing, *Memphis* (MSN)
The University of Tennessee, College of Nursing, *Knoxville* (MSN)

Texas
The University of Texas at Austin, School of Nursing, *Austin* (MSN, MSN/MBA)

Washington
Pacific Lutheran University, School of Nursing, *Tacoma* (MSN)
University of Washington, School of Nursing, *Seattle* (MN, MN/MPH, MSN/MHA)

Wisconsin
Marquette University, College of Nursing, *Milwaukee* (MSN, MSN/MBA)

Quebec
McGill University, School of Nursing, *Montréal* (M Sc)

Master's for Nurses with Non-Nursing Degrees

Alabama
University of South Alabama, College of Nursing, *Mobile* (MSN)

California
California State University, Bakersfield, Program in Nursing, *Bakersfield* (MSN)
California State University, Dominguez Hills, Program in Nursing, *Carson* (MSN)
California State University, Fresno, Department of Nursing, *Fresno* (MSN)
California State University, Sacramento, Division of Nursing, *Sacramento* (MS)
Dominican University of California, Program in Occupational Therapy, *San Rafael* (MSN)
Loma Linda University, School of Nursing, *Loma Linda* (MS, MS/MA, MS/MPH)
Samuel Merritt College, School of Nursing, *Oakland* (MSN)
San Francisco State University, School of Nursing, *San Francisco* (MSN)
University of California, San Francisco, School of Nursing, *San Francisco* (MS)
University of San Diego, Hahn School of Nursing and Health Sciences, *San Diego* (MSN, MSN/MBA)
University of San Francisco, School of Nursing, *San Francisco* (MSN)

Connecticut
Sacred Heart University, Program in Nursing, *Fairfield* (MSN, MSN/MBA)
Saint Joseph College, Department of Nursing, *West Hartford* (MS)
University of Hartford, College of Education, Nursing, and Health Professions, *West Hartford* (MSN, MSN/MSOB)

Florida
Florida Atlantic University, College of Nursing, *Boca Raton* (M Sc N)
Florida International University, School of Nursing, *Miami* (MSN)
University of South Florida, College of Nursing, *Tampa* (MS, MSN/MPH)

Georgia
Georgia Southern University, School of Nursing, *Statesboro* (MSN)

Illinois
DePaul University, Department of Nursing, *Chicago* (MS)
Rush University, College of Nursing, *Chicago* (MSN, MSN/MBA)
Saint Francis Medical Center College of Nursing, Baccalaureate Nursing Program, *Peoria* (MSN)
Saint Xavier University, School of Nursing, *Chicago* (MSN, MSN/MBA)
University of St. Francis, College of Nursing and Allied Health, *Joliet* (MSN)

Indiana
University of Saint Francis, Department of Nursing, *Fort Wayne* (MSN)

Iowa
Allen College, Program in Nursing, *Waterloo* (MSN)

Kentucky
Bellarmine University, Donna and Allan Lansing School of Nursing and Health Sciences, *Louisville* (MSN, MSN/MBA)

Louisiana
Loyola University New Orleans, Program in Nursing, *New Orleans* (MSN)

Maine
Husson College, School of Nursing, *Bangor* (MSN)
Saint Joseph's College of Maine, Department of Nursing, *Standish* (MSN, MSN/MA)

Maryland
University of Maryland, School of Nursing, *Baltimore* (MS, MS/MBA)

Massachusetts
MGH Institute of Health Professions, Program in Nursing, *Boston* (MS)
Salem State College, Nursing Department, *Salem* (MSN, MSN/MBA)
Simmons College, Department of Nursing, *Boston* (MS, MSN/MS)
University of Massachusetts Amherst, School of Nursing, *Amherst* (MS, MS/MPH)
Worcester State College, Department of Nursing, *Worcester* (MS)

Michigan
Grand Valley State University, Russell B. Kirkhof School of Nursing, *Allendale* (MSN, MSN/MBA)
University of Detroit Mercy, McAuley School of Nursing, *Detroit* (MSN)

Minnesota
Concordia College, Department of Nursing, *Moorhead* (MS)
Metropolitan State University, School of Nursing, *St. Paul* (MSN)
Minnesota State University Moorhead, Tri-College University Nursing Consortium, *Moorhead* (MS)

Missouri
Graceland University, School of Nursing, *Independence* (MSN)
Saint Louis University, School of Nursing, *St. Louis* (MSN, MSN/MPH)

New Hampshire
Rivier College, Department of Nursing and Health Sciences, *Nashua* (MS, MS/MBA)
University of New Hampshire, Department of Nursing, *Durham* (MS)

New Jersey
The College of New Jersey, School of Nursing, *Ewing* (MSN)
Fairleigh Dickinson University, Metropolitan Campus, Henry P. Becton School of Nursing and Allied Health, *Teaneck* (MSN)
Kean University, Department of Nursing, *Union* (MSN, MSN/MPA)
Monmouth University, Marjorie K. Unterberg School of Nursing, *West Long Branch* (MSN)
Saint Peter's College, Nursing Program, *Jersey City* (MSN)
William Paterson University of New Jersey, Department of Nursing, *Wayne* (MSN)

New Mexico
University of New Mexico, College of Nursing, *Albuquerque* (MSN, MSN/MALAS, MSN/MPA, MSN/MPH)

New York
Adelphi University, School of Nursing, *Garden City* (MS, MS/MBA)
College of Mount Saint Vincent, Division of Nursing, *Riverdale* (MSN)
Mercy College, Program in Nursing, *Dobbs Ferry* (MS)
Pace University, Lienhard School of Nursing, *New York* (MS)
University of Rochester, School of Nursing, *Rochester* (MS, MSN/PhD)

North Carolina
East Carolina University, School of Nursing, *Greenville* (MSN)
The University of North Carolina at Chapel Hill, School of Nursing, *Chapel Hill* (MSN, MSN/MS)

Ohio
Case Western Reserve University, Frances Payne Bolton School of Nursing, *Cleveland* (MSN, MSN/MA, MSN/MBA, MSN/MPH, MSN/PhD)
Wright State University, College of Nursing and Health, *Dayton* (MS, MS/MBA)

Oregon
University of Portland, School of Nursing, *Portland* (MS)

Pennsylvania
Bloomsburg University of Pennsylvania, Department of Nursing, *Bloomsburg* (MSN, MSN/MBA)
Thomas Jefferson University, Department of Nursing, *Philadelphia* (MSN)
University of Pittsburgh, School of Nursing, *Pittsburgh* (MSN)

Tennessee
The University of Memphis, Loewenberg School of Nursing, *Memphis* (MSN)
The University of Tennessee, College of Nursing, *Knoxville* (MSN)

Texas
Texas A&M International University, Canseco School of Nursing, *Laredo* (MSN)
The University of Texas at Austin, School of Nursing, *Austin* (MSN, MSN/MBA)

Vermont
University of Vermont, Department of Nursing, *Burlington* (MS)

Virginia
Jefferson College of Health Sciences, Nursing Education Program, *Roanoke* (MSN)

Washington
Gonzaga University, Department of Nursing, *Spokane* (MSN)
Intercollegiate College of Nursing/Washington State University, *Spokane* (MN)
Pacific Lutheran University, School of Nursing, *Tacoma* (MSN)
University of Washington, School of Nursing, *Seattle* (MN, MN/MPH, MSN/MHA)

Wisconsin
Marquette University, College of Nursing, *Milwaukee* (MSN, MSN/MBA)

University of Wisconsin–Madison, School of Nursing, *Madison* (MS)

Wyoming

University of Wyoming, Fay W. Whitney School of Nursing, *Laramie* (MS)

RN to Master's

Alabama

Samford University, Ida V. Moffett School of Nursing, *Birmingham* (MSN, MSN/MBA)
Troy University, School of Nursing, *Troy* (MSN)
The University of Alabama, Capstone College of Nursing, *Tuscaloosa* (MSN, MSN/MA, MSN/MBA)
The University of Alabama at Birmingham, School of Nursing, *Birmingham* (MSN, MSN/MPH)
The University of Alabama in Huntsville, College of Nursing, *Huntsville* (MSN)

Arkansas

University of Central Arkansas, Department of Nursing, *Conway* (MSN)

California

California State University, Bakersfield, Program in Nursing, *Bakersfield* (MSN)
Loma Linda University, School of Nursing, *Loma Linda* (MS, MS/MA, MS/MPH)

Colorado

University of Colorado at Denver and Health Sciences Center—Health Sciences Program, School of Nursing, *Denver* (MS, MSN/MBA)

Connecticut

Sacred Heart University, Program in Nursing, *Fairfield* (MSN, MSN/MBA)
Saint Joseph College, Department of Nursing, *West Hartford* (MS)
University of Connecticut, School of Nursing, *Storrs* (MS, MSN/MBA, MSN/MPH)
Yale University, School of Nursing, *New Haven* (MSN, MSN/MBA, MSN/MPH)

Delaware

University of Delaware, Department of Nursing, *Newark* (MSN)

District of Columbia

Georgetown University, School of Nursing and Health Studies, *Washington* (MS)

Florida

Florida Atlantic University, College of Nursing, *Boca Raton* (M Sc N)
Jacksonville University, School of Nursing, *Jacksonville* (MSN, MSN/MBA)
University of Central Florida, School of Nursing, *Orlando* (MSN)
University of North Florida, School of Nursing, *Jacksonville* (MSN)
University of South Florida, College of Nursing, *Tampa* (MS, MSN/MPH)

Georgia

Emory University, Nell Hodgson Woodruff School of Nursing, *Atlanta* (MSN, MSN/MPH)
Georgia College & State University, School of Health Sciences, *Milledgeville* (MSN, MSN/MBA)
Georgia Southern University, School of Nursing, *Statesboro* (MSN)
Georgia State University, School of Nursing, *Atlanta* (MS)
Medical College of Georgia, School of Nursing, *Augusta* (MSN)
Valdosta State University, College of Nursing, *Valdosta* (MSN)

Illinois

DePaul University, Department of Nursing, *Chicago* (MS)
Lewis University, Program in Nursing, *Romeoville* (MSN, MSN/MBA)
Loyola University Chicago, Marcella Niehoff School of Nursing, *Chicago* (MSN, MSN/MBA, MSN/MDIV)
Rush University, College of Nursing, *Chicago* (MSN, MSN/MBA)
Saint Francis Medical Center College of Nursing, Baccalaureate Nursing Program, *Peoria* (MSN)
Saint Xavier University, School of Nursing, *Chicago* (MSN, MSN/MBA)
University of St. Francis, College of Nursing and Allied Health, *Joliet* (MSN)

Indiana

Ball State University, School of Nursing, *Muncie* (MS)
Indiana University–Purdue University Indianapolis, School of Nursing, *Indianapolis* (MSN, MSN/MPH)
University of Southern Indiana, School of Nursing and Health Professions, *Evansville* (MSN)
Valparaiso University, College of Nursing, *Valparaiso* (MSN)

Kansas

Newman University, Division of Nursing, *Wichita* (M Sc N)
Pittsburg State University, Department of Nursing, *Pittsburg* (MSN)
Wichita State University, School of Nursing, *Wichita* (MSN, MSN/MBA)

Kentucky

Bellarmine University, Donna and Allan Lansing School of Nursing and Health Sciences, *Louisville* (MSN, MSN/MBA)
University of Kentucky, Graduate School Programs in the College of Nursing, *Lexington* (MSN)

Louisiana

Loyola University New Orleans, Program in Nursing, *New Orleans* (MSN)

Maine

Husson College, School of Nursing, *Bangor* (MSN)
Saint Joseph's College of Maine, Department of Nursing, *Standish* (MSN, MSN/MA)
University of Maine, School of Nursing, *Orono* (MSN)
University of Southern Maine, College of Nursing and Health Professions, *Portland* (MS, MS/MBA)

Maryland

University of Maryland, School of Nursing, *Baltimore* (MS, MS/MBA)

Massachusetts

Boston College, William F. Connell School of Nursing, *Chestnut Hill* (MS, MSN/MA, MSN/MBA)
MGH Institute of Health Professions, Program in Nursing, *Boston* (MS)
Northeastern University, School of Nursing, *Boston* (MS, MSN/MBA)
Regis College, Department of Nursing, *Weston* (MSN)
Salem State College, Nursing Department, *Salem* (MSN, MSN/MBA)
Simmons College, Department of Nursing, *Boston* (MS, MSN/MS)

Michigan

Grand Valley State University, Russell B. Kirkhof School of Nursing, *Allendale* (MSN, MSN/MBA)
Saginaw Valley State University, Crystal M. Lange College of Nursing and Health Sciences, *University Center* (MSN)
University of Michigan, School of Nursing, *Ann Arbor* (MS, MS/MBA, MS/MPH)
University of Michigan–Flint, Department of Nursing, *Flint* (MSN)

Minnesota

Metropolitan State University, School of Nursing, *St. Paul* (MSN)
Winona State University, College of Nursing, *Winona* (MS)

Mississippi

University of Mississippi Medical Center, Program in Nursing, *Jackson* (MSN)
University of Southern Mississippi, School of Nursing, *Hattiesburg* (MSN)

Missouri

Graceland University, School of Nursing, *Independence* (MSN)
Jewish Hospital College of Nursing and Allied Health, Division of Nursing, *St. Louis* (MSN)
Maryville University of Saint Louis, Nursing Program, School of Health Professions, *St. Louis* (MSN)
Saint Louis University, School of Nursing, *St. Louis* (MSN, MSN/MPH)
Southwest Missouri State University, Department of Nursing, *Springfield* (MSN)
University of Missouri–St. Louis, College of Nursing, *St. Louis* (MSN)

Nebraska

University of Nebraska Medical Center, College of Nursing, *Omaha* (MSN)

Nevada

University of Nevada, Las Vegas, Department of Nursing, *Las Vegas* (MSN)

New Jersey

The College of New Jersey, School of Nursing, *Ewing* (MSN)
Fairleigh Dickinson University, Metropolitan Campus, Henry P. Becton School of Nursing and Allied Health, *Teaneck* (MSN)
Felician College, Department of Professional Nursing–BSN, *Lodi* (MSN)
Seton Hall University, College of Nursing, *South Orange* (MSN, MSN/MA, MSN/MBA)

New York

Daemen College, Department of Nursing, *Amherst* (MSN)
D'Youville College, Department of Nursing, *Buffalo* (MS)
Excelsior College, School of Nursing, *Albany* (MS)
Long Island University, Brooklyn Campus, School of Nursing, *Brooklyn* (MS)
New York University, Division of Nursing, *New York* (MA, MS/MA)
Pace University, Lienhard School of Nursing, *New York* (MS)
St. John Fisher College, Nursing Program, *Rochester* (MS)

North Carolina

Duke University, School of Nursing, *Durham* (MSN, MSN/MBA, MSN/MCM)
East Carolina University, School of Nursing, *Greenville* (MSN)
Gardner-Webb University, School of Nursing, *Boiling Springs* (MSN, MSN/MBA)
Queens University of Charlotte, Division of Nursing, *Charlotte* (MSN, MSN/MBA)
The University of North Carolina at Chapel Hill, School of Nursing, *Chapel Hill* (MSN, MSN/MS)
The University of North Carolina at Charlotte, School of Nursing, *Charlotte* (MSN, MSN/MHA)
The University of North Carolina at Wilmington, School of Nursing, *Wilmington* (MSN)

Ohio

Capital University, School of Nursing, *Columbus* (MSN)
Franciscan University of Steubenville, Department of Nursing, *Steubenville* (MSN)
The University of Akron, College of Nursing, *Akron* (MSN)
Xavier University, Department of Nursing, *Cincinnati* (MSN, MSN/MBA)

Pennsylvania

Bloomsburg University of Pennsylvania, Department of Nursing, *Bloomsburg* (MSN, MSN/MBA)

Carlow University, Division of Nursing, *Pittsburgh* (MSN)
College Misericordia, Department of Nursing, *Dallas* (MSN)
DeSales University, Department of Nursing and Health, *Center Valley* (MSN, MSN/MBA)
Drexel University, College of Nursing and Health Professions, *Philadelphia* (MSN)
Gannon University, Villa Maria School of Nursing, *Erie* (MSN)
Gwynedd-Mercy College, School of Nursing, *Gwynedd Valley* (MSN)
Indiana University of Pennsylvania, Department of Nursing and Allied Health, *Indiana* (MSN)
La Roche College, Department of Nursing and Nursing Management, *Pittsburgh* (MSN)
La Salle University, School of Nursing, *Philadelphia* (MSN, MSN/MBA)
Neumann College, Program in Nursing and Health Sciences, *Aston* (MS)
The Pennsylvania State University University Park Campus, School of Nursing, *State College, University Park* (MS)
Thomas Jefferson University, Department of Nursing, *Philadelphia* (MSN)
University of Pittsburgh, School of Nursing, *Pittsburgh* (MSN)
The University of Scranton, Department of Nursing, *Scranton* (MS)
Widener University, School of Nursing, *Chester* (MSN)
Wilkes University, Department of Nursing, *Wilkes-Barre* (MS)
York College of Pennsylvania, Department of Nursing, *York* (MS)

Rhode Island
University of Rhode Island, College of Nursing, *Kingston* (MS)

South Carolina
Clemson University, School of Nursing, *Clemson* (MS)
Medical University of South Carolina, College of Nursing, *Charleston* (MSN)

South Dakota
South Dakota State University, College of Nursing, *Brookings* (MS)

Tennessee
The University of Tennessee, College of Nursing, *Knoxville* (MSN)
The University of Tennessee Health Science Center, College of Nursing, *Memphis* (MSN)

Texas
Baylor University, Louise Herrington School of Nursing of Baylor University, *Dallas* (MSN)
Texas Christian University, Harris School of Nursing, *Fort Worth* (MSN)
Texas Woman's University, College of Nursing, *Denton* (MS, MSN/MHA)
The University of Texas at El Paso, School of Nursing, *El Paso* (MSN)
The University of Texas at Tyler, Program in Nursing, *Tyler* (MSN, MSN/MBA)
The University of Texas Health Science Center at San Antonio, School of Nursing, *San Antonio* (MSN, MSN/MPH)

Vermont
University of Vermont, Department of Nursing, *Burlington* (MS)

Virginia
George Mason University, College of Nursing and Health Science, *Fairfax* (MSN, MSN/MBA)
James Madison University, Department of Nursing, *Harrisonburg* (MSN)
Marymount University, School of Health Professions, *Arlington* (MSN)
Old Dominion University, Department of Nursing, *Norfolk* (MSN)
Shenandoah University, Division of Nursing, *Winchester* (MSN)
Virginia Commonwealth University, School of Nursing, *Richmond* (MS, MS/MPH)

Washington
Gonzaga University, Department of Nursing, *Spokane* (MSN)
Pacific Lutheran University, School of Nursing, *Tacoma* (MSN)

West Virginia
West Virginia University, School of Nursing, *Morgantown* (MSN)

Wisconsin
Marquette University, College of Nursing, *Milwaukee* (MSN, MSN/MBA)
University of Wisconsin–Eau Claire, College of Nursing and Health Sciences, *Eau Claire* (MSN)
University of Wisconsin–Milwaukee, College of Nursing, *Milwaukee* (MS, MSN/MBA)

Alberta
University of Calgary, Faculty of Nursing, *Calgary* (MN)

New Brunswick
Université de Moncton, School of Nursing, *Moncton* (M Sc N)

Quebec
Université du Québec à Chicoutimi, Program in Nursing, *Chicoutimi* (MSN)

Joint Degrees

Alabama
Samford University, Ida V. Moffett School of Nursing, *Birmingham* (MSN, MSN/MBA)
The University of Alabama, Capstone College of Nursing, *Tuscaloosa* (MSN, MSN/MA, MSN/MBA)
The University of Alabama at Birmingham, School of Nursing, *Birmingham* (MSN, MSN/MPH)

Arizona
Arizona State University, College of Nursing, *Tempe* (MS, MS/MPH)
University of Phoenix Online Campus, College of Health and Human Services, *Phoenix* (MSN, MSN/MBA)
University of Phoenix–Phoenix Campus, College of Health and Human Services, *Phoenix* (MSN, MSN/MBA)
University of Phoenix–Southern Arizona Campus, College of Health and Human Services, *Tucson* (MSN, MSN/MBA)

California
California State University, Long Beach, Department of Nursing, *Long Beach* (MSN, MS/MHSA)
Holy Names University, Department of Nursing, *Oakland* (MSN, MSN/MBA)
Loma Linda University, School of Nursing, *Loma Linda* (MS, MS/MA, MS/MPH)
University of California, Los Angeles, School of Nursing, *Los Angeles* (MSN, MSN/MBA)
University of Phoenix–Northern California Campus, College of Health and Human Services, *Pleasanton* (MSN, MSN/MBA)
University of Phoenix–Sacramento Campus, College of Health and Human Services, *Sacramento* (MSN, MSN/MBA)
University of Phoenix–San Diego Campus, College of Health and Human Services, *San Diego* (MSN, MSN/MBA)
University of Phoenix–Southern California Campus, College of Health and Human Services, *Costa Mesa* (MSN, MSN/MBA)
University of San Diego, Hahn School of Nursing and Health Sciences, *San Diego* (MSN, MSN/MBA)

Colorado
University of Colorado at Colorado Springs, Beth-El College of Nursing and Health Sciences, *Colorado Springs* (MSN, MSN/MBA)
University of Colorado at Denver and Health Sciences Center—Health Sciences Program, School of Nursing, *Denver* (MS, MSN/MBA)
University of Phoenix–Colorado Campus, College of Health and Human Services, *Lone Tree* (MSN, MSN/MBA)
University of Phoenix–Southern Colorado Campus, College of Health and Human Services, *Colorado Springs* (MSN, MSN/MBA)

Connecticut
Sacred Heart University, Program in Nursing, *Fairfield* (MSN, MSN/MBA)
University of Connecticut, School of Nursing, *Storrs* (MS, MSN/MBA, MSN/MPH)
University of Hartford, College of Education, Nursing, and Health Professions, *West Hartford* (MSN, MSN/MSOB)
Yale University, School of Nursing, *New Haven* (MSN, MSN/MBA, MSN/MPH)

Delaware
Wilmington College, Division of Nursing, *New Castle* (MSN, MSN/MBA, MSN/MS)

District of Columbia
The Catholic University of America, School of Nursing, *Washington* (MSN, MA/MSM)

Florida
Barry University, School of Nursing, *Miami Shores* (MSN, MSN/MBA)
Florida State University, School of Nursing, *Tallahassee* (MSN, MSN/MS)
Jacksonville University, School of Nursing, *Jacksonville* (MSN, MSN/MBA)
University of Florida, College of Nursing, *Gainesville* (MSN, MSN/MBA, MSN/MPH, MSN/PhD)
University of Phoenix–Fort Lauderdale Campus, College of Health and Human Services, *Fort Lauderdale* (MSN, MSN/MBA)
University of Phoenix–Jacksonville Campus, College of Health and Human Services, *Jacksonville* (MSN, MSN/MBA)
University of Phoenix–Orlando Campus, College of Health and Human Services, *Maitland* (MSN, MSN/MBA)
University of Phoenix–Tampa Campus, College of Health and Human Services, *Tampa* (MSN, MSN/MBA)
University of South Florida, College of Nursing, *Tampa* (MS, MSN/MPH)

Georgia
Armstrong Atlantic State University, Program in Nursing, *Savannah* (MSN, MN/MHSA)
Emory University, Nell Hodgson Woodruff School of Nursing, *Atlanta* (MSN, MSN/MPH)
Georgia College & State University, School of Health Sciences, *Milledgeville* (MSN, MSN/MBA)

Hawaii
Hawai'i Pacific University, School of Nursing, *Honolulu* (MSN, MSN/MBA)
University of Phoenix–Hawaii Campus, College of Health and Human Services, *Honolulu* (MSN, MSN/MBA)

Illinois
Lewis University, Program in Nursing, *Romeoville* (MSN, MSN/MBA)
Loyola University Chicago, Marcella Niehoff School of Nursing, *Chicago* (MSN, MSN/MBA, MSN/MDIV)
Northern Illinois University, School of Nursing, *De Kalb* (MS, MSN/MPH)
North Park University, School of Nursing, *Chicago* (MS, MSN/MA, MSN/MBA)
Rush University, College of Nursing, *Chicago* (MSN, MSN/MBA)

Saint Xavier University, School of Nursing, *Chicago* (MSN, MSN/MBA)
University of Illinois at Chicago, College of Nursing, *Chicago* (MS, MS/MBA)

Indiana
Anderson University, Department of Nursing, *Anderson* (MSN, MSN/MBA)
Indiana University–Purdue University Indianapolis, School of Nursing, *Indianapolis* (MSN, MSN/MPH)
University of Indianapolis, School of Nursing, *Indianapolis* (MSN, MSN/MBA)

Iowa
The University of Iowa, College of Nursing, *Iowa City* (MSN, MSN/MBA, MSN/MPH)

Kansas
University of Kansas, School of Nursing, *Kansas City* (MS, MS/MHSA, MS/MPH)
Wichita State University, School of Nursing, *Wichita* (MSN, MSN/MBA)

Kentucky
Bellarmine University, Donna and Allan Lansing School of Nursing and Health Sciences, *Louisville* (MSN, MSN/MBA)

Louisiana
University of Phoenix–Louisiana Campus, College of Health and Human Services, *Metairie* (MSN, MSN/MBA)

Maine
Saint Joseph's College of Maine, Department of Nursing, *Standish* (MSN, MSN/MA)
University of Southern Maine, College of Nursing and Health Professions, *Portland* (MS, MS/MBA)

Maryland
The Johns Hopkins University, School of Nursing, *Baltimore* (MSN, MSN/MBA, MSN/MPH, MSN/PhD)
University of Maryland, School of Nursing, *Baltimore* (MS, MS/MBA)

Massachusetts
Boston College, William F. Connell School of Nursing, *Chestnut Hill* (MS, MSN/MA, MSN/MBA)
Northeastern University, School of Nursing, *Boston* (MS, MSN/MBA)
Salem State College, Nursing Department, *Salem* (MSN, MSN/MBA)
Simmons College, Department of Nursing, *Boston* (MS, MSN/MS)
University of Massachusetts Amherst, School of Nursing, *Amherst* (MS, MS/MPH)

Michigan
Grand Valley State University, Russell B. Kirkhof School of Nursing, *Allendale* (MSN, MSN/MBA)
Madonna University, College of Nursing and Health, *Livonia* (MSN, MSN/MSBA)
University of Michigan, School of Nursing, *Ann Arbor* (MS, MS/MBA, MS/MPH)
University of Phoenix–Metro Detroit Campus, College of Health and Human Services, *Southfield* (MSN, MSN/MBA)
University of Phoenix–West Michigan Campus, College of Health and Human Services, *Grand Rapids* (MSN, MSN/MBA)

Minnesota
University of Minnesota, Twin Cities Campus, School of Nursing, *Minneapolis* (MS, MS/MPH)

Missouri
Saint Louis University, School of Nursing, *St. Louis* (MSN, MSN/MPH)

Nevada
University of Nevada, Reno, Orvis School of Nursing, *Reno* (MS, MSN/MPH)

New Hampshire
Rivier College, Department of Nursing and Health Sciences, *Nashua* (MS, MS/MBA)

New Jersey
Kean University, Department of Nursing, *Union* (MSN, MSN/MPA)
Rutgers, The State University of New Jersey, College of Nursing, *Newark* (MS, MS/MPH)
Seton Hall University, College of Nursing, *South Orange* (MSN, MSN/MA, MSN/MBA)

New Mexico
University of New Mexico, College of Nursing, *Albuquerque* (MSN, MSN/MALAS, MSN/MPA, MSN/MPH)
University of Phoenix–New Mexico Campus, College of Health and Human Services, *Albuquerque* (MSN, MSN/MBA)

New York
Adelphi University, School of Nursing, *Garden City* (MS, MS/MBA)
Columbia University, School of Nursing, *New York* (MS, MS/MBA, MS/MPH)
Hunter College of the City University of New York, Hunter-Bellevue School of Nursing, *New York* (MS, MS/MPH)
New York University, Division of Nursing, *New York* (MA, MS/MA)
The Sage Colleges, Division of Nursing, *Troy* (MS, MS/MBA)
State University of New York Downstate Medical Center, College of Nursing, *Brooklyn* (MS, MS/MPH)
University of Rochester, School of Nursing, *Rochester* (MS, MSN/PhD)

North Carolina
Duke University, School of Nursing, *Durham* (MSN, MSN/MBA, MSN/MCM)
Gardner-Webb University, School of Nursing, *Boiling Springs* (MSN, MSN/MBA)
Queens University of Charlotte, Division of Nursing, *Charlotte* (MSN, MSN/MBA)
The University of North Carolina at Chapel Hill, School of Nursing, *Chapel Hill* (MSN, MSN/MS)
The University of North Carolina at Charlotte, School of Nursing, *Charlotte* (MSN, MSN/MHA)
The University of North Carolina at Greensboro, School of Nursing, *Greensboro* (MSN, MSN/MBA)

Ohio
Case Western Reserve University, Frances Payne Bolton School of Nursing, *Cleveland* (MSN, MSN/MA, MSN/MBA, MSN/MPH, MSN/PhD)
Cleveland State University, Department of Nursing, *Cleveland* (MSN, MSN/MBA)
Kent State University, College of Nursing, *Kent* (MSN, MSN/MBA, MSN/MPA)
University of Cincinnati, College of Nursing, *Cincinnati* (MSN, MSN/MBA)
Wright State University, College of Nursing and Health, *Dayton* (MS, MS/MBA)
Xavier University, Department of Nursing, *Cincinnati* (MSN, MSN/MBA)

Oklahoma
Oklahoma City University, Kramer School of Nursing, *Oklahoma City* (MSN, MSN/MBA)
University of Phoenix–Oklahoma City Campus, College of Health and Human Services, *Oklahoma City* (MSN, MSN/MBA)
University of Phoenix–Tulsa Campus, College of Health and Human Services, *Tulsa* (MSN, MSN/MBA)

Oregon
Oregon Health & Science University, School of Nursing, *Portland* (MS, MSN/MPH)

Pennsylvania
Bloomsburg University of Pennsylvania, Department of Nursing, *Bloomsburg* (MSN, MSN/MBA)
DeSales University, Department of Nursing and Health, *Center Valley* (MSN, MSN/MBA)
Duquesne University, School of Nursing, *Pittsburgh* (MSN, MSN/MBA)
La Salle University, School of Nursing, *Philadelphia* (MSN, MSN/MBA)
University of Pennsylvania, School of Nursing, *Philadelphia* (MSN, MSN/MBA, MSN/MPH, MSN/PhD)
Waynesburg College, Department of Nursing, *Waynesburg* (MSN, MSN/MBA)

South Carolina
University of South Carolina, College of Nursing, *Columbia* (MSN, MSN/MPH)

Tennessee
Southern Adventist University, School of Nursing, *Collegedale* (MSN, MSN/MBA)
Vanderbilt University, School of Nursing, *Nashville* (MSN, MSN/MBA)

Texas
Texas Tech University Health Sciences Center, School of Nursing, *Lubbock* (MSN, MSN/MBA)
Texas Woman's University, College of Nursing, *Denton* (MS, MSN/MHA)
The University of Texas at Arlington, School of Nursing, *Arlington* (MSN, MSN/MBA, MSN/MPH)
The University of Texas at Austin, School of Nursing, *Austin* (MSN, MSN/MBA)
The University of Texas at Tyler, Program in Nursing, *Tyler* (MSN, MSN/MBA)
The University of Texas Health Science Center at Houston, School of Nursing, *Houston* (MSN, MSN/MPH)
The University of Texas Health Science Center at San Antonio, School of Nursing, *San Antonio* (MSN, MSN/MPH)
University of the Incarnate Word, Program in Nursing, *San Antonio* (MSN, MSN/MBA)

Utah
University of Phoenix–Utah Campus, College of Health and Human Services, *Salt Lake City* (MSN, MSN/MBA)

Virginia
George Mason University, College of Nursing and Health Science, *Fairfax* (MSN, MSN/MBA)
University of Virginia, School of Nursing, *Charlottesville* (MSN, MSN/MA, MSN/MBA, MSN/PhD, MSN/HSM)
Virginia Commonwealth University, School of Nursing, *Richmond* (MS, MS/MPH)

Washington
Seattle Pacific University, School of Health Sciences, *Seattle* (MSN, MN/MBA)
University of Washington, School of Nursing, *Seattle* (MN, MN/MPH, MSN/MHA)

Wisconsin
Marquette University, College of Nursing, *Milwaukee* (MSN, MSN/MBA)
University of Wisconsin–Milwaukee, College of Nursing, *Milwaukee* (MS, MSN/MBA)

Nova Scotia
Dalhousie University, School of Nursing, *Halifax* (MN, MN/MHSA)

Ontario
McMaster University, School of Nursing, *Hamilton* (M Sc, MSN/PhD)
University of Toronto, Faculty of Nursing, *Toronto* (MN, MN/MBA)

Concentrations within Master's Degree Programs

Case Management

California State University, Bakersfield, CA
California State University, Los Angeles, CA
California State University, San Bernardino, CA
Carlow University, PA
DePaul University, IL
Duke University, NC
Florida State University, FL
Gonzaga University, WA
Grand Valley State University, MI
The Johns Hopkins University, MD
Kent State University, OH
Lewis University, IL
Loyola University New Orleans, LA
Millersville University of Pennsylvania, PA
Northern Arizona University, AZ
Pacific Lutheran University, WA
Saint Peter's College, NJ
Samuel Merritt College, CA
San Francisco State University, CA
Seton Hall University, NJ
Shenandoah University, VA
Sonoma State University, CA
Université de Moncton, NB
The University of Alabama, AL
The University of Alabama at Birmingham, AL
University of Central Florida, FL
The University of Iowa, IA
University of Kentucky, KY
University of Nebraska Medical Center, NE
University of New Brunswick Fredericton, NB
The University of North Carolina at Chapel Hill, NC
University of Saint Francis, IN
University of San Francisco, CA
The University of Texas Health Science Center at Houston, TX
University of Wisconsin-Madison, WI
Ursuline College, OH
Valdosta State University, GA
Villanova University, PA
York College of Pennsylvania, PA

Clinical Nurse Specialist Programs

Acute Care

Arizona State University, AZ
California State University, Fresno, CA
Case Western Reserve University, OH
Colorado State University-Pueblo, CO
Duquesne University, PA
Emory University, GA
Georgia Baptist College of Nursing of Mercer University, GA
Grand Valley State University, MI
The Johns Hopkins University, MD
Liberty University, VA
Loyola University Chicago, IL
McGill University, QC
Medical College of Georgia, GA
New York University, NY
Pacific Lutheran University, WA
Samford University, AL
Texas A&M University-Corpus Christi, TX
Thomas Jefferson University, PA
Université de Sherbrooke, QC
Université du Québec à Chicoutimi, QC
University at Buffalo, The State University of New York, NY
University of Alberta, AB
University of Arkansas, AR
University of Arkansas for Medical Sciences, AR
University of Calgary, AB
University of California, Los Angeles, CA
University of Central Florida, FL
University of Cincinnati, OH
University of Colorado at Colorado Springs, CO
University of Connecticut, CT
University of Illinois at Chicago, IL
University of Kentucky, KY
University of Manitoba, MB
University of Massachusetts Boston, MA
University of Medicine and Dentistry of New Jersey, NJ
University of Miami, FL
University of Nebraska Medical Center, NE
University of Nevada, Reno, NV
University of New Brunswick Fredericton, NB
University of North Dakota, ND
University of Oklahoma Health Sciences Center, OK
University of Ottawa, ON
University of Pennsylvania, PA
University of South Alabama, AL
University of South Carolina, SC
The University of Tennessee Health Science Center, TN
The University of Texas Health Science Center at Houston, TX
The University of Texas Health Science Center at San Antonio, TX
University of Utah, UT
University of Virginia, VA
University of Washington, WA
Vanderbilt University, TN
Virginia Commonwealth University, VA
Wichita State University, KS
Yale University, CT

Adult Health

Angelo State University, TX
Arizona State University, AZ
Arkansas State University, AR
Armstrong Atlantic State University, GA
Azusa Pacific University, CA
Bloomsburg University of Pennsylvania, PA
Boston College, MA
California State University, Chico, CA
California State University, Long Beach, CA
California State University, Sacramento, CA
Case Western Reserve University, OH
The Catholic University of America, DC
Clemson University, SC
College Misericordia, PA
College of Mount Saint Vincent, NY
The College of New Jersey, NJ
The College of St. Scholastica, MN
College of Staten Island of the City University of New York, NY
Concordia College, MN
Dalhousie University, NS
DeSales University, PA
East Carolina University, NC
Eastern Michigan University, MI
Emory University, GA
Florida International University, FL
Florida State University, FL
Georgia College & State University, GA
Georgia State University, GA
Gonzaga University, WA
Governors State University, IL
Grand Valley State University, MI
Hampton University, VA
Indiana State University, IN
Indiana University-Purdue University Fort Wayne, IN
Indiana University-Purdue University Indianapolis, IN
The Johns Hopkins University, MD
Kennesaw State University, GA
Kent State University, OH
La Salle University, PA
Lehman College of the City University of New York, NY
Loma Linda University, CA
Long Island University, C.W. Post Campus, NY
Louisiana State University Health Sciences Center, LA
Madonna University, MI
Marquette University, WI
McGill University, QC
McNeese State University, LA
Medical College of Georgia, GA
Medical College of Ohio, OH
Medical University of South Carolina, SC
Minnesota State University Moorhead, MN
Molloy College, NY
Mount Carmel College of Nursing, OH
Mount Saint Mary College, NY
Murray State University, KY
New York University, NY
North Dakota State University, ND
Northern Illinois University, IL
Northwestern State University of Louisiana, LA
The Ohio State University, OH
Oregon Health & Science University, OR
Otterbein College, OH
Pacific Lutheran University, WA
The Pennsylvania State University University Park Campus, PA
Purdue University Calumet, IN
Radford University, VA
Saint Louis University, MO
Saint Xavier University, IL
Salem State College, MA
Samford University, AL
San Diego State University, CA
San Francisco State University, CA
Seattle Pacific University, WA
Southeast Missouri State University, MO
State University of New York Downstate Medical Center, NY
State University of New York Upstate Medical University, NY
Stony Brook University, State University of New York, NY
Texas Christian University, TX
Texas Woman's University, TX
Thomas Jefferson University, PA
Troy University, AL
Université du Québec à Chicoutimi, QC
The University of Akron, OH
The University of Alabama at Birmingham, AL
The University of Alabama in Huntsville, AL
University of Alberta, AB
University of Arkansas for Medical Sciences, AR
University of Calgary, AB
University of Cincinnati, OH
University of Colorado at Colorado Springs, CO
University of Colorado at Denver and Health Sciences Center—Health Sciences Program, CO
University of Connecticut, CT
University of Delaware, DE
University of Illinois at Chicago, IL
The University of Iowa, IA
University of Kansas, KS
University of Kentucky, KY
University of Louisiana at Lafayette, LA
University of Louisville, KY
University of Massachusetts Dartmouth, MA
University of Miami, FL
University of Minnesota, Twin Cities Campus, MN
University of Missouri-Columbia, MO
University of Missouri-St. Louis, MO
University of Nebraska Medical Center, NE
University of Nevada, Reno, NV
University of New Brunswick Fredericton, NB

University of New Hampshire, NH
University of New Mexico, NM
The University of North Carolina at Charlotte, NC
The University of North Carolina at Greensboro, NC
University of North Dakota, ND
University of North Florida, FL
University of Puerto Rico, Medical Sciences Campus, PR
University of St. Francis, IL
University of San Diego, CA
University of San Francisco, CA
The University of Scranton, PA
University of Southern Indiana, IN
University of Southern Mississippi, MS
The University of Tennessee, TN
The University of Texas at Austin, TX
The University of Texas Health Science Center at Houston, TX
The University of Texas–Pan American, TX
University of the Incarnate Word, TX
University of Utah, UT
University of Vermont, VT
University of Wisconsin–Eau Claire, WI
University of Wisconsin–Madison, WI
University of Wisconsin–Milwaukee, WI
Ursuline College, OH
Valdosta State University, GA
Valparaiso University, IN
Western Connecticut State University, CT
Widener University, PA
Winona State University, MN
Wright State University, OH
York College of Pennsylvania, PA

Cardiovascular

Case Western Reserve University, OH
Creighton University, NE
Duke University, NC
The Johns Hopkins University, MD
Loyola University Chicago, IL
McGill University, QC
The Ohio State University, OH
Oregon Health & Science University, OR
Samford University, AL
Seattle Pacific University, WA
Université du Québec à Chicoutimi, QC
University of Alberta, AB
University of Calgary, AB
University of California, San Francisco, CA
University of Illinois at Chicago, IL
University of Missouri–Columbia, MO
University of Nebraska Medical Center, NE
University of New Brunswick Fredericton, NB
University of North Florida, FL
University of Washington, WA
Vanderbilt University, TN
Yale University, CT

Community Health

Albany State University, GA
Arizona State University, AZ
Augsburg College, MN
Augustana College, SD
Bloomsburg University of Pennsylvania, PA
Boston College, MA
California State University, Bakersfield, CA
California State University, Fresno, CA
California State University, Sacramento, CA
California State University, San Bernardino, CA
Capital University, OH
Case Western Reserve University, OH
The Catholic University of America, DC
College Misericordia, PA
Creighton University, NE
Dalhousie University, NS
DePaul University, IL
D'Youville College, NY
East Carolina University, NC
Emory University, GA
Georgia Southern University, GA
Hampton University, VA
Hawai'i Pacific University, HI
Holy Family University, PA
Hunter College of the City University of New York, NY
Indiana State University, IN
Indiana University of Pennsylvania, PA
Indiana University-Purdue University Indianapolis, IN
Indiana Wesleyan University, IN
Intercollegiate College of Nursing/Washington State University, WA
Jacksonville State University, AL
The Johns Hopkins University, MD
Kean University, NJ
La Roche College, PA
Lewis University, IL
Liberty University, VA
Louisiana State University Health Sciences Center, LA
McGill University, QC
Medical College of Georgia, GA
Montana State University–Bozeman, MT
New Mexico State University, NM
Northern Illinois University, IL
North Park University, IL
The Ohio State University, OH
Olivet Nazarene University, IL
Oregon Health & Science University, OR
The Pennsylvania State University University Park Campus, PA
Rutgers, The State University of New Jersey, College of Nursing, NJ
Saint Xavier University, IL
Salem State College, MA
Samford University, AL
San Diego State University, CA
Seattle Pacific University, WA
Seattle University, WA
Southeastern Louisiana University, LA
Southern Illinois University Edwardsville, IL
State University of New York at Binghamton, NY
Stony Brook University, State University of New York, NY
Texas Woman's University, TX
Thomas Jefferson University, PA
Université de Moncton, NB
Université de Sherbrooke, QC
Université du Québec à Chicoutimi, QC
Université du Québec à Rimouski, QC
Université du Québec en Outaouais, QC
University of Alaska Anchorage, AK
University of Alberta, AB
University of Calgary, AB
University of California, San Francisco, CA
University of Central Arkansas, AR
University of Cincinnati, OH
University of Colorado at Colorado Springs, CO
University of Colorado at Denver and Health Sciences Center—Health Sciences Program, CO
University of Connecticut, CT
University of Illinois at Chicago, IL
The University of Iowa, IA
University of Kentucky, KY
University of Maryland, MD
University of Massachusetts Amherst, MA
University of Massachusetts Dartmouth, MA
University of Miami, FL
University of Michigan, MI
University of Nebraska Medical Center, NE
University of Nevada, Reno, NV
University of New Brunswick Fredericton, NB
The University of North Carolina at Charlotte, NC
University of North Dakota, ND
University of North Florida, FL
University of Ottawa, ON
University of Puerto Rico, Medical Sciences Campus, PR
University of South Alabama, AL
University of South Carolina, SC
University of Southern Mississippi, MS
The University of Texas at Austin, TX
University of Utah, UT
University of Vermont, VT
University of Virginia, VA
University of Washington, WA
University of Wisconsin–Milwaukee, WI
Virginia Commonwealth University, VA
Wayne State University, MI
Wesley College, DE
West Chester University of Pennsylvania, PA
Widener University, PA
William Paterson University of New Jersey, NJ
Worcester State College, MA
Wright State University, OH

Critical Care

California State University, Fresno, CA
Case Western Reserve University, OH
Duke University, NC
Emory University, GA
Georgetown University, DC
Gonzaga University, WA
Indiana University–Purdue University Fort Wayne, IN
The Johns Hopkins University, MD
La Roche College, PA
Marymount University, VA
McGill University, QC
Medical College of Georgia, GA
Murray State University, KY
New York University, NY
Northwestern State University of Louisiana, LA
Purdue University Calumet, IN
Rush University, IL
Seattle Pacific University, WA
Stony Brook University, State University of New York, NY
Thomas Jefferson University, PA
Université du Québec à Chicoutimi, QC
Université du Québec à Rimouski, QC
Université du Québec en Outaouais, QC
University at Buffalo, The State University of New York, NY
University of Alberta, AB
University of Calgary, AB
University of California, San Francisco, CA
University of Central Florida, FL
University of Colorado at Colorado Springs, CO
University of Connecticut, CT
University of Kentucky, KY
University of Massachusetts Boston, MA
University of Medicine and Dentistry of New Jersey, NJ
University of Missouri–Columbia, MO
University of Nebraska Medical Center, NE
University of New Brunswick Fredericton, NB
University of North Florida, FL
University of Puerto Rico, Medical Sciences Campus, PR
The University of Tennessee Health Science Center, TN
The University of Texas Health Science Center at San Antonio, TX
University of Toronto, ON
University of Washington, WA
Widener University, PA
Yale University, CT

Family Health

California State University, Sacramento, CA
Capital University, OH
Case Western Reserve University, OH
Dalhousie University, NS
Florida International University, FL
Florida State University, FL
Graceland University, IA
Grand Valley State University, MI
The Johns Hopkins University, MD
McGill University, QC
Mercy College, NY
Minnesota State University Mankato, MN
Olivet Nazarene University, IL
Pittsburg State University, KS
Point Loma Nazarene University, CA
Saint Joseph College, CT
Seattle Pacific University, WA

Southeastern Louisiana University, LA
Southern University and Agricultural and Mechanical College, LA
State University of New York at Binghamton, NY
State University of New York at New Paltz, NY
Stony Brook University, State University of New York, NY
Université de Moncton, NB
Université de Sherbrooke, QC
Université du Québec à Chicoutimi, QC
University of Alberta, AB
University of Calgary, AB
University of Central Arkansas, AR
University of Illinois at Chicago, IL
University of Miami, FL
University of Nebraska Medical Center, NE
University of New Brunswick Fredericton, NB
University of North Dakota, ND
University of San Francisco, CA
University of South Alabama, AL
University of Wisconsin–Eau Claire, WI
Ursuline College, OH
Valdosta State University, GA
Webster University, MO

Gerontology

Boston College, MA
California State University, Dominguez Hills, CA
California State University, Sacramento, CA
Case Western Reserve University, OH
Clemson University, SC
College of Mount Saint Vincent, NY
The College of St. Scholastica, MN
Creighton University, NE
Dominican University of California, CA
Duke University, NC
Emory University, GA
Florida Atlantic University, FL
Gonzaga University, WA
Grand Valley State University, MI
Gwynedd-Mercy College, PA
The Johns Hopkins University, MD
Kent State University, OH
La Roche College, PA
Lehman College of the City University of New York, NY
Marquette University, WI
Maryville University of Saint Louis, MO
McGill University, QC
Medical University of South Carolina, SC
Neumann College, PA
New York University, NY
Oregon Health & Science University, OR
The Pennsylvania State University University Park Campus, PA
Pittsburg State University, KS
Point Loma Nazarene University, CA
Radford University, VA
Rush University, IL
Saint Louis University, MO
San Diego State University, CA
San Jose State University, CA
Seattle Pacific University, WA
State University of New York at Binghamton, NY
State University of New York at New Paltz, NY
Université de Sherbrooke, QC
Université du Québec à Chicoutimi, QC
Université du Québec à Rimouski, QC
University at Buffalo, The State University of New York, NY
The University of Akron, OH
University of Alberta, AB
University of Calgary, AB
University of California, Los Angeles, CA
University of California, San Francisco, CA
University of Illinois at Chicago, IL
The University of Iowa, IA
University of Kansas, KS
University of Kentucky, KY
University of Manitoba, MB
University of Massachusetts Amherst, MA
University of Michigan, MI
University of Minnesota, Twin Cities Campus, MN
University of Missouri–Columbia, MO
University of Nebraska Medical Center, NE
University of Nevada, Reno, NV
University of New Brunswick Fredericton, NB
University of New Mexico, NM
University of North Dakota, ND
University of North Florida, FL
University of Oklahoma Health Sciences Center, OK
University of Puerto Rico, Medical Sciences Campus, PR
University of Rhode Island, RI
University of St. Francis, IL
University of South Alabama, AL
University of South Florida, FL
The University of Tennessee, TN
The University of Texas Health Science Center at Houston, TX
University of Washington, WA
University of Wisconsin–Madison, WI
Vanderbilt University, TN
Washburn University, KS
Wilkes University, PA

Home Health Care

California State University, San Bernardino, CA
Carlow University, PA
The Johns Hopkins University, MD
McGill University, QC
New York University, NY
Salisbury University, MD
Seattle Pacific University, WA
Thomas Jefferson University, PA
Université de Moncton, NB
Université du Québec à Chicoutimi, QC
University of Michigan, MI
University of Missouri–Columbia, MO
University of North Dakota, ND
University of Washington, WA

Maternity-Newborn

Case Western Reserve University, OH
Clemson University, SC
College Misericordia, PA
Dalhousie University, NS
Duke University, NC
The Johns Hopkins University, MD
Kent State University, OH
McGill University, QC
Northwestern State University of Louisiana, LA
Seattle Pacific University, WA
State University of New York Downstate Medical Center, NY
Temple University, PA
Troy University, AL
Université du Québec à Chicoutimi, QC
University of Alberta, AB
University of Calgary, AB
University of Illinois at Chicago, IL
University of Nebraska Medical Center, NE
University of New Brunswick Fredericton, NB
The University of North Carolina at Chapel Hill, NC
University of North Florida, FL
University of Puerto Rico, Medical Sciences Campus, PR
University of South Alabama, AL
The University of Tennessee, TN
University of Washington, WA
Vanderbilt University, TN

Medical-Surgical

Angelo State University, TX
Azusa Pacific University, CA
California State University, Sacramento, CA
Case Western Reserve University, OH
Colorado State University-Pueblo, CO
DePaul University, IL
Emory University, GA
Gannon University, PA
Gonzaga University, WA
Hunter College of the City University of New York, NY
The Johns Hopkins University, MD
Long Island University, C.W. Post Campus, NY
Malone College, OH
McGill University, QC
Montana State University–Bozeman, MT
Murray State University, KY
New Mexico State University, NM
Oregon Health & Science University, OR
Pacific Lutheran University, WA
Point Loma Nazarene University, CA
Rush University, IL
Saint Francis Medical Center College of Nursing, IL
Seattle Pacific University, WA
Southern Illinois University Edwardsville, IL
Texas Christian University, TX
Thomas Jefferson University, PA
Université du Québec à Chicoutimi, QC
University at Buffalo, The State University of New York, NY
University of Alberta, AB
University of Arkansas, AR
University of Calgary, AB
University of Central Arkansas, AR
University of Colorado at Colorado Springs, CO
University of Illinois at Chicago, IL
University of Kentucky, KY
University of Michigan, MI
University of Missouri–Columbia, MO
University of Nebraska Medical Center, NE
University of Nevada, Reno, NV
University of New Brunswick Fredericton, NB
University of North Florida, FL
University of Pittsburgh, PA
University of St. Francis, IL
University of Southern Indiana, IN
University of Southern Maine, ME
The University of Texas at Austin, TX
The University of Texas Health Science Center at San Antonio, TX
University of Washington, WA
University of Wisconsin–Madison, WI

Occupational Health

Capital University, OH
Seattle Pacific University, WA
Université de Moncton, NB
Université du Québec à Chicoutimi, QC
University of Alberta, AB
University of California, San Francisco, CA
University of Cincinnati, OH
University of Illinois at Chicago, IL
The University of Iowa, IA
University of Michigan, MI
University of Washington, WA

Oncology

Case Western Reserve University, OH
Duke University, NC
East Carolina University, NC
Emory University, GA
Gwynedd-Mercy College, PA
The Johns Hopkins University, MD
Loyola University Chicago, IL
McGill University, QC
The Ohio State University, OH
Seattle Pacific University, WA
Thomas Jefferson University, PA
Université du Québec à Chicoutimi, QC
University of Alberta, AB
University of California, Los Angeles, CA
University of California, San Francisco, CA
University of Kentucky, KY
University of Louisville, KY
University of Medicine and Dentistry of New Jersey, NJ
University of Missouri–Columbia, MO
University of Nebraska Medical Center, NE
University of Nevada, Reno, NV
University of New Brunswick Fredericton, NB
University of Pennsylvania, PA
University of South Florida, FL
The University of Texas Health Science Center at Houston, TX

University of Utah, UT
University of Washington, WA
Yale University, CT

Parent-Child

Azusa Pacific University, CA
California State University, Dominguez Hills, CA
California State University, Sacramento, CA
College Misericordia, PA
Dalhousie University, NS
Hunter College of the City University of New York, NY
The Johns Hopkins University, MD
Kent State University, OH
Lehman College of the City University of New York, NY
Loma Linda University, CA
Long Island University, C.W. Post Campus, NY
Louisiana State University Health Sciences Center, LA
McGill University, QC
Medical College of Georgia, GA
Medical University of South Carolina, SC
The Ohio State University, OH
Old Dominion University, VA
Rush University, IL
Seattle Pacific University, WA
Stony Brook University, State University of New York, NY
Université du Québec à Chicoutimi, QC
University of Alberta, AB
University of Calgary, AB
University of Kentucky, KY
University of Nebraska Medical Center, NE
University of Nevada, Reno, NV
University of New Brunswick Fredericton, NB
University of Oklahoma Health Sciences Center, OK
University of Wisconsin-Milwaukee, WI
Valparaiso University, IN

Pediatric

Arizona State University, AZ
Azusa Pacific University, CA
California State University, Fresno, CA
Case Western Reserve University, OH
The Catholic University of America, DC
Clemson University, SC
Dalhousie University, NS
Duke University, NC
Emory University, GA
Florida International University, FL
Georgia State University, GA
Grand Valley State University, MI
Gwynedd-Mercy College, PA
Indiana University-Purdue University Indianapolis, IN
The Johns Hopkins University, MD
Kent State University, OH
Loma Linda University, CA
Marquette University, WI
McGill University, QC
Medical College of Ohio, OH
New York University, NY
Rush University, IL
Saint Louis University, MO
Seattle Pacific University, WA
Stony Brook University, State University of New York, NY
Texas A&M University-Corpus Christi, TX
Texas Woman's University, TX
Thomas Jefferson University, PA
Troy University, AL
Université de Moncton, NB
Université du Québec à Chicoutimi, QC
The University of Akron, OH
University of Alberta, AB
University of Arkansas for Medical Sciences, AR
University of Calgary, AB
University of California, Los Angeles, CA
University of Delaware, DE
University of Illinois at Chicago, IL
The University of Iowa, IA
University of Kentucky, KY
University of Minnesota, Twin Cities Campus, MN
University of Missouri-Columbia, MO
University of Missouri-Kansas City, MO
University of Missouri-St. Louis, MO
University of Nebraska Medical Center, NE
University of New Brunswick Fredericton, NB
University of New Mexico, NM
The University of North Carolina at Chapel Hill, NC
University of North Florida, FL
University of Puerto Rico, Medical Sciences Campus, PR
University of South Alabama, AL
The University of Tennessee, TN
University of Washington, WA
University of Wisconsin-Madison, WI
Vanderbilt University, TN
Wichita State University, KS
Wright State University, OH

Perinatal

California State University, Sacramento, CA
Georgia State University, GA
The Johns Hopkins University, MD
McGill University, QC
McMaster University, ON
The Ohio State University, OH
Saint Louis University, MO
San Francisco State University, CA
Seattle Pacific University, WA
Stony Brook University, State University of New York, NY
Université du Québec à Chicoutimi, QC
University of Alberta, AB
University of Calgary, AB
University of California, San Francisco, CA
University of Illinois at Chicago, IL
University of Kentucky, KY
University of Manitoba, MB
University of Nebraska Medical Center, NE
University of Pennsylvania, PA
The University of Tennessee, TN
University of Washington, WA
University of Wisconsin-Madison, WI

Psychiatric/Mental Health

Arizona State University, AZ
Boston College, MA
California State University, Fresno, CA
California State University, Los Angeles, CA
California State University, Sacramento, CA
Case Western Reserve University, OH
The Catholic University of America, DC
Colorado State University-Pueblo, CO
Creighton University, NE
Dalhousie University, NS
Duquesne University, PA
Florida International University, FL
Georgia State University, GA
Gonzaga University, WA
Grand Valley State University, MI
Hampton University, VA
Hunter College of the City University of New York, NY
Husson College, ME
Immaculata University, PA
Indiana University-Purdue University Fort Wayne, IN
Indiana University-Purdue University Indianapolis, IN
Kent State University, OH
Louisiana State University Health Sciences Center, LA
McGill University, QC
Medical College of Georgia, GA
Medical College of Ohio, OH
Medical University of South Carolina, SC
MGH Institute of Health Professions, MA
New Mexico State University, NM
New York University, NY
Northeastern University, MA
Northwestern State University of Louisiana, LA
The Ohio State University, OH
Oregon Health & Science University, OR
Point Loma Nazarene University, CA
Rivier College, NH
Rush University, IL
Rutgers, The State University of New Jersey, College of Nursing, NJ
The Sage Colleges, NY
Saint Joseph College, CT
Saint Louis University, MO
Saint Xavier University, IL
Seattle Pacific University, WA
Southern Illinois University Edwardsville, IL
Stony Brook University, State University of New York, NY
Temple University, PA
Université de Moncton, NB
Université du Québec à Chicoutimi, QC
Université du Québec à Rimouski, QC
Université du Québec en Outaouais, QC
The University of Akron, OH
University of Alaska Anchorage, AK
University of Alberta, AB
University of Calgary, AB
University of California, San Francisco, CA
University of Central Arkansas, AR
University of Colorado at Denver and Health Sciences Center—Health Sciences Program, CO
University of Delaware, DE
University of Florida, FL
University of Hawaii at Manoa, HI
University of Illinois at Chicago, IL
The University of Iowa, IA
University of Kentucky, KY
University of Louisville, KY
University of Maryland, MD
University of Massachusetts Amherst, MA
University of Massachusetts Lowell, MA
University of Medicine and Dentistry of New Jersey, NJ
University of Miami, FL
University of Michigan, MI
University of Minnesota, Twin Cities Campus, MN
University of Nebraska Medical Center, NE
University of Nevada, Reno, NV
University of New Brunswick Fredericton, NB
University of New Mexico, NM
The University of North Carolina at Chapel Hill, NC
The University of North Carolina at Charlotte, NC
University of North Dakota, ND
University of North Florida, FL
University of Oklahoma Health Sciences Center, OK
University of Pennsylvania, PA
University of Pittsburgh, PA
University of Puerto Rico, Medical Sciences Campus, PR
University of Rhode Island, RI
University of San Francisco, CA
University of Saskatchewan, SK
University of South Alabama, AL
University of South Carolina, SC
University of Southern Maine, ME
University of Southern Mississippi, MS
University of South Florida, FL
The University of Tennessee, TN
The University of Tennessee Health Science Center, TN
The University of Texas Health Science Center at Houston, TX
The University of Texas Health Science Center at San Antonio, TX
University of Toronto, ON
University of Virginia, VA
University of Washington, WA
University of Wisconsin-Madison, WI
University of Wisconsin-Milwaukee, WI
Valdosta State University, GA
Virginia Commonwealth University, VA
Wayne State University, MI
Widener University, PA

Wilkes University, PA

Public Health

Augustana College, SD
Bloomsburg University of Pennsylvania, PA
California State University, Fresno, CA
Dalhousie University, NS
Drexel University, PA
Emory University, GA
The Johns Hopkins University, MD
La Salle University, PA
McGill University, QC
Northern Arizona University, AZ
The Ohio State University, OH
Oregon Health & Science University, OR
Rush University, IL
San Francisco State University, CA
Seattle Pacific University, WA
Thomas Jefferson University, PA
Université de Moncton, NB
Université du Québec à Chicoutimi, QC
University of Alberta, AB
University of Calgary, AB
University of Colorado at Denver and Health Sciences Center—Health Sciences Program, CO
University of Illinois at Chicago, IL
University of Kentucky, KY
University of Massachusetts Amherst, MA
University of Missouri–Columbia, MO
University of Nebraska Medical Center, NE
University of New Brunswick Fredericton, NB
University of Pennsylvania, PA
University of South Carolina, SC
The University of Texas at Austin, TX
The University of Texas at Brownsville, TX
University of Vermont, VT
University of Virginia, VA
Wright State University, OH

Rehabilitation

The Johns Hopkins University, MD
McGill University, QC
Salem State College, MA
Seattle Pacific University, WA
Université du Québec à Chicoutimi, QC
Université du Québec en Outaouais, QC
University of Calgary, AB
University of Missouri–Columbia, MO

School Health

Bloomsburg University of Pennsylvania, PA
California State University, Sacramento, CA
California State University, San Bernardino, CA
Capital University, OH
Colorado State University-Pueblo, CO
Intercollegiate College of Nursing/Washington State University, WA
The Johns Hopkins University, MD
Kean University, NJ
Loma Linda University, CA
San Diego State University, CA
San Jose State University, CA
Seattle Pacific University, WA
Université de Moncton, NB
Université du Québec à Chicoutimi, QC
University of Illinois at Chicago, IL
University of Massachusetts Amherst, MA
University of Missouri–Columbia, MO
University of Nevada, Reno, NV
University of New Brunswick Fredericton, NB
Wright State University, OH

Women's Health

Case Western Reserve University, OH
Colorado State University-Pueblo, CO
Drexel University, PA
Grand Valley State University, MI
The Johns Hopkins University, MD
Kent State University, OH
McGill University, QC
The Ohio State University, OH
Oregon Health & Science University, OR
Seattle Pacific University, WA
Stony Brook University, State University of New York, NY
Texas Woman's University, TX
Université du Québec à Chicoutimi, QC
University of Alberta, AB
University of Calgary, AB
University of Illinois at Chicago, IL
University of Kentucky, KY
University of Miami, FL
University of Missouri–Columbia, MO
University of Missouri–St. Louis, MO
University of Nebraska Medical Center, NE
University of New Brunswick Fredericton, NB
University of New Mexico, NM
The University of North Carolina at Chapel Hill, NC
University of North Florida, FL
University of South Alabama, AL
The University of Tennessee, TN
The University of Texas Health Science Center at Houston, TX
University of Toronto, ON
University of Washington, WA
University of Wisconsin–Madison, WI
University of Wisconsin–Milwaukee, WI
Valparaiso University, IN
Vanderbilt University, TN

Health-Care Administration

Athabasca University, AB
California State University, Long Beach, CA
Cleveland State University, OH
Colorado State University-Pueblo, CO
Daemen College, NY
Drexel University, PA
Duke University, NC
Emory University, GA
Excelsior College, NY
Georgetown University, DC
Gonzaga University, WA
Graceland University, IA
Grand Canyon University, AZ
Holy Family University, PA
Kean University, NJ
Kent State University, OH
Lamar University, TX
Lewis University, IL
Louisiana State University Health Sciences Center, LA
Loyola University New Orleans, LA
Mercy College, NY
Midwestern State University, TX
North Park University, IL
Old Dominion University, VA
Olivet Nazarene University, IL
Oregon Health & Science University, OR
Pacific Lutheran University, WA
Quinnipiac University, CT
Regis College, MA
Regis University, CO
Rivier College, NH
Salisbury University, MD
Seton Hall University, NJ
Simmons College, MA
Southern Illinois University Edwardsville, IL
Southern University and Agricultural and Mechanical College, LA
Towson University, MD
Université de Moncton, NB
The University of Alabama at Birmingham, AL
University of Alaska Anchorage, AK
University of Colorado at Colorado Springs, CO
University of Colorado at Denver and Health Sciences Center—Health Sciences Program, CO
University of Delaware, DE
University of Hawaii at Manoa, HI
University of Illinois at Chicago, IL
University of Kansas, KS
University of Maine, ME
University of Maryland, MD
University of Michigan, MI
University of Mississippi Medical Center, MS
University of Nebraska Medical Center, NE
The University of North Carolina at Charlotte, NC
University of Oklahoma Health Sciences Center, OK
University of Pennsylvania, PA
University of Phoenix–Colorado Campus, CO
University of Phoenix–Fort Lauderdale Campus, FL
University of Phoenix–Hawaii Campus, HI
University of Phoenix–Jacksonville Campus, FL
University of Phoenix–Louisiana Campus, LA
University of Phoenix–Metro Detroit Campus, MI
University of Phoenix–New Mexico Campus, NM
University of Phoenix–Northern California Campus, CA
University of Phoenix–Oklahoma City Campus, OK
University of Phoenix Online Campus, AZ
University of Phoenix–Orlando Campus, FL
University of Phoenix–Phoenix Campus, AZ
University of Phoenix–Sacramento Campus, CA
University of Phoenix–San Diego Campus, CA
University of Phoenix–Southern Arizona Campus, AZ
University of Phoenix–Southern California Campus, CA
University of Phoenix–Southern Colorado Campus, CO
University of Phoenix–Tampa Campus, FL
University of Phoenix–Tulsa Campus, OK
University of Phoenix–Utah Campus, UT
University of Phoenix–West Michigan Campus, MI
University of Portland, OR
University of Rochester, NY
University of San Diego, CA
University of San Francisco, CA
The University of Texas at Arlington, TX
University of Virginia, VA
The University of Western Ontario, ON
University of Wisconsin–Milwaukee, WI
Vanderbilt University, TN
Villanova University, PA
Viterbo University, WI
Wright State University, OH

Nursing Administration

Abilene Intercollegiate School of Nursing, TX
Adelphi University, NY
Albany State University, GA
Allen College, IA
American International College, MA
Anderson University, IN
Armstrong Atlantic State University, GA
Azusa Pacific University, CA
Ball State University, IN
Barry University, FL
Baylor University, TX
Bellarmine University, KY
Bellin College of Nursing, WI
Bethel University, MN
Bloomsburg University of Pennsylvania, PA
Bowie State University, MD
Bradley University, IL
California State University, Bakersfield, CA
California State University, Dominguez Hills, CA
California State University, Fullerton, CA
California State University, Los Angeles, CA
California State University, Sacramento, CA
Capital University, OH
Carlow University, PA
Case Western Reserve University, OH
The Catholic University of America, DC
Clarke College, IA
Clarkson College, NE
Clemson University, SC
College Misericordia, PA
College of Mount Saint Vincent, NY
The College of New Rochelle, NY
The College of St. Scholastica, MN
Delta State University, MS
DePaul University, IL

CONCENTRATIONS WITHIN MASTER'S DEGREE PROGRAMS

Nursing Administration

DeSales University, PA
Drexel University, PA
Duke University, NC
Duquesne University, PA
East Carolina University, NC
East Tennessee State University, TN
Edgewood College, WI
Emory University, GA
Fairleigh Dickinson University, Metropolitan Campus, NJ
Florida Atlantic University, FL
Florida International University, FL
Fort Hays State University, KS
Gannon University, PA
Gardner-Webb University, NC
George Mason University, VA
Georgia College & State University, GA
Gonzaga University, WA
Grand Valley State University, MI
Hampton University, VA
Holy Names University, CA
Idaho State University, ID
Illinois State University, IL
Immaculata University, PA
Indiana University of Pennsylvania, PA
Indiana University–Purdue University Fort Wayne, IN
Indiana University–Purdue University Indianapolis, IN
Intercollegiate College of Nursing/Washington State University, WA
Jacksonville University, FL
Jefferson College of Health Sciences, VA
The Johns Hopkins University, MD
Kean University, NJ
Kent State University, OH
La Roche College, PA
La Salle University, PA
Lehman College of the City University of New York, NY
Lewis University, IL
Loma Linda University, CA
Long Island University, Brooklyn Campus, NY
Louisiana State University Health Sciences Center, LA
Loyola University Chicago, IL
Madonna University, MI
Marquette University, WI
Marshall University, WV
Marywood University, PA
McNeese State University, LA
Medical University of South Carolina, SC
Metropolitan State University, MN
Midwestern State University, TX
Molloy College, NY
Monmouth University, NJ
Mountain State University, WV
Nebraska Wesleyan University, NE
New Mexico State University, NM
New York University, NY
Northeastern University, MA
Northern Kentucky University, KY
Northwestern State University of Louisiana, LA
The Ohio State University, OH
Ohio University, OH
Old Dominion University, VA
Oregon Health & Science University, OR
Otterbein College, OH
Pace University, NY
Pacific Lutheran University, WA
Queens University of Charlotte, NC
Regis College, MA
Regis University, CO
Research College of Nursing, MO
Sacred Heart University, CT
Saginaw Valley State University, MI
Saint Joseph's College of Maine, ME
Saint Xavier University, IL
Salem State College, MA
Salisbury University, MD
Samford University, AL
San Francisco State University, CA
San Jose State University, CA
Seattle Pacific University, WA
Seton Hall University, NJ
Sonoma State University, CA
South Dakota State University, SD
Southeastern Louisiana University, LA
Southern Connecticut State University, CT
Spalding University, KY
State University of New York at Binghamton, NY
State University of New York Institute of Technology, NY
Texas A&M University–Corpus Christi, TX
Texas Tech University Health Sciences Center, TX
Texas Woman's University, TX
Troy University, AL
Union University, TN
Université de Moncton, NB
The University of Akron, OH
The University of Alabama at Birmingham, AL
The University of Alabama in Huntsville, AL
University of Arkansas for Medical Sciences, AR
University of California, Los Angeles, CA
University of California, San Francisco, CA
University of Central Florida, FL
University of Cincinnati, OH
University of Colorado at Colorado Springs, CO
University of Colorado at Denver and Health Sciences Center—Health Sciences Program, CO
University of Connecticut, CT
University of Detroit Mercy, MI
University of Hartford, CT
University of Illinois at Chicago, IL
University of Indianapolis, IN
The University of Iowa, IA
University of Kansas, KS
University of Manitoba, MB
University of Maryland, MD
The University of Memphis, TN
University of Michigan, MI
University of Minnesota, Twin Cities Campus, MN
University of Mississippi Medical Center, MS
University of Missouri–Columbia, MO
University of Missouri–Kansas City, MO
University of Missouri–St. Louis, MO
University of Mobile, AL
University of Nebraska Medical Center, NE
University of New Brunswick Fredericton, NB
University of New Mexico, NM
The University of North Carolina at Chapel Hill, NC
The University of North Carolina at Greensboro, NC
University of North Dakota, ND
University of Pennsylvania, PA
University of Phoenix–Colorado Campus, CO
University of Phoenix–Fort Lauderdale Campus, FL
University of Phoenix–Hawaii Campus, HI
University of Phoenix–Jacksonville Campus, FL
University of Phoenix–Louisiana Campus, LA
University of Phoenix–Metro Detroit Campus, MI
University of Phoenix–New Mexico Campus, NM
University of Phoenix–Northern California Campus, CA
University of Phoenix–Oklahoma City Campus, OK
University of Phoenix Online Campus, AZ
University of Phoenix–Orlando Campus, FL
University of Phoenix–Phoenix Campus, AZ
University of Phoenix–Sacramento Campus, CA
University of Phoenix–San Diego Campus, CA
University of Phoenix–Southern California Campus, CA
University of Phoenix–Southern Colorado Campus, CO
University of Phoenix–Tampa Campus, FL
University of Phoenix–Tulsa Campus, OK
University of Phoenix–Utah Campus, UT
University of Phoenix–West Michigan Campus, MI
University of Pittsburgh, PA
University of Puerto Rico, Medical Sciences Campus, PR
University of Rhode Island, RI
University of Saint Francis, IN
University of South Alabama, AL
University of South Carolina, SC
University of Southern Indiana, IN
University of Southern Mississippi, MS
The University of Tennessee, TN
The University of Tennessee Health Science Center, TN
The University of Texas at Arlington, TX
The University of Texas at Austin, TX
The University of Texas at El Paso, TX
The University of Texas at Tyler, TX
The University of Texas Health Science Center at Houston, TX
The University of Texas Health Science Center at San Antonio, TX
University of Toronto, ON
University of Utah, UT
University of Virginia, VA
University of Washington, WA
The University of Western Ontario, ON
University of West Georgia, GA
University of Wisconsin–Eau Claire, WI
Valdosta State University, GA
Vanderbilt University, TN
Virginia Commonwealth University, VA
Washburn University, KS
Waynesburg College, PA
Western Kentucky University, KY
West Texas A&M University, TX
Wheeling Jesuit University, WV
Wichita State University, KS
Wilkes University, PA
William Paterson University of New Jersey, NJ
Wilmington College, DE
Winona State University, MN
Wright State University, OH
Xavier University, OH
York College of Pennsylvania, PA

Nurse Anesthesia

Arkansas State University, AR
Boston College, MA
Bradley University, IL
California State University, Fullerton, CA
Case Western Reserve University, OH
Columbia University, NY
DePaul University, IL
Drexel University, PA
Duke University, NC
East Carolina University, NC
Florida Gulf Coast University, FL
Florida International University, FL
Gannon University, PA
Georgetown University, DC
Jewish Hospital College of Nursing and Allied Health, MO
La Salle University, PA
Louisiana State University Health Sciences Center, LA
Medical College of Georgia, GA
Murray State University, KY
Newman University, KS
Northeastern University, MA
Oakland University, MI
Old Dominion University, VA
Rush University, IL
Samford University, AL
Samuel Merritt College, CA
Southern Illinois University Edwardsville, IL
State University of New York Downstate Medical Center, NY
University at Buffalo, The State University of New York, NY
The University of Akron, OH
University of Cincinnati, OH
The University of Iowa, IA
University of Maryland, MD
University of Medicine and Dentistry of New Jersey, NJ
University of Miami, FL

University of Minnesota, Twin Cities Campus, MN
The University of North Carolina at Charlotte, NC
The University of North Carolina at Greensboro, NC
University of North Dakota, ND
University of Pennsylvania, PA
University of Pittsburgh, PA
University of Puerto Rico, Medical Sciences Campus, PR
The University of Scranton, PA
The University of Tennessee, TN
The University of Tennessee at Chattanooga, TN
The University of Tennessee Health Science Center, TN
The University of Texas Health Science Center at Houston, TX
Villanova University, PA
York College of Pennsylvania, PA
Youngstown State University, OH

Nursing Education

Abilene Intercollegiate School of Nursing, TX
Albany State University, GA
Alcorn State University, MS
Allen College, IA
American International College, MA
Andrews University, MI
Angelo State University, TX
Arkansas State University, AR
Azusa Pacific University, CA
Ball State University, IN
Barry University, FL
Bellarmine University, KY
Bellin College of Nursing, WI
Bethel College, IN
Bethel University, MN
Bowie State University, MD
Briar Cliff University, IA
California State University, Chico, CA
California State University, Dominguez Hills, CA
California State University, Long Beach, CA
California State University, Los Angeles, CA
California State University, Sacramento, CA
California State University, San Bernardino, CA
Capital University, OH
Cardinal Stritch University, WI
Carson-Newman College, TN
The Catholic University of America, DC
Central Missouri State University, MO
Clarion University of Pennsylvania, PA
Clarke College, IA
Clarkson College, NE
Clemson University, SC
College Misericordia, PA
College of St. Catherine, MN
Colorado State University-Pueblo, CO
Concordia College, MN
Concordia University Wisconsin, WI
Creighton University, NE
Delta State University, MS
DePaul University, IL
DeSales University, PA
Drexel University, PA
Duke University, NC
Duquesne University, PA
D'Youville College, NY
East Carolina University, NC
East Tennessee State University, TN
Edgewood College, WI
Edinboro University of Pennsylvania, PA
Fairleigh Dickinson University, Metropolitan Campus, NJ
Florida Atlantic University, FL
Florida Gulf Coast University, FL
Florida State University, FL
Fort Hays State University, KS
Franciscan University of Steubenville, OH
Gannon University, PA
Gardner-Webb University, NC
Georgia Baptist College of Nursing of Mercer University, GA
Georgia College & State University, GA
Gonzaga University, WA
Graceland University, IA
Grambling State University, LA
Grand Valley State University, MI
Hampton University, VA
Holy Family University, PA
Idaho State University, ID
Immaculata University, PA
Intercollegiate College of Nursing/Washington State University, WA
Jacksonville University, FL
James Madison University, VA
Jefferson College of Health Sciences, VA
Jewish Hospital College of Nursing and Allied Health, MO
Lamar University, TX
Lehman College of the City University of New York, NY
Lewis University, IL
Louisiana State University Health Sciences Center, LA
Mansfield University of Pennsylvania, PA
Marian College of Fond du Lac, WI
Marshall University, WV
Marymount University, VA
McNeese State University, LA
Medical College of Ohio, OH
Medical University of South Carolina, SC
Mercy College, NY
Michigan State University, MI
Midwestern State University, TX
Minnesota State University Moorhead, MN
Molloy College, NY
Monmouth University, NJ
Mountain State University, WV
Nebraska Methodist College, NE
Nebraska Wesleyan University, NE
Neumann College, PA
New York University, NY
North Dakota State University, ND
Northern Arizona University, AZ
Northern Kentucky University, KY
Northwestern State University of Louisiana, LA
Oakland University, MI
Ohio University, OH
Old Dominion University, VA
Olivet Nazarene University, IL
Otterbein College, OH
Pace University, NY
Pacific Lutheran University, WA
Point Loma Nazarene University, CA
Regis University, CO
Research College of Nursing, MO
Rivier College, NH
Saginaw Valley State University, MI
Saint Francis Medical Center College of Nursing, IL
Saint Joseph's College of Maine, ME
Saint Louis University, MO
Salem State College, MA
Samford University, AL
San Jose State University, CA
Seattle Pacific University, WA
Seton Hall University, NJ
Simmons College, MA
Slippery Rock University of Pennsylvania, PA
Sonoma State University, CA
South Dakota State University, SD
Southeastern Louisiana University, LA
Southeast Missouri State University, MO
Southern Adventist University, TN
Southern Connecticut State University, CT
Southern Illinois University Edwardsville, IL
Southern Nazarene University, OK
Southern University and Agricultural and Mechanical College, LA
Southwest Missouri State University, MO
Spalding University, KY
State University of New York at Binghamton, NY
Tennessee Technological University, TN
Texas Tech University Health Sciences Center, TX
Towson University, MD
Troy University, AL
Union University, TN
Université de Moncton, NB
University at Buffalo, The State University of New York, NY
University of Arkansas, AR
University of Arkansas for Medical Sciences, AR
University of California, San Francisco, CA
University of Central Florida, FL
University of Hartford, CT
University of Indianapolis, IN
The University of Iowa, IA
University of Kansas, KS
University of Louisiana at Lafayette, LA
University of Maine, ME
University of Mary, ND
University of Massachusetts Worcester, MA
University of Medicine and Dentistry of New Jersey, NJ
The University of Memphis, TN
University of Minnesota, Twin Cities Campus, MN
University of Mississippi Medical Center, MS
University of Missouri–Columbia, MO
University of Missouri–Kansas City, MO
University of Missouri–St. Louis, MO
University of Mobile, AL
University of Nebraska Medical Center, NE
University of Nevada, Las Vegas, NV
University of Nevada, Reno, NV
University of New Brunswick Fredericton, NB
University of New Mexico, NM
The University of North Carolina at Chapel Hill, NC
The University of North Carolina at Greensboro, NC
The University of North Carolina at Wilmington, NC
University of North Dakota, ND
University of Northern Colorado, CO
University of Oklahoma Health Sciences Center, OK
University of Phoenix–Colorado Campus, CO
University of Phoenix–Fort Lauderdale Campus, FL
University of Phoenix–Hawaii Campus, HI
University of Phoenix–Jacksonville Campus, FL
University of Phoenix–Louisiana Campus, LA
University of Phoenix–Metro Detroit Campus, MI
University of Phoenix–New Mexico Campus, NM
University of Phoenix–Northern California Campus, CA
University of Phoenix–Oklahoma City Campus, OK
University of Phoenix Online Campus, AZ
University of Phoenix–Orlando Campus, FL
University of Phoenix–Phoenix Campus, AZ
University of Phoenix–Sacramento Campus, CA
University of Phoenix–San Diego Campus, CA
University of Phoenix–Southern Arizona Campus, AZ
University of Phoenix–Southern California Campus, CA
University of Phoenix–Southern Colorado Campus, CO
University of Phoenix–Tampa Campus, FL
University of Phoenix–Tulsa Campus, OK
University of Phoenix–Utah Campus, UT
University of Phoenix–West Michigan Campus, MI
University of Pittsburgh, PA
University of Portland, OR
University of Puerto Rico, Medical Sciences Campus, PR
University of Rhode Island, RI
University of St. Francis, IL
University of Saint Francis, IN
University of South Alabama, AL
University of South Carolina, SC
University of Southern Indiana, IN
University of South Florida, FL
The University of Tampa, FL
The University of Texas at El Paso, TX
The University of Texas at Tyler, TX

CONCENTRATIONS WITHIN MASTER'S DEGREE PROGRAMS

Nursing Education

The University of Texas Health Science Center at Houston, TX
The University of Texas Health Science Center at San Antonio, TX
University of Utah, UT
University of Washington, WA
The University of Western Ontario, ON
University of West Georgia, GA
University of Wisconsin–Eau Claire, WI
University of Wisconsin–Madison, WI
University of Wisconsin–Milwaukee, WI
University of Wyoming, WY
Valdosta State University, GA
Villanova University, PA
Viterbo University, WI
Wagner College, NY
Waynesburg College, PA
Webster University, MO
Western Carolina University, NC
Western Kentucky University, KY
Westminster College, UT
West Texas A&M University, TX
Wheeling Jesuit University, WV
Widener University, PA
William Carey College, MS
William Paterson University of New Jersey, NJ
Wilmington College, DE
Winona State University, MN
Xavier University, OH
York College of Pennsylvania, PA
Youngstown State University, OH

Nursing Informatics

Case Western Reserve University, OH
Duke University, NC
Excelsior College, NY
Fairleigh Dickinson University, Metropolitan Campus, NJ
Georgia College & State University, GA
New York University, NY
Pace University, NY
Pacific Lutheran University, WA
Saginaw Valley State University, MI
Thomas Jefferson University, PA
Troy University, AL
University at Buffalo, The State University of New York, NY
The University of Arizona, AZ
University of California, San Francisco, CA
University of Colorado at Denver and Health Sciences Center—Health Sciences Program, CO
University of Illinois at Chicago, IL
The University of Iowa, IA
University of Kansas, KS
University of Maryland, MD
University of Medicine and Dentistry of New Jersey, NJ
University of Michigan, MI
University of Nebraska Medical Center, NE
University of New Brunswick Fredericton, NB
The University of North Carolina at Chapel Hill, NC
University of Pennsylvania, PA
University of Pittsburgh, PA
University of San Francisco, CA
University of South Florida, FL
The University of Texas Health Science Center at San Antonio, TX
University of Utah, UT
Vanderbilt University, TN

Nurse Practitioner Programs

Acute Care

Arizona State University, AZ
Barry University, FL
California State University, Los Angeles, CA
Case Western Reserve University, OH
The College of New Rochelle, NY
Colorado State University-Pueblo, CO
Columbia University, NY
Dalhousie University, NS
Drexel University, PA
Duke University, NC
Emory University, GA
Georgetown University, DC
Grand Valley State University, MI
Husson College, ME
Indiana University–Purdue University Indianapolis, IN
The Johns Hopkins University, MD
Loyola University Chicago, IL
Marquette University, WI
Memorial University of Newfoundland, NL
MGH Institute of Health Professions, MA
New York University, NY
Northeastern University, MA
Northwestern State University of Louisiana, LA
Rush University, IL
Rutgers, The State University of New Jersey, College of Nursing, NJ
The Sage Colleges, NY
Saint Louis University, MO
San Diego State University, CA
Seton Hall University, NJ
Texas Tech University Health Sciences Center, TX
Thomas Jefferson University, PA
University at Buffalo, The State University of New York, NY
The University of Alabama at Birmingham, AL
The University of Alabama in Huntsville, AL
University of Arkansas for Medical Sciences, AR
University of Calgary, AB
University of California, Los Angeles, CA
University of California, San Francisco, CA
University of Cincinnati, OH
University of Connecticut, CT
University of Florida, FL
University of Illinois at Chicago, IL
University of Kentucky, KY
University of Maryland, MD
University of Massachusetts Worcester, MA
University of Medicine and Dentistry of New Jersey, NJ
University of Miami, FL
University of Michigan, MI
University of Mississippi Medical Center, MS
University of Nebraska Medical Center, NE
University of New Brunswick Fredericton, NB
University of New Mexico, NM
University of Pennsylvania, PA
University of Pittsburgh, PA
University of Rochester, NY
University of South Alabama, AL
University of South Carolina, SC
University of Southern Indiana, IN
University of South Florida, FL
The University of Tennessee Health Science Center, TN
The University of Texas at Arlington, TX
The University of Texas at Tyler, TX
The University of Texas Health Science Center at Houston, TX
The University of Texas Medical Branch, TX
University of Toronto, ON
University of Utah, UT
University of Virginia, VA
University of Washington, WA
University of Wisconsin–Madison, WI
Vanderbilt University, TN
Virginia Commonwealth University, VA
Wayne State University, MI
Wichita State University, KS
Wright State University, OH
Yale University, CT

Adult Health

Adelphi University, NY
Arizona State University, AZ
Armstrong Atlantic State University, GA
Azusa Pacific University, CA
Ball State University, IN
Bloomsburg University of Pennsylvania, PA
Boston College, MA
California State University, Long Beach, CA
California State University, Los Angeles, CA
Case Western Reserve University, OH
Clemson University, SC
College of Mount Saint Vincent, NY
College of St. Catherine, MN
The College of St. Scholastica, MN
College of Staten Island of the City University of New York, NY
Columbia University, NY
Creighton University, NE
Daemen College, NY
Dalhousie University, NS
DePaul University, IL
Duke University, NC
East Tennessee State University, TN
Emory University, GA
Fairfield University, CT
Fairleigh Dickinson University, Metropolitan Campus, NJ
Felician College, NJ
Florida Agricultural and Mechanical University, FL
Florida Atlantic University, FL
Florida International University, FL
Florida State University, FL
George Mason University, VA
Grand Valley State University, MI
Gwynedd-Mercy College, PA
Hunter College of the City University of New York, NY
Indiana University–Purdue University Indianapolis, IN
Indiana Wesleyan University, IN
Jewish Hospital College of Nursing and Allied Health, MO
The Johns Hopkins University, MD
Kennesaw State University, GA
Kent State University, OH
La Salle University, PA
Loma Linda University, CA
Long Island University, Brooklyn Campus, NY
Loyola University Chicago, IL
Loyola University New Orleans, LA
Marian College of Fond du Lac, WI
Marquette University, WI
Maryville University of Saint Louis, MO
McNeese State University, LA
Medical College of Ohio, OH
Medical University of South Carolina, SC
Mercy College, NY
Metropolitan State University, MN
MGH Institute of Health Professions, MA
Michigan State University, MI
Molloy College, NY
Monmouth University, NJ
Mount Saint Mary College, NY
New York University, NY
Northeastern University, MA
Northern Illinois University, IL
Northern Kentucky University, KY
North Park University, IL
Oakland University, MI
The Ohio State University, OH
Oregon Health & Science University, OR
Otterbein College, OH
Purdue University, IN
Quinnipiac University, CT
Regis College, MA
The Richard Stockton College of New Jersey, NJ
Rush University, IL
Rutgers, The State University of New Jersey, College of Nursing, NJ
The Sage Colleges, NY
Saint Joseph College, CT
Saint Louis University, MO
Saint Peter's College, NJ
San Diego State University, CA
Seattle Pacific University, WA
Seton Hall University, NJ
Simmons College, MA

Southeastern Louisiana University, LA
Southern Adventist University, TN
Southern Illinois University Edwardsville, IL
Spalding University, KY
State University of New York Institute of Technology, NY
State University of New York Upstate Medical University, NY
Stony Brook University, State University of New York, NY
Temple University, PA
Texas Woman's University, TX
Thomas Jefferson University, PA
Université de Moncton, NB
University at Buffalo, The State University of New York, NY
The University of Akron, OH
The University of Alabama at Birmingham, AL
The University of Arizona, AZ
University of Calgary, AB
University of California, San Francisco, CA
University of Central Arkansas, AR
University of Central Florida, FL
University of Cincinnati, OH
University of Colorado at Colorado Springs, CO
University of Colorado at Denver and Health Sciences Center—Health Sciences Program, CO
University of Connecticut, CT
University of Delaware, DE
University of Florida, FL
University of Hawaii at Manoa, HI
University of Illinois at Chicago, IL
The University of Iowa, IA
University of Kansas, KS
University of Kentucky, KY
University of Louisiana at Lafayette, LA
University of Louisville, KY
University of Maryland, MD
University of Massachusetts Boston, MA
University of Massachusetts Dartmouth, MA
University of Massachusetts Worcester, MA
University of Medicine and Dentistry of New Jersey, NJ
University of Miami, FL
University of Michigan, MI
University of Michigan–Flint, MI
University of Mississippi Medical Center, MS
University of Missouri–Kansas City, MO
University of Missouri–St. Louis, MO
University of Nebraska Medical Center, NE
University of New Brunswick Fredericton, NB
University of New Hampshire, NH
The University of North Carolina at Chapel Hill, NC
The University of North Carolina at Charlotte, NC
The University of North Carolina at Greensboro, NC
University of Pennsylvania, PA
University of Pittsburgh, PA
University of Rochester, NY
University of St. Francis, IL
University of San Diego, CA
University of San Francisco, CA
University of South Carolina, SC
University of Southern Maine, ME
University of South Florida, FL
The University of Tampa, FL
The University of Texas at Arlington, TX
The University of Texas at Tyler, TX
The University of Texas Health Science Center at Houston, TX
The University of Texas Medical Branch, TX
University of Utah, UT
University of Vermont, VT
University of Washington, WA
University of Wisconsin–Eau Claire, WI
University of Wisconsin–Madison, WI
University of Wisconsin–Oshkosh, WI
Ursuline College, OH
Vanderbilt University, TN
Villanova University, PA
Virginia Commonwealth University, VA
Viterbo University, WI
Washburn University, KS
Western Connecticut State University, CT
William Paterson University of New Jersey, NJ
Wilmington College, DE
Winona State University, MN
Yale University, CT

Community Health

Athabasca University, AB
DePaul University, IL
Eastern Kentucky University, KY
Emory University, GA
Hawai'i Pacific University, HI
Idaho State University, ID
The Sage Colleges, NY
State University of New York at Binghamton, NY
Université de Moncton, NB
Université Laval, QC
University of Massachusetts Worcester, MA
University of Miami, FL
University of Nebraska Medical Center, NE
University of New Brunswick Fredericton, NB
University of Pennsylvania, PA
University of Virginia, VA
Washburn University, KS

Family Health

Abilene Intercollegiate School of Nursing, TX
Albany State University, GA
Alcorn State University, MS
Allen College, IA
Arizona State University, AZ
Azusa Pacific University, CA
Ball State University, IN
Barry University, FL
Baylor University, TX
Belmont University, TN
Boston College, MA
Bowie State University, MD
Brenau University, GA
Briar Cliff University, IA
Brigham Young University, UT
California State University, Bakersfield, CA
California State University, Dominguez Hills, CA
California State University, Fresno, CA
California State University, Fullerton, CA
California State University, Long Beach, CA
California State University, Los Angeles, CA
California State University, Sacramento, CA
Carlow University, PA
Carson-Newman College, TN
Case Western Reserve University, OH
The Catholic University of America, DC
Central Missouri State University, MO
Clarion University of Pennsylvania, PA
Clarke College, IA
Clarkson College, NE
Clemson University, SC
College Misericordia, PA
College of Mount Saint Vincent, NY
The College of New Jersey, NJ
The College of New Rochelle, NY
The College of St. Scholastica, MN
Columbia University, NY
Concordia College, MN
Concordia University Wisconsin, WI
Coppin State University, MD
Creighton University, NE
Delta State University, MS
DePaul University, IL
DeSales University, PA
Dominican College, NY
Drexel University, PA
Duke University, NC
Duquesne University, PA
D'Youville College, NY
East Carolina University, NC
Eastern Kentucky University, KY
East Tennessee State University, TN
Edinboro University of Pennsylvania, PA
Emory University, GA
Fairfield University, CT
Felician College, NJ
Florida Atlantic University, FL
Florida Gulf Coast University, FL
Florida International University, FL
Florida State University, FL
Fort Hays State University, KS
Franciscan University of Steubenville, OH
Gannon University, PA
George Mason University, VA
Georgetown University, DC
Georgia College & State University, GA
Georgia Southern University, GA
Georgia State University, GA
Gonzaga University, WA
Graceland University, IA
Grambling State University, LA
Grand Canyon University, AZ
Grand Valley State University, MI
Hampton University, VA
Hawai'i Pacific University, HI
Holy Names University, CA
Howard University, DC
Husson College, ME
Idaho State University, ID
Illinois State University, IL
Indiana State University, IN
Indiana University–Purdue University Fort Wayne, IN
Indiana University–Purdue University Indianapolis, IN
Indiana Wesleyan University, IN
Intercollegiate College of Nursing/Washington State University, WA
The Johns Hopkins University, MD
Kennesaw State University, GA
La Roche College, PA
La Salle University, PA
Loma Linda University, CA
Long Island University, Brooklyn Campus, NY
Long Island University, C.W. Post Campus, NY
Loyola University Chicago, IL
Loyola University New Orleans, LA
Malone College, OH
Marshall University, WV
Marymount University, VA
McNeese State University, LA
Medical College of Georgia, GA
Medical College of Ohio, OH
Medical University of South Carolina, SC
Metropolitan State University, MN
MGH Institute of Health Professions, MA
Michigan State University, MI
Midwestern State University, TX
Millersville University of Pennsylvania, PA
Minnesota State University Mankato, MN
Minnesota State University Moorhead, MN
Mississippi University for Women, MS
Molloy College, NY
Monmouth University, NJ
Montana State University–Bozeman, MT
Mountain State University, WV
Murray State University, KY
North Dakota State University, ND
Northeastern University, MA
Northern Arizona University, AZ
Northern Illinois University, IL
Northern Kentucky University, KY
Northern Michigan University, MI
North Georgia College & State University, GA
Northwestern State University of Louisiana, LA
Oakland University, MI
The Ohio State University, OH
Ohio University, OH
Old Dominion University, VA
Oregon Health & Science University, OR
Otterbein College, OH
Pace University, NY
Pacific Lutheran University, WA
The Pennsylvania State University University Park Campus, PA
Pittsburg State University, KS
Prairie View A&M University, TX

Purdue University Calumet, IN
Quinnipiac University, CT
Radford University, VA
Regis College, MA
Regis University, CO
Research College of Nursing, MO
Rivier College, NH
Rush University, IL
Rutgers, The State University of New Jersey, College of Nursing, NJ
Sacred Heart University, CT
The Sage Colleges, NY
Saginaw Valley State University, MI
St. John Fisher College, NY
Saint Joseph College, CT
Saint Louis University, MO
Saint Xavier University, IL
Salisbury University, MD
Samford University, AL
Samuel Merritt College, CA
San Diego State University, CA
San Francisco State University, CA
San Jose State University, CA
Seattle Pacific University, WA
Seattle University, WA
Shenandoah University, VA
Simmons College, MA
Slippery Rock University of Pennsylvania, PA
Sonoma State University, CA
Southeast Missouri State University, MO
Southern Adventist University, TN
Southern Connecticut State University, CT
Southern Illinois University Edwardsville, IL
Southern University and Agricultural and Mechanical College, LA
Southwest Missouri State University, MO
Spalding University, KY
State University of New York at Binghamton, NY
State University of New York Downstate Medical Center, NY
State University of New York Institute of Technology, NY
State University of New York Upstate Medical University, NY
Stony Brook University, State University of New York, NY
Tennessee State University, TN
Tennessee Technological University, TN
Texas A&M International University, TX
Texas A&M University–Corpus Christi, TX
Texas Tech University Health Sciences Center, TX
Texas Woman's University, TX
Thomas Jefferson University, PA
Troy University, AL
Université de Moncton, NB
University at Buffalo, The State University of New York, NY
The University of Alabama at Birmingham, AL
The University of Alabama in Huntsville, AL
University of Alaska Anchorage, AK
The University of Arizona, AZ
University of Arkansas for Medical Sciences, AR
The University of British Columbia, BC
University of California, Los Angeles, CA
University of California, San Francisco, CA
University of Central Arkansas, AR
University of Central Florida, FL
University of Cincinnati, OH
University of Colorado at Colorado Springs, CO
University of Colorado at Denver and Health Sciences Center—Health Sciences Program, CO
University of Delaware, DE
University of Detroit Mercy, MI
University of Florida, FL
University of Hawaii at Manoa, HI
University of Illinois at Chicago, IL
University of Indianapolis, IN
The University of Iowa, IA
University of Kansas, KS
University of Kentucky, KY
University of Louisville, KY
University of Maine, ME
University of Mary, ND
University of Maryland, MD
University of Massachusetts Amherst, MA
University of Massachusetts Boston, MA
University of Massachusetts Lowell, MA
University of Medicine and Dentistry of New Jersey, NJ
The University of Memphis, TN
University of Miami, FL
University of Michigan, MI
University of Michigan–Flint, MI
University of Minnesota, Twin Cities Campus, MN
University of Mississippi Medical Center, MS
University of Missouri–Columbia, MO
University of Missouri–Kansas City, MO
University of Missouri–St. Louis, MO
University of Mobile, AL
University of Nebraska Medical Center, NE
University of Nevada, Las Vegas, NV
University of Nevada, Reno, NV
University of New Brunswick Fredericton, NB
University of New Hampshire, NH
University of New Mexico, NM
The University of North Carolina at Chapel Hill, NC
The University of North Carolina at Charlotte, NC
The University of North Carolina at Wilmington, NC
University of North Dakota, ND
University of Northern Colorado, CO
University of North Florida, FL
University of Oklahoma Health Sciences Center, OK
University of Pennsylvania, PA
University of Phoenix–Colorado Campus, CO
University of Phoenix–Fort Lauderdale Campus, FL
University of Phoenix–Hawaii Campus, HI
University of Phoenix–Jacksonville Campus, FL
University of Phoenix–Louisiana Campus, LA
University of Phoenix–Metro Detroit Campus, MI
University of Phoenix–New Mexico Campus, NM
University of Phoenix–Northern California Campus, CA
University of Phoenix–Oklahoma City Campus, OK
University of Phoenix Online Campus, AZ
University of Phoenix–Orlando Campus, FL
University of Phoenix–Phoenix Campus, AZ
University of Phoenix–Sacramento Campus, CA
University of Phoenix–San Diego Campus, CA
University of Phoenix–Southern Arizona Campus, AZ
University of Phoenix–Southern California Campus, CA
University of Phoenix–Southern Colorado Campus, CO
University of Phoenix–Tampa Campus, FL
University of Phoenix–Tulsa Campus, OK
University of Phoenix–Utah Campus, UT
University of Phoenix–West Michigan Campus, MI
University of Pittsburgh, PA
University of Portland, OR
University of Rhode Island, RI
University of Rochester, NY
University of St. Francis, IL
University of Saint Francis, IN
University of San Diego, CA
University of San Francisco, CA
The University of Scranton, PA
University of South Alabama, AL
University of South Carolina, SC
University of Southern Indiana, IN
University of Southern Maine, ME
University of Southern Mississippi, MS
University of South Florida, FL
The University of Tampa, FL
The University of Tennessee, TN
The University of Tennessee at Chattanooga, TN
The University of Tennessee Health Science Center, TN
The University of Texas at Arlington, TX
The University of Texas at Austin, TX
The University of Texas at El Paso, TX
The University of Texas at Tyler, TX
The University of Texas Health Science Center at Houston, TX
The University of Texas Health Science Center at San Antonio, TX
The University of Texas Medical Branch, TX
The University of Texas–Pan American, TX
University of Utah, UT
University of Vermont, VT
University of Virginia, VA
University of Washington, WA
University of Wisconsin–Eau Claire, WI
University of Wisconsin–Milwaukee, WI
University of Wisconsin–Oshkosh, WI
University of Wyoming, WY
Ursuline College, OH
Vanderbilt University, TN
Virginia Commonwealth University, VA
Wagner College, NY
Western Carolina University, NC
Western University of Health Sciences, CA
Westminster College, UT
West Texas A&M University, TX
West Virginia University, WV
Wheeling Jesuit University, WV
Wichita State University, KS
Widener University, PA
Wilmington College, DE
Winona State University, MN
Winston-Salem State University, NC
Wright State University, OH
Yale University, CT

Gerontology

Boston College, MA
California State University, Long Beach, CA
Case Western Reserve University, OH
The Catholic University of America, DC
Clemson University, SC
College of St. Catherine, MN
College of Staten Island of the City University of New York, NY
Columbia University, NY
Concordia University Wisconsin, WI
Creighton University, NE
Dalhousie University, NS
Duke University, NC
East Tennessee State University, TN
Emory University, GA
Florida Agricultural and Mechanical University, FL
Florida Atlantic University, FL
George Mason University, VA
Grand Valley State University, MI
Hampton University, VA
Hunter College of the City University of New York, NY
Indiana Wesleyan University, IN
James Madison University, VA
Jewish Hospital College of Nursing and Allied Health, MO
Kent State University, OH
Long Island University, Brooklyn Campus, NY
Marquette University, WI
Maryville University of Saint Louis, MO
Medical University of South Carolina, SC
MGH Institute of Health Professions, MA
Michigan State University, MI
Nazareth College of Rochester, NY
Neumann College, PA
New York University, NY
Northeastern University, MA
Northern Kentucky University, KY
Oakland University, MI
Oregon Health & Science University, OR
Rush University, IL
The Sage Colleges, NY
Saint Louis University, MO
San Diego State University, CA
Seattle Pacific University, WA
Seton Hall University, NJ
Simmons College, MA

State University of New York at Binghamton, NY
Texas Tech University Health Sciences Center, TX
University at Buffalo, The State University of New York, NY
The University of Akron, OH
University of Arkansas for Medical Sciences, AR
University of California, Los Angeles, CA
University of California, San Francisco, CA
University of Cincinnati, OH
University of Colorado at Colorado Springs, CO
University of Colorado at Denver and Health Sciences Center—Health Sciences Program, CO
University of Hawaii at Manoa, HI
University of Illinois at Chicago, IL
University of Indianapolis, IN
The University of Iowa, IA
University of Kansas, KS
University of Kentucky, KY
University of Louisville, KY
University of Maryland, MD
University of Massachusetts Boston, MA
University of Massachusetts Lowell, MA
University of Massachusetts Worcester, MA
University of Medicine and Dentistry of New Jersey, NJ
University of Michigan, MI
University of Minnesota, Twin Cities Campus, MN
University of Missouri–Columbia, MO
University of Nebraska Medical Center, NE
University of New Brunswick Fredericton, NB
The University of North Carolina at Greensboro, NC
University of Pennsylvania, PA
University of Rochester, NY
University of St. Francis, IL
University of San Diego, CA
University of South Alabama, AL
University of South Florida, FL
The University of Tennessee, TN
The University of Texas at Arlington, TX
The University of Texas at Tyler, TX
The University of Texas Health Science Center at Houston, TX
The University of Texas Health Science Center at San Antonio, TX
The University of Texas Medical Branch, TX
University of Utah, UT
University of Virginia, VA
University of Washington, WA
University of Wisconsin–Madison, WI
Vanderbilt University, TN
Villanova University, PA
Wayne State University, MI
Wilmington College, DE
Yale University, CT

Neonatal Health
Arizona State University, AZ
Baylor University, TX
Case Western Reserve University, OH
The College of New Jersey, NJ
College of St. Catherine, MN
Columbia University, NY
Creighton University, NE
Dalhousie University, NS
Duke University, NC
East Carolina University, NC
Indiana University–Purdue University Indianapolis, IN
Jewish Hospital College of Nursing and Allied Health, MO
Loma Linda University, CA
Louisiana State University Health Sciences Center, LA
McMaster University, ON
Medical University of South Carolina, SC
Northeastern University, MA
Northwestern State University of Louisiana, LA
The Ohio State University, OH
The Pennsylvania State University University Park Campus, PA
Regis University, CO
Rush University, IL
South Dakota State University, SD
Stony Brook University, State University of New York, NY
Thomas Jefferson University, PA
University at Buffalo, The State University of New York, NY
The University of Alabama at Birmingham, AL
University of Calgary, AB
University of California, San Francisco, CA
University of Cincinnati, OH
University of Colorado at Colorado Springs, CO
University of Connecticut, CT
University of Florida, FL
University of Louisville, KY
University of Maryland, MD
University of Mississippi Medical Center, MS
University of Missouri–Kansas City, MO
University of Nebraska Medical Center, NE
University of New Brunswick Fredericton, NB
The University of North Carolina at Chapel Hill, NC
University of Pennsylvania, PA
University of Rochester, NY
University of South Alabama, AL
The University of Tennessee, TN
The University of Tennessee Health Science Center, TN
The University of Texas Health Science Center at Houston, TX
The University of Texas Medical Branch, TX
University of Utah, UT
University of Washington, WA
Vanderbilt University, TN
Wayne State University, MI

Occupational Health
Simmons College, MA
The University of Alabama at Birmingham, AL
University of California, Los Angeles, CA
University of California, San Francisco, CA
University of Illinois at Chicago, IL
University of Pennsylvania, PA
University of South Florida, FL
University of the Sacred Heart, PR

Oncology
Columbia University, NY
Dalhousie University, NS
Duke University, NC
Emory University, GA
Jewish Hospital College of Nursing and Allied Health, MO
Thomas Jefferson University, PA
Université de Moncton, NB
University of California, Los Angeles, CA
University of California, San Francisco, CA
University of Florida, FL
University of Maryland, MD
University of Medicine and Dentistry of New Jersey, NJ
University of Nebraska Medical Center, NE
University of Pennsylvania, PA
University of South Florida, FL
The University of Texas Health Science Center at Houston, TX
University of Utah, UT
Yale University, CT

Pediatric
Arizona State University, AZ
Azusa Pacific University, CA
Boston College, MA
California State University, Fresno, CA
California State University, Long Beach, CA
California State University, Los Angeles, CA
Case Western Reserve University, OH
The Catholic University of America, DC
College of St. Catherine, MN
Columbia University, NY
DePaul University, IL
Duke University, NC
Emory University, GA
Florida International University, FL
Georgia State University, GA
Grand Valley State University, MI
Gwynedd-Mercy College, PA
Hampton University, VA
Hunter College of the City University of New York, NY
Indiana University–Purdue University Indianapolis, IN
The Johns Hopkins University, MD
Kent State University, OH
Lehman College of the City University of New York, NY
Loma Linda University, CA
Loyola University Chicago, IL
Marquette University, WI
McGill University, QC
Medical College of Georgia, GA
Medical College of Ohio, OH
Medical University of South Carolina, SC
Memorial University of Newfoundland, NL
MGH Institute of Health Professions, MA
Mississippi University for Women, MS
Molloy College, NY
New York University, NY
Northeastern University, MA
Northern Kentucky University, KY
Northwestern State University of Louisiana, LA
The Ohio State University, OH
Old Dominion University, VA
Oregon Health & Science University, OR
Regis College, MA
Rush University, IL
Rutgers, The State University of New Jersey, College of Nursing, NJ
Saint Louis University, MO
Seton Hall University, NJ
Simmons College, MA
Spalding University, KY
State University of New York Upstate Medical University, NY
Stony Brook University, State University of New York, NY
Temple University, PA
Texas Tech University Health Sciences Center, TX
Texas Woman's University, TX
Thomas Jefferson University, PA
University at Buffalo, The State University of New York, NY
The University of Akron, OH
The University of Alabama at Birmingham, AL
University of Arkansas for Medical Sciences, AR
University of California, Los Angeles, CA
University of California, San Francisco, CA
University of Central Florida, FL
University of Cincinnati, OH
University of Colorado at Colorado Springs, CO
University of Colorado at Denver and Health Sciences Center—Health Sciences Program, CO
University of Florida, FL
University of Illinois at Chicago, IL
The University of Iowa, IA
University of Kentucky, KY
University of Maryland, MD
University of Michigan, MI
University of Minnesota, Twin Cities Campus, MN
University of Missouri–Columbia, MO
University of Missouri–Kansas City, MO
University of Missouri–St. Louis, MO
University of Nebraska Medical Center, NE
University of New Brunswick Fredericton, NB
The University of North Carolina at Chapel Hill, NC
University of Oklahoma Health Sciences Center, OK
University of Pennsylvania, PA
University of Pittsburgh, PA
University of Rochester, NY
University of San Diego, CA
University of South Alabama, AL
University of South Carolina, SC
University of South Florida, FL

The University of Tennessee, TN
The University of Texas at Arlington, TX
The University of Texas at Austin, TX
The University of Texas at Tyler, TX
The University of Texas Health Science Center at Houston, TX
The University of Texas Health Science Center at San Antonio, TX
The University of Texas Medical Branch, TX
The University of Texas–Pan American, TX
University of Utah, UT
University of Virginia, VA
University of Washington, WA
University of Wisconsin–Madison, WI
Vanderbilt University, TN
Villanova University, PA
Virginia Commonwealth University, VA
Wayne State University, MI
West Virginia University, WV
Wichita State University, KS
Wright State University, OH
Yale University, CT

Primary Care

Arkansas State University, AR
Athabasca University, AB
Azusa Pacific University, CA
California State University, Los Angeles, CA
California State University, Sacramento, CA
Duke University, NC
George Mason University, VA
Gonzaga University, WA
Grand Valley State University, MI
Kennesaw State University, GA
Kent State University, OH
Loma Linda University, CA
Louisiana State University Health Sciences Center, LA
Madonna University, MI
Maryville University of Saint Louis, MO
MGH Institute of Health Professions, MA
New York University, NY
Northeastern University, MA
The Ohio State University, OH
Oregon Health & Science University, OR
Regis College, MA
Samford University, AL
Seton Hall University, NJ
Simmons College, MA
South Dakota State University, SD
State University of New York at Binghamton, NY
Université de Moncton, NB
The University of Alabama at Birmingham, AL
University of Central Arkansas, AR
University of Connecticut, CT
University of Hawaii at Manoa, HI
University of Manitoba, MB
University of Miami, FL
University of Michigan, MI
University of Nebraska Medical Center, NE
University of New Brunswick Fredericton, NB
University of New Mexico, NM
The University of North Carolina at Chapel Hill, NC
University of North Florida, FL
University of Ottawa, ON
University of Pennsylvania, PA
The University of Tennessee, TN
The University of Tennessee Health Science Center, TN
The University of Texas Medical Branch, TX
University of Virginia, VA
University of Washington, WA
Virginia Commonwealth University, VA
Wayne State University, MI
Western Kentucky University, KY
West Virginia University, WV

Psychiatric/Mental Health

Arizona State University, AZ
California State University, Long Beach, CA
Case Western Reserve University, OH
The College of St. Scholastica, MN
Columbia University, NY
Drexel University, PA
East Tennessee State University, TN
Fairfield University, CT
Fairleigh Dickinson University, Metropolitan Campus, NJ
Florida International University, FL
Gonzaga University, WA
Grand Valley State University, MI
Husson College, ME
Intercollegiate College of Nursing/Washington State University, WA
Medical University of South Carolina, SC
MGH Institute of Health Professions, MA
Molloy College, NY
New Mexico State University, NM
New York University, NY
Northeastern University, MA
The Ohio State University, OH
Oregon Health & Science University, OR
Regis College, MA
Rivier College, NH
Rush University, IL
The Sage Colleges, NY
Seattle University, WA
Shenandoah University, VA
South Dakota State University, SD
Stony Brook University, State University of New York, NY
University at Buffalo, The State University of New York, NY
The University of Akron, OH
University of Alaska Anchorage, AK
The University of Arizona, AZ
University of California, San Francisco, CA
University of Cincinnati, OH
University of Colorado at Colorado Springs, CO
University of Colorado at Denver and Health Sciences Center—Health Sciences Program, CO
University of Florida, FL
University of Illinois at Chicago, IL
University of Kansas, KS
University of Kentucky, KY
University of Louisville, KY
University of Maryland, MD
University of Massachusetts Amherst, MA
University of Massachusetts Lowell, MA
University of Medicine and Dentistry of New Jersey, NJ
University of Miami, FL
University of Michigan, MI
University of Michigan–Flint, MI
University of Mississippi Medical Center, MS
University of Missouri–Columbia, MO
University of Nebraska Medical Center, NE
University of New Brunswick Fredericton, NB
The University of North Carolina at Chapel Hill, NC
University of North Dakota, ND
University of Pittsburgh, PA
University of Rochester, NY
University of San Francisco, CA
University of Saskatchewan, SK
University of South Alabama, AL
University of South Carolina, SC
University of Southern Maine, ME
University of Southern Mississippi, MS
University of South Florida, FL
The University of Tennessee, TN
The University of Tennessee Health Science Center, TN
The University of Texas at Arlington, TX
The University of Texas Health Science Center at Houston, TX
The University of Texas Health Science Center at San Antonio, TX
The University of Texas Medical Branch, TX
University of Utah, UT
University of Virginia, VA
University of Washington, WA
University of Wisconsin–Madison, WI
Vanderbilt University, TN
Virginia Commonwealth University, VA
Wichita State University, KS
Winston-Salem State University, NC
Yale University, CT

School Health

The Catholic University of America, DC
Monmouth University, NJ
The Ohio State University, OH
Seton Hall University, NJ
Simmons College, MA
University of Illinois at Chicago, IL

Women's Health

Arizona State University, AZ
Boston College, MA
California State University, Fullerton, CA
California State University, Long Beach, CA
California State University, Los Angeles, CA
Case Western Reserve University, OH
Columbia University, NY
DePaul University, IL
Emory University, GA
Florida Agricultural and Mechanical University, FL
Georgia Southern University, GA
Georgia State University, GA
Grand Valley State University, MI
Hampton University, VA
Indiana University–Purdue University Indianapolis, IN
Kent State University, OH
Loyola University Chicago, IL
MGH Institute of Health Professions, MA
Northwestern State University of Louisiana, LA
The Ohio State University, OH
Old Dominion University, VA
Oregon Health & Science University, OR
Pace University, NY
Rutgers, The State University of New Jersey, College of Nursing, NJ
San Diego State University, CA
Seton Hall University, NJ
Simmons College, MA
State University of New York Downstate Medical Center, NY
Stony Brook University, State University of New York, NY
Texas Woman's University, TX
University at Buffalo, The State University of New York, NY
The University of Alabama at Birmingham, AL
University of Arkansas for Medical Sciences, AR
University of Cincinnati, OH
University of Colorado at Colorado Springs, CO
University of Colorado at Denver and Health Sciences Center—Health Sciences Program, CO
University of Illinois at Chicago, IL
University of Louisville, KY
University of Maryland, MD
University of Medicine and Dentistry of New Jersey, NJ
University of Miami, FL
University of Minnesota, Twin Cities Campus, MN
University of Missouri–Kansas City, MO
University of Missouri–St. Louis, MO
University of Nebraska Medical Center, NE
University of New Brunswick Fredericton, NB
The University of North Carolina at Chapel Hill, NC
University of Pennsylvania, PA
University of South Alabama, AL
University of South Carolina, SC
The University of Tennessee, TN
The University of Texas at El Paso, TX
The University of Texas at Tyler, TX
The University of Texas Health Science Center at Houston, TX
The University of Texas Medical Branch, TX
University of Utah, UT
University of Washington, WA
University of Wisconsin–Madison, WI
Vanderbilt University, TN
Virginia Commonwealth University, VA

Wayne State University, MI
Wilmington College, DE
Yale University, CT

Nurse-Midwifery

California State University, Fullerton, CA
Case Western Reserve University, OH
Columbia University, NY
East Carolina University, NC
Emory University, GA
Georgetown University, DC
Loyola University Chicago, IL
Marquette University, WI
Medical University of South Carolina, SC
New York University, NY
The Ohio State University, OH
Old Dominion University, VA
Oregon Health & Science University, OR
Radford University, VA
San Diego State University, CA
Shenandoah University, VA
State University of New York Downstate Medical Center, NY
Stony Brook University, State University of New York, NY
University of California, San Francisco, CA
University of Cincinnati, OH
University of Colorado at Denver and Health Sciences Center—Health Sciences Program, CO
University of Florida, FL
University of Illinois at Chicago, IL
University of Indianapolis, IN
University of Kansas, KS
University of Maryland, MD
University of Miami, FL
University of Michigan, MI
University of Minnesota, Twin Cities Campus, MN
University of New Mexico, NM
University of Pennsylvania, PA
University of Rhode Island, RI
The University of Texas Medical Branch, TX
University of Utah, UT
University of Washington, WA
Vanderbilt University, TN
Yale University, CT
York College of Pennsylvania, PA

Doctoral Programs

Alabama
The University of Alabama at Birmingham, School of Nursing, *Birmingham* (PhD)

Arizona
The University of Arizona, College of Nursing, *Tucson* (PhD)

Arkansas
University of Arkansas for Medical Sciences, College of Nursing, *Little Rock* (PhD)

California
Azusa Pacific University, School of Nursing, *Azusa* (DSN)
Loma Linda University, School of Nursing, *Loma Linda* (PhD)
University of California, Los Angeles, School of Nursing, *Los Angeles* (PhD)
University of California, San Francisco, School of Nursing, *San Francisco* (PhD)
University of San Diego, Hahn School of Nursing and Health Sciences, *San Diego* (PhD)

Colorado
University of Colorado at Denver and Health Sciences Center—Health Sciences Program, School of Nursing, *Denver* (PhD)
University of Northern Colorado, School of Nursing, *Greeley* (PhD)

Connecticut
University of Connecticut, School of Nursing, *Storrs* (PhD)
Yale University, School of Nursing, *New Haven* (DN Sc)

District of Columbia
The Catholic University of America, School of Nursing, *Washington* (DN Sc)

Florida
Barry University, School of Nursing, *Miami Shores* (PhD)
Florida Agricultural and Mechanical University, School of Nursing, *Tallahassee* (PhD)
Florida Atlantic University, College of Nursing, *Boca Raton* (DNS)
Florida International University, School of Nursing, *Miami* (PhD)
University of Central Florida, School of Nursing, *Orlando* (PhD)
University of Florida, College of Nursing, *Gainesville* (PhD)
University of Miami, School of Nursing, *Coral Gables* (PhD)
University of South Florida, College of Nursing, *Tampa* (PhD)

Georgia
Emory University, Nell Hodgson Woodruff School of Nursing, *Atlanta* (PhD)
Georgia State University, School of Nursing, *Atlanta* (PhD)
Medical College of Georgia, School of Nursing, *Augusta* (PhD)

Hawaii
University of Hawaii at Manoa, School of Nursing and Dental Hygiene, *Honolulu* (PhD)

Illinois
Loyola University Chicago, Marcella Niehoff School of Nursing, *Chicago* (PhD)
Rush University, College of Nursing, *Chicago* (DN Sc)
University of Illinois at Chicago, College of Nursing, *Chicago* (PhD)

Indiana
Indiana University–Purdue University Indianapolis, School of Nursing, *Indianapolis* (PhD)

Iowa
The University of Iowa, College of Nursing, *Iowa City* (PhD)

Kansas
University of Kansas, School of Nursing, *Kansas City* (PhD)

Kentucky
University of Kentucky, Graduate School Programs in the College of Nursing, *Lexington* (PhD)

Louisiana
Louisiana State University Health Sciences Center, School of Nursing, *New Orleans* (DNS)
Southern University and Agricultural and Mechanical College, School of Nursing, *Baton Rouge* (PhD)

Maryland
The Johns Hopkins University, School of Nursing, *Baltimore* (PhD)
University of Maryland, School of Nursing, *Baltimore* (PhD)

Massachusetts
Boston College, William F. Connell School of Nursing, *Chestnut Hill* (PhD)
University of Massachusetts Amherst, School of Nursing, *Amherst* (PhD)
University of Massachusetts Boston, College of Nursing and Health Sciences, *Boston* (PhD)
University of Massachusetts Lowell, Department of Nursing, *Lowell* (PhD)
University of Massachusetts Worcester, Graduate School of Nursing, *Worcester* (PhD)

Michigan
Michigan State University, College of Nursing, *East Lansing* (PhD)
University of Michigan, School of Nursing, *Ann Arbor* (PhD)
Wayne State University, College of Nursing, *Detroit* (PhD)

Minnesota
University of Minnesota, Twin Cities Campus, School of Nursing, *Minneapolis* (PhD)

Mississippi
University of Mississippi Medical Center, Program in Nursing, *Jackson* (PhD)
University of Southern Mississippi, School of Nursing, *Hattiesburg* (PhD)

Missouri
Saint Louis University, School of Nursing, *St. Louis* (PhD)
University of Missouri–Columbia, Sinclair School of Nursing, *Columbia* (PhD)
University of Missouri–Kansas City, School of Nursing, *Kansas City* (PhD)
University of Missouri–St. Louis, College of Nursing, *St. Louis* (PhD)

Nebraska
University of Nebraska Medical Center, College of Nursing, *Omaha* (PhD)

Nevada
University of Nevada, Las Vegas, Department of Nursing, *Las Vegas* (PhD)

New Jersey
Rutgers, The State University of New Jersey, College of Nursing, *Newark* (PhD)

New Mexico
University of New Mexico, College of Nursing, *Albuquerque* (PhD)

New York
Columbia University, School of Nursing, *New York* (DN Sc)
New York University, Division of Nursing, *New York* (PhD)
State University of New York at Binghamton, Decker School of Nursing, *Binghamton* (PhD)
Teachers College Columbia University, Department of Health and Behavioral Studies, *New York* (EdD)
University at Buffalo, The State University of New York, School of Nursing, *Buffalo* (PhD)
University of Rochester, School of Nursing, *Rochester* (PhD)

North Carolina
East Carolina University, School of Nursing, *Greenville* (PhD)
The University of North Carolina at Chapel Hill, School of Nursing, *Chapel Hill* (PhD)
The University of North Carolina at Greensboro, School of Nursing, *Greensboro* (PhD)

North Dakota
University of North Dakota, College of Nursing, *Grand Forks* (PhD)

Ohio
Case Western Reserve University, Frances Payne Bolton School of Nursing, *Cleveland* (PhD)
Kent State University, College of Nursing, *Kent* (PhD)
The Ohio State University, College of Nursing, *Columbus* (PhD)
The University of Akron, College of Nursing, *Akron* (PhD)
University of Cincinnati, College of Nursing, *Cincinnati* (PhD)

Oregon
Oregon Health & Science University, School of Nursing, *Portland* (PhD)

Pennsylvania
Duquesne University, School of Nursing, *Pittsburgh* (PhD)
The Pennsylvania State University University Park Campus, School of Nursing, *State College, University Park* (PhD)
University of Pennsylvania, School of Nursing, *Philadelphia* (PhD)
University of Pittsburgh, School of Nursing, *Pittsburgh* (PhD)
Villanova University, College of Nursing, *Villanova* (PhD)
Widener University, School of Nursing, *Chester* (DN Sc)

Rhode Island
University of Rhode Island, College of Nursing, *Kingston* (PhD)

South Carolina
Medical University of South Carolina, College of Nursing, *Charleston* (PhD)
University of South Carolina, College of Nursing, *Columbia* (PhD)

Tennessee
East Tennessee State University, College of Nursing, *Johnson City* (DSN)
The University of Tennessee, College of Nursing, *Knoxville* (PhD)
The University of Tennessee Health Science Center, College of Nursing, *Memphis* (PhD)

Vanderbilt University, School of Nursing, *Nashville* (PhD)

Texas

Texas Woman's University, College of Nursing, *Denton* (PhD)

The University of Texas at Arlington, School of Nursing, *Arlington* (PhD)

The University of Texas at Austin, School of Nursing, *Austin* (PhD)

The University of Texas at El Paso, School of Nursing, *El Paso* (DSN)

The University of Texas at Tyler, Program in Nursing, *Tyler* (DNS)

The University of Texas Health Science Center at Houston, School of Nursing, *Houston* (DSN)

The University of Texas Health Science Center at San Antonio, School of Nursing, *San Antonio* (PhD)

The University of Texas Medical Branch, School of Nursing, *Galveston* (PhD)

Utah

University of Utah, College of Nursing, *Salt Lake City* (PhD)

Virginia

George Mason University, College of Nursing and Health Science, *Fairfax* (PhD)

Hampton University, Department of Nursing, *Hampton* (PhD)

University of Virginia, School of Nursing, *Charlottesville* (PhD)

Virginia Commonwealth University, School of Nursing, *Richmond* (PhD)

Washington

University of Washington, School of Nursing, *Seattle* (PhD)

West Virginia

West Virginia University, School of Nursing, *Morgantown* (DSN)

Wisconsin

Marquette University, College of Nursing, *Milwaukee* (PhD)

University of Wisconsin–Madison, School of Nursing, *Madison* (PhD)

University of Wisconsin–Milwaukee, College of Nursing, *Milwaukee* (PhD)

Alberta

University of Alberta, Faculty of Nursing, *Edmonton* (PhD)

University of Calgary, Faculty of Nursing, *Calgary* (PhD)

British Columbia

The University of British Columbia, School of Nursing, *Vancouver* (PhD)

University of Victoria, School of Nursing, *Victoria* (PhD)

Nova Scotia

Dalhousie University, School of Nursing, *Halifax* (PhD)

Ontario

McMaster University, School of Nursing, *Hamilton* (PhD)

University of Ottawa, School of Nursing, *Ottawa* (PhD)

University of Toronto, Faculty of Nursing, *Toronto* (PhD)

The University of Western Ontario, School of Nursing, *London* (PhD)

Quebec

McGill University, School of Nursing, *Montréal* (PhD)

Université de Montréal, Faculty of Nursing, *Montréal* (PhD)

Université de Sherbrooke, Department of Nursing, *Sherbrooke* (PhD)

Université Laval, Faculty of Nursing, *Québec* (PhD)

Postdoctoral Programs

Alabama
The University of Alabama at Birmingham, School of Nursing, *Birmingham*

Arizona
The University of Arizona, College of Nursing, *Tucson*

California
University of California, Los Angeles, School of Nursing, *Los Angeles*
University of California, San Francisco, School of Nursing, *San Francisco*

Colorado
University of Colorado at Denver and Health Sciences Center—Health Sciences Program, School of Nursing, *Denver*

Connecticut
Yale University, School of Nursing, *New Haven*

Georgia
Emory University, Nell Hodgson Woodruff School of Nursing, *Atlanta*

Illinois
Rush University, College of Nursing, *Chicago*
University of Illinois at Chicago, College of Nursing, *Chicago*

Indiana
Indiana University-Purdue University Indianapolis, School of Nursing, *Indianapolis*

Iowa
The University of Iowa, College of Nursing, *Iowa City*

Maryland
The Johns Hopkins University, School of Nursing, *Baltimore*

Michigan
Michigan State University, College of Nursing, *East Lansing*
University of Michigan, School of Nursing, *Ann Arbor*
Wayne State University, College of Nursing, *Detroit*

Nebraska
University of Nebraska Medical Center, College of Nursing, *Omaha*

New York
University of Rochester, School of Nursing, *Rochester*

North Carolina
The University of North Carolina at Chapel Hill, School of Nursing, *Chapel Hill*

Ohio
Case Western Reserve University, Frances Payne Bolton School of Nursing, *Cleveland*

Oregon
Oregon Health & Science University, School of Nursing, *Portland*

Pennsylvania
The Pennsylvania State University University Park Campus, School of Nursing, *State College, University Park*
University of Pennsylvania, School of Nursing, *Philadelphia*
University of Pittsburgh, School of Nursing, *Pittsburgh*

Tennessee
Vanderbilt University, School of Nursing, *Nashville*

Texas
The University of Texas at Austin, School of Nursing, *Austin*

Utah
University of Utah, College of Nursing, *Salt Lake City*

Virginia
University of Virginia, School of Nursing, *Charlottesville*

Wisconsin
University of Wisconsin–Madison, School of Nursing, *Madison*

British Columbia
The University of British Columbia, School of Nursing, *Vancouver*

Quebec
Université de Sherbrooke, Department of Nursing, *Sherbrooke*

Distance Learning Programs

Baccalaureate Programs

Arkansas Tech University, AR
Armstrong Atlantic State University, GA
Athabasca University, AB
Bemidji State University, MN
Bloomfield College, NJ
Boise State University, ID
California State University, Bakersfield, CA
California State University, Dominguez Hills, CA
California State University, Fullerton, CA
California State University, Stanislaus, CA
California University of Pennsylvania, PA
Central Missouri State University, MO
Chicago State University, IL
Clarion University of Pennsylvania, PA
Clemson University, SC
The College of St. Scholastica, MN
Creighton University, NE
Daemen College, NY
Delta State University, MS
Drexel University, PA
D'Youville College, NY
East Carolina University, NC
East Central University, OK
Eastern Kentucky University, KY
Eastern New Mexico University, NM
East Tennessee State University, TN
Excelsior College, NY
Fairleigh Dickinson University, Metropolitan Campus, NJ
Florida Atlantic University, FL
Florida International University, FL
Florida State University, FL
Gannon University, PA
Graceland University, IA
Grand Canyon University, AZ
Grand Valley State University, MI
Idaho State University, ID
Indiana State University, IN
Intercollegiate College of Nursing/Washington State University, WA
Jefferson College of Health Sciences, VA
Kent State University, OH
Keuka College, NY
Kutztown University of Pennsylvania, PA
Lake Superior State University, MI
Lakeview College of Nursing, IL
Lewis-Clark State College, ID
Madonna University, MI
Mansfield University of Pennsylvania, PA
Marian College of Fond du Lac, WI
Marshall University, WV
Medical College of Georgia, GA
Medical College of Ohio, OH
Mesa State College, CO
Minnesota State University Moorhead, MN
Mississippi University for Women, MS
Montana State University–Bozeman, MT
Montana State University–Northern, MT
Morehead State University, KY
Mountain State University, WV
Murray State University, KY
Nebraska Methodist College, NE
New Mexico State University, NM
North Carolina Central University, NC
Northeastern State University, OK
Northern Arizona University, AZ
Northern Illinois University, IL
Northern Kentucky University, KY
Northwestern Oklahoma State University, OK
Northwestern State University of Louisiana, LA
Oklahoma Wesleyan University, OK
Old Dominion University, VA
Oregon Health & Science University, OR
Otterbein College, OH
Pace University, NY
Pennsylvania College of Technology, PA
The Pennsylvania State University University Park Campus, PA
Prairie View A&M University, TX
Presentation College, SD
Radford University, VA
The Richard Stockton College of New Jersey, NJ
Sacred Heart University, CT
Saginaw Valley State University, MI
Salve Regina University, RI
Seton Hall University, NJ
Slippery Rock University of Pennsylvania, PA
South Dakota State University, SD
Southeastern Louisiana University, LA
Southeast Missouri State University, MO
Southern Illinois University Edwardsville, IL
Southwestern Oklahoma State University, OK
Southwest Missouri State University, MO
State University of New York at Plattsburgh, NY
Tarleton State University, TX
Tennessee State University, TN
Texas A&M University–Corpus Christi, TX
Texas Christian University, TX
Texas Tech University Health Sciences Center, TX
Texas Woman's University, TX
Thomas Jefferson University, PA
Troy University, AL
Université du Québec à Chicoutimi, QC
The University of Akron, OH
The University of Alabama in Huntsville, AL
University of Arkansas for Medical Sciences, AR
University of Calgary, AB
University of Central Florida, FL
University of Colorado at Denver and Health Sciences Center—Health Sciences Program, CO
University of Connecticut, CT
University of Hawaii at Hilo, HI
University of Hawaii at Manoa, HI
University of Illinois at Chicago, IL
The University of Iowa, IA
University of Maine, ME
University of Maryland, MD
The University of Memphis, TN
University of Michigan, MI
University of Michigan–Flint, MI
University of Mississippi Medical Center, MS
University of Missouri–St. Louis, MO
University of Nebraska Medical Center, NE
University of New Brunswick Fredericton, NB
The University of North Carolina at Chapel Hill, NC
University of North Dakota, ND
University of Northern Colorado, CO
University of Oklahoma Health Sciences Center, OK
University of Ottawa, ON
University of Pittsburgh, PA
University of Saint Francis, IN
The University of Tennessee Health Science Center, TN
The University of Texas at Arlington, TX
The University of Texas at Brownsville, TX
The University of Texas at Tyler, TX
The University of Texas Health Science Center at Houston, TX
University of West Georgia, GA
University of Wisconsin–Eau Claire, WI
University of Wisconsin–Madison, WI
University of Wisconsin–Oshkosh, WI
University of Wyoming, WY
Valdosta State University, GA
Villa Julie College, MD
Weber State University, UT
Western Carolina University, NC
Western Kentucky University, KY
West Liberty State College, WV
West Virginia University, WV
Winona State University, MN
Winston-Salem State University, NC
Wright State University, OH
York College of Pennsylvania, PA

Master's Degree Programs

Abilene Intercollegiate School of Nursing, TX
Augustana College, SD
Azusa Pacific University, CA
Baylor University, TX
Bethel University, MN
California State University, Chico, CA
California State University, Dominguez Hills, CA
Central Missouri State University, MO
Clarion University of Pennsylvania, PA
Clemson University, SC
The College of St. Scholastica, MN
Creighton University, NE
Drexel University, PA
Duke University, NC
Eastern Kentucky University, KY
Excelsior College, NY
Fairleigh Dickinson University, Metropolitan Campus, NJ
Florida Atlantic University, FL
Florida Gulf Coast University, FL
Florida International University, FL
Gannon University, PA
Graceland University, IA
Grand Canyon University, AZ
Grand Valley State University, MI
Idaho State University, ID
Indiana State University, IN
Indiana University–Purdue University Fort Wayne, IN
Intercollegiate College of Nursing/Washington State University, WA
Jacksonville State University, AL
Jefferson College of Health Sciences, VA
Madonna University, MI
Marian College of Fond du Lac, WI
Marshall University, WV
McNeese State University, LA
Medical College of Georgia, GA
MGH Institute of Health Professions, MA
Minnesota State University Moorhead, MN
Montana State University–Bozeman, MT
Murray State University, KY
Nebraska Methodist College, NE
Northern Arizona University, AZ
Northern Illinois University, IL
Northern Kentucky University, KY
Northwestern State University of Louisiana, LA
Old Dominion University, VA
Oregon Health & Science University, OR
Otterbein College, OH
Pace University, NY
The Pennsylvania State University University Park Campus, PA
Purdue University Calumet, IN
Sacred Heart University, CT
Saint Louis University, MO
Samuel Merritt College, CA
Seton Hall University, NJ
Slippery Rock University of Pennsylvania, PA
Sonoma State University, CA
South Dakota State University, SD
Southeastern Louisiana University, LA
Southeast Missouri State University, MO
Southern Illinois University Edwardsville, IL
Texas A&M University–Corpus Christi, TX
Texas Christian University, TX
Texas Tech University Health Sciences Center, TX
Texas Woman's University, TX

DISTANCE LEARNING PROGRAMS

Master's Degree Programs

Thomas Jefferson University, PA
Troy University, AL
Université du Québec à Chicoutimi, QC
University at Buffalo, The State University of New York, NY
The University of Akron, OH
The University of Alabama in Huntsville, AL
University of Arkansas for Medical Sciences, AR
University of Central Arkansas, AR
University of Colorado at Denver and Health Sciences Center—Health Sciences Program, CO
University of Connecticut, CT
University of Hawaii at Manoa, HI
University of Illinois at Chicago, IL
The University of Iowa, IA
University of Kansas, KS
University of Louisiana at Lafayette, LA
University of Maryland, MD
University of Massachusetts Worcester, MA
The University of Memphis, TN
University of Michigan–Flint, MI
University of Missouri–Kansas City, MO
University of Missouri–St. Louis, MO
University of Nebraska Medical Center, NE
The University of North Carolina at Charlotte, NC
University of North Dakota, ND
University of Northern Colorado, CO
University of Oklahoma Health Sciences Center, OK
University of Ottawa, ON
University of Pennsylvania, PA
University of Pittsburgh, PA
The University of Tennessee Health Science Center, TN
The University of Texas at El Paso, TX
The University of Texas at Tyler, TX
The University of Texas Medical Branch, TX
University of Washington, WA
University of Wyoming, WY
Valdosta State University, GA
Vanderbilt University, TN
Wayne State University, MI
Western Carolina University, NC
Western Kentucky University, KY
West Virginia University, WV
Winona State University, MN
York College of Pennsylvania, PA

Doctoral Programs

Oregon Health & Science University, OR
The Pennsylvania State University University Park Campus, PA
Texas Woman's University, TX
The University of Arizona, AZ
University of Calgary, AB
University of Colorado at Denver and Health Sciences Center—Health Sciences Program, CO
University of Massachusetts Amherst, MA
University of Massachusetts Worcester, MA
University of Nebraska Medical Center, NE
University of North Dakota, ND
The University of Tennessee Health Science Center, TN
The University of Texas at El Paso, TX
The University of Texas at Tyler, TX
The University of Texas Health Science Center at San Antonio, TX
The University of Texas Medical Branch, TX
West Virginia University, WV

Continuing Education Programs

Alabama

Jacksonville State University, College of Nursing and Health Sciences, *Jacksonville*
Samford University, Ida V. Moffett School of Nursing, *Birmingham*
The University of Alabama, Capstone College of Nursing, *Tuscaloosa*
The University of Alabama in Huntsville, College of Nursing, *Huntsville*
University of Mobile, School of Nursing, *Mobile*
University of North Alabama, College of Nursing and Allied Health, *Florence*

Arizona

Arizona State University, College of Nursing, *Tempe*
Grand Canyon University, Samaritan College of Nursing, *Phoenix*
The University of Arizona, College of Nursing, *Tucson*
University of Phoenix–Phoenix Campus, College of Health and Human Services, *Phoenix*

Arkansas

University of Arkansas, Eleanor Mann School of Nursing, *Fayetteville*

California

Azusa Pacific University, School of Nursing, *Azusa*
Biola University, Department of Nursing, *La Mirada*
California State University, Chico, School of Nursing, *Chico*
California State University, Dominguez Hills, Program in Nursing, *Carson*
California State University, Fresno, Department of Nursing, *Fresno*
California State University, Sacramento, Division of Nursing, *Sacramento*
Dominican University of California, Program in Occupational Therapy, *San Rafael*
Pacific Union College, Department of Nursing, *Angwin*
Point Loma Nazarene University, School of Nursing, *San Diego*
San Diego State University, School of Nursing, *San Diego*
San Francisco State University, School of Nursing, *San Francisco*
University of California, Los Angeles, School of Nursing, *Los Angeles*
University of San Francisco, School of Nursing, *San Francisco*

Colorado

Colorado State University-Pueblo, Department of Nursing, *Pueblo*
University of Colorado at Colorado Springs, Beth-El College of Nursing and Health Sciences, *Colorado Springs*
University of Colorado at Denver and Health Sciences Center—Health Sciences Program, School of Nursing, *Denver*

Connecticut

Quinnipiac University, Department of Nursing, *Hamden*
University of Connecticut, School of Nursing, *Storrs*
University of Hartford, College of Education, Nursing, and Health Professions, *West Hartford*

Delaware

Wesley College, Graduate Nursing Program, *Dover*

District of Columbia

Georgetown University, School of Nursing and Health Studies, *Washington*

Florida

Florida Agricultural and Mechanical University, School of Nursing, *Tallahassee*
Florida Atlantic University, College of Nursing, *Boca Raton*
Florida Gulf Coast University, School of Nursing, *Fort Myers*
Florida State University, School of Nursing, *Tallahassee*
St. Petersburg College, Department of Nursing, *St. Petersburg*
University of Miami, School of Nursing, *Coral Gables*
University of South Florida, College of Nursing, *Tampa*

Georgia

Georgia Baptist College of Nursing of Mercer University, Department of Nursing, *Atlanta*
Georgia Southwestern State University, School of Nursing, *Americus*
Kennesaw State University, School of Nursing, *Kennesaw*
Valdosta State University, College of Nursing, *Valdosta*

Idaho

Lewis-Clark State College, Division of Nursing and Health Sciences, *Lewiston*

Illinois

Lewis University, Program in Nursing, *Romeoville*
Rush University, College of Nursing, *Chicago*
Saint Xavier University, School of Nursing, *Chicago*
Southern Illinois University Edwardsville, School of Nursing, *Edwardsville*
University of Illinois at Chicago, College of Nursing, *Chicago*

Indiana

Indiana State University, School of Nursing, *Terre Haute*
Indiana University Kokomo, Indiana University School Of Nursing, *Kokomo*
Indiana University–Purdue University Fort Wayne, Department of Nursing, *Fort Wayne*
Indiana University–Purdue University Indianapolis, School of Nursing, *Indianapolis*
Purdue University, School of Nursing, *West Lafayette*
University of Southern Indiana, School of Nursing and Health Professions, *Evansville*
Valparaiso University, College of Nursing, *Valparaiso*

Iowa

Allen College, Program in Nursing, *Waterloo*
Briar Cliff University, Department of Nursing, *Sioux City*
Grand View College, Division of Nursing, *Des Moines*
Iowa Wesleyan College, Division of Health and Natural Sciences, *Mount Pleasant*
Luther College, Department of Nursing, *Decorah*
Mount Mercy College, Department of Nursing, *Cedar Rapids*
The University of Iowa, College of Nursing, *Iowa City*

Kansas

MidAmerica Nazarene University, Division of Nursing, *Olathe*
Pittsburg State University, Department of Nursing, *Pittsburg*
University of Kansas, School of Nursing, *Kansas City*
Washburn University, School of Nursing, *Topeka*

Kentucky

Bellarmine University, Donna and Allan Lansing School of Nursing and Health Sciences, *Louisville*
Berea College, Department of Nursing, *Berea*
Midway College, Program in Nursing (Baccalaureate), *Midway*
Murray State University, Department of Nursing, *Murray*
Spalding University, School of Nursing, *Louisville*
University of Kentucky, Graduate School Programs in the College of Nursing, *Lexington*
Western Kentucky University, Department of Nursing, *Bowling Green*

Louisiana

Louisiana State University Health Sciences Center, School of Nursing, *New Orleans*
McNeese State University, College of Nursing, *Lake Charles*
Nicholls State University, Department of Nursing, *Thibodaux*
Northwestern State University of Louisiana, College of Nursing, *Shreveport*
University of Louisiana at Lafayette, College of Nursing, *Lafayette*
University of Louisiana at Monroe, Nursing, *Monroe*

Maine

Saint Joseph's College of Maine, Department of Nursing, *Standish*
University of New England, Department of Nursing, *Biddeford*
University of Southern Maine, College of Nursing and Health Professions, *Portland*

Maryland

Columbia Union College, Nursing Department, *Takoma Park*
The Johns Hopkins University, School of Nursing, *Baltimore*
University of Maryland, School of Nursing, *Baltimore*

Massachusetts

Anna Maria College, Department of Nursing, *Paxton*
Atlantic Union College, Department of Nursing, *South Lancaster*
Boston College, William F. Connell School of Nursing, *Chestnut Hill*
Curry College, Division of Nursing, *Milton*
Elms College, Division of Nursing, *Chicopee*
Endicott College, Major in Nursing, *Beverly*
MGH Institute of Health Professions, Program in Nursing, *Boston*
Northeastern University, School of Nursing, *Boston*
Regis College, Department of Nursing, *Weston*
Salem State College, Nursing Department, *Salem*
Simmons College, Department of Nursing, *Boston*
University of Massachusetts Amherst, School of Nursing, *Amherst*
University of Massachusetts Boston, College of Nursing and Health Sciences, *Boston*
University of Massachusetts Dartmouth, College of Nursing, *North Dartmouth*
University of Massachusetts Worcester, Graduate School of Nursing, *Worcester*

Michigan

Grand Valley State University, Russell B. Kirkhof School of Nursing, *Allendale*
Madonna University, College of Nursing and Health, *Livonia*
Michigan State University, College of Nursing, *East Lansing*

Northern Michigan University, College of Nursing and Allied Health Science, *Marquette*
Oakland University, School of Nursing, *Rochester*
Saginaw Valley State University, Crystal M. Lange College of Nursing and Health Sciences, *University Center*
University of Michigan–Flint, Department of Nursing, *Flint*

Minnesota
Bemidji State University, Department of Nursing, *Bemidji*
Bethel University, Department of Nursing, *St. Paul*
Minnesota State University Mankato, School of Nursing, *Mankato*
University of Minnesota, Twin Cities Campus, School of Nursing, *Minneapolis*

Mississippi
University of Mississippi Medical Center, Program in Nursing, *Jackson*

Missouri
Missouri Western State College, Department of Nursing, *St. Joseph*
Saint Louis University, School of Nursing, *St. Louis*
Southwest Missouri State University, Department of Nursing, *Springfield*
University of Missouri–Columbia, Sinclair School of Nursing, *Columbia*

Montana
Carroll College, Department of Nursing, *Helena*
Montana State University–Northern, College of Nursing, *Havre*

Nebraska
Clarkson College, Department of Nursing, *Omaha*
Midland Lutheran College, Department of Nursing, *Fremont*
Nebraska Methodist College, Department of Nursing, *Omaha*
University of Nebraska Medical Center, College of Nursing, *Omaha*

Nevada
University of Nevada, Las Vegas, Department of Nursing, *Las Vegas*

New Hampshire
Saint Anselm College, Department of Nursing, *Manchester*

New Jersey
College of Saint Elizabeth, Department of Nursing, *Morristown*
Kean University, Department of Nursing, *Union*
Monmouth University, Marjorie K. Unterberg School of Nursing, *West Long Branch*
Rutgers, The State University of New Jersey, College of Nursing, *Newark*
Seton Hall University, College of Nursing, *South Orange*
University of Medicine and Dentistry of New Jersey, School of Nursing, *Newark*

New Mexico
New Mexico State University, Department of Nursing, *Las Cruces*

New York
Adelphi University, School of Nursing, *Garden City*
Columbia University, School of Nursing, *New York*
Elmira College, Program in Nursing Education, *Elmira*
Hunter College of the City University of New York, Hunter-Bellevue School of Nursing, *New York*
Mercy College, Program in Nursing, *Dobbs Ferry*
Molloy College, Department of Nursing, *Rockville Centre*
Nazareth College of Rochester, Department of Nursing, *Rochester*
New York University, Division of Nursing, *New York*
Pace University, Lienhard School of Nursing, *New York*
Roberts Wesleyan College, Division of Nursing, *Rochester*
State University of New York at Binghamton, Decker School of Nursing, *Binghamton*
State University of New York at Plattsburgh, Department of Nursing, *Plattsburgh*
State University of New York Downstate Medical Center, College of Nursing, *Brooklyn*
State University of New York Institute of Technology, School of Nursing and Health Systems, *Utica*
State University of New York Upstate Medical University, College of Nursing, *Syracuse*
Stony Brook University, State University of New York, School of Nursing, *Stony Brook*
University of Rochester, School of Nursing, *Rochester*
Utica College, Department of Nursing, *Utica*

North Carolina
The University of North Carolina at Chapel Hill, School of Nursing, *Chapel Hill*
The University of North Carolina at Charlotte, School of Nursing, *Charlotte*
Winston-Salem State University, Department of Nursing, *Winston-Salem*

North Dakota
North Dakota State University, Tri-College University Nursing Consortium, *Fargo*

Ohio
Case Western Reserve University, Frances Payne Bolton School of Nursing, *Cleveland*
Cleveland State University, Department of Nursing, *Cleveland*
Kent State University, College of Nursing, *Kent*
Malone College, School of Nursing, *Canton*
Medical College of Ohio, School of Nursing, *Toledo*
Otterbein College, Program in Nursing, *Westerville*
Shawnee State University, Department of Nursing, *Portsmouth*
The University of Akron, College of Nursing, *Akron*
University of Cincinnati, College of Nursing, *Cincinnati*
Wright State University, College of Nursing and Health, *Dayton*

Oklahoma
Oklahoma City University, Kramer School of Nursing, *Oklahoma City*

Oregon
Linfield College, School of Nursing, *McMinnville*
Oregon Health & Science University, School of Nursing, *Portland*

Pennsylvania
Alvernia College, Nursing, *Reading*
Carlow University, Division of Nursing, *Pittsburgh*
DeSales University, Department of Nursing and Health, *Center Valley*
Drexel University, College of Nursing and Health Professions, *Philadelphia*
Duquesne University, School of Nursing, *Pittsburgh*
Eastern University, Program in Nursing, *St. Davids*
Gwynedd-Mercy College, School of Nursing, *Gwynedd Valley*
Holy Family University, School of Nursing and Allied Health Professions, *Philadelphia*
Immaculata University, Department of Nursing, *Immaculata*
Kutztown University of Pennsylvania, Department of Nursing, *Kutztown*
La Roche College, Department of Nursing and Nursing Management, *Pittsburgh*
La Salle University, School of Nursing, *Philadelphia*
Millersville University of Pennsylvania, Department of Nursing, *Millersville*
Moravian College, St. Luke's School of Nursing, *Bethlehem*
Mount Aloysius College, Department of Nursing, *Cresson*
The Pennsylvania State University University Park Campus, School of Nursing, *State College, University Park*
Thomas Jefferson University, Department of Nursing, *Philadelphia*
University of Pennsylvania, School of Nursing, *Philadelphia*
University of Pittsburgh, School of Nursing, *Pittsburgh*
Villanova University, College of Nursing, *Villanova*
Wilkes University, Department of Nursing, *Wilkes-Barre*

Puerto Rico
Universidad Adventista de las Antillas, Department of Nursing, *Mayagüez*
University of Puerto Rico, Mayagüez Campus, Department of Nursing, *Mayagüez*
University of Puerto Rico, Medical Sciences Campus, School of Nursing, *San Juan*

Rhode Island
Salve Regina University, Department of Nursing, *Newport*

South Carolina
Clemson University, School of Nursing, *Clemson*
Medical University of South Carolina, College of Nursing, *Charleston*

South Dakota
South Dakota State University, College of Nursing, *Brookings*

Tennessee
Middle Tennessee State University, School of Nursing, *Murfreesboro*
Southern Adventist University, School of Nursing, *Collegedale*
Tennessee State University, School of Nursing, *Nashville*
Union University, School of Nursing, *Jackson*
The University of Tennessee, College of Nursing, *Knoxville*
The University of Tennessee at Chattanooga, School of Nursing, *Chattanooga*
The University of Tennessee at Martin, Department of Nursing, *Martin*
The University of Tennessee Health Science Center, College of Nursing, *Memphis*
Vanderbilt University, School of Nursing, *Nashville*

Texas
Abilene Intercollegiate School of Nursing, *Abilene*
East Texas Baptist University, Department of Nursing, *Marshall*
Lamar University, Department of Nursing, *Beaumont*
Midwestern State University, Nursing Program, *Wichita Falls*
Southwestern Adventist University, Department of Nursing, *Keene*
Tarleton State University, Department of Nursing, *Stephenville*
Texas A&M International University, Canseco School of Nursing, *Laredo*
Texas A&M University–Corpus Christi, School of Nursing and Health Sciences, *Corpus Christi*
Texas Christian University, Harris School of Nursing, *Fort Worth*
Texas Tech University Health Sciences Center, School of Nursing, *Lubbock*
University of Mary Hardin-Baylor, College of Nursing, *Belton*

The University of Texas at Arlington, School of Nursing, *Arlington*
The University of Texas at El Paso, School of Nursing, *El Paso*
The University of Texas at Tyler, Program in Nursing, *Tyler*
The University of Texas Health Science Center at Houston, School of Nursing, *Houston*
The University of Texas Health Science Center at San Antonio, School of Nursing, *San Antonio*
The University of Texas Medical Branch, School of Nursing, *Galveston*

Virgin Islands

University of the Virgin Islands, Division of Nursing, *Saint Thomas*

Virginia

George Mason University, College of Nursing and Health Science, *Fairfax*
Jefferson College of Health Sciences, Nursing Education Program, *Roanoke*
Old Dominion University, Department of Nursing, *Norfolk*
Shenandoah University, Division of Nursing, *Winchester*

Washington

Gonzaga University, Department of Nursing, *Spokane*
Intercollegiate College of Nursing/Washington State University, *Spokane*
Pacific Lutheran University, School of Nursing, *Tacoma*
University of Washington, School of Nursing, *Seattle*

West Virginia

Fairmont State University, School of Nursing/Allied Health Adm., *Fairmont*
Mountain State University, Program in Nursing, *Beckley*
Shepherd University, Department of Nursing Education, *Shepherdstown*
West Virginia Wesleyan College, Department of Nursing, *Buckhannon*

Wisconsin

Alverno College, Division of Nursing, *Milwaukee*
Concordia University Wisconsin, Division of Nursing, *Mequon*
Marquette University, College of Nursing, *Milwaukee*
University of Wisconsin–Eau Claire, College of Nursing and Health Sciences, *Eau Claire*
University of Wisconsin–Madison, School of Nursing, *Madison*
University of Wisconsin–Milwaukee, College of Nursing, *Milwaukee*
University of Wisconsin–Oshkosh, College of Nursing, *Oshkosh*

Alberta

University of Alberta, Faculty of Nursing, *Edmonton*
University of Calgary, Faculty of Nursing, *Calgary*

British Columbia

British Columbia Institute of Technology, School of Health Sciences, *Burnaby*
University College of the Cariboo, School of Nursing, *Kamloops*
The University of British Columbia, School of Nursing, *Vancouver*

Manitoba

University of Manitoba, Faculty of Nursing, *Winnipeg*

New Brunswick

Université de Moncton, School of Nursing, *Moncton*
University of New Brunswick Fredericton, Faculty of Nursing, *Fredericton*

Nova Scotia

St. Francis Xavier University, Department of Nursing, *Antigonish*

Ontario

Laurentian University, School of Nursing, *Sudbury*
Ryerson University, Program in Nursing, *Toronto*
University of Windsor, School of Nursing, *Windsor*
York University, School of Nursing, Atkinson Faculty of Liberal and Profesional Studies, *Toronto*

Quebec

Université du Québec à Rimouski, Program in Nursing, *Rimouski*
Université Laval, Faculty of Nursing, *Québec*

Saskatchewan

University of Saskatchewan, College of Nursing, *Saskatoon*

Alphabetical Listing of Institutions

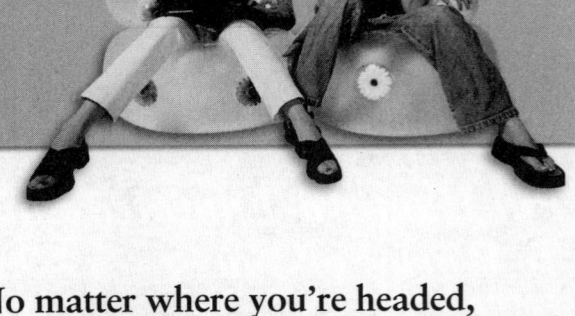

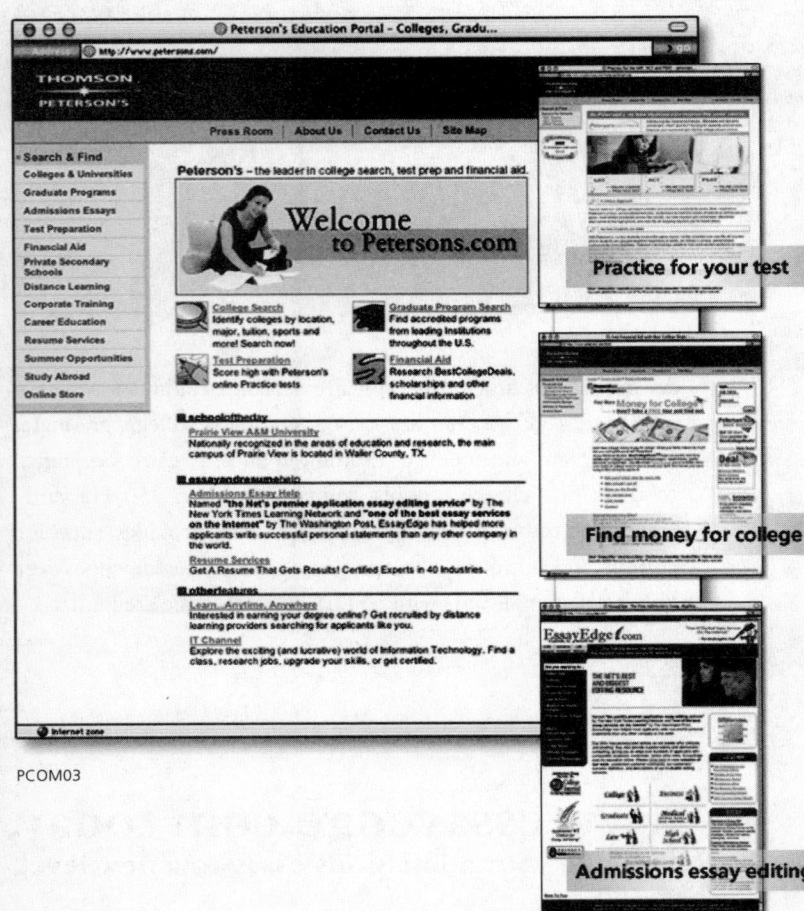